CAMBRIDGE LIBRARY COLLECTION

Books of enduring scholarly value

History of Medicine

It is sobering to realise that as recently as the year in which On the Origin of Species was published, learned opinion was that diseases such as typhus and cholera were spread by a 'miasma', and suggestions that doctors should wash their hands before examining patients were greeted with mockery by the profession. The Cambridge Library Collection reissues milestone publications in the history of Western medicine as well as studies of other medical traditions. Its coverage ranges from Galen on anatomical procedures to Florence Nightingale's common-sense advice to nurses, and includes early research into genetics and mental health, colonial reports on tropical diseases, documents on public health and military medicine, and publications on spa culture and medicinal plants.

The Elements of Materia Medica and Therapeutics

After training as an apothecary and surgeon, Jonathan Pereira (1804–53) taught materia medica for many years. His lectures at the medical school in London's Aldersgate Street were highly successful and formed the basis for the first edition of his major encyclopaedic work on medicinal substances. A pioneering text in the field of pharmacology, Pereira's work, which he subsequently updated in further editions, provided pharmacists and medical professionals with a more rigorous scientific understanding of the drugs and remedies they prescribed. After Pereira's death, medical jurist Alfred Swaine Taylor (1806–80) and physician George Owen Rees (1813–89) prepared this revised and expanded fourth edition, interspersed with instructive woodcuts. Volume 2 is divided into two parts. Part 1 (1855) continues with articles on special pharmacology, moving on from inorganic compounds to discuss the medicinal properties of organic compounds.

Cambridge University Press has long been a pioneer in the reissuing of out-of-print titles from its own backlist, producing digital reprints of books that are still sought after by scholars and students but could not be reprinted economically using traditional technology. The Cambridge Library Collection extends this activity to a wider range of books which are still of importance to researchers and professionals, either for the source material they contain, or as landmarks in the history of their academic discipline.

Drawing from the world-renowned collections in the Cambridge University Library and other partner libraries, and guided by the advice of experts in each subject area, Cambridge University Press is using state-of-the-art scanning machines in its own Printing House to capture the content of each book selected for inclusion. The files are processed to give a consistently clear, crisp image, and the books finished to the high quality standard for which the Press is recognised around the world. The latest print-on-demand technology ensures that the books will remain available indefinitely, and that orders for single or multiple copies can quickly be supplied.

The Cambridge Library Collection brings back to life books of enduring scholarly value (including out-of-copyright works originally issued by other publishers) across a wide range of disciplines in the humanities and social sciences and in science and technology.

The Elements of
Materia Medica
and Therapeutics

VOLUME 2 – PART 1

JONATHAN PEREIRA

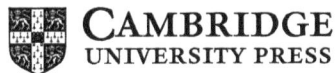

CAMBRIDGE
UNIVERSITY PRESS

University Printing House, Cambridge, CB2 8BS, United Kingdom

Published in the United States of America by Cambridge University Press, New York

Cambridge University Press is part of the University of Cambridge.
It furthers the University's mission by disseminating knowledge in the pursuit of
education, learning and research at the highest international levels of excellence.

www.cambridge.org
Information on this title: www.cambridge.org/9781108068833

© in this compilation Cambridge University Press 2014

This edition first published 1855
This digitally printed version 2014

ISBN 978-1-108-06883-3 Paperback

ELEMENTS

OF

MATERIA MEDICA.

LONDON
WILSON and OGILVY,
Skinner Street.

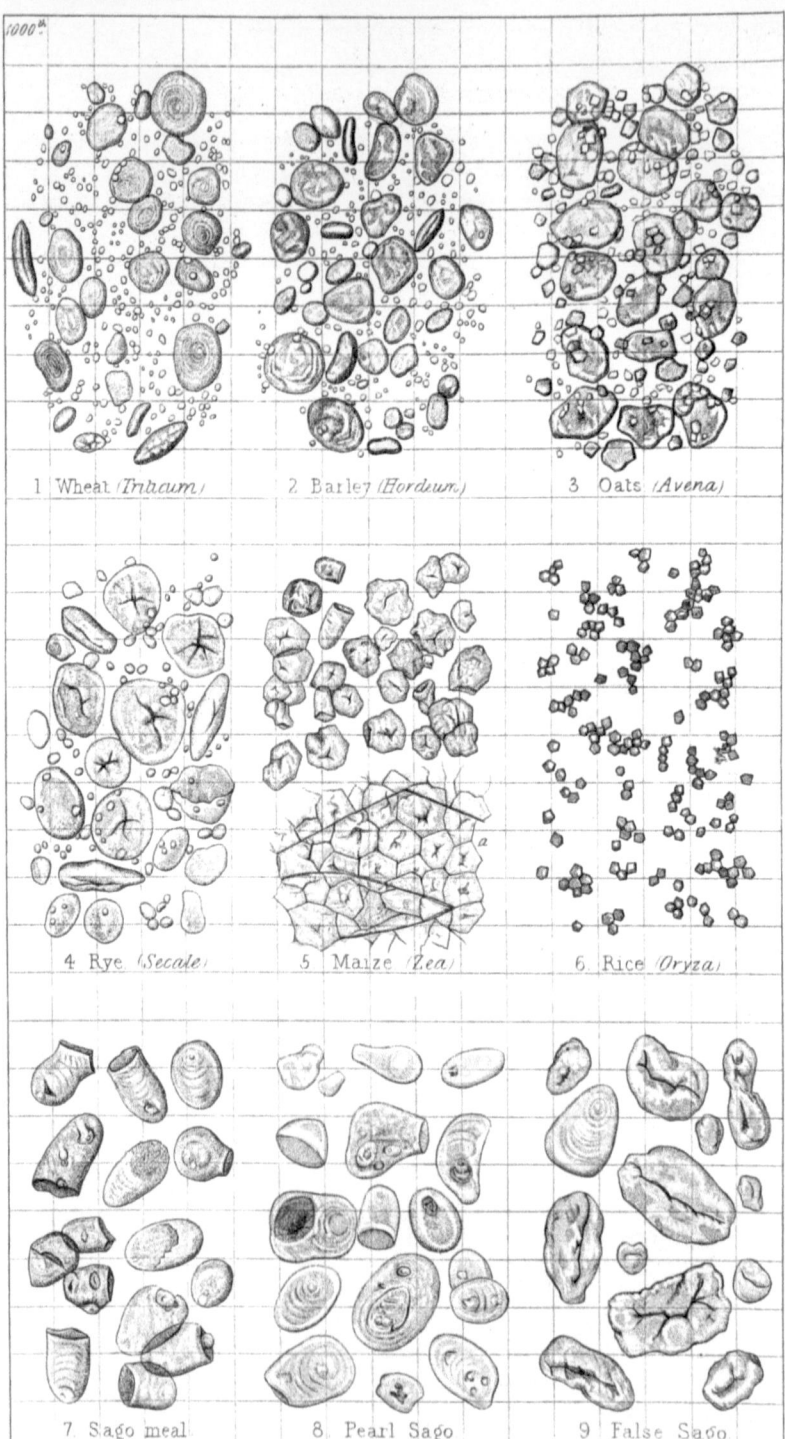

1. Wheat *(Triticum)*   2. Barley *(Hordeum)*   3. Oats *(Avena)*

4. Rye *(Secale)*   5. Maize *(Zea)*   6. Rice *(Oryza)*

7. Sago meal   8. Pearl Sago   9. False Sago

S. W. Leonard delt.   H. Adlard. sc

London, Longman & Cº.

THE

ELEMENTS

OF

MATERIA MEDICA

AND

THERAPEUTICS.

BY

JONATHAN PEREIRA, M.D. F.R.S. & L.S.

FELLOW OF THE ROYAL COLLEGE OF PHYSICIANS IN LONDON:
ASSOCIATE OF THE COLLEGE OF PHYSICIANS OF PHILADELPHIA:
HONORARY MEMBER OF THE PHARMACEUTICAL SOCIETIES OF GREAT BRITAIN, ST. PETERSBURG,
AND PORTUGAL; OF THE PHYSICO-MEDICAL SOCIETY OF ERLANGEN;
AND OF THE ASSOCIATION OF HESSIAN PHYSICIANS:
CORRESPONDING MEMBER OF THE SOCIETY OF PHARMACY OF PARIS:
EXAMINER IN MATERIA MEDICA AND PHARMACY TO THE UNIVERSITY OF LONDON:
PROFESSOR OF MATERIA MEDICA TO THE PHARMACEUTICAL SOCIETY;
AND PHYSICIAN TO THE LONDON HOSPITAL.

Fourth Edition,

ENLARGED AND IMPROVED,

INCLUDING

NOTICES OF MOST OF THE MEDICINAL SUBSTANCES IN USE IN THE
CIVILISED WORLD,

AND FORMING AN

Encyclopædia of Materia Medica.

VOL. II. PART I.

LONDON:

LONGMAN, BROWN, GREEN, AND LONGMANS.

1855.

PREFACE

TO THE FOURTH EDITION.

———

ALTHOUGH but a few years have elapsed since the publication of the First Part of the Second Volume of the ELEMENTS OF MATERIA MEDICA, it has been found necessary to make numerous additions and alterations. Many of the preparations of the LONDON COLLEGE have required revision; and the whole of those of the DUBLIN COLLEGE, some of which were inserted in a Supplement by the author, have now been incorporated with the text. In addition to these changes, the editors have considered it advisable to append to many of the articles various useful preparations of the UNITED STATES PHARMACOPŒIA. Some of the illustrations have been re-engraved, and others have been added to the new, as well as to the original articles of the author.

In making those additions which the progress of Pharmacy and Chemistry had, in their judgment, rendered necessary, the editors have carefully abstained from interfering with the opinions of the learned author, and they have adhered to the plan which they have adopted in editing other parts of this valuable work,—namely, of placing within brackets, those paragraphs which it has been found necessary to add to the text.

The additions made have been selected from authentic sources, and from a large body of materials. For great and valuable assistance in this part of their labours, the editors have to acknowledge their obligations to the Rev. J. M. Berkeley, Mr. Daniel Hanbury, Mr. A. Faber, and Mr. Jacob Bell. About eighty pages have been added to the volume; and, for the convenience of reference, a distinct Index is appended to this Part.

The editors, in the preface to the fourth edition of the First Volume, have expressed their opinion of the great value, in a medical and scientific point of view, of the literary labours of the late Dr. Pereira. With the completion of this Part, the three large volumes now constituting the ELEMENTS OF MATERIA MEDICA, have gone through an entire edition within the short period which has elapsed since his death,—a proof that the value in which the work was held during the author's life, has not diminished.

ALFRED SWAINE TAYLOR.
GEORGE OWEN REES.

LONDON: *October* 1855.

CONTENTS.

II.—ORGANIC BODIES.

I. Vegetabilia.—Vegetables.

I. Cryptogamia.—Cryptogams or Flowerless Plants.

Class I. Thallogenæ.—Thallogens.

Class II. Acrogenæ.—Acrogens.

II. Phanerogamia *Auct.*—Phanerogams or Flowering Plants.

Class III. Endogenæ.

Sub-class I. *Glumaceæ.*

b

Sub-class II. *Petaloideæ* vel *Floridæ.*

Sub-division I.

Perianth absent, squamiform, or glumaceous.

Sub-division II.

Perianth proper, often corolline.
1. Leaves straight-veined or curved-veined.
† Flowers sessile, spadiceous.

†† Ovary superior.

Class IV. Exogenæ.

Sub-class I. *Gymnospermæ.*

LIST OF WOODCUTS.

EXPLANATION OF PLATE.

This plate represents the appearance of starch-grains when moistened with water, and viewed by a power capable of magnifying 250 diameters. In order that the reader may compare the sizes of the different grains, the micrometer lines are faintly indicated: each of the square spaces between the lines represents the $\frac{1}{1000}$th part of a square inch.

1. *Wheat Starch.*—Most of the larger particles present their flattened faces to the observer. Three particles, seen edgeways, have a stronger lateral shading. (For a description of the grains, see p. 94–5.)

2. *Barley Starch.*—As wheat starch. (See p. 83.)

3. *Oat Starch.* (See p. 78.)

4. *Rye Starch.* (See p. 101.)

5. *Maize Starch.*—The upper portion represents isolated grains. The lower portion (*a*) represents a mass of grains, as seen in the outer or horny portion of the cells, the albumen with the cells *in situ*. (See p. 76.)

6. *Rice Starch.* (See p. 73.)

7. *Sago Meal.* (See p. 145.)

8. *Starch-grains of Pearl Sago.* (See p. 147.)

9. *Starch-grains of False Sago made from Potato Starch.*—One of the grains has escaped the action of the heating process to which they have been subjected: all the others have been ruptured. Chiefly taken from a specimen of Planche's "*Sagou de la Nouvelle Guinée.*" (See p. 148.)

CORRIGENDA.

Page 207, 7th line from top, *after* "none" *insert* "Distilled Water, ℥xij."

" 236, 24th line from top, for "*zerumber*" read "*zerumbet.*"

" 294, 19th line from top, *for* "Oiij." *read* "Ciij."

" 377, 7th line from bottom, *for* "Tinctura Lupinæ" *read* "Tinctura Lupulinæ."

" 397, 11th line from bottom, *for* "℥ss." *read* "℥ss."; and in line 6 from bottom, *for* "℥j. to ℥ij." *read* "℥j. to ℥ij."

" 415, in heading of page, and also in 23d line from top, *for* "Bush" *read* "Bark."

" 434, 23d line from top, *dele* "D."; the preparation not being in the Dublin Pharmacopœia.

" 465, 17th, 4th, and 3d lines from bottom, *for* "Roder" *read* "Rodier."

" 511, 18th line from top, *dele* "Water, Oj."

" 639, 27th line from bottom, *for* "Pareira" *read* "Pereira."

" 686, 17th line from top, for "*Gumma-resin*" read "*Gamma-resin.*"

ELEMENTS

OF

MATERIA MEDICA.

II. ORGANIC BODIES.

UNDER this division are included those vegetables and animals, with their educts and products, which are employed in medicine.

I adopt L. Gmelin's definition of an organic compound, which I have already stated (see Vol. i. p. 271, *foot-note*).

Certain medicinal compounds, which consist of an organic acid and an inorganic base, have been referred to the first division of this work, which treats of inorganic bodies.

I. Vegetabilia.—Vegetables.

These may be conveniently arranged in four classes, as follows :—

I. *Cryptogamia ;* acotyledonous, flowerless .	{ Stem and leaves undistinguishable... 1. *Thallogenæ.* { Stem and leaves distinguishable .... 2. *Acrogenæ.*
II. *Phanerogamia ;* flowering................	{ Cotyledons solitary or alternate; wood of stem youngest in the centre... 3. *Endogenæ.* { Cotyledons opposite or verticillate ; wood of stem youngest at the circumference .... 4. *Exogenæ.*

I. Cryptogamia, *Linn.*—Cryptogams or Flowerless Plants.

ACOTYLEDONES, *Jussieu,*—EXEMBRYONATÆ or ARHIZÆ, *Richard ;* AGAMÆ or ATHEOGAMÆ *Auctorum ;* NEMEÆ, *Fries.*

CHARACTERS.—Reproduction taking place either by *spores,* which are enclosed in cases called *thecæ,* imbedded in the substance of the plants, or borne at the tips of certain privileged cells (*sporophores*) ; or else by a mere dissolution of the utricles of cellular tissue. *Spores* destitute of embryo and cotyledons, germinating for the most part at no fixed point,[1] but at any part of their surface.

---

[1] [In many of the Uredineæ, as for example in Coleosporium, germination takes place at definite points, very much after the manner of pollen grains.—ED.]

B

Class I. Thallogenæ.—Thallogens.

ANANDRÆ, *Link;* ACOTYLEDONEÆ, *Agardh;* HOMONEMEÆ, *Fries;* CRYPTOPHYTA, *Link;* THALLOPHYTA, *Endlicher;* AMPHIGENÆ, *Ad. Brong.*

CHARACTERS.—*Substance of the plant* composed chiefly of cellular tissue, devoid of spiral vessels.[1] *Cuticle* destitute of stomata, or breathing pores. *Stem* and *leaves* undistinguishable. No opposition of stem and root.

This class includes three orders:—

I. Thallogens nourished through their whole surface by the medium in { Aquatic ...... 1. *Algæ.* which they vegetate... { Aërial......... 2. *Lichenes.*
II. Thallogens nourished through their thallus (spawn or mycelium) by juices derived from the matrix.. 3. *Fungi.*

ORDER I. ALGÆ, *DC.*—ALGALS.

CHARACTERS.—Cellular flowerless plants, nourished through their whole surface by the medium in which they vegetate; living in water, or very damp places; propagated by zoospores, coloured spores, or tetraspores.

PROPERTIES.—None of the plants of this order are poisonous. Some of them are nutritious, emollient, and demulcent: these properties they owe to the presence of mucilage[2] (*carrageenin*), starch, sugar (*mannite*), and a little albumen. The peculiar *mucilage* of sea-weeds will be more fully noticed hereafter (see *Chondrus crispus*). It differs, says Dr. Stenhouse, from ordinary gum, for, when digested with nitric acid, it yields oxalic, but neither mucic nor saccharic acids.

Mannite is probably obtainable in greater or less quantity from most if not all sea-weeds. It was procured from eight out of nine species examined by Dr. Stenhouse.[3] He could not detect it in *Ulva latissima.* The following is a list of the Algæ which he examined, arranged in order, according to the quantity of mannite which they severally yielded:—

1. Laminaria saccharina (12·15 per cent. of mannite).
2. Halidrys siliquosa (5 or 6 per cent.)
3. Laminaria digitata.
4. Fucus serratus.
5. Alaria esculenta.
6. Rhodomenia palmata (2 or 3 per cent.)
7. Fucus vesiculosus (1 to 2 per cent.)
8. Fucus nodosus.

FIG. 1.

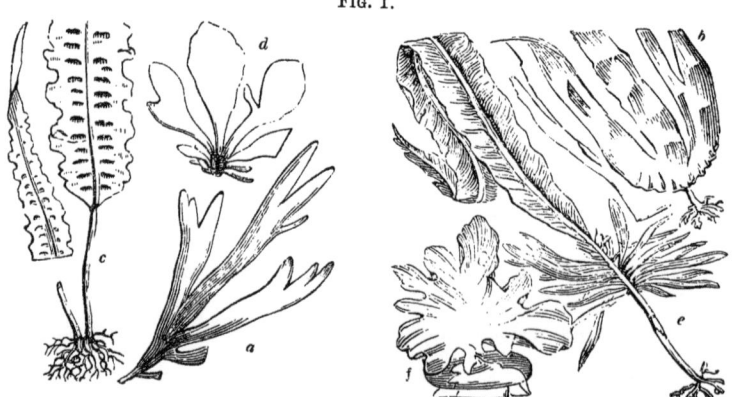

Esculent Sea-Weeds.

a. Rhodomenia palmata (or Dulse).
b. Laminaria digitata.
c. Laminaria saccharina.
d. Iridæa edulis.
e. Alaria esculenta.
f. Ulva latissima.

---

[1] [In a few fungi, as Trichia, Batarrea, Podaxon, &c. there are true spiral vessels analogous to the Elaters of Jungermanniæ.—ED.]
[2] *On the Mucilage of the Fuci, with Remarks on its Application to Economical Ends,* by Mr. S. Brown, jun., in Jameson's *Edinb. New Phil. Jour.* vol. xxvi. p. 409, 1839.
[3] *Memoirs and Proceedings of the Chemical Society of London* for 1844.

On the two first of these plants, when dried, the mannite often forms crystalline incrustations, which by some have been erroneously supposed to be common salt. Dr. Stenhouse thinks that mannite might be more economically procured from sea-weeds than from manna.

The alterative and resolvent virtues ascribed to sea-weeds, and their presumed beneficial effects in scrofulous affections and glandular enlargements, are referable to the inorganic constituents; such as iodine, bromine, the phosphates, and the alkaline substances. The following table shows the composition and proportion of ash of certain sea-weeds :—

	Laminaria saccharina. North Sea.	Fucus serratus. North Sea.	Laminaria latifolia.	Furcellaria fastigiata.	Chondrus crispus.	Iridæa edulis.	Polysyphonia elongata.	Delesseria sanguinea.	Fucus digitatus. From the mouth of the Clyde.	Fucus nodosus. From the mouth of the Clyde.	Fucus serratus. From the mouth of the Clyde.	Approximate mean.
Potash	24·77	16·02	16·91	21·36	18·00	23·42	21·23	13·72	22·40	10·07	4·51	17·50
Soda	1·84	6·01	..	24·77	19·47	16·06	5·06	21·34	8·29	15·80	21·15	12·70
Lime	6·50	7·05	8·28	6·02	7·11	10·23	2·92	2·30	8·79	10·98	11·09	7·39
Magnesia	8·13	7·59	6·80	11·04	11·80	..	20·56	5·94	7·44	10·93	11·66	9·89
Chloride of sodium	33·72	38·72	26·92	..	..	1·66	13·85	..	28·39	20·16	18·76	16·56
Chloride of potassium	..	..	10·18	..	..	..	..	..	..	..	..	0·93
Iodide of sodium	4·70	0·27	..	..	..	..	..	..	3·62	0·54	1·33	0·95
Phosphate of lime	8·41	4·95	12·80	3·96	0·76	23·23	2·99	3·90	5·63	3·34	9·67	7·24
Phosphate of iron	0·75	0·64	..	..	..	..	..	..	..	..	..	..
Oxide of iron	..	..	..	..	..	..	..	..	0·62	0·29	0·34	0·24
Oxide of manganese	..	..	..	0·22	..	..	..	..	..	..	..	..
Sulphuric acid	10·60	18·35	12·63	32·63	42·86	25·19	28·66	40·42	13·26	26·69	21·06	24·76
Silica	0·58	0·40	0·69	..	..	..	2·83	12·38	1·56	1·20	0·43	1·82
	100^1	100^1	^{0}95·21	100^2	100^2	^{2}99·79	^{0}98·10	100^2	100^3	100	100^3	99·98
Per-centage of ash in weed dried at 212° F.	9·78	25·83	13·62	18·92	20·61	9·86	17·10	13·17	20·40	16·19	15·63	16·46

The presence of so large a proportion of potash and phosphoric acid in plants growing in sea-water, which contains so small a proportion of these ingredients, is very remarkable. There is reason, however, to believe that the quantity and constitution of the ash are liable to very considerable variation, depending on the locality, season, and the age of the plant. A vermifuge property has been ascribed to some algals.

Laennec[4] tried the influence of an artificial " marine atmosphere" (air impregnated with the vapour of fresh sea-weed) on consumptive patients, and was impressed with an idea of its efficacy; but experience has not confirmed his favourable opinion of its beneficial influence : moreover, the inhabitants of sea-coasts, like those of inland districts, are the subjects of phthisis.

Sub-order I. CONFERVACEÆ, *Endl.*—CONFERVALS.

CHARACTERS.—Vesicular, filamentary, or membranous algals, propagated by sporidia (endogenous cells, or a gelatinous substance which is ultimately formed into cells), which are produced at the expense of the endochrome of one or more cells, or sometimes by the copulation of distinct individuals, and discharged by the opening or absorption of the mother cell.

PROPERTIES.—These are similar to those of the Order, and which I have already noticed.

1. Confervals of mineral waters.—Confervals are peculiarly abundant in both hot and cold sulphureous springs. *Calothrix nivea* (fig. 2), the Conferva nivea of Dillwyn,[5] has

---

[1] Schweitzer.
[2] Forchhammer.
[3] Gödechens, *Annal. der Chemie und Pharm.* liv. p. 352.
[4] *Treat. on Diseases of the Chest*, by Dr. Forbes, p. 369.
[5] *British Confervæ*, p. 54.

been found in the sulphur springs of Yorkshire, Durham, and Aix-la-Chapelle.[1] The same, or an allied species, was found by Dr. Daubeny[2] in the hot sulphur springs of Greoulx, in Provence. *Oscillaria labyrinthiformis*—the Tremella thermalis of some writers—is one of the most common species in the hot sulphur springs and other thermal waters of Germany, France, and Italy. In the Karlsbad waters, *Sphærozyga Jacobi* (fig. 3), and several species of *Oscillaria*, have been detected.[3] Humboldt found *Oscillaria calida* in the thermal waters of New Granada.

Fig. 2.

Fig. 3.

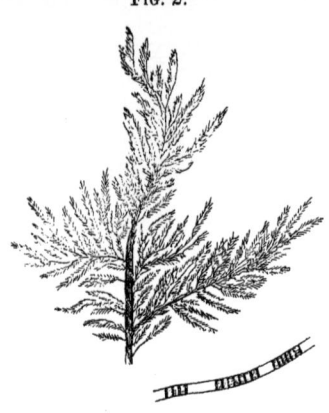

Calothrix nivea.

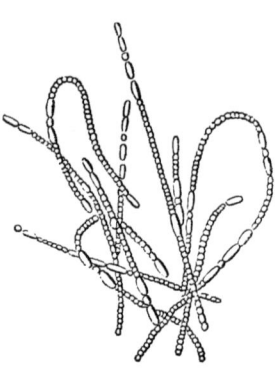

Sphærozyga Jacobi.

The organic substance found in mineral waters, and variously called *barégine* by Long-champ, *zoogen* by Gimbernat, *theiothermin* by Monheim, and *glairine* by Anglada, derives its origin from confervals. It is a glairy or mucus-like substance, which is said to communicate the flavour and odour of flesh-broth to the water in which it is contained. In the preparation of artificial sulphur-baths, animal gelatine is sometimes used to represent the barégine (see Vol. i. p. 501).

The confervals, under the influence of light, decompose water, retain the hydrogen, and evolve the oxygen. Robiquet[4] obtained from the Néris water, gas containing 44 per cent. of oxygen, derived from the Oscillatoria labyrinthiformis; and he ascribed the medicinal qualities of these waters to the presence of this very oxygenated air. "Dr. Edwards," says Robiquet, "has shown that the air contained in water has a great influence over the life of batrachians, and it is probable that, in some cases, our organs may also be more or less influenced by it."

2. Confervals employed in medicine.—*Yeast* is referred to Algæ by Kützing,[5] who calls it *Cryptococcus Fermentum.* It is more commonly, however, regarded as a fungus, and as such will be noticed hereafter. (See *Fungi.*) With this doubtful exception, none of the Confervals are employed, at the present day, in medicine. *Nostoc commune*, or star-jelly, of which formerly the most extraordinary superstitions were entertained,[6] and *Conferva rivularis*, or crow silk, recommended by Murray[7] for trial in asphyxia, asthma, and phthisis, on account of its evolving oxygen in solar light, have never been used in rational medicine.

---

[1] Daubeny, *Linn. Trans.* vol. xvi. p. 587, 1831.

[2] *Op. citato.*

[3] Endlicher, *Genera Plant.* Supp. 3me ; Geiger's *Handb. d. Pharm.* 2te Aufl. Ergängsheft, 1843.

[4] *Journ. de Pharmacie*, t. xxi. p. 583, 1835.

[5] *Phycologia generalis.*

[6] See the articles "*Nostoch*" in the *Dict. Univ. de Mat. Méd.* t. iv. p. 635, 1832 ; and "*Cœlifolium*" in James's *Medicinal Dictionary*, vol. ii.

[7] *Appar. Medicaminum*, t. v. p. 550, 1790.—Pliny (*Hist. Nat* lib. xxvii cap. 45) says he knew a labourer who fell from the top of a tall tree, and thereby broke nearly every bone in his body, and who being covered with a river conferva, kept moist by his own water, was cured in an incredibly short space of time! He adds, that the term *conferva* is derived from "*conferruminando*," in allusion to the supposed consolidating properties of this plant.

3. Confervals developed in pharmaceutical and other liquids.—The vesicular and filamentous plants which grow in various chemical solutions,[1] and to the naked eye appear like gelatinous or cottony masses, are considered by some botanists to be Algals. Kützing refers them to the genera *Cryptococcus, Ulvina, Hygrocrocis, Sirocrocis, Leptomitus,* and *Chamænema.*

FIG. 6.

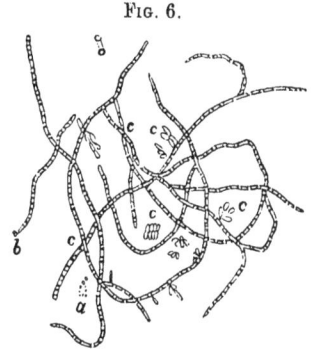

FIG. 4.

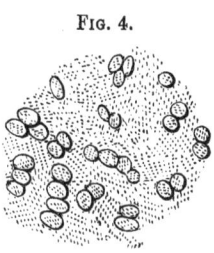

Cryptococcus inæqualis
(in aqua calami).

FIG. 5.

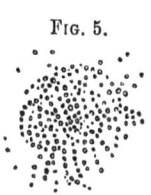

Ulvina myxophila
(in mucilage of
quince seed).

Hygrocrocis cuprica[2]
(in a solution of polychrome mixed
with sulphate of copper).

FIG. 8.

FIG. 7.

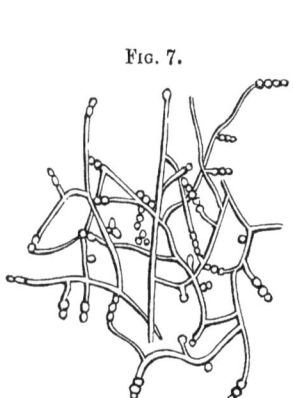

Sirocrocis stibica
(in a solution of emetic tartar).

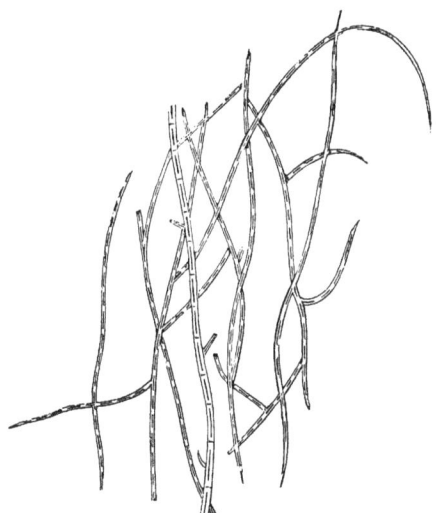

Leptomitus phosphoratus
(in phosphoric acid from bones).

But these minute plants are regarded by some eminent authorities as the spawn or mycelium of various moulds, or, in other words, as imperfect mucedinous fungi. " It is

---

[1] For some notices of these plants, the reader is referred to my paper *On the Microscopic Vegetations developed in Pharmaceutical Liquids,* in the *Pharmaceutical Journal,* vols. vii. and viii. 1848.

[2] [For a curious account of the Cryptogam, which is a pest in the electrotyping department of the Coast Survey Office at Washington, see Harvey, *Nereis Boreali-Americana,* Part 1, p. 6, 1852.—ED.]

true," says the Rev. M. J. Berkeley, "that moulds will vegetate in fluids, but as soon as they assume their normal form there is a distinction between the immerged and free portion."

4. Esculent Confervals.—Some few of the Confervals are cooked and brought to table under the name of *laver ;* but the amount of nourishment which they contain is very small. They are species of *Porphyra* and *Ulva.*

1. Porphyra laciniata, *Agardh.*—Laciniated Purple Laver.

Fig. 9.

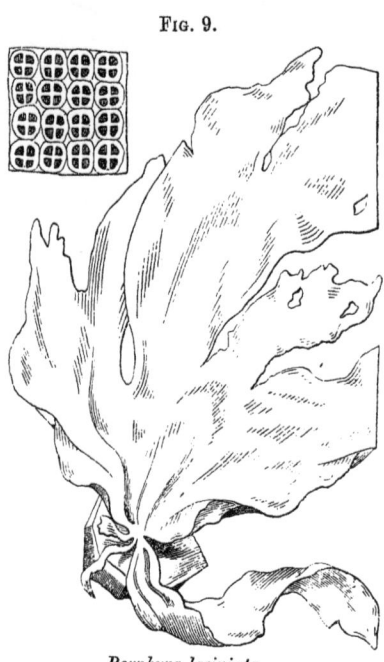

Porphyra laciniata.

a. Small portion of the frond, showing the quaternate granules (*magnified*).

Porphyra umbilicalis, Kützing; *Ulva umbilicalis,* Eng. Bot.—The fronds are delicately membranaceous, deeply and irregularly cleft into several broad segments. Their colour is deepish purple, but, when not in a state of perfection, it tends to livid olive. "Under the microscope the whole frond appears to be divided into squares, in the manner of a tessellated pavement, and within each square are four purple granules or spores, which constitute the fructification and the whole colouring matter of the frond"[1] (see fig. 1, *a*). Abundant on all our shores. This plant is pickled with salt, and sold in London as *laver.* The London shops are said to be supplied with it from the coast of Devonshire. When stewed, it is brought to the table and eaten with pepper, butter, or oil, and lemon-juice or vinegar. Some persons stew it with leeks and onions. It is generally taken as a luxury; but it might be employed with advantage, by scrofulous subjects, as an alterative article of diet. In the absence of other vegetables, it might be valuable as an antiscorbutic to the crews of our whaling vessels cruising in high latitudes, where every marine rock at half-tide abundantly produces it.

2. Ulva latissima, *Greville.*—Broad Green Laver.

Ulva Lactuca var. *latissima,* Lightf.; *Green Sloke ; Oyster Green.*—The fronds are bright herbaceous green, becoming tinged with brown in old age and decay. They are oblong or roundish, waved, and very tender (see fig. 1, *f.*) The granules are quaternate, and densely cover the whole frond. It is said to be used at table under the name of *green laver,* being cooked in the same way as the *Porphyra laciniata,* to which it is greatly inferior. It is rarely taken when the latter can be procured. I have never found it in the London shops.

Sub-order II. Phyceæ, *Endl.*—Sea Wracks.

Fucaceæ, *Lindl.* ; Aplosporeæ, *Decaisne.*

Characters.—Cellular or tubular algals propagated by spores (endogenous cells), contained in superficial, often bladdery (*utricles*) cells, produced singly out of endo-

---

[1] Harvey, *Phycologia Britannica,* vol. i. pl. xcii. 1846.

chrome, consisting of a simple nucleus clothed by its proper cellular membrane (*epispore*), and discharged by the opening of a transparent mother cell (*perispore*).

PROPERTIES.—Similar to those of the Order (see *ante*, p. 2). To this order several esculent species belong: such as *Laminaria digitata*, called by the English *sea-girdles*, by the Scotch, *Tangle ;* and *Alaria esculenta* (fig. 1, *e*), termed *Badderlocks, Hen-ware*, or *Honey ware*. These, as well as several other species of this order, viz. *Laminaria saccharina* (fig. 1, *c*), and *Halidrys siliquosa*, have been already referred to as containing mannite (see *ante*, p. 2).

The only species used for medicinal purposes which it will be necessary to notice is *Fucus vesiculosus*.

3. FUCUS VESICULOSUS, *Linn.*—COMMON SEA WRACK.

Sex. Syst. Cryptogamia, Algæ.

(Herba cum fructu, *Offic.*)

HISTORY. — Theophrastus[1] mentions several species of Algæ (φῦκος). Fucus vesiculosus is sometimes termed *quercus marina, bladder fucus*, and *common sea-ware, kelp-ware*, and *black tang*.

FIG. 10.

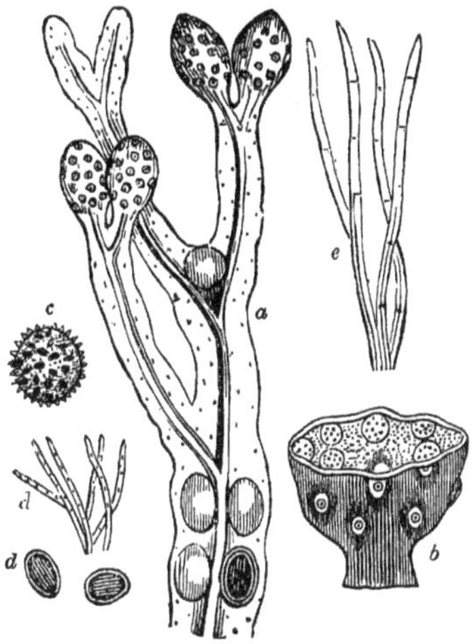

Fucus vesiculosus.

a. Upper part of a frond, with air-vessels and receptacles.

b. Section of a receptacle.

c. Conceptacle.

d. Filaments and spores, of which the conceptacles are composed.

e. Filaments, which issue from the pores on the surface of the frond.

BOTANY.   **Gen. Char.** — *Frond* linear, either flat, compressed, or cylindrical, dichotomous (rarely pinnated), coriaceous. *Air-vessels* [*vesiculæ*] when present innate, simple. *Receptacles* either terminal or lateral, filled with mucus, traversed by a network of jointed fibres, pierced by numerous pores, which communicate with immersed spherical *conceptacles*, containing parietal *spores*, or *antheridia*, or both (*Harvey*).

Sp. Char. — *Frond* plane, linear, dichotomous, entire at the margin. *Air-vessels* roundish-oval in pairs. *Receptacles* mostly elliptical, terminating the branches (*Greville*).

Very variable; but the varieties pass so insensibly into each other that it is difficult to define them strictly.

Hab.—Sea-shores. Very common everywhere.

PHYSICAL PROPERTIES.—Its substance is thickish, flexible, but very tough. Its colour is dark, olivaceous, glossy green, paler at the extremities, and becomes black by drying. Its odour is strong ; its taste nauseous.

COMPOSITION. — It has been analysed by Stackhouse,[2] by Gaultier de Claubry,[3] by John,[4] and by Fagerstrom.[5] The following appear to be its

---

[1] *Hist. Plant.* lib. iv. cap. vii.
[2] *Dict. Scien. Nat.* xviii. 500.
[3] *Ann. Chim.* xciii. 116
[4] *Schweigger's Journ.* xiii. 464.
[5] Gmelin, *Handb. d. Chem.* Bd. ii. S. 1354.

constituents :—*Cellulose, mucilage* (carrageenin), *mannite, odorous oil, colouring* and *bitter matters,* and various *salts.*

The following table shows the composition and proportion of ash of Fucus vesiculosus of different localities :—

	Mouth of the Clyde.	Mouth of the Mersey.	North Sea.	Denmark.	Greenland.	Mean.
Potash	15·23		17·68	9·03	17·86	11·96
Soda	11·16	15·10	5·78	7 78	21·43	12·25
Lime	8·15	16·77	4·71	21·65	3·31	10·92
Magnesia	7·16	15·19	6·89	10·96	7·44	9·53
Chloride of sodium	25·10	9·89	35·38	3·53	25·93	19·82
Iodide of sodium...	0·37		0·13			0·25
Phosphate of iron and phosphate of lime	2·99		5·44	9·67	10·09	5·64
Oxide of iron......	0 33	4·42				0·95
Sulphuric acid	28·16	30·94	23·71	26·34	13·94	24·62
Silica..............	1 35	7·69	0·28	11·04		4·06
	100·1	100·2	100·3	100·4	100·4	100·
Per-centage of ash (calculated dry)	16·39	13·22	20·56		16·22	16·60

Chemical Characteristics. — By treating the distilled water of Fucus vesiculosus with ether, *a semi-solid white oil* is extracted, which is the odorous principle. The aqueous decoction of this plant is neutral, and contains in solution mucilage (see Carrageenin) and various salts. It yields, with chlorine and starch, faint traces only of iodine, sometimes none at all. But if alcohol be added, by which the mucilage and a part of the sulphates are thrown down, the alcoholic·liquor evaporated, and the residue mixed with potash, then calcined, and afterwards treated with hydrochloric acid to disengage hydrosulphuric acid, we may sometimes detect iodine in the filtered liquor by the deep blue colour formed on the addition of starch and chlorine.[5] By combustion in the open air, this plant yields the ash called *kelp ;* and by incineration in a covered crucible it gives a charcoal, termed *vegetable ethiops.*

Physiological Effects.—During the winter, in some of the Scottish islands, horses, cattle, and sheep are fed on it.[6] Its local action is detergent, and perhaps discutient. Its remote effects are probably analogous to those caused by small doses of iodine, modified by the influence of salts of sodium and calcium.

Uses.—Frictions of the plant, with its contained mucilage, were employed, with supposed advantage, by Dr. Russell,[7] in glandular enlargements and other scrofulous tumors : the parts were afterwards washed with sea-water.

---

[1] Gödechens, *Annal. der Chemie und Pharm.* liv. p. 352.
[2] James, *ibid.*
[3] Schweitzer.
[4] Forchhammer.
[5] Guibourt, *Hist. des Drog.* 4me éd. ii. 46.
[6] Greville, *Algæ Brit.* xx.
[7] *Dissertation on the Use of Sea-water,* 5th ed. 1769, pp. 41 and 44.

He also gave internally the expressed juice of the vesicles in glandular affections.[1]

ÆTHIOPS VEGETABILIS ; *Vegetable Ethiops.*—This is prepared by incinerating Fucus vesiculosus in a covered crucible. It is composed of *charcoal* and various *salts* (see *supra*). When hydrochloric acid is added to it, traces of sulphuretted hydrogen are frequently evolved. By digesting the ethiops in water, and testing the solution with nitric acid and starch, I have sometimes failed to obtain the blue colour indicative of the presence of iodine. It has been exhibited in bronchocele and scrofulous maladies. Dr. Russell[2] says it far exceeds burnt sponge in virtue. It has been employed also as a dentifrice. The dose of it is from ten grains to two drachms.

Sub-order III. FLORIDEÆ, *Endl.*—ROSE-TANGLES.

CERAMIACEÆ, *Lindl.* ; CHORISTOSPOREÆ, *Decaisne.*

CHARACTERS.—Cellular or tubular algals propagated by thecæ (*favellæ* vel *favellidia*, *coccidia* vel *keramidia*), composed of granules [spores ?] contained within a cellular or gelatinous perisporangium, and by sphærospores (or *tetraspores*), composed of four (or three) spores in a transparent perispore.

PROPERTIES.—Several species of this sub-order are esculent. They owe this property to the mucilage, starch, mannite, and perhaps a little albumen, which they contain. Besides the species presently to be described, *Iridæa edulis* (fig. 1, *d*), and *Rhodomenia palmata* (fig. 1, *a*), which is cried about the streets of Edinburgh under the name of *dulse,* may be mentioned as illustrative examples of esculent species.

4. CHONDRUS CRISPUS, *Grev.*—CARRAGEEN OR IRISH MOSS.

Sex. Syst. Cryptogamia, Algæ.

(Planta, *Offic.*)

SYNONYMES.—*Chondrus polymorphus,* Lamour ; *Sphærococcus crispus,* Agardh ; *Curled Chondrus* (chondrus, from χόνδρος, *cartilage*).

HISTORY.—*Carrageen, Irish,* or *pearl moss* was introduced into medicine by Mr. Todhunter, of Dublin.[3]

BOTANY. **Gen. Char.**—*Frond* cartilaginous, nerveless, compressed or flat, flabelliform, dichotomously cleft : formed internally of three strata ; the *inner,* of densely packed, longitudinal fibres ; the *medial,* of small, roundish cells ; the *outer,* of vertical, coloured, moniliform filaments. *Fructification :*—1, prominent *tubercles* (*nemathecia*) composed of radiating filaments, whose lower articulations are at length dissolved into *spores* (?) ; 2, *tetraspores* collected into sori, immersed in the substance of the frond (*Harvey*).

Sp. Char.—*Frond* stipitate, thickish, cartilaginous, flat or curled, segments wedge-shaped, very variable in breadth ; apices truncate, submarginate, or

---

[1] *Op. cit.* p. 99.
[2] *Op. cit.* p. 98.
[3] Reece's *Monthly Gazette of Health,* Jan. 1831.

cloven ; axils obtuse ; sori elliptical or oblong, concave on one side (*Harvey*). *Fronds* from 2 or 3 to 10 or 12 inches long : their *substance* cartilaginous, in some varieties approaching to horny, flexible and tough ; their *colour* deep purple-brown, often tinged with purplish-red, paler at the summit, becoming greenish, and at length white in decay.

This, says Dr. Greville, is the Proteus of marine Algæ. The varieties are innumerable, and pass into one another so insensibly, that it is almost impossible to define them.

Mr. D. Turner[1] enumerates the following varieties :—

FIG. 11.

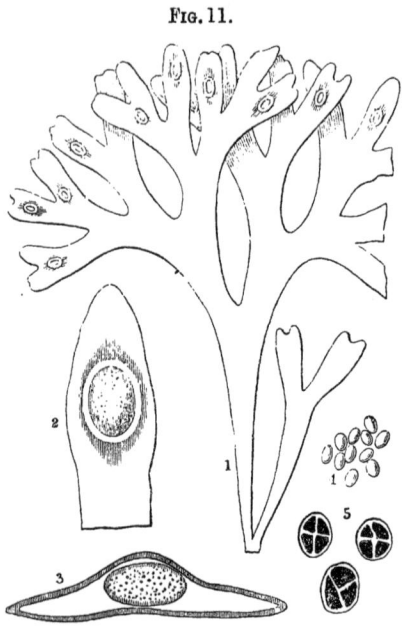

Chondrus crispus.

1. Plant with sori (*natural size*).
2. Segment with sorus.
3. A segment and sorus vertically divided.
4. Seeds or spores.
5. Tetraspores from the sorus (*magnified*).

β. *virens ;* frond submembranaceous, branches dilated upwards, flattish, extreme segments long and acuminated.

γ. *stellatus ;* frond submembranaceous, branches dilated upwards, divided at their apices into very numerous clustered short laciniæ.

δ. *equalis ;* frond cartilaginous, thick, all the branches equal, linear, the extreme segments obtuse.

ε. *filiformis ;* frond cartilaginous, sub-cylindrical, branches nearly linear, apices long and acuminated.

ζ. *patens ;* fronds subcartilaginous, channelled on one side, dichotomous, angles of the dichotomies patent.

η. *lacerus ;* frond cartilaginous, compressed, apices very narrow, elongated, branched.

θ. *sarniensis ;* frond between coriaceous and cartilaginous, branches slightly channelled on one side, dilated upwards, apices rounded and emarginate.

ι. *planus ;* frond subcoriaceous, flat, wide, branches linear, apices obtuse.

κ. *geniculatus ;* frond cartilaginous, compressed, branches nearly linear, tubercles subglobose, black, frond bent, and often broken at the tubercles.

According to Ormancey,[2] carrageen is a zoophyte, which he proposes to call *Antipathes polymorphus.* Unlike the fuci, he says, it has no canal, nerves, or roots ; but, like the zoophytes, it has voluntary motion of tentaculæ, sensibility, and two distinct bodies, one secreted by the other, simulating a plant.

Hab.—On rocks and stones on the sea-coast : very common.—Perennial : spring.

PREPARATION.—For dietetical and medicinal uses it is collected on the west coasts of Ireland (especially in Clare) ; likewise, according to Kohl,[3] in Antrim ; washed, bleached (by exposure to the sun), and dried. In Ireland it is sometimes employed by painters and plasterers as a substitute for size.

---

[1] *Fuci ; or, Figures and Descriptions of the Plants referred by botanists to the genus Fucus,* Lond. 1808–12, 4to.

[2] *Journal de Pharmacie et de Chimie,* 3me sér. t. xii. p. 265, 1847.

[3] *Ireland,* p. 247.

Along with *Chondrus crispus,* other allied species, especially *Ch. mamillosus,* are sometimes collected (see fig. 13).

PHYSICAL PROPERTIES.—The carrageen or Irish moss of commerce (*muscus carragenicus*) consists of fronds, which are usually from two to three or four inches long, dry, crisp, mostly yellowish or dirty white, but intermixed with purplish-red portions, inodorous or nearly so, with a mucilaginous taste. The frond is formed internally of three strata : the inner, of densely-packed, longitudinal fibres; the medial, of small, roundish cells ; the outer, of vertical, coloured, moniliform filaments.[1]

FIG. 12.

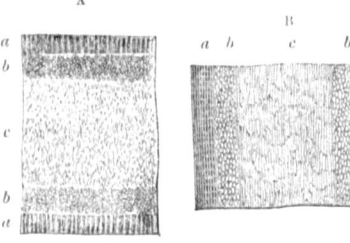

Chondrus crispus.

A. Transverse section of the frond } both
B. Longitudinal section of the frond } magnified.
a, a. Outer strata.
b, b. Medial strata.
c. Inner stratum.

In warm water, the dried commercial frond swells up, and, when boiled, almost entirely dissolves. If the swollen and partially dissolved frond be examined by the microscope, it is seen to consist of very minute, somewhat fusiform cohering cells. A calcareous meshy crust (consisting of various species of *Flustra*) is frequently found on the frond.

Chondrus mamillosus is found in commercial carrageen. Some samples I found to be principally composed of this species.[2] The frond of this plant is more or less channelled; but the species is best distinguished by the fructification : in *Ch. crispus* the subhemispherical capsules are imbedded in the disc of the frond, producing a depression on the opposite side (see fig. 11); in *Ch. mamillosus,* the spherical capsules are scattered over the disc of the frond, and are supported on little short stalks (fig. 13).

FIG. 13.

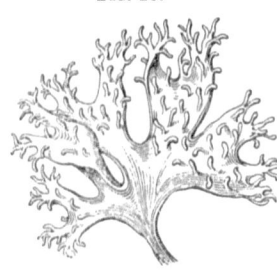

Chondrus mamillosus.

Portion of the channelled frond bearing the pedicellate capsules.

COMPOSITION.—It has been analysed by Herberger[3] and by Feuchtwanger.[4]

Herberger.	
Vegetable jelly [carrageenin]	79·1
Mucus	9·5
Two resins	0·7
Fatty matter and free acids	*traces*
Chlorides of sodium and magnesium	2·0
Fibre, water, and loss........................	8·7
No traces of iodine or bromine could be recognised.	
	100·0

Feuchtwanger.	
Jelly ... { Pectin [carrageenin] (a large portion). { Starch.	
Oxalate of lime.	
Compounds of sulphur, chlorine, and bromine.	
No fungic, boletic, or lichenic acids.	

[1] *Phycologia Britannica,* vol. i. pl. lxiii. Lond. 1846.
[2] See also Henschel, in Dierbach, *Die neuesten Entdeck. in d. Mat. Med.* Bd. ii. S. 276, 1843.
[3] Buchner's *Repertorium,* Bd. xlix. S. 200, 1834.
[4] *American Journal of Science and Arts,* xxvi.

Subsequently iodine has been detected in it by Sarphati,[1] and both iodine and bromine by Grosse.[2] (For the composition of the ashes, see p. 3.)

CARRAGEENIN.[3]—The mucilaginous constituent of carrageen moss is termed by some writers *vegetable jelly*, or *vegetable mucilage*, by others *pectin*. It appears to me to be a peculiar modification of mucilage, and I shall therefore call it *carrageenin*. It is soluble in boiling water, and its solution forms a precipitate with diacetate of lead and silicate of potash, and, if sufficiently concentrated, gelatinises on cooling. Carrageenin is distinguished from ordinary gum by its aqueous solution not producing a precipitate on the addition of alcohol; from starch, by its not assuming a blue colour with tincture of iodine; from animal jelly, by tincture of nutgalls causing no precipitate;[4] from pectin, by acetate of lead not throwing down anything, as well as by no mucic acid being formed by the action of nitric acid.

According to Schmidt,[5] the cell-walls of carrageen do not essentially differ from the contents of the cells; for when the plant is boiled in water, the whole swells up and forms a mucilage, which may be expressed through a linen cloth, leaving behind the *Flustræ* and smaller crustaceans with which this alga is covered. By digestion for a short time with dilute sulphuric acid in a water-bath, the whole plant is converted into sugar and gum.

The composition of carrageenin dried at 212° F., according to Schmidt, is represented by the formula $C^{12} H^{10} O^{10}$; so that it appears to be identical with starch and sugar. Mulder,[6] however, represents it by the formula $C^{24} H^{19} O^{19}$.

CHEMICAL CHARACTERISTICS.—The presence of carrageenin in the decoction is demonstrated by the tests before enumerated. No iodine is recognisable by nitric acid and starch. Oxalate of ammonia detects lime (or calcium) in solution, while nitrate of silver points out the presence of chlorine. Guibourt[7] could recognise neither sugar nor magnesia.

PHYSIOLOGICAL EFFECTS.—Carrageen moss is nutritive: its mucilaginous matter acts as an element of respiration (see Vol. i. p. 64), while its inorganic constituents (phosphate of lime, potash salts, &c.) may also serve some useful purpose in the animal economy. It is generally regarded as being readily digestible. Medicinally, it is emollient and demulcent (see Vol. i. pp. 170-1).

USES.—It is a popular remedy for pulmonary complaints (especially those of a phthisical character), chronic diarrhœa and dysentery, scrofula, rickets, enlarged mesenteric glands, irritation of bladder and kidneys, &c. As a culinary article it has been employed as a substitute for animal jelly, in the preparation of *blanc-mange*, jellies, white soup, &c. A thick mucilage of carrageen scented with some prepared spirit is sold as *bandoline, fixature*, or *clysphitique*, for stiffening the hair and keeping it in form.

ADMINISTRATION.—It is usually exhibited in the form of decoction or jelly. It has also been employed in combination with chocolate or cocoa.

1. DECOCTUM CHONDRI; *Decoction of Carrageen or Irish Moss.*—

Macerate half an ounce of carrageen in cold or warm water, during ten minutes; then boil in three pints of water for a quarter of an hour. Strain

---

[1] *Commentatio de Iodio*, Lugd. Bat. 1835.

[2] *Pharmaceutisches Central-Blatt für* 1839, S. 159.

[3] [This substance was called by Kützing *Gelin* (1843). See *Grundzüge der philosophischen Botanik*, vol. i. p. 190, 1851, where several modifications are enumerated.—ED.]

[4] *Berlin. Jahrb.* xxxiv. Abth. i. 1834.

[5] *Ann. der Chemie u. Pharm.* Bd. li. S. 29, 1844.

[6] *Pharmaceutisches Central-Blatt für* 1838, S. 500; and *The Chemistry of Animal and Vegetable Physiology*, by Fromberg and Johnston, Part ii. p. 239.

[7] *Journ. de Chim. Méd.* viii. 663.

through linen. When properly flavoured, it may be used as a *tisan* or common drink. By doubling the quantity of carrageen, a *mucilage* (*mucilago chondri*) is procured. Milk may be substituted for water when the decoction is required to be very nutritious. A preparation of this kind has been called *lac analepticum*. Sugar, lemon-juice, tincture of orange-peel, essence of lemon, or other aromatics, as cinnamon or nutmeg, may be employed as flavouring ingredients.

2. GELATINA CHONDRI; *Carrageen Jelly.*—This may be prepared by adding sugar to the strained decoction, and boiling down until the liquid is sufficiently concentrated to gelatinise on cooling; or by employing a larger quantity of carrageen. If milk be substituted for water, *carrageen blancmange* is obtained. Sugar and other flavouring ingredients may be employed, as above mentioned.

3. PASTA CACAO CUM CHONDRO; *Pasta Cacao cum Lichene Carragheno*, Ph. Dan.; *Carrageen Cocoa.* (The Danish Pharmacopœia gives the following directions for its preparation :—Roasted an l decorticated Cacao Seeds reduced to a very subtile mass in a warm iron mortar ; Powdered White Sugar, of each lb. ij.; Powdered Carrageen, ʒiij. Mix, and form into quadrangular sticks. Clarus and Radius[1] direct *carrageen*, or *white chocolate*, to be prepared as follows :—Cocoa Paste, ʒiv.; Powdered Carrageen, ʒvj.; White Sugar, ʒiv. ; Flour, q. s. (ʒvj.) Mix.)—These pastes are to be used like common cocoa or chocolate.

5. PLOCARIA CANDIDA, *Nees.*—CEYLON MOSS.

Sex. Syst. Cryptogamia, Algæ.

(Planta, *Offic.*)

SYNONYMES.—*Gracilaria lichenoides*, Greville; *Sphærococcus lichenoides*, Agardh; *Gigartina lichenoides*, Lamouroux; *Fucus lichenoides*, Turner; *Fucus amylaceus*, O'Shaughnessy; *Jaffna Moss; Edible Moss.*—According to Rumphius, it is called by the Malays *Sajor carang* and *Agar agar carang*: at Amboyna it is termed *Aysana* and *Aytsana* (h. e. *arbuscula ramosa*), and *Rume yar waccar;* at Java, *Bulung;* at Macassar, *Dongi dongi;* and at other places, *Lottu lottu* and *Collocane.*

HISTORY.—It seems to have been long known and used in the East. It has been described by Rumphius,[2] Gmelin,[3] Turner,[4] Nees,[5] and Agardh.[6] About the year 1837 it was introduced into England by Mr. Previtè ; and in the year 1840 public attention was drawn to its useful properties by Messrs. Sigmond and Farre.[7]

BOTANY.   **Gen. Char.**—*Frond* composed of large oblong-cylindrical cells containing granular endochrome, those of the surface forming moniliform,

---

[1] Dierbach, *Die neuesten Entdeck. in d. Mat. Med.* Bd. ii. S. 276, 1843.
[2] *Herb. Amboin.* Pars vi. lib. xi. cap. lvi. p. 181; *Alga coralloides*, tab. lxxvi. 1750.
[3] *Hist. Fucorum*, p. 113, 1768.
[4] *Fuci*, vol. ii. p. 124.
[5] *Hort. Physic. Berol.* 42, t. vi.
[6] *Syst. Algarum*, p. 233.
[7] *The Ceylon Moss*, Lond. 1840.

densely packed filaments. *Fructification* of two kinds: 1. hemispherical, *coccidia*, containing a glomerule of oblong spores on a central placenta, within a pericarp of moniliform, densely crowded filaments; 2. oblong *tetraspores* imbedded in cells of the surface (*Endlicher*).

Sp. Char.—*Frond* cartilaginous, cylindrical, filiform, much and irregularly branched; branches smooth, spreading, acute, somewhat fastigiate. *Coccidia* sessile, scattered.

Rumphius mentions four kinds of *Alga coralloides*, which he distinguishes as the *prima, secunda, tertia,* and *quarta;* and he has figured three kinds. Nees figures two plants,—one fertile, the other sterile. Turner notices two varieties: β *edulis* is a smaller variety, and has a remarkably flexuose frond, more thin and less branched than a: its colour is quite white.

Fig. 14.

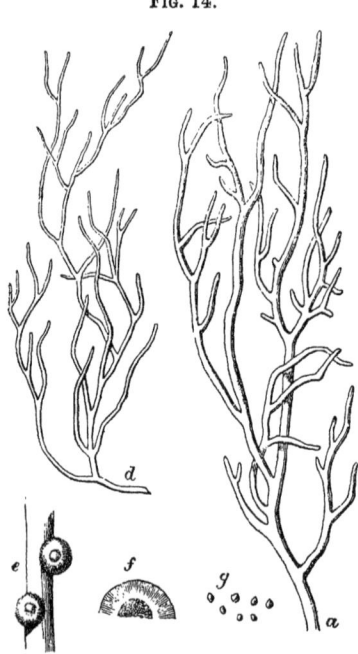

Plocaria candida.

a. Plocaria candida (nat. size).
d. Variety β edulis.
e. Part of frond with the coccidia (magnified).
f. Section of coccidium.
g. Spores.

Hab.—Ceylon at Jaffnapatam; the islands of the Indian Archipelago.

Commerce.—It is exported to China by the islands of the Indian Archipelago. Mr. Crawfurd[1] says that it forms a portion of the cargoes of all the junks; the price on the spot where it is collected seldom exceeding from 5s. 8d. to 7s.6¾d. per cwt. The Chinese use it in the form of jelly with sugar, as a sweetmeat, and apply it in the arts as an excellent paste. The gummy matter which they employ for covering lanterns, varnishing paper, &c. is made chiefly, if not entirely, from it.

[It would appear that under the name of Agar agar, or Ceylon moss, two very different articles are imported. Thus Mr. Archer has shown that specimens received at Liverpool consisted of Fucus spinosus, and contained no portion of Plocaria candida. It is certain, however, that this latter is also imported. The analyses which are here quoted seem to show that the specimen analysed by O'Shaughnessy, and by Bley, were different plants.[2]—Ed.]

Physical Properties.—Ceylon moss is in whitish or yellowish-white ramifying filaments of several inches in length. At the base the largest fibres do not exceed in thickness a crowquill; the smallest fibres are about as thick as fine sewing thread. To the naked eye the filaments appear almost cylindrical and filiform; but, when examined by a microscope, they appear shrivelled and wrinkled. The branchings are sometimes dichotomous, at other times irregular. Dr. Farre states that in a bale

[1] *History of the Indian Archipelago,* vol. iii. p. 446, 1820.
[2] *Pharm. Journ.* vol. xiii. p. 312, 447.

opened at Mr. Battley's, about $\frac{1}{15}$th appeared to bear fructification. The tubercles (*coccidia*) are inconspicuous when dry, but when moist are readily seen. They are hemispherical, about the size of a poppy-seed, and contain, according to Rumphius, a mass of minute, oblong, dark-red spores. The consistence of Ceylon moss is cartilaginous. Its flavour is that of sea-weed, with a feebly saline taste.

COMPOSITION.—This algal has been examined chemically, in 1834, by Dr. O'Shaughnessy ;[1] in 1842, by Guibourt ;[2] and in 1843, by Wonneberg and Kreyssig,[3] by Bley,[4] and by Riegel.[5]

O'Shaughnessy's Analysis.		*Bley's Analysis.*		*Riegel's Analysis.*	
Vegetable jelly	54·50	Pectin	37·5	Soluble gelatine	78·5
True starch	15	Lichen	3·85	Starch	6·0
Ligneous fibre	18	Ligneous fibre	16·08	Starchy skeleton	12·1
Gum	4	Gum	1·2	Resin	0·63
Wax	a trace	Albumen	0·9	Chloride of sodium	1·85
Sulphate and muriate of		Fatty matters	19·95	Chloride of magnesium ..	0·54
soda	6·50	Lichenic acid	0·05	Sulphate of soda	0·38
Sulphate and phosphate		Chloride of calcium	0·20		
of lime	1	Chloride of sodium	1·72		100·00
Iron	a trace	Water	18·5		
				The ashes of the skeleton con-	
	99		99·95	tained sulphate of lime,	
Assume the traces of the		The ashes of the ligneous fibre		phosphate of lime, and mag-	
wax and iron, and the		contained chloride of so-		nesia.	
loss, at	1	dium, sulphates of lime and			
		of magnesia, carbonates of			
Total	100	lime and magnesia, oxide of			
		iron, silica, and iodic salt.			

1. MUCILAGINOUS MATTER (*Carrageenin ?*) ; *Vegetable Jelly ; Pectin ; Soluble Gelatine.* —The mucilaginous or gelatinising principle of Ceylon moss appears to me to agree very closely, if indeed it be not identical, with carrageenin. It has not hitherto been analysed.

2. STARCHY MATTER.—This resides chiefly in the cortical portion of the algal. But the internal cell-walls become deeply stained purplish-brown on the addition of iodine, as if they were composed of a starchy substance (*starchy skeleton*).

CHEMICAL CHARACTERISTICS.—By moistening Ceylon moss with a weak solution of ioduretted iodide of potassium, the plant acquires a purplish-brown or red colour; the younger and more delicate fibres becoming almost black. The change of colour is most intense in the cortical portion, but the internal cell-walls also become stained. By digestion in warm water, the plant softens and swells up. By boiling it in water, and then compressing and rubbing it gently between two plates of glass, the larger spheroidal cells are readily separated from each other : they are stained purplish-brown by iodine. The aqueous decoction is mucilaginous and, when sufficiently concentrated, gelatinises on cooling. Iodine colours it a dull or purplish-brown, and gives an intense dark purplish colour to the undissolved residue of the plant. If the plant be immersed in diluted hydrochloric acid, slight effervescence occurs,

[1] Sigmond and Farre. *The Ceylon Moss*, p. 74, 1840.
[2] *Journ. de Chimie Méd.* t. viii. 2nde sér. p. 368, 1842.
[3] *Pharmaceutisches Central-Blatt für* 1843, p. 252.
[4] *Ibidem*, p. 409.
[5] *Ibidem.*

owing to the escape of carbonic acid evolved by the action of the hydrochloric acid on carbonate of lime.

Physiological Effects.—These are similar to those of *Chondrus crispus*. Ceylon moss, therefore, may be denominated nutritive (chiefly as an element of respiration, see Vol. i. p. 64), emollient, and demulcent. By the continued use of it at the table, the saline constituents of the plant would not be without some influence on the system.

Uses.—In the form of decoction or jelly, it is employed as a light and readily digestible article of food for invalids and children. The residue of the decoction is not devoid of nutritive matter, and might be served and eaten like cabbage or leguminous substances; especially when the alterative influence of the saline constituents is desired. The decoction or jelly of Ceylon moss may be employed in irritation of the mucous surfaces, and in phthisis. It is not apt to occasion thirst, sickness, flatulence, heartburn, acidity, or diarrhœa.

Administration.—It may be administered in the form of decoction or jelly. Dr. O'Shaughnessy recommends that it should be steeped for a few hours in cold rain water, as the first step to its preparation: this removes a large portion of the sulphate of soda. It should then be dried by the sun's rays, and ground to a fine powder; for cutting or pounding, however diligently performed, still leaves the amylaceous matter so mechanically protected that the boiling may be prolonged for hours without extracting the starch. This grinding process, however, is seldom employed, the prepared plant being in general merely cut into very small pieces.

1. DECOCTUM PLOCARIÆ CANDIDÆ ; *Decoction of Ceylon Moss.*—This is prepared by boiling the prepared moss in water, milk, or whey. One drachm of the plant will give a mucilaginous quality to eight ounces of water. Milk, sugar, orange- or lemon-juice and peel, wine, cinnamon, or other aromatics, may be used to communicate flavour. This decoction may be taken *ad libitum.*

2. GELATINA PLOCARIÆ CANDIDÆ ; *Jelly of Ceylon Moss.*—Mr. Previtè's directions for its preparation are the following:—Boil half an ounce of the prepared moss in a quart of boiling water for twenty-five minutes, or until a spoonful of the liquid forms into a firm jelly within two or three minutes after it is removed from the boiler. Flavour with wine, a little cinnamon, lemon- or orange-juice and peel, and sweeten according to taste. Boil the whole for five minutes, and pass it two or three times through a jelly-bag or doubled muslin. Leave it undisturbed, and it will become a firm jelly in ten minutes. If it be required perfectly clear for table use, add the white of two eggs beaten up into a whip before the second boiling, and allow it to stand for a few minutes away from the fire, with some hot coals on the top of the boiler. When clear, pass it through the jelly-bag, and leave it to congeal. Should the jelly be required particularly firm, add an ounce of moss to the quart of water.

6. PLOCARIA HELMINTHOCORTON, *Endl.*—CORSICAN MOSS.

Sex. Syst. Cryptogamia, Algæ.

(Planta, *Offic.*)

HISTORY.—This plant has been in use for several centuries, among the natives of Corsica, as a remedy for intestinal worms. In 1756, Vaucher sent it to Paris.[1]

BOTANY. **Gen. Char.**—See *Plocaria candida.*

Sp. Char.—*Frond* cartilaginous, terete, tufted, entangled. *Stem* filiform, creeping; branches setaceous, somewhat dichotomous, marked indistinctly with transverse streaks.

Hab.—The Mediterranean Sea, on the shores of Corsica.

PHYSICAL PROPERTIES.—Under the name of Corsican moss is sold in the shops a mixture of various marine vegetables and animals. The essential, though usually smaller, part of the mixture is the Plocaria Helminthocorton; the remainder consists of Corallines, Sertularias, and Ceramiums, to the number of twenty species.[2] Lamouroux states he found the remains of eighty species of marine plants.[3] (See also T. C. Martius.[4])

The structure of the frond of Plocaria Helminthocorton is "very peculiar, being exceedingly lax and cellular, with a consistence similar to that of the stems and leaf-stalks of some aquatic herbaceous phænogamous plants, and having the appearance of articulations which do not actually exist."[5] The fructification is scarcely ever seen. The plant has a reddish-grey colour externally, but is whitish internally. Its odour is strong, marine, and disagreeable: its taste is saline.

COMPOSITION. — Bouvier[6] obtained from 100 parts of Corsican moss, *vegetable jelly* [mucilage? carrageenin?], 60·2; *vegetable fibre*, 11·0; *chloride of sodium*, 9·2; *sulphate of lime*, 11·2; *carbonate of lime*, 7·5; *iron*, *manganese*, *silica*, and *phosphate of lime*, 1·7. Straub[7] and Gaultier de Claubry[8] have subsequently detected iodine, but the quantity is small.

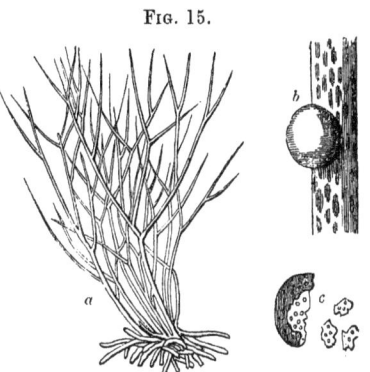

FIG. 15.

Plocaria Helminthocorton

a. The plant (natural size).

b. A small stony coral attached to the thallus, and which may be readily mistaken for the fructification.

c. The same, broken and magnified to show the pores.

---

[1] J. P. Schwendimann, in Schlegel's *Thesaurus Mat. Med.* t. iii. p. 181.

[2] De Candolle, *Essai sur les Propriétés Méd.* p. 348, 2d ed.

[3] Fée, *Cours d'Hist. Nat.* i. 147.

[4] *Grundriss d. Pharmakog.* 12.

[5] Greville, *Algæ Brit.* p. 146.

[6] *Ann. de Chim.* ix. 83, 1791.

[7] *Gilbert's Ann.* Bd. lxvi. S. 242.

[8] *Ann. de Chim.* xciii. 134.

CHEMICAL CHARACTERISTICS.—Corsican moss effervesces with acids, owing to the carbonate of lime which it contains. The brown watery infusion is deepened in colour by sesquichloride of iron, and lets fall some brown flocculi. Tincture of galls does not alter it. Nitric acid and starch give no indication of iodine.

PHYSIOLOGICAL EFFECTS.—Its effects are not very obvious. The vegetable jelly (mucilage) must render it somewhat nutritive; the iodine and saline matters alterative. Mr. Farr[1] says, that after using the decoction for six or seven days, it acts as a diuretic and diaphoretic, and occasionally produces nausea and giddiness: after some time the stools become darker, present greenish specks, and are sometimes slimy.

USES.—It has been principally celebrated as an anthelmintic against the large round worm (*Ascaris lumbricoides*). Bremser[2] ascribes its efficacy to chloride of sodium.

In 1822, Mr. Farr brought it forward as a remedy for cancer. He was led to try it from the circumstance of Napoleon Bonaparte having stated to Barry O'Meara that it was used in Corsica for dispersing tumors. Experience does not warrant us in ascribing any benefit to its employment in this disease.

ADMINISTRATION.—In *powder*, it is given in doses of a scruple to two drachms, mixed with honey or sugar; but the more usual mode of exhibiting it is in the form of *decoction*, prepared by boiling from four to six drachms of it in a pint of water; of this the dose is a wine-glassful, three times daily.

ORDER II. LICHENES, *Juss.*—LICHENS.

LICHENALES, *Lind.*

CHARACTERS.—*Perennial*, aërial thallogens, nourished through their whole surface by the medium in which they vegetate; always constituting a *thallus, crust*, or *frond* (*receptaculum universale; blastema*), formed of a cortical and a medullary layer, of which the former is simply cellular, the latter cellular and filamentous [producing here and there moniliform threads consisting of green globose cells (*gonidia*). Below the medullary layer is a third, closely resembling the first, and often producing on its surface filamentous or fibrous processes, by which it adheres to the matrix.—ED.] *Apothecia* (*fructus*) consisting of a *receptacle*, and a *proligerous layer* (*lamina proligera*) composed of *spores* (*sporæ*) naked or enclosed in *spore cases* (*asci; thecæ*), united to form a *nucleus*, or disposed on a *disc* (*discus*). [*Pycnidia* (*fructus secundarius*) subglobose, producing minute oblong naked spores (*spermatia*).—ED.]

PROPERTIES.—The tissue of lichens consists of *cellulose*. Many of them contain *amylaceous matters* (*lichenin* or *feculoid*, and *inulin*) and their congeners *gum* and *sugar*, which render them nutritive, emollient, and demulcent. *Bitter principles* (*cetraric acid; picrolichenin*) are sometimes found in lichens: these confer slight tonic properties. *Colouring matters* (*thallochlor, chrysophanic acid*, &c.) are frequently present. *Colorific principles* (*orcellic, erythric, lecanoric*, and other *acids*), or principles which, under the combined influence of ammonia and oxygen, form colouring matters (*orceine*, &c.), render some of the lichens valuable in the arts. Besides the before-mentioned bodies, several other *vegetable acids* (as the *tartaric, oxalic, tannic*, and *lichestearic*) are found in the lichens. The oxalic acid is found in combination with lime: one lichen (*Variolaria faginea*) contains 47 per cent. of calcareous oxalate. The *ashes* of the lichens constitute

---

[1] *A Treatise explanatory of a Method whereby occult Cancers may be cured*, 2d ed. 1825.
[2] *Sur les Vers Intestin.* 414.

about 8 per cent. of the dried plants, and consist principally of the earths: the ashes of lichens growing on siliceous rocks contain more silica than those of lichens growing in other situations. It is deserving of especial notice that not a single poisonous lichen is known.

The lichens which I shall have to notice may be conveniently divided, according to their uses, into the esculent, the medicinal, and the tinctorial lichens.

1. LICHENES ESCULENTI ET MEDICINALES.—EDIBLE AND MEDICINAL LICHENS.

The only lichen employed medicinally by British practitioners is Iceland moss (*Cetraria islandica*). But several other lichens, whose medicinal qualities are in reality similar to, though much feebler than, Iceland moss, are still kept in the London herb-shops, being occasionally employed as popular remedies. Those which I have met with are *Peltidea canina, Scyphophorus pyxidatus*, and *Sticta pulmonaria*. These, as well as *Gyrophora, Parmelia parietina*, and *Cladonia rangiferina*, require a short notice.

7. Peltidea canina, *Ach.*—Ash-coloured Ground Liverwort.

PELTIDEA CANINA, Ach. Syn. p. 239 ; *Lichen caninus*, Linn.; *Lichen cinereus terrestris*, Woodville, Med. Bot. vol. iv.; *Ash-coloured Ground Liverwort*.

This species, and also *Peltidea rufescens*, Ach., are sold in the herb-shops as *Ground Liverwort*. It formerly was in repute as a preservative against the bite of a mad dog,[1] and mixed with half its weight of black pepper it formed the *pulvis anti-lyssus* (ἀντί, against, and λύσσα, canine madness) of the London Pharmacopœia for 1721.

FIG. 17.

FIG. 16.

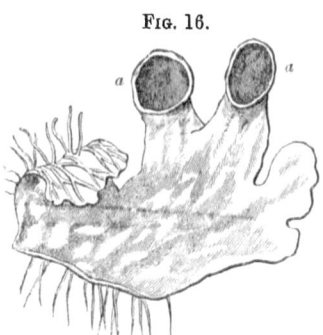

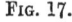

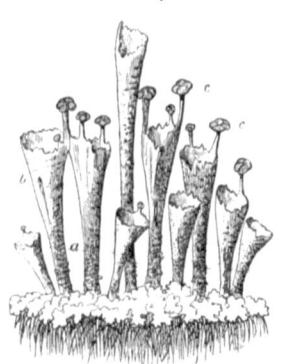

Peltidea canina.
Portion of the thallus, with the apothecia, *a a.* (Natural size.)

Scyphophorus pyxidatus.
a. The podetium. *b.* The cup or scypha. *c c.* The apothecia.

8. Scyphophorus pyxidatus, *Hook.*—Cup-moss.

SCYPHOPHORUS PYXIDATUS, Hook. Engl. Fl. vi. p. 238 ; *Cenomyce pyxidata*, Ach. Syn.; *Cladonia pyxidata*, Schær. Lich. Helv. Spicil. p. 26; *Lichen pyxidatus*, Linn.; *Muscus*

---

[1] *Phil. Trans.* vol. xx. p. 49; Mead, *A Mechan. Account of Poisons*, 5th ed. p. 165, Lond. 1756.

pyxidatus, Dale, Pharm.; *Cup-moss.*—This species (frequently mixed with *S. fimbriatus,* Hook., and sometimes with *S. cocciferus,* Hook.) is the Cup-moss of the shops. It was recommended by Dr. Willis[1] as a remedy for hooping-cough.[2] He gave it in drachm doses, in the form of powder, decoction, and syrup.

9. Sticta pulmonaria, *Hook.*—Tree Lungwort.

Sticta pulmonaria, Hook. Engl. Fl.; *St. pulmonacea,* Ach. Syn. p. 233; *Lichen pulmonarius,* Linn.; *Muscus pulmonaria,* Dale, Pharm.; *Tree Lungwort; Oak-lungs.*— This lichen has been analysed by John,[3] who found it to contain *resinous chlorophylle,* 2; *bitter extractive,* 8; *lichen starch,* 7; *insoluble matters,* 80; *salts,* &c. 3. Its virtues are dependent on the bitter and amylaceous matter, and are similar, but inferior, to those of Iceland moss. It has been esteemed as a pectoral in pulmonary affections, as an astringent in internal hemorrhages, and as a remedy for jaundice. It has been given in doses of a drachm, in the form of powder or decoction. In Siberia, where the plant seems to be more bitter than in this country, it is employed as a substitute for hops in brewing.[4]

10. Gyrophora.

Several species of Gyrophora (as *G. proboscidea* β *arctica, G. hyperborea, G. Pennsylvanica,* and *G. Muhlenbergii*) are employed by the hunters of the Arctic regions of America as articles of food, under the name of *tripe de roche.* All four species were eaten by Captain Franklin and his companions in 1821, when suffering great privations in America; and to its use may their preservation be in part ascribed.[5] But not having the means of extracting the bitter principle, these lichens proved noxious to several of the party, producing severe bowel complaints.

Fig. 18.

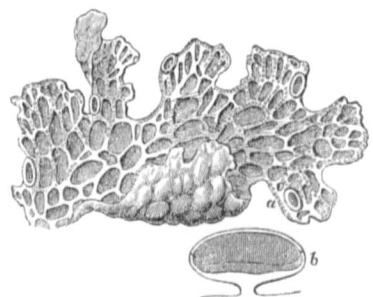

Fig. 19.

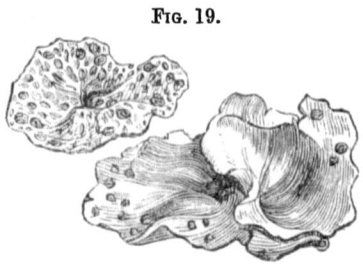

Sticta pulmonaria.
Portion of the thallus with the apothecia
(*scutellæ*).

a. Cyphellæ.
b. Section of the apothecium.

Tripe de Roche.
(Gyrophora.)

---

[1] *Pharmaceutice Rationalis,* pars 2da, p. 49, 1678.
[2] See also Dillenii *Dissertatio de Lichene Pyxidato,* in Schlegel's *Thesaurus Materiæ Medicæ,* t. i. p. 307, Lipsiæ, 1793.
[3] L. Gmelin, *Handb. d. th. Chem.* Bd. ii. S. 1351, 1829.
[4] Murray, *App. Medicam.* vol. v. p. 520.
[5] Franklin's *Narrative of a Journey to the Shores of the Polar Sea,* 1823.

11. Cladonia rangiferina, *Hoffm.*—Rein-deer Moss.

CLADONIA RANGIFERINA, Hoffm.; *Cenomyce rangiferina*, Ach. Syn. p. 277 ; *Lichen rangiferinus*, Linn.; *Rein-deer Moss.*—This lichen has become celebrated on account of the beautiful description of it, and of its uses, given by Linnæus, in his *Flora Lapponica*, p. 332. It is this plant which, for the greatest part of the year, and especially during the winter season, is the support of the vast heards of rein-deer, wherein consists all the wealth of the Laplanders.

I have frequently bought this lichen, with others, of the London herbalists, who, however, are unacquainted with its real name, but who sell various species of lichens under the denomination of "*mosses*," for the use of bird-stuffers, who decorate the inside of their cases with them.

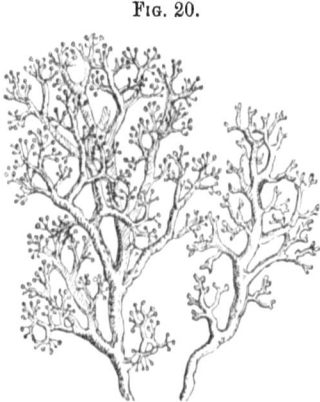

FIG. 20.

Cladonia rangiferina.

12. CETRARIA ISLANDICA, *Ach.*—ICELAND MOSS.

Sex. Syst. Cryptogamia, Algæ.
(Planta, *Offic.*)

HISTORY.—The medicinal properties of this plant (usually termed *Lichen islandicus*) were probably first known to the natives of Iceland. According to Borrichius, the Danish apothecaries were acquainted with them in 1673. In 1683, Hiärne spoke favourably of its effects in hæmoptysis and phthisis.

BOTANY. **Gen. Char.**—*Thallus* foliaceous, cartilagino-membranaceous, ascending and spreading, lobed and laciniated, on each side smooth and naked. *Apothecia* orbicular, obliquely adnate with the margin of the thallus, the lower portion being free (not united with the thallus) ; the disc coloured, plano-concave, with a border formed of the thallus, and inflexed (*Hooker*).

FIG. 21.

Sp. Char.—*Thallus* erect, tufted, olive-brown, paler on one side, laciniated, channelled, and dentatociliated, the fertile lacinia very broad. *Apothecia* brown, appressed, flat, with an elevated border (*Hooker*).

Hab.—Dry mountainous districts of the new and old continents. Although met with in considerable abundance in Scotland, it is never gathered there as an article of commerce.

The word *cetraria* is derived from *cetra* or *caetra* (καιτρεα, Hesych), an ancient shield made of leather, which the apothecia are supposed to resemble.

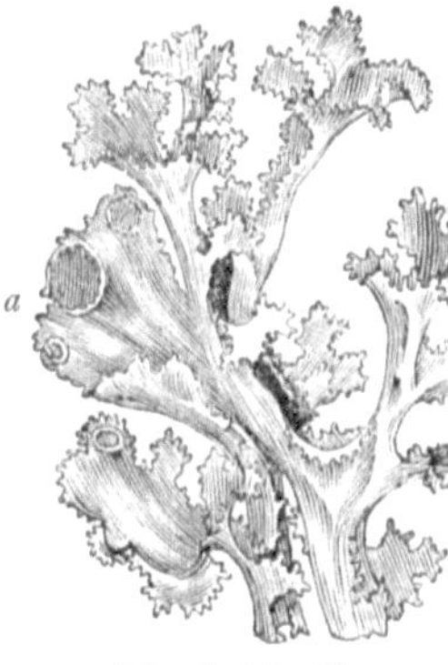

Cetraria islandica.

a. The *apothecia* on the larger lobes of the thallus.

COLLECTION.—The lichen should be collected on dry and clear days, carefully deprived of all foreign matter by hand-picking, and dried in the sun.

PHYSICAL PROPERTIES.—The Iceland moss of commerce (*muscus islandicus; lichen islandicus*) is in general brownish or greyish-white; the upper surface darker, towards the base sometimes marked with blood-red spots; the under surface paler, whitish, with white spots which have a chalky or mealy appearance, are lodged in little depressions of the thallus, and when submitted to microscopic examination appear warty, pearl-white masses. Apothecia are rather rare on the commercial lichen. When quite dry, the lichen is crisp, cartilaginous, and coriaceous. It is almost odourless, and has a bitter mucilaginous taste. Its powder (*farina*) is whitish-grey.

COMMERCE.—It is imported in barrels and bags from Hamburgh and Gottenburgh, and is said to be the produce of Norway and Iceland. In 1836, 20,599 lbs. paid duty; in 1837, 12,845 lbs.; in 1838, 6179 lbs.; in 1839, 15,933 lbs.; and in 1840, 6462 lbs.

COMPOSITION.—It was analysed by Berzelius[1] in 1808, who obtained the following products from 100 parts:—*green wax*, 1·6; *yellow extractive matter*, 7·0; *bitter matter*, 3·0; *uncrystallisable sugar*, 3·6; *gum*, 3·7; *starch*, 44·6; *starchy skeleton*, 36·2; *gallic acid*, trace; *bitartrate of potash, tartrate of lime*, and a little *phosphate of lime*, 1·9 (=101·6).

In 1844-5 it was examined by Messrs. Schnedermann and Knopp.[2]

The following figures represent the microscopic appearances of sections of the lichens:—

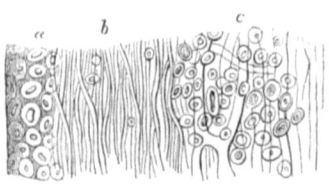

FIG. 22.

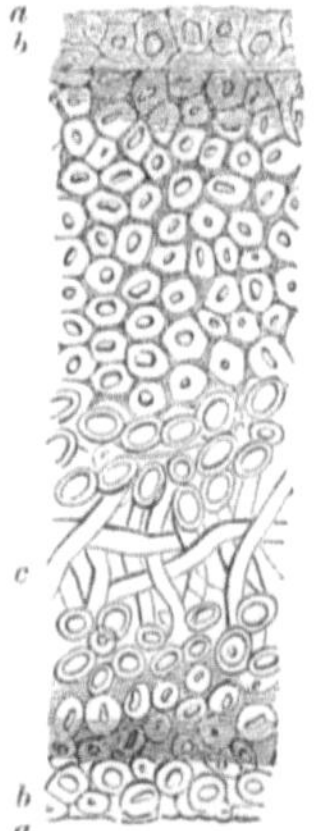

FIG. 23.

FIG. 24.

Longitudinal section of the thallus.

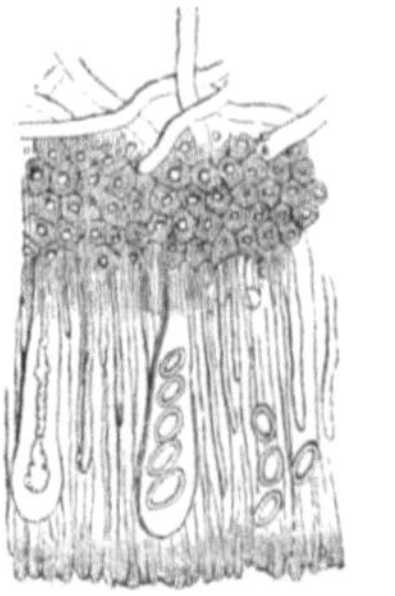

Longitudinal section of the apothecium, with the thecæ and the adherent filamentous layer.

Transverse section of the thallus.

Sections of Cetraria Islandica (highly magnified).

  a. External or cortical layer, which does not become blue by the addition of the tincture of iodine.
  b. Subcortical layer (*stratum gonimicum*, Wallroth; *stratum fæculare*, Wahlenberg), which becomes blue on the addition of tincture of iodine.
  c. Medullary layer, composed of felted filaments or tubes (*tela contexta*, Schleiden) and intermixed nucleated cells (*annuli*, Link; *gonidia*, Fr.)

1. AMYLACEOUS MATTER.—Cetraria islandica contains at least two kinds of amylaceous matter; namely, one which is coloured blue by iodine (*lichen-starch*), and one which does not become blue with this agent (*inuline*). Link[3] states that the amylaceous matter of

[1] *Ann. de Chim.* xc. 277.
[2] *Annal. der Chim. u. Pharm.* Bd. lv. S. 144, 1845; *Pharm. Journ.* vol. v. p. 427, 1846.
[3] *Icones selectæ Anatomico-Botanicæ*, Fascic. iii. Berlin, 1841.

Cetraria does not occur in a globular form. If by amylaceous matter is to be understood starch-grains, which are rendered blue by iodine, my observations confirm his statement. Payen,[1] however, says he has seen the starch of Iceland moss in the form of little balls; but he has probably mistaken the cells for starch-grains. When a thin section of the thallus has been soaked in cold water, and then placed under the microscope, a general blue tint is communicated to the subcortical layer (see figs. 22 and 23), on the addition of tincture of iodine: but none of the cells or granules become blue. A starchy non-granular matter, rendered blue by iodine, appears to reside in the intercellular tissue of the subcortical layer. My friend Mr. Henry Deane has traced this amylaceous matter to the surface of the apothecia, which appears to be deficient in the cortical non-amylaceous layer. Moreover, iodine colours sections of the apothecia in stripes, rendering blue the starchy matter between the thecæ and elongated cells (see fig. 24). I have sometimes seen the nucleated cells of the medullary layer (see fig. 23) assume an amber colour when treated with iodine. Is this owing to the presence of inuline?

α. *Lichen Starch.*—This becomes blue on the addition of iodine. According to Schnedermann and Knopp, hydrochloric acid converts it into a transparent jelly. Its formula, according to Mulder, is $C^{12}H^{10}C^{10}$. Even after very prolonged boiling in water, the tissue of Iceland moss still retains the property of being tinged blue by iodine; hence it has been called *amylaceous tissue, starchy skeleton,* &c. Mulder says that when boiled sufficiently, and acted on by solvents, the final residue of it is nothing but *cellulose :* it is improper, therefore, to call it amylaceous tissue.

β. *Inuline.*—This, according to Payen and others, is a constituent of Iceland moss. It is tinged yellow by iodine. When insoluble in cold water its formula is probably $C^{12}H^{10}O^{10}$. Mulder is of opinion that the chief part of lichen starch must be composed of a starch which, like inuline, is turned yellow by iodine, and, like common starch, can be precipitated by basic acetate of lead.

2. CETRARIC ACID; *Cetrarin ; Bitter Principle of Iceland Moss.*—This resides in the cortical portion of the thallus. It exists there for the most part in the state of free cetraric acid, and not as a cetrarate. In the pure state the acid occurs in the form of shining minute acicular crystals. It is intensely bitter, not volatile, and is infusible without decomposition. It is almost insoluble in water, which, however, acquires a bitter taste when boiled with the acid. It is soluble in boiling alcohol, but crystallises in great part on cooling. It is slightly soluble in ether, and is quite insoluble in the fixed and volatile oils. Its formula is $C^{34}H^{16}O^{15}$. It is dissolved both by the caustic and carbonated alkalies, and is precipitated from its solution by acids. *Cetrarate of ammonia* $(2NH^3,C^{34}H^{16}O^{15})$ is a beautiful yellow salt, having a faint ammoniacal odour, and being soluble in water. By exposure to the air it gradually becomes brown. Schnedermann explains the production of the brown colour of Iceland moss, by supposing that the cetraric acid of the thallus absorbs atmospheric ammonia, and the cetrarate of ammonia thus formed becomes brown by exposure to the air. The alkaline cetrarates yield a red colour (*cetrarate of iron*) with the salts of the peroxide of iron. Now as the ashes of Iceland moss contain iron, Schnedermann thinks it not improbable that the red spots which are sometimes found at the base of the lichen may be due to the presence of cetrarate of iron, produced by the action of cetrarate of ammonia (formed as above explained) on the ferruginous constituent. *Cetrarate of lead* $(2PbO,C^{34}H^{16}O^{15})$ forms a yellow flocculent precipitate.

3. LICHESTEARIC ACID (so called from λειχήν, *lichen ;* and στέαρ, *fat*).—When pure it is perfectly white, and consists of pearly crystalline plates. It is odourless, but has an acrid taste. It is soluble in alcohol, ether, and the volatile and fatty oils, but is insoluble in water. At 248° F. it melts, and on cooling congeals into a crystalline mass. It cannot be volatilised without decomposition. Its formula is $C^{29}H^{25}O^6$. It is dissolved by alkalies, and is precipitated from its alkaline solution by acids. *Lichestearate of potash* is a white indistinctly crystalline powder; *lichestearate of silver* $(AgO,C^{29}H^{24}O^5)$ is greyish-white; *lichestearate of lead* $(PbO,C^{24}H^{24}O^5)$ is white ; *lichestearate of baryta* is greyish-white; *lichestearate of ammonia* is crystallisable.

4. FUMARIC ACID; *Lichenic Acid.*—This acid was discovered in Iceland moss by Pfaff.

5. A neutral substance, called provisionally "*the body* C," is mentioned by Schnedermann as being contained in tolerable quantity in the lichen. It is white, tasteless, insoluble in water, ether, oils, alkalies, and acids, and difficultly soluble in hot spirit.

---

[1] *L'Institut de* 1837, p. 145.

6. Chlorothalle; *Thallochlor.*—This is the green colouring matter. It is soluble in ether, alcohol, and petroleum. It has the properties of a weak acid, and is distinguished from chlorophylle by being little or not at all soluble in hydrochloric acid.

Chemical Characteristics.—Iceland moss swells up in cold water, to which it communicates some portion of bitterness, and a very little mucilage. If to the moistened thallus some tincture of iodine be added, the tissues become intensely blackish-blue; but the white chalky- or mealy-looking spots, before mentioned, are unaltered by iodine, and appear more brilliantly white, in consequence of the black ground on which they are placed.

By prolonged boiling in water, the lichen yields a mucilaginous decoction, which, when sufficiently concentrated, gelatinises on cooling. A solution of iodine communicates a blue colour (*iodide of starch*) to the cold decoction.

When the decoction has been imperfectly prepared, in consequence of being weak, and insufficiently boiled, it yields a dingy green colour with iodine. The green colour depends on the mixture of two coloured substances,—one yellow, the other blue. "If," says Mulder, "a diluted decoction of Iceland moss, after being coloured with iodine, is allowed to settle for a while, the layer at the bottom is yellow, and that immediately above is blue."[1]

The decoction yields with the basic acetate of lead a copious whitish precipitate (*amylate of lead*); and with a mixture of sulphate of copper and potash, a green precipitate (*cetrarate of copper*).[2] The sesquisalts of iron communicate a red colour (*cetrarate of iron*) both to the decoction and to an alcoholic tincture of Iceland moss (prepared by digesting ℥ij. of the lichen in f℥vj. of rectified spirit).

In strong hydrochloric acid the thallus swells up, owing to the gelatinisation of the starch contained in the intercellular spaces.

Physiological Effects. *a. On Animals.*—In Carniola, pigs, horses, and oxen are fattened by it.[3]

β. On Man.—It is a mucilaginous or demulcent tonic, without any trace of astringency. If the bitter matter (*cetraric acid*) and extractive be removed, it is nutritive, emollient, and demulcent, like ordinary starch, over which it has no advantage. Captain Sir John Franklin and his companions tried it as an article of food, when suffering great privations in America, but its bitterness rendered it hardly eatable.[4]

[Recent Arctic voyagers have met with an Alga, *Nostoc arcticum*, Berk., which is far superior to the Tripe de roche.[5]]

Uses.—Iceland moss is well adapted to those cases requiring a nutritious and easily-digested aliment, and a mild tonic not liable to disorder the stomach. It has been principally recommended in chronic affections of the pulmonary and digestive organs, particularly phthisis, chronic catarrh, dyspepsia, chronic diarrhœa, and dysentery; but its efficacy has been much exaggerated.

---

[1] [According to our observation, the colour struck by iodine is rather a dingy purple-black colour. In the decoctions of some samples no change indicative of the presence of starch has been produced.—Ed.]

[2] Herberger, *Journ. de Pharm.* xxii.

[3] Murray, *App. Med.* v. 506.

[4] *Narrative of a Journey to the Shores of the Polar Sea*, p. 414, 1823.

[5] [Sutherland, *Journal of a Voyage in Baffin's Bay*, &c. p. cxiv.—Ed.]

ADMINISTRATION.—It is best exhibited in the form of decoction. When employed as an alimentary substance merely, the bitter matter should be extracted before ebullition. This is effected by digesting the lichen in a cold weak alkaline solution (composed of water 300 parts, and carbonate of potash 1 part), and afterwards washing it with cold water.[1] But the subsequent washing will not remove the whole of the alkaline salt. Instead, therefore, of using an alkali, distilled water may be used to extract the bitter principle. The lichen should be heated once or twice in water up to about 180° F., by which the lichen will be deprived of most of its bitterness. It is then to be boiled in water or milk. When the decoction is sufficiently concentrated it gelatinises on cooling. It may be flavoured with sugar, lemon-peel, white wine, or aromatics, and then forms a very agreeable kind of diet.

DECOCTUM CETRARIÆ, L.; *Decoctum Lichenis Islandici,* D.; *Decoction of Iceland Moss.* (Iceland Moss, ʒv.; Water, Oiss. Boil down to a pint, and strain. The *Dublin College* orders Moss, ʒj.; Water, Oiss. Wash the moss in cold water to remove impurities, then boil it for ten minutes in a covered vessel, and strain while hot. The product should measure about one pint.)—Dose fʒj. to fʒiv. every four hours.

13. Parmelia parietina, *Ach.*—Common Yellow Wall Lichen.

PARMELIA PARIETINA, Ach.; *Lobaria parietina,* Hoffm.; *Lichen parietinus,* Linn.; *Common Yellow Wall Lichen.*—Usually sold in the herb-shops under the name of *common yellow wall moss.* Χρυσοφύλλον, hodie in Zacyntho, *Sibth.* Thallus foliaceous, membranaceous, orbicular, bright yellow : the lobes marginal, radiating, rounded, crenate, and crisped, granulated in the centre, beneath paler and fibrillose. Apothecia deep-orange, concave with an entire border (*Hooker*).—This lichen has been the subject of repeated chemical investigation. According to Herberger,[2] it contains *two* beautiful colouring matters (parmelia-yellow and parmelia-red), several alimentary principles (gliadin, sugar, starch, and gum), and three medicinal substances (soft resin, bitter matter, and volatile oil); besides wax, stearine, chlorophylle, and woody fibre. Rochleder and Heldt[3] give the name of *chrysophanic acid* ($C^{10}H^8O^3$) to the golden-yellow crystallisable colouring matter, which, more recently, Schlossberger and Doepping[4] have found to be identical with the yellow colouring matter of rhubarb (*rheine, rheumine, rhabarbaric acid*). In 1815, this lichen was lauded by Dr. Sander[5] as a valuable substitute for cinchona bark in intermittents. He also gave it with success in hemorrhages and fluxes. Haller had previously spoken favourably of it as a tonic in diarrhœa and dysentery ; and Willemet had found it useful in contagious autumnal fluxes. Subsequent experience, however, has not confirmed the favourable reports made of its medicinal power. The dose of it in powder is from Ɖj. to ʒj. It may also be given in the form of decoction, tincture, and extract. Dr. R. D. Thomson[6] has proposed it as a test for alkalies, which communicate to its yellow colouring matter (called by him *parietin*) a beautiful red tint.

---

[1] Dr. Davidson, in a paper *On the Removal of the Bitter Taste and Lichenous Odour of Iceland Moss* (Jameson's *Edinb. New Phil. Journ.* vol. xxviii. p. 260, 1840), recommends a solution of caustic potash for extracting the bitter taste of this lichen. A pound of carbonate of potash (rendered caustic by a pound of lime) is sufficient for 28 lbs. of the plant.

[2] Buchner's *Repertorium,* Bd. xlvii. S. 179, 1834.

[3] *Ann. d. Chem. u. Pharm.* Bd. xlviii. S. 12, 1843 ; and *Chem. Gazette,* vol. ii. p. 162, 1844.

[4] *Ibid.* Bd. i. S. 295, 1844 ; *Pharm. Journal,* vol. iv.

[5] *Die Wandflechte, ein Arzneymittel, welches die peruv. Rinde nicht nur entbehrlich macht, sondern sie auch an gleichart. Heilkräften übertrifft,* 4to. Sondershausen, 1815.

[6] *Lond. Ed. and Dub. Phil. Mag.* July 1844.

2. Lichenes tinctorii.—Tinctorial Lichens.

1. Number and Variety.—A considerable number of lichens have been employed by man on account of the colouring matter which they yield him. Some of them (e. g. *Parmelia parietina* and *Evernia vulpina*) contain colouring principles (e. g. *chrysophanic* and *vulpinic acids*). Others (e. g. several species of *Roccella*, of *Lecanora*, of *Variolaria*, &c.) contain principles (e. g. *orsellic, erythric, lecanoric*, and *gyrophoric acids*) which are colourless while in the plant, but which, under the influence of alkalies and atmospheric oxygen, yield colouring matters (e. g. *orceine*). Such principles I shall distinguish as *colorific* or colour-making.

2. Colours.—Lichens furnish four principal colours, viz. brown, yellow, purple, and blue.

a. Brown colours are yielded by *Gyrophora pustulata* and *Sticta pulmonaria* (see *ante*, p. 20). The latter lichen, says Professor Guibourt,[1] produces on silk, by using as mordants bitartrate of potash and chloride of tin, a very fine and durable carmelite colour. For use in France it is principally collected in the Vosges.

β. Yellow colours are yielded by *Parmelia parietina* (see *ante*, p. 25) and *Evernia vulpina*. The former lichen contains, as its yellow colouring principle, *chrysophanic acid;* the latter, according to M Bebert,[2] contains a yellow crystallisable acid called *vulpinic acid.*

γ and *δ. Purple* and *blue* colours are yielded by a considerable number of lichens. In this country purple colours (*orchil* and *cudbear*) only are obtained from them; but in Holland a blue colour (*litmus*) is also prepared from these. It appears that the same lichens yield either the one or the other colour, according to the method of treatment.

The orchil or archil makers of this country call the cylindrical and flat pieces of Roccella used in the manufacture of orchil and cudbear, *weeds* or *orchella weeds,* and distinguish them according to the countries yielding them (e. g. *Angola weed, Canary weed,* &c.); while the crustaceous and foliaceous lichens, employed for similar purposes, they term *mosses* (e. g. *tartareous moss, pustulatous moss, rock moss,* &c.) A similar distinction is made in French commerce; the term *herbe* being applied to what the English call a *weed,* while the name of *lichen* is given to what our dealers term a *moss.*

The following is a list of the principal lichens employed by British manufacturers of orchil and cudbear, with their commercial names :—

Orchella Weeds.	*Mosses.*
Angola Orchella weed (*R. fuciformis*).	Tartareous moss (*Lecanora tartarea*).
Madagascar　" 　(*R. fuciformis*).	Pustulatous moss (*Gyrophora pustulata*).
Mauritius　"	Canary Rock moss (*Parmelia perlata ?*).[3]
Canary　"　(*R. tinctoria*).	Corsica and Sardinia Rock moss.
Cape de Verde "　(*R. tinctoria*).	Norway Rock moss.
Azores　"　(*R. tinctoria*).	
Madeira　" (*R. tinctoria & R. fuciformis*).	
South American (Lima), large and round　"	
(*R. tinctoria ?*).	
"　"　" small and flat　"	
(*R. fuciformis*).	
Cape of Good Hope　"　(*R. hypomecha*).	
Barbary (Mogadore)　"　(*R. tinctoria*).	
Corsican and Sardinian (*R. tinctoria*).	

Mr. Harman Visger, of Bristol, informs me that " every lichen but the best orchella weed is gone or going rapidly out of use; not from deterioration of their quality, for

---

[1] *Hist. Nat. des Drog. simpl.* t. 2me, p. 77, 4me éd. 1849.

[2] *Journ. de Pharm.* t. xvii. p. 696.

[3] I have not met with the Canary Rock moss in fructification, and cannot, therefore, positively state its botanical name. I found a similar lichen in commerce under the name of British Rock moss. The thallus of both corresponds to that of *Parmelia perlata*, Ach. [The Canary moss (Musgo or Muscus of the inhabitants of the islands) is undoubtedly *P. perlata.* See *Hist. Nat. des Isles Canaries*, par Webb et Berthelot, vol. iii. Part 2, p. 108.—Ed.]

being allowed to grow, they are finer than ever; but because the Angola weed is so supe
rior in quality, and so low-priced and abundant, that the product of a very few other
lichens would pay the expense of manufacture." In France the *Variolaria dealbata*,
De Cand. and *V. oreina*, Ach. (the *Parelle d'Auvergne*), are employed in the production of
orchil. These two lichens constitute the *V. corallina*, Ach., which must be confounded
neither with *Lecanora parella*, Ach., nor with *Isidium corallinum*, Ach.

3. COLORIFIC PRINCIPLES.—These in most, if not in all cases, are organic acids: *e. g.*
alpha orsellic, beta orsellic, erythric, lecanoric, gyrophoric, evernic, usnic, &c. acids.

Under the united influence of water, atmospheric oxygen, and ammonia, these colorific
principles yield coloured products, which, though probably not identical, pass under the
general name of *orceine*. The precise chemical changes which these colorific principles
undergo when exposed to the joint action of water, air, and ammonia, are not definitely
known. Some of these principles are not directly converted into coloured substances, but
into intermediate colourless substances. Thus *lecanoric acid* becomes first *orcine*, and
then *orceine*. Liebig, adopting the formulæ which have been given for these three bodies
respectively by Schunck, Will, and Dumas, has given the following explanation of the
changes:—Lecanoric acid, $C^{18}H^8O^8$, gives out two atoms of carbonic acid, C^2O^4, and
becomes anhydrous orcine, $C^{16}H^8O^4$, which, with three atoms of water, H^3O^3, yields one
atom of crystallised orcine, $C^{16}H^{11}O^7$; and one atom of crystallised orcine, $C^{16}H^{11}O^7$, with
one atom of ammonia, NH^3, and five atoms of oxygen, yield one atom of orceine,
$C^{16}H^9NO^7$, and five atoms of water; but the accuracy of the formulæ has been called in
question.

4. TEST OF THE COLORIFIC PROPERTY OF LICHENS.—Hellot's test is maceration in a
weak solution of ammonia (see *Roccella tinctoria*). Another method is by testing an
alcoholic tincture of the lichen with a solution of hypochlorite of lime. If the lichen
possess any colorific power, a fugitive red colour is produced.

Dr. Stenhouse[1] proposes to estimate the quantity of colorific matter in lichens by means
of a solution of hypochlorite of lime. Any convenient quantity of the lichen (say one
hundred grains) may be cut into very small pieces, and then macerated with milk of
lime till all the colouring principle is extracted. Three or four macerations are quite
sufficient for this purpose, if the lichen has been sufficiently comminuted. The clear
liquors should be filtered and mixed together. A solution of bleaching powder of
known strength should then be poured into the lime-solution from a graduated alkalimeter.
The moment the bleaching liquor comes in contact with the lime-solution of the lichen,
a blood-red colour is produced, which disappears in a minute or two, and the liquid has
only a deep yellow colour. A new quantity of the bleaching liquid should then be poured
into the lime-solution, and the mixture carefully stirred. This operation should be repeated so long as the addition of the hypochlorite of lime causes the production of the red
colour; for this shows that the lime-solution still contains unoxidised colorific principle.
Towards the end of the process, the bleaching solution should be added by only a few
drops at a time, the mixture being carefully stirred between each addition. We have
only to note how many measures of the bleaching liquor have been required to destroy
the colouring matter in the solution, to determine the amount of the colorific principle it
contained. The following are the results of trials with the same test liquors upon four
varieties of lichen :—

	Measures.
Angola lichen required	200 = 1·00
American lichen	120 = 0·60
Cape lichen..	035 = 0·17
Lecanora tartarea, from Germany near Giessen...........	025 = 0·12

The amount of colorific principle in a lichen may also be directly determined by extracting the lichen with milk of lime, by precipitating by means of acetic acid, collecting
the precipitate on a weighed filter, drying it at the ordinary temperature, and then
weighing it.

5. MODE OF EXTRACTING THE COLORIFIC PRINCIPLES FOR TRANSPORT.—Dr. Stenhouse
suggests the following method:—Cut the lichens into small pieces, macerate them in
wooden vats with milk of lime, and saturate the solution either with hydrochloric or acetic
acid. The gelatinous precipitate is then to be collected on cloths, and dried by a gentle

---

[1] *Phil. Trans.* for 1848.

heat. In this way almost the whole colorific matter can be easily extracted, and the dried extract transported at a small expense from the most distant inland localities, such as the Andes or the Himalayas.

Dr. Stenhouse has kindly furnished me with the following table of the lichens and their colorific principles and coloured products :—

LICHENS.		COLORIFIC PRINCIPLES.		COLOURING PRINCIPLES.		Authority.
Commercial Names.	Locality.	Names.	Formulæ.	Names.	Formulæ.	
S. American Orchella weed..............	Lima, &c. ...	Alpha Orsellic acid	$C^{32}H^{15}O^{13}$ + HO	Orceine	$C^{18}H^{10}NO$	Stenhouse.
Cape Orchella weed .	Cape G. Hope	Beta Orsellic acid	$C^{34}H^{18}O^{14}$ + HO	Ditto...	Ditto......	Stenhouse.
Angola Orchella weed	Angola, Africa	Erythric acid......	$C^{20}H^{10}O^9$ + HO	Ditto...	Ditto......	Stenhouse.
Perelle Moss (*Lecanora parella*) ...	Switzerland .	Lecanoric acid ...	$C^{18}H^8O^8$.........	Ditto...	Ditto......	Schunck.
Tartareous Moss (*L. tartarea*)	Norway	Gyrophoric acid .	$C^{36}H^{18}O^{15}$	Ditto...	Ditto......	Stenhouse.
Pustulatous Moss (*Gyrophora pustulata*)	Norway	Ditto..............	Ditto	Ditto...	Ditto......	Stenhouse.
Ragged hoary Lichen (*Everniaprunastri*)	Scotland	Evernic acid......	$C^{34}H^{15}O^{13}$ + HO	—	—	Stenhouse.
Usnea (*florida, plicata,* and *hirta,* &c.)	Germany......	Usnic acid.........	$C^{38}H^{17}O^{14}$	—	—	Rochleder and Heldt.
Rein-deer Moss (*Cladonia rangiferina*)	—	Ditto..............	Ditto	—	—	Rochleder and Heldt.
Ramalina (*fastigiata* [*calicaris*])	—	Ditto..............	Ditto	—	—	Rochleder and Heldt.

14. ROCCELLA TINCTORIA, *De Cand.*—DYER'S ORCHELLA WEED.

Sex. Syst. Cryptogamia, Algæ.

HISTORY.—Theophrastus,[1] Dioscorides,[2] and Pliny,[3] notice a plant which they respectively call πόντιον φύκος, φύκος θαλάσσιον, and *phycos thallassion,* i. e. *fucus marinus.* They state that it grew near the ground on the rocks of Crete, and was used for dyeing purple; and Dioscorides says that some persons imagine that the paint (*fucus*) used by women was this plant, but, he adds, it was a root bearing the same name.[4]

The phycos thallassion has been usually assumed to be *Roccella tinctoria,* and not, as the ancients state, a sea-weed.[5]   Bory de St. Vincent[6] even thinks that the ancients made their celebrated purple dye, brought from the isles of Elishah,[7] with the *R. tinctoria,* which he therefore calls *R. purpura*

---

[1] *Hist. Plant.* lib. iv. cap. vii. p. 82, ed. Heinsii, 1613.
[2] Lib. iv. cap. c. p. 283, ed. Saraceni, 1598.
[3] Lib. xxvi. cap. lxvi. ; and lib. xxxii. cap. xxii. ed. Valpy.
[4] Endlicher (*Enchiridion Botanicum,* p. 4, 1841) says that one of the Algæ, viz. *Rytiphlæa tinctoria,* Ag. yields a red colour, the *fucus* of the ancients.
[5] Beckmann, *Hist of Invent. and Discov.* translated by Wm. Johnston, vol. i. p. 59, 1797.
[6] *Essais sur les Isles Fortuneés,* 1803 ; *Dict. Classiq. d'Hist. Nat.* xiv. 1828.
[7] *Ezekiel,* ch. xxvii. v. 7.

antiquorum. Early in the 14th century the art of dyeing wool with *Roccella tinctoria* was made known at Florence by one of the descendants of a German nobleman named Ferro or Fredrigo. It is said that he accidentally discovered, in the Levant, the colour obtained by the action of urine on this plant, there called *respio* or *respo,* and in Spain *orciglia;* and that his family received the name of *Oricellarii,* altered to *Rucellai,* from this useful invention. From the latter term the generic name *Roccella* is supposed to be derived.[1]

BOTANY. **Gen. Char.**—*Thallus* coriaceo-cartilaginous, rounded or plane, branched or laciniated. *Apothecia* orbicular, adnate with the thallus; the disk coloured, plano-convex, with a border at length thickened and elevated, formed of the thallus, and covering a sublentiform, black, compact, pulverulent powder concealed within the substance of the thallus (*Hooker*).

Sp. Char.—*Thallus* suffruticose, rounded, branched, somewhat erect, greyish-brown, bearing powdery warts [*soredia*]. *Apothecia* flat, almost black and pruinose, with a scarcely prominent border (*Hooker*).

β. *R. tinctoria* β *hypomecha,* Ach.; *R. hypomecha,* Bory. — Thallus terete, filiform, very long, simplish, subconjugate, prostrate, pendulous.— Cape of Good Hope; Mauritius.—2 to 5 inches long: the thallus geniculate where the apothecia are developed (*Bory*): the apothecia by age lose the thalloid margin and become convex, naked, smooth, and black (*Ach.*)

γ. *R. dichotoma,* Ach. has a terete ash-grey, brownish thallus, with longish dichotomous branches.

Hab.—Maritime rocks of the eastern Atlantic islands (the Madeira Isles, the Azores, the Canaries, and the Cape de Verde Isles); western coast of South America (on porphyry near Riobamba in Colombia, and on the sea-shore near Chancay in Peru,—Humboldt);[2] Bourbon; extreme south of England, Guernsey, Portland Island, and the Scilly Islands.

In commerce several other species, or varieties of the above species, are met with. The most important are the following:—

R. FUCIFORMIS, *De Cand.; Ach. Syn.,* p. 244; *Hooker, Engl. Fl.,* vol. v. part 1, p. 222; Lichen fuciformis, *Linn.;* Flat-leaved Orchella Weed.—*Thallus* flat, branched, nearly upright, greyish-white, bearing powdery warts. *Apothecia* pruinose, bordered (*Hooker*). Maritime rocks with R. tinctoria; Canaries; from Cherbourg to Mogadore; St. Malo; South of England.

R. fuciformis β *linearis, Ach.*—Spain, Sumatra, the Dezertas (Madeira).

R. phycopsis, Ach., is also perhaps a variety of R. fuciformis. It is intermediate in character between the latter and R. tinctoria. Its thallus is somewhat flattened (terete-compressed), and much branched; the divisions being somewhat fastigiate, rarely more than an inch long, and very farinaceous.

R. FLACCIDA, Bory.—Branches somewhat cylindrical, filiform, very broad, pendulous, whitish. Mauritius.

R. MONTAGNEI, *Belanger, Voy. aux Indes Orient.* pl. 13, fig. 4, [no date].—*Thallus* coriaceous, flaccid, flat, entire and broad at the base, at length dichotomously (rarely trichotomously) laciniate, pale, glaucous, sorediferous. *Apothecia* marginal, somewhat pedicellate, with a black convex pruinose disc and persistent margin.—On the trunks of Mango trees (*Mangifera indica*) in India; especially at Pondicherry. This species, and *R. Pygmæa,* D. R. and Mont., which occurs in Algeria, are remarkable for growing on the trunks of trees; the others are found on maritime rocks.

---

[1] Beckmann, *op. citato.*
[2] *Synops. Plant. Æquin.* i. 50.

Fig. 25.   Fig. 26.   Fig. 27.   Fig. 28.

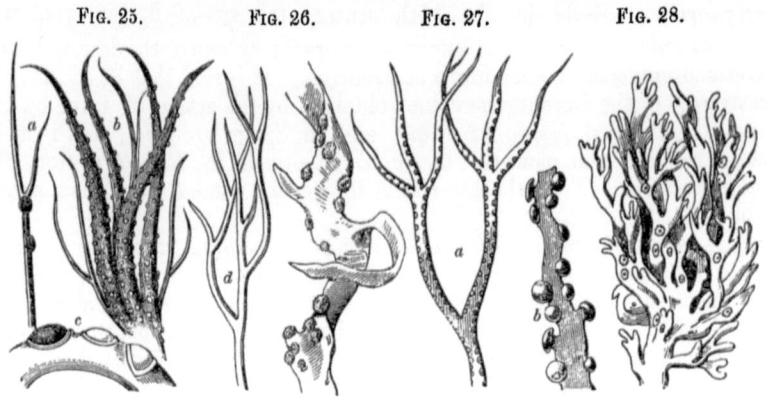

Roccella or *Orchella Weed.*

Fig. 25. Roccella tinctoria.
  a. Thallus with apothecia.
  b. Ditto with soredia.
  c. Portion of thallus with three more
    developed apothecia.
  d. R. tinct. var. dichotoma.

Fig. 26. Roccella fuciformis.
Fig. 27. Roccella Montagnei.
  a. Thallus with soredia.
  b. Ditto ditto (magnified).
Fig. 28. Roccella phycopsis with soredia.

COMMERCE.—All the species and varieties of Roccella found in commerce bear the general appellation of *Orchella weed ;* but they are distinguished by the name of the country from which they are imported.   The following is a list of the sorts which, within the last few years, have been found in the London market ; those marked with the asterisk (*) I have myself examined and possess samples of :—

*Angola Orchella weed.
 Mauritius   "
*Madagascar   "
*Barbary (Mogadore) ditto.
*Cape of Good Hope ditto.

*Canary Orchella weed.
 Cape de Verde   "
*Western Island "
*Madeira (Dezertas) ditto.

*Lima (thick) Orchella weed.
*Lima (thin)   "
 Corsica and Sardinia "

In 1838, 567 cwts.; in 1839, 6494 cwts.; and in 1840, 4175 cwts. of Orchella weed paid duty.

PHYSICAL PROPERTIES.—Having fully described the botanical characters of the different species of Roccella, it will be unnecessary here to describe minutely the different commercial sorts.[1]

The commercial kinds of Orchella weed may be conveniently arranged in three divisions, as follows :—

1. *Orchella weeds having a cylindrical tapering thallus.*—These consist usually of *Roccella tinctoria,* and perhaps R. *flaccida,* Bory.   In one case (Cape of Good Hope Orchella) the plant is R. *hypomecha,* a mere variety of R. *tinctoria.*   Occasionally flattened Orchella weeds are found intermixed : these may be regarded as accidental.

  a. Canary Orchella Weed ; Roccella tinctoria.—Formerly the most esteemed sort of Orchella. Thallus filiform, seldom exceeding in thickness a pin, and in length an inch and a half.   Colour from pale yellowish-grey to dark brown.

---

[1] For figures of the microscopic structure of the Roccella tinctoria, the reader is referred to Link's *Icones Selectæ Anatomico-Botanicæ,* Berl. 1841, 3tes Heft, Taf. vi.

β. *Western Island Orchella Weed ; St. Michael's Orchella Weed ; Roccella tinctoria.*—Similar to the preceding ; but less valuable as a dye-stuff.

γ. *Barbary Orchella Weed ; Mogadore Orchella Weed ; Roccella tinctoria.*—Somewhat smaller than the preceding sorts, and less valuable as a dye.

δ. *Lima thick Orchella Weed ; South American thick Orchella Weed ; Roccella tinctoria ? R. flaccida,* Bory ?—A very handsome lichen, brought from Lima and other parts of the west coast of South America. Distinguished from the other sorts by its large size : usually several, sometimes six or eight, inches long : its thickness from that of a crow-quill to that of a goose-quill. Thick tubercular excrescences are frequently found on it. It has a very leathery, sometimes a cartilaginous whitish appearance. Its quality as a dye is considered good, and superior to the preceding sorts.

ε. *Cape of Good Hope Orchella Weed ; R. tinctoria β hypomecha,* Ach.—A large lichen, though rather smaller than the preceding. Remarkable for its white or grey-white appearance : many of the divisions of the thallus are geniculated. As a dye its quality is very bad.

2. *Orchella weeds having a flat (plane) or compressed thallus.*—These consist of *R. fuciformis,* and perhaps, in some cases, of *R. Montagnei.*

ζ. *Angola Orchella Weed ; R. fuciformis.*[1]—Thallus very flat, seldom exceeding an inch and a half or two inches in length : in breadth (except at the fork or division) rarely more than one-sixth of an inch. Colour greenish or yellowish grey. As a dye stuff it is the most valuable of all the Orchella weeds.

η. *Madagascar Orchella Weed ; R. fuciformis.*—Smaller, but in other respects similar to the preceding sort. Somewhat less valuable than the Angola sort.

θ. *Lima thin Orchella Weed ; R. fuciformis ?*—Somewhat more rounded or less flat than the preceding, which it in other respects very much resembles.

3. *Mixed Orchella Weeds, consisting of both flat and round Orchella Weeds.*

ι. *Madeira Orchella Weed ; R. tinctoria* and *R. fuciformis β linearis,* Ach.—Gathered on the Dezertas, near Madeira. The round and terete thalli resemble the Canary Orchella. The flattened thalli are thicker than those of the Angola sort.

COMPOSITION.—A qualitative analysis of Roccella tinctoria was made by Fr. Nees v. Esenbeck,[2] who found in it a *brown resin* (soluble in alcohol and ether, and becoming brownish-red with ammonia), *wax, glutinous matter, insoluble starch, yellow extractive, yellowish-brown gummy matter, lichen starch, tartrate* and *oxalate of lime,* and *chloride of sodium* from the adherent sea-water.

The nature of the colorific principles of the Orchella weeds (Roccella) of commerce has been the subject of several analytical investigations, the most important of which are those of Heeren,[3] in 1830 ; of Kane,[4] in 1840 ; of Schunck,[5] in 1841, and also in 1846 ; of Rochleder and Heldt,[6] in 1843 ; of Knopp,[7] in 1844, and of Stenhouse,[8] in 1848.

---

[1] Dr. Scouler (in Dr. Stenhouse's paper on the Lichens in the *Phil. Trans.* for 1848, p. 72) has pronounced the Angola Orchella Weed to be *R. Montagnei* of Belanger. My own examination of it led me to believe that it was *R. fuciformis.* I therefore submitted samples of it to Sir W. Hooker and Mr. Bennett of the British Museum, both of whom have declared it to be one of the numerous varieties of *R. fuciformis.* [*R. Montagnei* is not regarded as a good species by the best modern lichenologists.—ED.]

[2] Brandes's *Archiv d. Apothekerverein,* Bd. xvi. S. 135.

[3] Schweigger's *Jahrb. d. Chem.* Bd. lix. S. 313, 1830 ; Buchner's *Repertorium,* Bd. xxxviii. S. 21.

[4] *Phil. Trans.* for 1840, p. 273.

[5] *Ann. d. Chem. u. Pharm.* Bd. xli. S. 157, 1842 ; and *Memoirs of the Chemical Society of London,* vol. iii. p. 144, 1846.

[6] *Ann. d. Chem. u. Pharm.* Bd. xlviii. S. 1, 1843.

[7] *Ibid.* Bd. xlix. S. 102, 1844.

[8] *Phil. Trans.* for 1848, p. 63.

Robiquet[1] has thrown much light on the subject by his investigations into the nature of the colorific principle of *Varioluria dealbata.*

The only constituents of the Orchella weeds which will require separate notice are the colorific principles; and in describing these I shall follow Stenhouse.

1. ALPHA-ORSELLIC ACID (*Stenhouse*); *Colorific Principle of Lima thick Orchella Weed* (*Roccella tinctoria*).—Obtained by macerating the lichen in milk of lime, and then adding excess of hydrochloric acid to the filtered solution. A white gelatinous precipitate is obtained, which, when washed, dried, dissolved in warm alcohol, and the solution allowed to cool, yields stellate prismatic crystals of alpha orsellic acid. It is nearly insoluble in cold water, but sparingly soluble in boiling water; pretty soluble in cold alcohol and ether, and readily so in boiling alcohol. It reddens litmus, and forms crystallisable salts with the alkalies and earths. Its most characteristic reaction, by which its presence can be very readily detected, is the deep blood-red colour which it instantly strikes with a solution of hypochlorite of lime: the colour soon changes to yellow, which gradually also disappears. A solution of orsellic acid in ammonia, on exposure to the air, soon assumes a bright red colour, which gradually becomes darker and purple coloured. The rational formula for alpha-orsellic acid is $C^{32}H^{15}O^{13} + HO$.

2. BETA-ORSELLIC ACID (*Stenhouse*); *Colorific Principle of Cape of Good Hope Orchella Weed* (*Roccella hypomecha*).—Is intermediate in its properties between alpha-orsellic acid and erythric acid, but approaches the former more closely. It is crystallisable, and its solution yields a fugitive blood-red colour with hypochlorite of lime. Its ammoniacal solution also becomes red in the air. The rational formula of the hydrated acid is $C^{34}H^{17}O^{14} + HO$.

3 ERYTHRIC ACID (*Schunck* and *Stenhouse*); *Colorific Principle of Angola and Madagascar Orchella Weeds* (*Roccella fuciformis*).—By macerating the lichen in milk of lime, as before stated, Stenhouse obtained 12 per cent. of crude erythric acid. It is a feebler acid than alpha- and beta-orsellic acids; but it agrees with these acids in being crystallisable, and in yielding red coloured compounds with ammonia, and also in its reaction with hypochlorite of lime. The formula of the hydrated acid is $C^{20}H^{10}O^{9} + HO$.

CHEMICAL CHARACTERISTICS.—The aqueous decoction of Orchella weed forms a copious precipitate with diacetate of lead, and has its colour deepened by alkalies. Digested in a weak solution of ammonia, in a corked phial, at a heat not exceeding 130° F., the plant yields a rich violet-red colour. This is *Hellot's test* for the discovery of a colorific property in lichens.[2] By adding a solution of hypochlorite of lime to an alcoholic tincture, or to an alkaline infusion of the lichen, a fugitive blood-red colour is produced.

PHYSIOLOGICAL EFFECTS.—Mucilaginous, emollient, and demulcent.

USES.—In the Mauritius it is employed in decoction to alleviate cough. In Europe it is only employed as a colorific agent.

1. LACMUS.—LITMUS.

SYNONYMES.—*Turnsole in cakes* (*tournesol en pains; tournesol en pierre*); *Dutch turnsole; lacca musica, musiva,* vel *musci; lacca cœrulea.*

HISTORY.—The manufacture of litmus was probably discovered by the Dutch about the latter end of the seventeenth century.[3]

---

[1] *Journ. de Chim. Méd.* t. v. p. 324, 1829; *Journ. de Pharm.* t. xxi. pp. 269 and 387, 1835.

[2] Berthollet *On Dyeing*, by Ure, vol. ii. p. 184; also *Proceedings of Comm. of Agricult. of Asiatic Society*, April 8th, 1837.

[3] Litmus is not mentioned by, and therefore was probably unknown to, Caspar Bauhin (*Pinax*, 1671), and to Dale (*Pharmacologia*, 3tia ed. 1737). The earliest authors in whose works I have found it mentioned, are Pomet (*History of Drugs*, Eng. ed. 1712) and Valentine (*Hist. Simpl.* 1716).

PREPARATION.—Litmus is obtained by the united influence of water, air, ammonia, and either potash or soda, on any of the tinctorial lichens capable of yielding orchil. If the potash or soda be omitted, the product is not litmus, but orchil. The manufacture of litmus has been described by Ferber,[1] by an anonymous writer,[2] by Morelot,[3] and by Amédée Gélis.[4] From their accounts it appears that the lichen is macerated for several weeks, with occasional agitation in a mixture of urine, lime, and potashes, in a wooden trough under shelter. A kind of fermentation takes place, and the lichen becomes first reddish, and subsequently blue. When the pulp has acquired a proper blue colour, it is placed in proper moulds, and the cakes thus procured are subsequently dried.

The moulds are either of steel or brass, and consist of two parts : the lower one, divided into rectangular cells, and the upper one, supporting a series of metallic rods bearing small metallic disks, so arranged as to accurately fit the cells of the lower piece. The lower piece is immersed in the pulp with which they are filled, and the excess of pulp is then scraped off by means of a wooden spatula. The upper piece being then applied, the discs enter the cells, and force out the moulded cakes of litmus.[5]

[Dr. de Vry, of Rotterdam, describes the manufacture of litmus as follows :— "Different species of Roccella from the Mediterranean, the Canary Islands, &c., are ground, and the powder mixed with weed ashes and water to make a pasty mixture, which is allowed to ferment. After some time, putrid urine and American potash are added to the mixture. When the paste has assumed a good blue colour, it is formed into quadrangular cakes, which are dried and sold, or, when they are of an inferior quality, are shaken with indigo or litmus powder of superior quality. It is very difficult to obtain accurate information about this manufacture, which is kept very secret. The makers say that they can use the urine of men only, and not that of women. This urine is sold in some benevolent institution, where old people are maintained by public charity. Litmus is made during the summer only, and its manufacture appears to be affected by the state of the weather, for the makers are much afraid of thunder; so it would seem that the electricity of the air has some influence over the process."

According to Dr. de Vry, the Dutch cheeses are coloured by litmus, obtained from the turnsole rags (tournesol en drapeaux) which are imported from France.[6]—ED.]

It appears from Gélis' experiments, that any of the lichens which serve for the production of orchil may be used in the preparation of litmus.[7]

---

[1] *Neue Beytrage zur Mineralgeschichte verschiedener Länder*, Bd. i. S. 378, Mietau, 1778. Ferber describes the process as practised at Amsterdam. He says that the pulp is ground in a mill, and forced through a hair cloth, before it is placed in the moulds.

[2] Nicholson's *Journal of Nat. Phil. Chem. and the Arts*, vol. ii. p. 311, 1799. The notice of litmus is a translation from an article in the *Journal du Commerce*. The lichen is said to be ground in a mill, and sifted through a brass wire sieve before maceration. The moulds are described as being 1¼ inches by 8-10ths of an inch.

[3] *Mémoire sur le Lichen Français*, vulgò *tournesol en pain*, in the *Mém. de la Soc. Méd. d'Emulation*, t. v. p. 281.

[4] *Journ. de Pharm.* t. xxvii. p. 476, 1840.

[5] [Dr. J. Müller, of Berlin, states that the great secret of obtaining good litmus is to employ Carrara marble and a potash made in Germany which contains a peculiar constituent (*Archiv der Pharm.* 2te Reihe, Bd. lxx. H. 3, p. 287.—ED.]

[6] *Pharm. Journ.* vol. x. p. 325.

[7] Ferber saw the *Roccella* lichen used at Amsterdam. Morelot stated that *Variolaria orceina* yielded it. Nees and Ebermaier (*Handb. d. med.-pharm. Bot.* Bd. i. S. 49), and Thomson (*Org.*

The urine serves for the production of carbonate of ammonia, and the lime employed abstracts the carbonic acid.

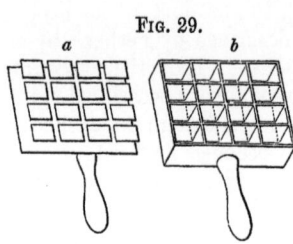

FIG. 29.

a. b.

Moulds used in making Litmus.

a. The lower or cell-piece.
b. The upper piece.

The Dutch manufacturers add chalk or sulphate of lime, and some siliceous or argillaceous substance, to give body and weight to the litmus. [With respect to the presence of indigo in litmus cake, it appears present only in the inferior qualities, and is not a constant ingredient, as was once believed.

There are as many as 19 sorts of litmus of varying quality kept by the Dutch manufacturers: some of these are more than six times the value of others, notwithstanding that, according to the observations of Mr. D. Hanbury, there is by no means a corresponding difference in richness or intensity of colour.[1]—ED.]

DESCRIPTION.—Litmus is imported from Holland in the form of small, rectangular, light, and friable cakes of an indigo-blue colour. Examined by the microscope, we find sporules, and portions of the epidermis and mesothallus of some species of lichen, moss leaves, sand, &c. The odour of the cakes is that of violets. The violet odour is acquired while the mixture is undergoing fermentation, and is common to all the tinctorial lichens. It has led some writers into the error of supposing that the litmus-makers use Florentine orris in the manufacture of litmus. The indigo odour occasionally observed depends on the presence of indigo in the litmus cakes of inferior quality.

COMPOSITION.—An accurate and complete analysis of litmus is yet a desideratum. In 1840, Dr. Kane[2] submitted it to examination, and obtained from it four colouring principles, to which he gave the names of *erythrolein, erythrolitmine, azolitmine,* and *spaniolitmine.* These, in their natural condition, are red, and the blue of litmus, he says, is produced by combination with a base. "There are, properly speaking," he adds, "only two characteristic colouring matters in litmus—the erythrolitmine and the azolitmine; for the erythrolein is coloured crimson-purple only by alkalies, and the spaniolitmine occurs but very seldom. In the litmus of commerce these colouring substances are combined with *lime, potash,* and *ammonia,* and there is mixed up in the mass a considerable quantity of *chalk* and *sand.*"

Gélis[3] has published some interesting observations on litmus. He says that litmus owes its colour to *four different coloured products,* which he designates by the letters A, B, C, and D. The ash of litmus he found to contain *carbonate of potash, carbonate* or *sulphate of lime, alumina, silica, traces of oxide of iron, chlorine, sulphuric acid,* and *phosphoric acid.*

Chemistry, p. 284), on the other hand, say that *Lecanora tartarea* is employed.—An orchil-maker under my care in the London Hospital told me that he had been accustomed to make litmus of pipe-clay, starch, soda, and orchil-liquor ; and he gave me some specimens of it thus prepared. Gélis prepared it with *Roccella tinctoria* (in the scutelliferous state), *Roccella fuciformis,* and the mixture of *Lecanora parella β pallescens* and *Isidium corallinum,* sold under the name of *Orseille d'Auvergne ;* but the last-mentioned plants yielded a less fine product than the others.

[1] *Pharm. Journ.* vol. x. p. 325.
[2] *Phil. Trans. for* 1840, p. 298.
[3] *Journ. de Pharmacie,* t. xxvii. p. 483, 1840.

In the commoner varieties of the litmus cakes of commerce there are at least two colouring matters, viz. 1st, the proper colouring matter of litmus derived from the lichen, and which I shall provisionally call *lichen-blue ;* and 2dly, *indigo.* The existence of the last-mentioned substance was for some time entirely overlooked.

1. Lichen-blue ; *Litmus-blue.* — By these terms I understand the peculiar blue colouring matter of litmus, which is soluble in water, and is reddened by acids. It is probably either some modification of *orceine,* or some allied principle. It may perhaps be a mixture or compound of several colouring principles. It is soluble in both water and spirit, yielding a coloured solution, which, in the concentrated state, has a purple colour when viewed by transmitted light; but in the dilute state it is pure blue. Viewed by transmitted candle-light, it has a reddish colour. An aqueous infusion of litmus neither reddens turmeric paper nor occasions a precipitate with a solution of chloride of calcium. It contains, therefore, no free alkali or alkaline carbonate. It is reddened by acids, and also by many of the metallic salts,—as corrosive sublimate, sulphate of copper, sulphate of iron, &c. The infusion of litmus which has been reddened by acids has its blue colour restored by alkalies, alkaline earths, the alkaline and earthy sulphurets, the alkaline carbonates, the soluble borates, the tribasic phosphate of soda, and the alkaline cyanides.

An infusion of litmus is decolorised by chlorine and by the alkaline hypochlorites. Certain deoxidising agents also deprive it of colour; as sulphuretted hydrogen, hydro-sulphuret of ammonia, sulphurous acid, the hyposulphites, nascent hydrogen (obtained by adding hydrochloric acid and zinc to an aqueous infusion of litmus), and the protosalts of iron. If an infusion of litmus be left in contact with sulphuretted hydrogen, in a well-stopped bottle, for a few days, the liquid is decolorised, but reacquires its colour by exposure to the air or oxygen gas. [We have found that a strong solution of litmus long kept in a well-closed bottle spontaneously undergoes changes by which the rich blue is converted to a dingy red-brown colour. It also acquires a very offensive smell. On exposure to air in a plate or dish for a short time, it loses the offensive odour, and the blue colour is restored. This restoration is evidently owing to oxidation.—Ed.]

2. Indigo.—The presence of indigo in common litmus cakes is proved by their odour; by the coppery lustre which they acquire when rubbed with the nail; by digesting them in oil of vitriol, by which a blue solution of sulphate of indigo is obtained; and by heating them in a watch-glass or platinum capsule, by which indigo vapour (characterised by its well-known odour and reddish-violet colour) and crystals of indigo are obtained.

Characteristics.—The lichen-blue is an aqueous infusion of litmus, is distinguished from other vegetable blues by the action of acids and alkalies on it (see *supra*) ; for most vegetable blues and purples (as red cabbage-juice, syrup of violets, &c.) are changed to green by alkalies, whereas lichen-blue does not undergo this change. The presence of indigo in some litmus cakes is shown by the tests above stated.

If a lump of moistened litmus be laid on turmeric paper, the latter is reddened by it ; but by the application of heat the redness disappears.[1]

When litmus cakes are thrown into diluted hydrochloric acid, a copious effervescence ensues, and a solution of chloride of calcium is obtained.[2]

If a cake of litmus be ignited in the outer cone of the flame of a candle, a whitish-violet tint is communicated to the flame, indicative of the presence of potash.

If the ashes of litmus be thrown into diluted hydrochloric acid, violent effervescence takes place : a solution of chloride of calcium is obtained, and a quantity of siliceous sand remains undissolved.

---

[1] [This shows the presence of ammonia or its carbonate.—Ed.]
[2] [This effect is only observed when the litmus cake is improperly mixed with carbonate of lime.—Ed.]

Uses.—Litmus is employed as a test for acids and alkalies. The former communicate a red colour to blue litmus; the latter restore the blue colour of reddened litmus. (The action of various salts on litmus has been before stated.) If the litmus present be reddened by an unboiled, but not by a boiled, water, we may infer that the acid present is a volatile one; probably carbonic acid, or perhaps sulphuretted hydrogen. Reddened litmus may have its blue colour restored not only by alkalies, &c., as before mentioned, but also by carbonate of lime dissolved in water by a considerable excess of carbonic acid.

1. TINCTURA LACMI; *Tincture of Litmus.* (Litmus, *one part*; Distilled Water, *twenty-five parts.* M.)—Though called *tincture,* it is in reality an *infusion* of litmus. In order to preserve it, a portion (about $\frac{1}{10}$th part) of spirit may be added to it. If required to be more concentrated, the proportion of litmus should be augmented. Some persons first bruise the litmus in a mortar, and then tie it up in a linen bag before steeping it in the water. By keeping in a closely-stopped bottle, its blue colour disappears, but is shortly restored on the admission of atmospheric air.

2. CHARTA EXPLORATORIA CŒRULEA; *Blue Test Paper; Blue Litmus Paper.*—This is prepared by dipping slips of paper in a strong and clear infusion of litmus; or by brushing the infusion over the paper.

Bibulous or unsized paper is usually preferred, on account of the facility with which it imbibes the liquid to be tested; and also because the alum which frequently enters into the composition of the size affects the colour of litmus. Professor Graham, however, recommends good letter-paper; or, if the infusion is applied to one side only, thin and sized drawing-paper. Faraday[1] recommends the infusion to be prepared from an ounce of litmus and half a pint of hot water. The Prussian Pharmacopœia of 1827 orders one part of litmus and four parts of water. Others employ one part of litmus and six parts of water.

In order to obtain *extremely delicate* test paper, the alkali, if present in the litmus, is to be almost neutralised by a minute portion of acid. To effect this, divide the filtered infusion of litmus into two parts; stir one portion with a glass rod which has been previously dipped into very dilute sulphuric acid, and repeat this until the liquid begins to look reddish; then add the other portion of liquid, and immerse the paper in the mixture. Good litmus paper should be of a uniform blue tint, and neither very light nor very dark. When it has a purplish tint it is a more delicate test for acids than when its colour is pure blue. When carefully dried, it may be preserved by wrapping it in stiff paper, and keeping it in well-stopped vessels in a dark cupboard or drawer. Books of test-papers, bound up like bankers' cheque-books, are sold in the shops, and are very convenient. They are about $1\frac{3}{4}$ inches long and $\frac{3}{8}$ths of an inch wide. To preserve them they are kept in leathern cases.

Blue litmus paper is used to detect the presence of acids and of certain salts which react as acids.

3. CHARTA EXPLORATORIA RUBEFACTA; *Reddened Test Paper; Red Litmus Paper.*—This is prepared with an infusion of litmus which has been

---

[1] *Chemical Manipulation.*

slightly reddened by an acid. Blue litmus paper may be extemporaneously reddened by exposing it for a few seconds to the vapour of acetic acid; but for preserving, it is better to prepare the paper with litmus which has been reddened by a minute portion of dilute sulphuric acid, the acetic acid being objectionable on account of its volatility.

Red litmus paper is employed as a test for alkalies and certain salts (see *supra*) which react as bases.

2. ORCHILLA.—ORCHIL-LIQUOR.

Two kinds of liquid or thin pulp called Orchil or Archil are met with: one termed *blue orchil,* the other *red orchil.* They are prepared as follows: *Blue orchil* is procured by steeping the lichens before mentioned (see pp. 26 and 28) in an ammoniacal liquor in a covered wooden vessel. *Red orchil* is made with the same liquor in common earthen jars placed in a room heated by steam, and called *a stove.* In one manufactory which I inspected, the ammoniacal liquor was prepared by distillation from a mixture of lime, impure muriate or sulphate of ammonia obtained from gas-works, and water; but some makers still employ stale urine and lime. Both kinds of orchil sold in the shops are liquids of a deep reddish-purple colour and an ammoniacal smell. Red and blue orchils differ merely in the degree of their red tint.

According to Dr. Kane, orchil consists of *orcein, erythroleic acid,* and *azo-erythrine.* To these must be added *ammonia.*

Orchil is employed merely as a colouring agent. It is used for dyeing, colouring, and staining. It is sometimes used as a test for acids.

3. CUDBEAR.

Cudbear is called by the Germans *Persio.* The manufacture of this pigment was begun at Leith about the year 1777, by the late Mr. Macintosh, of Glasgow, under the management of Dr. Cuthbert Gordon. From the latter gentleman's name the term *cudbear* (at first *Cuthbert*) originated.

It is procured in the manner of Orchil, by the mutual action of some of the colorific lichens, air, and an ammoniacal liquor.

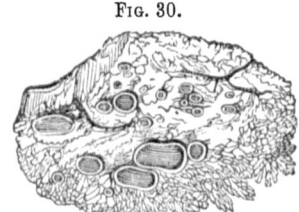

Fig. 30.

Lecanora tartarea.

White Swedish or *tartareous moss (Lecanora tartarea)* was formerly chiefly used in its manufacture. When the proper purplish-red colour has been developed, the mixture is dried in the air and reduced to powder.

I have found in the shops two kinds of powder of cudbear: one called *red cudbear,* the other *blue cudbear.* Both are purplish-red,—but one is redder than the other. I have likewise met with *red* and *blue cudbear pastes:* but the term Orchil might with more propriety apply to these.

Cudbear is employed as a purple dye for woollen yarn; but the colour which it yields is fugitive. It is sometimes used for colouring pharmaceutical preparations, and it may be employed also as a test.

Cudbear paper is sometimes used as a test for acids and alkalies. " A paper prepared from an infusion of the best cudbear, without the addition of either alkali or acid, has a purple colour, and is affected by both acids and alkalies.   It is convenient in alkalimetry, being already too red to be sensibly affected by carbonic acid, while it is distinctly reddened by the mineral acids."[1]

Order III. FUNGI, *Juss.*—FUNGALS.

Fungaceæ, *Lind.*

CHARACTERS.—Plants consisting of a congeries of cells or filaments, or both variously combined, increasing in size in the more perfect species by addition to their inside, their outside undergoing no change after its first formation; chiefly growing upon decayed organic substances, or soil arising from their decomposition, frequently ephemeral, and variously coloured, never accompanied, as in Lichens, by reproductive germs of a vegetable green called gonidia; nourished by juices derived from the matrix. *Fructification* either spores attached externally, and often in definite numbers, to the cellular tissue, and frequently on peculiar cells called *sporophores* or *basidia*, which are in many cases surmounted by fine processes which immediately support the *spores*, and called *spicules* or *sterigmata*; or inclosed in membranous sacs or *asci*, and then termed *sporidia* (*Berkeley*, in Lindley's *Vegetable Kingdom*).   [Many fungi produce secondary forms of fruit, like the pycnidia or spermatogonia of lichens, besides reproductive naked deciduous cells, known under the name of *conidia*. If *Saprolegnia* is a true fungus, for which opinion very weighty reasons may be adduced, there is at least one genus which produces zoospores. *Endodromia* is probably a second instance.—ED.]

PROPERTIES.—Variable: we have esculent, medicinal, and poisonous species; and unfortunately there are no anatomical characters by which the poisonous are to be distinguished from the edible fungi.

They are remarkable for containing a very large proportion of water; and for their dry matter being rich in nitrogen and phosphates. Among their proximate constituents are several alimentary principles (*e. g.* albumen, sugar, mannite, and mucilage), and some poisonous ones (*ergotin, tremellin,* and *amanitin*). The substance called *fungin,* formerly considered to be a nutritive principle, appears to agree with cellulose in its nature.

Sub-order I. GYMNOMYCETES, *Endl.*

CONIOMYCETES, *Fries.*

CHARACTERS.—*Sporidia* naked, without any hymenium, perithecium, or asci, produced beneath the epidermis of plants or within the matrix (*Fries*).

PROPERTIES.—No medicinal substances are obtained from this sub-order. The *yeast plant,* which Turpin refers to the genus *Torula* (from *torus,* a twisted cord), is an imperfect mucedinous fungus, and as such will be noticed hereafter (see Sub-order *Hyphomycetes*). The *ergot-mould,* called by the late Mr. E. J. Quekett, *Ergotætia abortifaciens,* and referred to this sub-order, is considered by Link and some other authorities to be a species of *Oidium,* and as such will be noticed subsequently (see Sub-order *Hyphomycetes*).

Sub-order II. HYPHOMYCETES, *Fries.*

CHARACTERS.—*Flocci* sporidiferous, naked (Fries).

PROPERTIES.—To this sub-order (which is closely allied to *Confervaceæ*) are referred the *yeast plant,* the *ergot-mould, mother of vinegar,* and some other plants interesting alike to the physician and pharmaceutist.

[The fungus found in vinegar has lately acquired some public notice under the name of the *Vinegar-plant,* and directions have been given in periodical works for the propagation

---

[1] Graham, *Elements of Chemistry,* p. 925.

of this plant as a source of the domestic manufacture of vinegar. Those who have ascribed some occult influence to this fungus in acetifying a saccharine fluid under favourable circumstances, have forgotten that vinegar itself is an excellent ferment for producing acetous fermentation, and that a porous fungous body, already saturated with vinegar, is in the condition of a sponge steeped in vinegar, and therefore in a most favourable state for causing the acetification of the sugar. The fine fibres or threads of the mould present a large surface to the fluid, and thus probably accelerate action. We are glad to have the support of the Rev. J. Berkeley in this view of the action of the so-called *Vinegar-plant*. A bottle or vessel rinsed with vinegar, and then filled with a saccharine fluid, would produce similar results, although, perhaps, more slowly.—ED.]

15. FERMENTUM CERVISIÆ.—BARM or YEAST.

HISTORY.—Leaven and ferment have been known from the most remote periods. *Leaven* (or *sour dough*), called in Hebrew *seor*,[1] and *ferment*, termed in Hebrew *khametz*,[2] are both referred to in the Old Testament: the one applies to solids, the other to both solids and liquids. In the common version, however, both these Hebrew words are translated leaven [3] The Greeks appear to have used the term ζύμη in a general sense, to include both leaven and ferment. Dioscorides[4] speaks of the medical properties of the *leaven of wheat* (ἄλευρων ζύμη), which Galen[5] and Paulus[6] simply call ζύμη. Pliny[7] distinguishes *leaven* (*fermentum*) from *beer-yeast* (*spuma cervisiæ*).

The history of the discovery of the vegetable nature of yeast is an interesting subject of inquiry. So long since as the year 1680, Leeuwenhoek[8] described and figured the globules of beer-yeast. He was fully aware of its vegetable nature, but was ignorant of its power of vegetating or growing, and, notwithstanding the high magnifying power which he used, he failed to detect the presence of the granules or nuclei in the interior of the yeast-cells.

In 1826, Desmazières[9] published some observations on Persoon's genus *Mycoderma*, which he defined anew, and referred to Gaillon's class of infusory animals, called *Nemazoaria* (now placed among Algæ). He described a *Mycoderma vini, glutinis farinulæ, malti-juniperini, malti-cervisiæ*, and *cervisiæ*. The latter is frequently considered to be the yeast-plant; but Desmazières confounded two things which deserve to be considered quite distinctly,—namely, the yeast-plant properly so called (the *Torula Cerevisiæ* of Turpin), and a larger filamentous confervoid plant, to which more strictly the name of *Mycoderma Cervisiæ* of Desmazières should be confined.

To Cagniard-Latour is due the credit of establishing the real nature of yeast.

---

[1] Hence the German *sauer* and English *sour*.

[2] The sour fermented mare's milk used by the Tartars appears to have derived its name, *koumiss*, from the Hebrew *khametz*.

[3] In *Exodus* xiii. 7, the terms *seor* and *khametz* occur together, and are evidently distinct. " *Unleavened things* (*matzah*) [ἄζυμα] shall be consumed during the seven days, and there shall not be seen with thee *fermented things* [ζυμωτόν], and there shall not be seen with thee *leavened mass* [ζύμη]" (*Biblical Cyclopædia*, vol. ii. pp. 236-7). The interpolated Greek words are from the Septuagint.

[4] Lib. ii. cap. 107.

[5] *De Simpl. Med. Facult.* lib. vi. § 3.

[6] Paulus Ægineta, trans. by F. Adams, Syd. Soc. ed. vol. iii. p. 126.

[7] *Hist. Nat.* lib. xviii. cap. 12 and 26; lib. xxii. cap. 82, ed. Valp.

[8] *Arcana Naturæ detecta*, p. 1, et seq. ed. nov. Lugd. Bat. 1722.

[9] Desmazières's observations were first published at Lisle. They were afterwards reprinted in the *Annales des Sciences Naturelles*, t. x. p. 42, 1827.

During the years 1835 and 1836 he communicated to the *Société Philomathique* some researches on ferments, which were published in the journal called *l'Institut* (Nos. 158, 159, 164, 165, 166, 167, 185, and 199); and on the 12th of June, 1837, he presented to the Academy of Sciences his *Mémoire sur la Fermentation Vineuse*, a notice of which appeared in the *Comptes rendus* of that period. The report[1] on this memoir, drawn up by Turpin in the name of himself, Thénard, and Becquerel, was made to the Academy in July 1838 (*Comptes rendus*); and the memoir itself was printed in the 68th volume of the *Annales de Chimie et de Physique*, 1838.

About the same time, Schwann[2] was occupied in investigations on this subject, but his observations were not published until 1837. He denied that the organised being found in fermenting liquids is one of the infusoria, as Desmazières had supposed, but asserted that it is undoubtedly a plant, and that it has great resemblance to many jointed fungi. Meyen, who examined it at Schwann's request, agreed as to its vegetable nature, and considered that the only doubt which could exist respecting it was, whether it was an algal or a fungus, but its deficiency in green pigment led him to regard it as a fungus. The filamentous fungus found in saccharine solutions which are undergoing fermentation Schwann therefore proposed to call the *sugar-fungus* (Zuckerpilz). Meyen[3] adopts Schwann's proposal, and refers to three species of *Saccharomyces*, viz. *S. vini*, *S. cerevisiæ*, and *S. pomorum*.

In 1837 Kützing[4] described and figured the yeast-plant.

On the 20th of August, 1838, Turpin[5] read to the Academy of Sciences at Paris his valuable *Mémoire sur la Cause et les Effets de la Fermentation Alcoolique et Acéteuse.* [In 1851 Dr. Hassall published some observations in the Lancet,—without, however, a knowledge of Turpin's paper,—tending to show that the yeast-plant is a mere form of some Penicillium. At the same period, Mr. Berkeley and Mr. G. H. Hoffman, without any knowledge of Dr. Hassall's investigation, examined several varieties of yeast furnished by Dr. Pereira; and, by causing them to germinate between slips of glass, proved that they are really a state of Penicillium, according with the figures of Turpin and Hassall. Their observations are embodied in the article Yeast of the Encyclopædia of Agriculture.—ED.]

The notion that yeast was an organised being, in fact a living plant, was at first strongly opposed by Berzelius and Liebig;[6] but was soon adopted by the eminent chemist Mitscherlich.[7]

---

[1] A translation of this report appeared in Jameson's *Edinburgh New Philosophical Journal*, vol. xxv.

[2] Poggendorff's *Annalen der Physik*, Bd. xli. p. 184, 1837.

[3] *Report on the Progress of Vegetable Physiology during the year* 1837, translated by W. Francis, p. 83–84, London, 1839.

[4] *Journal für praktische Chemie*, Bd. xi.

[5] *Mémoire de l'Académie Royale des Sciences*, t. xvii. 1840.

[6] In Liebig's *Annalen der Pharmacie*, vol. xxix. p. 100, 1839, a satirical paper (*The Mystery of Vinous Fermentation Unfolded*) was published, representing yeast to be an infusory animal which fed on sugar, and evacuated by the alimentary canal spirit of wine, by the urinary organs carbonic acid! In his *Chemistry in its Application to Agriculture and Physiology*, edited by Dr. Playfair, 2nd edition, 1842, Liebig declares yeast to be a body in a state of decomposition, and states that the idea of its reproducing itself, as seeds reproduce seeds, cannot for a moment be entertained. But in the third edition of his *Animal Chemistry* (edited by Dr. Gregory, 1846) he does not attempt to deny the vegetable nature of yeast, though he thinks that investigation into the nature of this substance is not yet completed.

[7] See the *Report of the Academy of Sciences at Berlin*, for February 1843, quoted in the trans-

BOTANY.—The substance called yeast is a mass of microscopic cryptogams.

The organisation and vitality of yeast are demonstrated by the *form* and *structure* of its particles, as determined by the microscope ; by their *chemical composition ;* by their *reproductive power,* as proved by the generation of yeast during the fermentation of beer ; and lastly, by the *effects* of mechanical injuries,[1] of heat and cold,[2] and of chemical and other poisons.[3]

Kützing,[4] who is a believer in the convertibility of some of the lower algals into species, or even genera, of a higher organisation, is of opinion that yeast is an algal in its lowest, but a fungus in its highest, grade of development.

When submitted to microscopic examination, yeast is found to consist of globose, or more or less ovoidal, ellipsoidal, or somewhat pyriform, transparent, nucleated cells, varying in size from $\frac{1}{7300}$ to about $\frac{1}{7800}$th of an English inch. The nucleus or protoplasm appears to me to consist of a mass of granules or nucleoli of unequal size : some of the larger ones are highly refractive, and probably contain oily or fatty matter. The nucleoli are called by Turpin *globuline.*

Turpin spent a night in a brewery to examine the changes which the yeast undergoes during the fermentation of beer. The fresh yeast had the appearance indicated in fig. 31. In one hour after it had been added to the wort he says that germination had commenced ; the maternal cells had produced one or two buds or young cells (see fig. 32). In three hours many of the cells were didymous, or double, the buds having attained the size of the maternal cells, and some of them had themselves begun to produce other buds or young cells (see fig. 33). In eight hours the cells were arranged in rows, forming moniliform mucedinous plants, composed of several cells or joints, which varied somewhat in diameter and shape. Terminal, and in some cases lateral, buds or young cells were observed, showing that the plants were about to ramify. Some of the smaller rows were seen to explode and emit a

---

lation of Link's *Report on the Progress of the Physiological Botany,* published by the Ray Society, p. 428, 1846.

[1] A very curious fact was mentioned to me by the importer of German and Dutch yeast in Finch Lane, Cornhill, London : it is, that mechanical injury kills or destroys yeast. Foreign yeast is imported in bags, and of these great care is requisite in their removal from place to place. If they be allowed to fall violently on the ground, the yeast is spoiled. A bruise, as a blow given to the bag, also destroys it. The men who make up the dried yeast into quarter-pound and half-pound balls for sale, are obliged to handle it very dexterously, or they injure and destroy it. In fact, falls, bruises, or rough handling, kill it, and the yeast which has thus been mechanically injured may be readily distinguished from good, unaltered yeast. Its colour becomes darker, somewhat like the change which an apple or pear undergoes when it becomes rotten ; and from being crumbly or powdery, it becomes soft, glutinous, sticky to the fingers, like flour-paste, and soon stinks. I have submitted some of this injured or dead yeast to microscopical examination, but have been unable to detect any difference in its appearance from healthy yeast. The effect of mechanical injuries is also noticed by several writers. Thus Liebig (*Chemistry in its Application to Agriculture,* by Dr. Playfair, p. 286, 3d ed. 1842) remarks that simple pressure diminishes the power of yeast to excite vinous fermentation.

[2] Boiling for a short period injures, and for a long period destroys the power of yeast to excite fermentation (*Berzelius*). Cold interrupts fermentation, apparently by rendering the yeast-plant torpid.

[3] The power of yeast to excite vinous fermentation is arrested or destroyed by alcohol, acids, alkalies, various salts (chloride of sodium, bichloride of mercury, nitrate of silver, &c.), volatile oils, excess of sugar, &c. (See Berzelius and Liebig ; also Quevenne, in the *Journ. de Pharmacie,* t. xxiv. p. 3334, 1838).

[4] The following are, according to Kützing, the generic and specific characters of the *yeast-plant,* which he calls *Cryptococcus Fermentum,* and refers to *Mycophaceæ* (Pilztange), a sub-order of Algæ.

CRYPTOCOCCUS.—Mucous hyaline globules collected in an indeterminate mucous stratum.

C. Fermentum.—Submersed ; globules elliptical, solid, in the centre 1- or 2-punctate.

fine powder, consisting of minuter globules (see fig. 34). Turpin placed some yeast-cells in an aqueous solution of sugar, and in three days observed that jointed filaments, with lateral branches, were produced (see fig. 35).

The Yeast-plant.

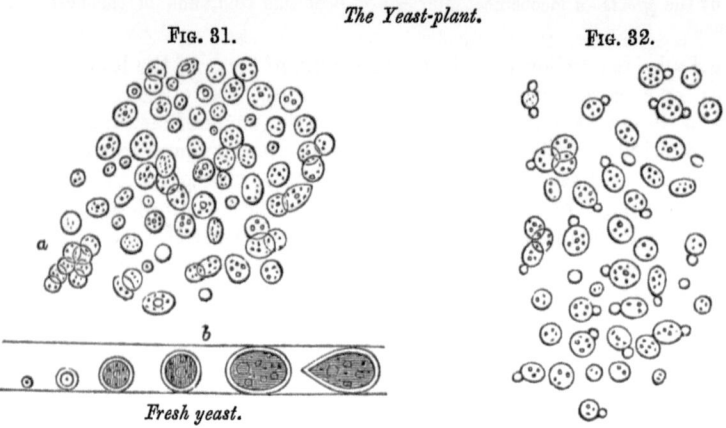

FIG. 31.

Fresh yeast.

a. Cells overlapping and showing their transparency.

b. Micrometer scale, indicating one-hundredth of a millimeter, with a progressive series of small seeds or seminules, the two first beginning to become vesicular at the centre, the two others showing the thickness of the cells, and their interior small granules of variable size.

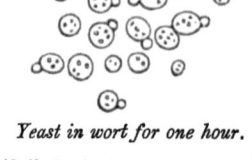

FIG. 32.

Yeast in wort for one hour.

(Cells beginning to germinate.)

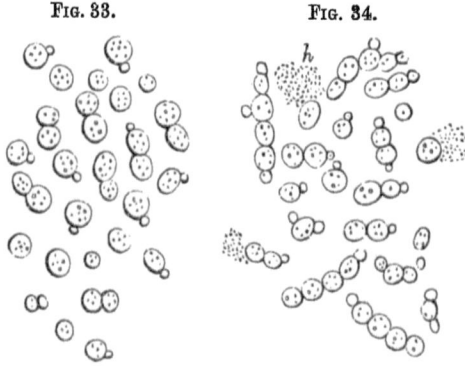

FIG. 33.

Yeast in wort for three hours.

(Cells double or didymous.)

FIG. 34.

Yeast in wort for eight hours.

(Cells united and converted into moniliform or jointed filaments.)

FIG. 35.

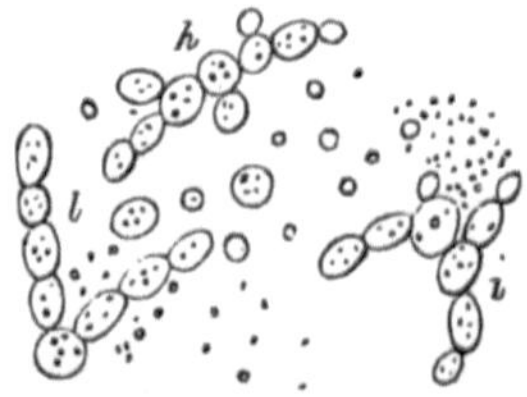

Yeast in a saccharine solution for three days.

h. The sporidia beginning to ramify and to evolve lateral buds.

i. Lateral branches composed of two joints.

l. An individual whose cell had evolved two branches.

The more or less small intermixed cells or granules are probably abortive.

I have myself examined yeast at Messrs. Hanbury and Buxton's brewery at various stages of the fermentation of both porter and ale, from a few hours to many days. In the more advanced stages of fermentation I observed the globules of yeast were frequently in strings or rows, apparently forming moniliform often branched plants. But as the cells or joints were very readily separable, I could not satisfy myself that the adhesion was otherwise than mechanical, such as we see between the blood-discs when they arrange themselves in series like money-rolls, and such as we sometimes perceive even in inorganic amorphous precipitates. My experience agrees precisely with that of Schlossberger,[1] who states that he "never could perceive a budding or bursting of the yeast-cells, accompanied by a discharge of their contents, nor could I ever produce this by compression. These curious brachial and other adjustments of the cells of yeast to each other, appeared to me the work of chance." [The yeast-grains certainly branch and produce short moniliform threads, but they are not always equally generated. Some specimens never exhibit more than a single new cell, which in turn generates another solitary cell. Others are far more prolific.—ED.] It is, however, proper to add that the artificial rupture of the cells has been effected by Mitscherlich, who also confirms Turpin's observation of the budding of the yeast-cells (see p. 41).

ORIGIN.—It is well known that a pure solution of sugar will not undergo fermentation when exposed to the air, but a saccharine vegetable juice, which contains albuminous matter (as the juice of the grape), suffers spontaneous fermentation, and this process always begins with the formation of yeast-cells.

By some it is assumed that these arise from yeast-germs floating in the air, and which, meeting with a fit receptacle for their development in the vegetable juice, germinate and grow, and effect vinous fermentation. By others their production is ascribed to a *generatio primitiva*.

Turpin was of opinion that there are three sources or modes of production of the yeast-plant:—1st, the transformation of globuline into yeast-cells; 2dly, budding, or the separation of the joints of moniliform stems; 3rdly, the escape of spores (*globulins seminulifères*) from the interior of the cells: Mitscherlich admits the two latter modes of growth.

The amylaceous particles contained in the cells of the albumen of barley (see figs. 36, 37) are called by Turpin *globuline*. The transformation of these into yeast-cells is, according to the same authority, the primitive origin of beer-yeast. Dr. Lindley[2] partly confirms Turpin, for he states that he has seen these smaller granules sprout during fermentation; and he adds that they have at that time lost all their starch, for iodine produces no sensible effect upon their colour.

FIG. 36.

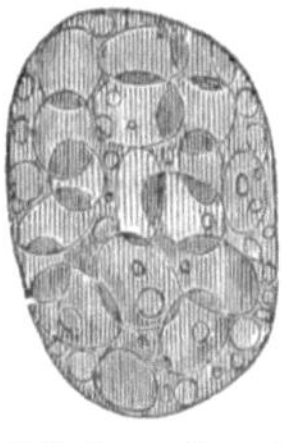

FIG. 37.

Cell from the albumen of barley, containing starch grains, called by Turpin globuline.

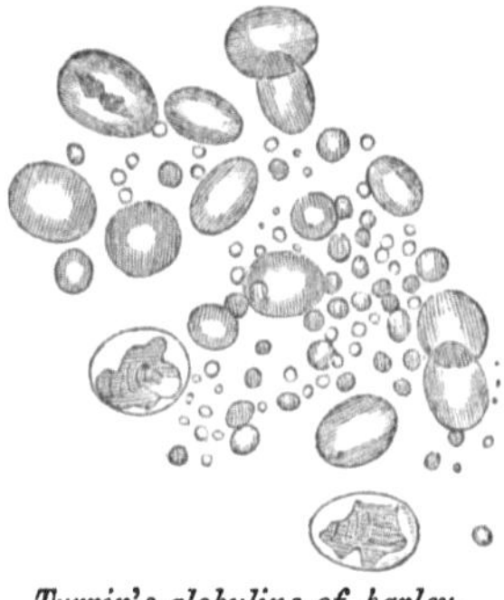

Turpin's globuline of barley.

Turpin states that 35 lbs. of dried or pressed yeast produced during the brewing of 5700 litres [about 14 butts] of beer 247 lbs. of dried or pressed yeast; that is, an actual increase of 212 lbs. of new yeast.

In the deposit from the porter refrigerator of Messrs. Truman and Han-

---

[1] *Pharmaceutical Journal*, vol. v. p. 131, 1845
[2] *Introduction to Botany*, p. 113, 4th ed. 1848.

bury's brewery I have observed the forms deposited in fig. 38, *c, d, e;* and *f.* These constitute the plant called by Desmazières the *Mycoderma Cervisiæ* [which is, however, a mere form of one and the same Penicillium with that produced by the yeast-globules.[1]—ED.]

OCCURRENCE IN THE HUMAN BODY.—Yeast-cells have been found in the human body. Hannover detected them in the black coating of the tongue of a typhoid patient. They have also been discovered in the liquids of the œsophagus, stomach, and intestine. In some cases probably they may have been introduced by the beer drunk by the patient; but, in other cases, their presence could not be accounted for in this way. As they are developed in the urine of diabetic patients, their occurrence in urine has been supposed to indicate the existence of sugar, but they have been found also in non-saccharine urine.[2]

FIG. 38.

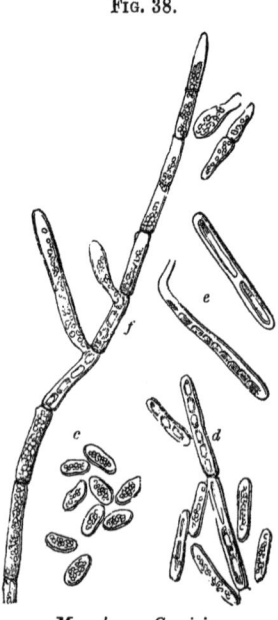

Mycoderma Cervisiæ,
Desmazières.

DESCRIPTION.—In commerce three varieties of yeast are known and distinguished. These are—brewers' yeast, dried yeast, and patent yeast.

Brewers' yeast.—In breweries two kinds of yeast may be distinguished; namely, *upper* or *top yeast,* and *lower* or *bottom yeast.* These have been described by Mitscherlich.[3]

Top yeast consists of large cells, at the extremities of which small ones are developed. It appears, therefore, to be produced by buds. In Berlin the most beautiful top yeast is obtained at a temperature of 77° F.

Bottom yeast consists of cells of various sizes, without any small globules attached to the large ones. It appears to be produced by the growth of small isolated granules (spores?) which Mitscherlich thinks have escaped from the yeast-cells which have burst and disburthened themselves of their contents. Bottom yeast is multiplied at a lower temperature than top yeast: Mitscherlich says that the bottom ferment of Bavarian beer is produced at a temperature which must not exceed 48° F. nor go below 32° F. The bottom yeast sold at breweries is generally impure.

Brewers and bakers distinguish yeast according to the quality of the beer from which it is obtained. *Ale-yeast* is the best and strongest, and is used for bread-making. *Porter-yeast* is objected to by bakers, but is used in distilleries. *Small-beer-yeast* is said to be weak, but rapid in its effects, and is sometimes used in making rolls.

2. *Dried yeast.*—Under this name is sold a granular or pasty mass of yeast-cells, which have been separated from mechanically admixed solids, as well as from the supernatant fermented liquid,—probably by filtration through linen

---

[1] [Other fungi occur in company with the Penicillium.—ED.]
[2] *Des Végétaux qui croissent sur les Hommes et sur les Animaux,* par M. Ch. Robin, Paris, 1847.
[3] Poggend. *Ann.* lix.; also *Chem. Gazette,* vol. i. p. 568, 1843.

cloths, and subsidence. That which is sold in London is imported from Holland, Belgium, and Germany, and is commonly called *German yeast*. It comes over in hempen bags, each holding half a hundredweight. If transported in casks it is apt to burst them, unless they are strongly iron-bound, by the quantity of carbonic acid which it evolves.

3. *Patent yeast.*—This might with more propriety be called *artificial yeast*. It is a watery liquid, containing yeast-cells, and which has usually been prepared purposely by the fermentation of an infusion of malt and hops. The hops probably contribute to prevent the liquid becoming rapidly sour. Turpin thinks that their oil may act as a stimulant in the development of the yeast-plant. I am informed by a baker that he prepares patent yeast for bread-making by mashing half a peck of ground malt with six gallons of water at 170° F.; then boiling the wort with half a pound of hops; and to the cooled liquid adding some brewers' yeast. In 24 hours the patent yeast is fit for use.[1] It rapidly turns sour in warm weather; and I am informed that bread made with it does not keep so well as that prepared with other kinds of yeast. It is in general use among bakers, especially those who use an inferior kind of flour. Mr. Fownes[2] describes the following mode by which he prepared some artificial yeast:—" A small handful of ordinary wheat-flour was made into a thick paste with cold water, covered with paper, and left for seven days on the mantel-shelf of a room where a fire was kept all day, being occasionally stirred. At the end of that period three quarts of malt were washed with about two gallons of water, the infusion boiled with some hops, and, when sufficiently cooled, the ferment added. The results of the experiment were a quantity of beer (not very strong, it is true, but quite free from any unpleasant taste), and at least a pint of thick barm, which proved perfectly good for making bread."

COMPOSITION.—Yeast has been analysed by Marcet,[3] by Dumas,[4] by Mitscherlich,[5] by Mulder,[6] and by Schlossberger.[7] It consists of two parts,— the *cell-walls*, composed of a kind of *cellulose ;* and the *contents of the cells*, composed of a *proteine substance*, and probably *fat*, or *oil*.

1. CELL-WALLS.—By digesting yeast in a weak solution of potash, the contents of the cells are removed, and the membranous matter composing the cell-walls is left. In its composition it approximates to *cellulose* or *starch*.

	Atoms.	Eq. Wt.	Per Cent.	Mulder.	Schlossberger.	
					With chromate of lead.	With oxide of copper and chromate of potash.
Carbon	12	72	44·44	45·00	45·45	45·09
Hydrogen	10	10	6·17	6·11	6·87	6·60
Oxygen	10	80	49·38	48·88	47·68	48·31
Cellulose of yeast	1	162	99·99	100·00	100·00	100·00

[1] Various receipts for making yeast are given in Webster's *Encyclopædia of Domestic Economy*, p. 760.

[2] *Pharmaceutical Journal*, vol. ii. p. 403, 1842.

[3] Quoted by L. Gmelin, *Handb. d. Chem.* Bd. ii. S. 1100.

[4] *Traité de Chimie appliquée aux Arts*, t. vi. p. 316, 1843.

[5] *Lehrbuch d. Chemie*, 4. Aufl. S. 370 (quoted by Schlossberger).

[6] *The Chemistry of Vegetable and Animal Physiology*, translated by Dr. Fromberg, p. 48; also *Pharm. Central-Blatt für* 1844, S. 891.

[7] *Ann. d. Chem. u. Pharm.* Bd. li. S. 193, 1844; also *Pharm. Journal*, vol. v. p. 42, 1846.

2. CONTENTS OF THE CELLS.—According to both Mulder and Schlossberger, yeast-cells contain a substance allied to the proteine bodies.

	Mulder.	Schlossberger.	
Carbon	43·35	55·53	55·53
Hydrogen	6·56	7·50	7·50
Nitrogen	12·68	14·01	13·75
Oxygen	37·41	22·96	23·22
	100·00	100·00	100·00

Besides traces of *phosphorus* and *sulphur*.

Mulder regards the contents of the cells as being the *hydrated oxide of proteine*, $C^{40}H^{37}N^{5}O^{26} = C^{40}H^{31}N^{5}O^{12} + O^{8} + 6HO$.

It is probable that, besides a proteine body, the cells contain a *fatty or oily substance.* Schlossberger states that he extracted a yellow oil from yeast by means of ether.

3. ASHES.—According to Schlossberger, the ashes of upper yeast amounted to 2·5 ; of lower yeast, to 3·5 per cent.

PHYSIOLOGICAL EFFECTS.—The effects of yeast on the animal economy are, if any, not very obvious. The constituent of the cell-walls is insoluble, and therefore inert. The contents of the cells may perhaps be slightly nutritive. To the evolved carbonic acid have been ascribed the topical antiseptic effects of yeast. The tonic and laxative effects ascribed to beer-yeast are probably referable to the fermented malt liquor in which the yeast-cells are usually contained and exhibited (see *Wort*).

USES.—Yeast is employed both for medicinal and chemical purposes.

As a medicine, yeast has been used both internally and externally. Internally it has been administered as a tonic and antiseptic in typhoid fevers. Dr. Stoker[1] states that it usually acts as a mild laxative, improves the condition of the alvine evacuations, and is more effectual in removing petechiæ and black tongue than any other remedy. It is admissible where cinchona and wine cannot be employed on account of the inflammatory symptoms. The dose of it is two table-spoonfuls every third hour, with an equal quantity of camphor mixture.. Enemata of yeast and assafœtida are said by the same writer to be efficacious against typhoid tympany.

Externally it has been used in the form of poultice. (See *Cataplasma Fermenti.*)

Yeast is an important agent in panification and brewing. In some cases of dyspepsia, unfermented bread appears to agree better with the stomach than fermented bread, which is supposed to derive an injurious quality from the yeast used in its preparation. Yeast is sometimes added to liquids to excite the vinous fermentation, and thereby to detect the presence of saccharine matter.

L. Gmelin[2] employed this test to detect sugar in the animal fluids after the ingestion of amylaceous food. Dr. Christison[3] found it so delicate that he could detect with it one part of sugar in 1000 parts of healthy urine of the sp. gr. 1·030. Messrs. Richard Phillips, Graham, and George Phillips[4] used it to detect the presence of saccharine matter in tobacco adulterated with this substance. (For the mode of using this test, see *Saccharum.*)

---

[1] *On Continued Fever*, p. 121, Dubl. 1829–30.
[2] *Recherches Expérimentales sur la Digestion*, Paris, 1826.
[3] *The Library of Practical Medicine*, vol. iv. art. *Diabetes*, p. 249.
[4] *Parliamentary Report.*

1. CATAPLASMA FERMENTI, L.; *Yeast Poultice.* (Flour, lb. j.; Yeast of Beer, and Water heated to 100°, of each ℥v. Mix, and apply a gentle heat until they begin to swell.)—It is applied, when cold, to fetid and sloughing sores as an antiseptic and stimulant : it destroys the fetor, often checks the sloughing, and assists the separation of the dead part. It should be renewed twice or thrice a day. I have frequently heard patients complain of the great pain it causes. The carbonic acid is supposed to be the active ingredient.

The following poultices are analogous in their nature and effects :—

2. CATAPLASMA FÆCULÆ CEREVISIÆ, Guy's Hospital Ph.; *Poultice of the Grounds of Beer.* (Grounds of Beer; Oatmeal; as much of each as may be required to make a poultice.)—It is applied cold twice or thrice a day, in the same cases as the preceding preparation, to which its effects are analogous. This poultice was formerly called[1] the *discutient cataplasm,* or *cataplasma discutiens,* and was applied to disperse tumours.

3. CATAPLASMA BYNES, Guy's Hospital Ph.; *Malt-meal and Yeast Poultice; Malt Poultice.* (Malt-meal and Beer-yeast, as much of each as may be required to make a poultice.)—This poultice is to be applied warm.

16. OIDIUM ABORTIFACIENS.—THE ERGOT-MOULD.

HISTORY.—Phillipar,[2] in 1837, recognised the joints or sporidia of this fungus on ergot. Phœbus,[3] in 1838, detected and figured these bodies, but did not consider them to be of a fungic nature. Mr. John Smith,[4] of the Kew Garden, in Nov. 1838, recognised them on various ergotised grasses. He considered them to be the joints of a minute articulated fungus, from whose action ergot resulted. In Dec. 1838, the late Mr. E. J. Quekett[5] gave an extended account of this fungus in a paper read before the Linnean Society. Mr. Quekett named the plant *Ergotætia abortans* (*Ergotætia,* from *Ergot,* and αἰτία, *origin; abortans,* in allusion to its destroying the germinating power of the grain of grasses, and also to the medicinal powers of ergot). Subsequently, at my suggestion, he substituted the word *aborti-faciens* for *abortans.*

Mr. Quekett at first[6] considered this fungus to belong to the sub-order *Hyphomycetes,* tribe *Mucedines ;* but after his paper had been read at the Linnean Society, and was returned to him for correction, he was led to suppose that the fungus belonged to the sub-order *Coniomycetes,* tribe *Spori-desmiei,* because its sporidia were produced beneath the epidermis of the grain. Both Link[7] and the Rev. M. J. Berkeley considered the ergot-mould to be a mucedinous fungus belonging to the genus *Oidium* (so called from ᾠόν, *an egg,* and εἶδος, *resemblance*), and I therefore called it, at the

---

[1] *Chirurgical Pharmacy,* p. 279, Lond. 1761.
[2] *Traité Organogr. et Physiologico-agric. sur l'Ergot,* Versailles, 1837.
[3] *Deutschl. kryptog. Giftgewachse,* Taf. ix. Berlin, 1838.
[4] *Trans. Linn. Society,* vol. xviii. p. 449.
[5] *Ibid.* vol. xviii. p. 453. An abridgment of this paper was published in the *Lond. Med. Gaz.* vol. xxiii. p. 606, Jan. 19, 1839.
[6] See the *Lond. Med. Gaz.* Jan. 19, 1839.
[7] *Report on the Progress of Physiological Botany* in 1841, published by the Ray Society, p. 91.

suggestion of the last-named eminent fungologist, *Oidium abortifaciens.*
Corda[1] has recently referred it to the genus *Hymenula,* of the sub-order
Hymenophycetes, and names it *Hymenula Clavus.*[2]   [Corda's *Hymenula
Clavus* is, in point of fact, not identical with the Oidium.—Ed.]

BOTANY.   **Gen. Char.**—*Sporidia* simple, more or less oval, arising from
the terminal moniliform joints of the flocci.   (*Berkeley.*)

Mr. Quekett's description of the ergot-mould (called by him *Ergotætia
abortifaciens*) is as follows :—Sporidia elliptical, moniliform, finally separating, transparent, sometimes slightly contracted about their middle, usually
containing one, two, or three, but occasionally as many as ten or twelve, well-
defined greenish granules.   They are, on the average, about 1-4000th of an
inch long, and 1-6000th of an inch broad.   When placed on glass and
moistened with water, they readily germinate or produce other plants, though
in various ways, as sometimes by emitting tubes (B), by the development of
buds (c), and by the formation of septa across their interior (E, F, G, H).

FIG. 39.

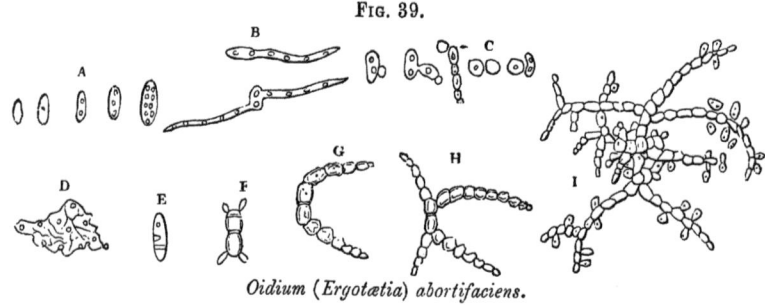

Oidium (Ergotætia) abortifaciens.

A, Sporidia.
B, C, E, F, G, H, Different modes of repro-
     duction in water.
D, Membrane of sporidium laid open.

I, The fungus assuming a radiated form,
     and beginning to develope sporidia
     upon its branches in water.

Hab.—Floral envelopes, and ovaria of grasses : Europe, America.
[This fungus often accompanies ergoted seeds, but it occurs on grasses
which are not ergoted.   Mr. Quekett supposed that it was the cause of the
ergot, but Tulasne's observations completely disprove it.—Ed.]   The
disease called the *ergot* or *spur* will be described hereafter (see *Secale
Cornutum*).   Mr. Quekett[3] states that the sporidia of this fungus are capable
of infecting healthy grains of corn, and of ergotising them ; [but as the conidia
of the Cordyceps are so often mixed with the spores of the Oidium, the error
was very easily committed.—Ed.]

---

[1] *Beitrag zur Kenntniss der Brandarten der Cerealien und des Mutterkorns,* in the *Oekonomische Neuigkeiten und Verdhandlungen,* No. 83, 1846 : a periodical publication.   I am indebted
to the Rev. M. J. Berkeley for the loan of Corda's paper.   A copy of Corda's figures, illustrating
the structure of the ergot of rye, and of the microscopic appearance of the fungus, will be given
hereafter (see *Secale Cornutum*).

[2] [Tulasne has lately published, in the *Annales des Sciences Naturelles,* a most interesting paper
showing that ergot is a diseased condition produced by the mycelium of one or more species of
Cordyceps.   If ergoted grains are deposited in soil, after a few months the perfect Cordyceps is
produced,—a fact confirmed, independently of each other, by Mr. Berkeley and Mr. Broome.   The
Hymenula Clavus of Corda is the conidiiferous state of this fungus, whereas the fungus of Quekett
appears to be of an entirely different nature.—Ed.]

[3] *Lond. Med. Gaz.* Oct. 8, 1841 ; and *Trans. of the Linn. Society,* vol. xix. p. 137.

PROPERTIES.—The chemical properties and physiological effects of this fungus are at present quite unknown. We have yet to learn whether the peculiar properties of ergotised grasses depend on the fungi, or on the morbid products of the ovarium.

Sub-order III. GASTEROMYCETES, *Endl.*

CHARACTERS.—*Sporidia* free or enclosed in asci within a closed receptacle (*peridium*), collected together in the centre, or immersed and concrete, intermixed with *flocci*, or contained in proper receptacles (*sporangia*).

17. Elaphomyces granulatus, *Fries.*—Granulated Elaphomyces.

Lycoperdon cervinum, Linn.; *Cervi Boletus*, J. Bauh.; *Elaphomyces officinalis*, Nees; *Tuber cervinum*, Nees; *Boletus cervinus*; *Hart's Truffles*; *Deer Balls.* Sold at Covent Garden Market as *Lycoperdon Nuts.* (Elaphomyces, from ἔλαφός, *a stag*; and μύκης, *a fungus*).—Rounded or oblong, from half an inch to two inches in diameter, brown, papilloso-verrucose, hard. Peridium internally white. Sporidia abundant, globular, black, —Indigenous. Grows underground. [Another species often confounded with it, but doubtless similar in quality, is distinguished by its muricated surface and mottled flesh. This is *E. muricatus*, and is equally common. In both, the spores are originally contained in distinct asci, as in the Truffles.—ED.]

A very complete analysis has been made by Biltz.[1] The sporidia consisted of a disagreeable odorous *volatile substance, soft resin,* 0·325; *hard resin,* 0·052; *red colouring matter, uncrystallisable sugar,* with *fungic ozmazome,* 2·708; *gum,* 2·083; *inulin,* 8·333; *soluble albumen,* a trace; *fungin, red colouring* and *albuminous matter,* soluble in potash; *free vegetable acid,* vegetable salts of *ammonia, potash,* and *lime, sulphate* and *phosphate of lime, chloride of sodium, silica, manganese,* and *iron.* The ashes amount to 1·25. The peridium, deprived of its warty coat, consisted of *yellow rancid soft fat,* 0·33; *fungic ozmazome,* with *crystalline sugar,* 12·000; *gum,* 10·40; *albumen, fungin, gummy* and *albuminous matter,* soluble in potash; *free vegetable acid, vegetable salts of ammonia* and *lime, phosphate* and *sulphate of lime.* The ashes amount to 1·1. The warty coat contains *yellow bitter fat, colouring matter* soluble in water and alkalies, but not in alcohol or ether; *bitter* and *other substances,* but neither sugar nor inulin. The capillitium contains *sugar,* but no inulin.

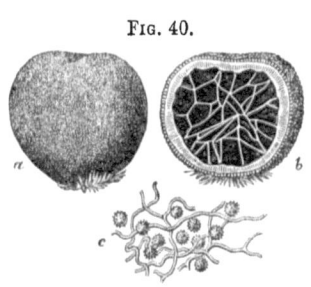

FIG. 40.

Elaphomyces granulatus.

a. The fruit with the mycelium (nat.
b. Vertical section of ditto. [size).
c. Sporidia, with flocci of the capillitium (magnified).

Though still retained in some of the best modern works on medical botany published on the continent, this subterranean fungus is no longer used in medicine, at least in England. As, however, I have met with it in the stock of a London herbalist, I presume at no very long period since it must have been in use. "It was formerly used by apothecaries for the preparation of the *balsamus apoplecticus;* and great power was ascribed to it in promoting parturition and the secretion of milk. Even now the country people in some places esteem it as an aphrodisiac, and prepare from it a spirituous tincture."[2] Parkinson[3] says the dose of it is one drachm and a half in powder, taken with sweet wine, or with such other things as provoke venery.

[1] Trommsdorff's *Neues Journ. d. Pharm.* Bd. xi.
[2] Gleditsch, quoted by Nees v. Esenbeck and Ebermaier, *Handb. d. med.-pharm. Botanik,* Bd. i. S. 28, 1832.
[3] *Theatrum Botanicum,* p. 1320, 1640.

18. Lycoperdon giganteum, *Batsch.*—Giant Puffball.

LYCOPERDON BOVISTA (GIGANTEUM), Fries; *Bovista gigantea*, Nees.—Sold in the London herb-shops as the *Common Puffball*, or simply as *Puffball*.—They are the *Fusseballs* of Parkinson.—In somewhat globular or obconical masses of variable size, sometimes one or two feet in diameter, and usually of a more or less yellow colour. *Peridium* very brittle, bursting in areolæ, evanescent, at length broadly open. *Capillitium* rare, evanescent together with the olive dingy-brown *sporidia*. This species, as well as *Lycoperdon cœlatum* of Bulliard, has been used in medicine under the name of *bovista, fungus chirurgorum*, and *crepitus lupi*. The spongy capillitium with the sporidia has been employed for staunching blood : thus it has been used as a plug in epistaxis, hemorrhage from the teeth, rectum, &c. The spongy base is employed as tinder. The fumes of this fungus, when burnt, are said to possess a narcotic quality, and have been employed to stupify bees, [and it has lately been proposed as a substitute for chloroform.—ED.]

19. Tuber cibarium, *Sibth.*—Common Truffle.

LYCOPERDON TUBER, Linn.; *Tubera*, Tourn.; *Tubera sincera*, Pliny, lib. xix. cap. 11.—Dr. Sibthorp (*Floræ Gr. Prodr.* ii. 352) considers it to be the ὕδνον of Diosc. lib. ii. cap. 175; its modern Greek name being ὕδνος ἤ ἴκνος : but Fries, while he admits, on the authority of Sprengel, that it is the ὕδνον of Theophrastus (*Hist. Pl.* lib. i. cap. 9), says it is certainly not the ὕδνον of Dioscorides.[1]

FIG. 41.   FIG. 42.

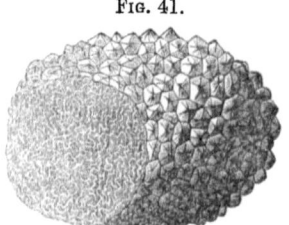

Tuber melanosporum.

A truffle (natural size) from which a slice has been cut to expose the internal structure.

A section of a truffle (magnified).
a a. Cells.
b b c. Pedicellated peridiola or sporangia containing sporidia.
d. A sporidium (or spore) more highly magnified.

The truffle of our markets occurs in rough rounded nodules, varying in size from a filbert to the fist, cracked into small subpyramidal warts. Internally it is marbled or veined. The white portions are filamentous, and are regarded by the Rev. M. J. Berkeley as constituting a sort of mycelium to the darker portions, which he calls the veins : the latter are cellular, and contain many subovate, shortly pedicellated *sporangia*, at first filled with a granular mass, which is ultimately collected into one or more globular yellowish reticulated *sporidia*. [These at first sight appear to be echinulated, as is the case in some species of Truffles, as in *T. melanosporum*, but the appearance arises from the membrane of the cells of the perisporium being overlooked, while the junctures of the cells themselves are visible.

[The species of Truffle are very numerous, and several occur in this country. Descrip-

<hr />

[1] *Systema Mycologicum*, vol. ii. 290, p. 1822.

tions will be found in Vittadini's Monograph, the magnificent work of Tulasne on Hypogæous Fungi, and in some papers by Mr. Berkeley and Mr. Broome in the Annals of Natural History. The two former are accompanied by beautiful figures, and the sixth posthumous fasciculus of Corda's Icones contains a large mass of information on the subject.—ED.]

Truffles grow a little below the surface of the ground in several parts of England. Covent Garden Market is chiefly supplied from the downs of Wiltshire, Hampshire, and Kent. Its odour is peculiar and penetrating, by which its presence is detected. In this country it is usually hunted by dogs trained for the purpose : in Italy, by pigs. [The principal species collected in England for sale is *Tuber æstivum*, but it does not vie in flavour with the pink-flesh *T. magnatum* of Italy, or the dark strong-scented *T. melanosporum*, which is the best truffle of the Paris markets, and is represented in our figure. *Melanogaster variegatus* is sometimes sold in the market at Bath, but it is very inferior to the real truffle.—ED.] Riegel[1] analysed the dried Perigord truffles, and found them to consist of a *brown fat oil* (olein), with traces of *volatile oil*, an acrid *resin*, *osmazome*, *mushroom sugar*, *nitrogenous matter* insoluble in alcohol, *fungic acid*, *boletic acid*, *phosphoric acid*, *potash*, *ammonia*, *vegetable mucus*, *vegetable albumen*, *pectine*, and *fungine* (fungic skeleton).

Truffles are a highly esteemed luxury at the table, being used as a seasoning or flavouring ingredient for ragouts, sauces, and stuffings. They are considered to possess aphrodisiac properties ; and an Italian physician essayed to prove that births were more numerous in those years which correspond to the more abundant production of truffles !

Sub-order III. PYRENOMYCETES.

CHARACTERS.—*Perithecium* indurated, at first closed up, then perforated by a pore or irregular laceration, inclosing a softer nucleus. *Sporidia* immersed in mucus or inclosed in *asci*, which are attached by their base.

20. Sphæria Sinensis, *Berk.*[2]

Hia Tsao Tom Tchom, Reaumur, Mém. de l'Acad. des Sc. 1726, p. 302, tab. 16 ; *Hia Tsao Tong Tchong*, Du Halde, Descr. Géogr. et. Hist. de la Chine, vol. iii. p. 490, 1770 ; *Totsu Kaso*, Thunberg, Travels in Europe, Asia, &c. between 1770 and 1779, vol. iii. p. 68 ; *Hiastaotomtchom*, Rees's Cyclop. ; *Tong Chong Ha Cho*, Reeves ; *Summer-Plant-Winter Worm*, Pereira, Pharm. Journ. vol. ii. p. 590, 1843 ; *Hea Tsaou Taong Chung*, Westwood, Ann. of Nat. Hist. vol. viii. p. 217 ; *Sphæria Sinensis*, Rev. M. J. Berkeley, in Hooker's London Journ. of Botany, vol. ii. p. 207, 1843.

This remarkable production is a highly esteemed article of the Chinese Materia Medica. It consists of a caterpillar or larva of a lepidopterous insect (probably a species of *Agrotis*), from whose neck projects the fungus called by the Rev. M. J. Berkeley *Sphæria Sinensis*.

SPHÆRIA, Fries.—*Perithecia* rounded entire, furnished at the apex with a minute orifice. *Asci* converging, at length dissolving.

S. Sinensis, Berkeley.—Brown ; stem cylindrical, somewhat thicker downwards ; head cylindrical, confluent with the stem, pointleted.

Du Halde says that it is produced in Thibet, and also on the frontiers of the province of Se-tchuen, which borders on Thibet, or Laza. It is brought to Canton in bundles tied up in silk (see fig. 43), each bundle containing about one dozen individuals.

Each individual (see fig. 44) is about three inches long, half being the caterpillar ; the other half, projecting from the back of the neck, is the club-shaped fungus, attached by

---

[1] *Pharmaceutisches Central-Blatt für* 1844, p. 17 ; also *Chem. Gaz.* vol. ii. p. 137.
[2] [The enormous genus *Sphæria* is now broken up into numerous genera. The present species is assigned to the genus *Cordyceps*, to which also belongs the fungus whose mycelium produces the disease known by the name of Ergot.— ED.]

slender filaments, which spread over the surface of the larva. The substance of the caterpillar is replaced by a mass of fine branched threads, mixed with globules of oil. In none of the specimens examined by Mr. Berkeley were the perithecia developed.

Fig. 43.

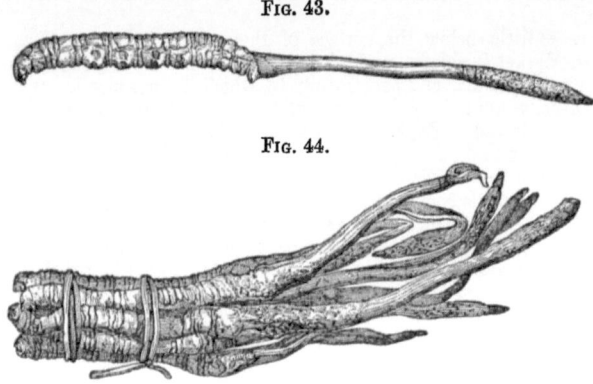

Fig. 44.

Sphæria Sinensis.

Fig. 43, Isolated individual.   Fig. 44, Bundle.

(Natural size.)

In China it is reputed as a strengthening and renovating substance, and is supposed to possess properties similar to those ascribed to ginsing. It is recommended in cases where the powers of the system have been reduced by over-exertion or sickness. But on account of its scarcity it is only used in the palace of the Emperor. The mode of employing it is curious. The belly of a duck is to be stuffed with five drachms of this fungus, and the animal roasted by a slow fire. The virtue of the fungus is supposed to pass into the flesh of the animal, which is to be eaten twice daily for eight or ten days!

Sub-order IV. Hymenomycetes.

Characters.—*Spores* generally quaternate on distinct *sporophores* (*basidia*). *Hymenium* naked.

21. Exidia Auricula Judæ, *Fries.*—Jew's Ear.

Tremella Auricula Judæ, Linn.; *Peziza Auricula,* Linn.—This fungus grows on living trees, especially the elder; whence its name *fungus sambuci* vel *sambucinus.* It is still professed to be kept in the London herb-shops; but in its place I find that *Polyporus versicolor,* Fries, is usually sold for it. Dr. Martiny[1] states that other species—namely, *Polyporus adustus,* Fries, *Polyporus zonatus,* Fries (especially when this is strongly dried and half charred), and *Dædalea unicolor,* Fries, are substituted for the genuine plant. All these adulterations or substitutions may be readily detected by immersing the dried fungus in water: the genuine Exidia Auricula Judæ softens and swells up so as to resume its natural gelatinous condition, whereas the others do not soften in water. It was formerly in repute as a topical astringent and discutient, and was employed in the form of decoction or infusion (made with water, rose-water, vinegar, or milk), and cataplasm made with milk and water. It has been used in sore-throat, sore-eyes, and deafness.[2] On account of its absorbing and retaining liquids, it has been soaked in collyria, and applied to the eyes, as a substitute for sponge.

---

[1] *Encyklop. d. Naturalien u. Rohrwaarenk,* Bd. i. S. 911, 1843.
[2] For further details respecting it, consult Alston's *Lect. on the Mat. Medica,* vol. i. p. 851, 1770; and Murray, *App. Medicaminum,* vol. v. p. 583.

22. Morchella esculenta, *Linn.*—Common Morell.

Phallus esculentus, Linn.; *Helvella esculenta*, Sowerby; *Fungus faginosus*, Lobel., Gerarde, Parkinson; *Merulius*, J. Bauh. Hist. Pl.

This fungus is sold at the Italian warehouses, and at Covent Garden Market, in the dried and shrivelled state; and, though a native of this country, is usually imported from the Continent. In the fresh state it is from 2 to 5 inches high, and hollow (see fig 45). The *stem* is white, from 1 to 3 inches long, ½ to 1 inch in diameter. The *pileus*, which is confluent with the stem, varies in size from that of a pigeon's egg to that of a swan's egg; is deeply pitted or formed in irregular areolæ, divided by anastomosing ribs, and varies in colour from a pale yellowish-brown to olivaceous and smoke-grey. The *hymenium* covers the whole pileus. The *thecæ*, when unruptured, contain eight elliptic *spores*.

The Morell is a highly-esteemed luxury at table. It usually enters into ragouts or other dishes; but is sometimes cooked by itself, being either stewed, or stuffed and dressed between thin slices of bacon. Though considered to possess nutritive qualities, it is employed at the table as a flavouring ingredient. Virey[1] enumerates it among aphrodisiacs.

23. Polyporus officinalis, *Fries.*—Larch Agaric.

SYNONYMES.—*Boletus Laricis*, Jacq., Misc. ii. p. 164; Ph. Boruss.; *Boletus purgans*, Pers. Syn. p. 531; *Boletus officinalis*, Villars, Delph. p. 1041; *Polyporus Laricis*, Roques.

HISTORY.—This fungus was used by the ancients. It is described by Dioscorides[2] under the name of 'Αγαρικόν. In the modern Greek Pharmacopœia it is termed 'Αγαρικόν τὸλευκόν, its Turkish name being Κατρὰν μανταρί.

BOTANY. **Gen. Char.**—*Hymenium* concrete with the substance of the pileus, consisting of subrotund pores with their simple dissepiments (*Berkeley*).

Sp. Char.—*Pileus* corky-fleshy, ungulate, zoned, smooth. *Pores* yellowish (*Fries*).

HAB.—South of Europe and Asia, on the Larch.

COMMERCE.—The best agaric is brought from Asia and Carinthia. A small and inferior kind is collected in Dauphiné. I was informed by the late Mr, Butler, of Covent Garden Market, that the London shops were supplied from Germany. Levant Agaric (an inferior sort of which is known at Marseilles by the name of *cucumule*) is exported from Smyrna. The Russian larch agaric exported from Archangel is the product of *Larix sibirica*.[3]

COLLECTION.—It is collected in the months of August and September, decorticated, dried, and bleached in the sun. Martiny states that it is beaten with wooden hammers to make it soft. But that which I have found in English commerce has neither been decorticated nor beaten.

DESCRIPTION.—This fungus is still kept in the herb-shops, being sold under the name of *agaric, white agaric (agaricus albus)*, or *larch* or *female agaric (fungus laricis)*. It occurs in masses varying in size from that of the fist to that of a child's head. The most usual shape which I have found is that of a horse's hoof, or of half a cone (divided by a plane passing

---

[1] *Bull. de Pharm.* t. v. p. 201, 1813.
[2] Lib. iii. cap. 1.
[3] Martius, in Buchner's *Repertorium*, N. S. Bd. xli. S. 92, 1846.

through both the apex and the base).[1] Externally it is yellowish or reddish-grey; internally it is white. It has a very feeble odour, and a bitter acrid taste. It is liable to be attacked by a beetle, the *Anobium festivum*, Panz.

Fig. 45.	Fig. 46.

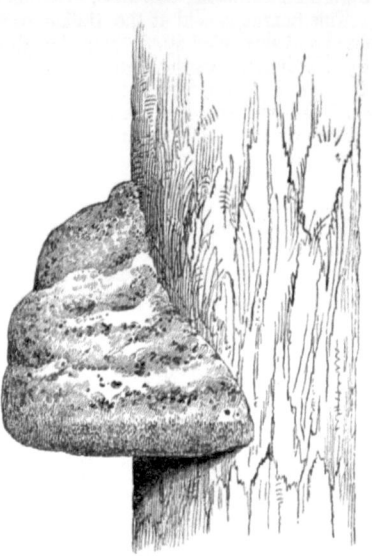

Morchella esculenta.

1. Morchella esculenta (nat. size).
2. A section of ditto.
3. Thecæ and sporules magnified.

Polyporus officinalis.

(Represented as growing on the stem of a tree.)

COMPOSITION.—It has been analysed by Bouillon-La Grange;[2] by Bucholz;[3] by Braconnot,[4] and by Bley.[5]

The constituents, according to Bley, are *resin*, 33·1; *extractive*, 2; *gum* and *bitter extractive*, 8·3; *vegetable albumen*, 0·7; *wax*, 0·2; *fungic acids*, 0·13; *boletic acid*, 0·06; *tartaric* and *phosphoric acids*, 1·354; *potash*, 0·329; *lime*, 0·16; *ammonia* and *sulphur*, traces. The following substances were obtained by the action of caustic potash and hydrochloric acid :—*coagulated albumen*, 0·4; *artificial gum*, 15·5; *artificial resin*, soluble in ether, 9·5; residual *fibre* called *fungine* (cellulose), 15; *moisture*, 11, and *loss*, 2·367 = 100·000.

The active principle of agaric has been usually said to reside in the resin; but Martius[6] states that it is a peculiar substance, which he proposes to call *laricin*. This is a white amorphous powder, possessing a bitter taste, soluble in alcohol and oil of turpentine, and forming with boiling water a paste. It

[1] The specimen from which fig. 46 was taken, was kindly lent me by the Rev. M. J. Berkeley. I have had it represented as growing on the stem of a tree.

[2] *Ann. de Chimie*, t. li. p. 76, 1808; also Thomson's *Chemistry of Organic Bodies—Vegetables*, p. 939, 1838.

[3] *Berlin. Jahrbuch für* 1808, p. 111.

[4] *Bull. de Pharm.* t. iv. p. 304, 1812.

[5] Trommsdorff's *N. Journ.* Bd. xxv. S. 119, 1832; Martiny, *Encyklop. d. Natur*, S. 909.

[6] Buchner's *Repertorium*, Bd. xli. S. 93, 1846.

has been analysed by Dr. Will, who found that its formula was $C^{14}H^{12}O^4$. The *resin* of agaric possesses purgative qualities, and was formerly employed for the adulteration of jalap resin.[1]　It probably contains laricin.

EFFECTS.—Larch agaric is an acrid substance.　Its dust irritates the eyes, and causes sneezing, cough, and nausea.　When swallowed in the dose of a drachm or two, this fungus excites nausea, vomiting, griping, and purging, and is said to check sweating.

USES.—It has been employed internally as an emetic, cathartic, discutient, and to check colliquative sweating: externally, as an astringent.　De Haen reported favourably of it as an anti-sudorific in phthisis, and Barbut confirms his statements.　Favourable reports of it were also made by Toel, Neumann, Kopp, Burdach, Andral, and others.　Subsequently, however, Andral has expressed an opinion that little benefit is to be derived from it.

ADMINISTRATION.—The dose of it is from ʒss. to ʒj. as a purgative; and from gr. iij. to gr. viij., taken before going to sleep, to check sweating.[2]

24. Polyporus igniarius, *Fries.*—Hard Amadou Polyporus.

Boletus igniarius, Linn.—An indigenous fungus found on willow, cherry, plum, and other trees, and commonly known by the names of *Agaric of the Oak* (*Agaricus* seu *Fungus Quercûs; Agaricus Quernus*), or *Surgeons' Agaric* (*Agaricus Chirurgorum*); *Spunk ; Touch-wood.* Formerly used in surgery as a mechanical styptic, and still retained in some foreign pharmacopœias (e. g. *Pharm. Castrenis Ruthenica*, 1840). It is prepared by decorticating it, cutting into thin slices, and beating it with a mallet until it has become sufficiently soft. Its action in restraining hemorrhages is mechanical, like lint.[3]　In some places, both it and the following species are employed in the preparation of Amadou or tinder.

25. Polyporus fomentarius, *Fries.*—Real Amadou.

Boletus fomentarius, Linn.—Another indigenous fungus, found on the oak, birch, and other trees. Its uses are similar to the preceding, and it might, with more propriety, be called *Agaric of the Oak*, or *Surgeons' Agaric*. The substance sold in the shops as *Amadou*, or *German tinder*, is prepared from this, as well as the preceding species, by cutting the fungus in slices, beating it, and then soaking it in a solution of nitre, and afterwards drying it.　When impregnated with gunpowder, it is called *black amadou.* Amadou, or German tinder, has been recommended by Mr. Wetherfield[4] as an elastic medium for applying support and pressure, and as a defence to tender and delicate parts; as in the form of a graduated compress, in umbilical hernia of new-born infants, and as a compress over fistulous ulcers of the groin.　It does not lose its elasticity, like lint.

26. Agaricus campestris, *Linn.*—Mushroom.

Agaricus edulis, Roques.—Fries[5] considers this species to be the μύκης ἐδώδιμος of Dioscorides (lib. i. cap. 109); the *Fungi qui rubent callo* of Pliny (*Hist. Nat.* lib. xxii. cap. 47); Μανιτάρι *hodiè Gr.* Sibth.

---

[1] Jacquin, *Diss. de Agarico Offic.* Vind. 1778 (Richter's *Arzneimittellehre*, Bd. ii. S. 275).

[2] For further details respecting its medical uses, see Murray, *App. Med.* vol. v. p. 573 ; Riecke, *Die neuern Arzneimitt. ;* and Dunglison, *New Remedies ;* and for formulæ for its preparation, see Jourdan's *Pharmacopée Universelle.*

[3] *Phil. Trans.* vols. xlviii. and xlix.; Warner's *Cases in Surgery*, p. 338 ; Murray, *App. Medicam.* vol. v.

[4] *Lond. Med. Gaz.* Nov. 26, 1841, p. 337.

[5] *Systema Mycologicum*, vol. i. p. 281, 1821.

AGARICUS, Linn.—*Hymenium* consisting of plates radiating from a common centre, with shorter ones in the interstices, composed of a double closely connected membrane, more or less distinct from the pileus. *Veil* various or absent.—Named from *Agaria*, a region of Sarmatia (*Berkeley*).

A. campestris, Linn.—Pileus fleshy, dry, subsquamose or silky, gills pink free ventricose, at length brown, stem stuffed furnished with a ring white (*Berkeley*).

Pileus or cap 2-5 inches broad, at first convex, then plano-convex, white or light brown, silky or clothed with reddish-brown adpressed fibrillæ collected into little fascicles ; *epidermis* easily peeled off, projecting beyond the gills, and often curled back, fleshy; *flesh* firm, thick, white, more or less stained with reddish brown, especially when bruised. *Gills* very unequal, at first of a beautiful pink, free, obtuse, and sometimes forked behind, broad in the middle ; at length dark, mottled with brownish-purple; the edge white, and minutely denticulate. *Spores* minute, elliptical, purplish-brown, immediately supported on *spicules* (*sterigmata*), which surmount the *sporophores* (*basidia*). *Root* consisting of branched fibres (*mycelia*). When quite young, there is a fine silky universal veil (*Berkeley*, with additions).

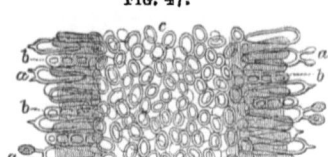

FIG. 47.

Section of one of the gills of A. campestris.

a a a, Sporophores surmounted by spicules bearing spores. Link[1] terms these bodies small tubes with stalked granules (*antheridia*).

b b b. Small tubes with transverse septa. According to Link they become spores. [This notion is, however, altogether erroneous, as indeed is the figure as far as these tubes are concerned.—ED.]

c c. The central vesicular tissue.

If the pileus be cut through, the fleshy part soon turns pink, and drops of pink juice may be squeezed out of it if young; but if old, the cut part, as well as the juice, are rather inclining to brown, but the *Agaricus Georgii*, Sow. (not of Clusius) turns yellow. The whole plant is rather brittle, and has a fine scent peculiar to itself (*J. Sowerby, jun.*)

The mushroom is artificially produced either with or without spawn. *Mushroom spawn* is the name given by gardeners to the white branching cottony fibres (*mycelium*), which form the so-called *root* of the mushroom, and upon which, at short intervals, are many very small round buds (the infant state of the plant). This spawn is collected and saved by gardeners, and at the commencement of autumn is planted on beds of dung, and covered with straw : in about two months the mushrooms come up, and rapidly increase. Mixed with dung, and made up into rectangular cakes, it forms what are called *spawn-cakes* or *spawn-bricks*. These are sold at Covent Garden Market, and are planted in beds.

Mushrooms are also propagated without spawn. The principal ingredient employed in preparing the compost used for this purpose is horse-droppings.[2] "The artificial production of this species without the aid of spawn," says the Rev. M. J. Berkeley,[3] "has been frequently brought forward as an argument for the equivocal generation of fungi. But when it is considered how many millions of these sporules must be devoured together with the herbage by the animal, whose dung is a principal material in the compost, much of the force of this argument vanishes."

The young mushroom is gathered while the margin of the pileus is connected with the stalk by the veil, and at this period it is commonly called the *button mushroom* (fig. 48, A *a*). The mature mushrooms are collected and sold as *full-grown* or *flap mushrooms* (fig. 48, B). Dr. Badham[4] mentions a very large variety commonly called by peasants the *ox-mushroom*.

The mushroom was analysed by Vauquelin,[5] who found in it a *brown-red fat*, a *spermaceti-like fat, mushroom sugar, peculiar animal matter, osmazome, albumen, fungine* [cellulose], *acetate of potash*, and *other salts*.

This species is esculent, and in general wholesome ; but it is employed at table for its savory, rather than for its nutritive qualities. At times it proves indigestible and

---

[1] *Icones Selectæ Anatomico-Botanicæ*, Fasc. iii. Berlin, 1841.
[2] See Loudon's *Encyclopædia of Gardening*.
[3] *English Flora*, vol. v. part ii. p. 107.
[4] *Treatise on Esculent Funguses*, p. 85, 1847.
[5] *Ann. de Chimie*, lxxxv. 5, 1813.

unwholesome,—occasionally, perhaps, from some peculiarity in the quality of the mushroom, or from the mode of cooking it; but frequently from idiosyncrasy on the part of the sufferer. The particular circumstances, however, which render it unwholesome, are very obscure. Its use should be avoided by dyspeptics, by persons liable to pruriginous, exanthematous, and scaly diseases of the skin, and by those who have a highly susceptible nervous system. The juice of the mushroom, flavoured with salt and aromatics, constitutes the sauce called *ketchup* (a word said to be derived from the Japanese *kit-jap*), which, though in common use at table, rarely produces any unpleasant effects when used in small quantities.

AGARICUS GEORGII, Withering.—This species, called *St. George's Mushroom*, because it grows up about St. George's day (April 23d), is said by the Rev. Mr. Berkeley to be frequently sold in London under the name of *White Caps*. But I have inquired for it by this name among the dealers of Covent Garden Market, but cannot meet with any one acquainted with it (fig. 48, C).

FIG. 48.

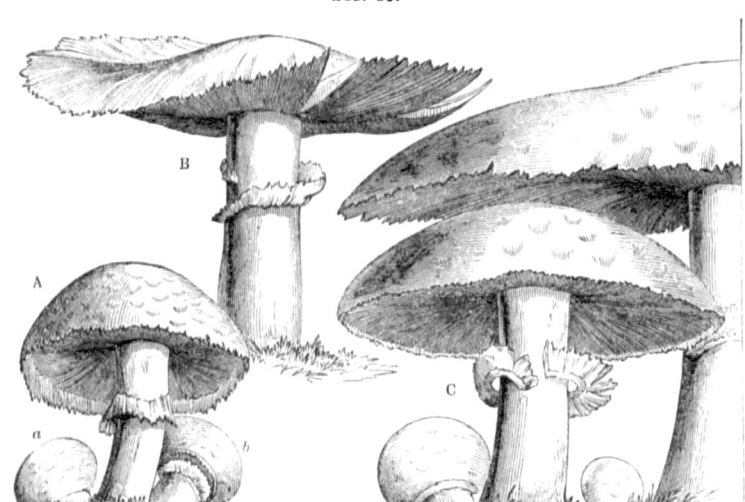

A. *Agaricus campestris.*
  a. Button.
  b. Ditto; the annulus splitting from
    pileus.

B. *A. campestris* (flap or full-grown
    Mushroom).
C. *A. Georgii,* Sow.

It is larger than the common mushroom (*A. campestris*), which it resembles in shape. When bruised or injured it soon turns yellow, and by this character may be readily distinguished from the common mushroom, which turns pink when cut. Its smell is strong and unpleasant. It contains but little juice, and that of a yellow colour, and is, therefore, not adapted for making ketchup. Although not poisonous, it is less wholesome than the preceding species, and is usually rejected by housekeepers. It is very tough, and difficult of digestion.

27. Agaricus oreades, *Bolton.*—Champignon.

Agaricus oreades, Withering, Brit. Pl., vol. iv.; *A. pratensis,* J. Sowerby, Eng. Fungi; J. Sowerby, jun., The Mushroom and Champignon Illustrated; *A. Pseudo-Mousseron,* Bulliard; *Fairy-Ring Agaric; Scotch Bonnets.*—This indigenous plant occurs in pastures, and is one of several fungi which grow in circles forming what have been termed *Fairy-rings.* It is commonly sold in the shops for use at table, and is liable to be mistaken for several other species of Agaricus, viz. *A. dealbatus, dryophilus, semiglobatus,* and *fœnisecii.* Of these, A. dealbatus is the only one which, like the true champignon, forms " fairy-rings."

The fungus varies in colour from a pale to a deep buff or nankeen colour. The *stem* is 1 or 2 inches high, and 2 or 3 lines thick, round, solid, often slightly twisted, readily splitting longitudinally into silky fibres, and is of the same colour as the gills. The *pileus* or cap is from ½ to 1 inch in diameter, irregularly round, convex, most elevated in the centre, tough and coriaceous. The gills free, distant, waved at the edges, often lacerated, paler than the pileus. " If the pileus be cut through (fig 49, *b*) the gills will not be found to separate from it, but the fleshy part runs down the middle of each gill, which is covered by the continuation of the same buff-coloured coat that lines the under surface of the pileus between the gills,—a structure widely different from the poisonous one [*Ag. semi-globatus*]."[1] *Taste* and *odour* agreeable.

FIG. 49.

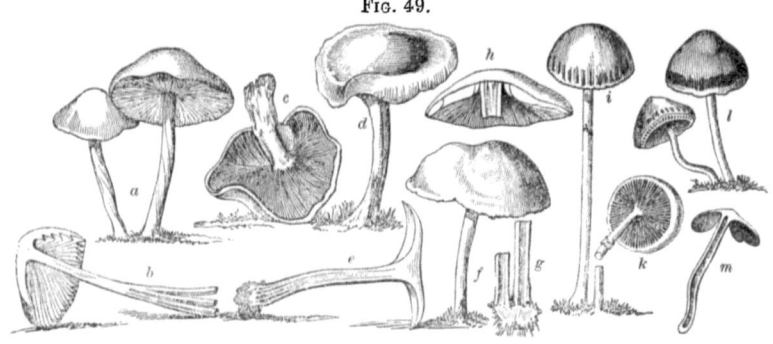

Agarici.[2]

a b. A. oreades.	*f g h.* A. dryophilus.	*l m.* A. fœnisecii.
c d e. A. dealbatus.	*i k.* A. semiglobatus.	

A. DEALBATUS, Sowerby (fig. 49, *c d e*) is distinguished from the champignon by the *margin of the pileus being at first rolled inwards,* by *its very fine dingy whitish gills,* by its becoming *grey-brown in zones* when soaked in water, and by its *disagreeable odour.* This species, according to Mrs. Hussey, resembles the champignon more than any other, and, like it, also grows in fairy-rings.

A. SEMI-GLOBATUS, Batsch. (fig. 49, *i k*) (*A. virosus* of Sowerby) is distinguished from the champignon by its *dark-coloured gills,* its *hollow stem,* and *shining glutinous pileus.* When young, this species has an *annulus* or *ring,* but this commonly disappears when the plant has attained its full size.

A. FŒNISECII, Persoon (fig, 49, *l m*), is distinguished from the champignon by its *dark-coloured gills,* its *hollow stem,* and its *umber purple spores.*

A. DRYOPHILUS, Bulliard (fig. 49, *f g h*), is distinguished from the champignon by its *fine close gills,* its *hollow stem,* and its *reddened swollen base.*

Like the Agaricus campestris, or mushroom, the A. oreades, or Champignon, is used at table on account of its savory qualities, and not for its nutritive power, which is probably very slight.

28. Fungi venenati.—Poisonous Fungi; Toadstools.

Many fungi are poisonous, and a still larger number frequently prove indigestible and unwholesome. The same species which may be taken with impunity by one individual, will excite in another various inconveniences, such as nausea, vomiting, griping, and diar-

---

[1] Sowerby, jun., *The Mushroom and Champignon Illustrated.*

[2] In the above cut, the figures marked *a* and *b* are from Mr. J. Sowerby, jun.'s *Mushroom and Champignon Illustrated;* the others from Mrs. Hussey's *Illustrations of British Mycology,* part xiii. pl. xxxix. 1848.

rhœa. Dyspepsia, and a highly susceptible condition of the nervous system, such as that called the hysterical constitution, dispose to those ill effects, which, in other cases, are ascribed to idiosyncrasy of constitution.

It must be obvious from these remarks that there can be no absolute anatomical characters by which the unwholesome can be distinguished from the wholesome species ; the effects greatly depending on the constitution of the eater, or on some other insufficiently determined circumstances. An illustrative fact of the truth of this statement has been adduced in the case of a French officer and his wife, who died in consequence of break-fasting off some poisonous Agarics, which were nevertheless eaten by other persons in the house with impunity. These and other circumstances have led to a general distrust of all fungi, except the cultivated ones; and so strongly was the late accomplished botanist, Professor L. C. Richard, impressed with this feeling, that, though no one was better acquainted with the distinctions of Fungi than he was, yet he would never eat any except such as had been raised in gardens in mushroom beds.

Of the genus *Agaricus*, most of the species which belong to the subgenus *Amanita* are either actually poisonous or highly suspicious. The characters of this subgenus are thus laid down by the Rev. M. J. Berkeley :—

AMANITA (a name given to some esculent Fungus by Galen). *Veil* double : one universal, covering the whole plant in a young state, distinct from the epidermis, at length burst by the protrusion of the pileus, part remaining at the base of the stem, part either falling off, or forming warts on the pileus; the other partial, at first covering the gills, and afterwards forming a reflected subpersistent ring on the top of the stipes. *Stem* puffed, at length hollow, squamoso-fibrillose, thickened at the base. *Pileus* with the disc fleshy, the margin thin, campanulate, then plane ; viscid when saturated with moisture. *Gills* attenuated behind, free, broader in front, ventricose, close, but little unequal; when full-grown, denticulated.

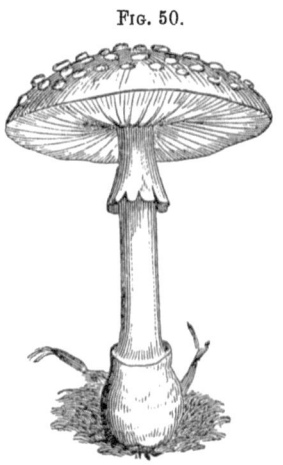

FIG. 50.

Agaricus muscarius.

One of the most remarkable species of this subgenus is the AGARICUS MUSCARIUS, Linn. (*Amanita muscaria*, Greville), the remarkable effects and uses of which have been already noticed (see Vol. i. p. 108).

The Russians, who eat no less than sixteen species of Agaricus,[1] never employ any belonging to the subgenus *Amanita*.[2]

Besides the species of the subgenus Amanita, many other Agarici are poisonous or suspicious.

The symptoms produced by poisonous fungi are those indicating gastro-intestinal irritation (nausea, vomiting, purging, and abdominal pain), and a disordered condition of the nervous system (delirium, stupor, blindness, convulsions, muscular debility, paralysis, and drowsiness). In some cases the power of the vascular system is remarkably depressed, the pulse being small and feeble, the extremities cold, and the body covered with a cold sweat. At one time, local irritation only ; at another, narcotism alone is produced.[3] In some cases the active principle of poisonous fungi seems to be a *volatile acrid principle;* in other instances it is a brown, uncrystallisable solid, called by Letellier *amanitin.*

No specific antidote is known. The first object, therefore, is to expel the poison from the stomach and bowels. The subsequent treatment will depend on the nature of the symptoms• which manifest themselves, and must be conducted on general principles.[4]

---

[1] For some remarks on the Fungi used as food by the Russians, see Lyall's *Character of the Russians, and a detached History of Moscow*, p. 556, Lond. 1823.

[2] Dr. Lefevre, *Lond. Med. Gaz.* xxiii. 414.

[3] For illustrations of the effects of particular species, consult Phœbus, *Deutschl. kryptog. Gift-gewächse*, 1838 ; and Letellier, *Journ. de Pharm.* Août 1837.

[4] For further information respecting poisonous fungi, consult Christison's *Treatise on Poisons.*

Class II. Acrogenæ, Ad. Brogniart.—Acrogens.

Pseudocotyledoneæ, Agardh; Heteronemeæ, Fries; Acrobrya, Mohl, Endlicher.

Characters.—*Substance of the plant* composed of cellular tissue chiefly, and, in the higher forms, of vessels. *Cuticle* bearing stomata or breathing pores. *Stem* and *leaves* distinguishable. Opposition of stem and root. Stem growing at the point only.

This class includes a number of Orders, of which two only (viz. *Lycopodiaceæ* and *Filices*) need be here noticed as yielding anything useful in medicine.

Order IV. FILICES, *Juss.*—FERNS.

(Filicales, *Lindley*.)

Fig. 51.

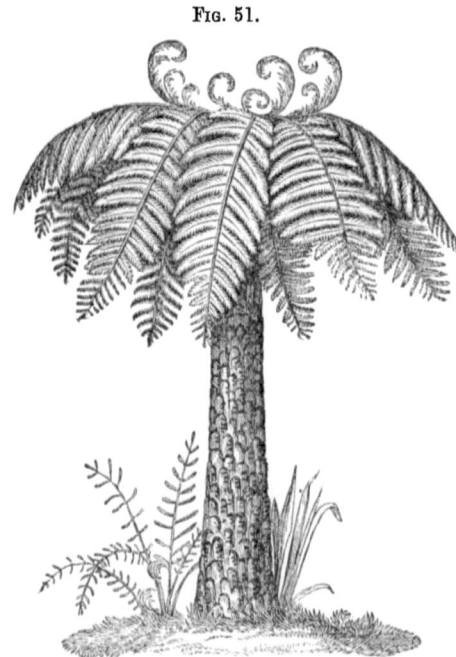

Cyathea glauca (a tree fern).

Character.—Herbaceous plants with a perennial *rhizome*, more rarely having an erect arborescent trunk [when they are called tree ferns, *filices arboreæ*, fig. 51]; *trunk* coated, of a prosenchymatous structure, with the entire cylinder of woody fasciculi divided into two concentric parts,—the one narrow, placed between the bark and the wood; the other larger, central, medullary, sending fasciculi of vessels towards the petioles, and communicating with the exterior by means of chinks in the woody cylinder. *Leaves* [*frondes*] scattered upon the rhizome or rosaceo-fasciculate on the apex of the caudex, with circinate vernation, annual or perennial, the base of the petioles persistent, growing to the caudex; simple or pinnate, entire or pinnatified, [equal-] veined (the veins composed of elongated cells), frequently having cuticular *stomata*. *Sporangia* [*thecæ*] placed on the veins of the back or margin of the leaves, collected in little naked heaps [*sori*], or covered with a membranous scale [*indusium*], or transmuted margin of the leaf, pedicellate [with the stalk (*seta*), passing round them in the form of an elastic ring (*annulus*)], or sessile, unilocular, indefinitely dehiscent. *Spores* [*sporules*] numerous, free, globose, or angular, in germination at first elongated in every direction, throwing out radicles downwards, and the cauliculus upwards (*Endlicher*).

Properties.—The leaves are mucilaginous, and frequently slightly astringent and aromatic. The rhizomes contain *starch, saccharine matter,* and *gum,* usually *tannic* and *gallic acids,* with more or less *bitter matter,* and sometimes both *fixed* and *volatile oils, resin.* They are considered to possess astringent and tonic properties, and in some cases act as vermifuges. From the tuberous rhizomes of fern is obtained, in some of the Polynesian Islands, as well as in some other parts of the world, a farinaceous or ligneous matter, which is employed by the natives as a nutritive substance. The rhizomes are cooked by baking or roasting. In general, however, they are only resorted to in times of scarcity, when other and more palatable food cannot be obtained.[1]

Several ferns have been used in medicine. Those which I shall particularly notice are *Nephrodium Filix mas*, still retained in the British pharmacopœias, and used as a vermifuge, and *Adiantum* or *Maidenhair*, a syrup of which, or a substitute for it, is still found in the shops under the name of *capillaire*.

Ruiz[2] has written a memoir on three fern-roots sent from Peru, in South America, to Spain, under the name of *Calaguala* (more correctly *Ccallahuala*, from *ccallua*, a batten or trowel, and *hualas*, a boy, *i. e.* a boy's batten). The first, or the *Genuine Calaguala*, or *Ccallahuala*, or *Slender Calaguala*, is the rhizome of *Polypodium Calaguala*, Ruiz; the second, called *Thick Calaguala*, *Puntu puntu*, and sometimes *Deer's Tongue* (Lengua de Ciervo), is the rhizome of *Polypodium crassifolium*, Linn.; and the third, termed *Middling Calaguala*, *the Little Cord* (Cordoncillo), or *Huacsaro*, is the rhizome of *Acrostichum Huacsaro*, Ruiz. The first is the species which should be used in medicine : as, however, it is unknown in English commerce, I need not describe it. Professor Guibourt[3] has figured three sorts of the rhizome, but states that, judging from Ruiz's description, he has not seen the true Calaguala. He once found the *Maltese fungus* (*Cynomorium coccineum*) in some Calaguala which he received from Marseilles. Calaguala has been analysed by Vauquelin.[4] This rhizome is regarded in Peru as possessing deobstruent, sudorific, diuretic, anti-venereal, and febrifuge virtues ; and it is frequently used to thin the blood, to promote perspiration, and to mitigate rheumatic and venereal pains. It is commonly administered in the form of decoction, prepared by boiling one ounce of the fresh root in six pints of water to three pints. This decoction is taken *ad libitum* as a kind of diet drink.

29. NEPHRODIUM FILIX MAS, *Richard.*—MALE SHIELD FERN.

Sex. Syst. Cryptogamia, Filices.

(Rhizoma.)

SYNONYMES.—*Polypodium Filix mas,* Linn.; *Aspidium Filix mas,* Swartz.

HISTORY.—Fern-root was employed by the ancients in medicine. Theophrastus[5] notices two kinds of fern ; the male, which he calls πτέρις, and the female, termed θηλυπτερις. Dioscorides[6] also mentions these two ferns, and states that the πτέρις is by some persons called βλήκνον, by others πολύρριζον. Pliny[7] notices both ferns, and says the *pterin* is supposed to be the male fern (*filix mas*).

BOTANY. **Gen. Char.**—*Sori* roundish, scattered. *Indusium* orbiculari-reniform, fixed by the sinus.

Sp. Char.—*Fronds* bipinnate, pinnules oblong, obtuse serrated, their stalk and midrib chaffy. *Sori* near the central nerve (*Hooker*).

The rhizome is large, tufted, and scaly. The leaves grow in a circle to a height of 3 or 4 feet.

---

[1] Ellis, *Polynesian Researches*, vol. i. p. 363 ; Bennet, *Narrative of a Whaling Voyage*, vol. ii. p. 394, 1840.—Dieffenbach (*Travels in New Zealand*, vol. ii. 1843) says that the "*korau* or *mamako*, the pulpous stem of a tree-fern (*Cyathea medullaris*) is an excellent vegetable ;" and, he adds, "it is prepared by being cooked a whole night in a native oven."

[2] *Memoria sobre la legitima Calaguala y otras dos raices que con el mismo nombre nos vienen de la America Meridional*, Madrid, 1805. A translation of Ruiz's Memoir is contained in Lambert's *Illustration of the Genus Cinchona*, p. 98, 1821.

[3] *Hist. Nat. des Drogues simpl.* t. ii. p. 87, 4me éd. 1849.

[4] *Ann. Chimie*, t. lv. p. 22.

[5] *Hist. Plant.* lib. ix. cap. xx. and xxii.

[6] Lib. iv. cap. clxxxvi. and clxxxvii. Sibthorp (*Prodr. Fl. Græcæ*, vol. ii. p. 274) puts a query whether *Aspidium aculeatum*, Willd. be not the πτέρις of Dioscorides ? But in the *Pharmacopæa Græca* of 1837, πτέρις is given as the modern Greek name of *Aspidium Filix mas*.

[7] *Hist. Nat.* lib. xxvii. cap. lv.

Hab.—It is an indigenous plant, frequent in woods and in shady banks. It is a native of other parts of Europe, of Asia, of the North of Africa, and of the United States of America.

FIG. 52.

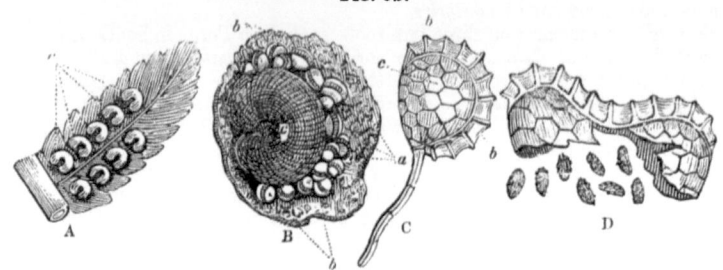

Nephrodium Filix mas.

A. Pinnule with nine sori (*a*).
B. Magnified portion of pinnule with the sporangia. *a.* Stomata. *b b.* Sporangia partially covered by *c.* the indusium.

C. Magnified sporangium. *a.* Stalk. *b.* Ring. *c.* Membranous sac.
D. Ruptured sporangium, with the spores escaping.

FIG. 53.

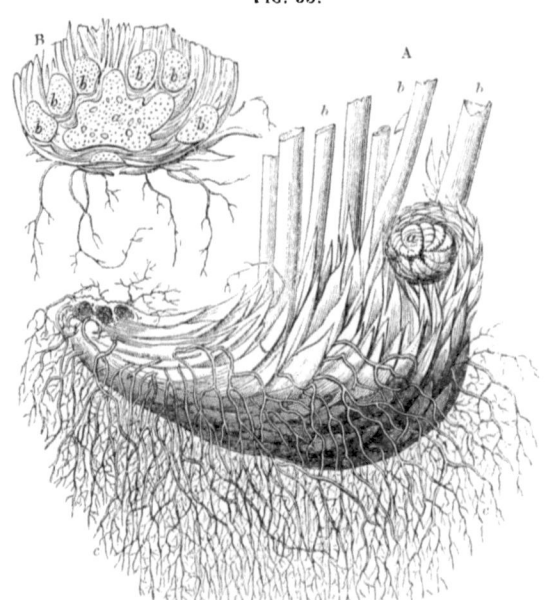

Nephrodium Filix mas.

A. Fresh rhizome entire. *a.* Spirally-coiled young frond. *b b b.* Leaf-stalks (*stipites*) cut off. *c c.* Root-fibres.

B. Transverse section of the fresh rhizome. *a.* Transverse section of the stem, with the vascular bundles. *b b b b b b.* Bases of the leaf stalks, called *phyllopodia.* They surround the stem in a circular manner, and are devoid of vascular bundles.

Description.—The subterraneous stem (*rhizoma ; caudex ; fern root, radix filicis,* officin.) lies obliquely in the ground. It varies in length and breadth, according to its age. For medical purposes it should be from three to six or more inches long, and from half an inch to an inch or more broad. It is almost completely enveloped by the thickened bases of the foot-stalks of the fallen leaves. These bases (*phyllopodia*) are arranged closely around the rhizome in an oblique direction, overlapping each other. They are one or two inches long, from three to five lines thick, curved, angular, brown, surrounded near their origin from the rhizome by two or more shining, reddish-yellow, thin, silky scales (*ramenta*). The radical fibres (root, properly so called) arise from the rhizome between these foot-stalks.

The *fern root of the shops* consists of fragments of the dried thickened bases of the footstalks (*phyllopodia*), to which small portions of the rhizome are found adhering, and of the root fibres. . Internally, the rhizome and foot-stalks are, in the recent state, fleshy, of a light yellowish-green colour ; but in the dried state, yellowish or reddish-white. Iodine colours the fresh rhizome bluish-black, indicating the presence of starch ; particles of which may be recognised by the microscope. In a transverse section of the rhizome we observe five or six, or more, bundles of woody fibres and scalariform ducts. These bundles are arranged in a circle, are of a reddish-white colour in the recent rhizome, but yellow in the dried one. The dried root has a feeble, earthy, somewhat disagreeable odour. Its taste is at first sweetish, then bitter astringent, and subsequently nauseous, like rancid fat.

COLLECTION.—The rhizome should be collected in the month of July, August, or September. The black portions, fibres, and scales, are to be removed, and the sound parts carefully dried and reduced to powder : this is of a yellowish colour, and is to be preserved in well-stoppered bottles. Both the whole rhizome and powder deteriorate by keeping.

Fern buds (*gemmæ filicis maris*), which are sometimes employed in medicine, are to be collected in the spring.

COMPOSITION.—Fern rhizome was analysed in 1805 by Vauquelin,[1] in 1821 by Gebhard,[2] in 1824 by Morin,[3] in 1826 by Wackenroder,[4] and by Geiger.[5] Subjoined are the results of the analyses of Geiger and of Morin :—

Geiger.		Morin.
Green fat oil	6·9	Volatile oil.
—— resin	4·1	Fixed oil (stearin and olein).
Uncrystallisable sugar } Easily oxidisable tannin }	22·9	Tannin. Gallic and acetic acids.
Gum and salts, with sugar and tannin	9·8	Uncrystallisable sugar.
Ligneous fibre and starch	56·3	Starch.
	——	Gelatinous matter, insoluble in water and alcohol.
	100·0	Ligneous fibre.
		Ashes (carbonate, sulphate, and hydrochlorate of potash, carbonate and phosphate of lime, alumina, silica, and oxide of iron).

The anthelmintic property of the rhizome resides in the oil (*oleum filicis maris*). Luck[6] obtained from the granular sediment which forms in oil of fern, tabular *rhombic plates*, whose formula was $C^{59}H^{38}O^{20}$ (probably

[1] *Ann. Chim.* iv. 31.
[2] *Diss. inaug.* in Pfaff's *Syst. d. Mat. Med.* 7er Bd. 219.
[3] *Journ. de Pharm.* x. 223.
[4] *De anthelm. regni vegetab.*
[5] *Handb. d. Pharm.* 1829.
[6] *Ann. der Chem. u. Pharm.* Bd. liv. 1845 ; also *Chem. Gazette*, vol. iii. p. 369.

it should be $C^{60}H^{36}O^{20}$), a *brown substance* soluble in alcohol and alkaline liquids, and whose formula was $C^{105}H^{54}NO^{45}$, and a *grey body*, insoluble in all solvents except caustic alkalies, and whose formula was $C^{24}H^{12}NO^{8}$. Batso[1] found a peculiar acid (*acidum filiceum*) and an alkali (*filicina*) in the rhizome. Fern buds contain, according to Peschier,[2] *a volatile oil, brown resin, fat oil, solid fatty matter, green colouring principle, a reddish-brown principle,* and *extractive.*

CHARACTERISTICS.—The presence of tannic acid in the aqueous decoction of fern rhizome is shown by the sesquisalts of iron producing a dark green colour (*tannate of iron*), and by a solution of gelatin causing a yellowish precipitate (*tannate of gelatin*). No indication of the presence of a vegetable alkali in the decoction can be obtained by tincture of nutgalls. If the rhizome be digested in alcohol, and afterwards boiled in water, the decoction, when cold, forms, with a solution of iodine, a dingy blue precipitate (*iodide of starch*).

PHYSIOLOGICAL EFFECTS.—These are not very obvious; but they are probably similar to those caused by other astringents. Large doses excite nausea and vomiting.

USES.—It is only employed as an anthelmintic. Theophrastus, Dioscorides, Pliny, and Galen, used it as such. The attention of modern practitioners has been directed to it principally from the circumstance of its being one of the remedies employed by Madame Nouffer, the widow of a Swiss surgeon, who sold her secret method of expelling tape-worm to Louis XVI. for 18,000 francs.[3] At the present time fern rhizome is but seldom employed in this country, partly because the efficacy of Madame Nouffer's treatment is referred to the drastics used, and partly because other agents (especially oil of turpentine) have been found more effectual. "It is an excellent remedy," says Bremser,[4] "against *Bothriocephalus latus* [the tape-worm of the Swiss], but not against *Tænia Solium* [the tape-worm of this country]; for though it evacuates same pieces of the latter, it does not destroy it."

ADMINISTRATION.—It may be administered in the form of powder, of oil or ethereal extract, or of aqueous decoction. The dose of the recently prepared powder is from one to three drachms. Madame Nouffer's *specific* was two or three drachms of the powder taken in from four to six ounces of water in the morning fasting, and two hours afterwards a *purgative bolus*, composed of calomel ten grains, scammony ten grains, and gamboge six or seven grains. The bolus was exhibited to expel the worm which the fern rhizome was supposed to have destroyed.

[Professor Albers has employed an extract of male fern, which he states is very efficacious, in Tænia. He keeps the patient on spare diet for three days, and then gives a dose of Glauber salts; next morning 30 grs. of extract are given, and the dose repeated in an hour's time. A dose of castor oil is then given after two hours more have elapsed. The fresh root should be used for this extract.[5]—Ed.]

The *Ethereal Tincture of Male Fern Buds* (prepared by digesting 1 part

[1] *Inaug. Diss.* 1826, quoted in Goebel and Kunze's *Pharm. Waarenk.*
[2] Quoted by Soubeiran, *Nouv. Traité de Pharm.* t. ii. p. 159, 2nde éd.
[3] *Trait. contre le Tænia,* &c. 1776, quoted by Bremser, *Sur les Vers Intest.*
[4] *Op. cit.* p. 422.
[5] [See Casper's *Wochenschrift,* 1850, No. 31.]

of the buds in 8 parts of ether) has been used with success by Dr. Peschier (brother of the chemist of that name) and by Dr. Fosbroke[1] as a vermifuge.

OLEUM FILICIS MARIS; *Oil of Male Fern.*—The impure oil of fern (called *oleum filicis Peschieri, extractum filicis æthereum,* seu *balsamum filicis*), recommended by Peschier,[2] is an ethereal extract, and is composed, according to its proposer, of a *fatty matter, resin, volatile oil, colouring matter, extractive, chloride of potassium,* and *acetic acid.* A pound of the rhizome yielded Soubeiran[3] an ounce and a half of thick black oil, having the odour of fern. It may also be prepared from the buds as above stated. The dose is from half a drachm to a drachm, in the form of electuary, emulsion, or pills : an hour afterwards, an ounce or an ounce and a half of castor oil should be exhibited. Numerous testimonies of its efficacy have been published.[4] I have tried it in several cases of tape-worm, but without success. By substituting alcohol for ether, twelve or thirteen drachms of oil can be obtained from $2\frac{2}{3}$ lbs. of the rhizome.[5] [Notwithstanding the doubt cast on this remedy by the late learned author, we must confess to much faith in the value of this oil as a destroyer and expeller of tape-worm. It has been used at Guy's Hospital with marked advantage.—ED.]

30. Adiantum, *Linn.*—Maidenhair.

HISTORY.—The term *Maidenhair* or *Capillary* (*Capillaris,* Apuleius ; *Capillaire,* Fr.) has been applied to several species of fern which have been used in medicine. Dioscorides (lib. iv. cap. 136 and 137) and Pliny (lib. xxii. cap. 30) notice two kinds, one termed *Adianton, Polytrichon,* or *Callitrichon* (ἀδίαντον, πολύτριχον, καλλίτριχον) ; the other called *Trichomanes* (τριχομανές). The former is supposed by Sibthorp[6] to be the *Adiantum Capillus Veneris,* Linn., or *True Maidenhair,* the latter the *Asplenium Trichomanes,* Linn., *Common Maidenhair Spleenwort* of modern botanists. In later times other ferns have been also employed under the name of Maidenhair ; especially *Asplenium Adiantum nigrum,* Linn., or *Black Maidenhair Spleenwort ; Asplenium Ruta muraria,* Linn., *Wall-rue* or *White Maidenhair,* formerly called *Salvia Vita ; Ceterach officinarum,* DC., or *Rough Spleenwort ;* and *Scolopendrium vulgare,* Smith, or *Common Hart's-tongue.* To these must be added *Adiantum pedatum,* Linn., or *Canadian Maidenhair,* and *Adiantum trapeziforme,* Linn., or *Mexican Maidenhair.*

The only species which it will be necessary here to notice are *Adiantum Capillus Veneris* and *A. pedatum.*

BOTANY. **Gen. Char.**—*Sporangia* placed on the distinct points of the veins in a linear or point-like receptacle, arranged in marginal *sori. Indusia* continuous with the edge of the frond, united to the receptacle, opening inward (*Endlicher*).

1. *A. Capillus Veneris,* Linn., Frond bipinnate, pinnules thin, membranaceous, obovate-cuneate inciso-sublobate, segments of the fertile pinnules terminated by a linear oblong sorus, sterile ones serrated (*Hooker*).—Indigenous. Perennial. May—September.

2. *A. pedatum,* Linn.—Frond pedate, divisions pinnate, pinnæ halved oblong lunate, incised at the upper edge, the sterile segments toothed ; sori linear ; petiole smooth.—North America.

DESCRIPTION.—The officinal part of Maidenhair is the frond, or rather the whole plant without the root.

[1] *Lancet,* for 1834–35, vol. ii. p. 597.
[2] *Journ. génér. de Méd.* 1825, p. 375.
[3] *Nouv. Traité de Pharm.* ii. 161, 2nde éd.
[4] Dierbach, *Neuesten Entd. in d. Mat. Med.* Band i. 1837.
[5] *Journ. de Chim. Méd.* t. v. 2nde sér. p. 68.
[6] *Prodr. Fl. Græcæ,* vol. ii.

The herb of *True Maidenhair* (*herba capillorum veneris*) is sold at herb-shops in the dried state. When rubbed, it has a feeble odour, and its taste is sweetish and bitterish.

The herb of *Canadian Maidenhair* (*herba capillorum veneris canadensis* vel *adianthi pedati*) is more aromatic than the preceding.

COMPOSITION.—No analysis has been made of these species of Adiantum. The most important constituents appear to be *tannic* or *gallic acid, bitter extractive*, and a *volatile oil*.

EFFECTS AND USES.—None of the sorts of Maidenhairs appear to be endowed with any active powers; though a great variety of imaginary properties have been ascribed to them. They are mucilaginous, bitterish, somewhat astringent, and aromatic substances; and in modern times have been used as pectorals in chronic catarrhs. The Canadian Maiden-hair (*Adianthum pedatum*, Linn.) is the most esteemed sort, on account of its stronger and more agreeably aromatic qualities.

A Syrup of Maidenhair (*Syrupus Adianthi ; Syrupus Capilli Veneris ; Sirop de Capil-laire*), prepared by adding sugar and orange-flower-water to an infusion of Maidenhair, has long been popular. Both Baumé and the French Codex direct it to be prepared with the Canadian Maidenhair. When diluted with water it forms a very refreshing beverage. But as the Maidenhair serves no essential purpose in this drink, it is usually omitted, and the syrup sold in the shops under the name of *capillaire* is nothing but clarified syrup flavoured with orange-flower-water. The Prussian and Hamburgh Pharmacopœias authorise this substitution by giving formulæ for a *syrupus florum aurantii* to be used " in loco syrupi capillorum veneris."

ORDER V. LYCOPODIACEÆ, *DC.*—CLUB-MOSSES.

CHARACTERS.—Herbaceous or shrubby vascular terrestrial *plants*. *Stem* terete, branched, leafy. *Leaves* inserted spirally on the stem, imbricated, simple, sessile or decurrent, never articulated. *Spore-cases* (*sporocarpia ; thecæ ; sporangia*) axillary, mostly uniform, sometimes on the same individuals biform ; some bivalved, containing a farina-ceous powder, composed of polygonal smooth or papillose-spinulous granules (*sporules ; pollen?*); others 3- 4-coccous, 3- 4-valved, containing a few (usually 3 or 4) somewhat globular corpuscles (*spores? gemmæ* or *buds?*) marked at the vertex with a 3-legged raphe.

PROPERTIES.—These are but little known.

An acrid principle resides in several species. Both *Lycopodium clavatum* and *L. Selago* act as emetics. The latter species, called *muscus catharticus* seu *erectus*, and supposed to be the *Selago*[1] of the Druids, has also been employed as a cathartic emmenagogue, and to produce abortion. In large doses it operates as a narcotico-acrid poison. A decoction of it is sometimes employed by the peasants of Sweden, and other places, as a lotion to destroy pediculi on the skin of horses, cows, pigs, &c.[2] Dr. Buchner[3] has recorded some cases of accidental poisoning by it, in which it caused staggering and sickness. *Lycopo-dium catharticum*, Hooker (*L. rubrum*, Chamisso), is also a violent purgative. Some species, e. g. *Lycopodium Phlegmaria*, Linn., and *Selaginella convoluta*, Spring (*L. hygro-metricum*, Mart.), are reputed aphrodisiacs.

31. Lycopodium clavatum, *Linn.*—Common Club-moss.
(Herba ; Sporulæ.)

HISTORY.—The earliest writers by whom the medicinal qualities of this plant are distinctly referred to, are the herbalists (Brunsfels, Tragus, Cordus, &c.) of the 16th century.

---

[1] Pliny, *Hist. Nat.* lib. xxiv. cap. 65.
[2] Murray, *App. Medicam.* vol. v. p. 493.
[3] *Repert. für d. Pharmacie*, Bd. xiv. S. 311, 1823.

BOTANY. **Gen. Char.**—*Spore-cases* unilocular, uniform or biform; the *fariniferous* ones subreniform, and bivalved ; the *globuliferous* ones somewhat globose, 3-4-lobed, 3-4-valved (*Endlicher, Gen. Pl.*)

Sp. Char.—*Stem* creeping; branches ascending; *leaves* linear-lanceolate, nerveless, terminating at the point in a bristle; *spikes* in pairs, stalked, cylindrical ; *bracts* ovate, acuminate, premorse, toothed (*Endl. Med. Pflanzen*).

FIG. 54.

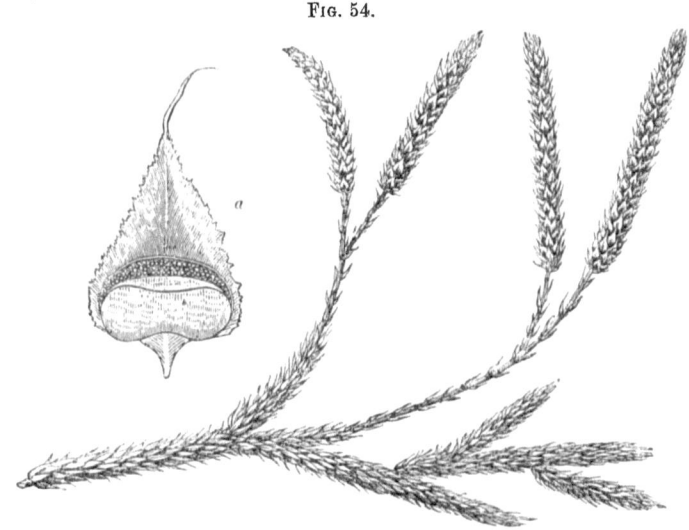

Lycopodium clavatum.

a. Scale of a spike with a capsule (magnified).

Roots of several strong scattered fibres. *Stems* procumbent, trailing, branching, leafy, several feet in length. *Leaves* crowded, curved upwards, linear-lanceolate, flat, ribless, smooth, deep green, partly serrated, tipped with a capillary point ; those of the branches erect; the upper ones loosely dispersed. *Spikes* terminal, usually in pairs, rarely one, or three, densely beset with shortened, dilated, ovate, entire, long-pointed *leaves* or *scales*, in whose bosoms the small, sulphur-coloured *capsules* [*thecæ*] are situated (*Smith*).

Hab.—Mountainous heaths and moors all over Europe. Indigenous. Perennial. July, August.

DESCRIPTION. 1.*SporulæLycopodii.*—The powder sold in the shops under the name of *lycopodium* (*pulvis, farina, pollen,* seu *semina lycopodii*), *witchmeal,* or *vegetable sulphur* (*sulphur vegetabile*), consists of granules, usually regarded as sporules, but by some considered to be grains of pollen. In both their physical and chemical properties they resemble the latter. They are gathered towards the end of the summer, and are separated from the capsules, &c. by sifting.

FIG. 55.

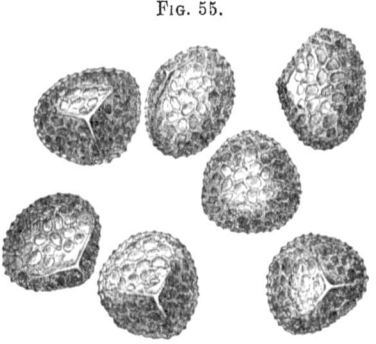

Sporules of Lycopodium clavatum
(highly magnified).

Lycopodium is a very fine, odourless, tasteless, and very mobile powder, of a pale yellow colour. It adheres to the fingers, but exhibits a repulsive force for water, and hence is with difficulty mixed with it. If strewed on this liquid it floats, and the hand may be dipped to the bottom without being moistened. If shaken up with water, a portion of it sinks, but the greater part floats. With spirit of wine it is readily miscible. It is tinged brown by iodine. When thrown into the flame of a candle it burns with great rapidity, producing an instantaneous flash of yellowish-white light. When moistened by spirit of wine, or, still better, by oil of vitriol, and examined by the microscope, the granules are found to have the shape of tetra-hedrons, with a convex base; or they may be described as spheroids, on a portion of whose surface there are three faces, or planes, uniting to form a three-sided pyramid. The faces appear to have been produced by the mutual pressure of the granules on each other while in the spore-cases. The external membrane forms reticulated elevations, with intervening depressions or pits, giving a cellular appearance to the surface of the granules. The three-legged mark, at the union of the three planes, appears to be formed by a cleft in the membrane.

2. *Herba Lycopodii* (*Herba musci clavati terrestris*).—This is odourless; at first sweetish, and then bitterish. Digested in water it yields a yellowish infusion, whose colour is deepened by sesquichloride of iron.

COMPOSITION.—Lycopodium sporules have been analysed by Bucholz[1] and by Cadet.[2] The former chemist obtained the following results:—*Fat oil,* 6·0; *sugar,* 3·0; *mucilaginous extract,* 1·5; and *pollenin,* 89·5. The substance called pollenin is, however, a complex organised body, and cannot be regarded as a proximate principle. By the action of caustic potash on lycopodium, Muspratt[3] has shown that acetic acid is obtained. The herb has not been analysed. It appears to contain some acrid principle.

ADULTERATION.—As met with in the London shops, I have never found lycopodium (the sporules) adulterated. The sporules of other species of *Lycopodium* are said to be sometimes substituted for those of *L. clavatum:* the microscope alone can detect the difference. The pollen of some plants, as of *Typha latifolia,* and of some coniferous plants, is said to be sometimes substituted for the lycopodium sporules. The microscope readily distinguishes the substitution. The shape, the size, the character of the surface, and the cohesion or isolation of the grains, must be attended to in distinguishing them. The pollen of coniferous plants is also sometimes recognisable by its terebin-thinate odour when rubbed in the hand: that of Typha latifolia is not so inflammable as genuine lycopodium meal.

Starch, talc, gypsum, chalk, and *boxwood powder,* have been reported as adulterating substances. By throwing the suspected lycopodium on water, the mineral substances present would readily fall to the bottom, and might be detected by their appropriate chemical tests. Iodine and the microscope will detect starch. Boxwood powder has been separated from lycopodium by a fine sieve, which let the genuine sporules through, but retained the wooden particles.

---

[1] *Berlin. Jahrb. für d. Pharm.* 1807, S. liv.; also L. Gmelin's *Handb. d. Chem.*
[2] *Bull. de Pharm.* t. iii. p. 31, 1811.
[3] *Pharmaceutisches Central-Blatt für* 1844, S. 904.

Once I have seen lycopodium infected by a fungus, the matted mycelium of which had a slate colour and a membranous or papery appearance.

EFFECTS.   1. *Of the sporules.*—Applied externally, lycopodium acts as an absorbent and desiccant.   Taken internally, it is reputed to possess demulcent, sedative, and diuretic properties : but these qualities are of doubtful existence.   2. *Of the herb.*—The herb appears to be endowed with some active properties.   It acts as an emetic and cathartic, and is reputed to possess diuretic and emmenagogue qualities.

USES.   1. *Of the sporules.*—Lycopodium is used both medicinally and pharmaceutically, as well as in the arts.   It is applied as a dusting powder to excoriated surfaces, especially the intertrigo of infants, and to parts affected with erysipelas, herpetic ulceration, eczema, &c.   It is sometimes used in the form of ointment.   In Poland it is popularly employed, as an external application, in plica polonica.   As an internal remedy its powers are very doubtful.   It has, however, been used by Wedelius and others,[1] and in later times by Hufeland, Jawandt, Rademacher, and Busser,[2] in the retention of urine and flatulent colic of infants, and in calculous complaints, hemorrhoids, and gout of adults.   In pharmacy it is used for enveloping pills and boluses.   It serves both to isolate the pills, and cover their taste.

But its principal use is at theatres, where it is employed for filling flash-boxes, and for producing artificial lightning.   It is also used in pyrotechny. Gray says that females employed in delicate works use it to keep their hands free from sweat.

2. *Of the herb.*—This is rarely employed.   It has been celebrated in the treatment of plica polonica, and in consequence has been called *plicaria*.   It was employed in the form of decoction both externally as lotion and liniment, and internally.[3]   More recently it has been recommended by Dr. Rodewald[4] in retention of urine from gravel or pus [!], in atony of the muscular coat of the bladder, in weakness and relaxation of the inner membrane of the bladder, and as a diuretic.   He states that he has used it for many years with great success.

ADMINISTRATION.—The *sporules* are administered internally in doses of from ten grains to a scruple, in the form of a mixture, or emulsion, made with syrup, mucilage, or yolk of egg.   Externally they are sometimes used in the form of ointment, composed of one drachm of lycopodium to an ounce of lard.   The *herb* is administered in the form of decoction or infusion. Two up-heaped tablespoonfuls, with a pint of water, are to be boiled to one-half; and of this decoction a teacupful may be taken every ten minutes, or at longer intervals.   In a more dilute state it may be drunk as tea.

---

[1] Murray, *App. Med.* vol. v.
[2] Hufeland's *Journal*, Bd. ii. iv. and xxxvi.
[3] Vicat, *Mémoire sur la Plique Polonoise* (Murray, *App. Med.*)
[4] No. 16, *Altenberger medicinische Zeitung*, 1833.   (Quoted by Dierbach, *Die neuesten Entd. in d. Mat. Med.* Bd. i. S. 56, 1837.)

II. Phanerogamia *Auct.*—Phanerogams or Flowering Plants.

Cotyledoneæ, *Juss.*—Embryonatæ, *Rich.*—Vasculares, *De Cand.*

Characters.—Substance of the plant composed of cellular tissue, woody fibre, ducts, and spiral vessels. *Leaves* usually present; *cuticle* with stomata. *Flowers* with perceptible stamens and pistils. *Seeds* with an embryo enclosed within a spermoderm, furnished with one or more cotyledons.

Class III.   Endogenæ, *DC.*—Endogens.

Monocotyledones, *Juss.*

Characters.—*Trunk* usually cylindrical, when a terminal bud only is developed, becoming conical and branched when several develope: consisting of cellular tissue, among which the vascular tissue is mixed in bundles, usually without any distinction of bark, wood, and pith, and destitute of medullary rays; increasing in diameter by the addition of new matter to the centre. *Leaves* frequently sheathing at the base, and not readily separating from the stem by an articulation, mostly alternate, generally parallel-veined, rarely netted. *Flowers* usually having a ternary division; the calyx and corolla either distinct or undistinguishable in colour and size, or absent. *Embryo* with but one cotyledon; if with two, then the accessory one is imperfect, and alternate with the other; *radicle* usually enclosed within the substance of this embryo, through which it bursts when germinating (*Lindley*, chiefly).

This class includes two sub-classes:—1. *Glumaceæ*, or glumaceous endogens. 2. *Petaloidæ*, or endogens whose floral envelopes, if present, are whorled.

Sub-class I. *Glumaceæ*, Endl.

Characters.—*Flowers* disposed in spikelets, and enclosed within imbricated bracts. *Ovary* free, unilocular, containing one erect *ovule*. *Fruit* a caryopsis. *Embryo* at the base of farinaceous albumen.

This class includes two orders:—1. *Gramineæ*, or glumaceous endogens with round stems, leaves having split sheaths, and embryo lying on the outside of the albumen. 2. *Cyperaceæ*, or glumaceous endogens with angular stems, leaves with entire sheaths, and embryo included within the albumen.

Order VI. GRAMINEÆ, *R. Brown.*—GRASSES.

Gramina, *Juss.*—Gramineæ, *Lind.*

Characters.—*Flowers* usually hermaphrodite, sometimes monœcious or polygamous; consisting of imbricated bracts, of which the most exterior are called *glumes*, the interior immediately enclosing the stamens *paleæ*, and the innermost at the base of the ovary *scales*. *Glumes* usually 2, alternate; sometimes single; most commonly unequal. *Paleæ* 2, alternate; the lower or exterior, simple; the upper or interior composed of 2, united by their contiguous margins, and usually with 2 keels, together forming a kind of dislocated calyx. *Scales* 2 or 3, sometimes wanting; if 2, collateral, alternate with the paleæ, and next the lower of them, either distinct or united. *Stamens* hypogynous, 1, 2, 3, 4, 6, or more, 1 of which alternates with the 2 hypogynous scales, and is, therefore, next the lower paleæ; *anthers* versatile. *Ovary* simple; *styles* 2 or 3, very rarely combined into 1; *stigmas* feathery and hairy; *ovule* ascending by a broad base, anatropal. *Pericarp* usually undistinguishable from the seed, membranous. *Albumen* farinaceous; *embryo* lying on one side of the albumen at the base, lenticular, with a broad cotyledon and a developed plumule; and occasionally, but very rarely, with a second cotyledon on the outside of the plumule, and alternate with the usual cotyledon.—Evergreen *herbs*. *Rhizoma* fibrous or bulbous. *Stems* cylindrical, usually fistular, closed at the joints, covered with a coat of silex, sometimes solid. *Leaves* narrow and undivided, alternate, with a split sheath, and a membranous expansion (*ligula*) at the junction of stalk and blade. *Flowers* in little spikes, called *locustæ*, arranged in a spiked, racemed, or panicled manner (*Lindley*).

PROPERTIES.—Considered with reference to their ultimate or mineral constituents, the grasses are remarkable for the large proportion of *silica, potash*, and *phosphoric acid*, and for the small proportion of *chlorine* which they contain. The silica predominates in the leaves and stem, the phosphoric acid in the seeds. The following table[1] represents the mean composition of the ashes of the most important cereal grains.

MEAN PER-CENTAGE COMPOSITION OF THE ASH OF THE FOLLOWING CEREAL GRAINS.

	Wheat.	Barley (with the husk).	Oat.	Rye.	Indian Corn.	Rice.
Potash	23·72	13·64 ⎱	26·18	⎱ 22·08	⎱ 32·48	⎱ 18·48
Soda	9·05	8·14 ⎰		⎰ 11·67	⎰	⎰ 10·67
Lime	2·81	2·62	5·95	4·93	1·44	1·27
Magnesia	12·03	7·46	9·95	10·35	16·22	11·69
Oxide of iron	0·67	1·48	0·40	1·36	0·30	0·45
Phosphoric acid	49·81	38·93	43·84	49·55	44·87	53·36
Sulphuric acid.............	0·24	0·10	10·45	0·98	2·77	......
Chlorine.....................	......	0·04	0·26	......	0·18	0·27
Silica	1·17	27·10	2·67	0·43	1·44	3·35
Alumina.....................	......	0·21	0·06	......	......	......
	99·50	99·72	99·76	101·35	99·70	99·54
Per-centage of Ash	about 2·0	2·84	2·18	2·425	about 1·5	1·00

The following table, drawn up by M. Payen,[2] shows the proportions of the proximate or immediate principles of the cereal grains:—

100 *parts of*	Starch.	Gluten, and other Azotised Matters.[3]	Dextrine, Glucose, or Congenerous Substances.	Fatty Matters	Cellulose.	Silica, Phosphates of Lime, Magnesia, and Soluble Salts of Potash and of Soda.
Wheat, hard, of Venezuela.........	58·12	22·75	9·50	2·61	4	3·02
" " of Africa	64·57	19·50	7·60	2·12	3·50	2·71
" " of Taganrog	63·30	20·00	8	2·25	3·60	2·85
" demi-hard, of Brie (France)	68·65	16·25	7	1·95	3·40	2·75
" white tuzelle	75·31	11·20	6·05	1·87	3	2·12
Rye	65·65	13·50	12	2·15	4·10	2·60
Barley	65·43	13·96	10	2·76	4·75	3·10
Oats	60·59	14·39	9·25	5·50	7·06	3·25
Maize...............................	67·55	12·50	4	8·80	5·90	1·25
Rice	89·15	7·05	1	0·80	3	0·90

[1] Drawn up from the calculated means contained in Johnston's *Lectures on Agricultural Chemistry and Geology*, 2d edit. 1847.

[2] *Précis de Chimie Industrielle*, p. 394, Paris, 1849.

[3] The proportions of azotised substances have been deduced from the elementary analysis by multiplying by 6·5 the weight of azote obtained.

Of the proximate or organic constituents of grasses, *starch* and *sugar* are found in large proportion,—the former in the seed, the latter in the stem. These constituents, with *proteinaceous matter* (gluten, albumen), to which may be added *gum*, confer on corn its valuable nutritive properties. (For the per centage proportion of starch and proteinaceous matter in corn, see Vol. i. p. 67.)

Fragrant volatile oils are obtained from herbaceous parts of some grasses. Several of these are employed in perfumery and in medicine (see the genus *Andropogon*).

The grasses are remarkable for their deficiency of pectin, as well as of pectic, tartaric, citric, and other vegetable acids commonly found in plants.

Considered with regard to their dietetical uses, the grasses are most important and valuable to man. They contain nitrogenised principles fitted for the production of the essential constituents of the blood and of the organised tissues, and also non-nitrogenised principles for the production of fatty matters, lactic acid, and, by combustion, of heat. The following table gives a general view of the uses which several constituents of grains of corn serve in the animal economy :—

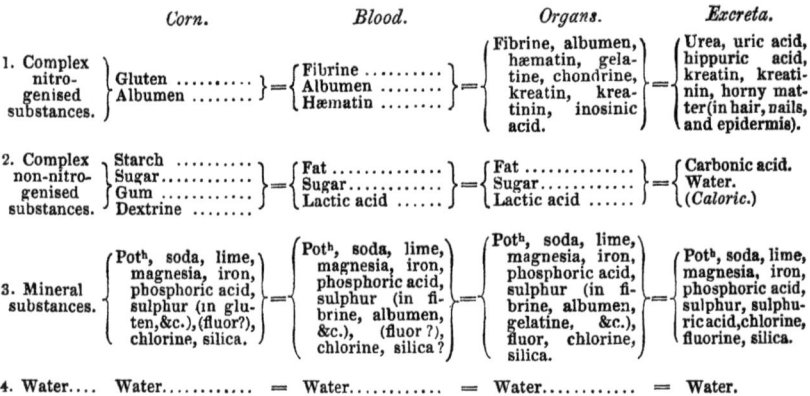

	Corn.	*Blood.*	*Organs.*	*Excreta.*
1. Complex nitrogenised substances.	Gluten .... Albumen	= Fibrine .... Albumen .... Hæmatin	= Fibrine, albumen, hæmatin, gelatine, chondrine, kreatin, kreatinin, inosinic acid.	= Urea, uric acid, hippuric acid, kreatin, kreatinin, horny matter (in hair, nails, and epidermis).
2. Complex non-nitrogenised substances.	Starch .... Sugar .... Gum .... Dextrine	= Fat .... Sugar........... Lactic acid	= Fat .... Sugar........... Lactic acid	= Carbonic acid. Water. (*Caloric.*)
3. Mineral substances.	Pot^h, soda, lime, magnesia, iron, phosphoric acid, sulphur (in gluten, &c.), (fluor?), chlorine, silica.	= Pot^h, soda, lime, magnesia, iron, phosphoric acid, sulphur (in fibrine, albumen, &c.), (fluor?), chlorine, silica?	= Pot^h, soda, lime, magnesia, iron, phosphoric acid, sulphur (in fibrine, albumen, gelatine, &c.), fluor, chlorine, silica.	= Pot^h, soda, lime, magnesia, iron, phosphoric acid, sulphur, sulphuric acid, chlorine, fluorine, silica.
4. Water....	Water............	= Water............	= Water............	= Water.

Almost every species of grass is wholesome. Some supposed exceptions to this statement have been already noticed (see Vol. i. pp. 85 and 86). Of these the best established is *Lolium temulentum*, which will be presently noticed. In a state of disease corn sometimes acquires most important and valuable medicinal properties. (See *Ergot.*)

Tribe I. Oryzeæ, *Endl.*

32. Oryza sativa, *Linn.*—Common Rice.

Sex. Syst. Hexandria, Digynia.

(Semina.)

Synonymes.—Όρυζον, Theophr. Hist. Plant. lib. iv. cap. 5 ; ὄρυζα, Dioscor. lib. ii. cap. 117 ; Galen, De simpl. med. facult. lib. viii. cap. xv. 16 ; *Oryza*, Pliny, Hist. Nat. lib. xviii. cap. 13.

Botany.—*Stems* numerous, 2 to 8 or 10 feet long. *Leaves* long and slender. *Panicle* diffuse thin, bowing when the seed is weighty. *Spikelet* hermaphrodite, 1-flowered ; *glumes* 2, small; *paleæ* 2 ; *scales* 2, smooth ; *stamens* 6 ; *ovary* sessile ; *styles* 2 ; *stigma* feathery. *Caryopsis* compressed, enclosed by the paleæ.—Originally a native of Asia. Extensively cultivated in India, China, the Indian Archipelago, and most other Eastern countries ; in the West Indies, Central America, and the United States ; and in some of the Southern countries of Europe. Forty or fifty varieties[1] are known to and cultivated

---

[1] Roxburgh, *Flora Indica*, vol. ii. p. 200, 1822.

by the Indian farmers: of these, some are awned, others are awnless. The kinds most esteemed in this country are the *Carolina* and *Patna rice*. Patna rice is imported in bags holding 1¼ cwt. each. It has usually been mixed with lime to prevent the attacks of insects. The grain whilst enclosed in the paleæ or husk is called *paddy* (*padi* or *paddie*) by the Malays, *bras* when deprived of the husk, and *nasi* after it has been boiled.

COMPOSITION.—Rice has been analysed by Vauquelin,[1] by Braconnot,[2] by Vogel,[3] and by D'Arcet and Payen[4] (see *ante*, p. 71). The composition of Carolina and Piedmont rice is, according to Braconnot, as follows:—

FIG. 56.

COMPOSITION OF RICE.

	Carolina Rice.	Piedmont Rice.
Starch	85·07	83·80
Parenchyma (woody fibre)	4·80	4·80
Glutinous matter	3·60	3·60
Rancid, colourless, tallowy oil	0·13	0·25
Uncrystallisable sugar	0·29	0·05
Gum	0·71	0·10
Phosphate of lime	0·40	0·40
Water	5·00	7·00
Acetic acid, phosphate of potash, chloride of potassium, and vegetable salts of potash and lime	traces	traces
	100·00	100·00

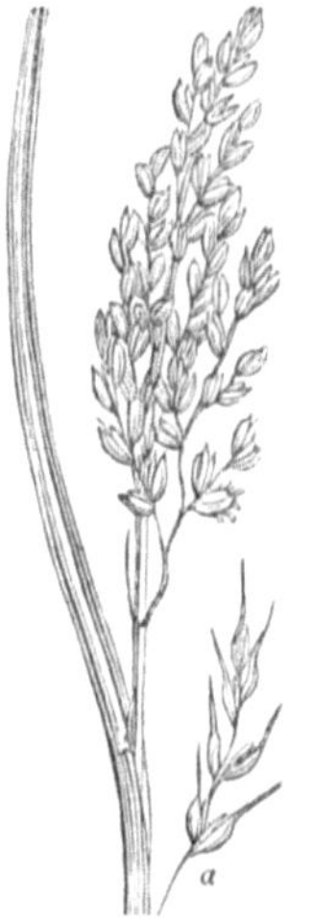

Oryza sativa.
a, Branch with awns.

The inorganic constituents of rice have been before stated (see *ante*, p. 71).

1. *Rice starch* is manufactured, under Mr. Orlando Jones's patent, as follows:—Patna rice is first freed from stones, dust, &c., by a process analogous to winnowing, and is then digested whole in a solution of caustic soda containing 200 grains of soda to the gallon. The solution being poured off, the grain, which has thus been deprived of part of its gluten, is ground in a mill, and the ground rice mixed with a solution of the same strength, so as to form a mixture having the consistence of thick cream. More lye is then added, and the mixture stirred up for a few hours, and then left to deposit: a heavy matter, called *fibre* (heavy starch), deposits, while the starch (lighter starch) remains suspended. The liquor is then run off into shallow vessels, where the starch deposits: the alkaline solution of gluten is then drawn off, and the starch repeatedly washed with water, and then allowed to deposit. The starch mass is now obtained of the consistence of clay. It is then usually mixed with blue colouring matter (smalt), to fit it for the use of the laundress, and removed to draining boxes, which are lined with cloth. These consist each of two cells, whose size is 3 feet long, 6 inches deep, and 6 inches broad. Here the starch forms a lump or mass of the shape and size of the cell, and is afterwards cut into 6 cubical blocks, which are placed on chalk stones to drain, and are then partially dried in a stove to produce what is called *crusting*. The crust is scraped off, the block wrapped in paper and returned to the stove to dry, when it splits into the columnar masses commonly known as the *race* of the starch. If, instead of crusting the lumps, the starch were slowly dried, decomposition is apt to take place; and, if rapidly dried, the races are apt to be small and needle-like. 100 lbs. of Patna rice, as it occurs in the market, yield from 80 to 85 lbs. of *good marketable starch*, 7·5 lbs. of *fibre*, the remainder being *gluten*, *gruff* or *bran*, and a small quantity of light starch, carried off in suspension in the alkaline liquor. Vogel states that from dried rice he obtained 96 per cent. of starch.

When examined by the microscope, the granules are observed to be polygonal, and

[1] *Mém. du Muséum d'Hist. Nat.* t. iii. p. 229, 1817.
[2] *Ann. Chim. Phys.* t. iv. p. 383, 1818.
[3] Quoted by L. Gmelin, *Handb. d. Chemie*, Bd. ii. S. 1345.
[4] *Journ. de Chimie Méd.* t. ix. p. 221, 1833.

very minute; their average diameter being about $\frac{1}{5263}$rd part of an inch.[1] They are the smallest granules of all the commercial starches. According to Vauquelin, rice starch begins to dissolve in water at from 122° to 132° F.

Two kinds of rice starch are found in the shops; one prepared under Orlando Jones's patent,—the other called *Mechlin glaze starch*, manufactured by Mottram, Rehè, and Co.

2. *Proteine matters.*—Rice contains a much smaller proportion of the so-called *gluten* than wheat does. According to Horsford[2] and Payen (see Vol. i. p. 67; and *ante*, p. 71), the quantity is about 7 per cent. The substance which the rice starch-makers term gluten is analogous to what Mulder calls proteine, being obtained by carefully neutralizing the alkaline solution in which rice has been digested, with an acid, by which a precipitate forms, which, when separated from the supernatant liquor, has a creamy consistence, an agreeable smell, and a bland taste, like pap. By evaporation it forms a dark-coloured hard mass. If kept for some time in the moist state, it undergoes decomposition, and evolves an odour somewhat like sour yeast. Mixed with eggs, I have employed it, in the form of a baked pudding, in diabetes.

3. *Fatty matters.*—The quantity of fatty matter contained in rice is smaller than in other varieties of corn. The outer part of the grain appears to contain more than the inner part.

EFFECTS.—Rice, though nutritious, is less so than wheat: this is proved by chemical analysis, which shows the much smaller proportion of glutinous or nitrogenous matter found in the former than in the latter grain (see Vol. i. p. 67; and *ante*, p. 71). "Rice," says Boussingault,[3] "is held up as a most nutritive food; but though I have lived long in countries which produce it, I am far from considering it as a substantial nourishment. I have always seen it, in ordinary use, replace bread; and when it has not been associated with meat, it has been employed with milk." The solid or dry part of rice does not materially differ from the solid or dry part of potatoes in the proportion of starch and gluten which it contains; and, therefore, as far as regards these two principles, the nutritive values of anhydrous rice and anhydrous potatoes are about equal. But, in some Union poor-houses, the substitution of an equal weight of boiled rice for potatoes was followed in a few months by scurvy.[4] Rice, when swallowed in the raw state, swells up in the alimentary canal, and acts injuriously by the mechanical distension it gives rise to. Mr. Hovell[5] has reported a case in which great pain, peritoneal inflammation, and death, arose from the ingestion of a tumblerful of raw rice.

"Rice," says Marsden,[6] "is the grand material of food, on which a hundred millions of the inhabitants of the earth subsist; and although chiefly confined by nature to the

---

[1] The following are measurements of the particles of rice starch made by my friend, Mr. Jackson :—

		Inches.
1.	....	·00027
2.	....	·00021
3.	....	·0002
4.	....	·00017
5.	....	·0001

$$5) \; ·00095$$

$$·00019 = \tfrac{1}{5268}$$

Most of the particles are angular; but the measurements were taken on those which most nearly approached the globular form.

[2] *Ann. Chem. u. Pharm.* Bd. xlviii. 1846.

[3] *Ann. Chim. et Phys.* lxvii. p. 413.

[4] *Provincial Medical and Surgical Journal*, June 1847. Dr. Garrod (*Monthly Journal of Medical Science*, January 1848) calculates that, prior to the substitution, the usual weekly food of the men in the Crediton Union contained 186 grains, and of the women 181 grains of potash; but, after the substitution, the weekly amount of potash taken by the men was about 51 grains, and by the women 46 grains, or a reduction of more than two-thirds : and he ascribes the occurrence of scurvy after the use of rice to the inferior proportion of potash which this grain contains in comparison with potatoes. We ought, however, also to take into consideration the fact that rice is deficient in certain vegetable acids found in the potato (see *ante*, p. 72).

[5] *Lancet*, April 10th, 1847, p. 390.

[6] *History of Sumatra*, p. 65, 3d ed. 1811.

regions included between, and bordering on the tropics, its cultivation is probably more extensive than that of wheat, which the Europeans are wont to consider as the universal staff of life."

Rice has less laxative powers than the other cereal grains. Indeed, it is generally believed to possess a binding or constipating quality; and, in consequence, is frequently prescribed by medical men as a light, digestible, uninjurious article of food in diarrhœa and dysentery. Various ill effects, such as disordered vision, have been ascribed to its use;[1] but, I believe, unjustly. Neither does there appear to me to be any real foundation for the assertions of Dr. Tytler,[2] that malignant cholera (which he calls the *morbus oryzeus*, or *rice disease*) is induced by it.

USES.—Rice is employed as a nutriment in a variety of forms; e. g. *boiled rice*, *rice milk*. *rice pudding*, *rice cakes*, &c. In China, *rice vermicelli* is prepared from it. This is sold in flat bundles (of about 5 inches long, and 1¼ inches broad), composed of a folded thread or filament made of rice paste. Medicinally, rice is employed as a demulcent, somewhat binding, nutritive substance in diarrhœa, &c. *Gardiner's alimentary preparation* is very finely ground rice meal.

TRIBE II. PHALARIDEÆ.

33. Zea Mays, *Linn.*—Indian Corn; Maize.

Sex. Syst. Monœcia, Triandria.

(Semina.)

HISTORY.—*Frumentum Indicum Mays dictum,* Casp. Bauhin, Pinax; *Frumentum* vel *Triticum Turcicum; Turkish Corn* or *Wheat.*—The first undoubted notice of this plant occurs in the works of Tragus,[3] who died in 1554; though by some writers it is thought to be referred to both in the Bible[4] and in the works of Greek and Roman authors.[5]

FIG. 57.

BOTANY.—*Stem* 2 to 10 feet high. *Leaves* broad, flat, entire, with a short ligula. *Flowers* monœcious: *males* terminal, racemose; *females* axillary, densely spiked. *Stamens* 3. *Ovary* sessile ovate. *Style* 1, long, capillary. *Stigma* ciliated. *Caryopsides* roundish or reniform, arranged on a large cylindrical receptacle or rachis, popularly called the *cobb*.—An annual plant, indigenous in tropical America, but cultivated in various parts of the world.

The ordinary colour of the ripe grains or caryopsides is yellow; but they are frequently met with white, party-coloured, red, purple, or even black.

Maize meal is sold in the shops under the name of *polenta.*

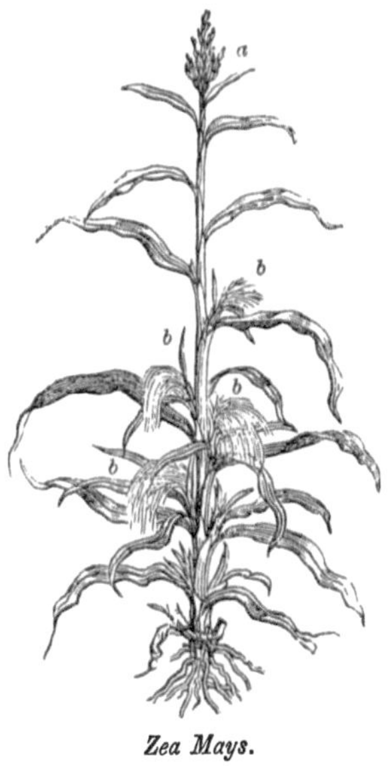

Zea Mays.

[1] Bontius, *Account of the Diseases, Natural History, &c. of the East Indies,* translated into English, 1769; also, Bricheteau, in Tortuelle's *Elém. d'Hygiène,* 4me éd.

[2] *Lancet,* 1833–34, vol. i.

[3] *De Stirpium Historia,* p. 651, 1532. (Sprengel, *Hist. Rei. Herb.* t. i. p. 320, 1807.)

[4] *Genesis,* ch. xli. ver. 5; *Leviticus,* ch. ii. ver. 14, ch. xxiii. ver. 14; *Matthew,* ch. xii. ver. 1, &c. See Cobbett's *Treatise on Cobbett's Corn,* ch. ii. 13, 1828.

[5] Both Theophrastus (*Hist. Plant.* lib. viii. cap. iv.) and Pliny (lib. xviii. cap. xiii.) mention a Bactrian corn of remarkably large size. Theophrastus says the grains were as large as olive-stones; and Pliny states that they were as large as the ears of our corn. Fraas (*Synopsis Plant. Floræ Class.* p. 312, 1845) suggests that the βόσμορον of Strabo (lib. xv.) may be our maize.

a. Male flowers.

b, b, b, b. Female flowers. (The styles which project beyond the enveloping sheaths form a kind of tassel, popularly called the *silks.*)

Composition.—Maize has been analysed by Dr. Gorham,[1] by Bizio,[2] and more recently by Payen, whose analysis may be considered to have superseded his predecessors.

1. *Maize starch* is not at present an article of commerce;[3] though a patent[4] has been taken out for its manufacture by fermentation as well as by the action of caustic and carbonated alkalies. The quantity of starch contained in dried maize is, in round numbers, about 67 per cent. (see Vol. i. p. 67; and *ante*, p. 71).

When examined by the microscope, the particles of maize starch are seen to be more or less rounded or ovoid, with a very distinct either circular or slit hilum, but with no visible rings or laminæ. Their shape is mostly somewhat irregular and knobby; some mullar-shaped. Owing to their mutual compression, many of the particles are angular or polyhedric: this is especially the case with those contained in the outer or horny portion of the albumen; while those found in the interior or farinaceous portion are more rounded. Occasionally particles are seen with a projection like a stalk. The particles of maize starch are mostly of the medium size[5] (·0005 to ·0007 of an inch). By polarised light they show very distinct crosses.

2. *Proteine matters.*—The quantity of *gluten* and other azotised constituents in maize is smaller than in wheat. Horsford[6] obtained 13·65 per cent. from maize meal, and 14·66 per cent. from maize grains. But Payen found only 12·5 per cent. Partly in consequence of this smaller proportion of gluten, and partly from some difference in the quality of this substance,[7] maize is less adapted for making bread than wheat.

3. *Fatty matters.*—Of all the cereal grains, maize appears to be the richest in *fatty matter*. MM. Dumas and Payen procured 2 per cent. of yellow oil from maize;[8] but Liebig[9] was able to obtain only 4·25 per cent. This oil consists, according to Fresenius, of *carbon* 79·68, *hydrogen* 11·53, and *oxygen* 8·79. More recently Payen[10] has given 8·80 per cent. as the proportion of oil found in maize.

Effects.—Maize agrees generally with the other cereal grains in its nutritive properties. It is remarkable for its fattening quality, and which probably depends on the larger amount of fatty matter contained in it than in other cereal grains. In those unaccustomed to its use it is considered apt to excite or keep up a tendency to diarrhœa.

Uses.—It is employed as an article of food. [Dr. W. F. Daniell states that on the gold coast, and several of the inland provinces of Western Africa, it is made into bread under the name of *kankié*, and is also fermented to form a beverage which goes by the name of *pitto* or *peto*.[11]—Ed.]

Tribe III. Avenaceæ.

34. AVENA SATIVA, *Linn.*—THE COMMON OAT.

Sex. Syst. Triandria, Digynia.

(Semina integumentis nudata, *L.*—Seeds, *E.*—Farina ex seminibus, *D.*)

History.—The oat is not mentioned in the Old Testament; but it is

---

[1] *Quarterly Journal of Science*, vol. ix. p. 206, 1821.

[2] L. Gmelin, *Handb. d. Chem.* ii. 1340.

[3] The substance usually sold in the shops as *Indian corn starch* is potato starch.

[4] *Repertory of Patent Inventions*, N. S. vol. xviii. p. 163, 1842.

[5] The following measurements of seven (including the largest and smallest) grains of maize starch were made by Mr. George Jackson:—

1. .... ·0010 of an English inch.		5. .... ·0003 of an English inch.	
2. .... ·0006 " "		6. .... ·0002 " "	
3. .... ·0005 " "		7. .... ·0001 " ..."	
4. .... ·0004 " "			

[6] *Ann. d. Chem. u. Pharm.* Bd. xlviii. 1846.

[7] M. Guibourt (*Hist. Nat. des Drog. simpl.* t. ii. p. 129, 4me éd. 1849) says that the gluten of maize contains less nitrogen than that of other grasses.

[8] *Comptes rendus*, Oct. 24, 1842.

[9] *Annalen der Chemie und Pharmacie*, Bd. xlv. S. 126, 1843.

[10] *Précis de Chim. Industrielle*, p. 394, 1849.

[11] [*Pharm. Journ.* vol. xi. p. 349.]

noticed by the ancient Greek[1] and Roman[2] writers, the former of whom called it βρόμος, the latter *avena*.

BOTANY. **Gen.. Char.**—*Spikelets* 3, many-flowered; flowers remote; the upper one withered. *Glumes* 2, thin, membranous, awnless. *Paleæ* 2, herbaceous; the lower one awned on the back, above the base, at the point almost bicuspidate; the upper one bicarinate, awnless; awn twisted. *Stamina* 3. *Ovarium* somewhat pyriform, hairy at the point. *Stigmata* 2, sessile, distant, villoso-plumose; with simple hairs. *Scales* 2-smooth, usually 2-cleft, large. *Caryopsis* long, slightly terete, internally marked by a longitudinal furrow, hairy at the point, covered by the paleæ, adherent to the upper one (?) (*Kunth*).

Sp. Char.—*Panicle* equal. *Spikelets* 2-flowered. *Florets* smaller than the calyx, naked at the base, alternately awned. *Root* fibrous, annual (*Kunth*).

Hab.—Cultivated in Europe.

A considerable number of varieties[3] of this species are cultivated: these may be arranged under the two heads of *white oats*, and the *red, dun,* or *black oats.*

FIG. 58.

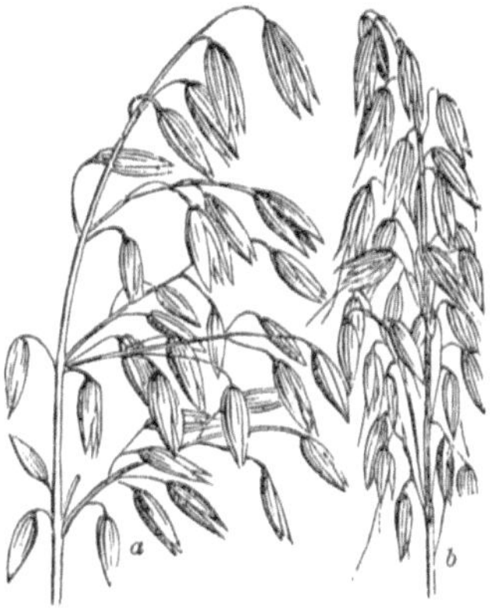

Avena.
a. The *white oat.*
b. *Siberian* or *Tartarian oat.*

The *white oats* have the paleæ of a whitish or straw colour. To this division belong the *potato oat,* the *Georgian oat,* the *Poland oat,* and the *Friezland* or *Dutch oat.*

The *red, dun,* or *black oats* are so called on account of their colour.

Besides the *Avena sativa,* several other species of Avena are cultivated as oats. The following are the chief:—

Avena orientalis, Kunth.—*Tartarian, Hungarian,* or 1-*seeded oat.* Cultivated in Europe.

Avena brevis, Kunth.—*Short oat.* Germany, Austria, and Hungary. Cultivated in France and Spain.

Avena nuda, Kunth.—*Naked oat.* Cultivated in Europe.

DESCRIPTION.—Oats (*caryopsides* vel *semina avenæ cruda*) are too well known to need description. As found in commerce, they are usually enclosed in the paleæ or husk. When deprived of their integuments, they are called *groats* (*semina integumentis nudata,* L.; *avena excorticata* seu *grutum*): these, when crushed, are denominated *Embden groats. Oatmeal* (*farina ex seminibus,* D.) is prepared by grinding the grains. It is not so white as wheaten flour, and has a somewhat bitterish taste.

COMPOSITION.—Oats have been analysed by Vogel,[4] by Payen,[5] and more

---

[1] Hippocrates, *De victûs ratione,* lib. ii. sect. iv. p. 356, ed. Fœs.; Theophrastus, *Hist. Plant.* lib. viii. cap. 9; Dioscorides, lib. ii. cap. 116, and lib. iv. cap. 140; Galen, *De Alim. Facult.* lib. i. cap. 14, p. 322, tom. vi.—Fraas (*Synops. Plant. Floræ Classicæ,* p. 303, 1845) considers that the term βρόμος includes both *Avena sativa* and *A. fatua,* Linn.

[2] Pliny, *Hist. Nat.* lib. xviii. cap. 44.

[3] For an account of the different sorts of cultivated oats, see *The Agriculturist's Manual,* by Peter Lawson and Son, 1836; and *Supplement,* 1842. Also, Loudon's *Encyclopædia of Agriculture.*

[4] Quoted by L. Gmelin, *Handb. d. Chemie,* Bd. ii. S. 1345.

[5] *Précis de Chimie Industr.* 1849.

recently by Messrs. Norton and Fromberg; and oatmeal by Dr. Christison.[1]
The results of Payen's analysis have been already stated (see *ante*, p. 71).

Four varieties of Scotch oats were analysed by Messrs. Norton and Fromberg[2]
with the following results :—

		HOPETON OATS.			POTATO OATS.
		Northumberland.	*Ayrshire.*	*Ayrshire.*	*Northumberland.*
	Starch	65·24	64·80	64·79	65·60
	Sugar	4·51	2·58	2·09	0·80
	Gum	2·10	2·41	2·12	2·28
	Oil	5·44	6·97	6·41	7·38
Proteine compounds	Avenin....	15·76	16·26	17·72	16·29
	Albumen	0·46	1·29	1·76	2·17
	Glatin	2·47	1·46	1·33	1·45
	Epidermis..............	1·18	2·39	2·84	2·28
	Alkaline salts and loss .	2·84	1·84	0·94	1·75
		100·00 N	100·00 F	100·00 F	100·00 N.

Oats consist of from 22 to 28 per cent. of *husks;* and of from 72 to 78
per cent. of grain.

The composition of the husk of the oat, according to Professor Norton, is
as follows :—

	HOPETON OAT.	POTATO OAT.
Oil	1·50	0·92
Sugar and gum	0·47	0·75
Gluten and coagulated albumen	1·88	1·88
Cellulose	89·68	89·46
Saline matter (ash)......................	6·47	6·99
	100·00	100·00

The husk of the oat, therefore, though nutritive, is less so than the bran of
wheat.

1. OAT STARCH, when examined by the microscope, is perceived to consist of small
particles, whose normal shape is round but which is modified by the mutual compression
of the particles,—some being mullar-shaped, from the mutual pressure of two particles,—
some being rounded at one end and dihedral at the other, from the mutual pressure of
three particles,—and others being polyhedric or many-angled, from the mutual pressure
of many particles. The hilum is tolerably distinct in the rounded granules, but rings or
laminæ are not visible. The great bulk of the granules are of the medium size[3] and polyhedral, frequently presenting a pentagonal outline. Unlike most other starches, little or
no variation is observed in their appearance when they are viewed by polarised light: no
crosses are visible.

2. AVENIN.—This is a protein compound analogous to casein or curd of milk, and on
it much of the nutritive value of oats depends. If oatmeal be washed on a sieve, and the
milky liquid which runs through be left till the starch is deposited, then heated to 200° F.
to coagulate the albumen, and to it, when cooled, acetic acid added, a white powder falls,
which is *avenin.*

CHEMICAL CHARACTERISTICS.—Iodine forms, when added to the cold
decoction of oats, the blue iodide of starch. Oatmeal, when mixed with

---

[1] *Dispensatory.*

[2] Johnston's *Lect. on Agricult. Chemistry*, p. 886, 2d edit. 1847.

[3] The following measurements of six (including large and small) grains of oat starch were made
by Mr. George Jackson :—

1. .... ·0010 of an English inch.	4. .... ·0003 of an English inch.
2. .... ·0006 " "	5. .... ·0002 " "
3. .... ·0004 " "	6. .... ·0001 " "

water, does not form a dough, as wheaten flour does; but by washing it with water on a sieve the whole of the meal, with the exception of the coarse parts, will be washed through.

PHYSIOLOGICAL EFFECTS.—Oatmeal is an important and valuable article of food. With the exception of maize or Indian corn, it is richer in oily or fatty matter than any other of the cultivated cereal grains; and its proportion of protein compounds exceeds that of the finest English wheaten flour. So that both with respect to its heat- and fat-making, and its flesh- and blood-making principles, it holds a high rank.

A diet of unfermented oat-bread is apt to occasion dyspepsia in those unaccustomed to its use; and it was formerly suspected of producing or aggravating chronic skin diseases, but without just grounds. Oatmeal porridge, taken at breakfast, sometimes relieves habitual constipation.

Intestinal concretions, composed of phosphate of lime, agglutinating animal matter, and the small stiff silky bristles seen at one end of the inner integument of the oat, are sometimes formed in those who habitually employ oats as food: forty-one specimens, collected by Dr. Monro secundus, are still in the anatomical museum of the University of Edinburgh. These formations are now comparatively rare,—probably because the oats are more perfectly deprived of their investing membranes before being ground (Christison).

USES.—The oat is employed dietetically and medicinally.

As a dietetical agent it is employed in the form of *oat-cake* or *unfermented oat-bread*, *oatmeal porridge* or *stir-about*, and *gruel*. The latter is sometimes given to infants as a substitute for the mother's milk. When there is a tendency to diarrhœa, either in adults or infants, it is advisable to substitute wheatmeal for oatmeal.

In medicine we employ *gruel*, prepared from groats or oatmeal, as a mild, nutritious, and, in most cases, easily-digested article of food in fevers and inflammatory affections. It is also in general use after parturition; and is the basis of *caudle*. In poisoning by acrid substances, it is employed as an emollient and demulcent. It is given after the use of purgatives, to render them more efficient and less injurious. It is frequently used, either alone or in conjunction with other agents, as a clyster. *Oatmeal* is used for making poultices.

Oats are also employed by distillers for the production of spirit (see *Alcohol*).

[It was formerly necessary to notice here the directions of the London and Dublin Pharmacopœias for making water gruel, and poultices. These unnecessary formulæ are now expunged from the above works. We simply give the author's formula for gruel.—ED.]

DECOCTUM AVENÆ; *Oatmeal Gruel; Water Gruel.*—This is usually prepared by boiling oatmeal or groats in water for about half an hour, and then straining. Dr. Cullen[1] directs it to be prepared by boiling an ounce of oatmeal with three quarts of water to a quart, constantly stirring; strain, and when cold decant the clear liquid from the sediment. Sugar, acids, or aromatics may be employed for flavouring.

---

[1] *Treatise of the Materia Medica*, p. 280.

Tribe IV. Hordeaceæ.

35. Lolium temulentum, *Linn.*—Bearded Darnel.

Sex. Syst. Triandria, Digynia.
(Semina.)

Synonymes.—Aἶρα, Dios. lib. ii. cap. 122; Galen, De simpl. med. fac. lib. vi. § 10, and De aliment. facult. lib. i. cap. 37; Paulus Æg. lib. vii. sect. iii.; *Lolium*, Pliny, Hist. Nat. lib. xxii. cap. 79; *Lolium infelix*, Virgil, Georg. i. 153.

History.—This grass was used medicinally by the ancient Greeks and Romans, though it is somewhat remarkable that it is mentioned neither by Hippocrates nor Celsus.

Botany.　**Gen. Char.**—*Spikes* many-flowered, distichous, sessile, contrary to the rachis. *Flowers* beardless at the base. *Glumes* 2, nearly equal, herbaceous, lanceolate, channelled, awnless; the lower or inner ones very often deficient in the lateral spikelets. *Paleæ* 2, herbaceous; the lower concave, awnless, or awned below the point; the upper bicarinate. *Stamens* 3. *Ovary* smooth; *styles* 2, very short, inserted below the point; *stigmas* feathery, with long, simple, finely-toothed, transparent hairs; *scales* 2, fleshy, smooth, acute, entire or 2-lobed. *Caryopsis* smooth, adhering to the upper paleæ (Kunth).

Fig. 59.

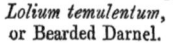

Sp. Char.—*Spikelets* about 6-flowered, equalling or shorter than the glume. *Outer palea* as long as its awn.—*Root* without barren shoots. *Stem* erect, 2 feet high, smooth and shining below, rough upwards. *Ligule* short. *Inner glume* usually present, often bifid.

Lolium temulentum β arvense (Babington, Brit. Bot.) is a variety of the above. It is usually smaller and smoother; its spikelets 4- or 5-flowered; its awns either absent or at most short, lax, and weak.

Europe (indigenous), Japan, New Holland, Chili, Monte Video.—Annual. —Fl. July.

Description.—The grain (*caryopsis*) enclosed in the husk is ovato-oblong, on one side flattened and furrowed,—on the other convex, greyish-brown; odourless, with a sweetish-bitterish, not disagreeable, taste. It yields a darkish meal or farina (called *ærina* by Pliny).[1]

Composition.—In 1827, Bizio[2] examined darnel, and discovered in the seeds two peculiar substances, which he called respectively *glajalico* and *lalico;* the latter he stated possessed a narcotic power similar to that of opium. In 1837, Muratori[3] analysed darnel seeds, and ascribed their poisonous properties to a peculiar acid. In 1834, Bley[4] examined them, and obtained the following substances:—Traces of *volatile oil, chlorophylle* 7·5, *soft resin* 3·5, *bitter extractive* with *chlorides* and *sulphates* 6·0, *gum* with *chloride of calcium* 6·0, *sugar* 0·7, *albumen* 0·65, *extractive* with *malate of lime* 1·55, *gum* with *sulphate* and *muriate of potash* 2·5, *gum* with *malate of potash* 3·0, *starch* 29·9, *artificial gum* and *coagulated albumen* 2·9, *gluten* 0·8, *vegetable fibre* 11·0, *moisture* 20·0 [loss 0·4?]. Bley concluded that the poisonous principle of darnel was extractable from the seeds by water. Subsequently[5] he procured from the watery extract of darnel seeds a peculiar substance, which he called *loliin.* 1000 grains of the seeds yielded him 294 grains of starch.

Loliin is a foliated or pulverulent dirty-white substance, soluble in hot and cold water and in hot alcohol. Its aqueous solution reddened litmus paper feebly. A tenth of a grain of loliin caused an acrid sensation in the throat, followed by an affection of the head and weakness of the whole body, which effects continued only for a short time.

Lolium temulentum, or Bearded Darnel.

---

[1] *Hist. Nat.* lib. xxii. cap. 58.
[2] Dierbach, *Die neuest. Entd. in. d. Mat. Med.* Bd. iii. S. 1139, 1847.
[3] Buchner's *Repert. für die Pharmacie*, 2te Reihe, Bd. xii. S. 181, 1838.
[4] *Ibid.* Bd. xlviii. S. 169, 1834.
[5] *Ibid.* 2te Reihe, Bd. xii. S. 175, 1838.

CHEMICAL CHARACTERISTICS.—According to Ruspini,[1] the presence of grains of Lolium temulentum in wheat-flour may be detected by digesting the suspected farina in rectified spirit. If the Lolium be present, the spirit immediately acquires a characteristic green tint, which gradually deepens; and the taste of the tincture is astringent, and so disagreeable that it may even excite vomiting. By evaporation it yields a green resin. But I have not succeeded in obtaining these results. By digesting bruised and coarsely powdered grains of Lolium temulentum in rectified spirit, the liquid had acquired in forty-eight hours a pale yellow colour and scarcely any flavour, and yielded, by spontaneous evaporation, a minute portion of yellowish residue with a saline taste.

PHYSIOLOGICAL EFFECTS. a. On Animals.—The effects of bearded darnel on animals have been examined by Seeger, Burghard, Mariotti, and Hertwig; and the general results establish the poisonous action of the seeds of this grass. Vomiting was a general effect; followed by tremblings, convulsions, insensibility, and augmentation of urine and sweat.[2]

β. On Man.—The ill effects of the seeds of bearded darnel on man were known to the ancient Greeks and Romans. The symptoms which they produce are twofold: those indicating gastro intestinal irritation,—such as vomiting and colic; and those which arise from disorder of the cerebro-spinal system,—such as headache, giddiness, languor, ringing in the ears, confusion of sight, dilated pupil, delirium, heaviness, somnolency, trembling, convulsions, and paralysis. These seeds, therefore, appear to be acro-narcotic poisons. According to Seeger, one of the most certain signs of poisoning by them is trembling of the whole body. Both Burghard and Schober (quoted by Wibmer) mention death as having resulted from their use. In Cordier's cases their ill effects were directly ascertained by experiments made upon himself; but in most other cases they were the results of accidental poisoning. In general they have arisen from the intermixture of bearded darnel seeds with other cereal grains.[3] In a prison at Cologne, sixty persons suffered from the use of a bread-meal containing a drachm and a half of Lolium temulentum in six ounces of meal.[4] [In January 1854, Dr. Kingsley, of Roscrea, communicated to one of us the particulars of some cases in which several families (including about thirty persons) suffered severely from the effects of bread containing, by accidental admixture, the flour of darnel seeds. The persons who partook of this bread staggered about as if intoxicated: there was giddiness, with violent tremors of the arms and legs, similar to those observed in delirium tremens, but of much greater intensity (the patients requesting those about them to hold them, and experiencing great comfort from this assistance being given to them); greatly impaired vision, everything appearing quite green to the sufferer; coldness of the skin, particularly of the hands and feet; great prostration of strength; and, in several cases, vomiting. Under the free use of stimulants and castor oil the whole of the patients were convalescent the following day, but much debilitated from the effects of the poison.—ED.]

Regarded in a medicinal point of view, bearded darnel appears to possess sedative and anodyne properties. Fantoni[5] and Giacomini consider it to be a direct hyposthenic (see Vol. i. p. 154), depressing the cerebral circulation and acting like aconite.

USES.—Darnel has been recently employed in headache, in rheumatic meningitis, and in sciatica. Fantoni used it with success in the case of a widow who, at the climacteric period, was affected with giddiness, headache, and epistaxis, which had resisted various other remedies. In a case of violent rheumatic meningitis, very great benefit was obtained from its use.

ADMINISTRATION.—The dose of powdered darnel is one or two grains every four or six hours, in the form of powder or pill. It may also be employed in the form either of decoction or of extract. The extract is given to the extent of half a grain or a grain in the day.

ANTIDOTES.—No specific chemical antidote is known. In the event, therefore, of a case of poisoning by darnel, our principal reliance must be on the use of evacuants and dynamical antidotes (see Vol. i. p. 163). After the removal of the poison from the stomach and bowels, stimulants (such as ammonia, coffee, &c.) may be administered to relieve the depression.

---

[1] Journ. de Pharm. et de Chimie, 3me sér. t. v. p. 297, 1844.
[2] Wibmer, Die Wirk. d. Arzneim. u. Gifte, Bd. iii. S. 237, 1837.
[3] See Christison On Poisons; and Wibmer, op. supra cit.
[4] Wibmer, p. 236.
[5] Annali universali di Medicina, Sept. 1848. (quoted by Dierbach).

G

36. HORDEUM DISTICHON, *Linn.*—TWO-ROWED OR LONG-EARED BARLEY.

Sex. Syst. Triandria, Digynia.

(Semina integumentis nudata, *L.*—Decorticated Seeds, *E.*—Semina decorticata, *D.*)

History.—Pliny,[1] on the authority of Menander, says barley (*hordeum*) was a most ancient aliment of mankind. It was cultivated in Egypt nearly 1500 years before Christ.[2] Hippocrates mentions three kinds of κριϑή or barley; namely, barley simply so called,[3] three-month barley,[4] and Achilles barley.[5] These probably were *H. vulgare, H. distichon, H. hexastichon.*

Botany. **Gen. Char.**—*Spikelets* 3 together, the lateral ones usually withered, 2-flowered, with an upper flower reduced to a subulate rudiment. *Glumes* 2, lanceolate-linear, with subulate awns, flattish, unequal-sided, at right angles [*contrariæ*], with the paleæ almost unilateral, turned inwards [*anticæ*], herbaceous, rigid. *Paleæ* 2, herbaceous; the inferior one (turned inwards) concave, ending in an awn; the superior one (turned outwards) contiguous to the rachis, bicarinate. *Stamina* 3. *Ovarium* hairy at the apex. *Stigmata* 2, sessile, somewhat terminal, feathery. *Scales* 2, entire or augmented by a lateral lobe, usually hairy or ciliated. *Caryopsis* hairy at the point, oblong, with a longitudinal furrow internally, adherent to the paleæ, rarely free (*Kunth*).

Sp. Ch.—The lateral *florets* male, awnless; the hermaphrodite ones distichous, close pressed to the stem, awned (*Kunth*).

β. With naked seeds : *H. nudum; Naked Two-rowed Barley.*—The grains of this variety separate from the paleæ or chaff-like wheat.

Fig. 60.

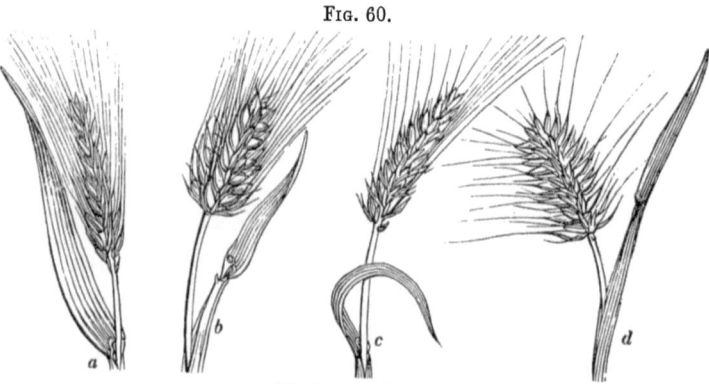

Hordeum or *Barley.*

a, H. vulgare.   *b,* H. hexastichon.   *c,* H. distichon.   *d,* H. zeocitron.

Hab.—A native of Tartary, cultivated in this country.

Several sorts of this species are in cultivation : such as the *common two-rowed* or *English barley,* the *Chevalier barley,* the *Annat barley, Dunlop*

---

[1] *Hist. Nat.* xviii. 14.
[2] *Exodus,* ix. 31.
[3] *De victûs rat.* lib. ii. p. 355, ed. Fœsii.
[4] *De morb. mul.* lib. i. p. 609.
[5] *De morbis,* lib. iii. p. 496.

barley, golden or *Italian barley,* and *black two-rowed barley* (*Hordeum distichon nigrum*).

Besides *H. distichon,* several other species of *Hordeum* are in cultivation —namely, *H. vulgare,* or spring barley; *H. hexastichon,* or six-rowed barley; and *H. zeocitron,* sprat or battledore barley.

DESCRIPTION.—The grains (*caryopsides* vel *semina hordei cruda*) are too well known to need description. As found in commerce, they are usually enclosed in the paleæ or husk. Deprived of their husk by a mill, they form *Scotch, hulled,* or *pot barley* (*hordeum mundatum*). When all the integuments of the grains are removed, and the seeds are rounded and polished, they constitute *pearl barley* (*hordeum perlatum*). The farina (*farina hordei*) obtained by grinding pearl barley to powder is called *patent barley.*

Three qualities of barley are distinguished in the market: the hard and flinty, fit for making pot barley; a softer kind, called malting barley, which is next in value; and feeding barley, which is adapted for neither of the uses of the two other kinds.

COMPOSITION.—According to Einhof,[1] barley has the following composition :—

The Ripe Seeds.		Barley-meal.	
Meal	70·05	Starch	67·18
Husk	18·75	Fibrous matter (gluten, starch, and lignin)	7·29
Moisture	11·20	Gum	4·62
	——	Sugar	5·21
	100·00	Gluten	3·52
		Albumen	1·15
		Phosphate of lime with albumen	0·24
		Moisture	9·37
		Loss	1·42
			——
			100·00

Payen's analysis of barley has been already given (see *ante,* p. 71), as also the proportion of starch and proteine constituents according to Krocker and Horsford (see Vol. i. p. 67). Mr. Johnston[2] gives the following as the average composition of fine barley-meal :—*Starch* 68; *gluten, albumen,* &c. 14; *fatty matter* 2; *saline matter* or *ash* 2; *water* 14 = 100.

1. PROTEINE COMPOUNDS.—The proportion of proteine matter in barley is much less than that in wheat, and its quality is very different. If barley dough be washed with water, nearly the whole is washed away, the husk alone excepted: it contains, therefore, little or no gluten properly so called. The milky liquid deposits starchy matter and an insoluble proteine matter (insoluble caseine?), while the clear liquid holds in solution a small quantity of albumen (coagulable by heat), and of caseine (precipitable by acetic acid). If the starchy deposit be digested with water containing ammonia, a solution of the proteine compound is obtained, from which a voluminous precipitate (caseine?) is thrown down by acetic acid (Johnston).

2. STARCH.—Barley-starch, like wheat-starch, consists principally of large and small grains, with but few of intermediate size: but the diameter of the largest grains is somewhat larger than that of the corresponding grains of wheat-starch.[3] The shape of the

---

[1] L. Gmelin's *Handb. d. Chemie,* ii. 1344.

[2] *Lect. on Agricultural Chemistry,* p. 881, 2d edit. 1847.

[3] The following measurements of seven (including the largest and smallest) grains of barley-starch were made by Mr. George Jackson :—

1.	0·0011 of an English inch.		5.	0·0005 of an English inch.	
2.	0·0010	" "	6.	0·0002	" "
3.	0 0009	" "	7.	0·0001	" "
4.	0 0008	" "			

larger grains is irregularly circular, or elliptical, or obscurely triangular, flattened or lenticular, the flattened surfaces being undulated or uneven : the smaller grains are globular, ellipsoidal, rarely angular or mullar-shaped. The hilum is scarcely, if at all, perceptible on the larger grains, and the rings are very faintly indicated: in these respects the grains of barley-starch differ remarkably from those of rye-starch. On the smaller grains, a hilum, or what appears to be such, is frequently perceptible. By polarised light the cross is less distinctly seen than in rye-starch. Barley-starch offers more resistance to the action of boiling water than some other starches; and the insoluble residue, after the prolonged ebullition of it in water, constitutes what Proust[1] called *hordeine*.

3. Fatty or Oily Matter.—Fourcroy and Vauquelin[2] detected a yellow, acrid, saponifiable, butyraceous oil, in barley.

Chemical Characteristics.—Iodine forms the blue iodide of starch, when added to the cold decoction of barley. Decoction of whole barley has an acrid bitter taste, which it derives from the husk.

Physiological Effects.—Barley is a valuable nutritive. Considered in relation to wheat, it offers several peculiarities. In the first place it contains much less proteine matter,—in other words, less of the flesh- and blood-making principles; though Count Rumford[3] considered barley-meal in soup three or four times as nutritious as wheat-flour. Secondly, its starch offers more resistance to the action of the gastric juice, in consequence of its more difficult solubility in water. Thirdly, its husk is slightly acrid ; and, therefore, this should be removed from barley intended for dietetical purposes, as in Scotch and pearl barley. Fourthly, barley-meal is more laxative than wheat-meal.

Uses.—Barley is employed both dietetically and medicinally ; as well also in the brewery and distillery.

Barley-meal is sometimes added to three times its weight of wheat-meal to form infants' food ; the addition of the barley-meal being intended to obviate the constipating effects of wheat-meal.

Scotch and *pearl barley* are employed to thicken soups, and to yield barley-water. It is frequently used in the dietaries of pauper establishments ; but when bowel complaints prevail, some other cereal grain (wheat, for example) should be substituted for it.

1. DECOCTUM HORDEI, L. D.; *Aqua hordeata ; Barley-water.*— (Barley [Pearl Barley, *D.*], ʒiiss. [℥iss. *D.*] ; Water, Oivss. [Oiss. *D.*] First wash away, with water, the foreign matters adhering to the barley-seeds ; then, half a pint of the water being poured on them, boil the seeds a little while. This water being thrown away, pour the remainder of the water, first made hot, on them, and boil down to two pints, and strain, *L.*—The process of the *Dublin Pharmacopœia* is not essentially different.)—This is a valuable demulcent and emollient drink for the invalid in febrile cases and inflammatory disorders, especially of the chest and urinary organs. It is sometimes given to children as a slight laxative. It is usually flavoured with sugar, and frequently with some slices of lemon. It is a constituent of the *Enema Aloës*, L., *Enema Terebinthinæ*, L., and *Decoctum Hordei compositum*, L.

2. DECOCTUM HORDEI COMPOSITUM, L.; *Mistura Hordei*, E.; *Decoctum Pectorale; Compound Decoction of Barley; Pectoral Decoction.*

---

[1] *Ann. Chim. Phys.* v. 339.
[2] *Ann. de Mus. d'Hist. Nat.* No. xxxvii. p. 8.
[3] *Essay on Feeding the Poor,* 1800.

(Decoction of Barley, Oij.; Figs, sliced, ℥iiss.; Fresh Liquorice [root] bruised, ʒv.; Raisins [stoned], ℥iiss.; Distilled Water. Oj. *L.*] Boil down to two pints, and strain.—The process of the *Edinburgh* Pharmacopœia is essentially the same).—This decoction is emollient, demulcent, and slightly aperient. It is employed in the same cases as the simple decoction.

3. BYNE (βύνη); *Brasium*;[1] *Maltum*; *Malt*.—This is barley which has been made to germinate by moisture and warmth, and afterwards dried, by which the vitality of the seed is destroyed. By this process part of the proteine matter of the barley is converted into *diastase*. This, although it does not constitute more than about $\frac{1}{500}$th of the malt, serves to effect the conversion of about 40 per cent. of the starch of the seed into *grape-sugar* and *gum* (dextrine). The grain loses by the operation of malting about 8 per cent. of its weight, and gains about $\frac{1}{11}$th or $\frac{1}{12}$th in bulk. This loss arises in part from the separation of the radicles in the form of malt-dust or cummins. The colour of the malt varies with the temperature at which it is dried. If the temperature does not exceed 100° F., the result is *pale malt*; if it be above this and does not exceed 180°, the result is *amber malt*. These varieties of malt yield fermentable infusions. *Brown* or *blown malt* dried at 260° F. is used to communicate flavour; while *roasted, burned,* or *high-dried malt,* which has been scorched, is employed for colouring porter.

[We append the microscopical characters of malt, on the authority of Drs. Lindley and Hooker :—

FIG. 61.

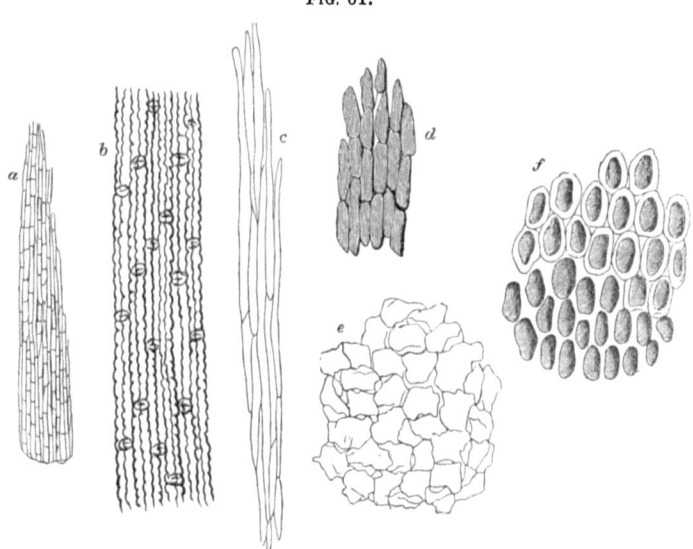

Microscopical Appearances of Malt.

---

[1] [The term "Brasin" was formerly applied to brewing, and "Brasin house" was the brewing house. Brazenose College, at Oxford, derives its name from its having been the site of the ancient brewing house of the University.—Ed.]

When malt is ground, it separates into several distinct forms of tissue; and, as it would not be practicable to separate the husk during grinding, the characteristic marks of the husk offer a certain means of detecting malt, whether for its identification, or for detecting it as an adulteration in coffee or other substances in the state of powder.

1. The *Husk* (*a*) consists of linear cells bounded by serrated lines (*b*), and marked abundantly by round spaces, which are the remains of the breathing pores.

2. *Cellular membranes,* some of which resemble fine parallel lines with indistinct appearances of serration (*c*); others consist of regularly prismatical vesicles, arranged with much uniformity (*d*); others of hexagonal cells with wavy margins (*e*).

In addition to these there occurs a thin skin (*f*), composed of minute roundish angular cells of a slightly opaque appearance, which readily detach themselves, and, when examined with a quarter-inch objective, are seen to owe their appearance to molecular matter of excessive fineness, with which they are filled : portions of this float abundantly in the water.—Ed.]

The *infusion of malt* (*infusum bynes*), commonly called *sweet-wort*, contains saccharine matter, starch, glutinous matter, and mucilage. It is nutritious and laxative, and has been used as an antiscorbutic and tonic. Macbride[1] recommended it in scurvy;[2] but it is apt to increase the diarrhœa. As a tonic it has been used in scrofulous affections, purulent discharges,—as from the kidneys, lungs, &c., and in pulmonary consumption.[3] The *decoction* (*decoctum bynes*) is prepared by boiling three ounces of malt in a quart of water. This quantity may be taken daily.

4. CERVISIA ;[4] *Ale and Beer.*—By the fermentation of an infusion of malt and hops, are obtained ale and beer. These liquids consist of *alcohol, sugar, mucilage,* an *extractive and bitter principle, fatty matter, aroma* (*volatile oil ?*), *glutinous matter, lactic and carbonic acids, salts,* and *water.* Common beer contains about 1 per cent., strong ale or beer about 4 per cent., best brown stout 6 per cent., and the strongest ale about 8 per cent. of spirit of sp. gr. 0·825. The ashes of beer consist of potash, soda, lime, chlorine, sulphuric acid, phosphoric acid, and silica.[5]

Beer is a thirst-quenching, refreshing, exhilarating, intoxicating, and slightly nutritious beverage.[6]

a. Ale[7] is prepared with pale malt. It is therefore, lighter coloured ; and, when made with an equal weight of malt, is richer in alcohol, sugar, and gum, than porter or stout. *Pale* or *bitter ale,* brewed for the India market, has been carefully fermented so as to be devoid of saccharine matter, and contains an extra quantity of the active principles of hops. It is frequently used as a restorative beverage for invalids and convalescents.

[In consequence of statements made by Mons. Payen, of Paris, in his public

---

[1] *Hist. Account of a New Method of Treating Scurvy,* 1767.

[2] See also a paper by Dr. Badenoch, *Med. Obs. and Inq.* vol. v. p. 61.

[3] Rush, *Med, Observ. and Inq.* iv. 367.

[4] Pliny (*Hist. Nat.* lib. xxii. cap. 82, ed. Valp.), in noticing the drinks prepared from corn, says that "*Zythum* is made in Egypt, *celia* and *ceria* in Spain, and *cervisia* and many more sorts in Gaul." For *cervisia,* some writers use the term *cerevisia.* *Zythum* (ζῦθος) was a kind of beer obtained by fermentation from barley. (See Herodotus, lib. ii. cap. 77.) As *cervisia* was made from unmalted barley, its colour would be pale, and it would, therefore, in this respect agree with our ale. But the ale and beer of the present day differ from the ancient *cervisia* in being flavoured with hops, and hence the phrase *cerevisia lupulata* which is sometimes applied to them.

[5] Dickson, *Phil. Mag. and Journal of Science,* vol. xxxiii. p. 341, 1848.

[6] For further details respecting the nutritive and dietetical properties of beer, see the author's *Treatise on Diet,* p. 415, et seq.

[7] *Ale,* in Saxon *eale* or *ealo* (probably from the word *celia,* before mentioned), is sometimes Latinised *ala* or *alla.*

lectures, a London journal adopted the charge that Messrs. Allsop and Co. used strychnia in order to give flavour to their bitter ales. A report was consequently published by Messrs. Graham and Hofmann, which showed that such neither was nor could be the case. The proportion of strychnia which they found necessary to flavour beer to the required degree of bitterness, was one grain to each gallon; so that a fatal dose would be taken in two pots of the ale, were strychnia present, and symptoms would occur on swallowing one pint. It is stated in the report that there exists a statute of Henry VII. forbidding the adulteration of ale by brimstone or hops,—a curious fact, showing how completely the present liquor differs from that formerly in use, when the bitterness of the ale is stated to have been produced by sage, chamomile, horehound, or other indigenous plants.[1]

It may be greatly doubted whether any benefit can be derived from swallowing the strongly bitter infusion now so largely consumed at meals, and whether positive mischief may not be done by mixing an active therapeutical agent with the gastric juice while the stomach is discharging its functions. The writer has had occasion to observe the evil occasionally resulting from the practice, and sincerely hopes that the present custom of ordering a powerful tonic with meals will soon fall into disuse.—ED.]

β. *Porter* (the stronger kinds of which are called *stout*) owes its dark colour to high-dried or charred malt. When fresh or new, it is said to be *mild;* and, when old and acid, is called *hard*. An extract of cocculus indicus, called *black extract* or *hard multum,* is occasionally used by dishonest dealers to augment its intoxicating quality. For medicinal purposes *bottled porter* (*cervisia lagenaria*) is usually preferred to draught porter. It is used as a restorative in the latter stages of fever, and to support the powers of the system after surgical operations, severe accidents, &c.

37. TRITICUM VULGARE, *Kunth.*—COMMON WHEAT.

Sex. Syst. Triandria, Digynia.

(Farina; farina seminum: Amylum; seminum fæcula, *L.*: Amylum; fecula of the seeds, *E.*: Farina seminum, *D.*)

HISTORY.—In the earlier ages wheat was an esteemed article of food,[2] and is frequently spoken of by Hippocrates,[3] who calls it πυρός, and mentions three kinds of it: wheat simply so called, three-month wheat, and Sitanian wheat. Pliny[4] describes several kinds of *triticum*.

BOTANY. **Gen. Char.**—*Spikelets* 3- or many-flowered; the fructiferous rachis generally articulated, flowers distichous. *Glumes* 2, nearly opposite, almost equal, awnless or awned, the upper one bicarinate; the keels more or less aculeato-ciliate. *Stamina* 3. *Ovarium* pyriform, hairy at the apex. *Stigmata* 2, terminal, subsessile, feathery; with long, simple, finely-toothed hairs. *Scales* 2, generally entire and ciliated. *Caryopsis* externally convex, internally concave, and marked by a deep furrow, distinct, or adhering to the paleæ (*Kunth*).

---

[1] [*Pharm. Journ.* vol. xi. 504].
[2] *Levit.* ii.
[3] *De victûs rat.* lib. iii. p. 374, ed. Fœsii.
[4] *Hist. Nat.* xviii. 12.

Sp. Char.—*Spike* 4-cornered, imbricated; with a tough rachis. *Spike-lets* generally 4-flowered. *Glumes* ventricose, ovate, truncate, mucronate, compressed below the apex, round, and convex at the back, with a prominent nerve. *Flowers* awned or awnless. *Grains* loose (*Kunth*).

a. æstivum,[1] Kunth; *T. æstivum*, Linn.; *Spring* or *Summer Wheat*.—Annual; glumes awned.—This variety includes a great many sorts known to farmers by different names, and which may be arranged in two divisions—viz. the *white-bearded* and the *red-bearded*.

β. hybernum,[1] Kunth; *T. hybernum*, Linn.; *T. compactum*, Host.; *T. velutinum*, Schuebl.; *T. erinaceum*, Hort. Hal.; *Winter Wheat*.—Biennial; glumes almost awnless. This variety also includes many sorts, which may be arranged in two divisions—viz. the *white beardless* and the *red beardless*.—Talavera wheat is a white beardless winter wheat. Mr. Hard, miller, of Dartford, tells me that "this kind (Talavera wheat) is far superior to any description of wheat, either foreign or English; and the great advantage it possesses consists in its strength, colour, and sweetness. The reason of there being so small a quantity at market arises from the fact of its being so unprofitable to the farmer, scarcely producing one crop in three, which I greatly regret, as it is the most valuable grain we have; and, technically speaking, if the flour is properly manufactured, 8 oz. will absorb as much liquor as 11 oz. of that used by the baker."

Hab.—It is a native of the country of the Baschkirs, and is cultivated in Europe.

Besides *T. vulgare*, other species of Triticum are cultivated. The following are the chief:—

T. TURGIDUM, Kunth; *Turgid Wheat*.—Some of the sorts of this species have smooth ears; others downy, woolly, or velvety ears. This species includes the *T. turgidum*, Linn., and *T. compositum*, Linn.

T. DURUM, Kunth; *Hard* or *Horny Wheat*.

T. POLONICUM, Kunth; *Polish Wheat*.

T. SPELTA, Kunth; *Spelt Wheat*.

T. MONOCOCCUM, Kunth; *One-grained Wheat*.

FIG. 62.

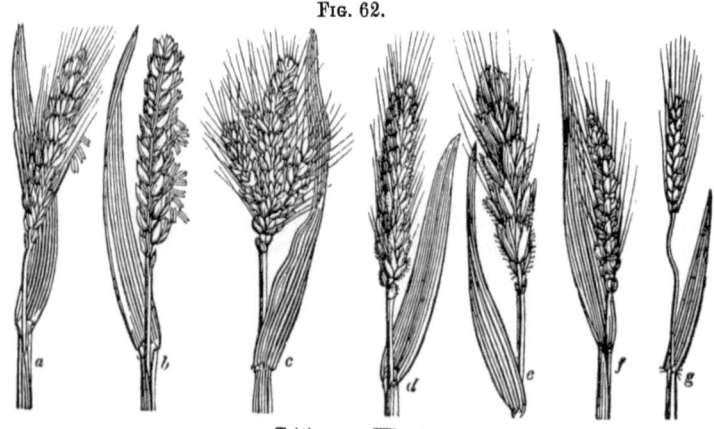

Triticum.—Wheat.

a. T. vulgare, *a.* æstivum.	*e.* T. polonicum.
b. T. vulgare, *β.* hybernum.	*f.* T. spelta.
c. T. turgidum (compositum).	*g.* T. monococcum.
d. T. turgidum.	

---

[1] The distinction of wheats into *summer* and *winter* wheats, or into those sown in the spring and those sown in the autumn, has been objected to on the ground that under the name of *T. hybernum* are included several of the earlier sorts of spring wheat, and under *T. æstivum* are included several wheats which require as long a time to arrive at maturity as the common winter sorts.

DESCRIPTION.—Wheat-grains (*caryopsides tritici; semina tritici*), as brought to market, are completely devoid of their paleæ (*chaff* or *husk*).

The number of parts into which millers separate wheat varies in different localities. According to Mr. Hard, miller, of Dartford, in Kent, the products obtained by grinding one quarter or eight bushels of wheat are as follows :—

PRODUCE OF ONE QUARTER OF WHEAT WEIGHING 504 lbs.

Flour	392 lbs.
Biscuit or fine middlings	10
Toppings or specks	8
Best pollard, Turkey pollard, or twenty-penny	15
Fine pollard	18
Bran and coarse pollard	50
Losses sustained by evaporation, and waste in grinding, dressing, &c.	11
	504 lbs.

Wheat-grains vary in size, smoothness, transparency, and hardness, and in the thickness of their integuments; and, consequently, the relative proportions of bran (and pollard) and flour which they yield, vary. The integument readily separates in soft-grained wheat, but with difficulty in the hard-grained: the former, therefore, yields more bran and less flour; while the latter produces flour of a lower quality, because it is intermixed with some of the ground integuments.

Semolina, Soujee, and *Manna Croup,*[1] are granular preparations of wheat deprived of bran.

I am indebted to Mr. Hard for the following notice (as well as for samples) of the products obtained in grinding wheat :—

" The wheat having been ground in the usual way, should be allowed to remain in the meal some time before dressing, which removes the heat caused by the process, and enables the miller to obtain more flour, and the baker a better quality, than if dressed immediately it is ground.

" The process of dressing is by a wire cylinder containing a certain number of sheets of different texture or fineness, which cylinder contains eight hair brushes attached to a spindle passed through the centre of the cylinder, and laid out so as to gently touch the wire: this cylinder is fed by a shoe with the meal; then the flour and offal, after passing through the wire in this way, are divided by wood partitions fixed close to the outside of the cylinder." The produce of wheat-meal dressed through the wire machine consists of— 1st, *Flour;* 2nd, *White Stuff,* or *Boxings,* or *Sharps;* 3rd, *Fine Pollard;* 4th, *Coarse Pollard,* or *Horse Pollard;* 5th, *Bran.* The second product (*i. e.* the White Stuff) is then submitted to another dressing through a fine cloth machine, and produces—1st, *Fine Middlings, for biscuits;* 2nd, *Toppings* or *Specks;* 3rd, *Dustings;* 4th, *Best Pollard, Turkey Middlings,* or *Coarse Middlings.*

COMPOSITION.—1. *Wheat-flour* has been analysed by Vogel,[2] by Proust,[3] by Henry,[4] and by Vauquelin.[5] The following are the results obtained by Vauquelin :—

---

[1] The term *Manna Croup* is probably derived from *Manna-Grout,* the name of a nutritious food prepared from the grain of *Glyceria fluitans.* (See Curtis, *Fl. Lond.* vol. i. pl. 7 ; also Tooke's *View of the Russian Empire,* vol. iii. p. 168, 2d edit. 1800.)

[2] Quoted by L. Gmelin, *Handb. d. Chem.* Bd. ii. S. 1341.

[3] *Ann. Chim. Phys.* t. v. p. 340.

[4] *Journ. de Pharm.* t. viii. p. 51, 1822 ; and t. xv. p. 127, 1829.

[5] *Ibid.* t. viii. p. 353, 1822.

COMPOSITION OF WHEAT-FLOUR.

	French Wheat.	Odessa Hard Wheat.	Odessa Soft Wheat.	Ditto.	Ditto.	Flour of Paris bakers.	Ditto, of good quality, used in public establishments.	Ditto, inferior kind.
Starch	71·49	56·5	62·00	70·84	72·00	72·8	71·2	67·78
Gluten.........	10·96	14·55	12·00	12·10	7·30	10·2	10·3	9·02
Sugar	4·72	8·48	7·56	4·90	5·42	4·2	4·8	4·80
Gum	3·32	4·90	5·80	4·60	3·30	2·8	3·6	4·60
Bran	—	2·30	1·20	—	—	—	—	2·00
Water	10·00	12·00	10·00	8·00	12·00	10·0	8·0	12·00
Wheat-flour	100·49	98·73	98·56	100·44	100·02	100·0	97·9	100·20

Payen's analysis of wheat has been already given (see *ante*, p. 71); as also the proportions of water, proteine matters, and starch, according to the investigations of Horsford and Krocker (see Vol. i. p. 67); and the composition of the ash of wheat (see *ante*, p. 71).

Mr. Johnston[1] found that in 20 samples of English flour the proportion of water varied from 15 to 17 per cent.

The proportion of the organic constituents of wheat is liable to considerable variation, according to soil, climate, variety of seed, mode of culture, time of cutting, and quality of manure.

2. The composition of *bran*, like that of wheat-flour, is subject to great variation; but the following is given by Mr. Johnston as the average:—

COMPOSITION OF BRAN.

Water..	13·1
Albumen (coagulated)	19·3
Oil..	4·7
Husk and a little starch	55·6
Saline matter (ash)...	7·3
Bran	100·0

1. STARCH.—As wheat-starch is an article of the materia medica, it will be noticed among the officinal preparations (see p. 94).

2. PROTEINE MATTERS.—The quantity of proteine matters in wheat has been already stated (see Vol. i. p. 67; and p. 71). Wheat contains at least four different proteine compounds; namely, *albumen, vegetable fibrine, glutin,* and *caseine.* They have an analogous composition, and contain each about 16 per cent. of nitrogen.

If wheaten dough be washed on a sieve by a stream of water, a milky liquid passes through, and a tenacious elastic mass is left behind, called *crude gluten,* or sometimes *Beccaria's gluten.* The milky liquid holds in solution gum, sugar, and albumen; and in suspension, starch: the crude gluten contains vegetable fibrine, glutin, caseine or mucine, and oil. According to Saussure,[2] crude gluten has the following composition:—

Glutin	20
Vegetable fibrine	72
Mucine (caseine ?)...	4
Oil...	3·7
Starch (accidental)	a small quantity
Crude Gluten.......................................	99·7

a. Vegetable Albumen.—Obtained by allowing the milky liquid above mentioned to deposit its starch, and then heating the supernatant liquor nearly to boiling: flakes of

---

[1] *Lectures on Agricultural Chemistry,* 2d edit. p. 867.
[2] *Bibliothèque universelle,* Sciences et Arts, t. liii. p. 260, 1833.

coagulated albumen are formed.   Its composition was found by Dr. Bence Jones[1] to be *carbon* 55·01, *hydrogen* 7·23, *nitrogen* 15·92, *oxygen, sulphur,* and *phosphorus* 21·84.

β. *Glutin; Gliadine* (from γλία, glue); *Pure Gluten.* — Obtained by boiling crude gluten in alcohol, which extracts glutin, caseine or mucine, and oil.   By cooling, the caseine is deposited.   The supernatant liquid is then evaporated to dryness, and the adhesive mass thus obtained digested with ether to extract the oil: the residue is glutin. Its composition has been before noticed (see Vol. i. p. 64).

γ. *Vegetable Fibrine ; Zymome* (from ζύμη, ferment).—This is the part of crude gluten which is insoluble in alcohol.   Mulder considers it to be coagulated albumen ; Liebig, as vegetable fibrine.   Johnston, on the other hand, thinks it different from both albumen and fibrine, and therefore calls it simply gluten.   When obtained as above described it much resembles the fibre of lean beef.   Dr. Bence Jones ascertained its composition to be *carbon* 55·22, *hydrogen* 7·42, *nitrogen* 15·98, *oxygen,* &c. 21·38.

δ. *Caseine.*—After the albumen has been separated by heat from the aqueous liquid before alluded to, the addition of acetic acid causes the separation of what is supposed to be caseine.   The white flocculent substance which deposits on cooling from the alcoholic liquor in which crude gluten has been boiled, and which has been called *mucine,* somewhat resembles caseine.

3. OIL.—Obtained by digesting wheat-flour in ether.   The quantity procured varies from 1½ to 3 per cent.   As bran yields about twice as much as fine flour, it follows that the oil exists in greater proportion in the outer than in the inner part of the grain.   The oil resembles the fatty oils or butter in its properties.   By washing wheat-dough, part of the oil is washed out, and part remains in the crude gluten.

4. WATER.—According to Johnston, English flour contains, on an average, from 15 to 17 per cent. of water.

5. MINERAL CONSTITUENTS. — The composition of the ashes of wheat has been already stated (see *ante*, p. 71).   The most important of these constituents are the alkaline and earthy phosphates.

CHEMICAL CHARACTERISTICS.—The cold decoction of wheat-flour forms with tincture of iodine the blue iodide of starch.   Nitric acid gives wheat-flour a fine orange-yellow colour.   Recently-prepared tincture of guaiacum forms a blue colour with good wheat-flour.

DISEASES OF WHEAT.[2]—Five principal diseases are produced in wheat by the attacks of parasitic fungi : namely, 1st, *bunt, smut-balls,* or *pepperbrand,* produced by *Uredo caries,* De Candolle ; 2ndly, *smut, dust-brand,* or *burnt-ear,* produced by *Uredo segetum ;* 3rdly, *rust, red-rag, red-robin,* or *red-gum,* caused, as Professor Henslow has shown, by the young state of *Puccinia graminis,* which was formerly supposed to form two distinct fungi, to which the names of Uredo rubigo and U. linearis had been given ; 4thly, *mildew,* produced by the *Puccinia graminis* in a more advanced period of its growth ; and 5thly, *ergot,* caused by the *Cordyceps purpurea* (see *ante,* p. 48).[3]

Two diseases of wheat are produced by parasitic animalcules ; namely, 1st, the *ear-cockle, purples,* or *peppercorn,* caused by a microscopic eel-shaped animalcule, called *Vibrio tritici ;* and, 2ndly, the *wheat-midge,* an abortion of the grain caused by a minute two-winged fly called *Cecidomyia tritici.*   Corn affected with any of these diseases is of course deteriorated in value ; but we have still to learn what are the precise effects on the animal economy of grain thus infected.   The *bunt* imparts to flour its disgusting odour, and makes it less fit for bread ; but flour thus tainted is used

---

[1] Liebig's *Animal Chemistry.*
[2] For an excellent account of the diseases of wheat, see the Rev. Professor Henslow's *Report* on this subject, in the *Journal of the Royal Agricultural Society of England,* 1841, vol. ii. part 1.
[3] [One or two other diseases of less importance are also produced by fungi.   (See Payen, *Maladies des Pommes de Terre,* p. 93, 1853 ; *Gardeners' Chronicle,* p. 601, 1845.)]

in the manufacture of ginger-bread. *Smut* does not give any unpleasant odour to corn, which, when infected with it, is frequently used for feeding fowls,—apparently without producing any ill effects. I have ascertained that *ergot of wheat* is as powerful in its action on the uterus as ergot of rye. It has been suggested that some remarkable cases of spontaneous gangrene which occurred at Wattisham, in Suffolk, in 1762, may possibly have arisen from the presence of ergot in the corn used by the persons affected; but of this there is no evidence.

Deterioration; Adulteration.—By exposure to a damp air, wheat-flour absorbs moisture, and after some time acquires a musty odour, and becomes mouldy; the gluten being the first to suffer change. In this state it may be readily conceived that wheat-flour would prove injurious to health. Wheat-flour is subject to adulteration with various vegetable and mineral substances. Among *vegetable* substances used for the purpose of adulterating wheat-flour the following have been named : Potato-starch, the meal of other cereal grains (viz. of maize, rice, barley, and rye), of buckwheat, and of certain leguminous seeds (viz. of beans, peas, and vetch).

In the detection of these adulterations, the microscope lends important assistance. It enables us to judge of the size and shape, the markings on, and the isolation and agglomeration of, the starch-grains, and thereby to distinguish the starch-grains of one meal from those of another. In some cases the microscopic examination of suspected flour is aided by the use of a solution of potash. Thus it enables us readily to detect the presence of either potato-starch or the meal of leguminous seeds. If a solution containing about $1\frac{3}{4}$ per cent. of potash[1] be added to a mixture of potato-starch and wheat-starch (or wheat-flour), the granules of potato-starch swell up, and acquire three or four times their original volume, while those of wheat-starch are scarcely affected by it. A solution of potash, containing about 12 per cent. of potash, dissolves all the varieties of starch, but not cellulose : hence, if to wheat-flour intermixed with the meal of some leguminous seed this solution be added, the starch-grains dissolve, and the hexagonal tissue of the adulterating leguminous seed is rendered very obvious.[2] Occasionally polarised light may be used to aid the microscope in detecting adulterations of wheat-flour. Thus, unlike wheat-starch, the starch of the oat produces no effect on polarised light, and presents no crosses when viewed by it.

In the detection of the meal of the leguminous seeds the odour and flavour of the suspected flour, and its chemical characters, aid in detecting the fraud. If the suspected flour be digested with twice its volume of cold water, the infusion filtered, and a few drops of acetic acid added to it, a precipitate of legumine (a kind of caseine) is produced, if the meal of a leguminous seed be present :[3] but wheat-flour treated in the same way yields a slight precipitate (of caseine), and, therefore, this test must not be relied on. Donny has pointed out a mode of detecting the meal of two leguminous seeds, viz.

---

[1] I find that a mixture of 1 measure of *liquor potassæ*, Ph. L., and 2 or 3 measures of distilled water, readily distinguishes potato-starch from wheat-starch.

[2] Donny, *Ann. de Chim. et de Phys.* 3me sér. t. xxi. p. 5, 1847 ; and *Journ. de Pharm. et de Chim.* 3me sér. t. xiii. p. 139, 1848. Also, Mareska, *Journ. de Pharm. et de Chim.* 3me sér. t. xii. p. 98, 1847; also, *Pharmaceutical Journal*, vol. vii. p. 394, 1848.

[3] *Journ. de Pharm. et de Chim.* 3me sér. t. xi. p. 322, 1847 ; also, *Pharmaceutical Journal*, vol. vii. p. 84, 1847.

the vetch (*Vicia sativa*), and beans (*Faba vulgaris*, common tick bean) : it consists in exposing the suspected flour to the successive action of the vapours of nitric acid and ammonia : wheat-flour, when thus treated, becomes yellow ; but the meals of the leguminous seeds just referred to become red, and hence wheat-flour adulterated with either of them becomes more or less spotted with red, according to the proportion of the leguminous meal present.

The *mineral* substances which have been used to adulterate wheat-flour are chiefly chalk and sulphate of lime (plaster of Paris). White clay and bone-ashes are also said to have been used. Sulphate of copper and alum are sometimes added to bad wheat-flour to improve its quality and render it more fitted for making bread. These different adulterations may be readily detected. Their quantity and nature may be judged of by incinerating the suspected flour, weighing the ash (which in genuine flour amounts to about 1 or 1¼ per cent.) and determining its nature. Flour mixed with chalk effervesces on the addition of hydrochloric acid, and yields a calcareous solution detect-able by a solution of oxalate of ammonia (see Vol. i. p. 617). Flour mixed with sulphate of lime, when digested in water, yields a solution which answers to the tests both for lime (see Vol. i. p. 617) and for sulphuric acid (Vol. i. p. 367). Pure wheat-flour is almost completely soluble in a strong solution of potash containing about 12 per cent. of alkali; but mineral substances used for the purpose of adulteration remain undissolved.

Physiological Effects.—The nutritive qualities of wheat are similar to those of the cereal grains generally, and which have been already noticed.

As it exceeds other kinds of corn in the proportion of proteine matters which it contains, so it surpasses them in its flesh- and blood-making qualities. But as it contains less starch and fatty matters than some other cereal grains, it is probably inferior to the latter as a fattening agent. The different parts of the grain differ in composition, and, therefore, in nutritive value. The external sub-epidermoid part contains a larger proportion of oil, of salts (chiefly phosphates), and albuminous and caseine matter, than the more internal and farinaceous portion ; and it is therefore probable that the finest flour, which has been freed as much as possible from all traces of bran, is actually some-what less nutritive than the coarser flour.

Wheat-flour, especially when baked, is rather constipating than purgative. In this it differs from both barley-meal and oat-meal. Infants who are fed on baked flour frequently suffer with constipation ; and to relieve this it is sometimes found necessary to substitute a portion of barley-meal for an equi-valent weight of wheat-flour. Wheat-flour yields the finest, whitest, lightest, and most digestible kind of bread. It owes its superiority in these respects to the large quantity of tenacious gluten which it contains. Undressed wheat-flour appears to act, by the bran which it contains, as a mechanical stimulant to the bowels ; and hence brown bread is resorted to for the purpose of counteracting habitual constipation.

Uses.—Wheat-flour is employed in medicine both as a therapeutical and a pharmaceutical agent. It is used with great advantage as a dusting powder in burns and scalds. It cools the part, excludes the air, and absorbs the discharge, with which it forms a crust which effectually protects the subjacent part. When the crust has become detached by the accumulation of purulent matter beneath, a poultice may be applied, and after the removal of the crust the exposed surface may be again dusted over with flour. A mixture of flour and water is used as a chemical antidote in poisoning by the salts of mercury, copper, zinc, silver, and tin, and by iodine (see Vol. i. p. 165).

Flour is a constituent of some poultices, as the *yeast-poultice* (see *ante*, p. 47), and the *mustard-poultice*.

It is used in pharmacy for enveloping pills.

1. AMYLUM TRITICI ; *Amylum; Wheat-starch.*—This starch was known to Pliny,[1] who says the discovery of it was first made in Chios, and that it received its name amylum (ἄμυλον ; from α, negative, and μύλος, *a mill*) because it was not prepared by grinding in a mill.

There are various modes of preparing it, but the method followed in this country is a mechanico-chemical one, the starch being separated from the other ingredients of wheat partly by mechanical agency, and partly by chemical means. The cellulose or woody fibre of the grain is separated by mechanical means ; the gum, sugar, albumen, and soluble salts, are dissolved out by cold water ; and the gluten is got rid of partly by allowing it to undergo decomposition, and partly by solution in the acetic acid which is developed by fermentation.

A mixture of coarsely-grained wheat is steeped in water in a vat for one or two weeks (according to the state of the weather), by which acetous fermentation is established. The acid liquor (called *sour water*, or simply *sours*) is drawn off, and the impure starch washed on sieves to separate the bran. What passes through is received in shallow vessels termed *frames.* Here the starch is deposited. The sour liquor is again drawn off, and the *slimes* removed from the surface of the starch, which is to be again washed, strained, and allowed to deposit. The liquid which is drawn off is called *green water.* If the operation of washing be again resorted to, the part washed off is called *white water* instead of slimes, the liquid itself being still termed green water. When, by these processes, the starch has become sufficiently pure, it is *boxed ;* that is, it is placed in wooden boxes perforated with holes and lined with canvas, where it drains. It is then cut in square lumps, placed on chalk stones or bricks, to absorb the moisture, and dried in a stove. By this process the blocks are *crusted.* The blocks are then scraped, papered, labelled, stamped, and returned to the stove. Here they split into columnar masses (like grain tin or basaltic columns), commonly called the *race.*

In commerce there are two kinds of wheat-starch—one *white*, the other *blue.*

1. *White wheat-starch* is the sort which should be employed for dietetical or medicinal purposes. What is sold under the names of *French starch* and *patent white starch* is of this kind.

2. *Blue wheat-starch* is used by the laundress for stiffening linen. It owes its colour to finely-powdered smalt or indigo, which has been introduced into it before the boxing process. The *Poland* and *glaze starches* of the shops are of this kind. They are not adapted for medicinal purposes. When examined by the microscope, wheat-starch is perceived to consist principally of

---

[1] *Hist. Nat.* lib. xviii. cap. 17, ed. Valp.

large and small grains, with but few of intermediate size.[1] The smaller particles appear to be spheroidal, or nearly so. The large ones are rounded, and flattened or lenticular. When at rest, they appear to be globular; but, by making them roll over in water, they are seen to be flattened, compressed, or lenticular; one of the flattened faces being sometimes a little more convex than the other. Viewed edgeways, the particles are strongly shaded. In the middle, or nearly so, of the flattened surface is the rounded, elongated, or slit hilum. This is surrounded by concentric rings, which extend frequently to the edge of the grains. When heated, the particles crack at the edges.

[Considerable discussion has of late taken place as to the structure of the starch-granule; some observers (among whom may be mentioned the late Dr. Pereira) being of opinion that it was composed of a number of overlapping scales or concentric layers of varying size, the edges of which being seen, produced the appearance of concentric rings. These he considered were invested by a thin transparent membrane. Other observers consider the starch-granule to be composed of this external membrane, containing within it a granular matter, and describe the concentric rings as produced by corrugations of the investing cell-walls.[2] —ED.]

When heated in a tray in an oven to 300° F., wheat-starch acquires a buff colour, and is converted into dextrine or *British gum*.

Boiled in water, wheat-starch yields a *mucilage*, which, when sufficiently concentrated, forms, on cooling, a *jelly* (*hydrate of starch*).[3] The consistence of this jelly is due to the mutual adhesion of the swollen hydrated integuments of the starch-grains. When submitted to prolonged ebullition in a large quantity of water, the granule almost entirely dissolves, and the decoction, on cooling, does not gelatinise. With iodine the decoction, when cold, forms the blue iodide of starch, the colour of which is destroyed by alkalies and by heat.

The composition of wheat-starch is $C^{12}H^{10}O^{10}$. [It is isomeric with gum and cane sugar.—ED.]

Wheat-starch is not employed alone as food. As found in commerce, its taste is somewhat disagreeable.

Starch-powder is used as a dusting powder to absorb acrid secretions and to prevent excoriation. Its decoction is used as an emollient and demulcent clyster in inflammatory conditions of the large intestines, and as a vehicle for the formation of other more active enemata. Starch is an antidote for poisoning by iodine, and is sometimes given in combination with this substance to

---

[1] The following measurements of the starch-grains of different sizes of common and spelt wheat were made by Mr. George Jackson :—

Common Wheat.			Spelt Wheat.		
1.	·0009	of an English inch.	1.	·0012	of an English inch.
2.	·0006	" "	2.	·0010	" "
3.	·0004	" "	3.	·0005	" "
4.	·0003	" "	4.	·0003	" "
5.	·0002	" "	5.	·0001	" "
6.	·0001	" "			

Pharm. Journ. Dec. 1854.

[The jelly of starch warmed for a few minutes with diluted sulphuric acid, or even saliva, is converted to glucose. A solution of starch has no power of redissolving oxide of copper when an excess of potash is present; and, until it has undergone the chemical conversion above mentioned, it will not reduce the oxide on boiling.—ED.]

prevent its local action (see Vol. i. p. 412). It enters into the composition of the *Pulvis Tragacanthæ compositus*, Ph. L.

2. DECOCTUM AMYLI, L. ; *Mucilago Amyli*, E. ; *Decoction* or *Mucilage of Starch.* (Starch, ʒiv.; Water, Oj. Rub the starch with the water gradually added, then boil for a short time.)—It is sometimes used alone as an enema in dysentery, irritation of the rectum, &c. It is a constituent of the *Enema Opii*, L.

3. FURFURES TRITICI ; *Bran.*—Decoction or infusion of bran is sometimes employed as an emollient foot-bath. It is also taken internally as a demulcent in catarrhal affections. Its continued use causes a relaxed condition of bowels. Bran poultices are applied warm in abdominal inflammation, spasms, &c. *Bran bread* is used in diabetes (see p. 97, foot-note).

4. FARINA TRITICI TOSTA ; *Baked Flour.*—Wheat-flour lightly baked, so as to acquire a pale buff tint, is an excellent food for infants, invalids, and convalescents. Unlike the more amylaceous substances (such as arrow-root, tapioca, sago, &c.), it contains flesh- and blood-making as well as fat-making ingredients. Moreover, it has no tendency to relax the bowels; on the contrary, I think it is somewhat constipating. Hence, therefore, it may be used with advantage where there is a tendency to diarrhœa. When employed as an infant's food, it may be sometimes desirable to mix it with a fourth of its weight of prepared barley-meal, to obviate its constipating effects. It is prepared by boiling it in milk or milk and water, and is taken as a kind of pottage or gruel.

Hard's Farinaceous Food is a fine wheat-flour, which has been subjected to some heating process. It is an excellent preparation.

5. TURUNDÆ ITALICÆ ; *Macaroni, Vermicelli,* and *Italian* or *Cagliari Paste* (in the form of stars, lentils, &c.)—These are pastes made with the finest and most glutinous wheat. By the artificial addition of wheat-gluten to the ordinary wheat, products may be obtained which rival the finest Italian pastes.[1] The *granulated gluten* (*gluten granulé*) of MM. Véron frères is a paste made in this way. These various preparations are agreeable and most nourishing foods. Boiled in beef-tea, or similar fluids, they may be taken with great advantage by invalids and convalescents.

6. PANIS TRITICEUS ; *Wheaten Bread.*—This is of two kinds,—fermented or leavened, and unfermented or unleavened.

a. Panis fermentatus ; *Fermented or Leavened Bread.*—The ingredients used in its manufacture are wheat-flour, salt, water, and yeast. In making the ordinary loaf-bread of London, the baker always employs a portion of potatoes,—not for adulteration, but to assist fermentation, and to render the bread lighter. Patent yeast (see *ante*, p. 45) is generally employed by him on the score of economy. The yeast excites the fermentation of the sugar, which it converts into alcohol and carbonic acid: the former is dissipated in the oven, and the latter, distending the dough, causes it to *rise*, and gives the vesicular character to bread. During the process, a portion of starch is converted into soluble gum (dextrine) and a small portion of sugar.

---

[1] Payen, *Précis de Chimie Industr.* p. 397, 1849.

The following table represents the comparative composition of the flour and bread of wheat, according to Vogel :[1]—

Flour.		Bread.	
Starch	68·0	Starch	53·5
Sugar	2·3	Sugar	3·6
Gum	2·5	Starch-gum	18·0
Moist gluten	24·3	Gluten, with some starch	20·75
Albumen	1·5	Carbonic acid, and the hydrochlorates of lime and magnesia.	
	98·6		95·85

Flour in baking takes up a considerable quantity of water, the absolute amount of which, however, depends on several circumstances. Home-made bread baked in separate tins contains about 44 per cent. of water, whereas the flour from which it is made contains only about 16 per cent. Ordinary bakers' bread, baked in united loaves, contains as much as 50 or 51 per cent. of water. Various additions made to wheat-flour enable it to take up more water [and to retain this water.] Common salt does this : in the language of the baker it gives stiffness or strength to the dough. Alum (used by bakers under the name of "*stuff*") has a similar effect : it also augments the whiteness and fineness of bread, and renders it less liable to crumble. It therefore enables the baker to use an inferior flour with less chance of detection. Sulphate of copper (in the proportion of one grain to two pounds of flour) has a like effect, and has been used in some parts of Belgium to adulterate bread. It is said to enable the latter to take up 6 per cent. more water without appearing moister.[2]

The general dietetical properties of bread resemble those of wheat-flour (see *ante*, p. 93). In diabetes its use is objectionable on account of its augmenting the saccharine condition of the urine.[3] In some forms of dyspepsia, fermented bread disagrees with the patient; and, in such, benefit is occasionally obtained by the substitution of unfermented bread. The use of *brown bread* as a preventive of habitual costiveness has already been referred to (see *ante*, p. 93). It, however, frequently fails to produce the desired effect.

Fermented bread is employed both in medicine and pharmacy. *Crumb of bread* (*mica panis*) is sometimes used in the formation of pills; but is objectionable for this purpose, on account of the pills thus made becoming

[1] Quoted by Gmelin, *Handb. d. Chem.* Bd. ii. S. 1341 and 1343 ; also, *Journ. de Pharm.* t. iii. p. 211, 1817.

[2] For further details respecting the chemistry of fermented bread, the reader is referred to Dumas, *Traité de Chimie appliquée aux Arts,* t. vi. 1843 ; Johnston's *Lectures on Agricultural Chemistry,* 2d edit. 1847 ; and Payen, *Précis de Chimie Industrielle,* 1849.

[3] Bourchardat (*Comptes rendus,* Nov. 1841, p. 942) suggested the use of a *gluten-bread,* in diabetes, as a substitute for the ordinary wheaten bread ; but in practice it has not been found available. When quite devoid of starch, it can be masticated only with extreme difficulty, and, in fact, is not edible.—*Bran-bread* is, perhaps, the best kind of bread for diabetic patients. Dr. Prout (*Stomach and Renal Diseases,* 5th edit. p. 44, 1848) has published a receipt for a bread of this kind, devised by his patient, the late Rev. J. Rigg. The following formula yields the best product which I have seen, and has proved highly useful in one case of diabetes :—Take coarse *wheat-bran ;* wash it thoroughly with water on a sieve, until the water passes through clear ; then dry it in an oven, and grind to a fine powder by a mill (the mill which was found to answer was made by White, in Holborn). Then take 7 eggs, 1 pint of milk, ¼ lb. of butter, a few caraways or some ginger, and make into a paste with a sufficiency of the bran-flour. Divide the mass into seven equal parts, and bake each separately, in a saucer, by rather a quick oven : the time required for baking is usually about twenty minutes.—Dr. Percy (*Chemical Gazette,* March 15, 1849) has published a receipt for a bread for diabetic patients made of the ligneous matter of potatoes (see the article *Solanum tuberosum*).

excessively hard by keeping. Furthermore, in some cases, the constituents of bread decompose the active ingredients of the pills. Thus the chloride of sodium of bread decomposes nitrate of silver. Crumb of bread is most valuable for the preparation of poultices. The *bread-and-water-poultice* is prepared by covering some bread in a basin with hot water : after it has stood for ten minutes, pour off the excess of water, and spread the bread about one-third of an inch thick on soft linen, and apply to the affected part. Sometimes lint dipped in oil is applied beneath the poultice.[1] Decoction of poppy, or Goulard's water, may be substituted for common water. This is a valuable application to phlegmonous inflammation. A *bread-and-milk-poultice*, to which lard is sometimes added, is also used to promote suppuration; but it should be frequently renewed, on account of its tendency to undergo decomposition. Both poultices are used in the treatment of irritable ulcers.

β. *Panis sine fermento; Panis azymus; Unfermented Bread.*—Of this there are two kinds ;—one compact and heavy, the other light and elastic.

Of the *heavy and compact* kind of unfermented bread we have an example in the common sea-biscuit or ship-bread (*panis nauticus*), which, on account of its hardness and compactness, must be more slowly permeated and acted on by the gastric juice than the ordinary light and porous fermented bread. These biscuits are frequently adulterated with chalk.[2] Some dyspeptics prefer the lighter kinds of biscuits (*panis biscoctus*) to fermented bread. *Biscuit powder* is frequently used for infants' food.

The *light and porous* kinds of unfermented bread owe their lightness and porosity to some volatile or gaseous body developed in the dough by either heat or chemical action. In the preparation of certain kinds of biscuits, solid sesquicarbonate of ammonia is used, to produce lightness. The heat of the oven volatilises the salt, the vapour of which distends the dough. Carbonic acid (developed by the action of an acid on an alkaline carbonate) is, however, the agent generally employed to give porosity to unfermented bread. The *patent unfermented bread* is a preparation of this kind. The following receipt yields an excellent product :—Take of Flour, lb.j.; Bicarbonate of Soda, 40 grains; Cold Water, half a pint, or as much as may be sufficient: Muriatic Acid of the shops, 50 drops; Powdered White Sugar, a tea-spoonful. Intimately mix the bicarbonate of soda and sugar with the flour, in a large basin, by means of a wooden spoon. Then gradually add the water with which the acid has been previously mixed, stirring constantly, so as to form an intimate mixture very speedily. Divide into two loaves, and immediately put them into a quick oven.—If any soda should escape the action of the acid, it causes one or more yellow spots, which, however, are more unsightly than detrimental. The sugar may be omitted if thought desirable. This kind of bread is well adapted for the use of invalids and dyspeptics. With the latter it sometimes agrees when ordinary fermented bread disagrees. It is superior to biscuits in lightness and porosity. It is a very convenient kind of bread for persons on ship-board and in other places where yeast cannot be procured.[3]

---

[1] Abernethy, *Lancet*, vol. v. 1824, p. 135.

[2] [We have found 10 per cent. of chalk in some biscuits intended for sea use, under a contract.—Ed.]

[3] The above formula yields a bread of excellent quality, as I can vouch from having repeatedly employed it. Various other formulæ have been published, many of which doubtless also yield

38. SECALE CEREALE, *Linn.*—COMMON RYE.

Sex. Syst. Triandria, Digynia.

(Semina, *Offic.*)

HISTORY.—Rye is mentioned in the English version of the Old Testament;[1] but in the opinion of Sprengel[2] spelt wheat is meant. The same writer also states that Theophrastus[3] is the earliest author who notices the *Secale cereale;* but the word τιφη, used by Theophrastus, is thought by Fraas[4] to refer to *Triticum monococcum*, and not to rye. Galen[5] mentions rye under the name of βριςα, the term by which, as well as by σικαλι, rye is known in modern Greece.[6] Pliny[7] speaks of *secale* or rye.

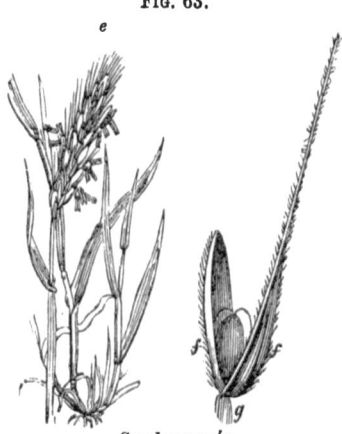

FIG. 63.

Secale cereale.

e, entire plant; *f f*, paleæ; *g*, receptacle.

BOTANY. **Gen. Char.** — *Spikelets* 2-flowered. *Florets* sessile, distichous, with the linear rudiment of a third terminal one. *Glumes* 2, herbaceous, keeled, nearly opposite, awnless or awned. *Paleæ*2,herbaceous; the lower one awned at the point, keeled, unequal sided, broadest and thickest on the other side; the upper shorter and bicarinate. *Stamina* 3. *Ovarium* pyriform, hairy. *Stigmata* 2, nearly sessile, terminal, feathery, with long, simple, finely-toothed

excellent products, The following are given in a little pamphlet entitled *Instructions for making Unfermented Bread*, by a Physician, 15th edit. 1848 :—

TO MAKE WHITE OR FLOUR BREAD.

Take of Flour, dressed or household	8 lbs. avoirdupoise.
Bicarbonate of soda, in powder	9 drachms, apothecaries' weight.
Hydrochloric (muriatic) acid	11¼ fluidrachms.
Water	about 25 fluidounces.

TO MAKE BROWN OR MEAL BREAD.

Take of Wheat-meal (that is, wheat well ground, as it comes from the mill, retaining the whole of the bran)	3 lbs. avoirdupoise.
Bicarbonate of soda, in powder	10 drachms, apothecaries' weight.
Hydrochloric (muriatic) acid	12½ fluidrachms.
Water	about 28 fluidounces.

In the shops are sold powders under various names (such as *Borwick's Original German Baking Powder for making Bread without Yeast;* and *Edwards's Egg Powder*), to enable persons to prepare a light bread without yeast, or even light puddings without eggs. They are usually mixtures of *tartaric acid* and *carbonate of soda*, with some farinaceous substance (*wheat-flour* and *potato-starch*); to which is sometimes added, a small portion of *alum*. They are very useful and convenient preparations [provided the proportions of the ingredients be properly adjusted.—ED.], and for employment on board-ship, and in various other situations, will be found very valuable.

[1] *Exodus*, ix. 32.
[2] *Hist. Rei Herb.* ii. 9, 1807.
[3] *Hist. Plant.* lib. viii. cap. 9.
[4] *Synops. Pl. Floræ Classicæ*, pp. 306 and 307, 1845.
[5] *De Alim. Facult.* lib. i. cap. xiii. tom. vi. p. 320.
[6] Fraas, *op. supra cit.* ; also, *Pharm. Græca*, pp. 501 and 540, 1837.
[7] *Hist. Nat.* lib. xviii. cap. 39 and 40, ed. Valp.

hairs. *Scales* 2, entire, ciliate. *Caryopsis* hairy at the point, loose (*Kunth*).

Sp. Char.—*Glumes* and *awns* scabrous (*Kunth*).

Hab.—The Caucasian-Caspian desert. Cultivated in Europe; but little in England; frequently on the continent.

Description.—Rye grains (*caryopsides* vel *semina secalis* vel *frumenti*), in external appearance, more resemble wheat than other cereal grains; but they are smaller and darker externally. Internally they are white and farinaceous: externally brownish. Like wheat, as found in commerce, they are devoid of their husk or paleæ.

In order that the changes which rye undergoes when it becomes ergotised may be better understood, Corda[1] has given the following description of the microscopic characters of healthy rye grains :—" When we submit a thin transverse section of a healthy grain of rye to microscopic examination, we perceive that the seed-coat (fig. 64, *a*) consists of three layers of thick-walled

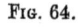

FIG. 64.   FIG. 65.   FIG. 66.

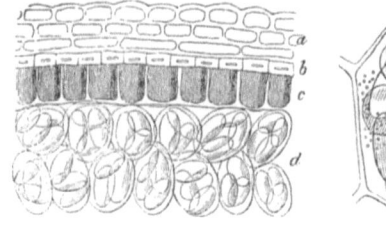
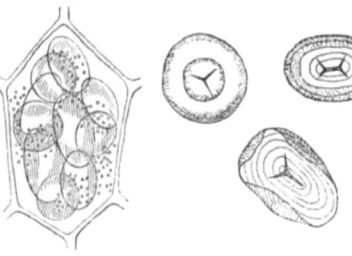

Microscopic appearance of a healthy Grain of Rye (highly magnified).

Fig. 64. A thin section of a ripe grain of rye. *a*, seed-coat; *b*, inner seed-coat; *c*, layer of gluten cells; *d*, cells of the albumen filled with starch grains.

Fig. 65. A single cell of the albumen more highly magnified, and showing the starch grains with which it is filled.

Fig. 66. Grains of rye starch very highly magnified (according to Corda).

cells, beneath which we find the second, properly the third, seed-coat (64, *b*) composed of a single layer of thick-walled cells, having scarcely any cavity. Next follows a layer of cells containing gluten (64, *c*); and afterwards the cellular tissue of the albumen (64, *d*). This consists of large roundish hexagonal cells, which contain grains of starch (fig. 65). The starch-grains (fig. 66) are roundish or ellipsoidal, and about the 0·000150 of the Paris line in length."

Composition.—Rye has been analysed by Einhof,[2] by Boussingault,[3] by Fuerstenburg,[4] and by Payen (see *ante*, p. 71). The proportion of starch and proteine compounds contained in it, as ascertained by Krocker and Horsford, have been before stated (see *ante*, Vol. i. p. 67).

[1] *Betrag zur Kenntniss der Brandarten der Cerealien und des Mutterkorns,* in the *Oekonomische Neuigkeiten und Verhandlungen,* No. 83, Vienna, 1846.
[2] L. Gmelin, *Handb. d. Chem.* Bd. ii. S. 1343.
[3] Quoted by Johnston, *Lectures on Agricultural Chemistry.*
[4] *Journ. f. pr. Chem.* Bd. xxxi. S. 195.

RYE-SEEDS.		
	Einhof.	Boussing.
Husk or bran	24·2	24
Pure meal	65·6	63·08
Moisture	10·2	12·92
	100·0	100·00

RYE-MEAL.		
	Einhof.	Boussing.
Starch	61·07	64·0
Gum	11·09	11·0
Gluten	9·48 ⎱	
Albumen	3·28 ⎰ ···	10·5
Saccharine matter	3·28	3·0
Husk	6·38 & salts	6·0
Undetermined acid and loss	5·42	2·0
Fatty matter	0·00	3·5
	100·00	100·0

The composition of the ashes of rye is stated at p. 71.

1. PROTEINE COMPOUNDS. *Fibrin, Glutin, and Albumen.*—The so-called gluten of rye differs from wheat-gluten. It is not cohesive, and is soluble in water and alcohol: but after it has been dissolved in alcohol it is insoluble in water. It agrees in its properties with the glutin of wheat (see Vol. i. p. 64; and *ante*, p. 90). Heldt[1] considers it to be identical in composition with the other proteine compounds of rye analysed by Dr. Bence Jones and Scheerer.

2. STARCH.—The starch of rye, like that of wheat, consists principally of large and small grains, with but few of intermediate size; the larger ones being, on the whole, somewhat larger than the corresponding ones of wheat.[2] The shape of the larger grains is circular, flat, or lenticular; of the smaller ones globular (chiefly), ellipsoidal or ovoidal, rarely angular or mullar-shaped. On the flattened surface of the larger grains is seen the central, rarely circular, usually slit, or 3-, 4-, or even 5-radiate hilum, sometimes surrounded by very faint concentric rings and delicate radiating lines. By polarised light the grains show a central cross.

CHEMICAL CHARACTERISTICS.—A cold decoction of rye forms with iodine the blue iodide of starch. By washing rye-dough with water, nearly the whole becomes diffused through the liquid, little more than husk or bran remaining behind. The milky liquid deposits on standing starch-grains, and the decanted portion yields on evaporation the so-called gluten; from which, sugar is extracted by water, and oil by ether: the residue (*glutin*) is soluble in alcohol.

PHYSIOLOGICAL EFFECTS.—In its nutritive qualities rye resembles wheat, especially in the fitness of its flour for making bread; but it contains less proteine matter and more sugar.

USES.—Rye is employed dietetically and medicinally; and also in the distillery and brewery.

Rye-bread (in Germany called *Schwartzbrod* or *black bread*) is in common use among the inhabitants of the northern parts of Europe, but in this country is rarely employed. It is said to be more laxative (especially to those unaccustomed to its use) than wheat-bread; and hence is sometimes taken to counteract habitual constipation. The *roasted seeds* (*semina secalis tosta*) have been employed as a substitute for coffee. On the continent *rye-flour* and *rye-bran* are applied to the same medicinal uses that wheat-flour and wheat-bran are applied in England. Rye pottage (*pulmentum* vel *jusculum secalinum*) is said to be a useful article of diet in consumptive cases.[3]

---

[1] *Ann. d. Chem. u. Pharm.* Bd. xlv. S. 198, 1843.

[2] The following measurements of eight (including the largest and smallest) grains of rye starch were made by Mr. George Jackson :—

1.	0·0016 of an English inch.		5.	0·0005 of an English inch.	
2.	0.0015	" "	6.	0·0003	" "
3.	0·0013	" "	7.	0·0002	" "
4.	0·0010	" "	8.	0·0001	" "

[3] Pearson, *Pract. Synop. of the Mat. Alim.* 91.

39. SECALE CORNUTUM.—SPURRED RYE OR ERGOT.

SYNONYMES.—*Clavi siliginis*, Lonicerus ; *Secalis mater*, Thalius ; *Secale luxurians*, Bauhin, Pinax, lib. i. sect. iv. p. 23 ; *Grana secalis degenerati*, Brunner ; *Secale cornutum*, Baldinger ; *Clavus secalis* vel *secalinus* ; *Secale maternum, turgidum* vel *temulentum* ; *Ergota*, Ph. Lond. et Ed. ; *Spur ; Spurred* or *horned Rye ; Ergot of Rye ; Cockspur Rye ; Cockspur.*

HISTORY.—No undoubted reference to ergot is found in the writings of the ancients. The disease produced by it is supposed to be referred to in the following passage:—" 1089. A pestilent year, especially in the western parts of Lorraine, where many persons became putrid, in consequence of their inward parts being consumed by St. Anthony's fire. Their limbs were rotten, and became black like coal. They either perished miserably, or, deprived of their putrid hands and feet, were reserved for a more miserable life. Moreover, many cripples were afflicted with contraction of the sinews [*nervorum contractio*]."[1]

The first botanical writer who notices ergot[2] is Lonicerus.[3] It seems to have been employed by women to promote labour pains long before its powers were known to the profession. Camerarius,[4] in 1683,[5] mentions that it was a popular remedy in Germany for accelerating parturition. In Italy and France, also, it appears to have been long in use.[6]

BOTANY.—The nature and formation of ergot are subjects on which botanists have been much divided in opinion.

1. **Some regard ergot as a fungus growing between the glumes of grasses in the place of the ovary.** — Otto von Münchausen,[7] Schrank,[8] De Candolle,[9] Fries,[10] Wiggers,[11] and formerly Berkeley, adopted this opinion, and described ergot as a fungus

---

[1] Extract from the works of Sigebert, in the *Recueil des Histoir. des Gauls et de la France*, t. xiii. p. 259. A passage somewhat similar to the above, with the addition of the following, " the bread which was eaten at this period was remarkable for its deep violet colour," is quoted by Bayle (*Biblioth. Thérap.* tom. iii. p. 374,) from *Mézerai, Abrégé Chronologique*. But I cannot find the passage in the first and best edition of Mezeray's *Abrégé Chron.*, 3 vols. 4to. 1668 ; or in his *Histoire de France ;* or in his *Mémoires Hist. et Critiques*. Whether or not it be in the second and less perfect edition of Mezeray's *Abrégé Chronologique*, I am unable to decide, not having seen this work.

[2] The etymology of the word *ergot* is very doubtful. Whiter (*Etymologicon Universale*, ii. 594,) thinks that it is derived from *arguo*, and is attached to such terms as *urgeo*. It was anciently written *argot*. [In the Dictionary of the Academy, ergot is given as the French name for the spur of a cock and the claws of a dog, and there are also an adjective, verb, and substantive of similar or metonymic signification. The disease is evidently called ergot from its resemblance to a cockspur. —ED.]

[3] *Kreuterbuch*, p. 885, Franckfort, 1582.

[4] *Actes des Curieux de la Nature*, art. 6, obs. 82, quoted by Velpeau.

[5] Dierbach, *Neuest Entd. in d. Mat. Med.* 130, 1837.

[6] Bayle, *Bibl. Thérap.* iii. 375. Velpeau, in his *Traité Complet de l'Art des Accouchemens*, gives an excellent literary history of ergot.

[7] *Hausvater*, i. 332, 1764-1773.

[8] *Baiersche Flora*, ii. 571, 1789.

[9] *Mém du Mus. d'Hist. Nat.* ii. 401, 1815.

[10] *Syst. Mycol.* ii. 268, 1822.

[11] *Inq. in Secale Corn.* Götting. 1831, in Christison's *Treatise*.

under the name of *Spermoedia Clavus*,[1] Fries (*Clavaria Clavus*, Münch.; *Sclerotium Clavus*, De Cand.) Fries and Berkeley, however, evidently entertained some doubts respecting its nature; for the first suggests that the genus Spermoedia consists of " *semina graminum morbosa*," and the second says " it appears to be only a diseased state of the grain, and has scarcely sufficient claim to be admitted among fungi as a distinct genus." The latest writer who has adopted this view is Guibourt,[2] who concludes that ergot is not an ovary or altered grain, but a fungus which, *after the destruction of the ovary*, is grafted in its place on the peduncle.

Against this opinion may be urged the circumstance noticed by Tessier,[3] that a part only of the grain may be ergotised. Moreover, the scales of the base of the ergot, the frequent remains of the stigma on its top, and the articulation of it to the receptacle, prove that it is not an independent fungus, but an altered grain.[4]

2. **Some regard ergot as a diseased condition of the ovary or seed.**—The arguments adduced against the last opinion are in favour of the present one. Though a considerable number of writers have taken this view of the nature of the ergot, there has been great discordance among them as to the causes which produce the disease.

α. *Some have supposed that ordinary morbific causes (such as moisture combined with warmth) were sufficient to give rise to this diseased condition of the grain.* Tessier[5] and Willdenow[6] appear to have been of this opinion.

β. *Some have ascribed the disease to the attack of insects or other animals.* Tillet, Fontana, Réad, and Field,[7] supported this view, which, I may add, has subsequently been satisfactorily disproved.

γ. *Some, dissatisfied with the previously assigned causes of the disease, have been content with declaring ergot to be a disease, but without specifying the circumstances which induce it.* Mr. Bauer,[8] who closely watched the development of ergot during eight years (1805–13), and has made some beautiful drawings of it in different stages, arrived at this conclusion; as also Phœbus.[9]

δ. *Others have referred the production of the disease to the presence of a parasitic fungus.* This opinion, which appears to me to be the correct one, and which must not be confounded with that entertained by De Candolle and others (vide *supra*), has been adopted and supported by Léveillé in 1826,[10] by Dutrochet,[11] by Mr. John Smith,[12] and by the late Mr. Edwin Quekett;[13] and more recently by Fée[14] and by Corda.[15] But though the writers just mentioned agree in considering ergot to be a disease of the ovary or seed, caused by a parasitic fungus, considerable difference exists among them as to the real nature of the parasite.[16]

The statements of Léveillé, Phillipar,[17] Smith, and Quekett, leave, I think, but little doubt that ergot is a disease of the grain caused by the presence of a parasitical fungus. This view is supported by the observations of Wiggers, that the white dust (*sporidia*, Quek.) found on the surface of ergot will

---

[1] Erroneously quoted in the *Pharm. Lond.* 1836 as *Acinula Clavus*.
[2] *Hist. Nat. des Drogues*, 4me édit. t. ii. p. 72, 1849.
[3] Quoted by De Candolle.
[4] Quekett, in *Proceedings of the Linn. Soc.* Dec. 4, 1838.
[5] *Mem. Soc. Roy. Médec.* 1776, p. 417; 1777, p. 587.
[6] In Christison's *Treatise on Poisons.*
[7] Referred to by Christison, *op. cit.*
[8] MS. *British Museum*; also, *Trans. of the Linn. Society*, vol. xviii.
[9] *Deutschl. kryptogam. Giftegewächse*, Berlin, 1838.
[10] *Ann. de la Soc. Linn. de Paris.*
[11] *Mémoires pour servir à l'Histoire anatomique et physiologique des Végét. et des Animaux*, vol. ii. p. 161, 1837.
[12] *Trans. Linn. Society*, vol. xviii.
[13] *Ibid.*
[14] *Mémoire sur l'Ergot du Seigle, et sur quelques Agames qui vivent Parasites sur les Epis de cette Céréale*, 1er Mém. Strasbourg, 1843. See *Pharm. Journ.* vol. v. p. 282, 1846.
[15] *Beitrag zur Kenntniss der Brandarten der Cerealien und des Mutterkorns*, in the *Oekonomische Neuigkeiten und Verhandlungen*, No. 83, published at Vienna, 1846.
[16] I have given an abstract of M. Fée's opinion in the *Pharmaceutical Journal*, vol. vi. p. 228.
[17] *Traité Organogr. et Phys.-Agr. sur la Carie, le Charbon, l'Ergot*, &c. 8vo. Versailles, 1837.

produce the disease in any plant (grass?) if sprinkled in the soil at its roots. Mr. Quekett infected grains of corn by immersing them in water in which the sporidia of the *Oidium abortifaciens* were contained. The plants which were produced by the germinations of the grains were all ergotised. Mr. Quekett, who most carefully examined the development of ergot, says that the first appearance of the ergot is observed by the young grain and its appendages becoming covered with a white coating composed of multitudes of sporidia mixed with minute cobweb-like filaments. This coating extends over all the other parts of the grain, cements the anthers and stigmas together, and gives the whole a mildewed appearance. When the grain is immersed in water, the sporidia fall to the bottom of the liquid. A sweet fluid—at first limpid, afterwards viscid—is found in the affected flower at this stage; and, when examined by the microscope, is found to contain the sporidia just referred to (Phillipar, Smith, Quekett). Phillipar says this fluid oozes from the floral centre; and Mr. Quekett, who at first thought that it had an external origin, was subsequently convinced that it escaped from the ergot or the parts around it.

Fig. 67.

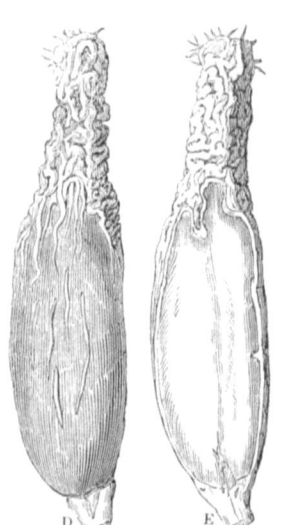

Ergot of Rye.

A. A side view of a longitudinal section of an infected grain, soon after fecundation, when the disease makes its first external appearance: magnified eight times in diameter.
B. Front view of a section of the above infected grain, cut at letter *a*: magnified sixteen times in diameter.
C. Ditto, cut at letter *b*: magnified sixteen times in diameter.

D. Side view of an unripe but advanced ergotised grain, at the upper part of which is the tuberculated portion, having a vermiform appearance, and constituting the fungus (*Sphacelia segetum*) of Léveillé.
E. Longitudinal section of the grain.
F. A full-grown ergot, within its floret, magnified twice its diameter.

If we examine the ergot when about half-grown (fig. 67), we find it just beginning to show itself above the paleæ, and presenting a purplish-black colour. By this time it has lost in part its white coating, and the production of sporidia and filaments has nearly ceased. At the upper portion of the grain, the coating now presents a vermiform appearance, which Léveillé[1] describes as constituting cerebriform undulations. These are beautifully depicted in Mr. Bauer's drawings (fig. 67, A D E). Léveillé regards this terminal tubercle of the grain as a parasitical fungus, which he calls the *Sphacelia Segetum*. But these undulations are merely masses of sporidia; for if a little be scraped off with a knife, then moistened and examined by the microscope, we find nothing but myriads of sporidia. The ergot now increases in a very rapid manner.

Corda has confirmed the observations of Messrs. Smith and Quekett; but, as I have already stated, he considers the fungus to be a new species of *Hymenula* (of the suborder *Hymenophycetes*), to which he has given the name of *H. clavus*.

[Tulasne, who has thrown so much light on many obscure points in the history of fungi, has at length shown, beyond the possibility of a doubt, that ergot is a diseased state of the grains, induced by the mycelium of Cordyceps purpurea Fr., and some other species. An elaborate memoir on the subject was published in 1853, in the *Annales des Sciences Naturelles*, from which it appears that if the ergoted grains are sown, after a few months the Cordyceps is developed from the mycelium, a fact which has been confirmed by Mr. Berkeley and Mr. Broome. The Hymenula of Corda is simply the spermatia of the Cordyceps, or, as Tulasne calls the genus, Claviceps. Whether the Oidium abortifaciens be a mere conidiferous state of the mycelium of the Cordyceps, or a distinct fungus, is at present uncertain. The ergot of the seed produces Cordyceps microcephala, as does that of Molinia cærulea; and the ergot of Scirpus produces Cordyceps nigricans.—ED.]

The accompanying figures (*a, b, c,* and *d,*) are after Tulasne.

FIG. 68.

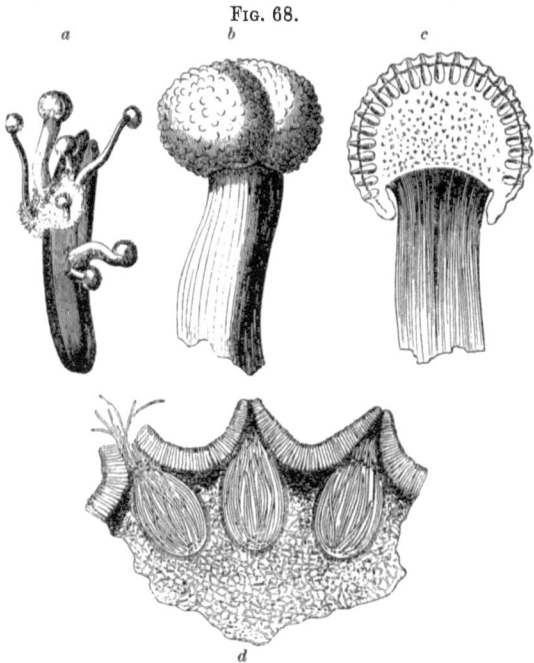

Specimens of Cordyceps purpurea.

a. An ergotised grain of rye, giving rise to a tuft of Cordyceps purpurea (nat. size.)

b. Upper part of stem and head slightly magnified. The perithecia project in consequence of a slight contraction of the substance.

c. Section of the same, showing the perithecia.

d. A portion of do. more highly magnified, showing the structure of the same, and the asci in the perithecia.

---

[1] Quoted by Richard, *Elém. d'Hist. Nat.* i. 332.

To the agriculturist, an important subject of inquiry is the predisposing causes of ergot. Very little of a satisfactory nature has, however, been ascertained on this point. One fact, indeed, seems to have been fully established —viz. that moisture, which was formerly thought to be the fertile source of the spur, has little, if any thing, to do with it.[1] Moreover, the disease is not peculiar to rye. Many other grasses (Phœbus has enumerated 31 species) are subject to it. In the summer of 1838 I found the following grasses, growing in Greenwich marshes, ergotised :—*Lolium perenne, Dactylis glomerata, Alopecurus pratensis, Festuca pratensis, Triticum repens,*

Fig. 69.

Arundo phragmites, Hordeum murinum, and *H. pratense.* Professor Henslow found it in wheat which had been sent to the miller.[2] I am indebted to him also for fine specimens of ergot on *Ammophila arundinacea.* But the disease is not confined to the *Gramineæ:* the *Cyperaceæ* are also subject to it, and perhaps, likewise, *Palmaceæ.*[3]

COMMERCE.—Ergot is imported from Germany, France and America. The late Mr. Butler, of Covent Garden Market, told me that about $1\frac{1}{2}$ tons were imported in the year 1839.

DESCRIPTION.—When we examine a number of ears of ergotised rye, we find that the number of grains in each spike which have become ergotized varies considerably: there may be 1 only, or the spike may be covered with them.[4] Usually the number is from 3 to 10.

The mature ergot (fig. 67) projects considerably beyond the paleæ. It has a violet-black colour, and presents scarcely any filaments and sporidia.

The spurred rye, or ergot

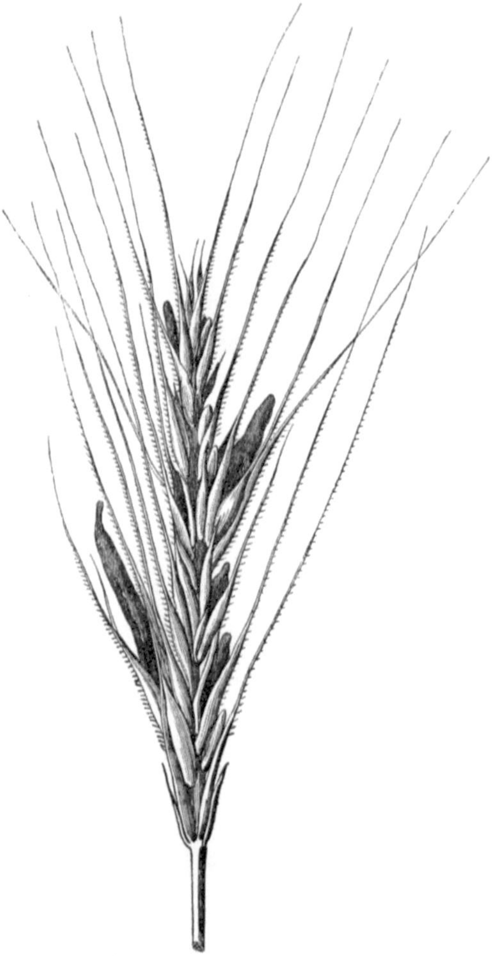

Full-grown Ear of Rye, strongly infected with ergot (nat. size).

---

[1] Phillipar, *op. cit.* 126 ; also, Bauer, *MSS.*
[2] *Report on the Diseases of Wheat,* p. 20, from the *Journal of the Royal Agricultural Society of England.*
[3] Phœbus, *op. cit.* 105.
[4] Phillipar, *op. cit.* p. 96.

(*ergota*) of commerce, consists of grains which vary in length from a few lines
to an inch, or even an inch and a half, and whose breadth is from half a line
to four lines. Their form is cylindrical or obscurely triangular, with obtuse
angles, tapering at the extremities (fusiform), curved like the spur of a cock,
unequally furrowed on two sides, often irregularly cracked and fissured. The
odour of a single grain is not detectable, but of a large quantity is fishy,
peculiar, and nauseous. The taste is not very marked, but is disagreeable, and
very slightly acrid. The grains are externally purplish-brown or black, more
or less covered by a bloom, moderately brittle, the fractured surface being
tolerably smooth, and whitish or purplish-white. Their sp. gr. is somewhat
greater than that of water, though, when thrown into this liquid, they usually
float at first, owing to the adherent air. The lower part of the grain is sometimes heavier than the upper.

When examined by the microscope, we find that the ergot consists of three
distinct parts :

1. The *internal part* or *body* of the ergot : this is composed of the hexagonal or rounded cellular tissue. The cells have the shape and regularity of the normal cells of the albumen, but they are considerably
   smaller (Corda says they are only $\frac{1}{35}$th of the size), and contain,
   instead of starch, from one to three globules of oil, which are lighter
   than water and soluble in ether (fig. 70 *d*, and 72). If the structure of ergot be examined after the grains have been dried and
   re-moistened, the tissue presents a very irregular appearance.

2. The *violet* or *blackish* coat of the ergot : this consists of a layer of
   longitudinally elongated delicate cells (see fig. 70 *c*).

3. The *bloom*, which to a greater or less extent covers the violet coat of
   the ergot : it resembles the bloom of plums, and may be readily wiped
   off. According to the late Mr. Quekett, it consists of the sporidia
   of the *Oidium abortifaciens*. But Corda describes it as consisting of two parts : a layer of cylindrical, undivided cells (*sporophores* or *basidia*, fig. 70, *b*) supporting the spores (fig. 70, *a*, and
   fig. 71).

FIG. 70.   FIG. 71.   FIG. 72.

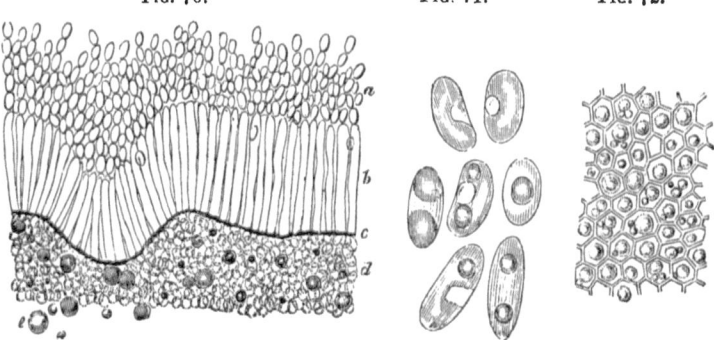

Microscopic appearance of Ergotised Rye (highly magnified) according to Corda.

Fig. 70. Thin transverse section of ergot of rye. *a*, layer of spores ; *b*, sporosphores or basidia ;
         c, epidermis of the receptacle ; *d*, body of the receptacle ; *e*, oil globules.
Fig. 71. Spores of the fungus very highly magnified. [It is probable that Corda confounded the
         Ergotætia of Quekett with the spermatia of Tulasne.—ED.]
Fig. 72. Body of the receptacle, with the cells containing oil.

In considering the metamorphosis which the normal rye-grains have undergone by becoming ergotised, it appears that the seed-coats and gluten-cells (fig. 64, *a b c*, p. 100) have been replaced by a layer of dark cells (fig. 70, *c*); that the large cells of the albumen (fig. 64, *d*, and fig. 65, p. 100) have been replaced by the small cells of the ergot (figs. 70, *d*, and 72); that the starch-grains of the cells of the albumen (fig. 65 and fig. 66) have been replaced by drops of oil in the cells of the ergot (fig. 70, *d*, and fig. 71); and that the little body at the top of the ergot (fig. 67, F *a*), which Phœbus calls the *Mützchen,* is the remains of the hairy crown of the grain, of the stigmata, and of the withered elevated pericarp.

Thus the entire organisation of the grains is changed, and at the same time their effects on the animal body are altered; for while sound rye is edible, nutritive, and healthy, ergotised rye is unwholesome and poisonous, producing raphania and abortion.

DETERIORATION.—The ergot of rye is fed on by a little acarus, which is about one-fourth of the size of a cheese-mite. This animal destroys the interior of the ergot, and leaves the grain as a mere shell. It produces much powdery excrementitious matter (Quekett). In four months $7\frac{1}{2}$ ounces of this fæcal matter of the acarus were formed in seven pounds of ergot. I have some ergot which has been kept for eleven years in a stoppered glass vessel without being attacked by the acarus, and it has all the characteristics of good ergot. It is advisable, however, not to use ergot which has been kept for more than two years.

COMPOSITION.—Ergot was analysed, in 1816, by Vauquelin;[1] in 1817, by Pettenkofer;[2] in 1826, by Winkler;[3] in 1829, by Maas;[4] in 1831, by Wiggers;[5] and more recently by Chevallier.[6] The results obtained by Chevallier were analogous to those of Wiggers.

Vauquelin's Analysis.	*Wigger's Analysis.*	
Pale yellow matter, soluble in alcohol, and tasting like fish-oil.	*Ergotin*	1·25
	Peculiar fixed oil	35·00
White bland oil, very abundant.	White crystallisable fat	1·05
Violet colouring matter, insoluble in alcohol, soluble in water.	Cerin	0·76
	Fungin	46·19
A fixed acid (phosphoric?).	Vegetable osmazome	7·76
Vegeto-animal or nitrogenous matter, prone to putrefaction, and yielding ammonia and oil by distillation.	Peculiar saccharine matter	1·55
	Gummy extractive, with red colouring matter	2·33
Free ammonia, disengaged at 212° F.	Albumen	1·46
	Superphosphate of potash	4·42
	Phosphate of lime, with trace of iron	0·29
	Silica	0·14
	Ergot	102·20

1. ERGOTIN was procured by digesting ergot with ether, to remove the fatty matter, and then in boiling alcohol. The alcoholic solution was evaporated, and the extract treated by water. The ergotin remained undissolved. It was brownish-red, with an acrid bitter taste, and, when warmed, had a peculiar but unpleasant odour. It was

[1] *Ann. Chim.* iii. 337.
[2] Buchner's *Repert.* iii. 65.
[3] Christison, *On Poisons.*
[4] Schwartze, *Pharm. Tabell.* 2er Ausg. 460.
[5] Phœbus, *Giftgewächse,* 102; *Journ. de Pharm.* xviii. 525, 1832.
[6] Dierbach, *Neuest. Entd. in d. Mat. Med.* 1837, p. 129.

soluble in alcohol, but insoluble in water or ether. It is probable, therefore, that it is a resinoid colouring matter. It proved fatal to a hen. Nine grains of it were equal to an ounce and a half of ergot. It appears, then, that though a poisonous principle, it is pro-bably not the agent which acts on the uterus, for the latter is soluble in water, whereas ergotin is not. It is possible, however, that it may be rendered soluble in water by com-bination with some other body.

[Winckler has succeeded in obtaining propylamine ($NH^3C^6H^6$) by distilling ergotin with potash. He considers it is present in combination with formic acid, and that it is not produced by the potash (as is the case when it is obtained by the action of potash on narcotina) but that it preexists, and is merely liberated from the formic acid by the alkali. He proposes that experiments be made to determine whether or not the thera-peutical action of ergot depends on propylamine; but it seems now clearly proved that the efficacy of ergot is altogether independent of ergotin, and that in all probability it entirely resides in the oily and fatty matters. Winckler's experiments of more recent date seem to have led him to believe that what he considered propylamine is really a new substance for which he proposes the name of secalin. There remains much yet to be done before we can feel much confidence in enunciating the chemistry of this subject.[1]—ED.]

2. OIL OF ERGOT.—As this is now used in medicine, its properties will be described hereafter.

There are no good grounds for suspecting the existence of either hydrocyanic acid or phosphate of morphia in ergot, as supposed by Pettenkofer.

CHEMICAL CHARACTERISTICS.—Ergot is inflammable, burning with a clear yellowish white flame. The aqueous infusion or decoction of ergot is red, and possesses acid properties. Both acetate and diacetate of lead cause precipitates in a decoction of ergot. Iodine gives no indication of the presence of starch. Nitrate of silver causes a copious precipitate soluble in ammonia, but insoluble in nitric acid. Tincture of nutgalls also produces a precipitate (*tannate of ergotin?*). Alkalies heighten the red colour of the decoction.

PHYSIOLOGICAL EFFECTS.—Great discrepancy is to be found in the accounts published respecting the influence of spurred rye on man and animals. While the majority of experimenters or practical observers concur in assigning to it energetic powers, others have declared it harmless.

a. On Vegetables.—Schübler and Zeller have tried its effects on plants, and I infer from their statements that they found it poisonous.[2]

β. On Animals.—Accidental observation and direct experiment concur in showing that in most instances spurred rye acts as a poison to the animal economy. But, as Phœbus correctly observes, we cannot call it a *violent* poison, since drachms and even ounces are required to destroy small animals (*e. g.* rabbits and pigeons). It has proved poisonous to flies, leeches, birds (geese, ducks, pigeons, common fowls, &c.), and mammals (dogs, cats, pigs, sheep, rabbits, &c.) Birds and mammals refuse to take it, even mixed with other kinds of food. Diez[3] gives the following as the symptoms produced by it in dogs who are compelled to swallow it :—" Great aversion to it, discharge of saliva and mucus from the mouth, vomiting, dilatation of the pupil, quickened respiration and circulation, frequent moanings, trembling of the body, continual running round, staggering gait, semi-paralysis of the extremities, especially the hinder ones, sometimes diarrhœa ; sometimes hot anus, increased formation of gas in the alimentary canal; faintness and sleepiness, with great thirst, but diminished appetite. Death followed under gradually

---

[1] *Pharm. Journ.* vol. xii. p. 42, vol. xiii. p. 86.
[2] Marx, *Die Lehre v. d. Giften*, ii. 107.
[3] Quoted by Phœbus, *op. cit.* p. 106.

increasing feebleness, without being preceded by convulsions. To the less constant symptoms belong inflammation of the conjunctiva, and the peculiar appearance of turning round in a circle from right to left." Similar observations as to its injurious operation have been made by Robert.[1] In some cases abscess and gangrene of various parts of the body, with dropping off of the toes and convulsions, have been noticed. A strong decoction injected into the vein of a dog caused general feebleness, paralysis of the posterior extremities, vomiting, and death.[2]

But there are not wanting cases apparently shewing that spurred rye has no injurious action on animals. The most remarkable and striking are those related by Block.[3] In 1811, twenty sheep ate together nine pounds of it daily for four weeks without any ill effects. In another instance, twenty sheep consumed thirteen pounds and a half daily, for two months, without injury. Thirty cows took together twenty-seven pounds daily, for three months, with impunity; and two fat cows took, in addition, nine pounds of ergot daily, with no other obvious effect than that their milk gave a bad caseous cream, which did not yield good butter. These statements furnish another proof to the toxicologist that the ruminants suffer less from vegetable poisons than other animals.

Another interesting topic of inquiry is the action of ergot on the gravid uterus of mammals. Chapman[4] says "it never fails, in a short time, to occasion abortion." We have the testimony of Percy and Laurent, that a decoction injected into the veins of a cow caused the animal to calve speedily; and in one out of three experiments, Mr. Combes has stated, the ergot caused abortion in the case of a bitch.[5] Diez[6] found that it caused uterine contractions in dogs, rabbits, and sows. Large doses given to bitches induced an inflammatory condition of the uterus, and destroyed both mother and her young. However, in opposition to these statements, we have the evidence of Chatard, Warner, Villeneuve, and others, who failed in producing abortion with it.[7]

I am indebted to the late Mr. Youatt, formerly Veterinary Surgeon to the Zoological Society, for the following note respecting the effects of ergot on animals :—" I have, for the last six or seven years, been in the habit of administering the ergot of rye to quadrupeds in cases of difficult or protracted parturition, in order to stimulate the uterus to renewed or increased action. In the *monogastric*, if I may venture to use the term, I have never known it fail of producing considerable effect, even when the uterus has been previously exhausted by continued and violent efforts. In the *ruminant*, with its compound stomach or stomachs, I have witnessed many a case of its successful exhibition. I have had recourse to it in the cow, the sheep, and the deer, both foreign and domestic. Parturition has not always been accomplished, from false presentation or other causes, but the uterus has in every case responded—it has been roused to a greater or less degree of renewed action. On the other hand, there are cases recorded by veterinary practi-

---

[1] Christison, *op. cit.*
[2] Gaspard, *Journ. de Phys. expér.* ii. 35.
[3] Phœbus, *op. cit.* p. 107.
[4] *Elem. of Therap.* i. 489, 4th edit.
[5] Neal, *Researches respecting Spur or Ergot of Rye*, p. 90.
[6] Phœbus, p. 106.
[7] Neal, *op. cit.*

tioners, in which it has been given in very large quantities without producing the slightest effect. I have always attributed this to a certain degree of forgetfulness of the construction of the stomachs of ruminants. If the medicine, as is too often the case, is poured hastily down, and from a large vessel, it breaks through the floor of the œsophagean canal and falls into the rumen, and there it remains perfectly inert. But if it is suffered to trickle down the œsophagean canal, although a portion of it may still enter the rumen, the greater part will flow on through the œsophagean canal and the manyplies into the fourth or villous stomach, and produce the desired effect."

γ. *On Man.*—These may be noticed under two heads : 1, effects of single doses; 2, effects of its continued use as an article of food.

1. *In single or few doses.*—Hertwig,[1] Lorinser,[2] Jörg,[3] and Diez,[4] who have endeavoured to ascertain the effects of ergot by experiment, agree in stating that, in doses of from half a drachm to two drachms, nausea, inclination to vomit, dryness of the throat, great thirst, aversion to food, uneasiness or actual pain in the abdomen, occasionally alvine evacuations, weight and pain in the head, giddiness, in some cases stupor and dilatation of pupils, have resulted from its use. It deserves, however, to be noticed, that these effects have not been observed by some experimenters.[5] The effects produced by the use of a single or a few doses of ergot may be conveniently arranged under four heads.

a. Effects on the uterine system. (Uterine contractions.)—The action of spurred rye on the uterus, *when labour has actually commenced,* is usually observed in from ten to twenty minutes after the medicine has been taken, and is manifested by an increase in the violence, the continuance, and the frequency of the pains, which usually never cease until the child is born ; nay they often continue for some minutes after, and promote the speedy separation of the placenta and the firm contraction of the uterus in a globular form. The contractions and pains caused by ergot are distinguished from those of natural labour by their continuance ; scarcely any interval can be perceived between them, but a sensation is experienced of one continued forcing effort. If from any mechanical impediment (as distortion) the uterus cannot get rid of its contents, the violence of its contraction may cause its rupture, as in the cases alluded to by Dr. Merriman,[6] Mr. Armstrong,[7] and Mr. Coward.[8] Ergot sometimes fails to excite uterine contractions. The causes of failure are for the most part conjectural. The quality of the ergot, peculiarities on the part of the mother, and death of the fœtus, have been assigned as such. The two first will be readily admitted ; but why the remedy should be altogether inert " where the fœtus has been for some time dead, and putrefaction to any extent taken place,"[9] cannot be readily explained. Its

---

[1] Sundelin, *Heilmittell.* i. 513, 8te Aufl.
[2] *Edin. Med. and Surg. Journ.* xxvi. 453.
[3] *Gebrauch inn. Reizm. z. Beförd. d. Geburt.* 1833.
[4] Phœbus, *op. cit.*
[5] Keil, *Diss. inaug. de Secali Cornuto,* Berol. 1822, quoted in Sundelin, *Heilmittell.;* also, Dr. Chapman, *Elem. of Therap.* vol. i. p. 488, 4th edit.
[6] *Syn. of Diff. Part.* p. 197, 1838.
[7] *Lond. Med. Gaz.* Aug. 4, 1838.
[8] *Ibid.* Nov. 27, 1840. Did the ergot cause the rupture, in the case related in the *Lancet,* vol. i. 1836-7, p. 824, by Mr. Hooper?
[9] Dr. Bibby, in Merriman's *Synopsis,* p. 198.

occasional failure has been urged by the late Dr. Hamilton[1] as an argument in favour of his notion that ergot acts " in no other way than by influencing the imagination." But on the same ground the sialogogue power of mercury might be denied. Dr. Hamilton's erroneous estimate of the power of ergot is referable to a want of experience of its use ; for he admits that he has only had two opportunities in practice of making a fair trial of it.

There is usually much less hemorrhage after delivery, when ergot has been employed, than where it has not been exhibited. The lochial discharges are also said to be less : but this is certainly not constantly the case. Moreover, it has been asserted " that the menstrual discharge has not recurred after the use of the ergot in certain cases of protracted parturition."[2] But the inference intended to be conveyed here, viz. that ergot caused the non-recurrence, is not correct ; at least, I am acquainted with several cases in which this effect did not follow the employment of spurred rye, and I know of none in which it did. Ergot has been charged with causing the death of the child ; but the charge has been repelled by some experienced practitioners as being devoid of the least foundation. " The ergot," says Dr. Hosack,[3] " has been called in some of the books, from its effects in hastening labour, the *pulvis ad partum;* as it regards the child, it may with almost equal truth be denominated the *pulvis ad mortem ;* for I believe its operation, when sufficient to expel the child, in cases where nature is alone unequal to the task, is to produce so violent a contraction of the womb, and consequent convolution and compression of the uterine vessels, as very much to impede, if not totally to interrupt, the circulation between the mother and child." However, Dr. Chapman[4] strongly denies this charge, and tells us that in 200 cases which occurred in the practice of himself and Drs. Dewees and James, the ergot was used without doing harm in any respect ; and he adds, " no one here believes in the alleged deleterious influence of the article on the fœtus." It is not improbable, however, where the impediment to labour is very great, that the violent action of the uterus may be attended with the result stated by Dr. Hosack. Dr. F. H. Ramsbotham[5] has suggested that the poisonous influence of ergot may be extended from the mother to the fœtus, as in the case of opium. He also states,[6] that of 36 cases in which he induced premature labour by puncturing the membranes, 21 children were born alive; while in 26 cases of premature labour induced by ergot only, 12 children only were born alive. This fact strongly favours the notion of the deleterious influence of the ergot on the fœtus.

Given to excite abortion, or premature labour, ergot has sometimes failed to produce the desired effect. Hence many experienced accoucheurs have concluded, that for this medicine to have any effect on the uterus it is necessary that the process of labour should have actually commenced.[7] But while we admit that it sometimes fails, we have abundant evidence to prove that it frequently succeeds ; and most practitioners, I think, are now satisfied

---

[1] *Pract. Observ. relating to Midwifery,* part ii. p. 84, 1836.
[2] Dr. J. W. Francis, in the 3d American edition of Deuman's *Midwifery,* 1829.
[3] *Essays,* vol. ii. 296.
[4] *Elem. of Therap.* i. 488, 4th edit.
[5] *Lond. Med. Gaz.* vol. xiv. p. 84.
[6] *Ibid.* June 15, 1839.
[7] Bayle, *Bibl. Thérap.* ii. 550.

that in a large number of cases it has the power of originating the process of accouchement. Cases illustrating its power in this respect are referred to by Bayle;[1] and others are mentioned by Waller,[2] Holmes,[3] Ramsbotham,[4] Müller,[5] and others.[6]

The action of ergot *on the unimpregnated uterus* is manifested by painful contractions, frequently denominated "bearing-down pains," and by the obvious influence which it exercises over various morbid conditions of this viscus; more particularly by its checking uterine hemorrhage, and expelling polypous masses. Tenderness of the uterus, and even actual metritis, are said to have been induced by it.[7]

β. Effects on the Cerebro-Spinal System. (*Narcotism*).—Weight and pain in the head, giddiness, delirium, dilatation of pupil, and stupor, are the principal symptoms which indicate the action of ergot of rye on the brain. Dr. Maunsell[8] has published five cases (viz. two which occurred to Dr. Churchill, one to Dr. Johnson, and two to Dr. Cusack), in which delirium or

---

[1] *Op. cit.* p. 550.

[2] *Lancet*, 1826, vol. x. p. 54.

[3] *Ibid.* 1827–28, vol ii. pp. 794.

[4] *Lond. Med. Gaz.* xiv. pp. 85 and 434; also, *Ibid.* June 15, 1839.

[5] Dierbach, *Neuesten Entd. in d. Mat. Med.* i. 139, 1837.

[6] [On trials for criminal abortion perpetrated or attempted, a medical witness must be prepared for a close examination on the specific emmenagogue properties of the drug administered. A very instructive case, which occurred a few years since (*Reg.* v. *Calder*, Exeter Lent Assizes, 1844), has been ably reported, with comments, by Dr. Shapter (*Prov. Med. Journal*, April 10, 1844.) It was alleged in this case, that savin, cantharides, and ergot, had been respectively given by the prisoner, a medical man, for the purpose of procuring miscarriage. The prosecutrix was a woman of notoriously bad character, and the prisoner was acquitted. There were three medical witnesses who agreed that savin and cantharides were only likely to occasion abortion indirectly, *i. e.* by powerfully affecting the system—the view commonly entertained by professional men. Some difference of opinion existed with regard to *ergot*. Dr. Shapter stated in his evidence, that he did not think the ergot would act unless the natural action of the uterus had commenced,—a statement supported by a number of authorities. Subsequently to the trial, he collected the observations of many obstetric writers, and so far modified his opinion as to admit that the ergot might *occasionally* exert a specific action on the uterus, in cases of advanced pregnancy, even when uterine action had *not* already commenced. His summary on this subject is one of the best which has been published. Dr. Ramsbotham has reported three cases, from which it would appear that the ergot may in some instances exert a direct action on the impregnated uterus. In these instances, the females were in or about the *eighth* month of pregnancy. (*Med. Gaz.* xiv. 434.) This observation has been fully confirmed by further experience on the use of the drug (*Med. Times and Gaz.* Jan. 7, 1854, p. 8. See also his *Obstetric Med. and Surg.* 198.) Dr. J. H. Davis believes that it is a specific excitant of uterine action, and points out the cases in which, in his opinion, it may be safely employed. (*Lancet*, Oct. 11, 1845, 393.) Mr. Whitehead, who has had considerable experience on this subject, has found that its action is very uncertain. In a case under his care, that of a woman with deformed pelvis, it was considered advisable to procure abortion in the fifth month of pregnancy; the ergot alone was employed, and at first with the desired effect. It was given in three successive pregnancies; and in each instance labour-pains came on after eight or ten doses had been administered, and expulsion was effected by the end of the third day. It was perseveringly tried in a fourth pregnancy in the same female, and failed completely. (*On Abortion*, 224.) It also failed in a recent case in the hands of Dr. Oldham. (*Med. Gaz.* vol. xliv., p. 49.) Nevertheless, the balance of evidence is now decidedly in favour of its specific action; and, according to Dr. Griffiths, this is so well known to the inhabitants of the United States, that it is in very frequent use as a popular abortive. Perhaps the differences which have been observed in its action may depend, in some cases, on the period at which it has been administered to a pregnant woman. Admitting that the uterus is subject to periodical excitement, corresponding to the menstrual periods, it is probable that the action of the ergot may be more powerfully abortive at these than at other times. The reader will find a large collection of cases, illustrating the properties of this drug, in Wibmer (*Arzneimittel und Gifte*, ii. 80: *Sphacelia Segetum.*)—ED.]

[7] Dr. Negri, *Lond. Med. Gaz.* xiv. 369.

[8] *Lond. Med. Gaz.* xvi. 606.

stupor resulted from the use of ergot (in half-drachm and two-drachm doses), and was accompanied by great depression of pulse.[1] Trousseau and Pidoux[2] found that under the repeated use of ergot, dilatation of pupil was the most common symptom of cerebral disorder. It began to be obvious in from twelve to twenty-four hours after the commencement of the use of the medicine, and sometimes continued for several days after its cessation. The cerebral disorder is frequently preceded by the uterine contractions, and usually remains for some time after these have subsided.

Effects of ergot on the circulatory system.—I have known increased frequency and fulness of pulse, copious perspiration, and flushed countenance, follow the use of ergot during parturition. But in most instances the opposite effect has been induced : the patient has experienced great faintness, the pulse has been greatly diminished in both frequency and fulness, and the face has become pale or livid. In one case, mentioned by Dr. Cusack,[3] the pulse was reduced from 120 to 90. Dr. Maunsell has referred to four other cases. These effects on the circulatory system were accompanied with cerebral disorder, of which they were probably consequences. Similar observations, as to the power of ergot to diminish the frequency of the pulse, have been noticed by others.[4]

δ. *Other effects of ergot.*—Nausea and vomiting are not uncommon consequences of the exhibition of ergot when the stomach is in an irritable condition. Various other symptoms have been ascribed to the use of ergot; such as weariness of the limbs and itching of the skin.[5]

2, *Effects produced by the continued use of ergot as an article of food* (*Ergotism*, Fr. ; *Raphania*, Linn. Vog. Cull. Good ; *Convulsio raphania, and Eclampsia typhodes*, Sauv. ; *Morbus Spasmodicus*, Rothm. ; *Morbus convulsivus, malignus, epidemicus, cerealis, &c.* Alt. ; *Krieblekrankheit, or the creeping sickness*, Germ.)—Different parts of the continent, *e. g.* France (especially in the district of Sologne), Silesia, Prussia, Bohemia, Saxony, Denmark, Switzerland, and Sweden, have been, at various periods, visited with a dangerous epidemic (known by the names above mentioned), which affected, at the same time, whole districts of country, attacking persons of both sexes and of all ages.[6] So long back as 1597, (Tissot), the use of ergotized rye was thought to be the cause of it. Various circumstances have appeared to prove the correctness of this opinion,[7] which has been further confirmed by the effects of ergot on animals, as well as by the occurrence of a disease similar to, if not identical with, ergotism, in consequence of the use of damaged wheat.[8] Yet several intelligent writers have not acquiesced in this view ; and the circumstances mentioned by Trousseau,[9] and by Dr. Hamilton,[10] are certainly calculated to throw some doubts over the usually received opinion.

---

[1] See also Dr. Cusack, in *Dubl. Hosp. Rep.* vol. v. p. 508.
[2] *Traité de Thérap.* i. 546.
[3] Dr. Maunsell, *Lond. Med. Gaz.* xiv. 606.
[4] Merriman, *Synopsis*, pp. 201 and 203, 1838 ; Trousseau and Pidoux, *Traité de Thérap.* i. 547.
[5] Trousseau and Pidoux, *op. cit.* i. 547.
[6] Tissot, *Phil. Trans.* vol. lv. ; Rothman, *Amœn. Acad.* vi. 430.
[7] *Mém. de la Soc. Roy. de Méd.* i. 1777.
[8] *Phil Trans.* for 1762 ; Henslow, *op. supra cit.*
[9] *Traité de Thérap.* i. 527.
[10] *Practical Observations relative to Midwifery*, part ii. p. 85.

Ergotism assumes two types ; the one of which has been denominated the *convulsive*, the other the *gangrenous ergotism.* Whether these arise from different conditions of the ergot, or from peculiarities on the part of the patient, or from the different quantity of the ergot taken, we are hardly prepared now to say. In *convulsive ergotism*, the symptoms are weariness, giddiness, contraction of the muscles of the extremities, formication, dimness of sight, loss of sensibility, voracious appetite, yellow countenance, and convulsions, followed by death. In the *gangrenous ergotism* there is also experienced formication ; that is, a feeling as if insects were creeping over the skin, voracious appetite, coldness and insensibility of the extremities, followed by gangrene.[1]

USES.—To Dr. Stearns, of the United States, is due the credit of introducing ergot of rye to the notice of the profession as an agent specifically exciting uterine contractions.[2] In 1814, a paper was published by Mr. Prescot,[3] on the effects of it in exciting labour-pains, and in uterine hemorrhage. It was not employed in England until 1824. The following are the principal uses of it :—

1. *To increase the expulsatory efforts of the womb in protracted or lingering labours.*—When the delay of delivery is ascribable solely to the feeble contractions of the uterus, ergot is admissible, provided, first, that there be a proper conformation of the pelvis and soft parts ; secondly, that the os uteri, vagina, and os externum, be dilated, or readily dilatable, and lubricated with a sufficient secretion ; and, lastly, that the child be presenting naturally, or so that it shall form no great mechanical impediment to delivery. A natural position of the head is not an absolute essential for the use of ergot, since this medicine is admissible in some cases of breech presentation.[4] The circumstances which especially contraindicate or preclude the use of this medicine are those which create an unusual resistance to the passage of the child : such are, disproportion between the size of the head and of the pelvis, great rigidity of the soft parts, and extraneous growths. Moreover, " earliness of the stage" of labour is laid down by Dr. Bigelow[5] as a circumstance contraindicating the use of ergot. The proper period for its exhibition is when the head of the child has passed the brim of the pelvis. Some practitioners assert that a dilated or lax condition of the os uteri is not an essential requisite for the exhibition of ergot. It has been contended that one of the valuable properties of this medicine is to cause the dilatation of the uterine orifice ; and cases are not wanting to confirm these statements.[6]

2. *To hasten delivery when the life of the patient is endangered by some alarming symptoms.*—Thus, in serious hemorrhages occurring during labour, after the rupture of the membranes, and where the placenta is not situated over the os uteri, the ergot is especially indicated.[7] It has also been

---

[1] Christison, *Treatise on Poisons;* Orfila, *Toxicol. Gén. ; Phil. Trans.* 1762 ; Henslow's *Report on the Diseases of Wheat,* in the *Journal of the Royal Agricultural Society of England,* vol. ii. 1841.

[2] *New York Med. Repos.* vol. xi. 1807 ; quoted in the *United States Dispensatory.*

[3] *Med. and Phys. Journ.* vol. xxxii. p. 90, 1815.

[4] Dr. F. H. Ramsbotham, *Lond. Med. Gaz.* xiv. 86.

[5] *Quarterly Journal of Literature, Science, and Arts,* ii. 63.

[6] Bayle, *op. cit.* p. 539.

[7] Dr. Blundell, *Lancet* for 1827-28, vol. i. p. 805 ; Dr. F. H. Ramsbotham, *Lond. Med. Gaz.* vol. xvi. pp. 86 and 692.

employed to accelerate delivery in puerperal convulsions.   Five successful
cases of its use are recorded by Bayle,[1] on the authority of Waterhouse,
Mitchell, Roche, Brinkle, and Godquin.   But the narcotic operation of ergot
presents a serious objection to its use in cerebral affections.

3. *To provoke the expulsion of the placenta when its retention
depends on a want of contraction of the uterus.*—In such cases ergot
has often proved of great advantage.[2]   When the hemorrhage is excessive
the ergot must not be regarded as a substitute for manual extraction, since,
during the time required for its operation, the patient may die from
loss of blood.[3]   In retention of the placenta from spasmodic or irregular
contraction of the uterus, as well as from morbid adhesion, ergot is improper
or useless.[4]

4. *To provoke the expulsion of sanguineous clots, hydatids, and
polypi from the uterus.*—Coagula of blood collected within the womb after
delivery may sometimes require the use of ergot to excite the uterus to expel
them, as in the case mentioned by Mackenzie.[5]   Ergot is also valuable in
promoting the expulsion of those remarkable formations called uterine hydatids,[6]
and which are distinguished from the acephalocysts of other parts of the body
by their not possessing an independent life, so that when separated from
their pedicles they die.[7]   A successful case of the use of ergot in this affection has been published by Dr. Macgill.[8]   In uterine polypus, ergot has been
exhibited with the view of hastening the descent of the tumour from the uterus
into the vagina, so as to render it readily accessible for mechanical extir-
pation ;[9] for it is well known that until this is effected the patient is con-
tinually subject to hemorrhage, which in some cases proves fatal.   In some
instances ergot has caused the expulsion of a polypus.[10]

5. *To restrain uterine hemorrhage, whether puerperal or non-puer-
peral.*—Ergot checks hemorrhage from the womb, principally, if not solely,
by exciting contraction of the muscular fibres of this viscus, by which its
blood-vessels are compressed and emptied, and their orifices closed.   The
experience of physicians and surgeons in all parts of the civilised world has
fully and incontestably established the efficacy of ergot as a remedy for uterine
hemorrhage.[11]   Maisonneuve and Trousseau[12] have shewn that the beneficial
influence of ergot is exerted equally in the unimpregnated as in the impregnated state ; proving, therefore, that the contrary statement of Prescott and
Villeneuve is incorrect.   Even in a case of cancer of the uterus they have
found it check the sanguineous discharge.   In females subject to profuse
uterine hemorrhages after delivery, ergot may be administered as a pre-

---

[1] *Bibl. Thérap.* iii. 448 and 548.
[2] Dr. Blundell, *Lancet*, 1827-28, vol. ii. 259 ; Bayle (*Bibl. Thérap.* vol. iii. 541) has recorded
nine cases, from Balardini, Bordol, Davies, Duchâteau, and Morgan ; and many others will be found
in the medical journals.
[3] Dr. F. H. Ramsbotham. *Lond. Med. Gaz.* xiv. 738.
[4] Dr. Jackson, *Lond. Med. Gaz.* iv. 105.
[5] Neal, *Researches*, p. 88.
[6] *Acephalocystis racemosa*, H. Cloq.
[7] Cruveilhier, *Dict. de Méd. et de Chir. prat.* art. Acéphalocystes, p. 260.
[8] Bayle, *op. cit.* p. 471.
[9] Dr. H. Davies, *Lond. Med. and Phys. Journ.* vol. liv. p. 102, 1825.
[10] *Lancet*, 1828-29, vol. i. p. 24.
[11] See the list of cases in Bayle's *Bibl. Thérap.* iii. 543.
[12] *Bull. de Thérap.* t. iv. ; also, Trousseau and Pidoux, *Traité de Thérap.* i. 540.

ventive, just before the birth of the child.[1] Even in placenta presentations, a dose or two of ergot may be administered previously to the delivery being undertaken.[2] To restrain excessive discharge of the lochia or catamenia, this remedy is sometimes most beneficial.

6. *To provoke abortion, and to promote it when this process has commenced and is accompanied with hemorrhage.*—Under certain circumstances the practitioner finds it expedient to produce abortion : as in serious hemorrhage during pregnancy, and in deformed pelves which do not admit the passage of a full-grown fœtus. In such cases the ergot may be employed with great advantage.[3] When abortion has already commenced, ergot may be employed to quicken the process and check hemorrhage.

7. *In leucorrhœa and gonorrhœa.*—Ergot was first given in leucorrhœa by Dr. M. Hall ;[4] and was subsequently employed by Dr. Spajrani[5] with success ; and in eight cases by Dr. Bazzoni,[6] seven of these were cured by it. Dr. Negri[7] published seven successful cases of its use. Its efficacy has been confirmed by many other practitioners. Dr. Negri also used it with apparent benefit, in gonorrhœa, in both the male and female. He concludes that " secale cornutum has a peculiar action on the mucous membranes ; but if exhibited when there is a state of acute inflammation, their morbid secretions may be considerably increased ; on the contrary, when a more chronic form of inflammation exists, the secale cornutum may have a beneficial influence in arresting their preternatural discharge."

8. *In hemorrhages generally.*—The power possessed by ergot of exciting uterine contractions, readily explains the efficacy of this agent in restraining sanguineous discharges from the womb ; but it has also been used to check hemorrhage from other organs. In these cases it can only act as a sedative to the circulation, in a similar way to foxglove. A considerable number of cases have been published in proof of its power of checking hemorrhage from other organs (as the nose, gums, chest, stomach, and rectum).[8] But having found it unsuccessful in my own practice, seeing that in the hands of others it has also failed,[9] and knowing how difficult it is to ascertain the influence of remedies on hemorrhages, I think further evidence is required to prove the anti-hemorrhagic powers of ergot.

9. *In amenorrhœa.*—Some few cases have been published tending to show that ergot possesses emmenagogue properties.[10] It appears to me to be more calculated to cause than to relieve amenorrhœa.

10. *In other diseases.*—Ergot has been employed in various other diseases with apparent success ; viz. intermittent fever,[11] paraplegia,[12] &c.

---

[1] Roche, *Dict. de Méd. et Chir. prat.* art. Ergot, p. 455.
[2] Dr. F. H. Ramsbotham, *Lond. Med. Gaz.* xiv. 660.
[3] *Ibid.* p. 434 ; also, Dr. Weihe, in *op. cit.* vol. xviii. 543.
[4] *Lond. Med. and Phys. Journ.* May 1829.
[5] *Lancet,* Feb. 5th, 1831.
[6] *Bayle,* p. 509.
[7] *Lond. Med. Gaz.* xiii. p. 369.
[8] See the cases of Drs. Spajrani, Pignacco, and Gabini, in the *Lancet* for 1830 and 1831 ; of Dr. Negri, in the *Lond. Med. Gaz.* xiii. 361.
[9] Trousseau and Pidoux, *Traité de Thérap.* i. 546.
[10] Neal, *Researches,* p. 79.
[11] Dierbach, *op. cit.* p. 444.
[12] Bayle, *op. cit.* p. 548.

Administration.—Ergot is usually given in the form either of powder or infusion. The decoction, less frequently the tincture, and still more rarely the extract, are also used. Latterly the ethereal oily extract or tincture, and oil, have been used.

1. PULVIS SECALIS CORNUTI; *Pulvis Ergotæ; Powdered Ergot.*—This powder is only to be prepared when required for use. The dose of it, for a woman in labour, is twenty grains, to be repeated, at intervals of half an hour, for three times; for other occasions (as leucorrhœa, hemorrhages, &c.) five to ten or fifteen grains, three times a day : its use should not be continued for any great length of time. It may be taken mixed with powdered sugar. It has had the various names of *pulvis parturiens* (more correctly *parturi-faciens*), *pulvis ad partum, pulvis partem accelerans, obstetrical powder,* &c.

2. INFUSUM ERGOTÆ, D.; *Infusion of Ergot.* (Ergot, in coarse powder, ʒij.; boiling water, fℨix. ; infuse for one hour in a covered vessel, and strain. The product should measure about eight ounces.)—The dose for a woman in labour is one-sixth or one-fourth of this quantity, to be repeated at intervals of half an hour, until the whole be taken. Sugar, aromatics (as nutmeg or cinnamon), or a little wine or brandy, may be added to flavour it.

3. DECOCTUM SECALIS CORNUTI; *Decoctum Ergotæ; Decoction of Ergot.* (Ergot, bruised, ʒj.; water, ℨvj. Boil for ten minutes in a lightly covered vessel, and strain.)—The dose is one-third of the strained liquor, to be repeated, at intervals of half an hour, until the whole be taken.

4. TINCTURA ERGOTÆ, D.; *Tincture of Ergot.*—Ergot in coarse powder, ℨviij.; Proof Spirit, Oij. Macerate for fourteen days, strain, express, and filter. Dr. Roberts[1] gave also a formula as follows :—Ergot, bruised, ℨss. ; Rectified Spirit, ℨvj. Digest for four days, and strain. The dose in lingering labours of both these preparations is a tea-spoonful. A tincture is recommended by Carus.[2] At Apothecaries' Hall, London, *tincture of ergot* is prepared by digesting ergot, ℨij. in proof spirit, Oj. Another formula has been published :[3] —Ergot, bruised, ℨj. ; boiling water, ℨij. Infuse for twenty-four hours, and add rectified spirit, ℨiss. Digest for ten days. Half a drachm of this tincture is said to be equivalent to ten grains of the powder. One or two spoonfuls of a tincture of ergot (prepared by digesting ℨss. of ergot in ℨiv. of rectified spirit) mixed with water, has been recommended as an injection into the uterus in difficult labour. It is to be introduced between the head of the child and the neck of the uterus.[5]

[**5. VINUM ERGOTÆ**, U. S.; *Wine of Ergot.* (Take of Ergot, bruised, ℨij.; White Wine, Oj. Macerate for fourteen days with occasional agitation : then express and filter through paper.)—This preparation is used as a substitute for the tincture.—Dose, ʒj. or ʒij.]

6. TINCTURA ERGOTÆ ÆTHEREA, L. (Take of bruised Ergot, ℨxv.; Ether, Oij. Macerate for seven days, then express and filter.)—This tincture may be

---

[1] Dierbach, *Neuesten Entd. in d. Mat. Med.* i. 147, 1838.
[2] *Lehrb. d. Gynäcologie,* i. 280, 1827.
[3] *Lancet,* 1827-28, vol. ii. p. 435.
[4] *Berlinisches Jahrbuch,* Bd. xxxviii. 234, 1837.

given in doses of ℥xv. to ʒss. every four hours in cases of hemorrhage of a slight character, but in order to exert ecbolic effects it must be given in doses of one drachm every half-hour for three or four doses; and this quantity is also required if we use the preparation to check violent internal hemorrhage.]

7. OLEUM ERGOTÆ ; *Oil of Ergot.*—The liquid sold in the shops under the name of *pure oil of ergot* is obtained by submitting the ethereal tincture of ergot to evaporation by a very gentle heat. Its colour is reddish brown. Mr. Wright[1] states that this depends on the age of the ergot, and that when obtained from recent specimens it is not unfrequently entirely free from colour. Its taste is oily and slightly acrid. It is lighter than water, and is soluble in alcohol and in solutions of the caustic alkalies. It is probably a mixture of several proximate principles. I made a guinea-pig swallow a fluidrachm of it : the only obvious effect was copious and frequent diuresis. Two fluidrachms diffused through water and injected into the jugular vein of a dog, caused trembling of the muscles, paralysis of the hind, and great weakness of the fore legs, which lasted for more than two days. The respiration and action of the heart were exceedingly rapid. The saliva streamed copiously from the mouth. The pupil was strongly dilated before the experiment, and no obvious change in it was induced by the oil. Mr. Wright found the oil very energetic. A drachm, he states, injected into the jugular vein caused dilatation of the pupil, feeble, slow, and intermittent action of the heart, deep and interrupted respiration, general paralysis, insensibility to punctures, and death in two hours and forty minutes. According to evidence adduced by Mr. Wright, the oil possesses the same influence over the uterus as that of the crude drug ; that is, it occasions powerful uterine contractions. To produce this effect it should be given in doses of from 20 to 50 drops in any convenient vehicle; as cold water, warm tea, or weak spirit and water.

The *ethereal solution of ergot* used by Dr. Lever[2] to promote uterine contraction is essentially a solution of the oil of ergot. It was prepared by digesting ℥iv. of powdered ergot in f℥iv. of ether during seven days. The tincture was submitted to spontaneous evaporation, and the residue dissolved in f℥ij. of ether. The dose of this solution is from ℥xv. to ℥xxx. on a lump of sugar.

8. EXTRACTUM SECALIS CORNUTI ; *Extractum Ergotæ; Bonjean's Ergotine.*—This is prepared by exhausting ergot of rye by means of water, and evaporating the liquors to the consistence of syrup. To this extract is to be added a considerable excess of alcohol, by which all the gummy matters and salts insoluble in alcohol are precipitated. The supernatant liquid is to be decanted and reduced in a water bath to the consistence of a soft extract. From 100 parts of ergot we obtain from 14 to 16 parts of extract, called, by Bonjean, *ergotine.* This extract is soft, reddish-brown, and homogeneous ; has an odour of roast meat, and a slightly piquant bitter taste. It may be employed medicinally in substance, made into pills, or dissolved in water. The dose of it is from five to ten grains. The aqueous solution of it is red, limpid, and transparent.

---

[1] *Ed. Med. and Surg. Journal*, vol. liv. p. 52.
[2] *Lond. Med. Gaz* new series, vol. ii. for 1839–40, p. 108.

ANTIDOTE.—The proper treatment to be adopted in a case of poisoning by an overdose of ergot has not been accurately determined. The first object would be, of course, to evacuate the poison from the alimentary canal by the use of emetics or purgatives. As chlorine decomposes ergotin, Phœbus recommends the employment of chlorine water. In the absence of this, nitro-hydrochloric acid (properly diluted) might be exhibited. The subsequent treatment should be conducted on general principles.

TRIBE V. ANDROPOGONEÆ, *Kunth.*

40. SACCHARUM OFFICINARUM, *Linn.*—THE SUGAR-CANE.

Sex. Syst. Triandria, Digynia.

(Sacchari fæx ; Saccharum : Succus præparatus, *L.*—Saccharum commune ; Sacchari fæx ; Saccharum purum, *E.*—Succus concretus, *a.* non purificatus, *b.* purificatus ; Syrupus empyreumaticus, anglice *molasses, D.*)

HISTORY.—The manufacture of sugar is said by Humboldt to be of the highest antiquity in China. Cane-sugar was known to the ancient Greeks and Romans, and was considered by them to be a kind of honey. Possibly, Herodotus[1] refers to it when he says that the Zygantes make honey in addition to that which they get from bees. Theophrastus[2] calls it *mel in arundinibus,* Dioscorides[3] terms it σάκχαρον; Pliny,[4] *saccharum.* Humboldt[5] adopts, too hastily I think, the opinion of Salmasius, that the latter writers meant the siliceous product of the Bamboo, viz. *Tabasheer ;* for, in the first place, as they arrange it with honey, it was probably sweet, which tabasheer is not; secondly, the Sanscrit name for sugar is *Sarkura ;*[6] thirdly, a passage in Lucan[7] seems distinctly to refer to the sugar cane—"Quique bibunt tenera dulces ab arundine succos." Surely no one will pretend to say that the bamboo is a "tenera arundo ?"[8]

BOTANY. **Gen. Char.**—*Spikelets* all fertile, in pairs, the one sessile, the other stalked, articulated at the base, 2-flowered, the lower floret neuter, with 1 palea, the upper hermaphrodite, with 2 paleæ. *Glumes* 2, membranous. *Paleæ* transparent, awnless, those of the hermaphrodite flower minute, unequal. *Stamens* 3. *Ovary* smooth. *Styles* 2, long ; *stigmas* feathered, with simple toothletted hairs. *Scales* 2, obscurely 2 or 3-lobed at the point, distinct. *Caryopsis* smooth (?), loose (?) (*Kunth*).

Sp. Char.—*Panicle* effuse. *Flowers* triandrous. *Glumes* obscurely 1-nerved, with very long hairs on the back (*Kunth*).

---

[1] Lib. iv. *Melpomene,* cap. cxciv.
[2] *De Melle.*
[3] Lib. ii. cap. civ.
[4] *Hist. Nat.* lib. xii. cap. xvii.
[5] *Journal of Science and Arts,* vol. v. p. 15.
[6] Royle's *Essay,* p. 83.—In his more recent work, called *Cosmos* (Sabine's translation, vol. ii. pp. 109 and xxvi.), Humboldt states that the Sanscrit name for sugar is the source of the Greek and Semitic names for it.
[7] Lib. iii. v. 237.
[8] References to passages in other ancient authors will be found in the notes to Valpy's edition of Pliny's *Hist. Nat.* vol. iv. 2193. See also Moseley's *Treatise on Sugar,* Lond. 1799.

The *stem* is solid, from six to twelve feet high. *Leaves* flat. *Panicle* terminal, from one to three feet long, of grey colour, from the long soft hair that surrounds the flower. *Paleæ* rose-coloured.

Kunth admits four varieties :—

α. *commune*, the *common yellow cane*, called by the Bengalees *Poori*, and by the West Indians the *Creole Cane* or *Native Cane*, from its having been the one originally introduced into the New World.

β. *purpureum*, the *purple cane*, called by the Bengalees *Kajooli*, and which is said to yield juice one-eighth richer than the yellow cane.

γ. *giganteum*, the *giant cane*, a large light-coloured cane, called by the Bengalees *Kullooa*. It grows in a low swampy soil, where the other two will not succeed. Its juice is weaker than that of the yellow cane, but the plant grows to a much larger size ; and it is, therefore, much cultivated in India.

δ. *tahitense*, the *Tahiti cane*, commonly called the *Otaheite cane*.

Hab.—It is cultivated in both Indies. Its native country is uncertain.

Two other species of *Saccharum* are cultivated for the sugar they produce :—
S. VIOLACEUM, Tussac, Antill. i. 160,—Kunth, Agrostogr. i. 474; *Violet Sugar-cane*. (By some authors considered to be identical with Tahiti sugar-cane, above mentioned.)— Cultivated in both Indies.
S. SINENSE, Roxb., Fl. Ind. ; *China Sugar-cane.*—Cultivated in China, where sugar is made from it.

COMPOSITION OF THE SUGAR-CANE.—Avequin[1] analysed the Tahiti and ribbon varieties of the fresh sugar-cane of Louisiana, and Dupuy[2] analysed the fresh sugar-cane at Guadaloupe. Peligot,[3] by combining the composition of cane-juice with that of the dried canes sent him from Martinique, has also deduced the composition of the fresh cane. More recently Casaseca[4] analysed the sugar-cane of Cuba.

	Dupuy.	Peligot.	*Avequin.*	
			Tahiti Cane.	Ribbon Cane.
Sugar	17·8	18·0		14·280	13·392
Cellulose	9·8	9·9		8·867	9·071
Mucilaginous, resinous, fatty, and albuminous matters ...	—	—		0·415	0·441
Salts	0·4	— { Salts, silica, and oxide of iron }	0·358	0·368
Water	72·0	72·1		76·080	76·729
Fresh Sugar-cane	100·0	100·0		100·000	100·001

The dried sugar-cane was analysed by O. Hervy.[5]

The composition of *sugar-cane ash* is an important consideration for the sugar-planter, as it enables him to deduce the most appropriate manure for promoting the growth of the cane.[6]

The sugar-cane, especially the violet variety, is coated by a glaucous powder of a peculiar kind of wax, which has been called *cerosine* or *sugar-cane wax*.[7] This is fusible at 180° F., and dissolves in boiling alcohol : the alcoholic solution, even when it contains but a small quantity of cerosine, gelatinises or solidifies on cooling like an alcoholic solution of soap. The composition of this wax is $C^{48}H^{50}O^2$ (Dumas).

[1] *Journ. de Chimie Méd.* t. ii. 2de sér. pp. 26 and 132, 1836.
[2] Quoted by Dumas, *Traité de Chimie*, t. vi. p. 209, 1843.
[3] *Journ. de Pharm.* t. xxvi. p. 154, 1840.
[4] *Ann. de Chim. et Phys.* 3me sér. t. xi. p. 39, 1844.
[5] *Journ. de Pharm.* t. xxvi. p. 569, 1840.
[6] For analyses of the ash of the entire sugar-cane, as well as of the crushed and pressed cane (*megass*), see Johnston's *Lectures on Agricultural Chemistry*, pp. 393 and 628, 2d edition, 1847. The same author also gives the formula for a special manure for the sugar-cane, deduced from the analyses of the ash (*op. cit.* p. 644).
[7] *Journ. de Pharm.* t. xxvi. p. 738, 1840.

EXTRACTION OF CANE-JUICE.—Cane-juice is generally extracted from the stems by means of the *sugar mill*. The canes, when ripe, are cut close to the ground, stripped of their leaves, and carried in bundles to the mill-house, where they are twice subjected to pressure between iron rollers, placed either vertically or horizontally. The residue of the canes which have been thus crushed and deprived of their juice is called *megass*.

Other methods of extracting the cane-juice have been suggested. The *hydraulic press* has been introduced into Jamaica and St. Vincent's. By *Michiel's patent* it is proposed to macerate thin slices of the cane in a mixture of lime and water, so as to coagulate the albuminous matters but to extract the sugar. It has also been proposed to extract the sugar in Europe from the canes imported in the dried state.[1]

PROPERTIES OF CANE-JUICE.—Cane-juice is pale yellowish-grey, and has an agreeable sweet taste and a faint fragrant odour. As it flows from the mill it is frothy, and, owing to the suspension in it of a finely-divided matter, is turbid or opalescent. Its sp. gr. ranges from 1·067 to 1·106 : the late Mr. Fownes[2] found it to be from 1·070 to 1·090. By boiling, its turbidity is commonly a little increased, and sometimes a few small flocks are separated from it. Both nitric acid and corrosive sublimate occasion after a time a very slight precipitate. A large addition of alcohol throws down flocks resembling gum or dextrine. A few drops of sulphate of copper, and an excess of caustic potash, occasion, on heating, a very abundant red precipitate of suboxide of copper, indicative of the presence of glucose or grape-sugar.

According to the late Mr. Fownes, the juice contains the following substances :—*Cane sugar* in great quantity, a notable amount of *glucose* or *grape-sugar, gum* or *dextrine, phosphates of lime and magnesia,* some *other salt of lime* and *magnesia, sulphates* and *chlorides, potash* and *soda,* and, lastly, *a peculiar azotised matter* belonging to the albuminous family, forming an insoluble compound with lime, not coagulable by heat or acids, and readily putrefiable. Of ordinary *vegetable albumen* there are but indistinct traces, and of caseine or legumine none. Avequin found a portion of *cerosine* or sugar-cane wax in cane-juice. It is detached from the canes in the mill.

Cane-juice has been analysed by Proust,[3] by Avequin,[4] by Peligot,[5] by Plagne,[6] and Casaseca.[7] The following are their more important results :—

	Avequin.		Peligot.		Plagne.		Casaseca.
Sugar	15·784	....	20·90	....	20·8000	....	20·94
Various organic matters ...	0·140	....	0·23	....	0·8317	....	0·12
Salts	0·236	....	0·17	...... small quantities		......	0·14
Water	83·840	....	78·70	....	78·3325	....	78·80
Cane-juice	100·000	....	100·00	....	99·9642	....	100·00

It appears, therefore, from these analyses that cane-juice contains about 20 per cent. of saccharine matter. Or assuming that the juice has an average sp.

---

[1] For further details, see Dr. Evans's *Sugar planter's Manual,* 1847.
[2] *Pharmaceutical Journal,* vol. viii. p. 15, 1848.
[3] *Ann. de Chim.* lvii. 181.
[4] *Journ. de Chim. Méd.* t. ii. 2de Sér. p. 26, 1836.
[5] *Journ. de Pharm.* t. xxvi. p. 154, 1840.
[6] *Ibid.* p. 248, 1840.
[7] *Ann. de Chim. et de Phys.* 3me Sér. t. xi. p. 39.

gr. of 1·073, the quantity will be 18 per cent.   Moreover, according to both Peligot and Casaseca, the whole of the saccharine matter is crystallisable, or true cane-sugar ; the uncrystallisable sugar, or molasses, which is obtained by evaporation from the juice, being the product of alterations effected in the crystallisable sugar by the operation ; but Mr. Fownes observed that this statement must be received with some reservation.

Of late years *concentrated West Indian cane juice* has been imported. It contains nearly half its weight of granular sugar, besides a variable amount of molasses.

CLARIFICATION OF CANE-JUICE.—The clarification or defecation of cane-juice is effected, usually in large copper vessels of the capacity of 300 or 400 gallons, by the combined use of heat and lime : the latter is technically called "the *temper.*"   The heat serves to coagulate any vegetable albumen which may be present.   The lime neutralises the free acid and combines with the peculiar albuminous or proteine body mentioned by Mr. Fownes, and forms a coagulum the separation of which is promoted by the heat.   Part of it rises to the top as a scum, and the remainder subsides as a thick muddy deposit. Various other substances[1] have been tried as a substitute for lime with more or less success.   Diacetate of lead has been employed for this purpose, but its use has been discontinued on account of a great number of persons having suffered the ill effects of this metal from partaking of sugar prepared with it.   [Considerable discussion has taken place, and great difference of opinion been expressed among chemists, as to the propriety of adopting a patent granted to Mr. Scoffern for refining sugar by means of diacetate of lead.   He proposes to remove the lead by precipitation with sulphurous acid, and subsequently to add lime in order to neutralise the acetic acid and excess of sulphurous acid left in the liquor.   There would appear a danger of contamination by lead, however, if this patent process be used.[2]—ED.]

CONCENTRATION OF THE CANE-JUICE.—The clarified juice should be filtered prior to evaporation.   This, however, is not usually practised.   It is generally drawn off from the clarifier into a copper *boiler*, where it is evaporated and skimmed.   It is then passed successively through a series of boilers, the last of which is called the *teache*.   When it has acquired a proper tenacity and granular aspect, it is emptied or "skipped" first into a copper cooler and afterwards into a wooden vessel, where it is allowed to crystallise or *grain*. The concrete sugar is then placed in casks (usually sugar hogsheads) perforated with holes in the bottom, each of which is partially closed by the stalk of a plantain leaf.   Here the sugar is allowed to drain for three or four weeks.   It is then packed in hogsheads and sent to this country under the name *muscovado* or *raw sugar*.   The drainings, or uncrystallised portion of sugar, constitute *molasses*.   This is received in an open cistern beneath.

The feculencies separated in the clarifying vessel, and the skimmings of the evaporating coppers, are employed in the manufacture of *rum*.

PROPERTIES OF RAW SUGAR.—Raw sugar is a mixture of crystallisable and uncrystallisable sugar, contaminated by various organic and mineral substances. Its mineral constituents are, according to Avequin, silica, phosphate and sub-phosphate of lime, carbonate of lime, sulphate of potash, chloride of potassium, and the acetates of potash and lime.   The raw sugar of the shops reddens

---

[1] See Dr. Evans's *Sugar-planter's Manual.*
[2] See *Pharm. Journ.* vol. ix. p. 220, and vol. x. pp. 150, 177, 245, 361.

litmus, and is not completely soluble in alcohol. Its aqueous solution yields precipitates with the diacetate of lead, oxalic acid, and caustic ammonia; and is frequently darkened by the addition of the sesquichloride of iron. By keeping, *strong* raw sugar becomes *weak*—that is, soft, clammy, and gummy. This change the late Mr. Daniell[1] ascribed to the action of the lime.

SUGAR-REFINING.—The following is a sketch of the process as usually practised in London:—Raw sugar is dissolved in water by the aid of steam (this process is technically called *blowing-up*). The liquid is then heated with bullock's blood[2] (technically called *spice*), and filtered through canvas bags (called *Schröder's bags*). The clear liquor is allowed to percolate slowly through enormous cylinders containing coarse-grained animal and fresh burnt charcoal. The depth of the bed of charcoal varies in different refining houses. I have seen it three feet deep; but I am told that some refiners employ a bed twenty feet in depth. The filtered liquor, which is nearly colourless, is conveyed to a copper vessel (Howard's *vacuum-pan*), where it is boiled by the aid of steam, under diminished atmospheric pressure, at a temperature of about 170° F.

FIG. 73.

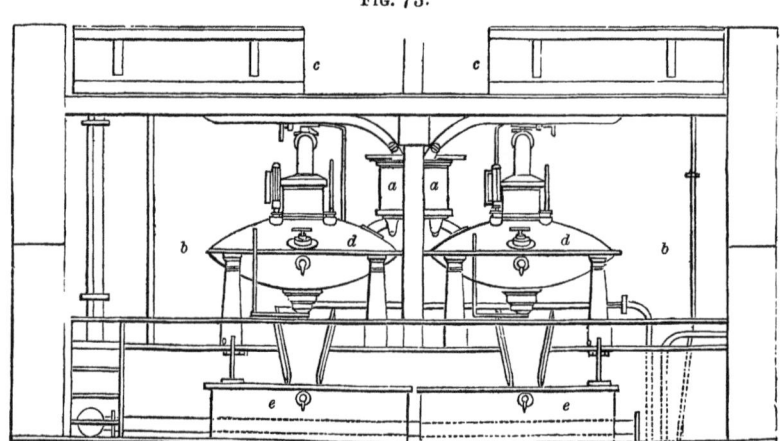

View of Two Vacuum Pans and their subsidiary apparatus.

a, a, Charging measures, supplied by pipes, which descend from *c, c,* the liquor cisterns. *d, d,* are the vacuum spheroidal pans, the lower half of each being supplied with a jacket, as a case for the steam. At the sides of the neck of each pan are a barometer and thermometer. Below the neck, and just above the horizontal line *b, b,* is the handle of the proof-stick, which appears like a stop-cock. When the syrup is sufficiently concentrated, it is discharged into the *heater, e, e.*

The consistence of the liquid is examined from time to time by taking out a sample by the *proof-stick,* which is so constructed as not to admit air.

When the requisite degree of concentration has been attained, a valve is opened in the bottom of the vacuum pan, and the syrup allowed to escape into a copper vessel (*heater*), enveloped by a jacket, so as to enable it to be heated by steam. The syrup is then transferred to conical moulds (made of

---

[1] *Quarterly Journal of Science,* vi. 38.
[2] At one time hydrate of alumina, under the name of *finings,* was used in addition to blood. [In some of the large sugar-refineries in London, blood is not used.—ED.]

earthenware or iron), whose orifices are closed by a paper plug, and the next morning, when solidified, these moulds are carried to the *curing-floor,* when the stoppers are withdrawn and the moulds placed in pots, in order to allow the *green syrups* to drain off : these are made into an inferior sort of refined sugar (*brown lumps*).   The loaves are then either *clayed* or *sugared,* generally the latter.

Claying[1] (which is now almost entirely out of use) consists in pouring clay and water on the base of the sugar-loaf : the water slowly percolating through the sugar, a portion of which it dissolves, carries with it the colouring matter and other impurities.   *Sugaring* is effected by substituting a saturated solution of pure sugar (called *liquor*), or rather a mixture of brown sugar and water, for the clay and water : it washes out the colouring matter, but does not dissolve the pure sugar.   The loaves are afterwards dried in a stove, and put in blue paper for sale.[2]

The following may be regarded as an approximation to the produce of 112 lbs. of raw sugar by the above process :—

Refined sugar	79 lbs.
Bastard	17
Treacle	16 (12 lbs. solid matter.)
Water	4
Raw Sugar	112

The animal charcoal used in sugar refining is changed every week, and of course is a more powerful decoloriser when fresh than when it has been used several times.   It follows, therefore, that the quality of the refined sugar obtained varies with the day of the week—that is, with the age of the charcoal.   At the commencement of the week, when the charcoal is fresh, the finest white *loaves* of sugar are made ; about the middle of the week *titlers* and *lumps* are obtained ; and, at the end of the week, *bastards*.

PROPERTIES.—Common or cane-sugar is the sweetest of all kinds of sugar. When pure, it is white and odourless.   It is very soluble in water, both hot and cold ; is soluble in rectified spirit, but not in ether.   Its watery solution, aided by heat, decomposes some of the metallic salts (as those of copper, mercury, gold, and silver) ; but several of them (as the diacetate of copper and nitrate of silver) require nearly a boiling temperature to change them. A dilute watery solution of common sugar, with a little yeast, undergoes the vinous fermentation.   Sugar promotes the solubility of lime in water, and forms both a soluble and an insoluble compound with oxide of lead. [A curious fact has lately been discovered by Mr. Barreswill, viz., that carbonate of lime unites with saccharate of lime to form a soluble double salt.[3] —ED.]   Cane-sugar is capable of existing either in the crystallised or amorphous state.   In this respect it resembles sulphur (see Vol. i. p. 353).

1. *Crystallised Cane-sugar.*—To this division are referred sugar-candy and the ordinary loaf and lump sugar of the shops.   By the slow cooling of a saturated aqueous solution of sugar, we obtain the large and fine crystals which

---

[1] " Claying sugar, as they report here, was first found out in Brazil : a hen having her feet dirty, going over a pot of sugar by accident, it was found under her tread to be whiter than elsewhere."— Sloane's *Jamaica,* vol. i. p. 61.

[2] For further details, consult a paper by Messrs. Guynne and Young, *Brit. Ann. of Med.* June 23, and July 13, 1837 ; also, Dr. Ure's *Dict. of Arts,* art. Sugar.

[3] *Journ. de Pharmacie ; Pharm. Journ.* vol. xi. p. 33.

constitute the commercial *sugar-candy* (*saccharum candum*), and of which three kinds are kept in the shops—namely, *white candy*, prepared from pure sugar ; *brown candy*, prepared from brown sugar ; and *pink* or *rose candy*, prepared from sugar artificially coloured (probably by cochineal). The crystals of sugar are doubly oblique prisms, and therefore have two axes of double refraction[1] (see Vol. i. p. 146). Their sp. gr. is 1·6065. Common crystallised sugar is permanent in the air, and phosphorescent in the dark when struck or rubbed. When heated, it melts and soon becomes coloured. By this process its tendency to crystallise is diminished or destroyed.

[M. Payen has shown that crystallised sugar is occasionally infested by a cryptogamic vegetation. This produces either furrows or round indentations in the sugar, at the bottom of which it flourishes. The fact was first observed in the sugar-refineries of Paris, producing in one case a reddish coloration in the sugar, and in another spots of a gray colour. The name proposed for these growths is respectively Glycyphila erythrospora, and G. elæospora. The genus forms part of the tribe Mucedineæ.—Ed.][2]

The commercial varieties of common crystallised cane-sugar are of two kinds —*white* or *brown*. The first is refined sugar.

1. Purified or Refined Sugar (*Saccharum*, L.; *Saccharum purum*, E.; *Succus concretus purificatus*, D.; *Saccharum purificatum*) is met with in the shops in conical loaves (*loaf sugar*) or truncated cones, called lumps (*lump sugar*), of various sizes and degrees of purity. Small lumps are called *titlers*. The finest refined sugar (*saccharum albissimum*) is perfectly white, and is termed *double refined* ; the inferior kind (*saccharum album*) has a slightly yellowish tint, and is called *single refined*. Both varieties are compact, porous, friable, and made up of small crystalline grains.

2. Brown Sugar (*Saccharum commune*, E.; *Saccharum fuscum*; *Succus concretus non purificatus*, D.) occurs in commerce in the form of a coarse powder composed of shining crystalline grains. It is more or less damp and sticky, and has a peculiar smell and a very sweet taste. Its colour is brownish-yellow, but varying considerably in intensity. *Muscovado*, or *raw sugar*, has the deepest colour, and is intermixed with lumps. *Bastard* is a finer kind, prepared from molasses and the green syrups. The *Demerara crystal sugar* is the finest : its colour is pale yellow, and its crystals are larger and more brilliant than the preceding varieties.

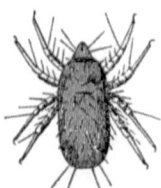

Fig. 74.

Acarus sacchari.

[The commoner and coarser brown sugars of the shops sometimes contain mites (Acari) in large numbers. These Acari are smaller in size than those observed in cheese, in meal, and in the itch pustule. Their length, according to the measurements of Mr. Jackson, is 0·08 parts of an English inch. The figure here given is taken from one in the *Pharmaceutical Journal* (see vol. x. page 396).—Ed.]

2. *Amorphous Cane-sugar.*—When syrup or a strong solution of crystallised cane-sugar is rapidly boiled down, and then poured out on a marble or metallic plate, it congeals in an amorphous, vitreous, more or less coloured mass, usually called *boiled sugar*, of which *barley-sugar* (*saccharum hordeatum*), *acidulated drops*, and *hard-bake*, are familiar examples. During the preparation of barley-sugar and acidulated drops, the confectioners usually add a small quantity of cream of tartar to the melted sugar, in order to destroy its tendency to crystallise. Vinegar and tartaric acid are mentioned by some writers as being used for this purpose. If when the melted sugar has partially

---

[1] Sugar-candy makes an interesting polariscope object. It is usually cut so as to show only one of its two systems of rings.

[2] *Pharm. Journ.* vol. xi. p. 311.

solidified, but while it is yet soft, it be hung on a hook and rapidly and repeatedly drawn out, it becomes opaque and white. This *pulled sugar* was formerly termed *sugar penides* (*saccharum penidium*).

When crystallised cane-sugar is subjected to a temperature of about 356° F., it melts; and, at a higher temperature, begins to give off water and to suffer decomposition. If the heat be gradually augmented, it becomes brown, evolves a remarkable odour, loses its sweet taste and acquires a bitter one. In this condition it is called *caramel* (from καίω, *I burn*, and μέλι, *honey*), or *burnt sugar* (*saccharum tostum*). It enjoys acid properties, and is composed, according to Peligot,[1] of $C^{24}H^{18}O^{18}$.

Molasses and Treacle.—These are viscid, dark brown, dense liquids, composed of amorphous or uncrystallisable sugar, crystallisable sugar, gum, extractive, various salts, and water. They are frequently confounded, but in trade are considered distinct.

1. MOLASSES (more correctly *Melasses*, from *mel*, honey, because it is soft and sweet, like honey) is the drainings from raw or muscovado sugar. *West India molasses* is occasionally imported for refining. It yields brown sugar, or bastard, and treacle.

2. TREACLE (*Theriaca; Fæx Sacchari*, L. E.; *Syrupus empyreumaticus, anglicè Molasses*, D.) is the viscid, dark brown, uncrystallisable syrup which drains from refined sugar in the sugar moulds. It is thicker than West Indian molasses, and has a somewhat different flavour. Its sp. gr. is generally 1·4; and it contains, according to Dr. Ure, on an average, 75 per cent. of solid matter. Payen says that it may be regarded as a saturated solution of crystallisable sugar, of which it contains from 40 to 50 per cent. of its weight. It is employed in the manufacture of gingerbread, and, by poor people, as a substitute for sugar. It is also sometimes used to yield, by fermentation, an alcoholic liquor,—either to be drank as a kind of beer, or to yield, by distillation, spirit. It is sold under the names of "*mélasse de la Cochinchine*" and "*prepared melasse*," to be taken with lentil-meal (sold as *ervalenta* or *revalenta arabica*), as a remedy for habitual constipation.

CHEMICAL CHARACTERISTICS.—As a species of sugar,[2] cane-sugar is known by its susceptibility of undergoing the vinous fermentation ; that is, of suffering a peculiar decomposition into alcohol and carbonic acid. For this purpose it is dissolved in water, and to the solution a small portion of yeast (dry yeast is to be preferred) is added, and the mixture exposed to a temperature of about 70° F. Effervescence soon takes place, carbonic acid is evolved, and a vinous or alcoholic liquor is produced. In this process the cane-sugar combines with water, and becomes grape sugar, $C^{12}H^{12}O^{12}$, which, by fermentation, is resolved into four atoms of carbonic acid, $4CO^2$, and two atoms of alcohol, $2C^4H^6O^2$.

The quantitative determination of sugar is effected by ascertaining the amount of carbonic acid evolved during fermentation. 171 grains of sugar-candy furnish 88 grains, or about 186·4 cubic inches of carbonic acid gas. At mean temperature and pressure, 100 cubic inches, or 47·2 grains, of carbonic acid gas are given out by 91·7 grains of sugar-candy. In round numbers, we may say that one cubic inch or half a grain of carbonic acid gas is equal to one grain of sugar-candy.[3]

---

[1] Peligot, *Ann. Chim. et de Phys.* lxvii. p. 175. [The equivalent now commonly adopted by chemists for *caramel* is one half of that above assigned, $C^{12}H^9O^9$. It is considered to be cane sugar deprived by heat of 2 eq. of water :—in other words, anhydrous sugar.—ED.]

[2] *Mannite, glycyrrhizin, glycerine*, and some other sweet substances, which were formerly called sugars, are, by modern chemists, excluded from the list of sugars properly so called, because they are incapable of undergoing the vinous fermentation.

[3] Full directions for the quantitative determination of sugar by fermentation are given by Dr. Miller, in the article *Organic Analysis* of the *Cyclopædia of Anatomy and Physiology*, vol. iii. p. 799.

Cane-sugar is distinguished from other kinds of sugar by the following characters :—Its crystallisability in prismatic crystals, its very sweet taste, its ready solubility in water, its solution being charred, and letting fall a brown or black powder when heated with a few drops of oil of vitriol, but being unchanged when treated in the same way with caustic potash,—and by the difficulty with which it reduces the blue hydrated oxide of copper to the orange suboxide.

[The property of reducing the oxide of copper, more especially resides in what has been denominated grape sugar and glucose,—terms, however, which have confused two distinct varieties of saccharine matter. Thus, if we extract the sugar contained in acid fruits, we obtain a mass of a gummy appearance, which, if placed in contact with ferments, very rapidly decomposes into alcohol and carbonic acid. Its constitution is $C^{12}H^{12}O^{12}$, and the first action of a ferment on cane sugar is to convert it into this body. If this gummy sugar from acid fruits be exposed for some days, we observe a crystallisation to occur through parts of it; and if we collect these granular crystals we find we have obtained a sugar which differs from the mass from which the crystallisation took place. Its composition is $C^{12}H^{14}O^{14}$, and it is this which we may more properly designate as glucose. It appears identical with diabetic sugar, with the granular part of honey, and also with the product obtained by boiling dilute sulphuric acid on starch. This glucose differs from cane sugar in rapidly reducing the salts of copper.—Ed.] The mode of applying this test of its presence is as follows :—Add to the saccharine solution a small quantity of a solution of caustic potash, and then a few drops of a weak solution of sulphate of copper; taking care that the alkali is in excess. Then apply heat : if grape-sugar be present, an ochre-yellow or red precipitate of suboxide of copper is formed before ebullition takes place. Uncrystallisable sugar, as well as sugar of milk, also readily reduces the oxide; but this effect does not take place with crystallisable cane-sugar: or rather, a higher temperature or a longer action of the ingredients is required to produce the effect. This is called *Trommer's test.*

[Another test (*Moore's test*) consists in boiling a solution of caustic potash with a solution of this sugar, when, if glucose be present, the liquor gradually darkens, assuming a brown colour of greater or less intensity according to the quantity present.—Ed.]

Fig. 75.

Fig. 76.

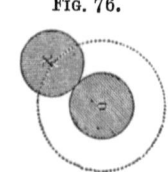

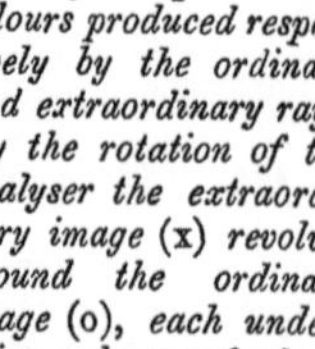

Representation of the two disks of complementary colours produced respectively by the ordinary and extraordinary rays. By the rotation of the analyser the extraordinary image (x) revolves around the ordinary image (o), each undergoing a change of colour.

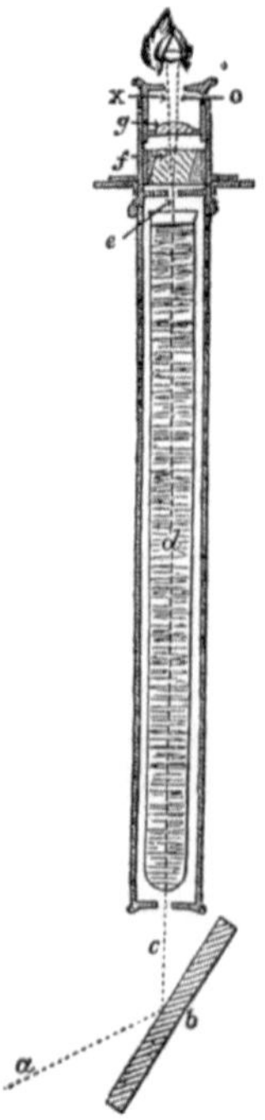

Plan of the Apparatus for showing the circular polarisation of liquids.

In this figure, g indicates a lens which is used to produce well-defined images.

A solution of crystallisable cane-sugar possesses the property of *right-handed* circular polarisation. If a ray of common light (fig. 75, a) be polarised by reflection at an angle of 56°·45 from the surface of glass[1] (b), the plane polarised ray (c), which is thus obtained, transmitted through a pure solution of crystallisable cane-sugar (d), and the emergent ray (e) analysed by a double refracting rhomb of calcareous spar (f), two coloured images are perceived (figs. 75 and 76); one (o) caused by ordinary refraction,

---

[1] The plane polarisation of the ray may be effected by a Nichol's prism instead of a glass-mirror. The use of a silvered glass-mirror is objectionable, on account of its producing elliptical polarisation.

the other (x) by extraordinary refraction. The colours of the images are complementary; that is, when one image is red, yellow, or blue,—the other is green, violet, or orange. By rotating the analyser (the rhomb of calcareous spar), the colours change : if the rotation be right-handed (that is, as we turn a screw or corkscrew to make it enter), the sequence of the colours is red, orange, yellow, green, blue, indigo, and violet.

SEQUENCE OF COLOURS FOR A SOLUTION OF CRYSTALLISABLE CANE-SUGAR, AS OBTAINED BY THE RIGHT-HANDED ROTATION OF THE ANALYSER.

Ordinary Image.	*Extraordinary Image.*
Red	Green.
Orange	Blue.
Yellow	{ Indigo. Violet.
Green	Red.
Blue	Orange.
Indigo } Violet }	Yellow.
Red	Green.

In one complete revolution of the analyser each of the colours of the spectrum occurs twice for each image.[1]

[Of the two varieties of sugar noticed above, constituted $C^{12}H^{12}O^{12}$ and $C^{12}H^{14}O^{14}$, the former polarises to the left, the latter to the right.—ED.]

COMPOSITION.—The following is the ultimate composition of sugar :—

	Atoms.	Eq.Wt.	Per Cent.		Atoms.	Eq.Wt.	Per Cent.
Carbon	12	72	47·05	Anhydrous sugar	1	153	89·47
Hydrogen	9	9	5·9	Water	2	18	10·53
Oxygen	9	72	47·05				
Anhydrous Sugar[2]	1	153	100·00	Crystallised Sugar...	1	171	100·00

ADULTERATION ; PURITY.—The purity of genuine sugar is readily judged of by its physical or sensible qualities. The impurities may also be detected by chemical means, but it is rarely necessary to resort to these. A solution of pure sugar is colourless, and yields no precipitate with oxalic acid, diacetate of lead, or caustic ammonia. Pure sugar is completely soluble in rectified spirit. Various adulterations have been practised on sugar. The most important of these is the intermixture of *starch-sugar*. A few years ago I inspected an extensive manufactory of sugar from potato-starch at Stratford, in Essex : the sugar obtained was sold for the adulteration of brown sugar, and the molasses produced was consumed in an oxalic acid manufactory. Brown cane-sugar adulterated with starch-sugar is less sweet, less readily soluble in water, and less

---

[1] The nature of the present work does not admit of a further elucidation of circular polarisation, which I have here introduced as an aid in the qualitative determination of a saccharine solution. Biot has applied it to the quantitative determination of sugar. To his various papers contained in the *Mémoires de l'Académie des Sciences*, and especially to his *Instructions Pratiques sur l'Observation et la Mesure des Propriétés Optiques appellées rotatoires*, Paris, 1845, the reader is referred for further information.—A popular sketch of the subject will be found in my *Lectures on Polarised Light*, published by Messrs. Longman and Co.—A very admirable report on this and other methods of effecting the qualitative and quantitative analysis of sugars, syrups, and molasses, by Professor R. S. M'Culloch, is contained in a *Letter from the Secretary of the* [United States] *Treasury to the United States Senate*, read Feb..21,1845. [See also *Pharm. Journ.* vol. xii. pp. 348 and 393.—ED.]

[2] Peligot, *Ann. de Chem. et de Phys.* lxvii. p. 124.

crystalline and sparkling, than pure brown cane-sugar. Moreover, potato-sugar always contains sulphate of lime, the detection of which (see the tests for sulphuric acid and lime, Vol. i. pp. 367 and 616) in a suspected sample of sugar is, therefore, of some value. It has been proposed to detect the presence of potato-sugar by Trommer's test (see *ante*, p. 128) and by caustic potash. But though Trommer's test readily detects starch-sugar in a solution of white cane-sugar, the detection is not so easily effected by it in a solution of brown cane-sugar, because the uncrystallisable cane-sugar, or treacle, which is present readily reduces the blue hydrate of copper to the orange suboxide,—acting thus like starch-sugar. Chevallier[1] proposes to detect starch-sugar in cane-sugar by means of Moore's test : Boil the suspected sugar in a ley of caustic potash : if no starch-sugar be present, the liquor remains colourless ; but, on the contrary, it becomes brown if starch-sugar be present. But this test, like the last one, is better adapted for detecting starch-sugar in white cane-sugar than in the ordinary brown cane-sugar of the shops.[2] Farinaceous substances and dextrine may be detected by boiling the suspected sugar in water, and testing the decoction, when cold, with iodine, which causes a blue colour with starch and a purplish colour with dextrine.

Gum is distinguished from sugar by its insolubility in rectified spirit.

Various other substances have, it is said, been used for the adulteration of sugar, as finely-powdered marble, chalk or whiting, sand, bone-dust, and common salt. With the exception of salt, all the substances here mentioned are insoluble in water, and by this character, therefore, may be readily separated from sugar. Common salt may be detected in a solution of the suspected sugar by the ordinary tests for that substance (see Vol. i. p. 586).

PHYSIOLOGICAL EFFECTS.—Sugar, considered as an article of food, is an alimentary principle which belongs to the class of "elements of respiration" (see Vol. i. p. 64). It contributes to the formation of fat and of lactic acid, and by its oxidation furnishes heat. It has recently been detected in the tissue of the liver, but in no other organ.[3] It disagrees with some dyspeptics, and is reputed to have a tendency to cause flatulency and preternatural acidity (by the formation of lactic acid?) of the *primæ viæ*. Treacle, and therefore raw sugar, check the tendency to constipation.

USES.—Sugar is used dietetically, medicinally, and pharmaceutically. *Medicinally*, it is but little employed. In the form of lozenges, sugar-candy, &c., it is slowly dissolved in the mouth to allay tickling cough. As a chemical antidote, it has been recommended in poisoning by the salts of copper, mercury, silver, gold, and lead.[4] But any advantage procured by its use in these cases is referable to its demulcent and emollient properties, and not to its chemical influence. The same remark may be made with respect to the benefit said to have been obtained by the use of the juice of the sugar-cane in poisoning by arsenious acid.[5] Powdered white sugar is sometimes sprinkled over ulcers, to

---

[1] *Journ de Chim. Méd.* t. viii. 2de sér. p. 472, 1842.

[2] On a trial for the recovery of excise duties on potato-sugar, it was stated that this sugar possessed only three-fifths of the sweetening properties of genuine cane-sugar, and that it was mixed with whiting, bone-dust, &c. previous to its being offered for sale. (*Pharm. Journ.* vol. i. p. 603, 1842.)

[3] *Comptes rendus*, xxvii. p. 514 ; *Chemical Gazette*, March 1, 1849.

[4] Vogel and Buchner, in *Schweigger's Journ.* xiii. 162 ; xiv. 224.

[5] Chisholm, *Quarterly Journal of Science*, x. 193.

remove spongy granulations, denominated proud flesh. The same remedy has also been employed for the removal of specks on the cornea.

In *pharmacy* the uses of sugar are much more extensive. It serves to preserve, to give flavour, bulk, form, colour, cohesiveness, and consistence; to sub-divide and to suspend oily substances in aqueous liquids. To fulfil one or more of these objects, it is a constituent of *syrups, elæosacchara, conserves, electuaries, confections, lozenges,* some *pills* and *powders,* &c. For making pills, treacle serves to give cohesiveness, to preserve the pill-mass soft, prevent mouldiness, and in some cases to check chemical changes. As an antiseptic, it is used for the preservation of various medicinal organic substances. It acts at least in two ways,—by excluding air, and by absorbing moisture (see Vol. i. pp. 167 and 168); and perhaps also in some other way, as when it promotes the solidification of pectine. Sugar is also useful in preserving some inorganic compounds: thus it checks, though it does not absolutely prevent, the higher oxidation of some of the protosalts of iron: hence its use in the *ferri carbonas saccharatum* (see Vol. i. p. 828), and *syrupus ferri iodidi* (see Vol. i. p. 850). It is employed in the manufacture of oxalic acid; and it is sometimes used in distilleries to yield, by fermentation, alcohol. The Edinburgh College directs it to be used in the rectification of sulphuric acid (see Vol. i. p. 369).

As a test, it is sometimes used in the laboratory, in conjunction with oil of vitriol, to detect the cholic acid of bile.

1. SYRUPUS, L.; *Syrupus simplex,* E. D.; *Syrup; Simple Syrup.* (Sugar, lb. iij. [lb. v. *D.*]; Distilled Water, Oj. [Oij. *D.*] Dissolve the sugar in the water by a gentle heat.)—By keeping for several months, syrup undergoes some molecular changes, by which its power of producing right-handed circular polarisation is considerably diminished.

The proportion of water and sugar used by the Edinburgh College is, by weight, water 1 part, sugar 2·1942 parts; or very nearly water 1 part, sugar 2¼ parts.

In order to yield a clear and bright syrup, distilled water and well-refined sugar should be employed. Ordinary spring-water becomes turbid by boiling, owing to the precipitation of carbonate of lime.[1] The sp. gr. of boiling syrup should be 1·264 (equal to 30° of Beaume's areometer). When it has cooled down to 60° F., its sp. gr. should be 1·321 (equal to 35° of Beaume's areometer).

Syrup is used in medicine to give flavour, cohesiveness, and consistence.

2. LIQUOR SACCHARI TOSTI; *Caramel; Burnt Sugar.*—This is a useful innocuous colouring agent. It is prepared by melting half a pound of brown sugar in an iron pot, and applying heat until the liquid acquires a deep brown colour, then adding a gallon of boiling water.

---

[1] See some observations by Mr. Savory, on the preparation of syrup, in the *Pharmaceutical Journal,* vol. ii. p. 452, 1843.

41. Andropogon muricatus, *Retz.* (Anatherum muricatum, *Pal.*)—Vittie-vayr, or Cuscus.

Sex. Syst. Triandria, Digynia.

(Radix.)

Virana, Asiat. Res. iv. 306; *A. squarrosus,* Linn., Suppl. 433; *Philaris zizanoides,* Linn., Syst. Veg. v. 104; *Anatherum muricatum,* Beauv., Agrost. 128, t. xxii. f. 10; *Vetiveria odorata,* Virey, Journ. de Pharm. xiii. 499; *Bena* (Bengalee), Roxburgh, Fl. Ind. i. 265; *Vittie-vayr* (Tamool), Ainslie, Mat. Indica, ii. 470; *Woetiwear* (Tamool), Roxb., op. supra cit.—Coromandel, Bengal: very common on every part of the coast.—Its root, called *cuscus,* or *khus-khus (radix vetiveriæ),* is imported from Bombay: it is long, fibrous, brownish or yellowish-white; has a fragrant aromatic odour,[1] and a feeble bitterish, aromatic taste. Iodine colours it bluish-black. In 1809, Vauquelin[2] analysed it under the name of *schœnanthus.* It was analysed in 1828 by Henry,[3] and in 1831 by Geiger:[4] the latter found *volatile oil, resin, bitter extractive, starch,* traces of *hydrochloric* and *calcareous salts,* and *woody fibre.* Cap[5] submitted the root to distillation with water, and obtained two volatile oils: one limpid, amber-coloured, and lighter than water; another in larger quantity, which was heavier than water, opaque, and adhered to the bottom of the receiver. The dried roots, when slightly moistened, emit a pleasant kind of fragrance, and are employed in India for making *vissaries* (large fans) and door- and window-screens (composed of a frame-work of bamboo covered by cuscus root). During the hot winds, the outsides of these screens are kept watered by natives, and the air that passes through is thereby rendered both cool and fragrant. Cuscus root is imported into England for perfumery purposes. It serves to make scented baskets, and is put into drawers to guard linen and woollen goods from the attacks of insects. This root has also been employed in medicine. It acts as a gentle excitant and diaphoretic. In India an infusion of it is used as a diaphoretic and gentle stimulant in febrile cases. The warm infusion has been employed as an antispasmodic, diaphoretic, diuretic, and emmenagogue. An ointment of the root has also been applied to destroy pediculi on the heads of children.[6] In 1831 it was used in Paris as a preservative against the cholera: it was worn by the ladies; bundles of it were hung up in the rooms; and fumigations were prepared with it.[7] In Hamburgh it was used by Dr. Buchheister[8] and others in cholera. A weak infusion has been used by Foy[9] in rheumatism and gout. It may be employed in the form of powder, infusion, tincture, or volatile oil. The dose of the powder (*pulvis vetiveriæ*) is about a scruple, in the form of pills. A weak infusion or tea is prepared with one or two drachms of the root and two pints of water: this may be drunk *ad libitum.* A strong infusion, prepared with one ounce of the root to half a pint of water, may be administered in doses of a table-spoonful. A tincture (*tinctura vetiveriæ*), made with one ounce of the root and half a pint of proof spirit, is given in doses of a tea-spoonful.

[Dr. Hooker, in his *Himalayan Journal* (p. 42), states that the *Andropogon muricatus* yields a favourite fragrant oil, used as a medicine in India. We are informed on good authority that it is unknown in this country under the name of *Kuskus-oil.* It may be the *Grass-oil* mentioned by the author in the following article. In commerce from India the oils chiefly received are *lemon-grass oil, citronelle, rose geranium, and ginger-grass-oil.* The latter varies greatly in quality.—Ed.]

---

[1] The odour is said by Martius (Buchner's *Repertorium,* Bd. xxxix. S. 230, 1831) to be between that of galbanum and of violet-root, and to approach that of serpentary; while Geiger considers it to be between that of calamus and of yellow water iris-root, and similar to myrrh.

[2] *Ann. du Muséum,* xiv. 28; and *Ann. de Chimie,* lxxii. 302.

[3] *Journ. de Pharm.* tom. xiv. p 57, 1828.

[4] Quoted by Goebel, *Pharm. Waarenkunde,* Bd. ii. S. 265.

[5] *Journ. de Pharm.* t. xix. p. 48, 1833.

[6] Lemaire-Lisancourt, *Bull. de la Soc. Phil.* vii. 43, 1822.

[7] Kunze, *Pharm. Central-Blatt für* 1831, S. 660.

[8] *Bull. gén. de Thérap.* Fev. 1834.

[9] Dierbach, *Die neuest. Ent. in d. Mat. Med.* Bd. i. S. 166, 1837.

42. Andropogon Iwarancusa, *Roxburgh.*

Sex. Syst. Triandria, Digynia.

(Radix.)

Ibharankusha, Iwarankusha, Kurankusha, Beng. and Hind.; *Iwarancussa,* Asiat. Res. iv. 109; *Terankus,* Blane, Phil. Trans. vol. lxxx. p. 286, 1790 : Sir G. Blane considered that it might be the *Nardus Indica,* or *Spikenard,* of the ancients : Mr. Hatchett[1] supposed it to be the source of the *grass-oil of Nemaur,*—an opinion which Dr. Royle[2] has declared to be incorrect.—This fragrant grass, which has a bitter, warm, pungent taste, is a native of the skirts of the northern mountains of India; between the river Rapty and the northern mountains, and about Hurdwar. It comes remarkably near *A. Schœnanthus* both in habit and taste. It is employed by the natives in fevers, whether continued or intermittent. They infuse about a drachm of it in half a pint of hot water, with a small quantity of pepper, and give this for a dose thrice daily. The virtues almost entirely reside in the larger parts of the roots, marked with annular cicatrices.

43. Andropogon Calamus aromaticus, *Royle.*

Sex. Syst. Triandria, Digynia.

(Oleum volatile.)

According to Dr. Royle,[3] the *grass-oil of Nemaur* is obtained from a new species of Andropogon, to which he has given the name of *A. Calamus aromaticus.* He says that it is "found in Central India, extends north as far as Delhi, and south to between Godavery and Nagpore, where, according to Dr. Malcolmson, it is called *spear-grass :* it may be the *A. Martini* of Roxburgh, as I believe it is also thought to be by Dr. Wight, though it has been named *A. Nardoïdes* by Nees von Esenbeck." Dr. Royle examined Mr. Hatchett's specimens of the grass, obtained from Mr. Swinton, as the source of the grass-oil, and found them to be identical with his *A. Calamus aromaticus,* though Mr. Hatchett's figure of the plant (copied from the *Phil. Trans.* vol. lxxx.) actually represents another species, viz. *A. Iwaruncusa.* Dr. Wallich[4] examined a specimen of the plant from which the grass-oil is obtained, and declared it to be either *A. Iwaruncusa* or perhaps *A. Martini,* Roxburgh. Dr. Royle[5] considers this species to be the *sweet calamus*[6] and *sweet cane*[7] of Scripture,—the κάλαμος ἀρωματικός of the ancient Greeks.[8]

GRASS-OIL OF NEMAUR; *Roosa-ke-tel,* Hind.; *Oleum graminis Indici.*—This oil is imported from India under the name of *grass-oil* or *ginger-grass-oil.*[9] In 1845, I obtained from a merchant in London a sample of essential oil which agreed in its sensible qualities with the grass-oil of Nemaur given me by Dr. Royle. With it I received the following notice :—" A sample of three canisters of essential oil imported from Bombay, under the name of *ginger-grass-oil,* and, according to the importer, used by the natives against rheumatism, and by them called *rosa oil.* The grass grows, according to the same authority, fifty or sixty miles from Bombay, in the jungle, and is there called *rosa grass.* It smells, as you will perceive, of ginger and turpentine." Grass-oil of Nemaur is commonly known to the perfumers by the name of *oil of geranium.* I have been informed

---

[1] *On the Spikenard of the Ancients* [by C. Hatchett, F.R.S. Lond. 1836. 4to.]
[2] *Essay on the Antiquity of Hindoo Medicine,* pp. 34 and 82.
[3] *Ibid.* pp. 33 and 82, 1837 ; and *Illustrations of the Botany, &c. of the Himalayan Mountains,* p. 425, 1839.
[4] *Transactions of the Medical and Physical Society of Calcutta,* vol. i. p. 368, Calcutta, 1825.
[5] In Kitto's *Cyclopædia of Biblical Literature,* vol. ii. p. 195, 1845.
[6] *Exodus,* ch. xxx. ver. 23. It is here called *Kaneh Bosem,* literally *reed of fragrance.*
[7] *Jeremiah,* ch. vi. ver. 20. It is here denominated *Kaneh Hattob,* or *good reed.*
[8] Dioscorides, lib. i. cap. 17.
[9] Ainslie (*Mat. Indica,* vol. ii. p. 401) applies the names of *ginger-grass, spice-grass, false spikenard, sukkunaro-pilloo* (Tamool), to the *Andropogon Nardus* (?) of Dr. Rottler, which he says is common in the Cautalum hills and in the Tinnevilly district ; but he puts a query whether it may not be the fragrant grass described by Mr. Maxwell in the *Transactions of the Medical Society of Calcutta,* vol. i. p. 367, 1825.

that it is sometimes called *oil of rose geranium*.   It is occasionally sold by druggists as *oil of spikenard*.

Under the name of "*Ol. Palm. ros.*" [sic], a volatile oil has been sent from a merchant in Constantinople to his correspondent in London, as an oil used for reducing (that is, adulterating) otto of roses; and in the accompanying letter it was stated that if genuine otto be mixed with from 20 to 30 per cent. of this oil, it would be still equal to the finest commercial otto.   By the dealers in London this oil was called *oil of geranium*.[1]   It is almost colourless, and is clearer, brighter, and more fragrant and roseate, than ordinary grass-oil; but its odour is, I think, essentially that of the latter.   Is it rectified grass-oil? It is remarkable that Dioscorides (lib. i. cap. xvi.) states that σχοῖνος (a native of Arabia) has the odour of the rose.

Grass-oil of Nemaur is, according to Mr. Forsyth,[2] procured at the foot of the Vindhya range of hills, in the vicinity of Jaum Ghat, and thirty miles further west, near Naleha. It is obtained by distillation.   When the plant begins to flower, it is cut and bound in small bundles or maniples, 250 or 300 of which are introduced into a wrought-iron boiler fitted over an earthen fireplace.   Water being added, ebullition is promoted.   The oil, with water, distils over into two large copper receivers immersed in cold water.   The process occupies about six hours.   After the product has stood for some time, the oil is skimmed off the surface by a small shallow spoon.   Commercial grass-oil of Namaur is of a light straw colour, and has a fragrant aromatic roseate odour, with taste which is not very dissimilar to that of oil of lemons.   It floats on water.   Dr. Stenhouse[3] found that it is usually a mixture of a pure volatile oil (C^4H^5), and of about half its bulk of a fluid resin, the latter probably being the product of the oxidation of the oil.

In India the grass-oil is frequently adulterated; usually, according to Mr. Forsyth, with the *ol. sesami*.   As this is a fixed oil, the sophistication is readily detected by dropping the suspected grass-oil into rectified spirit: if pure, it dissolves; but if it be mixed with a fixed oil, the spirit becomes milky.

Grass-oil is chiefly employed in perfumery; but it is also employed in medicine.   Its medicinal properties are similar to those of other aromatic fragrant volatile oils, and are those of a stimulant and diaphoretic.   It is highly esteemed in India for the cure of the more chronic forms of rheumatism.   It is applied as a liniment.   A couple of drachms of it are rubbed into the affected part in the heat of the sun, or before the fire, twice daily. It causes a sense of warmth and pricking, which lasts for two hours or longer.   It is also employed to excite diaphoresis in slight catarrhal affections; and for this purpose it is rubbed into the soles of the feet and wrists.

44. Andropogon Schœnanthus, *Linn.*

Sex. Syst. Triandria, Digynia.

I suspect that under this name three species of Andropogon have been confounded.
1. Rumphius's *Schœnanthum Amboinicum*, called by the natives of Amboyna *Siree*.   Its odour is that of a mixture of roses and fresh-mown hay.   As Linnæus, in the later editions of his *Systema Plantarum*, cites Rumphius's figure,[4] we may take this species as the genuine *Andropogon Schœnanthus* of Linnæus[5]   It has been recently very fully described by the late celebrated Professor Th. F. L. Nees von Esenbeck.[6]   Rumphius proposes to call it *Schœnanthum Indicum sterile*, to distinguish it from the Arabian plant.

---

[1] Recluz (*Journ. de Pharm.* t. xiii. p. 529, 1827) obtained from *Pelargonium odoratissimum* var. *odore rosato* (Persoon) a concrete volatile oil, which he calls *volatile oil of geranium with the odour of the roses* (huile volatile du Géranium à odeur de roses).   It must not be confounded with the so-called oil of geranium alluded to in the text.   [The various oils referred to in the text require a careful re-examination.   It is extremely difficult to obtain genuine samples, and, as we are informed, there is much mystery among dealers in reference to these articles.—ED.]

[2] *Transactions of the Medical and Physical Society of Calcutta*, vol. iii. p. 213, Calcutta, 1827.

[3] *Memoirs and Proceedings of the Chemical Society of London*, vol. ii. p. 122, 1845.

[4] *Herbarium Amboinense*, pars v. lib. viii. cap. 24, page 181, tab. lxxii. fig. 2.

[5] In the *Linnean Herbarium* there is a single specimen of *A. Schœnanthus*, but without any statement indicating its place of growth.

[6] Geiger's *Pharmacie*, 2te Aufl. von Th. F. L. Nees von Esenbeck, J. H. Dierbach, and Cl. Marquart, Bd. ii. 1te Hälfte, S. 145, 1839.

2. The *Arabian Schœnanthus* is said by Hasselquist[1] to grow plentifully in the deserts of both the Arabias, and to be gathered near Limbo, a port of Arabia Petræa, and exported to Egypt. The Arabians call it *Helsi Meccavi* and *Idhir Mecchi*. It is said that in the deserts between Syria and Egypt there is no grass but this, which camels eat : hence it has received the name of *fœnum* vel *stramen camelorum*, or *camel's hay* or *straw*. It was formerly in the London Pharmacopœia, and was called *schœnanthus*, *squinanthus*, vel *juncus odoratus ;* its vernacular name being *squinanch*, or *sweet-smelling rush*. The herbs (stem, leaves, and sometimes the flowers) were brought from Turkey and Arabia tied up in bundles about a foot long. The stem, which resembled a barley-straw, was filled with a pith like those of our common rushes : the flowers were of a carnation colour, striped with light purple.[2]

It was considered to possess stimulant and diaphoretic properties, and was commended in hiccup, vomiting, flatulent colic, and female obstructions ; but was little used, except in the *mithridatium* and *theriaca*. It was administered to the extent of one or two drachms in the form of infusion or tea.

It is not improbable that this plant may be the σχοῖνος εὔοσμος of Hippocrates,[3] the σχοῖνος of Dioscorides ;[4] for the last-mentioned writer states that the most esteemed sort grew in that part of Arabia called Nabatæa, which agrees with the statement of Hasselquist.

3. The *Andropogon citratum*, De Cand.—As this is undoubtedly the source of the oil of lemon-grass of the shops, it deserves a separate notice.

45. Andropogon citratum, *De Cand.*—Lemon-grass.

Although all the Anglo-Indian botanists whose works I have consulted consider the *Lemon-grass* of India to be identical with the *Andropogon Schœnanthus* of Linnæus, yet various circumstances have long since led me to suspect that they are in error. Its citron or lemon odour is so very strong and remarkable, that any one familiar with the plant, or its volatile oil, could not overlook or mistake it. Yet not one of the authorities quoted by Linnæus, nor any of the pharmacologists of the last century who were familiar with the Linnæan plant, mention it. Rumphius,[5] whose figure of the plant is referred to by Linnæus, says the odour of the Amboyna plant is similar to that of roses mixed with that of new-mown hay. Dale[6] describes the odour of Schœnanthus as being sweet and very fragrant, and Lewis[7] simply says it is agreeable.

The first botanical writer who notices the peculiar citron odour of lemon-grass is De Candolle,[8] who states that under the name of *Andropogon citratum* there was frequently met with in botanical gardens a grass which had very much the habit of *A. Schœnanthus*, but was larger, did not require a hot-house, and was most distinctly characterised by the citron-odour of the bruised leaves. The late eminent botanist Professor Th. Fr. L. Nees von Esenbeck[9] pointed out some botanical characters which distinguish the two plants. Thus he states that the leaves of A. citratum, De Cand. are much broader, *flat*, of a strong bluish-green colour, and both above and at the margin are very rough when drawn backwards through the fingers ; whereas the leaves of A. Schœnanthus are narrow (half a line in breadth), *completely keeled*, like those of the sedges, bluish-green, and somewhat sharp at the margin when drawn backwards through the fingers. Moreover,

---

[1] *Voyages and Travels in the Levant in the years* 1749, 50, 51, 52, Lond. 1766.—It is remarkable that Forskäl, in his *Flora Arabico-Yemen*, does not mention, in his list of odorous plants (p. xcv.), a single odorous grass as growing in Arabia Felix.

[2] Lewis's *New Dispensatory*, 5th ed. 1785, p. 160.

[3] *De Morb. Mul.* lib. ii. sect. v. p. 673, ed. Fœsii.

[4] Lib. i. cap. 16.

[5] *Herb. Amboinense*, pars v. lib. viii. cap. 24, p. 181, tab. lxxii. fig. 2, Amstel. 1750.

[6] *Pharmacologia*, 3tia ed. p. 258, 1737.

[7] *Experimental History of the Materia Medica*, 4th ed. vol. ii. p. 20, 1791.

[8] *Catalogus Plantarum Horti Botanici Monspeliensis*, p. 78, Monspelii, 1813. Link (*Hort. Berol.* i. 242, 1827), and, following him, Kunth (*Enum. Plant.* i. 493, 1843), in quoting this work, have substituted the name *A. citriodorus* for *A. citratum :* the former name does not occur in De Candolle's Catalogue.

[9] Geiger's *Pharmacie*, 2te Aufl. by Th. F. L. Nees von Esenbeck, J. H. Dierbach, and C. Marquart, 2te Abth. 1te Hälfte, S. 147, 1839.

the hairs of the rachis of the spikelets of the A. citratum are much shorter than those of A. Schœnanthus.

Lemon-grass is a native of the continent of India and of Ceylon. It was introduced into the West Indies towards the latter part of the last, or beginning of the present century.[1] The peculiar characteristic of this species of Andropogon is its odour, which, when the grass is fresh, is very distinctly citron-like; or rather, especially when the plant is dry, resembles that of balm,—the *Melissa officinalis*, Linn., called by the French *Citronnelle*. The lemon-grass yields, by distillation, an essential oil, which is imported from Ceylon, Bombay, Cochin (Malabar coast), and Madras, under the name of *lemon-grass oil*. It is yellow, and has a fragrant citron-like odour. It is much used in perfumery under the name of *oil of verbena*. It is frequently adulterated with a fixed oil, and when thus sophisticated it forms a milky liquid when dropped into rectified spirit; whereas the pure oil dissolves and yields a transparent solution.

The lemon-grass is employed in the form of infusion, in both the East and West Indies, as a mild diaphoretic in slight colds. The fresh leaves are sometimes used as a substitute for tea, and the white succulent centre of the leaf-bearing stems serves to give an agreeable flavour to curries. In Martinique it is reputed poisonous, or, at least, as capable of producing abortion both in animals and the human species.[2]

Order VII. CYPERACEÆ, *R. Brown.*—SEDGES.

Characters.—The plants in this order closely resemble grasses (see *ante*), from which they are distinguished by their *embryo* being inclosed within the base of the albumen; by their *leaf-sheaths* being whole or entire, not slit; and by their *stems* being solid, angular, and without joints or diaphragms.

Properties.—These plants are remarkable for their deficiency of those organic principles which render the grasses so valuable and important to man (see *ante*).— The so-called roots (rhizomes) of several species of *Cyperus* (e. g. *longus*, *rotundus*, and *esculentus*) were formerly employed in medicine.—They are mild aromatics, stomachics, and diaphoretics. The roasted roots of *C. esculentus* have been used as a substitute for coffee. The rhizomes of *Carex arenaria* have been employed as a substitute for sarsaparilla, under the name of *bastard* or *German sarsaparilla* (*radix sarsaparillæ germanicæ* vel *radix graminis major*).

Sub-class II. *Petaloidæ* vel *Floridæ*.

Characters.—Floral envelopes, if present, whorled.

This sub-class includes all the remaining orders of endogens, which may be arranged in two sub divisions.

SUB-DIVISION I.

Floral envelopes absent ; or, if present, imperfect, squamiform, sometimes more or less glumaceous.

Order VIII. AROIDEÆ, *Endl.*

Araceæ and Orontiaceæ, *Lindl.*

Characters. — *Flowers* generally unisexual, rarely hermaphrodite, arranged upon a *spadix*, in the axil of a *spathe*. *Perianth* either none, or, in the hermaphrodite flowers,

---

[1] Hamilton, *Pharmaceutical Journal*, vol. vi. p. 369, 1846.
[2] Guibourt, *Hist. Nat. des Drogues*, 4me édit. t. ii. p. 114, 1849.

rudimentary and scaly. *Stamens* numerous, or definite and opposite to the segments of the perianth: *anthers* opening outwards. *Ovaries* free, 1-, 3-, or many-celled. *Fruit* succulent or dry, indehiscent. *Seeds* usually with fleshy or mealy albumen, rarely with none.—Usually herbaceous plants with either subterranean tubers (cormi) or a creeping rhizome.

PROPERTIES.—The fresh plants of this order are frequently remarkable for acridity, which especially resides in the tubers and rhizomes, and often renders them violent poisons. This is especially remarkable in *Dieffenbachia Seguina*, or the Dumb Cane, a native of the West India Islands, two drachms of whose juice have been known to prove fatal in two hours. The acrid principle (which, perhaps, may be a sulphurated volatile oil) is in many cases readily dissipated or decomposed, and rendered inert, by cooking. Even drying seems to injure or destroy it. As it is soluble in water, washing removes it from the starch. The useful qualities of the order depend on *starch* and *aromatic volatile oil:* on the former depend the esculent properties of some species, and on the latter the medicinal properties of some.

Colocasia esculenta (also called *Caladium esculentum* or *Arum esculentum*) is used in some parts of the world as food. Its large fleshy and farinaceous tubers are called *yams* in Madeira, from whence they were sent me by Mr. Nobrega. I find that when boiled they form a very agreeable substitute for potatoes.

Colocasia Antiquorum is cultivated in Egypt and other parts of the world for the nutritious matter yielded by the tubers.

Sub-order I. ARACEÆ, *Endl.*

Flowers naked, unisexual.

46. Arum maculatum, *Linn.*—Cuckow-pint.

Sex. Syst. Monœcia, Polyandria.
(Tuber.)

ARUM VULGARE, Lam.; *Common Cuckow-pint; Wake Robin; Lords and Ladies.*—A well-known indigenous, acrid, and poisonous plant, which, by drying or by the aid of heat, loses its acridity. From the underground tubers is manufactured, in the island of Portland, a starch called *Portland arrow-root* or *Portland sago* (*fæcula ari; farina ari*). It is procured by cleansing the roots (tubers), pounding them in a stone mortar with water, and then straining. The starch subsides from the strained liquor, and, the super-natant water being poured off, is collected and dried.[1] Care is requisite in the pounding of the roots, on account of their acridity. From a peck of the roots about a pound of starch is procured. [Mr. Groves states that scarcely any Portland arrow-root is now manufactured. The yield, according to his informant (an old woman, and the only arrow-root manufacturer now on the island), is 3 lbs. from a peck of roots.[2]—ED.]

Portland arrow-root is a white amylaceous powder. Examined by the microscope, its particles are found to be exceedingly small,[3] circular, mullar-shaped, or polyhedral. The

---

[1] Mrs. Gibbs, *Transactions of the Society of Arts*, vol. xv. p. 238, 1797.
[2] [*Pharm. Trans.* vol. xiii. p. 60.]
[3] The following measurements of five particles were made by Mr. Jackson:—

1.	0·0004	of an English inch.
2.	0·0003	" "
3.	0·00022	" "
4.	0·00013	" "
5.	0·0001	" "

5) 0·00115

Average.............. 0·00023

The average size, therefore, is the $\frac{1}{4348}$th of the inch in diameter.

angular appearance of some of them arises from compression. The hilum is circular, and apparently lies in a small depression. It cracks in a linear or stellate manner. The dietetical uses of this starch are similar to those of other starches, as of the West Indian arrow-root. It makes very agreeable puddings. The roasted tubers are esculent.

The fresh plant is an acrid poison; causing burning and swelling of the throat, vomiting, colic, diarrhœa, and convulsions. By drying, the activity of the plant is in a great measure destroyed. Medicinally, the tubers were formerly used as diuretics in dropsies, and as expectorants in chronic catarrhs.[1]

47. Arisæma atrorubens, *Blume.*—Dragon-root.

Sex. Syst. Monœcia, Polyandria.
(Tuber.)

ARISÆMA ATRORUBENS, Blume, Rumphia, i. 97; *Arum triphyllum*, Linn.; *Dragon-root; Indian Turnip; Wake Robin.*—A native of the United States of America. Its properties agree closely with Arum maculatum, and, like the latter, it yields a pure white fecula. The tuber is used in America as a stimulant to the secretions in chronic bronchial affections, rheumatism, &c., in doses of from ten grains to a scruple. The powder made into a paste with honey has been beneficially applied to the mouth and throat of children in aphthæ.[2]

Sub-order II. CALLACEÆ, *Endl.*

Perfect stamens associated with ovaries in hermaphrodite florets.

48. ACORUS CALAMUS, *Linn.*—COMMON SWEET FLAG.

Sex. Syst. Hexandria, Monogynia.
(Rhizoma, *L.*—Rhizome, *E.*)

HISTORY.—This is probably the ἄκορον of Dioscorides.[3] Dr. Royle says that in Persian works *akoron* is given as its Greek appellation. It must not be confounded with the κάλαμος ἀρωματικός of Dioscorides, which, according to Dr. Royle,[4] is *Andropogon Calamus aromaticus,* Royle (see *ante,* p. 1025).

BOTANY. **Gen. Char.**—*Flowers* arranged upon a *spadix. Spathe* replaced by a 2-edged leaf-blade. *Perianth* of 6 pieces or scales, inferior, persistent. *Stamens* 6, filiform. *Stigma* sessile. *Ovaries* 2—3-celled. *Berries* 1-celled, 1—3-seeded. *Seeds* albuminous.

Sp. Char.—*Spathe,* a continuation of the 2-edged *scape,* rising much above the spadix.

Rhizome thick, rather spongy, with many long roots, aromatic, like every part of the herbage, but much more powerfully so. *Leaves* erect, two or three feet high, bright green, near an inch broad. *Stalk* like the leaves, except being thicker below the *spadix,* and not quite so tall. *Spadix* about a foot above the root, a little spreading, two or three inches long, tapering,

---

[1] See Murray, *App. Med.* vol. v. p. 44, 1790; and Alston's *Lectures on the Materia Medica,* vol. i. p. 387.

[2] Carson, in the American edition of my *Elements of Materia Medica;* also Wood and Bache's *United States Dispensatory.*

[3] Lib. i. cap. 2.

Essay on the Antiq. of Hindoo Med. p. 33.

covered with a mass of very numerous, thick-set, pale green *flowers*, which have no scent except when bruised. A very narrow wavy membrane may be observed at the base of the spadix, which perhaps ought to be taken into the generic character as a *spathe* (*Smith*).—Perennial ; flowers in June.

Hab.—It is a native of this country, growing in watery places about the banks of rivers, and is very plentiful in the rivers of Norfolk , whence the London market was formerly supplied. It grows also in other countries of Europe, in Asia, and in the United States.

Description.—The dried underground stem (*rhizoma*, L.; *radix acori, veri* seu *radix calami aromatici*, offic.) occurs in the shops in flattened pieces four or five or more inches long, and about as broad as the thumb ; jointed, somewhat curved, of a spongy or corky texture internally ; of a yel-lowish-brown or fawn colour externally, and buffy, with a slight roseate hue, internally. Their fracture is short : their upper surface is marked transversely with the vestiges of the leaves which were attached to it; the lower surface has numerous dark points, surrounded by small light-coloured elevated circles, from which the roots arise. Their taste is warm and bitter ; their odour is aromatic. In Germany the rhizome is usually peeled before drying it (*rhizoma decorticata*) ; but the operation is unnecessary and wasteful. In this state the rhizome is greyish-white and easily pulverisable.

The rhizome should be gathered in spring or late in the autumn, and dried quickly. It is usually gathered on the banks of the Thames about May, for the London market. The fresh rhizome is employed for distillation. The pieces are sometimes fourteen or fifteen inches long, and one inch wide. The rhizome of the Yellow Water Iris (*Iris pseudo-acorus*) is said to be some-times substituted for that of the true Acorus.

Composition.—The fresh rhizome was analysed by Trommsdorff,[1] who ob-tained the following results :—*Volatile oil*, 0·1 ; *soft resin*, 2·3 ; *extractive, with a little chloride of potassium*, 3·3 ; *gum, with some phosphate of potash*, 5·5 ; *starchy matter* (like inulin), 1·6 ; *woody fibre*, 21·5 ; and *water*, 65·7. Meissner found traces of copper in the ashes. The active con-stituents are the oil, the resin, and the extractive.

Oil of the Common Sweet Flag (*oleum acori calami*, called in the shops *oleum calami aromatici*) is obtained by distilling the fresh rhizome with water. Its odour is similar to, though less agreeable than, that of the rhizome. Its colour is yellow. It is bought by snuff-makers, so that it is used, I presume, for scenting snuff. It is also employed in the preparation of *aromatic vinegar*.

Chemical Characteristics.—Iodine blackens the rhizome (especially when it has been boiled), thereby indicating the presence of starch. The cold decoction of the rhizome forms with a solution of iodine the blue *iodide of starch*. Acetate and diacetate of lead, and protonitrate of mercury, cause pre-cipitates with the decoction. These precipitates consist principally of metallic oxides or subsalts, and the substance called extractive. Nitrate of silver pro-duces a precipitate (*chloride of silver*), which is insoluble in nitric acid, but soluble in ammonia. The decoction reddens litmus.

Physiological Effects.—It is an aromatic stimulant and mild tonic. Vogt[2] arranges it with the *excitantia volatilia*, and regards it as approaching

---

[1] Gmelin, *Handb. d. Chem.* ii. 1339.
[2] *Lehrb. d. Pharmakodyn.* i. 454, 2te Aufl.

angelica root on the one hand, and cascarilla and angustura barks on the other.

Uses.—It is rarely employed by medical practitioners, though it might be frequently substituted, with good effect, for the more costly oriental aromatics. It is a useful adjunct to other stimulants and tonics. It has been employed in continued asthenic fevers accompanied with much prostration of strength and greatly weakened digestive power. For the cure of ague, the dried root powdered is used by the country people in Norfolk.[1] It is well adapted for dyspeptic cases accompanied with, or dependent on, an atonic condition of the digestive organs, and is especially serviceable in gouty subjects. It has also been used as a local agent, viz. in the formation of aromatic baths, poultices, and gargles, as an application to foul-conditioned ulcers, &c. It is employed, I am informed, by some rectifiers to flavour gin.

Administration.—In *powder*, the rhizome may be given in doses of from a scruple to a drachm. The *infusion* is perhaps the most eligible preparation : it is made by digesting ℥j. of the rhizome in ℥xij. of boiling water ; the dose is two or three table-spoonfuls. The *decoction* is an objectionable preparation, as the oil of the rhizome is dissipated by boiling. The *tincture* (Ph. Bor.) is procured by digesting ℥ij. of the rhizome in ℥xij. of spirit (sp. gr. 0·900) ; the dose is a tea-spoonful.

SUB-DIVISION II.

Flowers with a proper, often corolline perianth, usually hermaphrodite.

1. Leaves with parallel veins, either proceeding from the base to the apex (*straight-veined*), or curved and proceeding from the midrib to the margin (*curved-veined*).

† Flowers sessile on a branched scaly spadix, usually unisexual.

Order IX. PALMÆ, *Juss.*—THE PALM TRIBE.

Palmaceæ, *Lindl.*

Characters.—*Flowers* hermaphrodite, or frequently polygamous. *Perianth* 6-parted, in two series, persistent ; the three outer segments often smaller, the inner sometimes deeply connate. *Stamens* inserted into the base of the perianth, usually definite in number, opposite the segments of the perianth, to which they are equal in number, seldom 3 ; sometimes, in a few polygamous genera, indefinite in number. *Ovary* 1, 3-celled, or deeply 3-lobed ; the lobes or cells 1-seeded, with an erect ovule, rarely 1-seeded. *Fruit* baccate or drupaceous, with fibrous flesh. *Albumen* cartilaginous, and either ruminate or furnished with a central or ventral cavity ; *embryo* lodged in a particular cavity of the albumen, usually at a distance from the hilum, dorsal, and indicated by a little nipple, taper- or pulley-shaped ; *plumule* included, scarcely visible ; the cotyledonous extremity becoming thickened in germination, and either filling up a pre-existing cavity, or one formed by the liquefaction of the albumen in the centre.—*Trunk* arborescent, simple, occasionally shrubby and branched, rough, with the dilated half-sheathing bases of the leaves or their scars. *Leaves* clustered, terminal, very large, pinnate or flabelliform, plaited in vernation. *Spadix* terminal, often branched, enclosed in a 1- or many-valved spathe. *Flowers* small, with bractlets. *Fruit* occasionally very large. (*R. Brown*, 1810.)

---

[1] Sir J. E. Smith, *Engl. Flora*, ii. 158.

PROPERTIES.—Palms, considered in a dietetical and medicinal point of view, are of the highest importance to the inhabitants of tropical regions. Their *stems* yield starch (sago), sugar, and wax; their *terminal leaf-buds* are boiled and eaten as a kind of cabbage; their *fruits* yield oil, sugar, and resins; and their *seeds* form articles of food, and yield, by pressure, fixed oil.

In the abundance of *sugar* and *starch* which the palms yield, this family resembles the grasses. But they are distinguished from the latter in containing in some cases a large quantity of fixed *oil*. To these three principles are chiefly due the nutritive qualities of palms. But these substances being non-nitrogenised, are merely fat-making and heat-yielding, and without the addition of *proteine compounds* (found in the seeds, and probably in other edible parts of palms), would be insufficient to support life.

Palm sugar in the crude state is called *jaggary*. By fermentation, it yields *toddy* or *palm wine*, from which, by distillation, an ardent spirit (*arrack* or *rack*) is obtained. *Date sugar*, and also other kinds of palm sugar, are imported into England, and are used by grocers for mixing; but, being deficient in what in trade is called "strength," they do not pay for refining.[1]

Wax, astringent matter (tannin), and *resinous principles*, are useful products obtained from palms; but they are of less frequent occurrence than the substances before mentioned. Still less frequently met with are *acrid* principles. The ashes obtained by the combustion of palm leaves yield *potash*.

1. PALMÆ FARINIFERÆ.—SAGO PALMS.

The farinaceous substance called *sago* is obtained from the stems of several palms. Those of the genera *Sagus* and *Saguerus* are the most important, and will be separately noticed.

The trunk of old trees of *Caryota urens*, called, by Robinson,[2] the *Sago palm of Assam*, yields a sago which both Roxburgh[3] and Robinson consider to be very little if at all inferior to the sago of the Malay countries. From *Phœnix farinifera*, which grows in the Coromandel coast, is likewise obtained a sago, but which is less nutritious and palatable than the common sago.[4] *Corypha umbraculifera*, or the Talipat palm, yields sago in Ceylon; which would appear from the statement of Bennett[5] to be of inferior quality.

Japan Sago is said to be obtained from several species of *Cycas*. None of this, however, reaches England. (See Order CYCADEÆ.)

49. SAGUS, *Gærtner.*

Sex. Syst. Monœcia, Hexandria.

Metroxylon, Rottb.

GEN. CHAR.—*Flowers* hermaphrodite or polygamo-monœcious on the same spadix. *Spadix* much branched, sheathed by many incomplete spathes. *Amenta* terete. *Bract* squamiform: *bractlets* very densely villose-bearded, connate like a cupule. *Calyx* 3-cleft. *Corolla* 3-partite. *Stamens* 6: filaments subulate, connate at the base; *anthers* affixed by the back. *Ovary* subtrilocular: stigmata 3, connate in a pyramid. Berry coated by reversed scales, 1-seeded. *Albumen* ruminated or uniform. *Embryo* dorsal. (*Blume,* Rumphia.)

---

[1] *Pharmaceutical Journal*, vol. v. p. 64, 1845.
[2] *A Descriptive Account of Asam*, p. 56, Calcutta, 1841.
[3] *Flora Indica*, vol. iii. p. 626.
[4] *Ibid.* p. 786.
[5] *Ceylon and its Capabilities*, p. 95, Lond. 1843.

1. Sagus lævis, Rumph. i. 76, tab. 86 and 126-127 (nomíne S. Rumphii).; Blume, Rumphia, vol. ii. p. 147; Jack, in Comp. Bot. Mag. i. 266; *Sagus inermis*, Roxb. Fl. Ind. iii. 623; *Metroxylon læve*, Mart. Gen. et Sp. Plant. p. 215, 2; Kunth, Enum. Plant. iii. 214, 2; *Metroxylon Sagus*, Rottb.; *Rambia* or *Rambija* of the Malays; the *Unarmed Sago-Palm*.

Stem tallish. Petioles, rachides, and spathes, unarmed. Fruit somewhat globose, and depressed on both sides. (*Blume,* in Rumphia, p. 147.)

Islands of the Indian Archipelago, Sumatra and Borneo, and the islands between them, growing spontaneously in low swampy lands.

A large quantity of granular sago is prepared from this species[1] in Sumatra especially, the peninsula of Malacca, and in Borneo. It is chiefly exported to Europe, Bengal, and China. The farina which is brought from Siak, on the northern coast of Sumatra, although inferior in whiteness to that of Borneo, is much sought after, on account of its being less friable. It commonly fetches twice the price of the latter.[2] The quantity of sago yielded by this palm is prodigious: Crawfurd[3] says 500 or 600 lbs. is not an unusual produce for one tree: and Blume mentions 600 to 800 lbs. as the quantity obtained from a single tree when mature.

2. Sagus genuina, Rumph. (ex parte); Blume, Rumphia, vol. ii. p. 150; *Sagus Rumphii*, Roxb. Fl. Ind. iii. p. 623 (excel. synon.); *Sagus spinosus*, Roxb. ibid.; *Metroxylon Rumphii*, Mart. Gen. et Sp. Palm. p. 214, tab. 102 and 159.

Stem of middling height. Petioles, rachides, and spathes prickly; the prickles scattered or confluent. Fruit somewhat globose, depressed on both sides (*Blume*).

Islands of the Indian Archipelago. Abounds in the Malacca islands, especially where the nutmeg and clove grow naturally.

"This, the Malay Sago Palm, is the tree the pith of which is the staff of life to the inhabitants of the Moluccas" (*Roxburgh*).

The stature of this tree seldom exceeds thirty feet. Before maturity, and previous to the formation of the fruit, the stem consists of a thin hard wall about two inches thick, and of an enormous volume of tissue (commonly termed the *medulla* or *pith*), from which the farina, called sago, is obtained. As the fruit forms, the farinaceous medulla disappears; and when the tree attains full maturity, the stem is no more than a hollow shell. The utmost age of the tree does not exceed thirty years.[4]

50. SAGUERUS SACCHARIFER, *Blume.*—THE GOMUTO PALM.

Sex. Syst. Monœcia, Polyandria.

Synonymes.—*Palma Indica vinaria secunda, Saguerus,* sive *Gomutus Gomuto,* Rumph. Amb. i. p. 57, t. 13; *Anau,* Marsden, Hist. Sum. p. 88, 3d ed.; *Saguerus Rumphii,* Roxb. Fl. Ind. iii. 626; *Arenga saccharifera,* Mart. Gen. et Sp. Palm. p. 191, tab. 108.

---

[1] Roxburgh (*Flora Indica,* vol. iii. p. 623) says that from the pith of this tree "the granulated sago which we meet with in Europe is made."
[2] Blume, *Rumphia,* vol. ii. p. 148.
[3] *History of the Indian Archipelago,* vol. i. p. 393.
[4] Crawfurd, *op. cit.* vol. i. p. 384.

BOTANY. **Gen. Char.**—*Flowers* monœcious by abortion, on separate spadices, sessile, the female ones between two males. *Spadices* simply branched. *Spathes* many incomplete. *Calyx* 3-cleft, with imbricated leaflets. *Corolla* 3-petalous, with valvate æstivation. MALES: *Stamina* indefinite : *filaments* filiform : *anthers* linear, cuspidate. FEMALES : *Ovary* trilocular, with the *Ovule* affixed at the bottom of the internal angle. *Stigmata* 3, acute, connivent. *Berry* 3- or, by abortion, 2-seeded. *Albumen* uniform. *Embryo* dorsal (*Blume.*)

Sp. Char.—Petioles unarmed. Segments of the fronds linear-lanceolate, at the base 1- or sub-2-auriculate, beneath whitish. Branches of the spadices elongated, fastigiate, pendulous. Berry turbinate-globose (*Blume*).—From 20 to 25 feet high : readily distinguished by its rude and wild aspect.

Hab.—Very common in the islands of the Indian Archipelago, the Moluccas, and the Philippines.

A saccharine juice called *nera* or toddy is obtained in large quantities by wounding the spadices and receiving the liquor in earthenware pots or bamboos closely fastened beneath.[1] This juice yields by boiling a coarse dark kind of sugar (*jaggary*), and by fermentation an intoxicating beverage; wine, which is used by the Chinese residing in the Indian islands in the preparation of Batavian arrack.[2] When the trees are exhausted by the incessant draining of their juices, sago of good quality is obtained from the trunk,—as much as 150 to 200 lbs. weight from a single tree.[3]

The flesh of the fruit is acrid, and affords a juice which, when applied to the skin, occasions great pain and inflammation. The inhabitants of the Moluccas were in the practice of using in their wars, in the defence of posts, a liquor afforded by the maceration of the fruit which the Dutch denominated *hell water* (*aqua infernalis*).[4]

SAGO.

HISTORY.—Sago does not appear to have been known to the Greeks, Romans, or Arabians. The preparation of sago-meal and sago-bread, as carried on at Fanfur (Kampar, in Sumatra ?), was first described by Marco Polo[5] in the thirteenth century. Sago-bread was described and figured by Clusius.[6]

Granulated sago was not known until a later period. It is said[7] to have been introduced into England in 1729, into France in 1740, and into Germany in 1744. Rumphius[8] states that in Borneo grains of the size of a coriander seed are made from the farina of the Saguerus (*Saguerus saccharifer,*

---

[1] Marsden's *History of Sumatra*, p. 88, 3d edit. 1811.
[2] Crawfurd's *History of the Indian Archipelago*, vol. i. p. 399, 1820.
[3] Blume, *Rumphia*, vol. ii. p. 126.
[4] Crawfurd, *op. cit.*
[5] *Travels in the Eastern Part of the World in the Thirteenth Century*, translated from the Italian, with Notes, by W. Marsden, p. 614, 4to, Lond. 1818.
[6] *Exotic.* lib. i. cap. iii. p. 5, 1605.
[7] Steck, quoted by J. A. Murray, *App. Medicam.* vol. iv. p. 17, 1790.
[8] *Herbarium Amboin.* pars 1ma, p. 64, Amst. 1750. " .... in Borneo ex eadem conficiunt farina rotunda grana Coriandri semen magnitudine et forma referentia." I have given the words of Rumphius, because some highly respectable authorities (J. A. Murray and Guibourt) have overlooked this passage, and assumed that Rumphius does not mention granulated sago..

Blume). The word *sagu* (also written by some of the earlier authors *zagu* and *saga*[1]) is the Malay name both for the palm and its farina :[2] it is also used in Java to signify the bread made from the farina.[3]

COMMERCE.—[Sago is brought to England from Singapore in boxes and bags, chiefly the former. The quantities on which duty was paid from 1848 to 1853 are, in cwts., as follows :—

	Cwts.		Cwts.		Cwts.
1848	64,103	1850	67,651	1852	87,166
1849	63,199	1851	70,464	1853	65,545—Ed.]

Newbold[4] gives the following as the quantities imported into Singapore in 1836 :—

	Bundles.
Sago from Sumatra	157750
" West Side Peninsula	140
" Borneo, 1308 piculs	140560
" North Islands, 140 piculs	15251
Total imported	313701

The quantity exported from Singapore in the same year was 28,764 piculs.

MANUFACTURE. a. *Of Raw Sago-meal.*—The manufacture of sago-meal varies somewhat in different localities. In the Moluccas it is procured as follows :—When the tree is sufficiently mature, it is cut down near the root, and the trunk subdivided into portions of six or seven feet long, each of which is split into two parts. From these the medullary matter is extracted, and with an instrument of bamboo or hard wood is reduced to powder, like sawdust. To separate the farina from the accompanying bran and filaments, it is mixed with water, and the mixture then strained by a sieve. The strained liquor deposits the farina, which, after two or more edulcorations, is fit for use. This is *raw sago-meal.*[5]

b. *Of Sago-bread.*—In the Moluccas sago-cakes are made by throwing the dry meal into heated earthenware moulds : a hard cake is formed in a few minutes, so that one heating of the mould serves to bake several series of cakes.[6]

c. *Of Granulated Sago.*—To prepare this the meal is mixed with water and made into a paste, which is then granulated. Forrest says that in New Guinea granulated sago is made by mixing the sago-meal with water and passing the paste through a sieve into a very shallow iron pot held over a fire, by which it is made to assume a globular form ; so that, he adds, our grained sago is half baked and will keep long. This, according to Blume, is the process which is followed by the Chinese colony in Singapore ; the meal being first repeatedly worked and dried. Blume adds, that during the heating

---

[1] See the authorities quoted in C. Bauhin's *Pinax.*

[2] Crawfurd, *History of the Indian Archipelago,* vol. i. p. 387, 1820.

[3] Sir F. Drake, iu Hakluyt's *Principal Navigations, Voyages,* &c. vol. iii. p. 742.

[4] *Political and Statistical Account of the British Settlements in the Straits of Malacca,* vol. i. p. 304, Lond. 1839.

[5] Crawfurd, *op. supra cit.* vol. i. p. 390. Mr. Crisp (*Asiat. Researches,* vol. vi. 1799) has described the mode of preparing sago-meal in the Poggy Islands, lying off Sumatra. See also Forrest's *Voyage to New Guinea,* 2d edit. 1780, pp. 39–41, for the method of preparing it by the Papuans.

[6] Forrest (*op. supra cit.*) has figured a mould which he calls the *Papua oven.*

process the grains are constantly turned, and that, though quite white at the commencement, they become hard and somewhat pellucid during the process.

One kind of pearl sago of the shops has been obviously subjected to some heating process: this is the *Tapioka-sago* of Guibourt; but the application of heat must have been most carefully regulated, for charred sago is unknown to commerce. Some of the granulated sago of the shops presents no evidence of having been heated; and it has, therefore, been supposed that its granulation must have been effected by a mill.

DESCRIPTION OF SAGO.—Sago occurs in commerce in two states,—pulverulent and granulated.

1. Pulverulent Sago; *Sago-meal; Sago-flour (Farina Sagi).*—This is imported in the form of a fine amylaceous powder. It is whitish, with a buffy or reddish tint. Its odour is faint, but somewhat unpleasant and musty. Viewed by a powerful pocket-lens, it presents a glistening granular appearance. Examined by the microscope, it is found to consist of irregularly elliptical or oval, more or less ovate, usually isolated particles,[1] which are often somewhat narrowed or tapered at one extremity. Owing to their mutual pressure, many of them appear as if truncated, either by a single plane perpendicular to the axis of the particle, in which they are more or less mullar-shaped,—or by two inclined planes, giving the particles a dihedral extremity. Some of them resemble in form a caoutchouc bottle cut off at the neck. From their strong lateral shading they are obviously convex. Many of the particles are more or less broken. Most of them have an irregular or tuberculated surface, as if eroded. The hilum, when perfect, is circular; but it cracks in the form of a single slit, or of a cross, or in a stellate manner. The surface of the particles presents the appearance of a series of concentric rings or annular lines, which, however, are much less distinct than in potato-starch. These lines are indicative of the concentric layers of which each particle is composed. When examined by the polarising microscope, the particles show a black cross, the centre of which is the hilum.

I have met with sago-meal in commerce under different names. Once I received a sample from Cockermouth, in Cumberland, where it was sold as "*Food for the People.*" A sample of a fine white and carefully-prepared sago-meal was given me under the name of *arrow-root.* I shall distinguish it as *refined sago-meal.* The following information respecting the mode of refining sago-meal was furnished me by a starch-manufacturer :—" By sifting and washing, the best sago-meal loses about one-fifth of its weight in the form

---

[1] The following measurements, in parts of an English inch, of the particles of starch of sago-meal, brown sago, and pearl sago, were made for me by Mr. George Jackson :—

Particles.	Sago-meal.		Brown Sago.		Pearl Sago.	
	Long diam.	Short diam.	Long diam.	Short diam.	Long diam.	Short diam.
1.	0·0022	0·0016	0·0026	0·00155	0·0031	0·0019
2.	0·00195	0·00135	0·0020	0·0014	0·0022	0·0015
3.	0·0017	0·0013	0·0017	0·0015	0·0021	0·0014
4.	0·0014	0·0014	0·0017	0·0012	0·0018	0·0013
5.	0·0013	0·00095	0·0013	0·0010	0·0018	0·0012
6.	0·0012	0·00095	0·0009	0·0006	0·0017	0·0012
7.	0·0005	0·0008	0·00·8	0·0008	0·0012	0·0008
8.	....	....	0·0075	0·0006	0·0008	0·00075

of earthy matter and woody fibre. The meal thus sifted and washed is then bleached by means of chloride of lime and sulphuric acid. The bleached meal is afterwards washed in successive waters until a perfectly pure product is obtained. In this state it serves as a food for infants and invalids. Coloured by turmeric, and flavoured by the essential oils of cassia and bitter almonds, it forms a *custard powder.* Without the colouring matter it serves as a *blanc-mange powder.*"

2. Granulated Sago; *Grain Sago* (*Sagus granulosa*); *Grana Sagi.*—The grains are more or less rounded masses of variable size and colour. Examined by a microscope with a low object-glass (say of 2- or 3-inch focus), they are seen to be masses of glistening particles. There are two kinds of granulated sago,—brown sago, and pearl sago.

a, *Common or Brown Sago* (*Sagus fusca*); *Sagou gris des Moluques,* Planche and Guibourt.—This is the only kind of sago which was known in English commerce prior to the introduction of pearl sago. It occurs in somewhat irregularly rounded or globular masses or grains, which are whitish on one side, and greyish-brown on the other. The ordinary brown sago of the shops consists of grains which are usually about the size of the grains of pearl barley. This may be termed the *smaller* or *ordinary brown sago.* It is the *sagou gris des Moluques* of both Planche and Guibourt. But there is another variety, the globular masses of which are larger, sometimes as large as grey peas. To distinguish it from the smaller sort just mentioned, I shall call it *large brown sago.* I received it first from Dr. Douglas Maclagan, of Edinburgh, and subsequently from Professor Guibourt, who terms it *gros sagou gris de Moluques.* The smaller masses of it are about equal in size to the larger masses of the former sort of brown sago. Except in the size of the grains or masses, the two sorts are identical.

Examined by the microscope, the grains of brown sago are found to consist of particles like those of sago-meal, but somewhat more broken and less regular in their shape. Some of them present the appearance of containing in their interior a smaller particle, or rather perhaps an air-cavity, which, when examined by polarised light, forms the centre of the black cross. Intermixed with the starch particles is a yellowish-brown substance, which gives colour to the sago.

[This is known here as "Borneo sago," and as now imported includes all sizes, from a mustard-grain to that of a small pea, in the same bag : it is usually very dusty, say 25 per cent. The sorts called by the author "smaller or ordinary brown" and "large brown" are not now imported.—Ed.]

β. *Pearl Sago* (*Sagus perlata*).—The manufacture of this kind of sago is comparatively recent. Crawfurd,[1] who wrote in 1820, says, " within the last few years the Chinese of Malacca have invented a process by which they refine sago so as to give it a fine pearly lustre. . . . A small quantity of it, exposed for sale in the London market in 1818, sold for about thrice the price of ordinary [that is, brown] sago." The sago used by the Chinese at Malacca in the manufacture of pearl sago, is, according to Newbold,[2] brought from Sumatra. Pearl sago is also prepared at Singapore.[3]

---

[1] *History of the Indian Archipelago,* vol. iii. p. 349, 1820.
[2] *Political and Statistical Account of the British Settlements in the Straits of Malacca,* vol. i. p. 243-4, 1839.
[3] Blume, *Rumphia,* vol. ii. p. 148.

Pearl sago occurs in pearl-like grains, which vary in size from that of poppy-seeds to that of white mustard-seeds, or even somewhat larger than these. The shape of the larger grains is more or less globular, that of the smaller ones being often much less regular. The surface of the larger grains is smooth, even, and regular; that of the small grains often rough, uneven, and somewhat tuberculated. Occasionally two or three of the smaller grains adhere together. Some samples are white, some brownish-yellow, pink, or roseate. The coloured grains are not of uniform tint over the whole of their surface; often being on one side white, on the other coloured. By the aid of a solution of chloride of lime, the coloured kinds can be bleached and rendered perfectly white (*bleached pearl sago*). When submitted to microscopic examination, pearl sago is found to consist of the same kind of starch-particles as sago-meal, but all more or less ruptured, and presenting indistinct traces of rings. These peculiarities are doubtless produced by the process of granulation.

αα. White Pearl Sago.—Grains smaller than white mustard-seeds; opaque and white on one side, pearly on the other. The filtered cold aqueous infusion does not strike a blue colour with tincture of iodine. The whiteness of this kind of pearl-sago has probably been produced by bleaching.

ββ. Coloured Pearl Sago.—Grains of different size. Those of some sorts are not larger than poppy-seeds (*small coloured pearl sago*), while those of other sorts are nearly as large, or even somewhat larger, than white mustard seeds (*large coloured pearl sago*). The colour varies in intensity, and slightly in shade also; but the prevailing tint is that of bran, or sometimes pinkish-brownish yellow. Some sorts are as pale as ground, unsifted, wheat-flour (*pale coloured pearl sago*); others are nearly as deep coloured as bran itself. Some of the larger sorts have a greyish or brownish colour (*greyish* or *brownish pearl sago*); but, like all kinds of coloured sago, the tint is not uniform on different parts of the same grain; being deep on one side and pale on the other.

The filtered cold aqueous infusion of some sorts does not strike a blue colour with tincture of iodine. This kind corresponds to the *Sagou rosé des Moluques* of Planche and Guibourt. The filtered cold aqueous infusion of other sorts yields a blue colour on the addition of tincture of iodine, showing that a higher temperature has been employed in the preparation of it than of other sorts. This corresponds to the *Sagou-tapioka* or *Tapioca-sago* of Guibourt. When examined by the microscope, the particles are found to be more ruptured and torn,—an obvious effect of heat on them. This sort of pearl sago is often not distinguishable by its external appearance from that of the *Sagou rosé des Moluques* of Planche and Guibourt.

Under the name of *damaged pearl sago* I have received a sample of coloured pearl sago, some of the particles of which are yellow (from sulphur-yellow to orange-coloured). When bleached by means of chloride of lime, it becomes quite white (*bleached pearl sago*).

[Within the last three or four years a new sort of sago has been introduced from Singapore, which is called "Tapioca-sago." It is made in various sizes (the same as pearl sago), but is very much finer and brighter, and fetches more money. It has been observed that some of this sago has a curious flavour—somewhat tallowy.—ED.]

FACTITIOUS SAGO.—This is prepared in both Germany and in France (at Gentilly, near Paris) with potato-starch. It occurs both white and coloured.

There are two kinds of *white factitious sago*,—one small-grained, the grains of which are scarcely so large as white mustard-seeds; the other large-grained, the grains of which are intermediate in size between white mustard-seeds and coriander-seeds. The first I met with in English commerce; for the other I am indebted to Professor Guibourt. I have also two kinds of *coloured factitious sago*, both large-grained,—one red,[1] the other brownish,[2] and somewhat resembling brownish pearl sago. For both of these I am indebted to Professor Guibourt. The white and the red sorts are remarkable for being spherical and smooth.

The microscope can alone distinguish factitious sago from the real sort. The difference in the size, the shape, and other characters, between the particles of sago-starch and the unaltered particles of potato-starch, readily distinguish the one from the other. (See also *Potato-starch*). But many of the starch-particles of potato-sago are ruptured by the influences to which they have been subjected during the preparation of the sago. They have become swollen, ruptured in the direction of their long axis, and by drying have shrivelled, leaving a long, linear, sometimes curved or even-branched line with incurved or involuted edges, indicating the situation of the rupture.

I have received from Professor Guibourt samples of "*Sagou des Maldives* de Planche, donné par lui," and "*Sagou de la Nouvelle Guinée* de Planche,[3] donné par lui," and find them to be fictitious sagos made from potato-starch. The grains of New Guinea sago are undistinguishable externally, and by the microscopic examination of their starch-particles form red-coloured "*Sagou de fécule de pomme de terre*," also sent me by Professor Guibourt. Both are bright red on one side, and whitish on the other. Most of their starch-grains are ruptured and shrivelled, as above described. The Maldive Sago is paler-coloured, and some of its starch-particles are little or not at all altered; others are ruptured and shrivelled.

COMPOSITION.—Sago has not been analysed. The pure starch, of which it essentially consists, doubtless has the same composition as other amylaceous substances, viz. $C^{12}H^{10}O^{10}$. Sago-meal is contaminated with various impurities (see *ante*, p. 146). Granulated sago contains some colouring matter, particles of which may readily be detected by the microscope.

CHEMICAL CHARACTERISTICS.—Sago possesses the general characters of an amylaceous substance.

Sago-meal is insoluble in cold water; but, by boiling in water, it almost entirely dissolves, and yields a tolerably clear solution. The decoction, when cold, strikes a blue colour with tincture of iodine.

Granulated sago swells up in cold water, but does not completely dissolve by boiling; a more or less considerable amount of insoluble matter remaining behind. The remarkable difference in the action of boiling water on sago-meal, and on different kinds of granulated sago, leads me to suspect that some substance of difficult solubility in water is used in the preparation of the paste for making granulated sago. The filtered cold aqueous infusion of some sorts of pearl sago (*Sagou-tapioka* of Guibourt) strikes a blue colour with tincture of iodine. The cold infusion of brown sago is rendered milky

[1] This is, perhaps, the kind mentioned by Planche (*Journ. de Pharm.* t. xxiii. p. 305, 1837) as being "falsified sago coloured by cochineal."
[2] This, perhaps, is the brown sort of German sago made from potato-starch, and said by Dierbach (*Synopsis Materiæ Medicæ*, Abt. i. S. 27, 1841) to be coloured by burnt sugar.
[3] *Journ. d. Pharm.* tom. xxiii. p. 155, 1837.

by nitrate of silver, diacetate of lead, and protonitrate of mercury; but the cold infusions of pulverulent and of pearl sago are scarcely affected by these tests.

PHYSIOLOGICAL EFFECTS.—It is nutritive and easy of digestion, and is an important article of food in some parts of the East. "The Malay sago palm," says Dr. Roxburgh, "is the tree the pith of which is the staff of life to the inhabitants of the Moluccas." It is probable that this pith contains some nitrogenised nutritive substance in addition to the amylaceous matter.

USES.—Sago puddings are occasionally brought to table. But the principal use of sago is to yield a light, nutritious, easily digestible, and non-irritating article of food for the invalid in febrile and inflammatory cases. For this purpose it should be boiled in water (in some cases milk is preferred), the solution strained, and flavoured with sugar and spices, or even with a little white wine, when the use of this is not contraindicated.

2. PALMÆ OLEIFERÆ.—OIL PALMS.

Oil is obtained from the fruit of some, and from the seeds of many palms. Two oils obtained from palms are found in commerce: they are palm oil, and cocoa-nut oil; the one obtained from a species of Elæis, the other from a Cocos.

51. Elæis, *Jacquin.*—The Guinea Oil Palms.

Sex. Syst. Diœcia, Hexandria.
(Fructûs oleum.)

Palm oil is obtained from two species of Elæis, both natives of Guinea, and to both of which the name of Guinea Oil Palm is equally applicable. The oil resides in the fleshy portion of the fruit, which, in this respect, resembles the olive.

1. ELÆIS GUINEENSIS, Jacquin; *The True Guinea Oil Palm; The Palm Oil-tree,* Sloane's Jamaica, vol. ii, p. 113, 1725; *Avoira,* Aubl., Pl. de la Guiane, 1775.—A native of Guinea; cultivated in tropical America. The drupes are about the size of pigeons' eggs, ovate, somewhat angular, deep orange-yellow, collected in heads. They have a thin epicarp, a fibrous, oily, yellow sarcocarp, which covers and closely adheres to the hard stony putamen or endocarp, within which is the seed. From the sarcocarp is procured *palm oil* (*oleum palmæ*). This is obtained by boiling the pulp in water, by which the oil separates and floats on the surface.

2. ELÆIS MELANOCOCCA, Gaertner.—The drupes are somewhat smaller than those of the preceding species. Some time since I received from Mr. Warrington a bunch of them, which had been recently brought from Guinea as the fruit from which palm oil is obtained. The flesh of the fruit is oily, and has the well-known odour and colour of palm oil. Gaertner[1] thought that it might be only a variety of *E. guineensis;* but Von Martius,[2] who has fully described it, regards it as a distinct species.

At the ordinary temperatures of this country it is solid, and might, therefore, with more propriety be termed *palm butter.* It is said that, when quite fresh, it fuses at 81° F.; but that, by keeping, its fusing point rises. Stenhouse[3] found that very old palm oil required a temperature of 98½° F. to fuse it. Palm oil has a rich orange-yellow colour, a sweetish taste, and an agreeable odour resembling that of the rhizome of the Florentine orris. It is soluble in boiling alcohol and in ether. By exposure to solar light it becomes white. Palm oil requires to be bleached for various uses in the arts, and there are several

---

[1] *De Fructibus et Semin. Plant.* vol. i. p. 18, 1801.
[2] *Palmæ Brasil.* p. 62, tab. 54–56.
[3] *Ann. d. Chemie u. Pharm.* Bd. xxxvi. S. 50.

agents which are used for decolourising it—viz. chlorine, oxygen, powerful acids (sulphuric, nitric, or chromic acid), and the combined influence of air, heat, and light.[1]

Palm oil consists of *oleine, palmitine,* and *colouring matter.* As found in commerce, it usually contains also *free fatty acids* (oleic and palmitic) and *free glycerine,* and, therefore, may be said to be rancid. The cause of the separation of these acids from the glycerine has not been satisfactorily explained. The quantity of them increases with the age of the oil, and, according to Pelouze and Boudet,[2] varies from 33 to 80 per cent. of the entire oil. In proportion as the quantity increases, the fusing point of the oil rises. The glycerine which is set free gradually becomes converted into *sebacic acid,* which is also found in old palm oil. These various changes seem to be effected by a kind of fermentation, to the commencement of which, according to Guibourt,[3] the presence of atmospheric air is necessary.

Palmitine is a white solid fat, which is resolved, by saponification and by the fermentation just alluded to, into *palmitic acid* ($C^{32}H^{31}O^3+HO$), considered by Dumas to be identical with ethalic acid,—and *glycerine* (oxide of glycerule).

The Africans use palm oil as a kind of butter. It is now rarely employed in medicine. By the public it is occasionally used by way of friction in bruises and sprains. It is a constituent of the common black bougie. Its ordinary use in this country is in the manufacture of soap and candles.[4] It readily becomes rancid.

The *seeds* of both species of Elæis are nutritive. They yield by pressure a fixed oil (*palm-seed oil; oleum palmæ seminis*), which is solid at ordinary temperature. It is devoid of the orange-yellow colour and orris odour of palm oil. It is said to be used in Africa as a kind of butter. It is rarely brought to Europe; but a few years since I obtained from Africa a specimen of it, with a sample of the seeds from which it was procured.

52. Cocos nucifera, *Linn.*—The Cocoa-nut Tree.

Sex. Syst. Monœcia, Hexandria.
(Semina.)

Tenga, Rheede, Hort. Malab. i. t. 1, 2, 3, 4; *Calappa,* Rumph., Herb. Amb. i. t. 1, 2.— A native of tropical countries, but does not thrive except near the coast. It is one of the most important and valuable palms. Five varieties of it are indigenous to Ceylon.[5] Its stem yields *porcupine wood.* A powerful oil is extracted from the bark, which is used by the Cingalese in the form of ointment in cutaneous diseases. By incision into the spathe at the top of the leaves, *sweet toddy* is obtained, which, by fermentation, yields *palm wine,* from which *arrack* is procured by distillation. The fruit, the *cocoa-nut in the shell* of the shops, is a drupe, the fibrous portion of which yields *coir,* which is used for making ropes, mats, &c., and is also employed, as a substitute for horse-hair, for stuffing mattresses. Within the *cocoa-nut* is the nucleus or kernel (in the dried state called *copra* in commerce), consisting of the albumen (the edible portion), within which is the unsolidified liquor amnii (called *cocoa-nut milk*) and the embryo, which is lodged in a small cavity at the base of the albumen. The albumen and cocoa-nut milk have been analysed by Brandes,[6] Buchner,[7] and Bizio.[8] According to the latter authority, 100 parts of cocoa-nut milk contain—water, 95; crystallisable glycine (identical with orcine and granatine), 3·825; zymome, 0·75; and mucilage, 0·25 [loss, 0·175]. In 100 parts of the albumen he found 71·488 of oil; 7·665 of zymome; 3·588 of mucilage; 1·595 of crystallisable glycine; 0·325 of yellow colouring matter; and 14·950 of woody fibre [loss, 0·392].[9] There are

---

[1] Knapp's *Chemical Technology,* vol. i. p. 431, 1848.
[2] *Journ. de Pharm.* t. xxiv. p. 385, 1838.
[3] *Hist. Nat. des Drogues simples,* 4me édit. t. ii. p. 142, 1849.
[4] [It is also used in the manufacture of anti-attrition grease. A compound of palm oil and soda is now extensively employed in the attrition boxes of railway carriages.—Ed.]
[5] *The Coco-nut Palm, its Uses and Cultivation,* by J. W. Bennett, 2d edit. Lond. 1836.
[6] Quoted by L. Gmelin, *Handb. d. Chemie,* Bd. ii. S. 1338.
[7] *Repert. für die Pharm.* Bd. xxvi. S. 337, 1827.
[8] *Journ. de Pharm.* t. xix. p. 455, 1833.
[9] [A more recent analysis will be found in the *Pharm. Journ.* vol. xi. p. 513. No fact of interest, however, has been elicited on this subject, excepting the formation of metacetonic acid during the decomposition of the cocoa-nut milk.—Ed.]

two modes, practised at Malabar and Ceylon, of obtaining *cocoa-nut oil* or *cocoa-nut butter :* the one is by pressure, the other by boiling the bruised nut and skimming off the oil as it forms on the surface. It is a white solid, having a peculiar odour, like that of the flowers of furze (*Ulex europæus*), and a mild taste. It fuses at a little above 70° F., readily becomes rancid, and dissolves easily in alcohol. It consists of a solid fat called *cocin* or *cocinine* (a combination of glycerine and cocinic or coco-stearic acid, $C^{27}H^{26}O^3+2HO$), and of a liquid fat or oleine, which has not been much examined. Cocoa-nut oil is used in the manufacture of candles and soap.[1] It serves particularly for the manufacture of marine soap, which forms a lather with sea-water. Cocoa-nut oil has been used for medicinal purposes. Loureiro considered it, when fresh, not inferior to olive oil. On the continent of India, as well as in Ceylon, it is used as a pomatum for promoting, preserving, and softening the hair. Mr. Bennett thinks that if it were perfumed, and used for this purpose by Europeans, it would soon display its virtues to such advantage as to ensure its general use. But the great drawback to its medicinal employment in pomatums and unguents is its odour, and the facility with which it becomes rancid.

3. PALMÆ CERIFERÆ.—WAX-BEARING PALMS.

The only palm wax which has been brought to Europe as an article of commerce is the produce of the following palm :—
CORYPHA CERIFERA, Mart., Gen. et Sp. Palm. tab. 49 and 50; *Caranaiba* and *Ananachi cariri*, Piso et Marcgrave, pp. 62 and 130, 1648; *Carnauba*, Brande, Phil. Trans. 1811, and Virey, Journ. de Pharm. t. xx. p. 112, 1834.—Grows on the shores of the Rio Francesco, in the Brazils.[2] In the axillæ of the leaves waxy scales are secreted, which are collected and melted by the Indians. The wax thus obtained is imported into this country from Rio Janeiro under the names of *Carnauba Wax, Brazilian Wax,* or *Palm Wax.* It was submitted to chemical examination by Mr. Brande, and has subsequently been analysed by Lewy, who found it to consist of $C^{36}H^{36}O^2$. The fusing point of this wax is 180° F. It is, therefore, less fusible than bees' wax, whose melting point is about 150° F. Being a genuine wax, it is applicable to some of the purposes for which common bees' wax is now employed.

4. PALMÆ RESINIFERÆ.—RESIN-BEARING PALMS.

The only resinous substance used in medicine and the arts, and which is obtained from the palms, is Dragon's Blood, the produce of Calamus Draco.

53. Calamus Draco, *Willd.*—The Dragon's Blood Calamus.

Sex. Syst. Diœcia, Hexandria.
(Resina ; Sanguis Draconis.)

Palma Juncus Draco, Rumph., Herb. Amb. pars v. p. 114, t. lviii. fig. 1.—A native of the islands of the Indian Archipelago. The berry, which is round, pointed, and about the size of a cherry, yields a resinous substance called in commerce *dragon's blood* (*sanguis draconis*)—a term which is also applied to a product of the *Dracæna Draco* (vide LILIACEÆ), and likewise to a substance obtained from the *Pterocarpus Draco* (vide LEGUMINOSÆ). Lieut. Wellstead says that in Socotra dragon's blood exudes spontaneously from the stem of a tree.[3] The following are the kinds of it which I have met with :—

---

[1] Knapp's *Chemical Technology*, vol. i. p. 468, 1848.
[2] The stems of this palm are sold at Haynes's timber-yard, Long Lane, Smithfield, London, under the name of *Palm Wood.*
[3] *Athenæum*, May 16, 1835 ; also, *Journal of Royal Geographical Society.*

1. *Dragon's blood in the reed ; Dragon's blood in sticks ; Sanguis Draconis in baculis.*—This occurs in dark reddish-brown sticks of from twelve to eighteen inches long, and from a quarter to half an inch in diameter, enveloped with the leaf of the Talipat palm (*Corypha umbraculifera*), and bound round with slender slips of cane (probably the stem of *Calamus petræus*). It is supposed to be obtained from a species of *Calamus*, perhaps *C. Draco.*

2. *Dragon's blood in oval masses ; Dragon's blood in drops ; Sanguis Draconis in lachrymis*, Martius.—This occurs in reddish-brown lumps of the size and shape of an olive, enveloped with the leaf of *Corypha umbraculifera* or *Corypha Licuala*, which thus connects them together in a row, like the beads of a necklace. This kind is rare in English commerce. It is obtained, according to Rumphius, by rubbing or shaking the fruit of *Calamus Draco* in a bag. A resinous exudation is by this means separated, and is afterwards softened by heat, and made up in these masses.

3. *Dragon's blood in powder.*—This is a reddish powder of very fine quality, imported from the East Indies. It is probably the dust obtained from the fruit of the *C. Draco*, in the way just described.

4. *Dragon's blood in the tear ; Sanguis Draconis in granis*, Martius.—It occurs in irregular pieces, some as large as the fist. T. W. C. Martius[1] says pieces of the fruit of the Calamus Rotang are frequently found intermixed.

5. *Lump Dragon's blood ; Sanguis Draconis in massis.*—[Dragon's blood in lump varies very much in quality from fine to very ordinary, and occurs in pieces of all sizes and shapes.

6. *Dragon's blood in cakes* occurs in flat, oblong pieces, half the size of a brick, and mostly fine in quality.—ED.]

Other varieties of Dragon's blood are described, but I have never met with them. Guibourt mentions a *dragon's blood in cakes*, and a *false dragon's blood* in oval masses.

Dragon's blood is composed of *red resin* (called *draconin*) 90·7, *fixed oil* 2·0, *benzoic acid* 3·0, *oxalate of lime* 1·6, *phosphate of lime* 3·7.[2] According to Johnstone,[3] the resin of *lump dragon's blood* has the formula $C^{40}H^{21}O^8$; that of *reed dragon's blood*, $C^{40}H^{20}O^9$.

It is inert, or nearly so, but was formerly reputed an astringent. It is a constituent of some tooth-powders and tinctures, but is never prescribed by medical practitioners. Its principal consumption is for colouring spirit and turpentine varnishes.

5. PALMÆ TANNINIFERÆ.—TANNIN-BEARING PALMS.

The only palm which yields any officinal astringent substance is the Areca Catechu.

54. ARECA CATECHU, *Linn.*—CATECHU PALM.

Sex. Syst. Monœcia, Hexandria.

(Semen.—Extract of the kernels, *E.*—Carbo seminis, *offic.*)

HISTORY.—Areca nuts are not mentioned in the writings of the ancient Greeks and Romans. Avicenna speaks of them under the name of *Fufel.*[4]

BOTANY. **Gen. Char.**—1. MALE : *Calyx* 3-parted. *Corolla* 3-petalled. 2. FEMALE : *Calyx* 3-leaved. *Corolla* 3-petalled ; *nectary* 6-toothed. *Ovarium* superior, 1-celled, 1-seeded ; attachment inferior. *Drupe* coriaceous. *Seed* single, ruminate. *Embryo* in the base of the albumen (*Roxburgh*).

Sp. Char.—*Trunk* straight and slender, from 40 to 50 feet high. *Fronds* pinnate ; *leaflets* compound, linear, opposite, premorse. *Spathe* erect,

---

[1] *Pharmakognosie.*
[2] Herberger, *Journ. de Pharm.* xvii. 225.
[3] *Phil. Trans.* for 1840, p. 384.
[4] Lib. ii. tract. ii. cap. 262, p. 306, Venet. 1564.

ramous. *Male flowers* hexandrous. *Seed* of a roundish conic form, and obtuse (*Roxburgh*).

Hab.—Cultivated in all the warmer parts of Asia.

1. DESCRIPTION AND USES OF THE SEEDS.—The fruit of the Catechu palm is about the size and shape of a small egg, yellowish, and smooth. Within the fibrous pericarp is the seed (*areca nut ; betel nut ; pinang*). This is about the size of a nutmeg, roundish conical, flattened at the base, hard, horny, inodorous, externally reddish-brown, internally brown with whitish veins. The principal part of the seed is the ruminate albumen, at the base of which is the embryo.[1] The varieties of this fruit are numerous : of these some have been figured by Blume,[2] viz. *Pinang Putie* (Areca alba), *Pinang Susu* (Areca lactea), *Pinang Betul* (Areca propria), and *Pinang Pict.*

According to Morin,[3] areca nuts (seeds) are composed of *tannin* (principally), *gallic acid, glutin, red insoluble matter, fixed oil, gum, oxalate of lime,* and *lignin*.

With lime and the leaves of *Piper Betel*, these nuts form the celebrated masticatory of the East, called *betel*. They are usually cut into four equal parts, one of which is rolled up with a little lime in the leaf of the Piper Betel, and the whole chewed. The mixture acts as a sialogogue, and tinges the saliva red. The Indians have an idea that by this means the teeth are fastened, the gums cleansed, and the mouth cooled. Peron[4] was convinced that he preserved his health, during a long and difficult voyage, by the habitual use of the betel, while his companions, who did not use it, died mostly of dysentery. In this country, *areca-nut charcoal* is used as a tooth-powder. I know of no particular value it can have over ordinary charcoal, except, perhaps, that derived from its greater hardness.

2. ARECA-NUT CATECHU.—In the southern parts of India, and probably in Ceylon, an extract called catechu is procured from areca nuts.[5] The mode of preparing it has been described by Herbert de Jäger[6] and Dr. Heyne.[7] The last-mentioned author states that it is largely procured in Mysore, about Sirah, in the following manner :—"Areca nuts are taken as they come from the tree, and boiled for some hours in an iron vessel. They are then taken out, and the remaining water is inspissated by continued boiling. This process furnishes *Kassu*, or most astringent terra japonica, which is black, and mixed with paddy husks and other impurities. After the nuts are dried, they are put into a fresh quantity of water, boiled again, and this water being inspissated, like the former, yields the best or dearest kind of catechu, called *coury*. It is yellowish-brown, has an earthy fracture, and is free from the admixture of foreign bodies."

---

[1] Roxburgh's *Plants of Coromandel*, pl. 75 ; *Flora Indica*, vol. iii. p. 615.

[2] *Rumphia*, vol. ii. p. 68, tab. 102, 1836.

[3] *Journ. de Pharm.* viii. 449.

[4] *Voyage aux Terres Australes.*

[5] Ainslie (*Mat. Indica*, vol. i. p. 65) notices two preparations of areca nuts, which he says have been confounded with the true or real catechu (*i. e.* catechu of the *Acacia Catechu*). One of these he calls *cuttacamboo* (in Tamool), the other *cashcuttie* (in Tamool) ; and he adds that both are brought to India from Pegu. It is probable, however, from his description, that by cuttacamboo he means *gambir* (an extract of Nauclea Gambir), and by cashcuttie, *Pegu cutch* (an extract of Acacia Catechu).—Blume (*Rumphia*, vol. ii. p. 67) denies that an extract called catechu is procured from areca nuts, and says that the error has arisen from the circumstance that old and dry areca nuts, broken in small pieces, are macerated in rose-water in which catechu has been dissolved.

[6] *Miscellanea curiosa*, Dec. ii. Ann. iii. p. 10, Norimb. 1685.

[7] Dr. Heyne, *Tracts, Historical and Statistical, on India.*

None of the extracts brought from India under the denomination of catechu are distinguished by any name by which they can be referred to the areca nut. It is probable, however, that some of them which come over in the form of *round and flat cakes,* and also *in balls,* and which are more or less covered with paddy husks (glumes of rice), are obtained from this seed. A decoction of some of these kinds of catechu yields, when cold, a blue colour on the addition of iodine, indicating the presence of starch. The presence of fatty matter in them is considered by Professor Guibourt[1] to be a proof that the areca nut has been employed in their production. It is probable that the *Colombo* or *Ceylon catechu* of commerce, in the form of round flat cakes, covered by paddy husks, is the *Kassu* of Heyne; and Professor Guibourt is of opinion that the *dull reddish catechu in balls* partially covered by paddy husks is the *Coury* of Heyne. (For further details, the reader is referred to the article *Acacia Catechu,* where a general notice will be given of all the commercial sorts of catechu.)

†† Flowers with a true perianth free from the ovary (*superior ovary*), usually hermaphrodite.

Order X. MELANTHACEÆ, *R. Brown.*

CHARACTERS.—*Perianth* inferior, petaloid, in six pieces, or, in consequence of the cohesion of the claws, tubular; the pieces generally involute in æstivation. *Stamens* 6; *anthers* mostly turned outwards. *Ovary* 3-celled; many-seeded; *style* trifid or 3-parted; *stigma* undivided. *Capsule* generally divisible into three pieces; sometimes with a loculicidal dehiscence. *Seeds* with a membranous testa; *albumen* dense, fleshy. (*R. Brown.*)

PROPERTIES.—Several violently poisonous alkaloids (*veratria, colchicina, sabadillina,* and *jervina*) are peculiar to this order. They exist in combination with organic acids. These bases, as well perhaps as resins, are the active principles of the order. The Melanthaceæ are acrids (emetics, purgatives, diuretics, and errhines) and sedatives (see Vol. i. p. 232). When acting as poisons, they are called narcotico-acrids (see Vol. i. p. 203).

55. COLCHICUM AUTUMNALE, *Linn.*—COMMON MEADOW SAFFRON.

Sex. Syst. Hexandria, Trigynia.

(Cormus et semina, *L. E. D.*)

HISTORY.—Dioscorides[2] speaks of *Colchicum* (κολχικόν), and states that it grows abundantly in Messenia and at Colchis (from which latter place it received its name). Dr. Sibthorp[3] found three species of Colchicum in Greece—viz. *C. autumnale, C. montanum,* and *C. variegatum;* and of these he considers the first to be the Colchicum of Dioscorides. In this opinion he is to a certain extent confirmed by the editors of the *Pharmacopœa Græca* (1837), who apply the modern Greek name of κολχικόν to C.

---

[1] *Journ. de Pharm. et de Chimie,* 3me sér. t. xi. p. 363, 1847.
[2] *Lib. iv. cap.* 84.
[3] *Prodr. Fl. Græcæ,* i. 250.

autumnale. But there is reason to doubt the accuracy of this opinion : for this species is only found in Greece, on this side of the Sperchius, at an elevation of at least 3500 to 4000 feet,—at Parnassus, and Thymphrastus ; whereas *C. variegatum*, which Fraas[1] thinks is the κολχικόν of Dioscorides, is common, and occurs on the Xirobuni,[2] at an elevation of only 1000 to 2000 feet, at Hymettus, Messapius, and Helicon.

For the introduction of Colchicum into modern practice we are chiefly indebted to Störk,[3] in 1763 ; but partly, also, to the opinion that it is the active principle of a celebrated French remedy (*eau médicinale*) for gout.

BOTANY. **Gen. Char.**—*Perianth* single, tubular, very long, rising from a spatha; limb campanulate, 6-partite, petaloid. [*Stamens* 6, inserted into the throat of the tube. *Ovarium* 3-celled. *Styles* 3, filiform, long. *Stigmas* somewhat clavate.] *Capsule* 3-celled : cells united at the base (*Hooker*, with some additions).

Sp. Char.—*Leaves* plane, broadly lanceolate, erect (*Hooker*).

Root fibrous. *Cormus* (improperly called *root* or *bulb*) ovate, fleshy, large, covered with a loose brown membrane. The *leaves* are produced in the spring along with the fruit, and disappear before the flower appears. *Flowers* several, lilac or pale purple, arising from the cormus by a long narrow white tube.[4] *Fruit* oblong, elliptical, composed of three cells, which may be regarded as distinct follicles, with intermediate fissures. *Seeds* small, spherical, with a rough brown testa and large fleshy strophiola ; internally they are white, and consist of a minute embryo lodged in a horny elastic albumen. The flowers appear in September, and the fruit the following spring or summer.

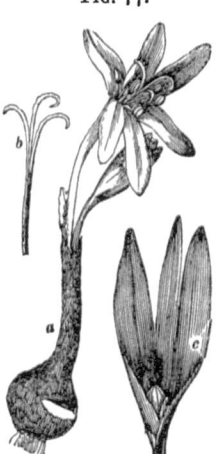

FIG. 77.

There is a variety, β *with late flowers* (*floribus serotinis*), growing near Devizes, in Wiltshire, which flowers in the spring.

Florists cultivate several sorts ; such as the *white*, the *striped-flowered*, the *striped-leaved*, the *broad-leaved*, the *many-flowered*, and the *double-flowered*.

Hab.—Moist rich meadows in many parts of England and in various countries of Europe.

The plant is propagated by seeds, by a single mature cormus, or by several immature or infant cormi.

COLLECTION OF THE CORMI.—The cormus is biennial. It first appears about the end of June or beginning of July : it flowers in the autumn, and produces its leaves in the spring, and its seeds in the June of the following year. It then begins to

Colchicum autumnale.

a. The flowering plant.
b. Stigmas, with a portion of the styles.
c. Leaves and fruit.

---

[1] *Synopsis Plant. Floræ Classicæ*, p. 284, 1845.

[2] Xirobuni, by Col. Baker called " Xezo Vouni" (*Journal of the Geographical Society*, vol. vii. p. 94, 1837).

[3] *Libellus quo demonstratur Colchici autumnalis Radicem non solum tuto posse exhiberi hominibus, sed et ejus usu interno curari quandoque morbos difficillimos, qui aliis remediis non cedunt*, 8vo. Vindob. 1763.

[4] Miller says that in Warwickshire the flowers are called *naked ladies*, because they appear without leaves.

shrivel, becomes leathery, and finally disappears in the succeeding spring or summer.[1]

The activity of the cormus varies at different seasons of the year. It is usually considered to be greatest when the cormus is about a year old—that is, about the month of July, between the withering of the leaves and the sprouting forth of the flower of the young cormus. At this period the cormus is fully developed, and has not exhausted itself by the production of the young one. But many of the cormi brought to market have already pushed forth their flowers, which are broken off so as to prevent the circumstance from being observed. "I have seen many cwts.," says Dr. Lindley,[2] "sent to town in this state, which nevertheless found a ready sale, and at the best price."

Dr. Christison[3] has expressed some doubts as to the propriety of collecting the cormi in July; for though they are plumpest, firmest, and abound most in starch at this period, yet he has found the shrivelled cormi in the succeeding April to be equally if not more bitter; and he quotes the analyses of Stoltze to show that while the October cormus yields 2 per cent., the March cormus yields 6 per cent. of bitter extract. But there is an error in the quotation which vitiates the inference intended to be drawn from it. Stoltze found that the October cormus contained 2·17 per cent. of *bitter* extractive, and that the March cormus contained 5·91 of *sweet* extractive matter combined with some bitter extractive; and he concludes that the October cormus is much more active, and contains more bitter extractive, than the spring cormus.

The *seeds* should be gathered when fully ripe. The London market is principally supplied from Gloucestershire, but partly, also, from Hampshire and Oxfordshire.

DESCRIPTION.—The *cormus,* commonly called the *bulb* or *root* (*radix colchici,* offic.), when gathered at the proper season, is about the size of a chestnut, and somewhat resembles in external appearance the bulb of the common tulip (*Tulipa Gesneriana*) ; which, as well as other liliaceous bulbs, are distinguished from the cormus of colchicum by being composed of laminæ or scales, whereas the cormus of colchicum is solid.[4] It is rounded on one side, flattened on the other, where is perceived the fibrous germ of a new cormus, which, if allowed to grow, shoots up and bears the flower, while the old cormus wastes. It is covered by two coats—an inner reddish-yellow one, and an external brown one. Internally, the cormus is white, fleshy, solid; contains a milky juice, is very feculent, and has an acrid bitter taste. "Before drying the cormus, it should be cut transversely in thin slices, the dry coats being previously removed."[5] The slices are to be quickly dried, in a dark airy place, with a heat not exceeding 170° F.[6] The late Dr. A. T. Thomson[7] recommended the slices to be dried upon clean white paper *without artificial heat;* but the time required for this is an objection to it in practice. The dried slices (*radix siccata,* offic.) should be about the eighth or tenth of an

---

[1] [For figures of the appearances presented at different periods by the cormus, see *Pharm. Journ.* vol. xi. p. 417.—ED.]

[2] *Flora Medica,* p. 589.

[3] *Dispensatory,* 2d edit. p. 353.

[4] Some years ago a load of tulip bulbs was delivered at Apothecaries' Hall, London, for colchicum cormi. The late Mr. Anderson, gardener to the Apothecaries' Botanic Garden at Chelsea, for many years cultivated some of these tulips,—in commemoration, I suppose, of the attempted fraud.

[5] *Ph. Lond.* 1836.

[6] Battley, *Lond. Med. Rep.* xiv. 429.

Ibid. p. 344.

inch thick, rounded, oval, with one notch only on one part of their circumference (not fiddle-shaped), inodorous, of a greyish-white colour and an amylaceous appearance.

The *seeds* (*semina*) are about the size of those of black mustard, odourless, and have a bitter acrid taste. Their colour is brown, varying from pale to dark or blackish. They somewhat resemble several of the cruciferous seeds (black mustard, turnip, and rape), but are larger than these; moreover, the latter, being more oily, are more readily crushed. I have known colchicum seeds mistaken for grains of paradise.

COMPOSITION.—The colchicum cormus was analysed in 1810 by Melander, and Moretti;[1] in 1818 and 1819, by Stoltze;[2] and in 1820 by Pelletier and Caventou.[3]

ANALYSIS OF PELLETIER AND CAVENTOU.	STOLTZE'S ANALYSES.		
		Cormi gathered in March.	*Ditto in October.*
	Volatile acrid matter	trace	......................rather more
Fatty matter composed of { Olein. Stearin. Volatile acid.	Soft resin	0·04	.... 0·06
	Crystallisable sugar	0·41	.... 1·12
	Sweet extractive with some } bitter extractive .... }	5·91	{ Uncrystallisable sugar 2·72 { Bitter extractive ..... 2·17
Supergallate of *veratria*.	Difficultly soluble extractive	1·30	.... 0·52
Yellow colouring matter.	Gum, like tragacanth	0·81	.... 1·65
Gum.	Starch......................	7·46	.... 10·12
Starch.	Lignin	2·32	.... 1·61
Inulin in abundance.	Extractive, soluble in potash	0·61	.... 0·52
Lignin.	Water......................	81·04	.... 80·31
Ashes, a minute quantity.			
Colchicum cormus.	Colchicum cormus .... 99·90		......................100·80

The seeds have been submitted to chemical examination, in 1832, by L. A. Buchner, jun.,[4] who found in them *fixed oil, free acid, bitter extractive* (impure colchicina), and *resin*.

1. COLCHICINA; *Colchicia; Colchicene.*—The existence of this principle in colchicum seeds was announced by Geiger and Hesse.[5] They *prepared* it by digesting the seeds in boiling alcohol: this dissolved a supersalt, which was precipitated by magnesia, and the precipitate treated with boiling alcohol. By evaporation, colchicina was deposited. The following are said to be its *properties:*—It is a crystallisable alkaline substance, without odour, but having a bitter taste. Its hydrate is feebly alkaline, but neutralises acids, and forms crystallisable salts, having a bitter taste. It is soluble in water, and the solution precipitates the solution of chloride of platinum. Nitric acid colours colchicina deep violet, which passes into indigo blue, and quickly becomes, first green, and then yellow. Concentrated sulphuric acid colours it yellowish-brown. Colchicina is said to be distinguished from veratria by the following characteristics:—1st, it is soluble in water, whereas veratria is not; 2dly, it is crystallisable, whereas pure veratria is not; 3dly, it does not possess the acridity of veratria; and it differs from the latter in this, that when applied to the nose it does not excite sneezing, whereas the least portion of [impure] veratria occasions a most convulsive sneezing.

Colchicina is a powerful poison. One-tenth of a grain, dissolved in weak spirit, killed a young cat in about twelve hours. The symptoms were salivation, diarrhœa, vomiting, a staggering gait, cries, convulsions, and death. The stomach and intestines were violently inflamed, and had extravasated blood throughout their whole course.

---

[1] *Bull. de Pharm.* vol. ii. p. 217.
[2] *Berlinisches Jahrbuch für die Pharmacie*, Bd. xix. S. 107, 1818 ; and Bd. xx. S. 135, 1819.
[3] *Journ. de Pharm.* vi. 364.
[4] *Repert. für die Pharm.* Bd. xliii. S. 376, 1832.
[5] *Journ. de Chim.* x. 465.

2. STARCH.—The starch-grains of the cormus of colchicum are moderately uniform in size: though normally rounded, they present more or less flattened faces, produced by their mutual compression in the cells of the plant, by which they have acquired a polygonal appearance. Many are mullar-shaped, some are dihedral at one end, others trihedral; owing to the mutual pressure of two, three, or four particles. The hilum is usually stellate.

CHEMICAL CHARACTERISTICS. *α. Of the Cormi*.—The decoction of the fresh cormi, when cold, forms with a solution of iodine a deep blue precipitate (*iodide of starch*); with sesquichloride of iron, a faint bluish tint (*gallate of iron*); with diacetate of lead, or protonitrate of mercury, a copious white precipitate; with nitrate of silver, a precipitate which is at first white, but becomes in a few minutes black; with tincture of nutgalls, a very slight dirty-looking precipitate, which is somewhat diminished by the effect of heat [Pelletier and Caventou[1] regard this precipitate as a mixture of the *tannates of starch* and *inulin*[2] (and of veratrin?)]; and with a solution of gelatine, a slight haziness. Fresh-prepared tincture of guaiacum, with a few drops of acetic acid, produces a cerulean blue colour with the fresh cormus, indicating the presence of gluten.

β. Of the Seeds.—The decoction of the seeds, when cold, yields with oxalate of ammonia a white precipitate (*oxalate of lime*); with diacetate of lead, a copious white precipitate; and with nitrate of silver a precipitate. If the decoction be concentrated, and poured into alcohol, a gelatiniform precipitate is produced.

PHYSIOLOGICAL EFFECTS. *α. On Vegetables*.—Not yet determined.

β. On Animals.—Colchicum is a poison to animals. It acts as a local irritant, reduces the force of the circulation, and causes inflammation of the alimentary canal. Animals, for the most part, refuse to feed on it. It has, however, been eaten by deer and cattle, and proved poisonous to them.[3] It is said to prove injurious at spring-time only.[4] Moreover, we are told that when dry it may be eaten in hay with impunity. Störck[5] and Kratochwill[6] gave it to dogs, on whom it acted as an acrid poison, and caused death. Sir E. Home[7] injected 160 drops of a vinous infusion of colchicum into the jugular vein of a dog: all power of motion was instantly lost, the breathing became slow, the pulse hardly to be felt. In ten minutes it was 84, in twenty minutes 60, in an hour 115, with the respiration so quick as scarcely to be counted. In two hours the pulse was 150, and very weak. The animal was purged, vomited, and very languid: he died in five hours. On dissection, the internal coat of the stomach was found inflamed, in a greater or less degree, universally. From this experiment it appears that the action of colchicum on the alimentary canal is of a specific kind. In opposition to the above statements it deserves notice that Orfila[8] has frequently given to

---

[1] *Journ. de Pharm.* vi. 365.

[2] The precipitate produced in an amylaceous decoction by infusion of nutgalls disappears when the liquor is gradually heated to 122° F.; but if inulin be present, it does not disappear until the liquor has reached the boiling point.

[3] Wibmer, *Wirk. d. Arzn. u. Gifte*, Bd. ii. 150.

[4] Hacquet, in Wibmer, *op. cit.*; also, Want, *Lond. Med. and Phys. Journal*, vol. xxxii. p. 216.

[5] *Lib. de Colchico*, p. 17.

[6] Quoted by Wibmer.

[7] *Phil. Trans.* 1816.

[8] *Toxicol. Gén.*

dogs, in the month of June, two or three cormi without perceiving any sensible effects; from which he infers that climate and season of the year have great influence on their deleterious properties.

It has been said that horses eat colchicum with impunity; but it is probable that this statement is erroneous.   Withering[1] states, on the authority of Mr. Woodward, that "in a pasture in which were several horses, and eaten down nearly bare, the grass was closely cropped, even under the leaves, but not a leaf bitten."   Some further information on the effects of colchicum on dogs will be found in Sir C. Scudamore's *Treatise on Gout and Rheumatism*, 3d edit. p. 477, 1819.

γ. *On Man.*—Colchicum is acrid and sedative.   Taken internally, *in small and repeated doses*, it promotes the action of the secreting organs, especially the intestinal mucous membrane.   The kidneys, the skin, and the liver, are less certainly and obviously affected by it.   Salivation has been ascribed to it by Dr. Aldridge.[2]   The most constant effects observed from the use of *larger doses* are nausea, vomiting, and purging.   Reduction of the frequency of the pulse is a common, though not an invariable effect.   Mr. Haden[3] was, I believe, the first to direct attention to the advantages to be taken of this effect in the treatment of inflammatory diseases.   In some experiments made on healthy individuals by Dr. Lewins,[4] debility, a feeling of illness, and headache, were experienced.   This feeling of debility is not, however, to be referred to the evacuations produced; for, as Dr. Barlow[5] has observed, the number of motions is sometimes considerable without any proportionate depression of strength ensuing.   "I have known," says Dr. B., " even twenty stools occasioned by a single dose of colchicum, the patient not complaining of the least debility."   The action of colchicum on the secretory apparatus is not confined to that of the alimentary canal : after the use of three or four full doses of this medicine copious sweating is often produced, especially when the skin is kept warm.   On other occasions the kidneys are powerfully acted on.   In one case mentioned by Dr. Lewins seventy drops of *Vinum Colchici* caused the discharge of upwards of a pint of bile by vomiting.   Violent salivation resulted in a case recorded in an American journal.[6]   Chelius, of Heidelberg,[7] asserts that in gout and rheumatism colchicum occasions a striking increase in the quantity of uric acid contained in the urine : in one case it was nearly doubled in the space of twelve days.   But this effect is by no means constant, as Dr. Graves[8] has pointed out.   Indeed, it sometimes happens, in acute rheumatism, when the urine is loaded with uric acid or the urates, that under the use of colchicum the quantity of these matters in the urine is diminished; so that it would seem rather to prevent the formation of uric acid in the system than to provoke its elimination.

In excessive or *poisonous doses* colchicum acts as a powerful poison.   In a case related by Mr. Fereday,[9] where two ounces of the wine of the seeds of

---

[1] *Brit. Plants*, ii. 462, 7th edit. 1830.
[2] *Dublin Hospital Gazette*, p. 52, Oct. 1845.
[3] *Practical Observations on the Colchicum autumnale*, 1820.
[4] *Edinburgh Medical and Surgical Journal*, vol. xlvii. p. 345, 1837.
[5] *Cyclopædia of Practical Medicine*, art. *Gout*, vol. ii. p. 371.
[6] Wood and Bache's *United States Dispensatory*, 3d edit.
[7] *Lond. Med. Gaz.* vol. ii. p. 830.
[8] *Ibid.* vol. vii. p. 548.
[9] *Ibid.* vol. x. p. 160.

colchicum were swallowed, the symptoms were acute pain in the bowels, coming on in about an hour and a half after taking it, vomiting, acute tenesmus, small, slow, and feeble pulse, cold feet, and weakness of limbs. The nausea, vomiting, and pain in the stomach, continued with undiminished violence, the pulse became also imperceptible and intermitting, the urine was suppressed, the respiration hurried, purging of copious liquid stools came on, and loss of sight for a minute or two after getting out of bed. The patient died forty-seven hours after swallowing the poison. On a *post-mortem* examination, the skin of most parts of the body was found to be covered with a purple efflorescence : no inflammation was observed in the alimentary canal ; two red patches were found, one in the stomach, and the other in the jejunum. These were produced by the effusion of a small quantity of blood, in the one case between the muscular and mucous coats ; in the other, between the peritoneal and muscular coats. Ecchymosed spots were observed on the surface of the lungs, of the heart, and of the diaphragm. More recently a case of poisoning by a decoction of the seeds has been recorded ;[1] as also by the leaves of this plant. In Mr. Fereday's case the only indications of an affection of the nervous system were weakness of the limbs, the temporary loss of sight, and the slowness and feebleness of the pulse.

It is deserving of notice, that in this case, also in another related by Chevallier,[2] likewise in a third mentioned by Mr. Dillon,[3] and in Mr. Haden's case,[4] no convulsions were observed ; and in the three first cases no insensibility. In the last case, however, Mr. Haden mentions that at "ten P.M. she fell into an apoplectic kind of sleep, which terminated in death before morning." It is remarkable that convulsions are ascribed to veratria by Magendie, and to colchicina by Geiger and Hesse. In one case of fatal poisoning from an ounce and a half of the tincture of colchicum,[5] delirium occurred.

[In one instance a person recovered after swallowing an ounce of the tincture. There were cramps in the limbs, and twitchings of the tendons.[6] A case of poisoning by the medicinal administration of colchicum was communicated to us by Mr. Mann, of Bartholomew Close. Three and a half drachms of the wine of colchicum were taken in divided doses, and caused death on the fourth day. There was no inflammation of the mucous membrane, but simply extravasation of blood in the mucous follicles. A good summary of the action of colchicum has been published by Dr. Maclagan.[7]—ED.]

It is a popular notion that colchicum acts as an emmenagogue ; and hence it is sometimes used to produce abortion. Several cases of poisoning by its use for this purpose have occurred.

Some persons appear to be peculiarly susceptible of the influence of colchicum. In Mr. Haden's case, ʒiiss. of tincture of colchicum caused death in a female, whose mother was also exceedingly susceptible of the action of colchicum

---

[1] *Journ. de Chim. Méd.* t. vi. 2de série, p. 505. [Two fatal cases of poisoning by the fresh seeds are reported in the same journal for 1853, p. 421.—ED.]

[2] *Ibid.* viii. 351.

[3] Stephenson and Churchill's *Med. Bot.* vol. ii.

[4] *Magendie's Formulary*, by C. T. Haden.

[5] *Edinburgh Medical and Surgical Journal*, xiv. 262.

[6] See *L'Union Médicale*, Aug. 24, 1848.

[7] See *Edinburgh Monthly Journal* for December 1851.

in even very small doses. In a case related by Mr. Mann,[1] ʒiiiss. of the wine of colchicum in divided doses caused death on the fourth day.

The above account of the effects of colchicum applies both to the *cormi*, the *seeds*, and the *leaves*. The *flowers* are likewise poisonous, and a fatal case from their use is mentioned by Dr. Christison.[2] They have been recommended for medicinal use.

USES.—The following are the principal diseases in which the Meadow Saffron has been employed:—

1. *In gout.*—The circumstances which of late years have led to the extensive employment of colchicum in gout are the following:—About seventy years ago, M. Husson, a military officer in the service of the king of France, discovered, as he informs us, a plant possessed of extraordinary virtues in the cure of various diseases. From this plant he prepared a remedy called *Eau Médicinale*, which acquired great celebrity for abating the pain and cutting short the paroxysm of gout.[3] Various attempts were made to discover the nature of its active principle. In 1782, MM. Cadet and Parmentier declared that it contained no metallic or mineral substance, and that it was a vinous infusion of some bitter plant or plants. Alyon[4] asserted that it was prepared with Gratiola; Mr. Moore[5] that it was a vinous infusion of white hellebore with laudanum: Mr. Want[6] that it was a vinous infusion of colchicum. Although most writers have adopted Mr. Want's opinion, we should bear in mind that the proofs hitherto offered of its correctness, viz. analogy of effect, cannot be admitted to be conclusive, as is well shown by the fact that they have been advanced in favour of the identity of other medicines with the *Eau Médicinale*.

The power of colchicum to alleviate a paroxysm of gout is admitted by all; but considerable difference of opinion exists as to the extent of this power, and the propriety of employing it. Sir Everard Home,[7] from observation of its effects on his own person, regarded it as a specific in gout, and from experiments on animals concluded that its beneficial effects in this malady are produced through the circulation.

Dr. Paris[8] observes—"As a *specific* in gout its efficacy has been fully ascertained: it allays pain, and cuts short the paroxysm. It has also a decided action upon the arterial system, which it would appear to control through the medium of the nerves." But if by the word specific is meant a medicine infallibly, and on all patients, producing given salutary effects, and acting by some unknown power on the disease, without being directed by indications,[9] undoubtedly colchicum is no specific for gout. That colchicum alleviates a paroxysm of gout I have before mentioned; but that alleviation is palliative, not curative. It has no tendency to prevent a speedy recurrence of the attack; nay, according to Sir Charles Scudamore,[10] it renders the dispo-

---

[1] Taylor *On Poisons*.
[2] *Treatise on Poisons*, 3d edit. p. 792.
[3] Dr. E. G. Jones, *An Account of the Remarkable Effects of the Eau Médicinale d'Husson in the Gout.*
[4] *Elém. de Chimie.*
[5] *Two Letters on the Composition of the Eau Médicinale*, 2d edit. 1811.
[6] *Med. and Phys. Journal*, vol. xxxii. 1814.
[7] *Phil. Trans.* 1816.
[8] *Pharmacalogia*, 6th edit. vol. ii. p. 175.
[9] Vide Dr. Parr's *Lond. Med. Dict.* art. *Specifica.*
[10] *Treatise on Gout and Rheumatism*, 3d edit. p. 197.

sition to the disease much stronger in the system.   Furthermore, by repetition
its power over gouty paroxysms becomes diminished.

The *modus medendi* of colchicum in gout is an interesting though not very
satisfactory part of our inquiry.   I have already stated that some regard this
remedy as a specific ; that is, as operating by some unknown influence.   Others,
however, and with more propriety, refer its therapeutical uses to its known
physiological effects.   "Colchicum," says Dr. Barlow,[1] " purges, abates pain,
and lowers the pulse.   These effects are accounted for by assigning to it a
cathartic and sedative operation; and it is this combination perhaps to which
its peculiar virtues are to be ascribed."   The fact that a combination of a
drastic and a narcotic (as elaterium and opium, mentioned by Dr. Sutton,[2]
and white hellebore and laudanum, recommended by Mr. Moore,[3] has been
found to give, in several cases of gout, marked and speedy relief, seems to me
to confirm Dr. Barlow's opinion.   The idea entertained by Chelius, and adopted
by Dr. G. Hume Weatherhead,[4] that colchicum relieves gout by augmenting
the quantity of uric acid in the urine, is not supported by fact, as I have
already mentioned.   Whether it acts by preventing the formation of uric acid
in the system I am not prepared to say.

In acute gout occurring in plethoric habits, blood-letting should precede
the use of colchicum.   This medicine should then be exhibited in full doses,
so as to produce a copious evacuation by the bowels, and then the quantity
must be considerably diminished.   Though purging is not essential to the
therapeutical influence of colchicum, it is admitted by most that, in a large
number of cases at least, it promotes the alleviation of the symptoms.   Hence
many practitioners recommend its combination with saline purgatives, as
the sulphate of magnesia.   Sir Charles Scudamore has experienced "the most
remarkable success from a draught composed of *Magnesiæ* gr. xv. ad xx.;
Magnes. Sulphat. ʒj. ad ʒij.; *Aceti Colchici* ʒj. ad ʒij.; with any distilled
water the most agreeable, and sweetened with any pleasant syrup, or with
15 or 20 grains of Extract. Glycyrrhiz."

2. *In rheumatism.*— The analogy existing between gout and rheumatism
has led to the trial of the same remedies in both diseases.   But its
therapeutical powers in the latter disease are much less marked than in
the former.   Rheumatism may affect the fibrous tissues of the joints, the
synovial membrane, the muscles or their aponeurotic coverings, the periosteum, or the neurilemma, constituting thus five forms of the disease, which
may be denominated respectively the *fibrous* or *ligamentous ;* the *synovial,
arthritic,* or *capsular ;* the *muscular ;* the *periosteal ;* and the *neuralgic*
forms of rheumatism.[5]   Of these colchicum is said to produce its best effects
in the synovial form.   It is remarkable, however, that in all the severe cases
of this variety of rheumatism which have fallen under my notice, the disease
has proceeded unchecked, or was scarcely relieved by the use of colchicum.
In one instance, that of my much-lamented friend, the late Dr. Cummin (whose
case is noticed by Dr. Macleod, in the *Lond. Med. Gaz.* xxi. 358), the
disease proved fatal by metastasis to the brain.   In another melancholy but

---

[1] *Cyclopædia of Practical Medicine,* art. *Gout,* vol. ii. p. 372.
[2] *Tracts on Gout,* p. 201.
[3] *Op. cit.*
[4] *Treatise on Headaches,* p. 88, 1835.
[5] Dr. Macleod, *Lond. Med. Gaz.* xxi. 120.

not fatal case, the gentleman lost the sight of both his eyes, and has both knee-joints rendered stiff. In neither of these cases was colchicum of the slightest avail.

Of the mode of administering colchicum in "rheumatic gout," recommended by Mr. Wigan,[1] I have no experience. He gives eight grains of the powder in some mild diluent every hour until active vomiting, profuse purging, or abundant perspiration, take place; or at least till the stomach can bear no more. The usual quantity is eight or ten doses; but while some can take fourteen, others can bear only five. Though the pain ceases, the more active effects of the colchicum do not take place for some hours after the last dose. Thus administered, Mr. Wigan declares colchicum "the most easily managed, the most universally applicable, the safest, and the most certain specific, in the whole compass of our opulent Pharmacopœia." But its use in these large doses requires to be carefully watched.

3. *In dropsy.*—Colchicum was used in dropsy with success by Störck,[2] It has been employed in dropsical cases with the twofold view of purging and promoting the action of the kidneys. Given in combination with saline purgatives, I have found it beneficial in some cases of anasarca of old persons.

4. *In inflammatory diseases generally.*—Colchicum was recommended as a sedative in inflammatory diseases in general by the late Mr. C. T. Haden.[3] He used it as an auxiliary to blood-letting for the purpose of controlling arterial action; and gave it in the form of powder, in doses of six or seven grains, three or four times daily, in combination with purgatives, in inflammatory affections of the lungs and their membranes, and of the breasts and nipples. In chronic bronchitis it has also been found useful by Dr. Hastings.[4]

5. *In fevers.*—The late Mr. Haden,[5] and more recently Dr. Lewin,[6] have spoken favourably of the use of colchicum in fever. In my opinion it is only admissible in those forms of the disease requiring an active antiphlogistic treatment. In such it may be useful as an auxiliary to blood-letting and cathartics.

6. *In various other diseases.*—*For expelling tape-worm,* colchicum has been found efficacious by Chisholm and Baumbach. *In some chronic affections of the nervous system,* as chorea, hypochondriasis, hysteria, &c. Mr. Raven[7] employed it with advantage. *In humoral asthma, and other chronic bronchial affections,* I have found it of great service, especially when these complaints were accompanied with anasarcous swellings.

ADMINISTRATION.—The cormi and seeds of meadow saffron have been employed in substance, in a liquid form, and in the state of extract.

1. PULVIS CORMI COLCHICI.—Dose, from two to eight or nine grains. To preserve it, Mr. Wigan recommends it to be kept mixed with sugar.

2. PULVIS SEMINUM COLCHICI.—Dose the same as that of the cormus. The seeds are to be preferred to the cormi, as being more uniform in their properties.

---

[1] *Lond. Med. Gaz.* June 30, 1838.
[2] *Libellus.*
[3] *Practical Observations on the Colchicum autumnale,* 1820.
[4] *Treatise on Inflammation of the Mucous Membrane of the Lungs,* 1820.
[5] *Op. cit.*
[6] *Edinburgh Medical and Surgical Journal,* April 1837.
[7] *London Medical and Physical Journal,* Jan. 1817.

3. TINCTURA [SEMINUM] COLCHICI, L. Ed. ; *Tinctura seminum Colchici,* D. (Meadow Saffron seeds bruised [ground finely in a coffee-mill, *Ed.*], ʒv. ; Proof Spirit, Oij. Macerate for seven days and strain, *L.* (Fourteen days, strain, express, and filter, *D.*) " Percolation is much more convenient and speedy than digestion," *E.*)—Dr. Williams[1] objected to this preparation as being " turbid, unpalatable, and disposed to precipitation." The same writer[2] also asserts, that the active property of the seeds resides in their husk or cortical part, and, therefore, protests against bruising them. But were his assertion correct (and it is most improbable that the embryo is devoid of activity), bruising them cannot destroy or injure their activity. The average dose is from fʒss. to fʒj. I have repeatedly given fʒij. at a dose without any violent effect. Dr. Barlow, who prefers this to the other preparations of colchicum, advises that in gout a drachm, a drachm and a half, or two drachms of the tincture, should be given at night, and repeated the following morning. If this quantity fail to purge briskly, a third dose may be administered the ensuing night. Externally, the tincture has been employed as a liniment, to relieve rheumatic, gouty, venereal, and other pains.[3]

4. TINCTURA [SEMINUM] COLCHICI COMPOSITA, L. ; *Spiritus Colchici ammoniatus,* L. 1824. (Meadow Saffron Seeds, ʒv. ; Aromatic Spirit of Ammonia, Oij. Macerate for seven days, and strain. Dose, ♏xx. to fʒj.)—This preparation was recommended by Dr. Williams as being " of greater value when acidity or flatulence prevails, than the *Vin. Sem. Colchici,* and better adapted to the palates of those who object to the flavour of white wine." It is seldom employed. Mr. Brande[4] says, doubts are entertained as to the propriety of employing ammonia in it.

5. VINUM SEMINUM COLCHICI.—No formula for this exists in any of the British pharmacopœias. The following is Dr. Williams's formula :—Meadow Saffron seeds, dried, ʒij. ; Sherry Wine, Oj. (*wine measure*). Macerate for eight or ten [fourteen] days, occasionally agitating, then filter. The average dose is fʒss. to fʒj. I have given it to the extent of fʒij. Dr. Williams says it may be gradually increased to fʒiij.

6. VINUM [CORMI] COLCHICI, L. E. (Meadow Saffron Cormus, dried and sliced, ʒviij. ; Sherry Wine, Oij. Macerate for seven days [express strongly the residuum, *E.*], and strain). Average dose, fʒss. to fʒj.—Sir E. Home[5] thought that the second and subsequent deposits which take place from this wine contain the principle which acts on the stomach and bowels, while that which cures the gout is retained in permanent solution. But Sir C. Scudamore[6] found the sediment to be inert.

7. ACETUM [CORMI] COLCHICI, L. E. D. (Dried Meadow Saffron Cormus, sliced, ʒiiiss. ; Dilute Acetic Acid, Oj. ; Proof Spirit, fʒiss. Macerate the meadow saffron cormus with the acid, in a covered glass vessel, for three days ; afterwards press and strain the liquor, and set it by, that the dregs may sub-

[1] *Lond. Med. Rep.* vol. xiv. p. 93.
[2] *Op. cit.* vol. xv. p. 442.
[3] Laycock, *London Medical Gazette,* vol. xxiii. p. 899 ; and vol. xxiv. 388.
[4] *Dict. of Mat. Med.* 1839.
[5] *Phil. Trans.* 1837.
[6] *Treatise on Gout,* 3d edit. p. 513.

side : lastly, add the spirit to the clear liquor, L. The *Edin. Pharmacopœia* orders an ounce of the fresh cormus to ʒxvj. of distilled vinegar and ʒj. of proof spirit. The *Dublin College,* however, orders the dried cormus in the proportion of ʒj. to ʒiv. of acetic acid (sp. gr. 1044), and ʒxij. of distilled water). The three Colleges formerly ordered the *fresh* cormus to be used ; druggists, however, frequently prepared it with the *dried,* on account of the impossibility of procuring the fresh at all seasons of the year. Hence the London and Dublin Colleges have now directed the dried to be employed, to avoid variation in the mode of preparation. In practice, one part of the dried cormus may be considered equal to three parts of the fresh : for Mr. Battley[1] says the cormus loses about 67 per cent. of its weight in drying ; and Mr. Bainbrigge[2] obtained 2 lbs. 15 oz. of dried slices from 8 lbs. of fresh cormi. The proof spirit used in preparing the acetum is for the purpose of checking decomposition. By the action of the acetic acid on the colchicina of the cormus, an acetate of this alkaloid is obtained. Sir C. Scudamore[3] regards an acetic preparation of colchicum as milder than the wine or tincture made with the same relative weights of cormi and liquids, though it is a most efficient preparation in gout. He advises, as I have before mentioned, that it should be given in combination with magnesia, by which its acid menstruum is destroyed (acetate of magnesia being formed), and the active principle of the colchicum left in the most favourable state for administration. The average dose is from fʒss. to fʒij.

8. EXTRACTUM [CORMI] COLCHICI ACETICUM, L. E.

(Fresh Meadow Saffron Cormus, lb. j. ; Acetic [pyroligneous, *Ed.*] Acid, fʒiij. Bruise the cormus gradually sprinkled with the acetic acid, then press out the juice, and evaporate it in the undefecated state [over the vapour-bath, *Ed.*] to a proper consistence. The Dublin College orders ʒiv. of the dried root to ʒviij. of dilute acid, to be digested 14 days, filtered, and evaporated by water-bath to a soft extract.)—This compound contains the acetate of colchicina. It is a very favourite remedy in the treatment of gout and rheumatism, and was introduced into practice by Sir C. Scudamore. Dr. Paris[4] observes that he has "found it useful in promoting healthy discharges of bile." He occasionally combines it with blue pill, calomel, or potassio-tartrate of antimony. The dose is from gr. j. to gr. iij. twice or thrice a day.

[According to Mr. Southall, this extract when prepared without the starch being separated (as is directed by the London College), forms a spongy mass unfit for use. It would appear desirable to effect a change in the directions of the College in a future Pharmacopœia.[5]—Ed.]

9. EXTRACTUM COLCHICI CORMI, L.

(Fresh Meadow Saffron Cormus, lb.j. Remove the external coat of the cormus, and proceed as directed in preparing extract of Aconite.)—This is a favourite preparation with Dr. Hue, of St. Bartholomew's Hospital, in the early stage of acute rheumatism. The dose is gr. j. every four hours.

---

[1] *Lond. Med. Gaz.* xii. 463.
[2] Haden, *Practical Observations on Colchicum autumnale,* p. 77.
[3] *Observations on the Use of Colchicum.*
[4] *Appendix to the Eighth Edition of the Pharmacologia.*
[5] *Pharm. Journ.* vol. xiii. p. 62.

10. SUCCUS COLCHICI ; *Preserved Juice of Colchicum.*—I am informed that in one experiment from one cwt. of very fine cormi gathered at the end of August, and well bruised and pressed, four imperial gallons and f℥xij. of a light fawn-coloured juice were obtained. This juice becomes darker coloured by exposure to the air. After standing forty-eight hours the spirit is added to it. A large quantity of feculent deposit is formed, and the liquor acquires a paler tint. The deposit by boiling yields a coagulum. Exposure to light appears to render it somewhat paler. The smallest dose of succus colchici is five minims.

ANTIDOTE.—See VERATRUM ALBUM.

56. Hermodactylus *Auct.*—Hermodactyl.

HISTORY.—Among the later Greek and the Arabian physicians, a medicine called hermodactyl (ἑρμοδάκτυλος, from Ἑρμῆς, *Mercury* or *Hermes ;* and δάκτυλος, *a finger*) was in great repute as a remedy for arthritic diseases. It was first mentioned by Alexander of Tralles,[1] who flourished A.D. 560. Paulus Ægineta,[2] who lived A.D. 650, Avicenna,[3] Serapion,[4] and Mesue,[5] also speak of it. It is deserving of especial notice, that under the name of *Surugen* or Hermodactyl, Serapion comprehends the κολχικόν and ἐφήμερον of Dioscorides, and the ἑρμοδάκτυλος of Paulus. By some of the old writers hermodactyl was called *anima articulorum,* or *the soul of the joints.*

NATURAL HISTORY.—The cormi brought from Oriental countries in modern times under the name of hermodactyls, answer to the descriptions given of the ancient substance bearing this name. I am, therefore, induced to believe them to be identical with the latter. Their resemblance to the cormi of Colchicum autumnale leads me to reject the notion of Matthiolus, at one time entertained by Linnæus,[6] and adopted by Martius[7] and Fraas,[8] that they are produced by *Iris tuberosa.* That they are the underground stems of some species of colchicum can scarcely, I think, be doubted by any one who carefully examines them. Notwithstanding the statements of Mr. Want[9] and of Sir H. Halford,[10] I cannot admit the assumption that hermodactyls are the cormi of *Colchicum autumnale,* though this is the only species of *Colchicum* admitted into the new Greek Pharmacopœia. Though resembling the latter in several circumstances, they possess certain distinctive peculiarities. Some of the most eminent pharmacologists of Europe (*e. g.* Guibourt, Goebel, Geiger, Geoffroy, &c.) also regard them as distinct. The *Colchicum illyricum,* mentioned in many works as yielding hermodactyl, is unknown to modern botanists. The cormus of *Colchicum byzantinum* is too large to be confounded with hermodactyl. *Colchicum variegatum* has been supposed by several botanists and pharmacologists to be the source of hermodactyl, but further evidence is required to establish the opinion. This plant is a native of Sicily, Crete, Greece, and Portugal. Dr. Sibthorp[11] found it on Helicon, Parnassus, and other mountains of Greece. It is not improbable, I think, that *Colchicum bulbocodiodes* may yield hermodactyl, which Dale[12] tells us is brought from Syria. Dr. Lindley informs me that this species was found by Colonel Chesney near the Euphrates, where it was very common, flowering in March. The cormi were not brought

---

[1] Lib. xi.
[2] *Opera,* lib. iii. cap. 78 ; also, Adams's Translation for the Sydenham Society, vol. i. 660 and vol. iii. pp. 114 and 495.
[3] Lib. ii. cap. 352.
[4] *De simplicibus,* cap. 194.
[5] *Opera,* p. 37, ed. Bonon. 1484.
[6] Murray, *App. Med.* vol. v. p. 215.
[7] *Pharmakognosie,* 42.
[8] *Syn. Plant. Fl. Classicæ,* p. 293, 1845.
[9] *Med. and Phys. Journal,* vol. xxxii.
[10] *London Medical Gazette,* vol. viii. p. 318.
[11] *Prod. Fl. Græcæ,* ii. 250.
[12] *Pharmacologia,* p. 245, ed. 3tia.

over. Iris tuberosa was not found there.   Forskäl[1] found *Colchicum montanum* (which Sprengel, in his *Syst. Veg.*, regards as identical with C. bulbocodiodes) at Kurma, in Arabia.

DESCRIPTION.—Mesue says that hermodactyl is either long, like the finger, or round. Of the round, he adds, there are three kinds,—the white, the red, and the black; the white being the best. C. Bauhin[2] considered that the black and red hermodactyl of Mesue and Serapion are C. autumnale, or, as he terms it, "Colchicum commune;" but the white hermodactyl he regarded as a distinct kind, which he calls "Colchicum radice siccata alba." Through the kindness of my friend Professor Royle, I have had the examination of two kinds of hermodactyl, procured by him in the bazaars of Northern India, brought, he thinks, from Surat or Bombay, and probably imported there from the Red Sea.

1. *Tasteless Hermodactyl; Sorinjun sheeran* (i. e. sweet sorinjan), Royle; *Hermodactylus*, Auct. nostræ ætatis.—In their general form these cormi resemble those of Colchicum autumnale. They are flattened, cordate, hollowed out or grooved on one side, convex on the other. At their lower part (forming the base of the heart) is a mark or disk for the insertion of the root fibres. Their size varies: the specimens I have examined were from $\frac{3}{4}$ to $1\frac{1}{2}$ inches in length or height, 1 to $1\frac{1}{2}$ inches in breadth, and about $\frac{1}{2}$ an inch in depth. They have been deprived of their coats, are externally dirty yellow or brownish, internally white, easily broken, farinaceous, opaque, odourless, tasteless, or nearly so, and worm-eaten. They agree precisely with hermodactyls furnished me by Professor Guibourt. They are readily distinguished from the cormi of Colchicum autumnale by the following characters, which are correctly stated by Geoffroy:[3]—They are not rugose, are white internally, are moderately hard, easily broken, and form a whitish powder; whereas the dried cormi of Colchicum autumnale are rugose, softer, and have a reddish or greyish tint both internally and externally.

2. *Bitter Hermodactyl; Sorinjan tulkh* (i. e. bitter sorinjan), Royle; ? *Bulbs* [cormi] *of another Colchicum.*[4] ?? *Hermodactylus rubens et niger* (Avicenna and Mesue).—The cormi of this variety are distinguished from the preceding by their bitter taste, their smaller size, and by having externally a striped or reticulated appearance. Their colour for the most part is darker; in some specimens it is blackish. One cormus is ovate-cordate; 1 inch in height or length, $\frac{3}{4}$ of an inch broad, and about $\frac{1}{4}$ of an inch thick, grooved or hollowed on one side, convex on the other; of a brownish yellow colour, semi-transparent, has a horny appearance, and is marked by longitudinal stripes, indicating a laminated structure. A second is opaque, amylaceous, reticulated externally, white internally, less flattened, and of a remarkable shape, the concave or hollow side of the cormus being continued half an inch below the mark for the attachment of the root fibres. The other cormi are of the size and shape of a large orange-pip, but flattened or grooved on one side; some of them are worm-eaten, and one is blackish-brown externally.

COMPOSITION.—Lecanu[5] analysed hermodactyls (the *tasteless* variety), and obtained the following results :—*Starch* (forming the principal constituent of the hermodactyl), *fatty matter, yellow colouring matter, gum, supermalates of lime* and *potash,* and *chloride of potassium.* Is the absence of veratria or colchicina to be ascribed to the cormi having undergone decomposition by keeping? No inulin was detected.

CHEMICAL CHARACTERISTICS.—Both the *tasteless* and *bitter* hermodactyls are blackened by tincture of iodine, showing the presence of starch. A cold decoction of the *bitter* variety produced an intense blue precipitate (*iodide of starch*) with a solution of iodine. Tincture of galls, and solutions of protonitrate of mercury, and of diacetate of lead, caused a cloudiness in the cold decoction.

EFFECTS AND USES.—No modern experiments have been made to determine the activity of hermodactyl. The *tasteless* variety is probably inert, or nearly so; but the *bitter* variety, I suspect, possesses some activity. Is its operation analogous to that of the cormus of Colchicum autumnale? Speaking of the treatment of gout and arthritis, Paulus says, "some, in the paroxysms of all arthritic diseases, have recourse to purging with hermodactylus; but it is to be remarked, that the hermodactylus is bad for the

---

[1] *Fl. Ægypt. Arab.* p. 77.
[2] *Pinax,* p. 67, 1671.
[3] *Trait. de Mat. Méd.* t. ii. p. 79.
[4] Goebel, *Pharm. Waarenk.* p. 271.
[5] *Journ. de Pharm.* xi. 350.

stomach, producing nausea and anorexia, and ought, therefore, to be used only in the case of those who are pressed by urgent business ; for it removes rheumatism speedily, and after two days at most, so that they are enabled to resume their accustomed employment."[1]

57. VERATRUM ALBUM, *Linn.*—WHITE HELLEBORE.

Sex. Syst. Polygamia, Monœcia.
(Radix, *L. D.*—Rhizoma, *E.*)

HISTORY.—This is, I think, the ἐλλέβορος λευκὸς of Dioscorides (lib. iv. cap. 150), and probably, therefore, of other ancient writers, as Hippocrates and Theophrastus.   On this point, however, considerable difference of opinion has existed.   Schulze,[2] while he acknowledges the great similitude between *Veratrum album*, Linn. and the white hellebore of Dioscorides, is of opinion that the true hellebore (both white and black) of Theophrastus is wholly lost. And Dr. Sibthorp,[3] who found both *V. album* and *V. nigrum* in Greece,[4] regards *Digitalis ferruginea* as the white hellebore of Dioscorides,—an opinion from which Sir J. Smith, the editor of the Prodromus, expresses his dissent.[5]   The term *veratrum* is said by Lemery to be derived from *vere atrum* (*truly black*), in reference to the colour of the rhizome; but this etymology is improbable.

BOTANY.   **Gen. Char.**—*Flowers* polygamous.   *Perianth* 6-parted ; segments broad, concave, imbricating, nearly equal, striated, not excavated at the base.   *Stamens* 6, equal, inserted into the base of the segments ; *filaments* subulate ; *anthers* reniform, with confluent cells. *Ovary* with 3 divaricating *stigmas*.   *Capsule* 3-horned, separating into three many-seeded follicles. *Seeds* compressed, winged at the apex (*Lindley*).

Sp. Char.—*Panicle* decompound.   *Bracts* equalling the flowers.   *Pedicels* pubescent.   *Segments of the perianth* somewhat erect and obtuse, serrulate.   *Leaves* ovate-oblong, plaited (*Sprengel*).

Root composed of numerous fleshy, brownish-white fibres, arising from a perennial, cylindrical, fleshy, subterraneous stem or *rhizome*, which is brown externally, brownish-white internally, and is placed obliquely in the earth.   *Stem* 1 to 4 feet high.   The plant flowers from June to August.

Two varieties (by some considered distinct species) are included here :—

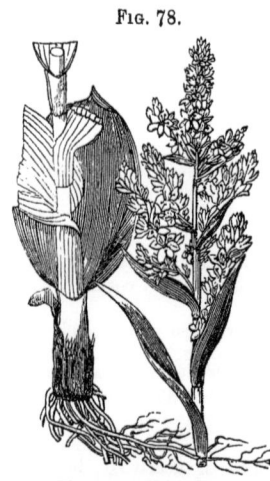

FIG. 78.

Veratrum album, Linn.
var. *albiflorum*.

α. *albiflorum* (*V. album*, Bernh.) with decompound raceme and white flowers.

β. *viridiflorum* (*V. lobelianum*, Bernh.) with compound raceme and greenish flowers.

---

[1] Adams's *Translation*, vol. i. p. 660, Sydenham Society's edition.

[2] *Diss. inaug. sist. Toxicol. Veterum*, Halæ, 1788.

[3] *Prod. Fl. Græcæ*, i. 489.

[4] Neither Fraas nor any other botanists whose collections in Greece he examined found either of the above mentioned species of veratrum.

[5] For some interesting information respecting the ancient hellebore, consult Dierbach, *Arzneimittel. d. Hippocrates*, p. 107.

Hab.—Mountainous regions of Europe. Abounds in the Alps and Pyrenees.
DESCRIPTION.—The *rhizome* or *cormus* (*radix veratri*, offic., *radix helle-bori albi*) is single-, double-, or many-headed, having the form of a cylinder, or, more frequently, of a truncated cone. It is from two to four inches long, and about one inch in diameter, rough, wrinkled, greyish or blackish-brown externally, whitish internally. Portions of the root fibres are usually attached to it, as well as some soft, fine, hair-like fibres. At the upper extremity of the rhizome we frequently observe the cut edges of numerous concentric, woody, or membranous scales : they are portions of the dried leaf-sheaths. When cut transversely, the rhizome presents a large central portion (frequently called *medulla*), which varies in its qualities; being woody, farinaceous, or spongy, in different specimens. This is separated by a brown fine undulating line from a thick woody ring, in which the root fibres take their origin. On the outside of this is a narrow but compact brown epidermoid coat. The odour of the dried rhizome is feeble ; the taste is at first bitter, then acrid. By keeping, the rhizome is apt to become mouldy.

The rhizome of *Veratrum viride* is used in the United States as a substitute for that of Veratrum album (see p. 172).

COMPOSITION.—White hellebore rhizome was analysed in 1820 by MM. Pelletier and Caventou,[1] who obtained the following results :—*Fatty matter* (composed of *olein, stearin,* and a *volatile* [cevadic?] *acid*), *supergallate of veratria, yellow colouring matter, starch, ligneous matter,* and *gum.* The ashes contained much *phosphate* and *carbonate of lime, carbonate of potash,* and some traces of *silica* and *sulphate of lime,* but no chlorides. They could not obtain the volatile [cevadic?] acid in a crystalline form.

1. VERATRIA. (See p. 177.)
2. JERVIN (so called from *Jerva,* the Spanish name for a poison obtained from the root of white hellebore) ;[2] *Barytin.*—A white crystalline, fusible, and inflammable substance, discovered by Simon.[3] It is soluble in alcohol, but not in water. With acetic and phosphoric acids it yields readily soluble salts ; but, on the contrary, with sulphuric, nitric, and hydrochoric acids, it forms difficultly soluble compounds.[4] On account of its resembling baryta in being precipitable from its solution in acetic acid by sulphuric acid, it was called at first *barytin.* Its composition, according to Will, is $C^{60}H^{45}N^2O^5$.

CHEMICAL CHARACTERISTICS.—A decoction of the rhizome undergoes, on the addition of a solution of gelatin, no change, shewing the absence of tannic acid ; but with the sesquichloride of iron, it becomes olive green (*gallate? of iron*). With tincture of galls it became slightly turbid (*tannates of veratria and starch*). With acetate and diacetate of lead, and protonitrate of mercury, it formed copious precipitates. Oil of vitriol reddens the concentrated decoction, owing to its action on the veratria. The rhizome left after the decoction had been prepared from it, becomes, on the addition of a solution of iodine, black (*iodide of starch*).
PHYSIOLOGICAL EFFECTS. α. On Vegetables.—Not ascertained.
β. *On Animals generally.*—" The best account of its effects is contained in a thesis by Dr. Schabel, published at Tübingen, in 1817. Collecting toge-

---

[1] *Journ. de Pharm.* vol. vi. p. 363.
[2] Bauhin's *Pinax,* p. 186.
[3] Poggendorff's *Annalen,* xli. 569 ; and *Pharmaceutisches Central-Blatt für* 1837, S. 191.
[4] *Pharm. Central-Blatt für* 1837, S. 753; also, *Berlinisches Jahrb. für d. Pharm.* Bd. xxxiii. S. 393; and *Lond. and Edinb. Phil. Mag.* vol. xii. p. 29.

ther the experiments previously made by Wepfer, Courten, Viborg, and Orfila, and adding a number of excellent experiments of his own, he infers that it is poisonous to animals of all classes—horses, dogs, cats, rabbits, jackdaws, starlings, frogs, snails, and flies; that it acts in whatever way it is introduced into the system—by the stomach, windpipe, nostrils, pleural membrane of the chest, on external wounds, or the veins; that it produces in every instance symptoms of irritation in the alimentary canal, and injury of the nervous system; and that it is very active, three grains of the extract applied to the nostrils of a cat having killed it in sixteen hours."[1]

γ. *On Man.*—Its *local* action is that of a powerful acrid. Applied to the Schneiderian membrane, it excites violent sneezing. Epistaxis even is said to have been induced by it. Its operation when swallowed, or placed in contact with the skin, is also that of an energetic irritant.

Its *remote* action is on the secretory apparatus, the stomach and intestines, and the nervous system. In *small* and *repeated doses* it promotes secretion from the mucous surfaces, the salivary glands, the kidneys and the uterus, and increases the cutaneous exhalation.[2] In *larger doses* it causes vomiting, purging, pain in the abdomen, tenesmus, and occasionally bloody evacuations, and great prostration of strength. In some instances a few grains even have had these effects. Schabel says there is no substance which so certainly and promptly provokes vomiting; and Horn[3] employed it as a sure emetic. In addition to the local action which it exercises, when swallowed, on the stomach and intestines, it possessss a specific power of influencing these viscera: for Etmuller[4] has seen violent vomiting result from the application of the rhizome to the abdomen; and Schröder[5] observed the same occurrence where the rhizome was used as a suppository. In *excessive doses* it operates as a narcotico-acrid poison, producing gastro-intestinal inflammation and an affection of the nervous system. The symptoms are, violent vomiting and purging (sometimes of blood), tenesmus, burning sensation of the mouth, throat, œsophagus, stomach, and intestines, constriction of the throat, with a sense of strangulation, griping pain in the bowels, small, and in some cases almost imperceptible pulse, faintness, cold sweats, tremblings, giddiness, blindness, dilated pupils, loss of voice, convulsions, and insensibility, terminating in death. A cutaneous eruption has in some instances followed the use of white hellebore.

I am indebted to Dr. Wm. Rayner, of Stockport, for notes of three cases of poisoning by infusion of white hellebore. The symptoms resembled those just mentioned, except that there was no purging. All three cases rapidly recovered.

Hutchinson[6] remarked, that when death did not occur, palpitation and intermitting pulse, besides dyspeptic and nervous symptoms, remained for some time. These effects were not observed in Dr. Rayner's cases.

In its action on the system, Veratrum album is more closely related to cebadilla and meadow saffron than to any other medicinal agents. It is more

---

[1] Christison's *Treatise on Poisons*, 3d edit. p. 790.
[2] Greding, *Sämmtl. med. Schrift.* Th. 1, S. 179.
[3] *Archiv*, B. x. H. 1, S. 161.
[4] *Opera omnia*, tom. ii. pt. ii. p. 144.
[5] Orfila, *Toxicol. Gén.*
[6] Schwartze's *Pharm. Tab.* 2te Ausg.

acrid and less stupifying than Helleborus niger, with which it has been so frequently compared both by ancients and moderns. Orfila[1] ascertained by experiment on animals that it is more active as a poison than the last mentioned substance. It exercises no known chemical influence over the tissues, by which it is distinguished from the mineral irritants, as baryta and emetic tartar, with which Schabel compared it.

USES.—It is but rarely employed, principally on account of the alleged uncertainty of its operation. But from the few trials which I have made with it, I suspect this uncertainty is much exaggerated, and is chiefly referable to the varying lengths of time during which the rhizome has been kept after its removal from the earth, for, like colchicum, it deteriorates by keeping. The following are the principal cases in which it has been employed:—

1. *In affections of the nervous system*, as melancholia, mania, and epilepsy.[2] As an emetic, purgative, and promoter of the secretions generally, we can easily understand that it may prove occasionally beneficial.

2. *In chronic skin diseases*, as herpes, Dr. C. Smyth[3] gave the tincture internally with benefit. As external applications, the decoction and ointment are used in scabies (hence the Germans call the rhizome *Kratzwurzel*, i. e. *itch-root*), tinea capitis, &c.; but their use is not quite free from danger.

2. *In gout*, it was given in combination with opium, by Mr. Moore,[4] as a substitute for, or in imitation of, the *Eau Médicinale*. The dose, in a paroxysm of gout, was from forty minims to two drachms of a mixture composed of three parts of *Vin. Veratri albi* and one part of liquid laudanum.

4. *In amaurosis* and *chronic affections of the brain* occurring in torpid habits, it is employed as an errhine or sternutatory (hence its German name, *Niesswurzell*, i. e. *sneeze-root*). It is usually diluted with some mild powder. The German snuff called *Schneeberger* is said to contain it.

5. *To destroy pediculi*, the decoction is used as a wash (*infra*).

6. *As an emetic*, it was employed by Horn.

ADMINISTRATION.—The following are the principal modes of exhibition:—

1. PULVIS VERATRI; *White Hellebore Powder.*—The dose of this at the commencement should not exceed one or two grains. This quantity will sometimes occasion nausea and vomiting; but Greding found that in some cases eight grains, and, in a few instances, a scruple of the bark of the rhizome in powder, were required to excite vomiting. As an errhine, not more than two or three grains, mixed with eight or ten of some mild powder (as starch, liquorice, Florentine orris, or lavender), should be employed at one time. It is a constituent of the *Unguentum Sulphuris compositum* (see Vol. i. p. 358).

2. VINUM VERATRI, L; *Tinctura Veratri albi; Tincture of White Hellebore.* (White Hellebore, sliced, ℥viij.; Sherry Wine, Oij. Macerate for seven days, and strain.)—As a substitute for colchicum in gout and rheumatism, the dose is ten minims twice or thrice daily. This quantity is to be gradually increased. A full dose acts as an emetic and cathartic.

---

[1] *Toxicol. Gén.*
[2] Greding, *Sämmtl. mediz. Schriften*, T. 1, S. 179.
[3] *Med. Communications*, vol. i. p. 207.
[4] *Two Letters to Dr. Jones*, 1811.

3. DECOCTUM VERATRI, P. L. 1836; *Decoction of White Hellebore.*
(White Hellebore, bruised, ℥x.; Distilled Water, Oij.; Rectified Spirit, f℥iij.
Boil the hellebore in the water down to a pint, and when it is cooled add the
spirit.)—This preparation is only used as an external application in skin
diseases (scabies, lepra, and tinea capitis), and to destroy pediculi. When
the skin is very irritable, the decoction will sometimes require dilution. If
the surface to which it is applied be denuded, absorption of the veratria may
occur, and constitutional symptoms be thereby induced; hence it is a dangerous
application, especially to children.

Antidotes.—Astringent solutions have been recommended; and in one
case which fell under my notice infusion of nutgalls seemed to give relief.
The supposed benefit has been referred to the union of tannic acid with
veratria, by which the solubility and activity of the latter are diminished; but
Schabel[1] found that three drachms of a tincture of white hellebore, given with
infusion of galls, to a cat, proved fatal in twenty minutes. Hahnemann recommends coffee, both as a drink and in clyster. Demulcent liquids, and in
some cases opiates, may be useful. The other parts of the treatment must
be conducted on general principles. Stimulants will be usually required on
account of the failure of the heart's action.

58. Veratrum viride, *Willd.*—American Hellebore.

Sex. Syst. Polygamia, Monœcia.

(Rhizoma.)

The Veratrum viride, U. S. (*Secondary List*), is known in the United States as
American Hellebore, Swamp Hellebore, Indian Poke, and *Itch Weed.* It has a perennial,
thick, fleshy root, tunicated at top, the lower part solid and sending off numerous white
or light-yellow radicles. The stem is annual, from 2 to 3 feet high, pubescent. Leaves
at base 6 inches to a foot long, broad, oval, nerved, acuminate, of a deep green colour,
and pubescent; those on the stem narrower, and, at the summit, bracteæform. Flowers
in panicles, terminal, and of a greenish-yellow tint. The calex is wanting; petals 6,
stamens 6, pistil a rudiment (*Willdenow*). Germs 3, when not rudimentary, on the lower
portion of the panicle.

The plant is found in many parts of the United States, from Canada to Carolina,
inhabiting damp places in the neighbourhood of streams and meadows. It appears early
in March.

The whole plant has an acrid and burning taste; the root only is officinal. This, when
dried, consists of a somewhat tunicated top, with a thick hard base, and numerous radicles
attached to it. The odour, disagreeable in the recent state, is lost by drying. The taste
is at first sweetish, then bitter, followed by an acrid burning sensation in the mouth,
which lasts for some hours after it has been chewed. When powdered, it acts as a sternutatory. For the composition of this root we are indebted to Mr. Henry Worthington,[2]
who found it to contain *gum, starch, sugar, bitter extractive, fixed oily matter, colouring
matter, gallic acid,* an ALKALOID SUBSTANCE identical with *veratria, lignin, salts of lime,*
and *potassa.* With regard to the alkaloid substance, he describes it as "nearly insoluble
in water, more soluble in ether, and entirely soluble in absolute alcohol. When exposed
to flame, it first melts, then swells up, and burns without residue. It produces a burning
acrid sensation in the mouth, which lasts for several hours. It acts powerfully as a
sternutatory, producing violent sneezing, which lasts for half an hour after it has been
applied to the nose." "In its chemical relations, the analogy is carried out by not being

---

[1] Quoted in Brandt and Ratzburg's *Giftgewächse*, Abt. 1, S. 28.
[2] *American Journal of Pharmacy*, vol. x. p. 97.

changed to a red colour by the action of nitric acid, and from its forming salts with the acids, none of which are crystallisable but the sulphate, tartrate, and oxalate."

That the framers of the United States Pharmacopœia have done well in the introduction of this article, is shown by the testimony in its favour as a potent medicine. Dr. Osgood[1] and Dr. Ware[2] have each instituted a course of experiments to test its remedial powers. The first found it an emetic; and the second met with a case where this effect on the stomach was produced by the application of the ointment to an ulcer on the leg. Mr. Worthington submitted himself to the test of its powers. He took the fourth of a grain of the *Alcoholic Extract*, which caused an acrid burning sensation in the mouth, and communicated to the throat and fauces a sense of dryness and heat, which finally reached the stomach. In the course of about an hour, this dryness and burning sensation in the throat and stomach became intense, and a disposition to hiccough was excited, which soon commenced, gradually increasing in frequency until it reached fifteen or twenty times per minute. This was attended with some sickness and retching until vomiting took place. This was violent, and seemed to come on about every ten or fifteen minutes for the space of an hour. During this time dizziness and tremor were created, which passed off with the effect of the dose. With the hiccough there was a copious secretion of saliva and discharge of mucus from the stomach and nose. During the action of this dose, the pulse was weakened so as to be scarcely perceptible, and reduced from sixty-eight to fifty-two pulsations per minute.[3]

The experiment just detailed was repeated three times, and in neither was there a disposition to catharsis. The effects are those of an acro narcotic, and not one of the least potent of this class of remedies. The uses and mode of administration are similar to those of the White Hellebore. In gout and rheumatism, the medical gentlemen before mentioned speak in its favour. A knowledge of it is stated to be possessed by the North American Indians.

59. Veratrum Sabadilla, *Retz.*

Sex. Syst. Polygamia, Monœcia.

(Semina.)

A native of Mexico and the Antilles. Its leaves are radical, oval-oblong, obtuse, ribbed. Its stem is almost leafless. The panicle is nearly simple. The flowers have short pedicels, and are nodding.

Its fruit and seeds are said to be brought from the Antilles, under the name of *cebadilla* (*semina sabadillæ caribææ*), but I have never met with them.

60. ASAGRÆA OFFICINALIS, *Lind.*—SPIKE-FLOWERED ASAGRÆA.

Sex. Syst. Hexandria, Trigynia.

(Semina; Sabadilla, *L.*—Sabadilla; Fruit of Veratrum Sabadilla,[4] of Helonias officinalis, and probably of other Melanthaceæ, *E.*)

Synonymes.—Veratrum officinale, *Schlecht ;* Helonias officinalis, *Don.*

History.—This plant was described by Schlechtendahl,[5] afterwards by Mr. Don,[6] and subsequently by Dr. Lindley.[7] The seeds were known to Monardes in 1573. They were called *sabadilla*, or *cevadilla*, or more

---

[1] *Am. Journ. of Pharm.* vol. vii. p. 202.
[2] Bigelow's *Med. Bot.* vol. ii. pp. 127, 132.
[3] *Op. cit.*
[4] See *supra.*
[5] *Linnea*, vi. 45.
[6] *Ed. New Phil. Journ.* Oct. 1839.
[7] *Bot. Reg.* June 1839.

properly *cebadilla* (from the Spanish *cebada, barley*), on account of the supposed resemblance of the inflorescence of the plant to that of *hordeum*.

BOTANY.　**Gen. Char.**—*Flowers* polygamous, racemose, naked. *Perianth* 6-partite; *segments* linear, veinless, almost equal, with a nectariferous excavation at the base, equal to the stamens. *Stamens* alternately shorter; *anthers* cordate, as if unilocular, after dehiscence shield-shaped. *Ovaries* 3, quite simple, attenuated into an obscure *stigma*. *Follicles* 3, acuminate, papery; *seeds* scimitar-shaped, corrugated, winged. *Bulbous herbs*, with grass-like *leaves*, and small, pale, densely-racemed *flowers* (*Lindley*).

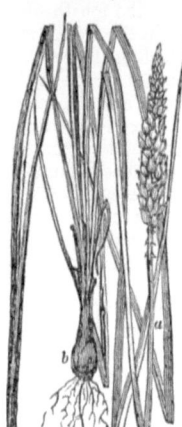

FIG. 79.

Asagræa officinalis.

a. Fruit-bearing stem.
b. Root, bulb, and leaves.

Sp. Char.—The only species known.

Leaves linear, acuminate, subcarinate, roughish at the margin, 4 feet long and 3 lines broad. *Scape* round, about 6 feet high. *Raceme* a foot and a half long, very dense, very straight, spiciform. *Flowers* white, with a bractea at the base. *Anthers* yellow.

Hab.—Eastern side of the Mexican Andes, near Barranca de Tioselo (*Schiede*). Neighbourhood of Vera Cruz (*Hartweg*).

DESCRIPTION.—The *cabadilla, cevadilla,* or *sabadilla* of the shops (*sabadilla; semina sabadillæ mexicanæ*) comes from Vera Cruz and Mexico. It consists of the follicles (some containing seeds, others empty), loose seeds, stalks, and abortive flowers of the Asagræa officinalis, and perhaps of Veratrum Sabadilla also.

The follicles, commonly termed capsules, rarely exceed, or even equal, half an inch in length, and are about one line or a line and a half in diameter. They are ovate-oblong, acuminate. Their colour is pale yellowish-brown, or reddish-grey. The coat of each is thin, dry, and of a papery consistence. Each fruit is composed of three follicles mutually adherent towards the base, open at the superior and internal part. The receptacle, fruitstalk, and the remains of the dried and withered calyx, are usually present in the cebadilla of the shops. Seldom more than one or two, though sometimes three, seeds are found in each follicle. The seeds are two or three lines long, scimitar-shaped, pointed, blackish-brown, shiny, wrinkled or corrugated, slightly winged. Internally they are whitish or horny. Embryo straight, next the hilum, lodged in fleshy albumen. They have little odour, but a bitter, acrid, persistent taste.

COMPOSITION.—Two analyses of cebadilla have been made about the same time (1819); one by Meissner,[1] and a second by Pelletier and Caventou.[2] The following are the results:—

---

[1] *Schweigger's Journ. f. Chem.* xxxi. 187.
[2] *Journ. de Pharm.* vi. 353.

MEISSNER'S ANALYSIS.		
Fatty matter (*olein* and *stearin*)	24·63
Wax (*myricin*)............................	0·10
Sabadillin (*veratria*).......................	0·58
Resin (soluble in ether)	1·45
Hard resin (insoluble in ether)	8·45
Bitter extractive with the acid which is united to the sabadillin	5·97
Sweet extractive	0·65
Extractive separable by alkalies	24·14
Gum	4·90
Vegetable jelly (*phyteumacolla*) with chloride of potassium and vegetable salts of potash	1·11
Oxalate of lime combined with bassorin	1·06
Lignin....................................	20·56
Water	6·40
Cebadilla	100·00

The ashes contained oxide of copper.

PELLETIER AND CAVENTOU'S ANALYSIS.
Fatty matter composed of { Olein. Stearin. Cevadic acid.
Wax.
Supergallate of *veratria*.
Yellow colouring matter.
Starch.
Lignin.
Gum.
Ashes composed of ...... { Carbonate of potash. " lime. Phosphate lime. Chloride potassium. Silica.
Cebadilla.

1. CEVADIC or SABADILLIC ACID.—This is a crystalline, fusible, volatile, fatty acid, having an odour analogous to butyric acid. It is soluble in water, alcohol, and ether. It is obtained by the saponification of the *oil of cebadilla* (fatty matter). Cevadate of ammonia causes a white precipitate with the persalts of iron. The composition of this acid is unknown.

Oil of cebadilla given me by Mr. Morson is green, lighter than water, and has a faint, somewhat rancid taste.

2. VERATRIC ACID, of Merck.[1]—This is a crystalline, fusible, volatile acid, soluble in alcohol, slightly so in water, but insoluble in ether. According to Schroetter it consists of $C^{18}H^9O^7$+aq.

3. RESINS.—The two *resins* found by Meissner, but overlooked by Pelletier and Caventou, are probably endowed with activity.

Couerbe obtained from cebadilla seeds, *sabadillina, helonin* or *resin of veratria*, and *gum resin of sabadillina*.

a. Sabadillina ia a white crystalline solid, possessing alkaline properties, being soluble in boiling water and in alcohol, but not in ether. In the fused state it consists of $C^{20}H^{13}NO^5$. It forms with acids crystallisable salts. It is said by Simon[2] to be merely a compound of resinate of soda and resinate of veratria. Dr. Turnbull found it inferior in activity to veratria.

β. Helonin or *resin of veratria* (*veratrin*, Couerbe; *pseudo-veratria*) is a brown solid, fusible at 365°. Insoluble in ether (by which it is distinguished from *veratria*) and in water. It combines with acids; but neither saturates them, nor forms with them any crystallisable salts. It consists of $C^{14}H^9NO^3$. Its action on the animal economy has not been determined.

γ. Gum-resin of sabadillina (*resinigomme*, Couerbe; *monohydrate of sabadillina*, Alter.) is a reddish solid, soluble in water and alcohol, but slightly so in ether. It saturates acids, but does not form crystalline compounds with them. Alkalies throw it down from its saline combinations. It consists of $C^{20}H^{14}NO^6$. Hence it differs from anhydrous *sabadillina* in containing an atom more water. Furthermore, it is distinguished from this alkali in not being crystallisable.

4. VERATRIA.—See p. 177.

CHEMICAL CHARACTERISTICS.—The brownish-coloured decoction of cebadilla reddens litmus, owing to the presence of free acid. Sesquichloride of iron deepens the colour of the decoction, and causes an olive-brown precipitate. Alkalies deepen, whilst acids diminish, the colour of the decoction (by their action on the yellow colouring matter, *Pelletier*). Acetate and diacetate of

---

[1] *Pharmaceutisches Central-Blatt für* 1839, S. 235.
[2] *Berl. Jahrb.* Bd. xxxix. S. 393.

lead, protonitrate of mercury, and sulphate of copper, form precipitates in the decoction. Oxalate of ammonia renders it turbid (*oxalate of lime*). Nitrate of silver forms a coloured precipitate, which is for the most part soluble in nitric acid : the insoluble portion is *chloride of silver*. Solutions of iodine and tincture of nutgalls have no obvious effect. Oil of vitriol reddens the decoction, owing to its action on the veratria.

Physiological Effects. *a. On Vegetables.*—Not ascertained.

β. *On Animals.*—Are similar to those of Veratrum album. Cebadilla has proved poisonous to dogs and cats.[1] A pinch of it produced violent spasms in cats ; half a drachm caused vomiting and convulsions in dogs. It is a poison to insects. Thus bugs die from it in convulsions : hence its use as a bug poison ![2] Its efficacy in destroying pediculi has long been known.

γ. *On Man.*—The action is probably similar to, though more acrid than, white hellebore. The effects of *small and epeated doses* have not been satisfactorily ascertained. *Large and poisonous doses* cause burning and pain in the throat and stomach, nausea, vomiting, purging, prostration of strength, convulsions, delirium, and sometimes a cutaneous eruption. Even the external application of the powder has caused dangerous effects. Plenck tells us of a young man who was rendered temporarily insane by the application of powder of cebadilla to his head. Lentin says an infant, whose nurse had sprinkled the powder in its hair, died in convulsions.[3] Rubbed on the skin, the tincture causes a stinging sensation similar to that produced by veratria. After its use for some days, a slight eruption appears on the skin. Rubbed over the cardiac region, it in some instances reduces the frequency and force of the pulse in a marked degree. The alcoholic extract has nearly the same effects, when taken internally, as veratria. It also induces sensations of heat and tingling on the surface of the skin, and sometimes acts as a diuretic.[4]

Uses.—Cebadilla has been employed internally, as an *anthelmintic,* in both thread-worms and tape-worms.[5] Dr. Turnbull[6] has given the extract with benefit in painful rheumatic and neuralgic affections. Though it is applicable in all the maladies for the relief of which veratria has been recommended, it is rarely administered by the mouth. *Externally* the powder of the seeds has been used to destroy pediculi; hence the Germans called the seeds *Läusesaamen,* or *lice-seeds.* But it cannot be applied with safety to children, and especially when the skin is broken. I have already referred to the dangerous consequences of its employment. The tincture has been used as a rubefacient in chronic rheumatism, and, rubbed over the heart, in some cases of nervous palpitation.[5] It may, in fact, be employed as a cheap though efficient substitute for the tincture of veratria.

The principal use of the seeds, for which indeed they have been introduced into the Pharmacopœia, is for yielding veratria.

Administration.—The following are the preparations of cebadilla which have been employed in medicine :—

---

[1] Willemet, *Nouv. Mém. de l'Acad. de Dijon,* 1782.
[2] Seeliger, in Schmucker's *Vermischt. chirurg. Schrift.* vol. ii. p. 272.
[3] Murray, *App. Med.* vol. v. p. 172.
[4] Turnbull, *On the Medicinal Properties of the Ranunculaceæ,* p. 7.
[5] Schmucker's *Verm. chirurg. Schrift.* Bd. ii. S. 271.
[6] *Op. cit.* p. 7.
[7] Turnbull, *op. cit.*

1. PULVIS SABADILLÆ; *Pulvis contra pediculos ; Poudre de Capucin ; Powder of Cebadilla.*—The dose for an adult is from two to six grains, gradually increased. In one case of tape-worm, half a drachm was taken daily for fourteen days.[1]

2. TINCTURA SABADILLÆ; *Saturated Tincture of Cebadilla,* Turnbull. (Cebadilla Seeds, freed from their capsules and bruised, *any quantity ;* Rectified Spirit, *as much as will cover them.* Digest for ten days.)—Used as a rubefacient liniment in chronic rheumatism and paralysis. It is rubbed over the heart in nervous palpitation.

3. EXTRACTUM ALCOHOLICUM SABADILLÆ; *Alcoholic Extract of Cebadilla.*—Evaporate the saturated tincture, with a very gentle heat, to a proper consistence. Dose, 1-6th of a grain, gradually increased. It is given, in the form of pill, in rheumatic and neuralgic cases.

4. VERATRIA, L. E.; *Veratrine; Veratrina,* Thomson ; *Sabadillin,* Meissner.—This vegetable alkaloid was discovered about the same time (1819) by Meissner in Germany, and by Pelletier and Caventou in France. Couerbe[2] probably was the first who obtained it pure.

PREPARATION.—The following process for making veratria, contained in the London Pharmacopœia for 1836, is nearly identical with that described by Soubeiran,[3] and is a modification of one given by Couerbe.

" Take of Cebadilla, bruised, lb. ij. ; Rectified Spirit, Cong. iij. ; Diluted Sulphuric Acid ; Solution of Ammonia ; Purified Animal Charcoal ; Magnesia ; each as much as may be sufficient. Boil the Cebadilla with a gallon of the spirit, for an hour, in a retort to which a receiver is fitted. Pour off the liquor, and boil what remains with another gallon of spirit and the spirit recently distilled, and pour off the liquor : and let it be done a third time. Press the Cebadilla and let the spirit distil from the mixed and strained liquors. Evaporate what remains to the proper consistence of an extract. Boil this three or more times in water to which a little diluted sulphuric acid has been added, and with a gentle heat evaporate the strained liquors to the consistence of a syrup. Into this, when cold, put the magnesia to saturation, frequently shaking [them] ; then press, and wash. Let this be done twice or thrice : then dry what remains, and digest with a gentle heat in spirit two or three times, and as often strain. Afterwards let the spirit distil. Boil the residue in water to which a little sulphuric acid and animal charcoal are added, for a quarter of an hour, and strain. Lastly, the charcoal being thoroughly washed, cautiously evaporate the [mixed] liquors until they have the consistence of a syrup, and drop into them as much ammonia as may be sufficient to throw down the veratria. Separate this, and dry it."

Dr. Christison[4] declares the process of the London College impracticable f⸳⸳ want of sufficient directions for reducing the seeds to a fine state of divisi⸳ and adds, that it gives no instructions for detaching the seeds from their follicles. But a manufacturer assures me he never separates the follicles from the seeds in making veratria.

[The London College now merely notices veratria in the Materia Medica, giving no process for its preparation, but appending the following note :—" It is slightly soluble in water, more so in ether, but most in rectified spirit. Odourless, irritating to the nares, and it tastes acrid. It is to be used with great caution."—ED.]

---

[1] Seeliger, in Schmucker, *op. cit.* vol. ii. p. 271.
[2] *Ann. de Chim. et de Phys.* t. lii. p. 368.
[3] *Nouv. Traité de Pharm.* t. ii. p. 190.
[4] *Dispensatory.*

The process of the Edinburgh Pharmacopœia is as follows :—

" Take any convenient quantity of Cevadilla: pour boiling water over it in a covered vessel, and let it macerate for 24 hours; remove the Cevadilla, squeeze it, and dry it thoroughly with a gentle heat. Beat it now in a mortar, and separate the seeds from the capsules by brisk agitation in a deep narrow vessel. Grind the seeds in a coffee-mill, and form them into a thick paste with rectified spirit. Pack this firmly in a percolator, and pass rectified spirit through it till the spirit ceases to be coloured. Concentrate the spirituous solutions, by distillation, so long as no deposit forms, and pour the residuum, while hot, into twelve times its volume of cold water. Filter through calico, and wash the residuum on the filter so long as the washings precipitate with ammonia. Unite the filtered liquid with the washings, and add an excess of ammonia. Collect the precipitate on a filter, wash it slightly with cold water, and dry it, first by imbibition with filtering paper, and then in the vapour-bath. A small additional quantity may be got by concentrating the filtered ammoniacal fluid, and allowing it to cool.

" Veratria thus obtained is not pure, but sufficiently so for medicinal use. From this coloured substance it may be obtained white, though at considerable loss, by solution in very weak muriatic acid, decolorisation with animal charcoal, and reprecipitation with ammonia."

Theory.—The following statement applies to the process formerly recommended by the London College, and is perhaps correct as far as it goes :— Cebadilla yields to rectified spirit veratria in combination with a vegetable acid. When the alcoholic extract is treated with water and sulphuric acid, an impure solution of the sulphate of veratria is obtained. Magnesia decomposes this, unites with the sulphuric and vegetable acids, and sets free the alkaloid, which is taken up by rectified spirit. The extract obtained by distilling off the spirit is then boiled in water with sulphuric acid and animal charcoal: the acid unites with the alkaloid, while the charcoal abstracts colouring matter. Ammonia being added to the strained solution, combines with the sulphuric acid, and occasions a precipitate, which, when dried, constitutes *commercial* or *medicinal veratria*. By Couerbe's process, a drachm of commercial veratria may, it is said, be procured from one pound of cebadilla.

Commercial veratria was said by Couerbe to be composed of *pure veratria, sabadillina, resin of veratria* (veratrin, *Couerbe*), and *gum-resin of veratria* (resinigomme, *Couerbe*). These are separated from each other by the successive action of water, ether, and alcohol, as shown by the following table :—

Commercial Veratria {
yields to boiling water ... {
1. *Sabadillina*, which crystallises on cooling.
2. *Resin of veratria*, left in the cold solution.

insoluble in boiling water {
3. *Veratria*, soluble in ether.
4. *Gum-resin of veratria*, insoluble in ether, but soluble in alcohol.

The nature of sabadillina has been already pointed out (p. 175).

Properties.—*Commercial veratria* is pulverulent, odourless, and brownish-white. All the samples I have tasted were bitter and acrid, and produced a feeling of numbness and tingling when applied to the tongue. But *pure veratria* is an almost white friable solid, having the aspect of a resin: it is uncrystallisable, odourless, has a very acrid taste, without any mixture of bitterness. It is fusible at 240° F. It is sparingly soluble in ether, readily so in alcohol, scarcely so in cold water. It possesses alkaline properties: thus it restores the blue colour of reddened litmus, and saturates acids. Its salts crystallise with difficulty: indeed, the *sulphate* and *hydrochlorate* alone have been obtained in the state of crystals.

Characteristics.—Veratria is known by the following characters:—Its alkalinity, its combustibility, its uncrystallisability, the difficult crystallisability of its salts, its solidity at ordinary temperatures, its ready solubility in alcohol, its being almost insoluble in water, and by the intense red colour which it assumes after some time when mixed with oil of vitriol. Pure veratria is readily soluble in ether; not so impure or commercial veratria. Nitric acid renders commercial veratria of a light-reddish colour, and forms ultimately a yellow solution with it (see *Morphia* and *Narcotina*). A solution of veratria in dilute acetic acid produces a whitish precipitate (*tannate of veratria*) with tincture of nutgalls, a white one (*hydrated veratria*) with ammonia, and an intense red colour with oil of vitriol. Carbazotic acid does not occasion a precipitate unless the solution be concentrated. [The following is the most convenient method of applying sulphuric acid as an aid to the detection of veratria :—Place a small quantity of the alkaloid on a glass slide, and add to it two or three drops of diluted sulphuric acid. Warm the glass by a spirit-lamp. The veratria is dissolved without change : but in a few minutes, by the slow evaporation of the water, the sulphuric acid begins to act, and a rich crimson colour is brought out, resembling that of murexid. If overheated, it is turned brown, and ultimately blackened. Concentrated sulphuric acid at first produces a yellowish-brown colour when added to veratria. By exposure to air, or by the addition of one or two drops of a solution of bichromate of potash, the mixture acquires a deep crimson-red colour. Some oxide of chrome is set free. The peroxide of lead produces a similar reaction. This can scarcely be regarded as a characteristic test for veratria, since gallic acid, essential oil of almonds, and other organic substances, produce a crimson-red colour when treated with sulphuric acid.—ED.] To these chemical peculiarities must be added those characteristics derived from its physiological effects :—A minute portion of veratria causes violent sneezing, and a small quantity of a solution of four grains of veratria in a fluidrachm of rectified spirit, rubbed on the wrist or forehead, produces, within three or four minutes, heat and tingling. Pure veratria is less apt to occasion sneezing, by handling, than the impure or commercial sort.

COMPOSITION.—The following is the composition of pure veratria, according to Couerbe :—

	Atoms.	Eq. Wt.	Per Cent.	Couerbe.
Carbon	34	204	70·83	70·786
Hydrogen	22	22	7·64	7·636
Nitrogen	1	14	4·86	5·210
Oxygen	6	48	16·67	16·368
Veratria	1	288	100·00	100·00

PHYSIOLOGICAL EFFECTS. *α. On Animals.*—Magendie[1] has shown that the local action of veratria is that of an irritant. Placed in the nostrils of a dog, the acetate of veratria provoked violent and continued sneezing. When introduced into the intestinal canal it caused inflammation. Applied to parts whence absorption goes on actively (as the pleura and tunica vaginalis), it occasions tetanus, and death in a few minutes. Forcke[2] gave moderate and

---

[1] *Formulaire*, p. 162, 8me édit.
[2] *Untersuch. über d. Veratrin*, 1837.

gradually increased doses ($\frac{1}{8}$ to $\frac{1}{4}$ of a grain) of veratria for twenty days. It caused vomiting, and occasionally foaming at the mouth. The stools continued hard. Dr. Bardsley[1] observed vomiting and giddiness (reeling) produced in animals to whom he gave veratria.

β. On Man.—Applied to the nose, a minute quantity excites excessive sneezing. Rubbed on the skin in the form of ointment, it causes a sensation of heat and tingling (called by Dr. Turnbull *electro-stimulation*). This effect is not confined to the part and its immediate neighbourhood where the application has been made, for somewhat similar sensations are occasionally experienced in distant parts. Taken internally, in *small* or *medicinal doses,* veratria excites a feeling of warmth in the stomach and bowels, which extends to the chest and extremities. Tingling and various anomalous sensations (as of a current of hot or cold air or water passing over the skin) are perceived in various parts of the body. Nausea and vomiting are occasionally excited by a full dose. On the secretions and exhalations its action is not very uniform. It frequently produces perspiration, and not unfrequently diuresis. Forcke[2] mentions increased secretion of saliva and of tears produced without the contact of the veratria either with the conjunctiva or mouth. The bowels are for the most part confined, so that purgatives are not unfrequently required during the use of it. Yet in some cases veratria has caused copious bilious evacuations. In some instances it has promoted, in others diminished, the appetite. Forcke mentions that a pustular eruption is sometimes induced by it. Dr. Bardsley generally found the pulse become slower and depressed after the use of veratria.

I am not acquainted with any cases of poisoning in the human subject by *excessive doses* of veratria. Vomiting and convulsions would probably be induced. [A case is recorded in the Pharm. Journ. vol. x. page 521, in which twenty-nine grains of veratria were swallowed in a liniment by mistake. The patient fortunately found medical aid at hand, and speedily rejected the poison by using emetics. The symptoms were a peculiar sense of oppression and anxiety in the head, and a sense of suffocation. In about half an hour after the rejection of the poison, violent sneezing occurred, and continued for an hour. The patient then slept, and woke perfectly well.

The late Mr. Callaway communicated to us the following case:—A physician prescribed for a female patient one grain of veratria, divided into fifty pills, and three of these were directed to be taken for a dose. Not long after the first dose had been swallowed, the patient was found insensible, the surface cold, the pulse failing, and there was every symptom of approaching dissolution. She remained some hours in a doubtful condition, but ultimately recovered. Supposing the pills to have been properly dispensed, not more than one-sixteenth of a grain of veratria was taken.—ED.]

USES.—Veratria is employed externally or internally,—sometimes in both ways at the same time. It has been tried in the following cases :—

α. In neuralgia it has been used by Dr. Turnbull, Dr. Ebers of Breslau,[3] and Dr. Forcke. It is applied in the form of ointment, containing from twenty to forty grains of veratria to an ounce of lard. The frictions are to be

---

[1] *Hosp. Facts and Observ.* 1829.
[2] *Op. cit.* p. 22.
[3] Dierbach, *Neuest. Entd. in d. Mat. Med.* 1837.

continued until the heat and tingling caused by the veratria have acquired a considerable degree of intensity. Though, according to my own experience, it fails to give relief in a large majority of cases, yet in some few its effects are highly beneficial, and in none is it injurious. As a remedy for neuralgia, it is, however, far inferior to *Aconitum* and its alkali *Aconitina*.

β. *In some nervous diseases* (Neuroses, *Cull.*)—Veratria has been extensively used in this class of diseases, but for the most part empirically. If it possess any therapeutical power, "a more extended experience is required to establish its claim to our regard."[1] Among the maladies against which it has been used (in some instances internally, but mostly externally) are,—nervous palpitation, paralysis, hooping-cough, epilepsy, hysteria, hypochondriasis, &c.[2]

γ. *In rheumatism and gout.*—Dr. Bardsley gave it internally in rheumatism, but with no remarkable results. More recently, however, M. Piédagnel[3] has found it serviceable in articular rheumatism. Externally it has been employed in the form of ointment by Sir C. Scudamore and Dr. Turnbull. It should not be applied while the inflammation is of an active kind. It would appear to be best adapted for the neuralgic forms of rheumatism.

δ. *In dropsy.*—Dr. Bardsley administered it internally in dropsy, but says it possesses "no *particular* claims to the attention of the profession." Ebers employed veratria endermically, and also, in the form of ointment, epidermically. It acted as a diuretic, and gave relief.[4]

ADMINISTRATION.—The ordinary veratria of the shops is administered in doses of one-sixth of a grain three times a day. On account of its acridity it should not be given in solution, but in the form of pills.

α. *Pilulæ Veratriæ ; Veratria Pills ;* Turnbull.—Veratria, gr. j. ; Extract of Hyoscyamus ; Liquorice Powder, aa. gr. xij. Let 12 pills be made, of which one may be taken every three hours.

β. *Tinctura Veratriæ ; Veratria Embrocation ;* Turnbull. — Veratria, ʒj. ; Rectified Spirit, ʒij. Dissolve. This embrocation is sometimes used as a substitute for the ointment. Magendie (*Formulaire*) directs a tincture of veratria to be prepared by dissolving four grains of the alkali in an ounce of alcohol. Of this from 10 to 25 drops are taken, in a cup of broth, as a substitute for the tincture of colchicum.

γ. *Unguentum Veratriæ ; Veratria Ointment ;* Turnbull.—Veratria, ʒss. ; Olive Oil, ʒj. ; Prepared Lard, ʒj. M.

δ. *Sales Veratriæ.*—The *sulphate* and *tartrate of veratria* (prepared by saturating veratria with sulphuric or tartaric acid) are sometimes used instead of the uncombined alkali. The dose and mode of administration are the same as for the latter.

ANTIDOTE.—*Vide* VERATRUM ALBUM.

ORDER XI. LILIACEÆ, *Lindl.*—LILYWORTS.

CHARACTERS.—*Calyx* and *corolla* both alike, coloured, regular, occasionally cohering in a tube. *Stamens* 6, inserted into the sepals and petals ; *anthers* opening inwards. *Ovary* superior, 3-celled, many-seeded ; *style* 1 ; *stigma* simple or 3-lobed. *Fruit* succulent, or dry and capsular, 3-celled. *Seeds* packed one upon another in one or two rows ; *embryo*

---

[1] Paris, *Appendix* to the 8th edit. of the *Pharmacologia*.
[2] See the treatises of Turnbull and Forcke, before referred to.
[3] *Annuaire de Thérapeutique*, 1853.
[4] See Forcke, *op. supra cit.*

with the same direction as the seed, in the axis of fleshy *albumen*, or uncertain in direction and position, occasionally very minute.—*Herbaceous* plants, shrubs or trees, with bulbs, or tubers, or rhizomes, or fibrous roots. *Leaves* narrow, with parallel veins, membranous, not articulated with the stem; either sessile or with a narrow leafy petiole.

PROPERTIES.—Not uniform. Mucilage, resinous matters, acrid volatile oils, and acrid extractive substances, are the organic principles to which the medicinal qualities of this order are chiefly referable. Their relative proportions, however, vary considerably in different species. The fleshy bulbs are usually more or less acrid. Those of the genus *Allium* owe their acridity to a volatile oil (*sulphuret of allyle*) whose composition is C^6H^5,S (see Vol. i. p. 225). Bundles of acicular crystals or *raphides;* usually considered to be phosphate, but by Schleiden declared to be oxalate of lime, are found in some of the cells of these bulbs.

61. ALOË, *Linn.*—ALOE.

Sex. Syst. Hexandria, Monogynia.
(Succusproprius spissatus foliorum ex variis Aloës speciebus.)

HISTORY.—Neither aloe plants nor the inspissated juice of their leaves are mentioned by Hippocrates or Theophrastus; but both are described by Dioscorides[1] and Pliny.[2]

BOTANY. **Gen. Char.**—*Perianth* tubular, 6-cleft, fleshy, nectariferous at the base, the sepals of the same form as the petals, and closely imbricating them. *Stamens* hypogynous, as long as the perianth, or even longer. *Capsule* membranous, scarious, 3-corned, 3-celled, 3-valved, with a loculicidal dehiscence. *Seeds* numerous, in 2 rows, roundish or angular (*Lindley*).—Succulent plants.

Species.—The following species furnish the greater part of the substance called in the shops *aloes :*—

1. ALOË VULGARIS, Lam. D.; *Aloë perfoliata* π *vera*, Linn.; *A. barbadensis*, Miller, Haworth, ’Αλόη, Dioscor., Sibth.—*Stem* woody, simple, cylindrical, short. *Leaves* fleshy, amplexicaul, first spreading, then ascending, lanceolate, glaucous, green, flat above, convex below, armed with hard, distant, reddish spines, perpendicular to the margin; a little mottled with darker colour; the parenchyma slightly coloured brown, and very distinct from the tough leathery cuticle. *Scape* axillary, glaucous reddish, branched. *Spike* cylindrical-ovate. *Flowers* at first erect, then spreading, afterwards pendulous, yellow, not larger than the stamens (*Lindley*).—East Indies, Barbary, Spain, Italy, Sicily, Malta, Greece, West Indies.

Specimens of this species are frequently brought to London from the West Indies by sailors, a tarred cloth being closely tied around the truncated stem, to prevent the escape of the juices of the plant. If suspended by a cord from the ceiling of a room, they continue to live for a considerable time, and throw out fresh leaves. I have had one in my possession for nearly two years, and it is still living and growing.

This species yields *Barbadoes aloes*. The brownish-yellow, bitter, resinous juice which by inspissation forms aloes, is contained in parallel greenish vessels beneath the epidermis of the leaves.

2. A. ABYSSINICA, Lam. is by some writers considered to be a variety of *A. vulgaris*. By Kunth it is regarded as a distinct species. Its flowers are greenish-yellow. It is a

---

[1] Lib. iii. cap. xxv.
[2] *Hist. Nat.* lib. xxvii. cap. v.

larger and more resinous species than the preceding, and was brought from Africa by Bruce. It may, perhaps, yield a portion of the aloes of commerce. It contains a very bitter juice, which becomes brown in the air.

3. ALOË SOCOTRINA, Lam., De Cand.—*Stem* woody, straight, one and a half feet high or more, naked below, where it is strongly marked with the scars of leaves. *Leaves* amplexicaul, ascending, ensiform, green, curved inwards at the point, convex below, rather concave above, marked with numerous small white marginal serratures, the parenchyma abounding in a bright brownish-yellow juice. *Raceme* cylindrical, unbranched. *Flowers* scarlet at the base, pale in the middle, green at the point. *Stamens* unequal, three of them longer than the flowers (*Lindley*).—Socotra ; also, according to Nees von Esenbeck, Cape of Good Hope.

FIG. 80.

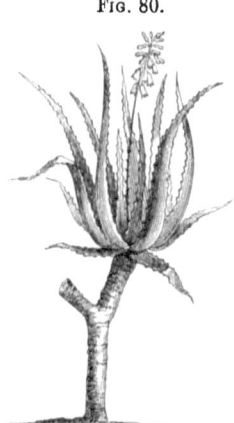

Aloë socotrina.

Lieut. Wellstead[1] says that the hills on the west side of Socotra are covered for an extent of miles with aloe plants ; and he observes that it is not likely, at any future period, that the whole quantity will be collected which might be required.

It is said to yield *socotrine* (and *real hepatic ?*) *aloes.*—Under the epidermis of the leaves are parallel greenish vessels containing the bitter resinous juice, as in the last-mentioned species. By drying, the leaves of *A. socotrina* (like those of *A. purpurascens*, but unlike those of *A. vulgaris*) acquire a purplish-red colour, which commences first in the parallel vessels, and is probably produced by the oxidation of the resinous juice contained in these vessels.

4. A. PURPURASCENS, Haworth.—This species has dark red flowers and glaucous leaves, which become purplish-red when drying. It has the same localities as the last-mentioned species. Its juice is very bitter and resinous, and becomes blood-red in the air.

5. ALOË SPICATA, Thunb., L. D.—*Stem* 3 to 4 feet high, as thick as a man's arm. *Leaves* thick, fleshy, broad at the base, gradually narrowing to the point, channelled, full 2 feet long, distantly toothed, with a few white spots ; their parenchyma almost colourless. *Spike* a foot long, very compact, with the flowers campanulate and horizontal. The three petals broader, ovate, obtuse, white, with a triple green line, the sepals narrower, less concave. *Stamens* much longer than the perianth. The flowers are filled with a purplish honey (*Lindley*). This species is a native of the interior of the Cape of Good Hope, and contributes to yield *Cape aloes.* Thunberg[2] states that it yields the best hepatic aloes ("succus Aloës hepaticus purus et optimus").

OTHER SPECIES.—It is probable that several other species contribute to the supply of the aloes of commerce. I have received four species from Mr. Dunsterville, of Algoa Bay, who writes that from all of them, as well as from other species, the so-called Cape aloes is obtained. Thunberg[3] states that *A. perfoliata* yields a large quantity of aloes at the Cape ; and he also says[4] that *A. linguæformis*, Linn. yields the best and purest sort.

---

[1] *Journal of the Royal Geographical Society*, vol. v.
[2] *Dissertatio Botanico-medica de Aloë*, 1785.
[3] *Ibid.* p. 10.
[4] *Ibid.* p. 7.

Dr. Christison[1] suggests that *A. Commelini* of Willdenow may yield some. He was informed by Mr. John Lyell, that at Swellenden and George (South Africa), aloes is obtained from *A. spicata, A. Africana* of Haworth, and varieties of these crossed with *A. ferox.* The last-mentioned species is now cultivated in Barbados, according to Schomburgk.[2]

In Arabia, Forskäl[3] found *A. officinalis* (*A. rubescens* of De Candolle ?), whose juice had the odour of the officinal socotrine aloes. Its flowers were red.

In India there is also a species with reddish flowers, which Dr. Royle[4] has called *A. Indica.* This, if known to Roxburgh, was probably included by him in *A. perfoliata.*

Nees von Esenbeck mentions the following species as being rich in a bitter resinous juice:—*A. humilis,* Lam.; *A. ferra,* De Cand.; *A. ferox,* Lam.; and *A. subferox,* Spreng. He also found that the following were feebly bitter, but in different degrees:—*A. glauca,* Mill.; *A. paniculata,* Jacq.; *A. saponaria,* Haw.; *A. cæsia,* S. D.; *A. plicatilis,* Mill.; *A. arborescens,* Mill.; and *A. frutescens,* S. D. He says that *A. glauca,* Mill. was also slightly bitter, but that the juice became dark brown in the air, which shows that this colouring matter is a peculiar principle originally different from the bitter matter.

[Dr. Pappe, in his *Floræ Capensis Medicæ Prodromus,* says that the *A. ferox* yields the best aloes at the Cape, and that, though the *A. Africana* yields a quality nearly as good, its juice is not so bitter nor so powerful a drastic as that of *A. ferox.* The *A. plicatilis,* he states, supplies most of the aloes used by the colonists: it is a milder purgative, and more like the Barbados aloes.—ED.]

PREPARATION.—The finest kind of aloes is obtained by evaporating the juice which flows spontaneously from the transversely-cut leaves. This juice is lodged in vessels running longitudinally beneath the epidermis. The exudation of it is promoted by gravity, by dipping the leaves in hot water, and by making fresh sections of the leaves. But if pressure be employed the proper aloetic juice becomes mixed with the mucilaginous liquid of the leaves, and thus an inferior kind of aloes is obtained. A still commoner variety is procured by boiling the leaves, from which the juice has been previously allowed to escape, in water.

a. Of Socotrine Aloes.—In the Island of Socotra the leaves are plucked at any period, and by anyone who chooses to take the trouble; and after being placed in a skin, the juice is allowed to exude from them.[5] The following mode of preparing Socotrine aloes, as related by Hermann, was communicated to Ray by Dr. Palmer :[6]—" When the leaves which have been pulled from the roots are gently compressed by the hand or an instrument, the juice drops from them into a receiving vessel ; and being allowed to stand during a night, deposits the grosser parts. The next day it is transferred to another vessel, in which it is exposed to the sun that it may harden and become dry, when it acquires a brownish-yellow colour."

β. Of Barbados Aloes.—In Barbados, the aloes is best procured in the month of March. It is obtained as follows :—" Every slave hath by him three or four portable tubs. The leaves being cut near the roots, are thrown into these with their broken ends downwards ; and as the leaves are full of large longitudinal veins or vessels, they yield an easy passage to the juice (which is of a greenish-yellow colour) to drip out. This being boiled for about five hours in a copper or kettle, the watery particles evaporate, and the

---

[1] *Dispensatory,* 2d edit.
[2] *Hist. of Barbados,* p. 590.
[3] *Flora Ægyptiaco-Arabica,* p. 73, 1775.
[4] *Illust. of the Botany of the Himalayan Mountains.*
[5] Wellstead, *op. citato.*
[6] Dale, *Pharmacologia.*

remainder comes to a consistency and thickening as sugar doth when sufficiently boiled. The way to know when it is enough boiled is to dip a stick in the liquor, and observe whether the aloe sticking to it, when cold, breaks short : if it doth, then it is boiled to perfection, and fit to be poured into gourds or calabashes, or other vessels, for use."[1]

Dr. Wright[2] says that in Jamaica the leaves contained in hand-baskets or nets are boiled in water, and the strained liquor evaporated to a proper consistence, and then poured into gourds or calabashes. Dr. Patrick Browne,[3] on the other hand, states that the sun-dried juice is called *Socotrine aloes ;* but the common aloes, he adds, is obtained by squeezing out the juice by the hand, adding water to it, and boiling down to a proper consistence.

γ. *Of Cape Aloes.*—The method of preparing aloes followed at the Cape of Good Hope has been described by Thunberg,[4] Lieut. Moody,[5] and others.[6]

Mr. George Dunsterville, surgeon of Algoa Bay, and formerly one of my pupils, has furnished me with the following information respecting the manufacture of Cape aloes :—" A shallow pit is dug, in which is spread a bullock's hide or sheep's skin. The leaves of the aloe plants in the immediate vicinity of this pit are stripped off, and piled up on the skin to variable heights. These are left for a few days. The juice exudes from the leaves, and is received by the skin beneath. The Hottentot then collects in a bucket or other convenient article the produce of many heaps, which is then put in an iron pot capable of holding 18 or 20 gallons. Fire is applied to effect evaporation, during which the contents of the pot are constantly stirred to prevent burning. The cooled liquor is then poured into wooden cases of about three feet square by one foot deep, or into goat or sheep skins, and is thus fitted for the market. In the colony, aloes realises about $2\frac{1}{4}$d. to $3\frac{1}{2}$d. per lb." Mr. Dunsterville also informs me that the Hottentots and Dutch boors employ indiscriminately different species of Aloë in the preparation of Cape aloes. He adds, that " the Cape aloes which is usually prized the highest in the English market, is that made at the Missionary Institution of Bethelsdorp (a small village about nine miles from Algoa Bay, and chiefly inhabited by Hottentots and their missionary teachers). Hence it is called *Bethelsdorp Aloes.* Its superiority arises, not from the employment of any particular species of Aloë, for all species are indiscriminately used ; but from the greater care and attention paid to what is technically called ' the cooking of the aloes,' that is, to the evaporation, and to the absence of all adulterating substances (fragments of limestone, sand, earth, &c.) often introduced by manufacturers."

DESCRIPTION AND VARIETIES.—I am acquainted with seven commercial varieties of aloes ; namely, *Socotrine, Hepatic, Barbados, Cape, Mocha, Caballine,* and *Indian.* To these must be added *Curacoa Aloes.*

---

[1] Hughes, *Natural History of Barbados,* p. 154, 1750. This account is further confirmed by that of Mr. Millington, *Lond. Med. Journ.* vol. viii. p. 422. But Dr. Christison states, the Barbados aloes of the present day is the extract of a decoction.

[2] *Lond. Med. Journ.* vol. viii. p. 219.

[3] *History of Jamaica,* p. 198, 1789.

[4] *Travels in Europe, Asia, and Africa, between the Years* 1770 *and* 1799, vol. ii. p. 49.

[5] *Ten Years in South Africa,* vol. ii p. 2, 1835.

[6] *Four Months in Cape Colony,* in Chambers's *Miscellany of Useful and Entertaining Tracts,* vol. xx. No. 173, Edinb. 1847 ; also Mr. John Lyell in Christison's *Dispensatory,* 2d ed.

The terms socotrine, hepatic, and caballine, have been used to indicate rather the quality and purity, than the origin, of aloes. Thus Thunberg[1] says, "Pro diversa puritate potius quam quidem sua origine, triplicem imprimis Aloës speciem in Pharmacopolis nostris introductam invenimus, scilicet *socotrinam, hepaticam*, et *caballinam*." And Jussieu[2] states that he saw all three varieties prepared at Morviedro, in Spain, from the Aloë vulgaris. The term *Aloë lucida*, or *clear aloes*, has been applied by Schröder,[3] Geoffroy,[4] Fée,[5] and others, to a clear or transparent aloes supposed to be formed by the concretion of the juice on the leaves after they have been incised. It is probable that by this term is meant the clearest and most transparent pieces of socotrine aloes. I have never met with, in English commerce, any aloes by this name; and a similar remark has been made by Alston.[6]

1. Socotrine Aloes (*Aloë socotrina ; Aloë socotorina* and *Aloë Indica*, E.[7])—A few years ago this kind of aloes was brought by way of Smyrna, and hence was frequently termed *Turkey aloes*. But since the expiration of the charter of the East India Company, it is usually brought by way of Bombay. [According to Dr. X. Landerer, much of the aloes employed in the East is produced in Arabia. The drug is rudely manufactured by the Arabs, and then carried to the bazaars of Alexandria, Smyrna, Cairo, &c.[8]—Ed.] Socotrine aloes is the kind sold at Apothecaries' Hall, London, and at other places, under the name of *extract of spiked aloes* (*extractum aloës spicatum*), although there is no evidence of its being obtained from Aloë spicata. It comes over in skins[9] contained in casks (holding from 11 to 15 cwt. each), kegs, and chests. Its consistence and colour are subject to considerable variation. The exterior portion of each skinful is usually hard, but the internal portion is frequently soft, or even semiliquid.

The hardened portions vary in colour in different parts of the same mass; sometimes they are garnet-red, at other times much paler, and when quite dry are golden-red, and yield a golden-yellow powder. By exposure to the air the colour is deepened. The fracture of fine selected pieces is smooth, glassy, and conchoidal; but socotrine aloes of excellent quality often breaks with a roughish fracture. The finest kind of socotrine which I have met with had the semitransparent red colour observed when we break a fine tear of myrrh. Thin films of pure and hardened socotrine aloes are usually translucent or nearly transparent. The fragments, which have a ruby colour, are called *aloë socotrina vera*. The odour of fresh-broken pieces (especially when breathed on) is very fragrant, and is much stronger in recent and soft specimens. The same agreeable odour is obtained by heating the aloes on a point of a knife in a candle. By distillation with water we obtain a liquid having the same odour, but free from any bitter taste. When fresh, socotrine aloes possesses considerable acidity, and the late Mr. Hennell informed me that in the preparation of the compound extract of colocynth he had fre-

---

[1] *Dissertatio Botanico-medica de Aloë*, 1785.
[2] *Elements of Chemistry*, by M. J. A. Chaptal, vol. iii. p. 86, 1791.
[3] *The Compleat Chymical Dispensatory*, p. 500, 1669.
[4] *Tractatus de Materia Medica*, t. ii. p. 649, 1741.
[5] *Cours d'Hist. Nat. Pharm.* t. i. p. 327, 1828.
[6] *Lectures on the Materia Medica*, vol. ii. p. 422, 1770.
[7] I have received from Dr. D. Maclagan, Lecturer on Materia Medica in Edinburgh, two specimens of aloes,—one marked "*True Socotrine Aloes garnet red in their fragments;*" the other "*Aloes given to me as True Socotrine, rough fracture nearly garnet red in thin fragments. Included under Aloë Indica*, Ed. Pharm." Both kinds are socotrine aloes.
[8] [*Pharm. Trans.* vol. xi. p. 300.]
[9] I am informed that they are the skins of the gazelle.

quently observed the fatty acid of the soap set free by the acid of the socotrine aloes. I have been shown samples of what was declared to be socotrine aloes, which was soft or semiliquid, and had a bright or palm-oil yellow
colour, and a very fragrant odour (see page 188).

When a package of socotrine aloes arrives at a druggist's warehouse, it is
usually garbled or sorted. The finest, clear, and hard pieces are separated
for sale. The soft portions are placed upon slabs or in shallow tin trays, or
other vessels, and exposed to a very gentle heat to harden them (*hardened
socotrine aloes*), and at the same time to preserve the favourite colour of this
kind of aloes. Mr. Whipple, who has had great experience in these matters,
informs me that " the loss would be frightful, if, after selecting or separating
the clean aloes, the skins were not washed and the aloes obtained by subsequent evaporation."

" It is brittle, bitter, of a reddish-brown colour and aromatic odour : translucent when
in fresh thin laminæ."—*Ph. L.*

In the Edinburgh Pharmacopœia the following characters are assigned to
the *Aloë socotrina* :—

"In thin pieces, translucent, and garnet red; almost entirely soluble in spirit of the
strength of sherry. *Very rare.*"

But socotrine aloes, as imported, is not " *in thin pieces ;*" this character
being given to it in the garbling process, or by drying the soft portions in
thin layers, as above mentioned. *Translucency* and a *garnet-red* colour are
qualities not possessed by many fine specimens of socotrine aloes. The
alcoholic strength of sherry is subject to variation, and, therefore, the
statement of the College as to the solubility of socotrine aloes is not very
definite. Lastly, as to socotrine aloes being *very rare*, I may observe that
the late Mr. Hennell, of Apothecaries' Hall, informed me (Dec. 21, 1841)
that he would be happy to take an order for 500 lbs. of it. The impure and
dirty pieces of socotrine aloes are sometimes melted and strained (*strained
socotrine aloes*), by which the colour and odour are impaired, and the other
qualities somewhat altered.

Socotrine aloes has long been regarded as the best kind of aloes, though
its commercial value is now below that of Barbados aloes. It is, I suspect,
inferior in activity. Socotrine aloes is mentioned by Avicenna and Mesue,
both of whom regarded it as the best kind. By Fée,[1] and some other continental writers, it is confounded with Cape aloes.

The aloes prepared in the Island of Socotra is probably procured from *Aloë
socotrina*, and perhaps also *A. purpurascens*. In 1833, the quantity exported from this island was 83 skins, or 2 tons. But a much larger quantity
might be procured if required.[2] Two samples (one of which I have in my
museum) brought direct from the island of Socotra by a friend of Professor
Royle, are largely intermixed with foreign substances, as sand, skins, &c.

Sir Whitelaw Ainslie[3] says that the greater part of the extract now sold
under the name of socotrine aloes is prepared in the kingdom of Melinda ;
and I am informed by an eminent drug-merchant, that both socotrine and
hepatic aloes have been imported into London directly from Zanzibar.

---

[1] *Cours d'Hist. Nat. Pharm.* t. i. p. 325.
[2] Wellstead, *Journ. Geograph. Soc.* vol. v.
[3] *Materia Indica*, vol. i. p. 9.

[The author published an interesting paper on the subject of the socotrine aloe, in the 11th volume of the *Pharmaceutical Journal;* and as the communication is replete with chemical, pharmaceutical, and commercial interest, we shall print it *in extenso.*—ED.]

It has long been known that the Socotrine aloes imported into England varies considerably in its consistency, and is sometimes met with in a soft or semifluid state. Frequently, on opening a package of this sort of aloes the interior is found to be quite soft, while the exterior is firm and hard. In general this arises from insufficient evaporation of the aloe juice.

In the third edition of my *Elements of Materia Medica,*[1] published in 1850, I have briefly referred to a soft or semiliquid Socotrine aloes, which had a bright or palm-oil yellow colour, and a very fragrant odour. At that time I had but little opportunity of investigating this very interesting drug; but a large importation of it having recently taken place, I have more fully examined it; and as it appears to me to be the raw or unboiled juice of the plant yielding what is known in commerce as Socotrine aloes, I propose to distinguish it from the ordinary soft Socotrine aloes by the name of "*Socotrine Aloe Juice.*"

Messrs. Horner, the holders of the whole of the present importation of this juice, inform me that it was purchased of the Arabs up the Red Sea by a merchant who was assured by the vendors that it was very fine aloe juice, and had not been boiled or otherwise altered. It was imported into London by way of Madras, in casks each containing six cwt. I am informed that the contents of some of the packages have undergone decomposition during the voyage.

Its consistence is that of treacle or very thin honey; its colour deep orange or palm-oil yellow; its odour powerful, fragrant, and resembling that of fine Socotrine aloes. By standing it separates into two parts,—an inferior, paler-coloured, opaque, finely granular portion, and a superior, darker-coloured, transparent liquid. The latter forms, however, a very small portion of the whole mass.

When the granular portion is submitted to microscopic examination, it is found that the opacity and granular appearance arise from myriads of beautiful prismatic crystals. If a temperature of 132° F. be applied to the juice, these crystals melt or dissolve, and the juice becomes deep red and transparent; and when the liquid becomes cold it retains its transparency, and does not deposit any crystals. By evaporation the juice yields a solid, transparent extract, having all the characters of fine Socotrine aloes, in which no trace of crystalline texture can be discovered. Mr. Jacob Bell has ascertained that 14lbs. of the juice yield 8lbs. 12ozs. of solid extract, or $62\frac{1}{2}$ per cent. When the juice is mixed with cold distilled water, it becomes opaque yellow, and renders the water turbid, but is not miscible with it. If, however, heat be applied, the juice dissolves in the water, forming an almost clear rich red liquid. As the solution cools, it at first becomes turbid, owing to the separation of an opaque yellow precipitate, which, apparently, is the crystalline principle in an amorphous form. This gradually separates from the liquid and collects as a clear resiniform mass (commonly called the *resin* of aloes) at the bottom of the vessel, leaving the supernatant liquid tolerably clear. If the juice be shaken up with rectified spirit of wine an uniform clear mixture is obtained, from which numerous yellow crystals rapidly fall to the bottom of the liquid. Similar results are obtained when we mix the juice with equal parts of rectified spirit of wine and water.

This crystalline constituent of Socotrine aloes is, doubtless, either the *aloin* described by Messrs. T. and H. Smith, of Edinburgh, and by Dr. Stenhouse, or a principle closely allied to it. Dr. Stenhouse, to whom I have given a sample of it, is now engaged in its investigation; and in a letter which I have received from him, he says, that though he has not been able to get the aloin ready for analysis, yet, from the experiments he has already made with it, he has scarcely a doubt that it will be found identical with that formerly obtained from Barbados aloes. It forms, he adds, a precisely similar combination with bromine, and, in short, agrees with it in every particular; I shall, therefore, provisionally term this crystalline principle the *aloin of Socotrine aloes*. On comparing it with a fine specimen of aloin kindly presented to me by Messrs. Smith, I find its crystals smaller and more tapering, the summits of the crystals being more acute.

---

[1] Vol. ii. part i. p. 1077 (page 187 of present volume).

In drying, the crystals of the Socotrine aloin have a strong tendency to break up; so that crystals which in the moist state are moderately large and regular, become small and pulverulent when dry. Like the aloin crystals of Messrs. Smith, the aloin crystals of Socotrine aloes strongly double refract and depolarise light, and are, therefore, beautiful objects when viewed by the polarising microscope.

FIG. 81.   FIG. 82.

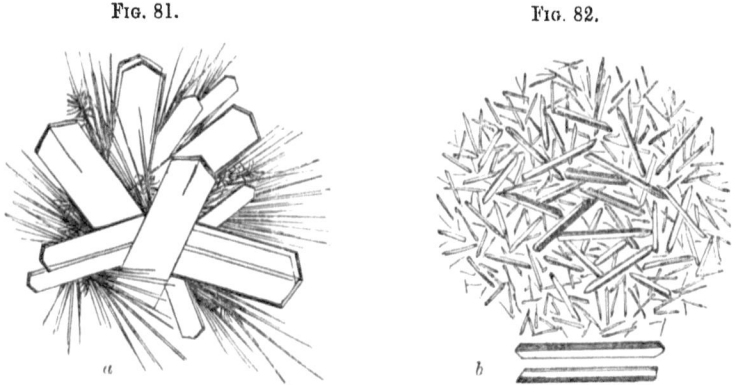

Microscopic Appearances of Crystals of Aloin.

a. Aloin prepared by Messrs. Smith.   *b.* Aloin contained in Socotrine aloe juice.
(The magnifying power used was the same in both cases.)

The crystals of aloin contained in Socotrine aloe juice cannot be confounded with the crystals of oxalate and phosphate of lime found in the juices of various plants, and which are called by botanists *raphides.* The appearance under the microscope of the former is very different from that of the latter. Moreover, the ready fusibility, solubility, and complete combustibility of aloin crystals easily distinguish them from the calcareous salts just referred to. On platinum foil the aloin burns without leaving any residue, except such as may arise from the presence of traces of some foreign matter.

Aloin may be readily obtained from the juice by mixing the latter with spirit (either rectified or proof), and collecting and drying the precipitate. When procured in this way it appears to the naked eye like a yellow powder; but when examined by the microscope it is found to consist of minute fragments of crystals.

The tincture from which the aloin has been separated, yields by distillation a spirit having the fragrant odour of the juice; showing that the latter contains some volatile odorous principle. By evaporation the tincture yields a resiniform extract.

In the first edition of my *Elements of Materia Medica,* published in 1840, I have stated, that by digesting hepatic aloes in rectified spirit of wine, a yellowish granular powder is obtained, which is insoluble in [cold] water, alcohol, ether, and dilute sulphuric acid, but is readily soluble in a solution of caustic potash, forming a red-coloured liquid. The powder-like residue here referred to is identical with the aloin of Socotrine aloes. When examined by the microscope, it is perceived to consist of very minute prismatic crystals, which depolarise polarised light like the larger crystals of aloin above referred to. I think, therefore, that it may be safely inferred that hepatic aloes has been prepared without the employment of artificial heat, and that its opacity is due to the presence of minute crystals of aloin.

When Socotrine aloes is digested in rectified spirit, an insoluble portion is also obtained; but its colour, instead of being yellow, as in hepatic aloes, is dark brown. On submitting this dark brown insoluble portion to microscopic examination, I find that it contains depolarising crystals.

Artificial Socotrine aloes (prepared by evaporating this aloe juice) also yields, when digested in rectified spirit, a dark brown insoluble portion.

I think, therefore, that Socotrine aloes differs from hepatic aloes in the circumstance of its having been prepared by the aid of artificial heat, by which its aloin constituent has become altered. This inference is further substantiated by the fact that after it has been melted hepatic aloes is found to have acquired the clearness and transparency of the Socotrine sort.

The clear supernatant portion of aloe juice, from which the above crystals have subsided, would probably also yield, by spontaneous evaporation, an extract resembling, or identical with, Socotrine aloes.

That Socotrine and hepatic aloes were obtained from the same plant, and were not different species of aloes, I have long suspected; and in the first edition of my work on Materia Medica, published in 1840, I have observed that "the similarity of the odour of Socotrine and hepatic aloes leads to the suspicion that they are obtained from the same plant; and which is further confirmed by the two being sometimes brought over intermixed, the Socotrine occasionally forming a vein in a cask of the hepatic aloes."

This intermixture of the two sorts of aloes in the same cask might be explained by supposing that the consolidation of the clear portion of the juice has produced the so-called Socotrine aloes; while the opaque aloin, containing no portion of juice, has yielded what is termed hepatic aloes.

In the third edition of my work above alluded to, I have stated that the name of *opaque liver-coloured Socotrine aloes* might with propriety be applied to hepatic aloes. But until the present time I have been unable to offer a plausible explanation of the cause of the difference in these two commercial kinds of aloes.

From the preceding remarks I think we may infer :—

1. That *aloin* pre-exists in a crystalline form in the juice of Socotrine aloes.

2. That the substance which deposits as a decoction of Socotrine aloes cools, and which is usually termed the *resin* or the *resinoid* of Socotrine aloes, is the aloin in a modified state.

3. That hepatic aloes[1] is the juice of the Socotrine aloes plant which has been solidified without the aid of artificial heat.

4. That hepatic aloes owes its opacity to the presence of minute crystals of aloin.

5. That the juice of Socotrine aloes yields, when evaporated by artificial heat, an extract possessing all the properties of commercial Socotrine aloes.

2. Genuine Hepatic Aloes; *Liver-coloured Socotrine Aloes (Aloë hepatica vera ; ? Aloë Indica,* E.)[2]— Aloes under this commercial name usually comes to London from Bombay (hence it is sometimes called *Bombay* or *East India Aloes*) in skins, contained in casks holding from 200 to 300 pounds,[3] or in kegs. Its odour is very much the same as that of the socotrine kind, or perhaps it is a little less fragrant. It is distinguished from the latter by its opacity and its liver colour, but comes almost certainly from the same plant (vide *supra*).

[" Opake, of a liver colour, bitter taste, and unpleasant odour."—*Ph. L.*]

3. Barbados Aloes; *Aloes in gourds (Aloë barbadensis,* Ph. Ed.)—This is the kind denominated by most continental writers (as Geiger, Theod. Martius, Pfaff, Fée, and others) *hepatic aloes (aloë hepatica),* but its colour is not constantly that of the liver. It is imported from Barbados or Jamaica usually in gourds (*Lagenaria vulgaris*), weighing from 60 to 70 pounds, or even more than this; and sometimes in cases or boxes holding 56 lbs. each. The hole in the gourd-shell is partially closed by a piece of gourd let in and covered by a portion of coarse cloth, which is nailed down over the aperture.

---

[1] By the term " *hepatic aloes*" I mean the opaque liver-coloured aloes imported into England from the East Indies (usually from Bombay). This sort of aloes is very different from the *hepatic Barbados aloes,* which formerly appears to have been exclusively called " hepatic aloes."

[2] I suspect hepatic aloes is included by the Edinburgh College under "*Aloë Indica;*" for in preparing Decoction of Aloes the College orders Socotrine or Hepatic Aloes, though the term hepatic does not occur in the list of Materia Medica.

[3] Mr. Whipple informs me that it is " received in packages varying from 56 lbs. to 12 cwt. casks, most commonly in firkins. Lately it has come over in boxes lined with tin, and holding about 56 lbs. All of these, except the last, contain the skin packages."

The finest Barbados aloes is the inspissated juice, which I have heard called by an inhabitant of the island *cold drawn Barbados aloes,* to distinguish it from the extract of the decoction, which is of inferior quality. Barbados aloes varies in colour from a dark brown or black (*brown* or *black Barbados aloes*) to a reddish-brown or liver colour (*liver-coloured* or *hepatic Barbados aloes*) : even in the same gourd a difference of colour is occasionally observed. The fracture also varies, sometimes being dull, at other times glossy, or even resinous. Its unpleasant odour (which is much increased by breathing on it) will always distinguish it from the foregoing kinds. Its powder is of a dull olive-yellow colour. This kind of aloes is obtained chiefly, if not exclusively, from the *Aloë vulgaris*.[1]

["Opake dull, of a liver colour, afterwards becoming blackish; of a nauseous bitter taste, and a very unpleasant odour."—*Ph. L.*]

The quantity of aloes annually exported from Barbados is stated by Sir R. H. Schomburgk (op. cit. pp. 149, 150, and 160) to be as follows :—

1740 to 1748 } average annually	327 gourds.
1792	515 gourds.
1841	1361 gourds.
1842	2956 gourds, 1 case, 1 package.
1843	4227 gourds, 8 puncheons, 27 boxes.
1844	2371 gourds, 2173 packages, and 78 boxes.
1845	1958 packages.

4. Cape Aloes (*Aloë capensis ; A. lucida* of Geiger).—This kind is imported, as its name indicates, from the Cape of Good Hope. It is brought over in chests and skins, the latter being preferred, as the aloes contained therein are usually purer and more glossy. It has a shining resinous appearance, is of a deep brown colour, with a greenish tint, and has a glossy or resinous fracture; its edges, or thin laminæ, viewed by transmitted light, have a yellowish-red or ruby colour ; its odour is stronger and more disagreeable than the Barbados aloes ; its powder is greenish-yellow. Some of the commoner kinds of Cape aloes have a rough fracture. The finest kind of Cape aloes is called *Bethelsdorp aloes* [which is imported from Algoa Bay, is more red and more transparent than that which is imported from Cape Town, but more liable to get soft, on account of its being less boiled.—ED.] Occasionally it has been imported of a reddish-brown colour, like that of the liver, and opaque (*liver-coloured* or *hepatic Cape aloes*). Some years since an experienced dealer bartered 3 lbs. of Cape aloes for 1 lb. of what he thought to be the genuine hepatic aloes, but which turned out to be a fine sort of Cape aloes. I presume this is the kind which Professor Guibourt,[2] to whom I sent a specimen of it, formerly termed *false hepatic aloes ;* and which more recently[3] he calls *opaque Cape aloes.* Its odour when breathed on instantly detects it.

---

[1] Dr. Maycock (*Flora Barbadensis,* 1830) notices no other species of Aloë indigenous, naturalised, or cultivated in Barbados. But Dr. Christison observes, that though at one time Barbados aloes was made only from A. vulgaris, he is assured by various pupils from that island, that, while this species is commonly used, others are likewise employed. Sir R. H. Schomburgk (*History of Barbados,* p. 590, 1847) mentions *A. ferox,* Lam., or Great Hedge-hog Aloe, as having been introduced from the Cape of Good Hope. Kunth (*Enum. Plant.*) says, but I know not on what authority, that A. socotrina is cultivated at Barbados.

[2] *Hist. des Drog. simpl.* 3me édit. t. ii. p. 418.

[3] *Ibid.* 4me édit. p. 168.

I have received four species of *Aloë* plants from Mr. Dunsterville, of Algoa Bay, and the four extracts which he was informed were obtained respectively from the species sent. Two of the plants were dead and rotten; and the others were unknown to the late Mr. Anderson, of the Chelsea Gardens. The four extracts are as follows:—

a. Ordinary Cape Aloes.—Dark, glossy, very resinous, with a strong disagreeable odour and greenish tint.

β. Socotrine Cape Aloes.—This in colour resembled socotrine aloes; but it was more glossy, brittle, and transparent. Its odour, though disagreeable, was less so than the first kind.

γ. Hepatic Cape Aloes.—This is an intermixture of an opaque liver-coloured extract (*hepatic Cape aloes*) with a dark, glossy, transparent extract.

δ. This very much resembled the preceding, and might equally claim for its opaque portion the name of *hepatic Cape aloes.*

Cape aloes is procured from *Aloë spicata* and other species (see *ante*).

5. Fetid, Horse, or Caballine Aloes (*Aloë caballina*).—I have never met with any particular kind of aloes under this name in English commerce; Barbados aloes being used in England for horses. From Prof. Guibourt I have received two substances, which he denominates *Aloès Caballin.*

a. One is *impure* or *foot Cape aloes.*

β. The other is in black opaque masses, intermixed with straws, pieces of bark, sand, charcoal, and other impurities. Its fracture is uniform. It is difficult to pulverise, adheres to the pestle, gives a greenish powder, has a very little odour, and yields a dark brown decoction. It is probably an extract prepared by boiling the leaves in water.

Guibourt says Caballine aloes is procured either in the countries which furnish ordinary aloes, or in Spain[1] or Senegal. [On the continent the inferior and impure qualities of any description of aloes are administered to horses, and pass there by the name Aloë caballina. Mocha aloes is mostly used for that purpose. This variety of aloes varies much in quality. It is generally very impure. The quantities of aloes on which duty was paid in three years were as follows:—

1842	223,597 lbs.
1843	248,441 lbs.
1844	202,294 lbs.]

6. Mocha Aloes (*Aloë de Mochâ*).—Under this name I found in a drug warehouse, where it had lain for many years, an impure kind of aloes, in large irregular masses, opaque, and black externally, intermixed with sand, strings, &c. In its brittleness, odour, and the pale colour of its decoction, it resembles Cape aloes. The interior of the mass is not uniform: in some places it is dark and opaque, somewhat like Barbados aloes; in other places it resembles socotrine aloes, and here and there we find portions having the transparency and resinous appearance of Cape aloes. Recently this kind of aloes has been imported, under the name of Mocha aloes, from Muscat, in chests containing nearly 2 cwt. each.[2] Dr. Christison thinks it is East India aloes of low

---

[1] Formerly the inhabitants of Morviedro, in Valencia, cultivated the aloe plant (*A. vulgaris*), and obtained from it three kinds of aloes, called respectively socotrine, hepatic, and caballine (Jussieu, in Chaptal's *Elements of Chemistry*, vol. iii. p. 86); but Laborde (*View of Spain*, vol. i. p. 302, 1809) says the cultivation is now neglected.

[2] Mr. Whipple tells me, that in dissolving and straining Mocha aloes he has never found less than 25 per cent. of impurities (sand, stones, &c.)

quality. It is described by Guibourt under the name of *blackish* or *fetid aloes* (*aloès noirâtre et fétide*).

7. Indian Aloes (*Aloë indica ;* not the Aloe indica of the Edinburgh Pharmacopœia).—Dr. O'Shaughnessy[1] mentions two kinds of Indian aloes : *Kurachee* aloes, nearly black, opaque, and soluble in water to the extent of 52 per cent.; and *Deckan* aloes, deep brown, and soluble to the extent of 98 per cent.

Through the kindness of Professor Royle, I have examined four kinds of aloes brought from the interior of India :—

a. Aloes from Northern India.—Is dull, black, and brittle, and has little odour. It came from the northern parts of India, where it is common in the bazaars (*Bazaar aloes*). It is probably the kind which Ainslie[2] says resembles Barbados aloes, and is brought to India from Yemen in Arabia. Is this the produce of *Aloe officinalis*, Forskäl?

β. Guzerat Aloes.—Is dark, more gummy in its appearance and feel, more difficult to fracture.

γ. Salem Aloes.—In blackish masses. It was brought from Salem. It is distinguished from all the preceding by the numerous large air-cavities observed in its interior. Its odour is analogous to that of socotrine aloes. Its price is marked one anna and nine pice [about twopence halfpenny] a pound.

δ. Trichinopoli Aloes.—Resembles Cape aloes in its brittleness, odour, and colour, but is more opaque. Its price is marked at two annas [about threepence] a pound.

These aloes are the produce, in part at least, of *Aloë indica ;*[3] a species with reddish flowers, common in dry situations in the north-western provinces of India, and which, if known to Roxburgh, was included by him in the *A. perfoliata*, Linn., and perhaps also of *A. vulgaris*, or the plant mentioned by Rheede.[4]

8. Curacoa Aloes.—This species of Aloes is not known in the London market, but a notice of it has been published by Mr. A. Faber.[5] It is the produce of the Dutch West India Island, Curacoa ; but as even in Holland it cannot be regularly obtained, it is probable that its production is scanty. It is most like Cape aloes, but does not possess the greenish colour which is sometimes perceived in the latter ; its appearance is more dull, and its colour is often that of the liver. From hepatic aloes it differs by its saffron-like odour. It is probably the produce of *A. vulgaris*.

Powdered Aloes.—In January 1846 the lecture assistant of the Pharmaceutical Society carefully powdered selected samples of five kinds of aloes in the Society's museum. The colour of the various powders was as follows :—

Powders.

No. 1. Cape aloes ... Lightest colour. Tint, pale yellow.
" 2. Hepatic aloes . ⎫ Nearly alike. Deeper coloured than No. 1. No. 2 had a reddish, No. 3 a
" 3. Barbados aloes ⎭ greenish tint.
" 4. Socotrine aloes ⎧ Both darker than the three preceding sorts. That of No. 4 had the tint of, but was less deep than, roasted chicory powder; that of No. 5 was olive or greenish. In twelve months No. 4 had become coherent and darkest of all.
" 5. Mocha aloes. Darkest colour ⎭

---

[1] *Bengal Dispensatory.*
[2] *Mat. Ind.* vol. ii. p. 10.
[3] Royle, *Bot. of the Himalayan Mountains.*
[4] *Hort. Malab.* ii. t. 3.
[5] *Pharmaceutical Journal,* vol. vii. p. 547, 1848.

O

Strained Aloes; Aloë colata.—In order to deprive aloes of the various foreign matters with which they are frequently mixed, the wholesale druggist purifies the extract by melting and straining it. The fusion is effected in a metallic vessel heated by steam or hot water, a hair or wire sieve being used for straining the liquor. By this process the aloes suffers a physical, and probably also a chemical change. It becomes darker-coloured, harder, and somewhat less odorous. It is probable that the deepened colour is produced by the action of atmospheric oxygen.

COMPOSITION.—Aloes has been analysed by Trommsdorff,[1] by Bouillon-Lagrange and Vogel,[2] by Braconnot,[3] and by Winkler.[4]

Trommsdorff.		Bouillon-Lagrange and Vogel.		Braconnot.		Winkler.	
Socotrine.	*Barbados.*		*Soc.*	*Bar.*	*Soc*		*Soc.*	*Bar.*
Saponaceous principle 75	81·25	Extractive 68	52	Bitter princip. 73	Bitter matter 50	60
Resin 25	6·25	Resin 32	42	Puce do. 26	Resin 50	35
Vegetable albumen.. 0	12·5	Vegetable } 0	6	Impurities .. 1	Albumen.... 0	5
Gallic acid ....trace	trace	albumen }				
Aloes.............. 100	100·00	100	100	100	100	100

1. ALOESIN, Pfaff (*SaponaceousMatter; Extractive; Bitter Principle of Aloes,* or *Aloe-bitter; Aloin*).—This is the principal constituent of aloes. It is contained in the cold infusion of aloes, and also in a decoction which has cooled: it may be obtained from either by evaporation. Thus procured, it is a brown and bitter mass, readily soluble in water, but difficultly so in spirit of wine. In pure alcohol or ether it is said to be insoluble, or nearly so. Besides *carbon, hydrogen,* and *oxygen,* it contains *nitrogen,* for it yields ammonia by destructive distillation, and furnishes carbazotic acid when treated by nitric acid. Aloesin is probably a mixture or compound of various proximate principles. Obtained as above, Braconnot says it contains some of the *puce-coloured principle,* which may be removed by oxide of lead.

2. ALOE RESIN.—The substance which deposits from a decoction of aloes as it cools is usually denominated resin. Braconnot says it is a mixture of aloesin and *puce-coloured principle;* while Berzelius regards it as *apothème* combined with unaltered extract. It is transparent, brown, fusible, soluble in alcohol, ether, and alkaline solutions. The *puce-coloured principle* of Braconnot is an odourless and tasteless powder, combustible, but not fusible; and is prepared by digesting aloes with water and oxide of lead: a compound of the puce principle and the oxide is procured, which is to be washed and decomposed by weak nitric acid: the oxide is dissolved, and the puce principle left. From Braconnot's observations, this principle seems to be rather oxidised extractive (*apothème,* Berz.) than resin.

3. VEGETABLE ALBUMEN.—This term is applied to a substance insoluble in both water and alcohol.

4. ALOESIC ACID.—This is the acid which Trommsdorff supposed to be *gallic acid.* A solution of aloes reddens litmus, darkens ferruginous solutions, but does not precipitate gelatin: hence Trommsdorff assumed the presence of gallic acid. But while gallic acid causes a blue colour with the persalts of iron, infusion of aloes produces an olive-brown one. Furthermore, if excess of diacetate of lead be added to this infusion, and sulphuretted hydrogen be passed through the filtered liquor, to throw down the excess of lead, the boiled and strained liquor possesses the property of becoming olive-brown on the addition of sesquichloride of iron. Hence it appears to me that the acid is a peculiar one, and I have accordingly termed it *aloesic acid.* It must not be confounded with an acid obtained by the action of nitric acid on aloes, and which has been termed aloetic acid.

---

[1] *Ann. de Chim.* t. lxviii. p. 11, 1808.
[2] *Ibid.* p. 155.
[3] *Journ. de Physiq.* t. lxxxiv. p. 334, 1817.
[4] Geiger, *Hand. d. Pharm.* Bd. ii. 782, 1829.

Meissner[1] has given the name of *Aloine* to a supposed alkali in aloes. Its solution was brown, and acted as an alkali on reddened litmus paper. With sulphuric acid, aloine formed a crystalline salt. [Dr. Stenhouse has described an aloine,[2] and the Messrs. T. and H. Smith have also given this name to what they believe the cathartic principle of aloes.[3] Dr. Stenhouse gives the formula $C^{34}H^{18}O^{14}+HO$ for aloine crystals.—ED.] Winkler[4] regards aloes as a neutral vegetable salt, composed of two peculiar basic substances (viz. a non-bitter resin, and a bitter substance) and an acid, viz. a colouring, non-bitter matter. Fabroni[5] obtained a fine violet colour from the recent juice of the Aloë, which has been proposed as a dye for silk. It is formed by the action of the oxygen of the air on the juice.

CHEMICAL CHARACTERISTICS.—Aloes is almost completely soluble in boiling water. When the decoction of aloes cools, the substance called *resin* is deposited. The clear cold solution (*aloesin*) reddens litmus, strikes a deep olive-brown tint (*aloesate of iron*) with sesquichloride of iron, is deepened in colour by alkalies, but is unchanged with gelatine. Diacetate of lead forms a copious yellow precipitate with it. The alcoholic tincture of aloes does not become turbid when mixed with water. When the ethereal tincture is poured in water, the ether evaporates, and leaves a film of resin.

The bitter principle of aloes (*aloesin*) is distinguished from that of rhubarb by its not striking a green colour with the salts of iron, and by its insolubility in ether.

The differential chemical characters of the various kinds of aloes are not constant. The following, however, are the results of some experiments :—

α. *Cape aloes*, when good, usually completely dissolves in boiling water, leaving no residuum of vegetable albumen, &c. The decoction is clear, usually paler than that of the other kinds, and deposits much of the so-called resin in cooling.

β. *Barbados aloes* sometimes leaves an insoluble residuum (vegetable albumen, &c.) when boiled in water. The decoction, when cold, is dark and usually turbid : generally it is darker than that of the other sorts, yet I have found it the palest. I have also observed that the decoction on cooling becomes turbid, and lets fall a yellow powder like that which I have seen in decoction of hepatic aloes.

γ. *Socotrine aloes* yields a decoction which, when cold, is dark and nearly clear.

δ. *Hepatic aloes* yields a decoction which, on cooling, frequently deposits a yellow powder.

Products of the decomposition of aloes by nitric acid.—When aloes is heated with nitric acid, nitrous fumes are evolved, and the principles of which aloes consist are oxidised. The residuum has an intensely bitter taste, and is termed *artificial aloe-bitter* (*künstliches Aloebitter.*) It is a mixture of several principles.

The products of the action of nitric acid on aloes have occupied the attention of several distinguished chemists; but the results of their experiments, though highly interesting, are not uniform. Braconnot[6] and Chevreul[7] examined the reaction. The former applied the term *aloetic acid* to the residual solid, which Liebig[8] subsequently declared to be a mixture of *nitric* or *nitrous acid, carbazotic acid, and a peculiar, non acid, resinous, red matter.* Boutin[9] has more recently examined the reaction of nitric acid on aloes, and he

---

[1] Pfaff's *Mat. Med.* vol. vii. p. 171.
[2] [*Phil. Mag.* Dec. 1850.]
[3] [Vide *Pharm. Trans.* vol. xi. p. 23 ; and also Dr. Pereira's paper quoted above.]
[4] Schwartz, *Pharm. Tabell.* p. 294, 2te Ausg.
[5] *Ann. de Chim.* xxv. 301.
[6] *Ibid.* lxviii. 28.
[7] *Ibid.* lxxiii. 46.
[8] Poggendorff's *Annalen*, xiii. 205 ; also Liebig and Poggendorff's *Handwörterbuch d. Chemie*, S. 268, 1837.
[9] *Journ. d. Pharmacie*, t. xxvi. p. 185.

states the products to be *polychromatic acid* (the aloetic acid of Braconnot), composed, according to Pelouze, of $C^{15}H^2N^2O^{13}$, *oxalic acid, carbazotic acid*, and *cyanile*. Schunk[1] states that by the action of nitric acid on aloes he obtained four peculiar acids, viz. *aloetic acid, aloëresinic acid, chrysammic acid*, $C^{15}HN^2O^{12}+HO$, and *chrysolepic acid*, $C^{12}H^2N^3O^{13}+HO$.

Mulder[2] has recently examined the products of the reaction of nitric acid on aloes. *Anhydrous chrysammic acid*, he says, consists of $C^{14}HN^2O^{11}$. The so-called *chrysolepic acid* he considers to be identical with nitropicric acid (*i. e.* carbazotic acid). He found the composition of the foliaceous crystals of this acid to be $C^{12}H^3N^3O^{14}$.

PHYSIOLOGICAL EFFECTS. *α. On Vegetables.*—Not ascertained.

β. On Animals.—Aloes is the ordinary purgative for solipedes (the horse, the ass, and the zebra), as it is both safe and sure. In horses, previously prepared by two or three bran-mashes to soften the dung, the dose is from five to seven drachms.[3] It acts slowly, requiring from eighteen to forty-eight hours for its operation.[4] Mr. Youatt informs me that aloes is a valuable purgative for the dog, in doses of from one to three drachms, and with the addition of from one to three grains of calomel. Barbados also is preferred by veterinarians, as being more effective than Cape aloes, in the ratio of about seven to five. Aloes proves purgative to oxen, sheep, and pigs, but, as in the other cases, it operates slowly.[5] Moiroud[6] injected into the veins of a horse four drachms of aloes dissolved in water with a little alcohol, and the next day an ounce more, without any other effect than the evacuation of a large quantity of urine. The dung, however, was enveloped by a thin pellicle formed by altered intestinal mucus. This was collected and analysed subsequent to the death of the animal (which followed three days after the injection) : it offered scarcely any traces of the constituents of the bile.

γ. On Man.—Taken internally *in small doses,* aloes acts as a tonic to the alimentary canal, assisting the digestive process, strengthening the muscular fibres, and promoting the secretions, especially that of the liver, which organ it is thought specifically to influence. *In large doses* it acts as a purgative. There are, however, some peculiarities attending its cathartic operation deserving of notice. In the first place, these effects are not so speedily produced as by some other purgatives; for eight, twelve, and sometimes twenty-four hours elapse before they are produced. Secondly, aloes acts especially on the large intestines, and a full dose is in some persons apt to produce heat and irritation about the rectum, and tenesmus ; and in those troubled with hemorrhoids it is said not unfrequently to increase, or even to bring on, the sanguineous discharge. Fallopius[7] tells us, that of one hundred persons who used aloes as a purgative, ninety were affected with the hemorrhoidal flux, which ceased when the use of aloes was omitted. But though this statement has been often quoted as an objection to the use of aloes, it is of little importance, as there is no evidence that the disease was brought on by aloes. The uterus, in common with all the pelvic viscera, is stimulated by aloes. A determination of blood towards these organs, and a

[1] *Ann. der Chemie*, Bd. xxxix.
[2] Buchner's *Repertorium*, 3te Reihe, Bd. ii. 1849.
[3] Youatt, *The Horse*, p. 211.
[4] Moiroud, *Pharm. Vétér.* p. 26.
[5] Wibmer's *Wirk. d. Arzneim.*
[6] *Op. cit.*
[7] *Opera omnia*, p. 109, Francof. 1600.

fulness of the blood-vessels (especially of the veins), are produced, and thus uterine irritation and menorrhagia are apt to be increased by aloes, while in amenorrhœa and chlorosis it may occasionally act as an emmenagogue. Dr. Wedekind[1] says that small doses of aloes often occasion erection, and increase the sexual feelings. The purgative effects of aloes do not arise merely from their local action on the alimentary canal, since this effect is sometimes produced when the medicine has been neither swallowed nor given by the rectum. Thus Monro *primus*[2] tells us that the tincture of aloes applied to a caries of the bone produced purging; and it is said[3] that an aloetic pill used as a stimulant to an issue had a similar effect; lastly, applied to a caries of the bone it produced purging; and it is said[3] that an aloetic pill used as a stimulant to an issue had a similar effect; lastly, applied to a blistered surface it has the same operation. So that the purgative action of aloes appears to be of a specific kind.

According to Dr. Wedekind,[4] the operation of aloes depends on the increased secretion of bile, which is produced by the specific action of this medicine on the liver. He founds this opinion on the results of various experiments. Thus he says that if aloes be added to purgatives (a laxative infusion and sulphate of soda), whose operation is speedy, its effects do not take place for some hours after those caused by the other purgatives; and he also asserts that the evacuations in the second purging differ from those of the first both in appearance and smell. Moreover, he found that as long as the stools were white or grey in icterus, the aloes did not purge even when exhibited in large doses; but the purgative effect supervened immediately after the fæcal matter began to contain bile, proving that the presence of bile in the intestinal canal is a necessary condition of the purgative effect of aloes. But in Moiroud's experiment above quoted, no effect seemed to be produced on the hepatic secretion. In all probability, the increased secretion of bile, the irritation about the rectum, the disposition to hemorrhoids, and the vascular excitement of the sexual organs, all of which are said to be produced by aloes, are the effects of a stimulant action exerted by this medicine over the venous system of the abdomen, and especially of the pelvis. Dr. Greenhow[5] ascribes a diuretic effect to aloes, and his statement is corroborated by Moiroud's experiment.

Socotrine aloes is said not to be so apt to occasion hemorrhoids as the Barbados kind. Some years since, Dr. Clutterbuck instituted numerous experiments at the General Dispensary, Aldersgate Street, which I witnessed, to determine the effects of the different kinds of aloes, but scarcely any difference in their operation on the human subject was perceptible. However, it is probable that Cape aloes is less powerful in its action on man, as it is on the horse, than the Barbados kind. But the difference is the less obvious in the human subject, on account of the comparative smallness of the dose required to produce the purgative effect. As a purgative, aloes holds an intermediate rank between rhubarb and senna. Vogt[6] places it between jalap

---

[1] Rust's *Magazin*, 1827, Bd. xxiv. Heft 2, S. 304.
[2] *Works*, p. 306, 1781.
[3] *Mém. de la Soc. Roy. de Méd. Paris*, tom. ii. p. 162.
[4] *Op. cit.*; also *Lancet*, vol. i. p. 347, 1827–8.
[5] *Lond. Med. Gaz.* vol. xix. p. 270.
[6] *Pharmakodynamik*, Bd. ii. S. 334, 2te Aufl.

and rhubarb. From rhubarb it is distinguished by its more stimulant influence over the large intestines and the pelvic organs : from senna by its feebler action as a purgative, by its slow operation, and by its tonic influence when given in small doses. It irritates less powerfully than either jalap or scammony : further, its influence over the blood-vessels of the pelvic viscera is greater than these.

Uses.—The uses of aloes may be readily inferred from the remarks already made. It is evidently not adapted for those cases in which a speedy effect is required; and it is therefore useless to add it to purgatives to quicken their operation. It is well fitted for cases of costiveness where there is a scanty secretion of bile, and for torpid conditions of the large intestines, especially when attended with deficient uterine action. Some of the ill effects ascribed to the use of aloes are probably imaginary, and others are much exaggerated.[1] It is, however, advisable to avoid the use of this purgative in inflammatory conditions and organic diseases of the liver, in biliary calculi, in mechanical impediments to the passage of the blood through the branches of the portal veins, in hemorrhage from any of the pelvic organs (as the uterus and rectum), in irritation of the rectum, prostate gland, or bladder, in pregnancy, &c. For we have many other equally efficient purgatives to the use of which, in these cases, no ill consequences have been ascribed. While, therefore, I concur with Dr. Fothergill[2] in advising that the exhibition of aloes should be avoided when the menses are about to cease, I am not prepared to admit that " the piles, strangury, immoderate discharges of the menses, racking pains in the loins, representing labour pains, and other similar complaints," are frequently induced by this medicine. On the contrary, I suspect this catalogue of the evils of aloetic purges to be much overcharged. " Aloetic medicines," says Dr. Denman,[3] "are forbidden during pregnancy, lest they should do mischief by their supposed deobstruent qualities ; but they are cheap and conveniently given in the form of pills, and I have not observed any bad effects from them." The emaciation, stricture of the rectum, and enteritis, referred by Dr. Greenhow[4] to the long-continued use of aloetic medicines, ought doubtless to be ascribed to other causes.

The following are some of the cases in which the use of aloes has been advised :—

1. *In loss of appetite and dyspepsia*, depending on a debilitated condition of the digestive organs, accompanied by costiveness, but unattended with any signs of local irritation, aloes may be given in small doses as a stomachic.

2. *In habitual costiveness*, depending on deficiency of bile, or on a sluggish condition of the large intestines—particularly in hypochondriacal or studious persons, or in those whose habits or occupations are sedentary—aloes, given in sufficient doses to purge, will be found a very useful medicine. A torpid state of the colon, with large fæcal accumulation, is not unusual in females.[5] In such the use of aloes is often attended with much benefit.

---

[1] *On the Use and Abuse of Aloes, London Medical Gazette*, vol. iv. p. 139.
[2] *Med. Obs. and Inq.* vol. v. p. 173.
[3] *Introd. to the Pract. of Midwifery.*
[4] *Lond. Med. Gaz.* vol. xix. p. 270.
[5] Copland, *Dictionary of Practical Medicine*, art. *Colon, Torpor of.*

3. *To excite the menstrual discharge* aloes is frequently employed. It has been supposed that by determining an afflux of blood to the pelvic organs, aloes would stimulate the uterine vessels, and thus relieve deficient menstruation connected with atonic conditions of the uterus. But it often fails : indeed Dr. Cullen[1] says that it rarely succeeds.

4. *To reproduce the hemorrhoidal discharge* aloes has been frequently employed in large doses. Serious affections of the head, or of other parts, have sometimes disappeared on the occurrence of the hemorrhoidal flux ; and therefore, in persons who have been subject to this discharge, but in whom it has stopped, it is advisable to attempt its re-establishment, with the view of relieving other more serious disorders.

5. *To promote the secretion of bile* where a deficiency of this fluid does not arise from hepatic inflammation ; as in some forms of jaundice which are unconnected with biliary calculi, inflammation, mechanical obstruction of the ducts, &c.

6. *In cerebral affections.*—The compound decoction of aloes is a most valuable stimulating purgative for elderly persons in whom a tendency to apoplexy exists, especially in cold and phlegmatic habits. It will frequently be necessary to conjoin other cathartics, as the infusion of senna.

7. *As an anthelmintic,* a decoction of aloes, used as an enema, has been efficacious in the small thread-worm (*Ascaris vermicularis*).

ADMINISTRATION.—On account of its nauseous taste, aloes is frequently given in the form of pill (*pilulæ aloeticæ* offic.) One or two grains seldom fail to produce one stool, which seems to be merely an evacuation of what may be supposed to have been present for the time in the great intestines (Cullen). The ordinary dose is five grains; but ten, fifteen, or even twenty grains, are sometimes given.

1. PILULÆ ALOËS COMPOSITÆ, L. D.; *Pilulæ Aloës,* E.; *Compound Pills of Aloes.* (Socotrine Aloes [hepatic, ℥ij. *D.*], powdered, ℥j. ; Extract of Gentian, ℥ss. [℥j. *D.*] ; Oil of Caraway, ♏xl. [℥j. *D.*] ; Treacle, as much as may be sufficient, *L.* [℥j. by weight, *D.*] ; beat them together until incorporated. The *Edinburgh College* orders of Socotrine Aloes and Castile Soap, *equal parts ;* Conserve of Red Roses, a sufficiency : beat them into a proper pill mass. This pill may be also correctly made with the finer qualities of East Indian Aloes, as the Socotrine variety is scarce ; and many, not without reason, prefer the stronger Barbados Aloes, *E.*)—This pill is a valuable purgative in habitual costiveness. Dose, five to fifteen grains.

2. PILULÆ ALOËS CUM MYRRHA, L. D.; *Pilulæ Aloës et Myrrhæ,* E.; *Pilulæ Rufi* offic.; *Pills of Aloes and Myrrh ; Rufus's Pills.* (Aloes, Socotrine or hepatic [hepatic, *D.* ; Socotrine or East Indian, *E.*], ℥ss. [*four parts,* E. ; ℥ij. *D.*] ; Saffron [*one part,* E.], Myrrh, Soft Soap, of each ℥ij. [*two parts,* E. ; Myrrh, ℥j. ; Saffron, ℥ss. *D.*] ; Treacle [Conserve of Red Roses, *E.*], as much as may be sufficient [℥iss. by weight, *D.*] Beat the whole together until incorporated. The *Dublin College* orders the Aloes, Myrrh, and Saffron to be triturated and sifted before incorporation.)—Used as a purgative in chlorosis and amenorrhœa. Dose, ten to twenty grains.

---

[1] *Treat. of the Mat. Med.*

3. PILULÆ ALOËS CUM SAPONE, L. Extract of Barbados Aloes, powdered; Soft Soap; Extract of Liquorice, equal parts; Treacle, as much as may be sufficient. Beat the extract of aloes with the soap, then, the rest being added, beat them together into a mass.

4. PILULÆ ALOËS ET ASSAFŒTIDÆ, E.; *Pills of Aloes and Assafœtida.* (Aloes [Socotrine or East Indian], Assafœtida, and Castile Soap, *equal parts.* Beat them, with Conserve of Red Roses, into a proper pill-mass.)— Used in dyspepsia attended with flatulence and costiveness. Dose, ten to twenty grains.

5. PILULÆ ALOËS ET FERRI, E.; *Pills of Aloes and Iron.* (Sulphate of Iron, *three parts;* Barbados Aloes, *two parts;* Aromatic Powder, *six parts;* Conserve of Red Roses, *eight parts.* Pulverise the aloes and sulphate of iron separately; mix the whole ingredients, and beat them into a proper mass, which is to be divided into five-grain pills.)—A valuable emmenagogue in atonic amenorrhœa and chlorosis. Dose, one to three pills.

6. PULVIS ALOËS COMPOSITUS, L.; *Compound Powder of Aloes.* (Aloes, ℥iss.; Guaiacum Resin, ʒj.; Compound Powder of Cinnamon, ℥ss. Rub the aloes and the guaiacum resin, separately, to powder; then mix them with the compound powder of cinnamon.)—Purgative and sudorific. Seldom used. Dose, ten to twenty grains.

7. PULVIS ALOËS CUM CANELLÂ; *Hiera Picra,* offic.; *Powder of Aloes and Canella.* (Hepatic Aloes, ℔ j.; Canella Bark, ℥iij. Powder them separately, and then mix.)—A popular emmenagogue. Dose, five to fifteen grains. [This was retained in the Dublin Pharmacopœia until 1850.—Ed.]

8. DECOCTUM ALOËS COMPOSITUM, L. D.; *Decoctum Aloës,* E.; *Compound Decoction of Aloes.* (Extract of Liquorice, ʒvij. [℥ss. *E. D.*]; Carbonate of Potash, ʒj. [ij. *E.;* Əij. *D.*]; Socotrine Aloes [hepatic, *D.,* or Socotrine, *E.*], powdered; Myrrh, powdered; Saffron, of each ℈iss. [ʒj. *E. D.*]; Compound Tincture of Cardamom, f℥vij. [f℥iv. *E.*]; Distilled Water, Oiss. [f℥xvj. *E.;* ℥xiv. *D.*] Boil down the liquorice, carbonate of potash, aloes, myrrh, and saffron, with the water, to a pint [f℥xij. *E.*], and strain; then add the compound tincture of cardamom. [The *Dublin College* orders as much Tincture of Cardamoms as may be necessary to make up the measure to f℥xvj. It directs the materials to be boiled ten minutes, cooled, and strained through flannel.)]—A most valuable preparation. A mild cathartic, tonic, antacid, and emmenagogue. Used in the before-mentioned cases in doses of f℥ss. to f℥ij. Acids, acidulous salts, and most metallic salts, are incompatible with it. If it be desirable to conjoin chalybeates with it, either the *Potassæ Ferro-Tartras* or the *Ammoniæ Ferro-Citras* may be added to the cold decoction without undergoing decomposition. The quality of the aloes used, the length of time the decoction is boiled, and the purity of the extract of liquorice, affect the transparency or turbidity of this decoc'ion, which is never so brigh‘ as tincture of aloes.[1]

9. EXTRACTUM ALOËS, L.; *Extractum Aloës Aquosum,* D.; *Extract of Aloes.* (Aloes, powdered, ℥xv.; Boiling Distilled Water, Cong. j. Macerate

---

[1] *Pharmaceutical Journal,* vol. i. p. 182, 1841.

for three days with a gentle heat; afterwards strain and set by, that the dregs may subside. Pour off the clear liquor, and evaporate it to a proper consistence. The *Dublin College* orders ℥iv. of Hepatic Aloes to be boiled in Oij. of Water till dissolved. The cold and clear liquor is then poured off and evaporated.) —It is intended to deprive the aloes of the substance called resin, on which its irritating and griping qualities have been supposed to depend.[1] Dose, five to fifteen grains.

[**10. EXTRACTUM ALOËS BARBADENSIS, L.**—This is to be prepared by the same process as the Extract of Aloes (*supra*).]

11. TINCTURA ALOËS, L. E.; *Tincture of Aloes.* (Aloes, Socotrine or hepatic [Socotrine or Indian, *E.*], coarsely powdered, ℥j.; Extract of Liquorice, ℥ij. Distilled Water, Oiss. [Oj. and f℥viij. *E.*]; Rectified Spirit, Oss. [f℥xij. *E.*] Macerate the aloes in the spirit and water for seven [with occasional agitation, *E.*] days, add the extract, and strain. This tincture cannot without difficulty and delay be prepared by percolation, *E.*)—Purgative and stomachic. Dose, ℨij. to ℥j.

12. TINCTURA ALOËS COMPOSITA, L.; *Tinctura Aloës et Myrrhæ*, E.; *Elixir Proprietatis* of Paracelsus; *Compound Tincture of Aloes.* (Aloes, Socotrine or hepatic [Socotrine or Indian, *E.*], coarsely powdered, ℥iv.; Saffron, ℥ij.; Tincture of Myrrh, Oij. Macerate for seven days, and strain, L. This tincture cannot be well prepared by percolation, *E.*)—Purgative, stomachic, emmenagogue. Used in cold sluggish habits. Dose, ℨss. to ℨj.

13. VINUM ALOËS, L. E.; *Tinctura Sacra; Wine of Aloes.* (Socotrine Aloes, rubbed to powder, ℥ij.; Canella, powdered, ℨiv.; Sherry Wine, Oij. Macerate for seven days, and strain. The *Edinburgh College* uses Aloes [Socotrine or East Indian], ℥iss.; Cardamom Seeds, ground; Ginger, in coarse powder, of each ℨiss.; Sherry, Oij. Digest for seven days, and strain through linen or calico.)—Wine of aloes is purgative in doses of f℥ss. to f℥ij.; stomachic in doses of fℨj. to ℨij.

Aloes is a constituent of several other preparations (as *Pilula Colocynthidis composita*, L. D., *Pilulæ Colocynthidis*, E.; *Pilulæ Rhei compositæ*, L. E.; *Pilulæ Cambogiæ*, E., *Pilula Cambogiæ composita*, L.; *Tinctura Rhei et Aloës*, E.), which will be described hereafter.

62. URGINEA SCILLA, *Steinheil.*—THE SEA ONION, OR OFFICINAL SQUILL.

Sex. Syst. Hexandria, Monogynia.
(Bulbus recens, *L.*—Bulbus, *D.*—Bulb, *E.*)

SYNONYMES.—*Urginea Scilla*, Steinheil;[2] *Scilla maritima*, Linn.; *Cepa marina*, Lobel.

---

[1] [This end is by no means answered, however, according to the statements of Winkler (*Pharm. Trans.* vol. x. p. 310.)—ED.]

[2] In 1834, Steinheil (*Ann. Sc. Nat.* t. i. p. 321, 2nde sér.) proposed the name *Urginea* for the genus to which squill (*Urginea Scilla*, Steinh.) belongs. Some objections having been raised to it, and no systematic writer having then adopted it, Steinheil in 1836 (*op. cit.* t. vi. p. 272) proposed to substitute the name of *Squilla* (σκίλλα) for Urginea; but subsequently some writers have adopted the term Urginea as the generic name.

HISTORY.—The Egyptians worshipped a bulbous plant called by Lucian Κρόμμυον, and which Pauw[1] asserts to be the squill, and further suggests that it was the red variety (? *Squilla Pancration* var. *a Bulbo rufo*, Steinheil) ; but by others it has been thought to be the onion (see *Allium Cepa*). Pythagoras[2] is said to have written a volume on the medicinal properties of squill, and to have invented the *acetum scillæ*. Hippocrates employed squill (σκίλλα) internally,[3] externally,[4] and as a pessary.[5] Pliny[6] says there are two medicinal sorts of squills,—one, which he calls the *male* with white leaves ; the other, or *female*, with black leaves : the former probably is white, the latter red squills.

BOTANY. **Gen. Char.**—*Sepals* 3, coloured, spreading. *Petals* very like them, and scarcely broader. *Stamens* 6, shorter than the perianth ; *filaments* smooth, somewhat dilated at the base, acuminate, entire. *Ovary* 3-parted, glandular and melliferous at the apex ; *style* smooth, simple ; *stigma* obscurely 3-lobed, papillose. *Capsule* rounded, 3-cornered, 3-celled. *Seeds* numerous, in two rows, flattened with a membranous testa (*Steinheil*).

Sp. Char.—*Leaves* very large, subsequently spreading. *Bracts* long. *Flowers* white ; flower-bud somewhat acute. *Anthers* yellow. *Ovarium* thick, yellowish. *Bulb* very large (*Steinheil*).

Bulb roundish-ovate, half above ground. The *leaves* appear after the flowers : they are broad, lanceolate, 12 to 18 inches long. *Scape* about 2 feet high, terminated by a dense long raceme.

Hab.—Shores of the Mediterranean, viz. Spain, France, Sicily, Africa, &c. Navarino has long been celebrated for its squills. In its native soil the plant flowers about August.

SQUILLA PANCRATION, Steinh. (Πανκράτιον, Dioscorides) is said by Steinheil to yield a small bulb of a reddish colour, found in commerce under the name of squill.

DESCRIPTION.—The fresh bulb (*bulbus recens*, L. ; *radix recens* offic.) is pyriform, of the size of the fist to that of a child's head, and is composed of thick, fleshy, smooth, shiny scales, attenuated at their edges, closely applied over each other, and attached to a conical disc (a rudimentary stem) which projects inferiorly, and gives origin to the root-fibres, the remains of which are to be frequently found in the bulbs of commerce. The outer scales are usually dry, thin, coloured, membranous, or papery. By cracking the inner or fleshy scales, numerous spiral vessels may be drawn out. On submitting the cuticle of the scales to a microscopic examination, numerous acicular crystals (*raphides*) are perceived in cells, which are distinguished from the surrounding angular cells by being larger and elliptical. The *pulvis scillæ* offic. contains nine or ten per cent. of these crystals. Two kinds of squills, both abounding in an acrid juice, and having a very bitter taste, are met with in commerce ; viz. the *white* (*squilla alba, mascula*, vel *hispanica*), and the *red* (*squilla rubra, fæmina*, vel *italica*),[7] both of which are so called from the colour of the scales. The white is preferred in England.

---

[1] *Phil. Diss. on the Egyptians and Chinese*, vol. i. p. 130, 1795.
[2] Pliny, *Hist. Nat.* lib. xix. cap. 30, ed. Valp.
[3] *De victûs ratione.*
[4] *De ulceribus.*
[5] *De nat. mul.*
[6] *Hist. Nat.* lib. xix. cap. 30, ed. Valp.
[7] Is the red kind the *Squilla Pancration* var. *a Bulbo Rufo*, Steinheil?

In the London Pharmacopœia the fresh bulbs are directed to be preserved in dry sand; and, before drying them, the dry rind is to be removed; they are then to be cut transversely into thin slices, and dried with a gentle heat at first, which is to be raised gradually to 150°.

Dried squill (*radix scillæ siccata* offic.) is, however, for the most part imported, in consequence of the duty being no higher for this than for the recent bulb. It occurs in white or yellowish-white, slightly diaphanous pieces, which, when dry, are brittle, but when moist are readily flexible. As their affinity for moisture is great, they should be preserved in well-stoppered bottles, or in a very dry place. Squill is imported from Malta, and other countries of the Mediterranean. Also from Petersburg and Copenhagen.[1]

COMPOSITION.—The more recent analyses of squill are those of Vogel, in 1812,[2] and of Tilloy, in 1826.[3] Buchner,[4] in 1811, examined the juice of the fresh bulb.

Vogel's Analysis of Squills dried at 212° F.		*Tilloy's Analysis of dried and fresh Squills.*	*Buchner's Analysis of fresh Squill bulb juice.*	
Scillitin with some sugar ...	35	Acrid bitter resinous extractive (*Scillitin*).	Peculiar bitter extractive	9·47
Tannin	24		Mucilage	3·09
Gum	6	Uncrystallisable sugar. Gum.	Gelatinous matter (*Tragacanthin?*)... }	0·94
Woody fibre and some citrate (and perhaps tartrate) of lime }	30	Fatty matter.	Phosphate of lime	0·31
Acrid volatile matter		Piquant, very fugacious matter.	Fibrous matter	3·38
Loss	5		Water	79·01
			Astringent acid	traces
			Loss	4·40
Squill bulb	100	Squill bulb.	Squill juice	100·60

1. ACRID, VOLATILE ? MATTER.—It is well known that squill, in the recent state, is very acrid, and, when applied to the skin, causes irritation, inflammation, and even vesication. By drying, the greater part of this acridity is got rid of; and hence the acrid principle is usually described as being of a volatile nature; and, in confirmation of its volatility, Athanasius[5] states that two ounces of water distilled from fresh squills caused the death of a dog in six hours. However, by others its volatility is denied; and Vogel says that six ounces of water distilled from fresh squills had no effect on dogs. Buchner[6] states that, besides the bitter scillitin, squill contains, according to his experiments, another principle, which is combined with phosphate of lime, and which is capable of exciting itching and inflammation. This acrid matter may be easily decomposed, but is not volatile, as is generally supposed.

[According to the experiments of Wittstein, this acrid matter combines with oxide of lead, forming an insoluble compound, and is not volatile. He further states, that in the analysis of Vogel, given above, the proportions of tannin and of gum should be reversed. Wittstein denies the *bitter* taste ascribed to this *acrid* matter, and says these two qualities are owing to the presence of perfectly different substances : the acrid matter being electro-negative, the bitter matter indifferent.[7]—ED.]

2. SCILLITIN (*Scillitite*, Thomson).—The substance to which Vogel gave the name of Scillitin is a whitish transparent deliquescent substance, which, when dry, has a resinous fracture, and may be easily rubbed to powder. Its taste is bitter and subsequently

[1] *Trade List*, Sept. 11, and Nov. 20, 1838. Sir James Wylie (*Pharm. Castren. Ruthenica*, p. 335, ed. 4to. 1840) gives North Russia as one of the habitats of this plant.

[2] *Ann. de Chim.* t. lxxxiii. p. 147.

[3] *Journ. de Pharm.* xii. p. 635.

[4] *Berl. Jahrb.* xv. p. 1.

[5] Pfaff, *Mat. Med.* Bd. v. S. 18.

[6] *Toxikologie*, 340.

[7] [*Pharm. Journ.* vol. x. p. 359.]

sweetish. It readily dissolves in water, spirit of wine, and acetic acid. The substance sold in the shops under the name of Scillitin is a thick treacle-like liquid. Landerer[1] obtained crystals of scillitin. He says they possessed alkaline properties. Lebordais,[2] on the other hand, says it is neutral and uncrystallisable. It obviously requires further examination.

3. RAPHIDES (*Phosphate of lime? Oxalate of lime?*).—The acicular crystals found in the cuticle of the scales of the bulb, as before mentioned, probably consist of phosphate of lime, or, according to Schleiden, of oxalate of lime. These, perhaps, are the needle-like crystals obtained by Vogel by evaporating the juice of the bulb, and which he regarded as citrate of lime. According to the late Mr. E. Quekett, they constitute about 10 per cent. of powdered squills.

CHEMICAL CHARACTERISTICS.—An aqueous decoction of squills is pale and very bitter. Sesquichloride of iron communicates an intense purplish-blue colour (*gallate of iron*) to it. (This test I have not found to succeed uniformly. The decoction of some specimens of squills scarcely becomes altered by the salts of iron.) Gelatin has scarcely any effect on it. Nitrate of silver forms a white precipitate (*chloride of silver*) soluble in ammonia, but insoluble in nitric acid. Oxalate of ammonia renders the decoction turbid, and after some time causes a white precipitate (*oxalate of lime*). Diacetate of lead and protonitrate of mercury form precipitates in the decoction. Tincture of nutgalls has little or no effect on it; it sometimes occasions a cloudiness. Starch is not recognisable in it by iodine. Alkalies heighten the colour of the decoction.

An infusion of squills in water acidulated with hydrochloric acid yields a white precipitate with oxalate of ammonia (*oxalate of lime*); and with caustic ammonia sometimes a precipitate (*phosphate of lime*), at others scarcely a cloud.

PHYSIOLOGICAL EFFECTS. *α. On Vegetables.*—Not ascertained.

β. On Animals.—An ounce of powdered squill acts as a diuretic on horses and other large animals; the same effect is produced on smaller animals by half a drachm.[3] When the dose is large, squill acts as a poison. It first causes local irritation; then its active principle becomes absorbed, affects the nervous system, and thereby quickens the respiration, causes convulsions and death.[4] Hillefeld[5] mentions paralysis produced in a rabbit by nineteen grains of powdered squill. Emmert and Hoering[6] state that squill juice introduced into the abdominal cavity became absorbed.

γ. On Man.—Squill is an acrid. *In small doses* it acts as a stimulant to the excretory organs. Thus it promotes secretion from the mucous membranes (especially the bronchial and gastro-intestinal) and the kidneys. Its most marked effect is that of a diuretic. Its expectorant effects are less obvious and constant. Sometimes, when it fails to act on the kidneys, it increases cutaneous exhalation. Its influence on secreting organs is probably to be referred to the local stimulus communicated to their vessels by the active principle of squill in its passage out of the system; for Emmert and Hoering[7] have shown that the juice is absorbed, so that squills may be regarded as an acrid even for

[1] Thomson's *Org. Chem.* p. 717.
[2] *Ann. de Chim. et de Phys.* xxiv. 58.
[3] Moiroud, *Pharm. Vétér.*
[4] Orfila, *Toxicol. Gén.*
[5] Marx, *Die Lehre von d. Giften*, vol. ii.
[6] Meckel's *Archiv*, B. iv. Heft 4, S. 527.
[7] *Op. cit.*

these remote parts.   When it proves diuretic in dropsies, it usually promotes the absorption of the effused fluid,—an effect which is, I think, indirect, and a consequence of the diuresis.   But Sundelin[1] observes of squill, that it promotes the secretion of urine less by its local irritation of the kidneys, than by its general excitement of the absorbent apparatus.

By the continued use of squill in gradually increased doses, it disturbs the functions of digestion and assimilation.

In full medicinal doses, squill excites nausea and vomiting.   Purging, also, is not unfrequently produced.   When squill proves emetic or purgative, its diuretic operation is much less obvious,—a circumstance which Cullen[2] refers to the squill being prevented reaching the blood-vessels and kidneys. Home,[3] however, alleges that the diuretic effects are not to be expected unless there be some operation on the stomach.   But the operation on the stomach may be, as Cullen suggests, a mere test of the activity of the squills.   However, that the effect of squill, in strong doses, is not confined to the alimentary canal, is proved by the fact that when the vomiting and purging were present the pulse has been observed to be reduced in frequency,—often to forty beats per minute (Home).

In excessive doses, squill acts as a narcotico-acrid poison, and causes vomiting, purging, griping pain, strangury, bloody urine, convulsions, inflammation and gangrene of the stomach and intestines.[4]   Twenty-four grains of the powder have proved fatal.[5]

Considered with reference to its diuretic effect, squill is comparable with foxglove.   But it exceeds the latter in its stimulant influence over the urinary organs.   On the other hand, foxglove is characterised by its powerfully sedative effect on the vascular system ; for though squill has, in some instances, reduced the frequency of the pulse, this effect is by no means common. Squill, says Vogt,[6] preponderates in its action on the inferior or vegetative [organic] life; foxglove, on the other hand, in its action on the higher or animal life.

USES.—The principal uses of squill are those of an emetic, diuretic, and expectorant.

1. *As a diuretic in dropsies.*—It is applicable to those cases of dropsy requiring the use of stimulating or acrid diuretics, and is improper in inflammatory cases.   It is an unfit remedy for dropsy complicated with granular kidney or vesical irritation ; but when these conditions are not present, it is adapted for torpid leucophlegmatic subjects.   Hence it is more serviceable in anasarca than in either ascites or hydrothorax.   It should be given so as to excite a slight degree of nausea (not vomiting), as recommended by Van Swieten.[7]   By this means its absorption is promoted.   The acetate or bitartrate of potash may be conjoined.   Calomel is usually regarded as a good adjunct for promoting the diuretic influence of squill.   When it does not purge it is beneficial, but its tendency to affect the bowels is an objection to its use.

---

[1] *Handb. d. sp. Heilm.* Bd. ii. S. 17.
[2] *Treat. of the Mat. Med.* p. 557.
[3] *Clinical Experiments,* 3d edit. p. 387, 1783.
[4] Murray, *App. Med.* vol. v. p. 97.
[5] Vogel, *Journ. de Phys.* lxxv. 194.
[6] *Pharmakodyn.* ii. 343, 2te Aufl.
[7] *Commentary upon Boerhaave's Aphorisms,* vol. xii. p. 435.

2. *As an expectorant in chronic pulmonary affections* admitting of the use of a substance stimulating the capillary vessels of the bronchial membrane. Thus in chronic catarrh, humid asthma, and winter cough, it is often employed with considerable benefit. It is of course improper in all acute cases accompanied with inflammation or febrile disorder. In old persons it is often combined with the *tinctura camphoræ composita,* and with good effect. The oxymel or syrup of squill may be given to relieve troublesome chronic coughs in children.

3. *As an emetic* it is occasionally used in affections of the organs of respiration requiring or admitting of the use of vomits. Thus the oxymel is given, with the view of creating sickness and promoting expectoration, to children affected with hooping-cough; and sometimes, though with less propriety, in mild cases of croup. The great objection to its use is the uncertainty of its operation : in one case it will hardly excite nausea, in another it causes violent vomiting. Furthermore, it is of course highly objectionable as an emetic for delicate children with irritable stomachs, on account of its acrid properties, and the irritation it is capable, in these cases, of setting up.

Administration.—The following are the preparations of squill usually employed :—

**1. PULVIS SCILLÆ; *Powdered Squill.*—The Dublin College formerly gave directions for the preparation of this as follows :—Remove the membranous integuments from the bulb of the squill, cut it into slices, and dry with an inferior heat (between 90° and 100° F.) ; then reduce them to powder, which ought to be kept in glass bottles with ground stoppers. The bulb loses about four-fifths of its weight by drying : so that six grains of the dry powder are equal to half a drachm when fresh. Powdered squill readily attracts water from the atmosphere, and becomes soft and mouldy; hence the necessity of preserving it in stoppered bottles and in a dry place. I have seen it become hard and massive like diachylon plaster. It is usually administered in the form of pill. The dose of the powder, as an emetic, is from six to fifteen grains; ten grains being the average. As an expectorant or diuretic we should commence with one grain, and gradually increase the dose until slight nausea is excited.

**2. PILULA SCILLÆ COMPOSITA, L.; *Pilulæ Scillæ compositæ,* D.; *Pilulæ Scillæ,* E.; *Compound Squill Pills.* (Squill, fresh dried and powdered, ʒj. [ʒiiss. *D.*] ; Ginger, powdered; Ammoniacum, powdered, each ʒij.; Soft Soap, ʒiij. [Castile Soap, ʒij. *D.*] ; Treacle, ʒj. [ʒss. by weight, *D.*] Mix the powders together; then beat them with the soap, and add the treacle so as to obtain a proper consistence. The *Edinburgh College* takes of powdered Squill, *five parts ;* powdered Ammoniac, and Ginger and Spanish Soap, each *four parts ;* Conserve of Red Roses, *two parts ;* and forms them into five-grain pills.)—Expectorant and diuretic. Principally used in chronic bronchial affections. Dose from five to twenty grains. It readily spoils by keeping.

**3. TINCTURA SCILLÆ, L. D. E.; *Tincture of Squills.* (Squill, fresh dried [in coarse powder, *E.*] ʒv. ; Proof Spirit, Oij. ; macerate for seven days, and strain, *L.* The directions of the *Dublin College* do not essentially differ from these. "Prepare this tincture by percolation, as directed for tincture of cinchona, but without packing the pulp firmly in the percolator. It may likewise be obtained by the process of digestion from the sliced bulb," *E.*)—Expectorant and diuretic. Used in chronic bronchial affections. Dose ♏x. to f℥ss.

4. ACETUM SCILLÆ, L. D. E. ; *Vinegar of Squills.* (Squill, fresh dried, ℥iiss. [℥ij. *D.*], Dilute Acetic Acid, Oj. [℥iv. sp. gr. 1044, *D.*] ; Proof Spirit, ℥iss. [none, *D.*] The relative proportions used by the Edinburgh College are the same as those of a former London Pharmacopœia, except that one-tenth less spirit is employed [viz. Squill, ℥xv. ; Distilled Vinegar, Ovj. ; Proof Spirit, ℥ix.] Macerate the squill with the vinegar, with a gentle heat, in a covered vessel, for three days [seven days, *D. Ed.*] ; afterwards press out [the liquor] and set it by, that the dregs may subside : lastly, add the spirit to the clear liquor.)—A most ancient preparation. Expectorant and diuretic. Used in chronic pulmonary affections and dropsies under the regulations before described. Dose ʒss. to ʒiss. in some aromatic water. It is a constituent of the *Mistura Cascarillæ composita,* Ph. L.

5. OXYMEL SCILLÆ, L. ; *Syrupus Scillæ,* E. D. ; *Oxymel of Squills ; Syrup of Squills.* (Honey, lb. v. ; Vinegar of Squill, Oiiss. Boil down the vinegar with a slow fire to ℥xij., and mix the honey warmed, *L.* The Dublin College orders ℥viij. of Vinegar of Squills to lb. j. of Sugar, and the Edinburgh, Vinegar of Squills, Oiij. ; Pure Sugar, lb. vij. Dissolve the sugar in the vinegar of squills with the aid of a gentle heat [and agitation, *E.*])—Used as an expectorant in chronic catarrhs and asthma, in doses of f℥j. or f℥ij. As an emetic it is sometimes given to children affected with hooping-cough or croup, in doses of a teaspoonful repeated every quarter of an hour until vomiting occurs.

[6. SYRUPUS SCILLÆ, U. S. ; *Syrup of Squills.*—This is directed to be prepared of Vinegar of Squills a pint ; Sugar two pounds. Add the sugar to the vinegar of squill, and proceed in the manner directed for syrup. This preparation is used in place of the preceding as an emetic and expectorant. In affections of the lungs, where squill is beneficial, it may be employed as an ingredient of cough mixtures, variously compounded. As a common remedy for children in cases of cough or cold, it is with safety directed to be used. The dose is f℥ss. to ʒj. or ʒij.

7. SYRUPUS SCILLÆ COMPOSITUS, U. S. ; *Compound Syrup of Squill ; Hive Syrup.*—Take of Squill bruised, Senega bruised, each four ounces ; Tartrate of Antimony and Potassa, forty-eight grains ; Sugar, three pounds and a half. Pour the water upon the squill and senega, and having boiled to one-half, strain, and add the sugar ; then evaporate to three pints, and, while the syrup is still hot, dissolve it in the tartrate of antimony and potassa. Another mode of preparation is, to take of squill in coarse powder, Senega in coarse powder, each four ounces ; Tartrate of Antimony and Potassa, forty-eight grains ; Alcohol, half a pint ; Water, a sufficient quantity ; Sugar, three pounds and a half. Mix the alcohol with two pints and a half of water, and macerate the squill and senega in the mixture for twenty-four hours. Put the whole in an apparatus for displacement, and add as much water as may be necessary to make the filtered liquor amount to three pints. Boil the liquor for a few minutes, evaporate to one-half, and strain ; then add the sugar, and evaporate until the resulting syrup measures three pints. Lastly, dissolve the tartrate of antimony and potassa in the syrup, while it is still hot.

This preparation is a modification of that made according to the formula given by Dr. J. R. Coxe, and which goes by the name *Coxe's Hive Syrup*. In the former editions of the Pharmacopœia, the formula of Dr. Coxe was adopted; and as honey was substituted for sugar, it had the officinal name of *Mel Scillæ compositum*. The formula above cited authorises the substitution of sugar for honey, as it is less liable, when prepared as directed, to undergo fermentation,—a great desideratum in hot weather. There is no difference between the proportions of the ingredients, so that an equal strength of the two preparations is obtained by both. The latter was introduced in accordance with the recommendation of the Committee of the Philadelphia College of Pharmacy.

This preparation combines the advantages of squill, senega, and tartarised antimony, and is an exceedingly active preparation. In sufficient doses, it operates upon the stomach, producing free vomiting and expectoration. It is used at the commencement of croup, hooping-cough, and catarrhal affections in children, with the view to its evacuant impression. In the inflammatory stages, as an expectorant and nauseant, it may also be employed with advantage, in reduced doses. The dose is from gtt. x. to f3j., according to the age of the child, repeated every ten or fifteen minutes until it vomits. As an expectorant for adults, the dose is gtt. xx. to gtt. xxx.]

ANTIDOTE.—No antidote is known for Squills. The first object, therefore, in a case of poisoning, is to evacuate the stomach; the second, to allay the inflammatory symptoms which may supervene.

63. ALLIUM SATIVUM, *Linn.*—COMMON OR CULTIVATED GARLIC.

Sex. Syst. Hexandria, Monogynia.

(Bulbus. *L. D.*—Bulb, *E.*)

HISTORY.—This plant was well known to the ancients. The Greeks called it σκόροδον;[1] the Romans *Allium*.[2] It was used by Hippocrates.[3]

BOTANY. **Gen. Char.**—*Flowers* umbellate, with a membranous *spathe*. *Perianth* 6-parted, permanent, equal. *Stamens* inserted into the base of the perianth; *filaments* either all alike, or every other one tricuspidate, with the *anther* on the middle point. *Style* subulate, *stigma* simple. *Capsule* usually obtusely 3-cornered, or 3-lobed, depressed, 3-celled, bursting into 3 valves through the dissepiments, and containing 2 or 1 black angular seed in each cell (*Lindley*).

Sp. Char.—*Bulb* surrounded by smaller ones. *Leaves* linear, entire. *Umbel* bulbiferous, globose. *Spathe* ovate, rounded. *Segments of the perianth* ovate, obtuse. *Pistil* and *stamens* exsert.[4] *Stem* about 2 feet high. *Flowers* whitish.

---

[1] Theophrastus, *Hist. Plant.* lib. vii. cap. iv. ; Dioscorides, lib. ii. cap. 182.
[2] Pliny, *Hist. Nat.* lib. xix. cap. 31, ed. Valp.
[3] *De victûs ratione in acutis,* p. 404, ed. Fœsii.
[4] De Candolle, *Bot. Gall.*

Hab.—? South of Europe. ? Egypt. ? Persia. Cultivated in kitchen gardens. It flowers in July.

DESCRIPTION.—The *bulb* (*bulbus allii*) is composed of *cloves* (*spicæ vel nuclei allii*), each furnished with its proper envelopes. Its odour is strong, irritating, and characteristic : its taste is acrid.

COMPOSITION.—Cadet[1] analysed garlic. He found the constituents to be *acrid volatile oil, extractive* (a little), *gum, woody fibre, albumen,* and *water.* The ashes contained alkaline and earthy salts. Bouillon-Lagrange has detected, besides these, *sulphur, starch,* and *saccharine matter.*[2]

OIL OF GARLIC (*Oleum Allii*) is a sulphuret of allyle, $AllS = C^6H^5,S$ (see Vol. i. p. 225). According to Wertheim,[3] oxide of allyle, $AllO = C^6H^5,O$, also exists in the crude oil. Oil of garlic has a very acrid taste, a strong smell, and a yellow colour. It is heavier than water, and is soluble in alcohol. As it contains sulphur, it produces, in burning, sulphurous acid. According to Cadet, 20 lbs. of garlic yielded only six drachms of essential oil ; Wertheim obtained between three and four ounces from 1 cwt. of garlic. It strikes a black colour when rubbed with oxide of iron. It is a powerful irritant, and when applied to the skin causes irritation. The Hindoos, according to Dr. Ainslie,[4] prepare a stimulating expressed oil from garlic, which they give internally in ague, and use externally in palsy and rheumatism.

PHYSIOLOGICAL EFFECTS.—Garlic is a local irritant. When swallowed, it operates as a tonic and stimulant to the stomach. Its volatile oil becomes absorbed, quickens the circulation, occasions thirst, and is thrown out of the system by the different excretories, the activity of which it promotes, and to whose excretions it communicates its well-known odour. Large doses occasion nausea, vomiting, and purging. Puihn[5] says the expressed juice has proved fatal.

USES.—Employed by the cook as a flavouring ingredient in various made-dishes, sauces, &c. Rarely used by the medical practitioner. Internally it has been exhibited as a stimulant and stomachic in enfeebled digestion; as an expectorant in old chronic catarrhs ; as a diuretic in atonic dropsies; and as an anthelmintic. Externally it has been employed as a resolvent in indolent tumours ; as a local irritant or rubefacient applied to the feet to cause revulsion from the head or chest; as an antispasmodic liniment (composed of oil and garlic juice) in infantile convulsions; as a remedy for some cases of deafness, a clove or a few drops of the juice being introduced into the ear.

ADMINISTRATION.—A clove may be swallowed either entire, or, more conveniently, cut into small pieces. The dose of the fresh bulbs is one or two drachms. The expressed juice mixed with sugar, the infusion of garlic, and a syrup, is sometimes employed.

[SYRUPUS ALLII.—Take of fresh Garlic, sliced, six ounces ; diluted Acetic Acid, a pint ; Sugar, two pounds. Macerate the garlic in the dilute acetic acid in a glass vessel for four days, then express the liquor, and set it by that the dregs may subside. Add the sugar to the clear liquor, and proceed in the manner directed for Syrup.

[1] Gmelin, *Handb. d. Chem.* ii. 1336.
[2] *Journ. de Pharm.* t. ii. p. 358.
[3] *Ann. d. Chem. u. Pharm.* Bd. li. S. 289, 1844 ; *Pharmaceutical Journal,* vol. iv. p. 325, 1845.
[4] *Materia Indica,* i. 151.
[5] Quoted by Wibmer, *Die Wirk. d. Arzneim.*

This formula was adopted upon the recommendation of Mr. Daniel B. Smith, of Philadelphia, who demonstrated the futility of the old method of preparing syrup of garlic, of which formula (*Journal of Philadelphia College of Pharmacy*, No. 1, p. 50) it is a modification. Dose, ʒj.]

64. ALLIUM CEPA, *Linn.*—THE ONION.

Sex. Syst. Hexandria, Monogynia.

(Bulbus, *D.*)

History.—The onion was known and used in the most ancient times. By Fraas[1] it is considered to be the κρόμμυον (see *ante,*) of Theophrastus[2] and Dioscorides.[3] The σητάνιον of Theophrastus was a variety of onion. By Pliny[4] the onion is called *cepa.* It was employed in medicine by Hippocrates. An onion taken from the hand of an Egyptian mummy, perhaps 2000 years old, has been made to grow.[5]

Botany. **Gen. Char.**—Vide *Allium sativum.*

Sp. Char.—*Stem* fistulous, ventricose beneath; longer than the terete, fistulous *leaves. Umbel* capsuliferous, globose. *Segments of perianth* linear-elliptic, obtuse, shorter than the stamens and pistil.[6] Biennial. *Flowers* whitish. July.

Loudon[7] enumerates eighteen varieties deserving of culture.

Hab.—Egypt. Cultivated in kitchen gardens.

Besides *A. sativum* and *A. Cepa*, various other species of *Allium* are also cultivated for culinary purposes; as *A. Porrum, the Leek; A. ascalonicum, the Shallot; A. Schœnoprasum, the Chive;* and *A. Scorodoprasum* or *Rocambole.* Their virtues are analogous to those of the onion and garlic.

Description.—The bulb (*bulbus*) is tunicated. When cut, it evolves an acrid principle having a well-known odour and a powerful action on the eyes, causing a flow of tears. Its taste is sweet and acrid. *Onion juice* is colourless, but by exposure to the air it becomes reddish.

Composition.—According to Fourcroy and Vauquelin,[8] the onion contains *an acrid volatile oil, uncrystallisable sugar, gum, woody fibre, albumen, acetic* and *phosphoric acids, phosphate* and *citrate of lime,* and *water.*

Oil of Onions (*Oleum Cepæ*) contains sulphur, and is probably similar in composition to oil of garlic, AllS=C⁶H⁵,S. It is acrid, piquant, and colourless.

Physiological Effects.—Analogous to those of garlic, but milder. The oil becomes absorbed, and communicates the well-known onion odour to the breath. By boiling onions the volatile oil is dissipated, and the bulb is deprived of its irritating qualities, and becomes a mild esculent substance.

Uses.—Extensively used as an article of food and as a condiment. It is very rarely employed in medicine, but is adapted to the same cases as garlic.

---

[1] *Synops. Plant. Fl. Class.* p. 291, 1845.
[2] *Hist. Plant.* lib. vii. cap. 4.
[3] Lib. ii. cap. 181.
[4] *Hist. Nat.* lib. xix. cap. 32, ed. Valp.
[5] Müller's *Physiol.* by Baly, vol. i. p. 29.
[6] *Botanicon Gallicum.*
[7] *Encyclopædia of Gardening.*
[8] *Ann. Chim.* lxv. 161, 1808.

Raw onions are occasionally taken as an expectorant, with advantage, by elderly persons affected with winter cough.

ADMINISTRATION.—A roasted onion is sometimes employed as an emollient poultice to suppurating tumours, or to the ear to relieve ear-ache. The expressed juice has been given to children, mixed with sugar, as an expectorant.

65. Asparagus officinalis, *Linn.*—Common Asparagus.

Sex. Syst. Hexandria, Monogynia.

(Turiones et Radix.)

A well-known indigenous culinary vegetable, which is extensively cultivated in gardens for its young succulent shoots (*turiones asparagi*), which, when boiled, form a much-admired article of food. These, as well as the root (*radix asparagi*), have been used in medicine.

The shoots have been chemically examined by Robiquet,[1] who found in their juice *asparagin, mannite, peculiar aqueous extractive, green acrid oleo-resinous matter, wax, gluten, albumen, colouring matter,* and *salts of potash and lime.*

Dulong[2] analysed the root, and found in it *albumen, gum, a peculiar matter* (precipitable by basic acetate of lead and protonitrate of mercury), *resin, saccharine matter* (reddened by oil of vitriol), and *salts of potash and lime.* He detected neither asparagin nor mannite.

Asparagin (also called *asparamid, althæin,* and *agédoil*) crystallises in right rhombic prisms,[3] whose formula is $C^8H^8N^2O^6+2HO$. When heated to 248° F. they lose 12 per cent. of water. They have a cooling, somewhat nauseous taste, are slightly soluble in cold water, more so in boiling water, but are insoluble in alcohol and ether. By the action of acids and alkalies, aided by heat, asparagin is resolved into *aspartic acid,* $C^8H^5NO^6$, and ammonia, NH^3. Asparagin is found in the urine of those who have swallowed it.

The young shoots act as diuretics, and communicate a peculiar fetid odour[4] to the urine. This is produced neither by the asparagin nor by the volatile matter contained in the distilled water of the shoots, but by something which resides in the aqueous extract.[5] Formerly an emmenagogue and aphrodisiac property was ascribed to asparagus.

The medicinal properties of the root are similar to those of the shoots. Like the latter, it communicates an unpleasant odour to the urine. It formed one of the *five greater aperient roots* (*radices quinque aperientes majores*) which were formerly used in visceral diseases. The other four were butcher's-broom (*Ruscus aculeatus*), celery or smallage (*Apium graveolens*), parsley (*Petroselinum sativum*), and fennel (*Fœniculum officinale*).

Though no longer contained in our Pharmacopœia, asparagus is still occasionally used as a popular remedy, chiefly as a diuretic in dropsies, and as a lithic.[6] For these purposes the shoots are boiled and used at table; or the root, which is considered superior to the shoots, is taken in the form of an infusion or decoction (prepared by boiling an ounce of the root in a quart of water), which may be taken as a common drink.

---

[1] *Ann. de Chim.* lv. 152; also Thomson's *Chemistry of Organic Bodies—Vegetables,* 1838.

[2] *Journ. de Pharm.* t. xii. p. 278, 1826.

[3] Mr. C. Brooke, *Pharm. Journ.* vol. vi. p. 560, 1847.

[4] Murray (*App. Med.* vol. v. p. 184, 1790) thinks the odour not dissimilar to that of Geranium robertianum.

[5] Plisson et Henry fils, in *Journ. de Pharm.* xvi. 725, 1830.

[6] For some experiments on the solvent power of asparagus juice for urinary calculi, see Lobb's *Treatise on Dissolvents of the Stone,* 1739.

66. Polygonatum vulgare, *Desf.*—Solomon's Seal.

Sex. Syst. Hexandria, Monogynia.

(Rhizoma.)

Convallaria polygonatum, Linn.—A well-known indigenous plant, whose rhizome (*radix polygonati*), though long banished from the Pharmacopœia, is still kept in the herb-shops and sold as *Solomon's Seal* (*Sigillum Salomonis*). I suspect that the rhizome of *P. multiflorum* is also sold under the same name. When neither species is to be obtained, bryony root is commonly substituted.

Solomon's seal is a white fleshy odourless rhizome, having a sweetish, mucilaginous, very slightly bitterish, acrid taste. Iodine applied to the fresh-cut surface of the rhizome gathered in September, does not darken it. In these properties the rhizomes of both the above-mentioned species of Polygonatum agree. Walz[1] examined chemically the herb, stem, and root of *P. multiflorum.* He found in them asparagin, uncrystallised sugar, starch, gum, gluten, peculiar nitrogenous matter, acrid resin, pectin, malic, citric, hydrochloric, and phosphoric acids, potash, magnesia, lime, and alumina.

Solomon's seal is a popular application to bruised parts (the eye, for example) to remove the marks. For this purpose it is scraped and applied to the parts. Gerarde[2] says it "taketh away in one night, or two at most, any bruse, blacke or blew spots gotten by falls or women's wilfulness, in stumbling upon their hastie husbands' fists."

67. Dracæna Draco, *Linn.*

Sex. Syst. Hexandria, Monogynia.

This tree, which has the habit of a palm, is a native of the Canary Islands. Its stem yields by incision a red juice, which concretes and forms a red resin resembling *dragon's blood* (see *ante*, p. 151), which appears to have been collected by the Spaniards when they took possession of those islands. Hence this species has usually passed for one of the sources of dragon's blood; but none of the commercial article is obtained from it. Indeed, Guibourt[3] states that at the present time it is impossible to obtain the smallest quantity of it at the Canary Islands.

One of the Dracæna trees growing at Orotava has long been celebrated for its great size and age; and next to the Baobab trees (*Adansonia digitata*), it is regarded as one of the oldest inhabitants of the earth.[4]

68. Xanthorrhœa, *Smith.*

Sex. Syst. Hexandria, Monogynia.

(Resina.)

The *Xanthorrhœas* or *Grass Trees* of Australia differ considerably in habit from the other Liliaceæ. Their stems are usually shrubby and resiniferous; their leaves long, narrow, grass-like, and in tufts; and their flowers small, white, and densely crowded on long cylindrical spikes like those of bullrushes (*Typha*). Mr. Brown[5] has described seven species, viz. *X. arborea, australis, Hastile, media, minor, bracteata,* and *Pumilio.* The two first are arborescent, the third and fourth have short stems, and the three last are stemless.

---

[1] *Jahrb. f. pr. Pharm.* vi. 15 ; vii. 17. (Wittstein's *Vollstand. etym. chem. Handwörterbuch,* Bd. i. S. 360, 1847.)

[2] *Herball.* 1633.

[3] *Hist. Nat. des Drogues,* 4ème édit. t. ii. p. 145.

[4] Humboldt, *Tabl. de la Nature.* See also *Ann. des Scien. Nat.* t. xiv. p. 137.

[5] *Prodromus Floræ Novæ Hollandiæ,* 1810. One of the arborescent species (probably *X. arborea*) is called *black boy* (Drummond, in Hooker's *Journal of Botany,* vol. ii. p. 344, 1840).

Two resins, both the produce of this genus, have been imported into this country—one yellow, the other red.

1. The *yellow resin of Xanthorrhœa*, known by the various names of *yellow resin of New Holland* (*resina lutea novi Belgii*), *Botany Bay resin*, and *acaroid resin* or *gum* (*resina* vel *gummi acaroides*), was first noticed by Governor Phillips,[1] in 1789. It is obtained from the trunk of one or more species[2] of Xanthorrhœa by spontaneous exudation.[3] It occurs in more or less rounded tears; in flattened pieces bearing on one side an impression of the stems to which they were attached, and intermixed with portions of wood, stalks, earth, &c.; and in masses of variable size and irregular shape, having, when fractured, a speckled or granitic character. The pure resin is reddish-yellow. Its fresh-fractured surface resembles that of gamboge: its powder is greenish-yellow. When heated, it emits a vapour having a fragrant odour like that of Tolu or storax. It has been repeatedly subjected to chemical examination; viz. by Lichtenstein,[4] Schrader,[5] Laugier,[6] Widmann,[7] Trommsdorff,[8] and more recently by Stenhouse.[9] It consists essentially of *resin, cinnamic acid*, a small quantity of *benzoic acid*, and a trace of *volatile oil*. Some samples contain a small quantity of *bassorine*. Heated with peroxide of manganese and oil of vitriol, it evolves the odour of the oil of bitter almonds. Its alcoholic solution yields, on the addition of water, a yellow precipitate soluble in caustic potash. By the action of nitric acid it yields so large a portion of carbazotic acid, that it is likely to prove the best source of that acid. As it sometimes resembles Tolu and storax in composition, so it probably resembles them also in its medicinal properties. Mr. Kite[10] employed it in several diseases. He says it neither vomits, purges, nor binds the belly; nor does it act materially as a diuretic or diaphoretic. More recently Dr. Fish[11] has employed it in the form of tincture, with opium, in *fluxus hepaticus* and the colliquative diarrhœa of phthisis. On account of its resemblance in composition to the balsams, it deserves a trial in chronic catarrhs. A *tincture* of New Holland resin is prepared by digesting the resin in rectified spirit: Kite used equal parts of resin and spirit; Fish, 2 ounces of resin to lb. j. of spirit. The dose of the tincture is ʒj. or ʒij. in milk or mucilaginous mixture.—It might be used as a substitute for, or mixed with, other substances in the preparation of fumigating pastiles.

2. The *red resin of Xanthorrhœa* is sometimes imported under the name of *black-boy gum*. In colour it somewhat resembles dragon's blood, or Botany Bay kino (*Eucalyptus resinifera*); but many of the pieces, like some of those of the yellow resin of Xanthorrhœa, are marked by the impression of the trunk to which they have adhered. When heated, it evolves a fragrant balsamic odour; and, with the exception of the intermixed and adherent ligneous matters, is completely soluble in rectified spirit. The source of this resin would appear to be *X. Hastile ;* for Viquet (quoted by Nees von Esenbeck[12]) says that this species yields a red resin which resembles dragon's blood.

---

[1] *Voyage to Botany Bay*, 1789.
[2] Smith (Rees's *Cyclop.* vol. xxxix. art. *Xanthorrhœa*) refers it to *X. Hastile* and some other species (see also Bennett's *Wanderings in New South Wales*, &c. 1834). On the other hand, L. Gmelin (*Handb. d. Chem.* ii. 618), on the authority of Sieber, and Mérat and De Lens (*Dict. Mat. Méd.* vi. 970, 1834), on the verbal authority of Mr. R. Brown, refer it to *X. arborea*.
[3] White, *Journal of a Voyage to New South Wales in 1787*, p. 235, 1790.
[4] Crell's *Journal*, ii. 242, 1799 ; also, Thomson's *Chemistry of Organic Bodies—Vegetables.* p. 532.
[5] Trommsdorff's *Journal*, v. 96.
[6] *Ann. de Chimie*, lxxvi. 265.
[7] Buchner's *Repertorium*, xxii. 198, 1825.
[8] *Taschenbuch*, 1826; also, Gmelin, *Handb. d. Chemie*, ii. 618.
[9] *Memoirs of the Chemical Society*, iii. 10, 1848.
[10] *Essays and Observations*, p. 141, 1795.
[11] Dierbach, *Die neuesten Entdeckungen in d. Materia Medica*, Bd. i. S. 225, 1837 ; from the *Boston Journal*, vol. x. p. 94.
[12] Geiger's *Pharmacie*, Bd. ii. S. 178, 2te Aufl. 1839.

††† Flowers with a true perianth adherent to the ovary (*inferior ovary*), usually hermaphrodite.

Order XII. IRIDACEÆ, *Lindl.*— IRIDS, OR CORN-FLAGS.

Irideæ, *Juss.*

Characters.—*Calyx* and *corolla* superior, confounded, their divisions partially cohering, or entirely separate, sometimes irregular, the three petals being occasionally very short. *Stamens* 3, arising from the base of the sepals; *filaments* distinct or connate; *anthers* bursting externally lengthwise, fixed by their base, 2-celled. *Ovary* 3-celled, cells many-seeded; *style* 1; *stigmas* 3, often petaloid, sometimes 2-lipped. *Capsule* 3-celled, 3-valved, with a loculicidal dehiscence. *Seeds* attached to the inner angle of the cell, sometimes to a central column, becoming loose; *albumen* horny, or densely fleshy; *embryo* enclosed within it.—*Herbaceous* plants, or very seldom *under-shrubs*, usually smooth; the hairs, if any, simple. *Roots* tuberous or fibrous. *Leaves* equitant, and distichous in most genera. *Inflorescence* terminal, in spikes, corymbs, or panicles, or crowded, sometimes radical. *Bracts* spathaceous, the partial ones often scarious; the *sepals* occasionally rather herbaceous (*Lindley*).

Properties.—The underground stems and roots usually abound in fecula and mucilage; but these nutritive substances are generally combined with an acrid principle, which excludes their employment as articles of food. However, *Moræa edulis, M. sisyrinchium, Gladiolus edulis*, and a species of *Tigridia*, have been used as esculent substances. The rhizomes of several species of *Iris* (as *I. pseudo-acorus, I. germanica, I. sibirica*, and *I. versicolor*) are remarkable, especially in the fresh state, for their acridity, in consequence of which some of them have been used as purgatives, sialogogues, or errhines, or for issue-peas. The rhizomes of some species (as *I. florentina* and *I. germanica*) have an agreeable smell. The colour and the odour of saffron are to be regarded as part of the petaloid qualities of the stigmata of *Crocus*. The effects of this medicine on the nervous system are regarded by De Candolle[1] as similar to those of [certain odorous] flowers.

69. CROCUS SATIVUS, *Allioni.*—THE SAFFRON CROCUS.

Sex. Syst. Triandria, Monogynia.
(Stigmata exsiccata, *L.*—Stigmata, *E. D.*)

History.—Saffron is mentioned in the Old Testament.[2] Homer[3] speaks of the *crocus* (κρόκος). Hippocrates[4] employed saffron in uterine and other maladies. The word *saffron* (*za'faran*) is probably of Persian origin.

Botany. **Gen. Char.**—*Perianth* [coloured], with a slender tube twice as long as the limb; limb 6-partite, equal, erect. [*Stamens* 3, inserted into the tube; *anthers* sagittate.] *Stigmas* 3, thick, convoluted, generally crested. *Capsule* under ground, elevated by a short peduncle from the root, which peduncle elongates after the decay of the flowers, and the capsules appear above ground (*Hooker*, with some additions).

Sp. Char.—*Stigma* protruded, drooping, in 3 deep linear divisions (*Hooker*).

Cormus roundish; its brownish coats reticulated, separating superiorly into distinct parallel fibres. *Leaves* linear, with a white central stripe, and

---

[1] *Essai sur les Propriétés Méd.*
[2] *Solomon's Song,* iv. 14.
[3] *Iliad,* xiv. 346.
[4] *Opera,* ed. Fœs. pp. 407, 575, 614, 626, and 876.

surrounded at their base with long membranous sheaths. *Flowers* light purple, shorter than the leaves, with a 2-valved membranous spathe. *Anthers* pale yellow. *Stigmas* deep orange-coloured.

Hab.—A native of Asia Minor. Now naturalised in England, France, and some other European countries. It is a doubtful native of the Eastern parts of Europe. It is said to have been introduced into Spain by the Arabs.[1] It flowers in September and October.

PREPARATION.—The flowers are gathered in the morning, and the stigmata, with a portion of the style, plucked out for use, the rest of the flower being thrown away. The stigmata are then dried on paper, either by means of portable kilns over which a hair-cloth is stretched,[2] or in a room by the sun.[3] When dried between paper under the pressure of a thick board and weights, the saffron is formed into cakes now no longer to be met with.

DESCRIPTION.—The only saffron now found in the shops is that called *hay saffron*. The article sold as *cake saffron* is in reality not saffron.

Hay saffron (*crocus in fœno*) consists of the stigmas, with part of the style, which have been very carefully dried. They are from an inch to an inch and a half long, thin, brownish-red ; the upper portion (stigma) is expanded, notched at the extremity ; the lower portion, which constitutes part of the style (called by Th. Martius[4] *Föminelle*) is narrow, capillary, yellowish. The odour is penetrating, aromatic, and, of large quantities, narcotic. The taste is bitter, somewhat aromatic. When chewed, saffron tinges the mouth and the saliva yellow. I find by careful examination that one grain of good commercial saffron contains the stigmata and styles of nine flowers ; hence 4,320 flowers are required to yield one ounce of saffron.

α. *English saffron* (*crocus anglicus*) is no longer found in commerce.

β. *Spanish saffron* (*crocus hispanicus*) constitutes the best saffron of the shops. It is imported from Gibraltar (principally), Cadiz, Denia, Santander, and Malaga. [For some years past the importations have been chiefly from Cadiz, and less frequently from the other ports mentioned by the author.—ED.] From the concurrent accounts of pharmacologists it would appear that formerly Spanish saffron was spoiled by being dipped in oil to preserve it. But the saffron now imported from Spain has not been subjected to this treatment. Occasionally Spanish, as well as any other kind of saffron, is oiled by the dealers to give it an appearance of freshness.

γ. *French saffron* (*crocus gallicus*) is usually considered in commerce to be of second quality. It is the produce of Gatinais ((*Gatinais saffron*) and Orléanais, which comprehend part of the departments of Seine-et-Marne and Eure-et-Loire, and the whole of the department of Loiret. The saffron of Angoulême is intermixed with the pale styles, and is the worst.[5] French saffron is shipped for England at Calais, Boulogne, and Havre.

[After the French saffron, by far the most important description is—

δ. The Neapolitan, which is cultivated in the province of Aquila, in consequence of which it is known in all the Italian markets by the name of *Aquila saffron*. It is rather more plump than the Spanish, but contains more yellow petals, and is therefore hardly as valuable. It is packed into small leather bags of 40 to 50 lbs.

ε. The produce of Austria and Bavaria is so small, that it is only to be met with in the locality of its growth.

ζ. The oriental saffron, on the continent known by the name of *Macedonian*, is very ordinary and coarse, and always quite wet, from honey being mixed with it. In conse-

---

[1] Dillon, *Travels through Spain.*
[2] Douglas, *Phil. Trans.* for 1728.
[3] Fiske, *Stephenson and Churchill's Med. Bot.* vol. iii.
[4] *Pharmakognosie*, 1832.
[5] Guibourt, *Histoire des Drog.* ii. 194, 4ème édit. 1849.

quence of its inferior quality it found at last no buyers, and the article may be considered obsolete.—Ed.]

Besides the preceding, several other varieties of saffron are mentioned by pharmacologists, but they are not distinguished in English commerce, and I am unacquainted with them. Such are *Austrian, Bavarian, Oriental,* and the *Sicilian saffron (C. austriacus, bavaricus, orientalis,* and *siciliensis)* mentioned by Murray,[1] Geiger,[2] and others. The saffron of Lower Austria is said to be the best and most costly in Europe, but the produce is scarcely sufficient for the home consumption; and, therefore, saffron is imported into Austria. Austrian saffron is chiefly produced at Ravelsbach, Meissau, Eggendorf, Kirchbeg, and Wagram.[3]

From the Customs report[4] it appears that saffron is occasionally imported into England from Hamburgh, Antwerp, Genoa, and Bombay; but I am ignorant of its place of growth and quality. According to Gussone,[5] *Crocus odorus* yields Sicilian saffron. Dioscorides[6] considered the saffron of Corycus (a mountain of Cilicia, in Asia Minor, now called *Curco*) to be the best, and that of Lycia and Olympus to be of second quality; while Cyrenaic saffron, as well as that from Centuripinum (*Centorbe*) in Sicily, he declares to be the worst.

[X. Landerer, of Athens, states that on the continent of Greece, as well as on the islands of the Archipelago, the stigmata of *Crocus Spruneri, sativus, vernus, luteus,* and *variegatus,* are gathered and sold as saffron (*safora*). In the whole of Greece about 30 to 40 lbs. are annually gathered; but much more is brought from Macedonia and Thracia, where the saffron is said to be taken from the *Crocus aureus,* but mixed with the petals of Crocus and Calendula.

It is sold in the bazaars of Smyrna, Thessalonica, and Gallipolis. A large quantity of saffron, about 30,000 litres annually, is brought by Persian small dealers to the so-called misir bazaars in Constantinople, *i. e.* the bazaars where all the products from the interior of Asia Minor, from Egypt and the Caucasus, are sold.[7]—Ed.]

Cake saffron (crocus in placentâ) was formerly prepared by compressing hay saffron. But the cakes now met with in the inferior shops are composed of Safflower (*Carthamus tinctorius*) and gum-water, made into a paste, and rolled out on a tin plate with a rolling-pin into oval cakes of 11 inches long, 10 inches broad, and about one-tenth of an inch thick. These are dried on brown paper in a stove. They are shining, and of a brownish-red colour. I can detect neither saffron nor marigolds (*Calendula officinalis*) in them. Their price is considerably less than that of good hay saffron. I am informed by a maker of cake saffron that there is only another person besides himself by whom this substance is made in London.

ADULTERATION.—To increase the weight of saffron, it is said to be sometimes intermixed with *sand* or *grains of lead.* To detect these it is sufficient to scatter the saffron loosely over a sheet of white paper, when the sand or grains of lead fall out.

To give saffron flexibility and an appearance of freshness, as well as to augment its weight, it is sometimes damped or oiled. To detect either *water* or *oil,* a small portion of saffron should be subjected to pressure between folds of white blotting paper: if this become either moistened or greased, the adulteration is obvious.

Another adulteration practised on saffron is intermixing it with the petals of some plant,—usually of *safflower (Carthamus tinctorius),* which is some-

[1] *App. Med.* vol. v.
[2] *Handb. der Pharm.*
[3] *Pharmaceutical Journal,* vol. viii. p. 171, 1848.
[4] *Trade List* for 1837-8-9.
[5] Lindley, *Flora Medica.*
[6] Lib. i. cap. xxv.
[7] [*Pharm. Journ.* vol. x. page 198.]

times called *bastard saffron*. The safflower readily escapes the eye of a superficial observer. If rubbed with the moistened finger on paper, it produces a slightly yellow mark only, whereas genuine saffron causes a very intense orange-yellow stain. The fraud may also be detected by carefully examining the suspected portion by a magnifying glass. The fraud is the more easily detected if the suspected saffron be previously macerated in hot water. Genuine saffron consists of a filiform style, divided at one extremity into 3 long, convoluted, deep orange stigmata, which are a little dilated upwards, and notched at the extremity. Safflower, on the other hand, is composed of florets, each consisting of a monopetalous, tubular, 5-toothed red corolla, inclosing 5 syngenesious stamina and a style. Moreover, the corolla is devoid of the softness and flexibility of the stigmata of saffron; but is, on the contrary, dry and brittle.

Other florets or strips of petals artificially dyed to give them colour, and greased with oil to render them supple, have been employed to adulterate saffron. Guibourt mentions the *marigold* (*Calendula officinalis*), *arnica*, and *soapwort* (*Saponaria*), as having been used for this purpose. By attention to the above-mentioned characters of saffron, the fraud may be readily detected. The dilated extremities of the stigmata of saffron are broader than the style; whereas the extremities of the divisions of a strip of a petal will usually be found narrower than the body of the strip.

Genuine saffron, from which the colouring matter has been extracted, is sometimes found in commerce.[1] The sample which I have seen had the essential characters of the stigmata of saffron, but wanted the softness and flexibility of good saffron, and was somewhat darker-coloured. It did not present the pale yellow filaments (styles) of ordinary saffron, and imparted no colour to spirit of wine.

Fibres of smoked beef are said to have been used for adulterating saffron.

COMMERCE.—[The quantity of saffron imported into England during the last few years will be seen from the following table :—

In 1849 .... 19,430 lbs. | In 1851 .... 9,538 lbs. | In 1853 .... 18,261 lbs.
" 1850 .... 16,575 " | " 1852 .... 23,554 " | " 1854 .... 5,300 "

It is brought over in cases, barrels, and boxes.—ED.]

COMPOSITION.—Saffron was analysed in 1811 by Vogel and Bouillon-Lagrange,[2] and in 1818 by Aschoff.[3]

	Vogel and Bouillon-Lagrange.	Aschoff.
Volatile oil	7·5	1·4
Wax	0·5	4·0
Polychroite..	65·0	52·0
Gum	6·5	10·4
Soluble albumen	0·5	—
Woody fibre	10·0	19·0
Water...	10·0	10·0
Balsamic matter, soluble in ether and alcohol...	—	2·0
Saffron.................................	100·0	98·8

[1] *Pharmaceutical Journal*, vol. iii. p. 341, 1843.
[2] *Bull. de Pharm.* iv. 89.
[3] Gmelin, *Handb. d. Chem.* ii. 1334.

1. Volatile Oil of Saffron (*Oleum Croci*).—Obtained by distilling saffron with water. It is yellow, heavier than water, has a burning, acrid, somewhat bitter taste, and is slightly soluble in water. By keeping, it becomes white, solid, and lighter than water. On it depend probably the medicinal properties of saffron.

2. Colouring Matter: *Polychroite* (so called from πολύς, *many*, and χρόα, *colour*, in consequence of its being susceptible of numerous changes of colour).—By digesting the aqueous extract of saffron in alcohol, and evaporating the tincture to dryness, a substance is obtained which Bouillon-Lagrange and Vogel called *polychroite*, but which Henry[1] has separated into volatile oil and a bitter red substance (*polychroite properly so called*). Pure polychroite is pulverulent, bitter, scarlet-red, odourless, slightly soluble in cold water, much more so in hot water, readily soluble in alcohol and oils (both fixed and volatile), slightly soluble in ether. Sulphuric acid turns it blue, then lilac. Nitric acid makes it green, but the colour is very fugitive. The hypochlorites destroy the yellow colour of a solution of polychroite.

Chemical Characteristics.—An aqueous infusion of saffron gives no indication of starch on the addition of a solution of iodine. The hypochlorites bleach it. Sulphuric and nitric acids act on it as on polychroite above mentioned. Acetate of lead causes no precipitate. By evaporation, the infusion yields an extract from which alcohol removes the colouring matter and leaves a gummy substance.

Physiological Effects.—Formerly saffron was considered to be cordial, aromatic, narcotic, and emmenagogue. Some[2] have accused it of causing laughing delirium; others[3] have ascribed to its use great mental dejection; and several[4] have declared that they have seen immoderate uterine hemorrhage produced by it, which, in the case referred to by Riverius, is said to have terminated fatally. But modern experience has proved that most of these statements are erroneous. Alexander[5] swallowed four scruples of saffron without perceiving any obvious effects therefrom; and Wibmer[6] took a drachm without observing the slightest effect.

By the long-continued use of saffron, the colouring particles become absorbed, and tinge the secretions, especially the urine and perspiration. In some instances the *fœtus in utero* has been stained by it.[7] The failure of Alexander to detect the yellow tinge in his secretions arose probably from the short time he had been using this medicine. Mr. Gibson[8] gave a considerable quantity of saffron to a pigeon, which thereby had its fæces tinged; yet no perceptible alteration was produced in its bones.

Headache, prostration of strength, apoplexy, and even death, have been ascribed to the inhalation of the vapour arising from large quantities of saffron;[9] and perhaps correctly so, for it is well known that the odours of other plants (as the rose, the pink, &c.) act on some individuals as narcotic poisons.[10]

Uses.—Saffron is employed, especially on the continent, as a flavouring and colouring ingredient in various culinary preparations, articles of con-

---

[1] *Journ. de Pharm.* vii. 397.
[2] Boerhaave, *Hist. Plant.* pars ii. p. 590.
[3] Bergius, *Mat. Med.* t. i. p. 38.
[4] Boerhaave, *op. cit.*; Riverius, *Op. Med.*
[5] *Experim. Essays*, p. 88, 1768.
[6] *Wirk. d. Arzneim.* Band ii. S. 204.
[7] Wibmer, *op. cit.*
[8] *Mem. of the Lit. and Phil. Soc. of Manchester*, 2d ser. vol. i. p. 148.
[9] See the *Reports* of Borellus, Tralles, Forster, and others, quoted by Wibmer and Murray, *op. cit.*
[10] Orfila, *Toxicol. Gén.*

fectionery, liqueurs, &c. It was used by the ancients as a perfume as well as a seasoning agent.[1]

In the modern practice of medicine it is used chiefly as a colouring ingredient. It is a popular remedy for assisting the eruption of exanthematous diseases,—on the same principle, I suppose, that bird-fanciers give it to birds when moulting. It was at one time esteemed as an antispasmodic in asthma, hysteria, and cramp of the stomach; and was formerly used as an emmenagogue, and to promote uterine contractions and the lochial discharge. Lastly, it has been employed as a stimulant to the nervous system in hypochondriasis.

ADMINISTRATION.—It may be given in doses of from ten grains to a drachm in the form of powder or pill. It is popularly used in the form of infusion or *tea*.

1. SYRUPUS CROCI, L. E. D.; *Syrup of Saffron.* (Saffron, ʒv.; Boiling Distilled Water, Oj.; Sugar, lb. iij.; Rectified Spirit, ʒiiss. Macerate the saffron in the water for twelve hours, in a vessel lightly covered; then strain the liquor, and proceed as ordered for the Syrupus Althææ. [The Edinburgh College orders ʒx. of Saffron to the Sugar, &c., as in the former London Pharmacopœia. The Dublin formula is as follows:—Saffron, ʒss.; Boiling Distilled Water, Oj.; Refined Sugar, a sufficiency. The saffron is ordered to macerate twelve hours, to be boiled five minutes, and strained by expression. The clear liquor is decanted, and twice its weight of sugar added and dissolved.]) —It is employed principally for its colour.

2. TINCTURA CROCI, E. D.; *Tincture of Saffron.* (Saffron chopped fine, ʒij.; Proof Spirit, Oij. [Oj. *D.*] This tincture is to be prepared like tincture of cinchona, either by percolation or by digestion, the former method being the more convenient and expeditious. [The Dublin College macerates the saffron fourteen days, and filters.])—Used as a colouring liquid. It is also employed as a stimulant and emmenagogue in doses of from fʒj. to fʒij.

As a colouring and flavouring ingredient, saffron is a constituent of several other preparations.

70. Iris florentina, *Linn.*—Florentine Orris.

Sex. Syst. Triandria, Monogynia.

(Rhizoma.)

The *orris root (radix iridis florentinæ)* of the shops consists of the rhizomes of three species of Iris; namely, *I. florentina, I. pallida,* and *I. germanica.*[2] They acquire their well-known violet odour while drying. They are brought to us in the decorticated state, in casks, from Leghorn and Trieste.

Orris root consists, according to Vogel,[3] of *volatile oil, acrid resin, astringent extractive, gum, starch,* and *ligneous matter.* Raspail[4] detected in it crystals, which he considered to

---

[1] Beckmann, *History of Inventions and Discoveries.* vol. i. p. 278.
[2] According to Savi, orris root is collected in Italy indiscriminately from the three species named in the text. (F. G. Hayne, *Getreue Darst. u. Beschreib. der in d. Arzneykunde gebraucht. Gewächse,* Bd. xi. 1830.)
[3] *Journ. de Pharm.* i. 481.
[4] *Chim. Organ.*

be those of *oxalate of lime.* The starch of orris root[1] consists of elliptical-shaped particles, which form interesting objects for the polarising microscope. Some of them consist of two mullar-shaped particles applied base to base. Most of them are cracked at the hilum, and even at their edges. Schleiden[2] describes the starch particles of *Iris florentina* and kindred species as being perfectly hollow, and apparently cup-shaped.

Orris root is an acrid substance, and in full doses causes vomiting and purging. It is principally used on account of its violet odour. Thus *hair* and *tooth powders, perfumed oils,* &c. are frequently scented with it. Issue peas (*pois d'iris*) have been made of it. During teething, infants are sometimes permitted to rub their gums with, and bite, the rhizome; but the practice is objectionable, since it is not unfrequently attended with irritation of the mouth, and disorder of the stomach and bowels. Furthermore, the danger of the rhizome getting into the œsophagus or trachea is not to be overlooked. One fatal case of this kind is recorded.[3] Powdered orris root is sometimes used as an errhine.

A *tincture of orris root* (*tinctura iridis florentinæ*), prepared by digesting one part of powdered orris root in eight parts of rectified spirit, is used as a scent, and is frequently sold as *essence of violets,* or *eau de violettes.*

ORDER XIII. TACCACEÆ, *Lindley.*

CHARACTERS.—A small and imperfectly-known order of endogenous plants, with tuberous *roots, leaves* with curved parallel veins, hermaphrodite regular *flowers,* a petaloid tubular, 6-parted *periunth,* 6 *stamens,* a 1-celled inferior *ovary,* and *seeds* with fleshy albumen.

PROPERTIES.—The tuberous roots are bitter and acrid, but by cultivation become larger and milder. They yield a large quantity of nutritive farina.

71. Tacca, *Forster.*

Sex. Syst. Hexandria, Monogynia.

(Radix; Farina.)

This genus contains two species, which deserve a short notice.

1. TACCA PINNATIFIDA, Roxb. Fl. Ind. ii. 172.—A native of the Moluccas and Malay countries. The tuberous roots are intensely bitter when raw, but yield a large quantity of beautifully white starch, used for puddings, cakes, and other articles of confectionary. The tubers "are the *tacca youy* of some navigators: they form an article of diet in China and Cochin China, as also in Travancore," where, according to Dr. Ainslie, they attain a large size, and are eaten by the natives with some acid, to subdue their acrimony.[4]

2. TACCA OCEANICA, Nuttal, Amer. Journ. of Pharm. vol. ix. p. 306.—A native of Tahiti and other islands of the South Sea. Until Mr. Nuttal pointed out its peculiarities, it was supposed to be identical with T. pinnatifida. Ellis[5] says that the "*pia,* or arrow root, *chailea tacca*" grows on the high sandy banks near the sea, or on the sides of the lower mountains.

---

[1] The following measurements, in parts of an English inch, of particles of starch of orris root were made for me by Mr. George Jackson :—

Particles.	Length.	Breadth.	Particles.	Length.	Breadth.
1	0·0011	0·0010	5	0·0004	0·0004
2	0·0012	0·0006	6	0·0003	0·0002
3*	0·0009	0·0006	7	0·0002	0·0002
4	0·0006	0·0004			

The most prevalent-sized particle is marked thus *.

[2] *Principles of Scientific Botany,* pp. 15–16, translated by Ed. Lankester, M.D. 1849.

[3] Kraus, *Heilmittellehre,* S. 541.

[4] Royle, *Illustrations of the Botany of the Himalayan Mountains,* p. 378.

[5] *Polynesian Researches,* vol. i. p. 361, 1829.

The tuberous roots yield a highly nutritious fecula. At Tahiti (Otaheite) this fecula is procured by washing the tubers, scraping off their outer skin, and then reducing them to a pulp by friction on a kind of rasp made by winding coarse twine (formed of the cocoa-nut fibre) regularly round a board.[1] The pulp is washed with sea-water through a sieve made of the fibrous web which protects the young frond of the cocoa-nut palm. The strained liquor is received in a wooden trough in which the fecula is deposited; and the supernatant liquor being poured off, the sediment is formed into balls, which are dried in the sun for 12 or 24 hours, then broken and reduced to powder, which is spread out in the sun to dry.[2]

Tacca starch, or *Tahiti arrow-root*, sometimes called *Otaheite salep*,[3] is imported into London, and sold as " Arrow-root prepared by the native converts at the Missionary stations in the South Sea Islands." It is a white amylaceous powder, with a slightly musty odour. Examined by the microscope, I find it to consist of particles[4] which appear circular, mullar-shaped, or polyhedral. Some of the mullar-shaped particles are slightly narrowed at the base. Moreover, the base of the mullar, instead of being flat, appears to me to be hollowed out. The hilum is small and circular; it cracks in a linear or stellate manner. The rings are few and not very distinct.

This fecula is used as a substitute for the West Indian arrow-root, to which it would probably be equal if it were prepared with equal care. Its composition, like that of other starches, is presumed to be $C^{12}H^{10}O^{10}$.

ORDER XIV. AMARYLLIDACEÆ, *Lindley.*—AMARYLLIDS.

None of the plants of this order are employed in England as articles of the Materia Medica. Yet many of them act powerfully on the system, and one of them (*Hæmanthus toxicarius*) is said to be used by the Hottentots to poison their arrow-heads. The prevailing property of the order is acridity, which is possessed principally by the bulbs, several of which (as those of *Pancratium maritimum* and *Hæmanthus coccineus*) seem to be endowed with properties very similar to those of squill. The leaves and flowers of *Narcissus pseudo-Narcissus* or *Daffodil* are enumerated among the simples of the French *Codex*. In doses of 20 or 30 grains they sometimes cause vomiting. They have been employed in spasmodic affections (as hooping-cough), in diarrhœa, and in agues.[5] Several other species of *Narcissus*, as *N. Tazetta* and *N. odorus*, also possess emetic properties.[6] *Narcissus Tazetta*, the *Italian* or *Polyanthus Narcissus*, is supposed by Dr. Sibthorp to be the Narcissus of the poets. The root and succulent leaves of the *Agava Americana*, or *American aloe*, a native of Tropical America, yield a saccharine juice which lathers like soap, and when fresh is said to be laxative, diuretic, and emmenagogue. By fermentation it yields an acid liquor. The ligneous fibres of the leaves and roots are used as a thread (*pita thread*).

---

[1] Ellis states that the rind of the root is scraped off by a courie shell, and the root then grated on a piece of coral.

[2] Matthews, *Gardener's Magazine*, vol. viii. p. 585, Lond. 1832.

[3] Rees's *Cyclopædia*, art. *Tacca pinnatifida*.

[4] The following measurements, in parts of an English inch, of the particles of Tacca starch, were made for me by Mr. George Jackson:—

Particles.	Length.	Breadth.	Particles.	Length.	Breadth.
1	0·0012	0·0009	4	0·0006	0·0005
2	0·0011	0·0009	5	0·0004	0·0004
3*	0·0008	0·0007	6	0·0003	0·0003

The most prevalent-sized particle is marked thus *.

[5] Mérat and De Lens, *Dict. de Mat. Méd.* t. iv.

[6] De Candolle, *Essai sur les Propriétés Méd.*

Order XV. MUSACEÆ, *Agardh.*

Characters.—*Leaves* with veins curved, and proceeding from the midrib to the margin (*curved-veined*). *Perianth* 6-parted, adherent, petaloid, irregular. *Stamens* normally 6, by abortion usually 5. *Anthers* 2-celled. *Ovary* inferior, 3-celled. *Fruit* 3-celled. *Seed* albuminous.

Properties—An important order of endogens whose fruits (bananas and plantains) form a valuable article of food in some tropical regions.

72. Musa sapientum, *Linn.*—Plantain ; Banana.

Sex. Syst. Pentandria, Monogynia.[1]

(Fructûs amylum.)

Plantains (*Musa paradisiaca*, Linn.) and Bananas (*Musa sapientum*, Linn.) are probably only varieties of the same species. The former have a stem wholly green, and persistent male flowers ; the latter have a spotted stem, deciduous male flowers, and shorter and rounder fruit. Numerous varieties of each are cultivated in the tropical parts of Asia, Africa, and America: the wild parent is found at Chittagong, and other parts of Tropical Asia. The fruit is a berry, and in the unripe state abounds in starch ; but during maturation this disappears, being converted into a mucilaginous substance, and this into sugar ; so that in the ripe fruit not an atom of starch can be detected.[2]

Fig. 83.   Fig. 84.

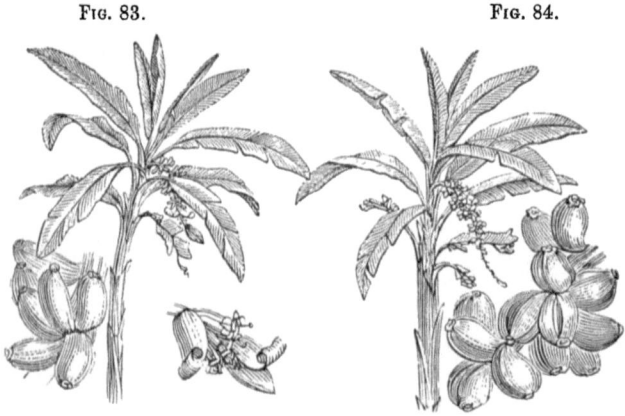

The Plantain.   *The Banana.*

Boussingault[3] analysed the ripe fruit of *Musa paradisiaca*, and found in it *sugar, gum, malic, gallic,* and *pectic acids, albumen,* and *lignin.*

Plantains and bananas form important and valuable articles of food to the inhabitants of many tropical regions. "But for plantains," says Dr. Wright,[4] "Jamaica would scarcely be habitable, as no species of provision could supply their place. Even flour, or bread itself, would be less agreeable and less able to support the laborious negro, so as to enable him to do his business, or to keep in health."

---

[1] I have followed Roxburgh (*Fl. Indica*, vol. i.) in referring this genus to Pentandria, Monogynia. In Reichard's edition of Linnæus's *Systema Plantarum* (1780), it is placed in Polygamia, Monogynia ; and in Loudon's *Encyclopædia of Plants* it is referred to Hexandria, Monogynia.

[2] Avequin, *Journ. de Pharm.* t. xxiv. p. 555, 1838.

[3] *Journ. de Pharmacie,* xxii. 385.

[4] *London Medical Journal,* vol. viii.

Humboldt[1] calculates that as 33 lbs. of wheat and 99 lbs. of potatoes require the same space as that in which 4000 lbs. of bananas are grown, the produce of bananas is consequently to that of wheat as 133·1, and to that of potatoes as 44·1.

Dr. Shier,[2] in an interesting report on the starch-producing plants of British Guiana, has given us some interesting details respecting the plantain. He states that " a new plantain-walk in this colony will yield 450 bunches of 50 lbs. each, of which, as nearly as possible, 50 per cent. will be core, containing 17 per cent. of starch, thus producing 17 cwt. of starch per acre." I am indebted to this gentleman for specimens of the *sliced plantain core dried, plantain meal,* and *plantain starch,* prepared in April 1847.

a. *Sliced Plantain Core.*—The sample sent to me by Dr. Shier was prepared in April 1847. It was obtained by stripping off the husk of the plantain, slicing the core, and drying it in the sun. The dried slices, as I have received them, are segments of circles from $\frac{1}{2}$ to $\frac{3}{4}$ of an inch in diameter, and $\frac{1}{8}$ to $\frac{1}{6}$ of an inch in thickness. Their prevailing tint is whitish, like that of dried slices of colchicum cormi, but marbled with reddish veins. Their odour is fragrant, and somewhat similar to that of orris root. Their taste is farinaceous.

β. *Plantain Meal; Conquin-tay.*—Obtained by powdering and sifting the thoroughly dried sliced plantain core. It is known among the creoles of the colony by the name of *Conquin-tay.* It is a whitish meal, speckled with minute dark-reddish spots. Its odour is fragrant, and similar to that of orris root (Dr. Shier says it resembles fresh hay or tea.) Its taste is bland, like that of common wheat flour. When examined by the microscope it is seen to consist chiefly of starch-grains. According to Dr. Shier's statement, plantain meal contains about 68 per cent. of starch. 100·0 parts of plantain meal yielded Dr. Shier 0·88 parts of nitrogen. If this number be multiplied by 6·5 (see *ante,* p. 71, foot-note), we have 5·72 as the per-centage amount of proteinaceous matter (albumen, gluten, &c.) contained in plantain meal.

It is obvious, therefore, that plantain meal must be greatly superior to the pure starches, inasmuch as it contains blood- and flesh-making principles, which the latter are devoid of. Dr. Shier states that it is easy of digestion, and that it is largely employed in British Guiana as the food of infants, children, and invalids; but it will not serve for the manufacture of maccaroni, as this, when made from it, falls to powder when put into hot water. The same authority tells us that the plantain yields about 20 or 25 per cent. of meal.

γ. *Plantain Starch.*—This is obtained from the plantain by rasping and washing; but owing to the flesh-coloured tissue in which the starch is imbedded being somewhat denser than the latter, it settles below the starch, and it is somewhat difficult to separate completely the finer parts of it from the starch; hence the latter is not perfectly white. The plantain yields about 17 per cent. of starch. Examined by the microscope, I find the starch-grains[3] to be flat transparent discs, like those of the starch of Zingiberaceæ : hence they have but little lateral shading, and, when superimposed, the contour of the lower grains can be seen through the upper ones. Their shape is more or less elliptical and ovate, the extremity at which the so-called nucleus or hilum is placed being narrower than the opposite one. When viewed edgeways their shape appears to be linear, and the lateral shading is stronger. The lines or segments of rings seen on the flat surfaces of the grains do not extend to the edges of the grain, nor do they surround the hilum. When examined by the polarising microscope, these grains present the well-known crosses. In its chemical, dietetical, and medicinal properties, the starch of the plantains agrees with those of other starches.

---

[1] Humboldt's *Pl. Æquinoc.* ; also, *Library of Entertaining Knowledge—Vegetable Substances.*

[2] *Report on the Starch-producing Plants of the Colony of British Guiana,* Demerara, 1847 ; also, *Pharmaceutical Journal,* vol. vii. p. 193, 1847.

[3] The following measurements, in parts of an English inch, of the particles of plantain starch (prepared by Dr. Shier, of Demerara), were kindly made for me by Mr. George Jackson : —

Particles.	Length.	Breadth.	Particles.	Length.	Breadth.
1	0·0020	0·0013	5*	0·0013	0·0008
2	0·0018	0·0009	6	0·0009	0·0006
3	0·0016	0·0010	7	0·0007	0·0005
4*	0·0014	0·0007	8	0·0005	0·0003

The most prevalent-sized particles are marked thus *.

Order XVI. MARANTACEÆ, *Lindl.*

Cannaceæ, *Agardh.*

CHARACTERS.—*Calyx* superior, of 3 sepals, short. *Corolla* tubular, irregular, with the segments in 2 whorls; the *outer* 3-parted, nearly equal, the *inner* very irregular; one of the lateral segments usually coloured, and formed differently from the rest; sometimes by abortion fewer than 3. *Stamens* 3, petaloid, distinct, of which one of the lateral and the intermediate one are either inactive or abortive, and the other lateral one fertile. *Filament* petaloid, either entire or 2-lobed, one of the lobes bearing the anther on its edge. *Anther* 1-celled, opening longitudinally. *Pollen* round (papillose in Canna coccinea, smooth in Calathea zebrina). *Ovary* 1-3-celled; *ovules* solitary and erect, or numerous and attached to the axis of each cell; *style* petaloid or swollen; *stigma* either the mere denuded apex of the style, or hollow, hooded, and incurved. *Fruit* capsular, as in Scitamineæ. *Seeds* round, without aril; *albumen* hard, somewhat floury; *embryo* straight, naked, its *radicle* lying against the hilum. *Herbaceous* tropical plants, destitute of aroma. *Rhizome* often tuberous, and abounding in starch. *Stem* often branching (*Lindley*).

PROPERTIES.—The rhizomes frequently abound in starch.

73. MARANTA ARUNDINACEA, *Linn.*—THE WEST INDIAN ARROW-ROOT.

Sex. Syst. Monandria, Monogynia.

(Arrow-root; Rhizomatis fæcula. *Lond.*—Fecula of the tubers; Arrow-root. *Ed.*)

HISTORY.—This plant was brought from the island of Dominica, by Colonel James Walker, to Barbados, and there planted. From thence it was sent to Jamaica. That gentleman observed that the native Indians used the root against the poison of their arrows, by mashing and applying it to the poisoned wounds.[1]

The valuable properties of the starch made from the root are mentioned by Hughes,[2] in 1751, and the mode of procuring it described by Browne,[3] in 1789.

BOTANY. **Gen. Char.**—*Corolla* unequal, one of the inner segments in the form of a lip. *Stamens* petaloid, with half an anther on its edge. *Style* hooded, adhering to the edge of a sterile filament. *Ovary* 3-celled, smooth: *ovules* solitary. *Fruit* even, dry, 1-seeded.—Caulescent plants with fleshy *rhizomata* or *tubers*. *Stems* branched, often dichotomous. *Inflorescence* terminal, panicled, jointed, with glumaceous, deciduous *bracts* (*Lindley*).

Sp. Char.—*Culm* branched, herbaceous. *Leaves* ovate, lanceolate, somewhat hairy underneath. *Peduncles* 2-flowered (*Willdenow*).

Rhizome white, articulated, tuberous, placed horizontally in the earth, and giving origin to several tuberous jointed stoles (*stolones tuberosi*), similar to itself, but covered with scales. These stoles are often more than a foot long, and curved, so that the points rise out of the earth and become new plants (*Nees* and *Ebermaier*). *Stem* 2 to 3 feet high. *Leaves* alternate, with long, leafy, hairy sheaths. *Flowers* white and small.

---

[1] Sloane's *Jamaica*, vol. i. p. 254.
[2] *The Natural History of Barbados*, p. 221, 1750.
[3] *The Civil and Natural History of Jamaica*, p. 112, 1789.

The *Maranta indica*, Tussac,[1] E., is characterised by its leaves being smooth on both sides, and by its seeds; those of *M. arundinacea* being violet. But, after a careful examination, Wickström declares that Tussac's plant is identical with the *M. arundinacea*, Linn.[2]

Hab.—West Indies. It is cultivated both in the West and East Indies, Ceylon, Sierra Leone, &c.

COMPOSITION OF THE ROOT.—According to P. C. Benzon,[3] the root of the Maranta has the following composition:—*Volatile oil*, 0·07; *gummy extract*, 0·50; *starch*, 26·00; *woody fibre*, 6·00; *albumen*, 1·58; *muriate of lime*, 0 25; and *water*, 65·600.

The per-centage quantity of starch obtained from the root has been thus stated by other authorities:—7·81 (Dr. J. Clark),[4] 12·5 (De Candolle),[5] 21·43 (Dr. Shier,[6] from roots scarcely ripe).

EXTRACTION OF THE FECULA.—The starch, or fecula, is extracted from the roots (tubers) when these are about ten or twelve months old. The process is entirely a mechanical one, and is performed either by hand or by machine.

In Jamaica it is procured as follows:—The tubers are dug up, well washed in water, and then beaten, in large, deep, wooden mortars, to a pulp. This is thrown into a large tub of clean water. The whole is then well stirred, and the fibrous part wrung out by the hands and thrown away. The milky liquor being passed through a hair-sieve, or coarse cloth, is suffered to settle, and the clear water is drained off. At the bottom of the vessel is a white mass, which is again mixed with clean water and drained; lastly, the mass is dried on sheets in the sun, and is pure starch.[7] In Bermuda[8] the roots are first deprived of their paper-like scales, and then rasped by a kind of wheel-rasp (something like fig. 85, p. 229), and the fecula well washed through sieves and carefully dried. Upon the Hopewell estate in the Island St. Vincent,[9] the carefully-skinned tubers are washed, then ground in a mill, and the pulp washed in tinned-copper cylindrical washing-machines. The fecula is subsequently dried in drying houses. In order to obtain the fecula free from impurity, pure water must be used, and great care and attention paid in every step of the process. The skinning or peeling of the tubers must be performed with great nicety, as the cuticle contains a resinous matter, which imparts colour and a disagreeable flavour to the starch. German silver palettes are used for skinning the deposited fecula, and shovels of the same metal for packing the dried fecula. The drying is effected in pans covered by white gauze, to exclude dust and insects.

COMMERCE.—Arrow-root is brought, in tin cases and in barrels and boxes from the West India Islands (Jamaica, Barbados, Antigua, St. Vincent Dominica, Bermuda, St. Kitts, Grenada, Demerara, and Berbice), Calcutta

---

[1] *Journ. Bot.* iii. 41.
[2] Nees v. Esenb. and Eberm. *Handb. d. med.-pharm. Bot.*
[3] Buchner's *Repertorium für die Pharmacie*, Bd. xvi. S. 255, 1823.
[4] *Medical Facts and Observations*, vol. vii. 1797.
[5] *Physiologie Végétale*, t. i. p. 187, 1832.
[6] *Report on the Starch-producing Plants of the Colony of British Guiana*, p. 11, Demerara, 1847.
[7] Wright, *London Medical Journal*, vol. viii.
[8] Cogswell, in Cormack's *Monthly Journal of Medical Science*, vol. v. p. 789, 1845.
[9] *Recent Improvements in Arts and Manufactures*, by A. Ure, M.D. 1844.

and Sierra Leone. The packages of West Indian arrow-root sent to this country are lined with paper attached with arrow-root paste. When sent to this country in the hold of the ship, their contents are easily tainted by noisome effluvia. Arrow-root is usually distinguished by the name of the island or place producing it; as *Bermuda arrow-root, St. Vincent's arrow-root, Jamaica arrow-root, African or Sierra Leone arrow-root,* &c. Bermuda arrow-root is the most esteemed variety. In 1845, about 400,000 lbs. were manufactured, of which more than three-fourths came to England. Dr. Ure says that the St. Vincent's arrow-root prepared on the Hopewell estate vies with the Bermuda sort.

In commerce the term *arrow-root* is frequently used generically to indicate a starch or fecula. The following are illustrations of its use in this way :—

Portland Arrow-root is obtained from *Arum maculatum* (see *ante,* p. 137).

East India Arrow-root is the fecula procured from *Curcuma angustifolia,* and will be described hereafter. But the West Indian plant (*Maranta arundinacea*) is also cultivated in the East Indies, and the fecula obtained therefrom is exported from thence, and might with equal propriety be called *East India arrow-root.*

Brazilian Arrow-root is the fecula of *Jatropha Manihot,* and will be noticed hereafter (vide Euphorbiaceæ).

Tahiti Arrow-root is the fecula of *Tacca oceanica,* and has already been noticed (see *ante,* p. 221).

Properties.—The starch or fecula (*amylum* vel *fæcula marantæ*) called in the shops *West Indian arrow-root,* or simply *arrow-root,* is white, odourless, and tasteless. It is in the form either of a light opaque white powder or of small pulverulent masses. When passed between the fingers it feels firm, and, when rubbed, produces a slight crackling noise. When viewed by a good pocket lens, it is seen to consist of glistening particles. When examined by a microscope, these are seen to be convex, more or less elliptical, and moderately uniform in size.[1] The shape is more or less irregular, but often oblong, or usually somewhat ovate-oblong, frequently obscurely triangular, or oyster-shaped, or mussel-shaped.[2] After having been digested for a short time in water, one or rarely two mamillary processes are, in some samples, seen projecting from the surface of some of the particles. In some specimens these processes have appeared like short spines. The rings are very distinct, though fine. The nucleus, central cavity, or hilum, is usually very distinct, generally towards one end of the particle normally circular, but frequently cracked in a linear or stellate manner. When viewed by the polarising microscope, the particles show very distinct crosses : the junction of the arms of the cross indicates the position of the hilum.

---

[1] The following measurements, in parts of an English inch, of the particles of West India arrow-root, were kindly made for me by Mr. George Jackson :—

Particles.	Length.	Breadth.	Particles.	Length.	Breadth.
1	0·0020	0·0013	4	0·0008	0·0005
2	0·0012	0·0009	5	0·0006	0·0004
3*	0·0010	0·0008	6	0·0005	0·0003

The most prevalent-sized particle is distinguished thus *.

[2] Schleiden (*Principles of Scientific Botany*) describes the granules as being compound, without evident central cavity, and always exhibiting the smooth connecting surfaces; but this description does not apply to commercial West Indian arrow-root.—Raspail has depicted the grains of the fecula of Convolvulus Batatas for arrow-root (see Payen, *Ann. Scien. Nat.* 2nde sér. t. x. Botanique, p. 18, 1838).

COMPOSITION OF THE STARCH.—Arrow-root has been analysed by Dr. Prout[1] and by Payen,[2] who obtained the following results :—

PROUT.				PAYEN.		
	Air Dried.	Dried between 200° and 212° for 20 hours.	Dried at 212° for 6 hours longer.		Portion most easily disaggregated, dried at 212° F.	Amidon intact purified by alcohol & water and dried at 382° F.
				Carbon.........	44·3	44·33
Carbon	36·4	42·8	44·4	Hydrogen......	6 2	6·25
Water	63·6	57·2	55·6	Oxygen.........	49·5	49·42
Arrow-root...	100·0	100·0	100·0	Arrow-root	100·0	100·00

The formula which agrees with Prout's third analysis is $C^{12}H^{10}O^{10}$.

Dr. Prout regards arrow-root as a low variety of starch analogous to the low sugar of honey; while wheat-starch he considers to be the most perfect form of starch, analogous to sugar-candy.

SUBSTITUTIONS, IMPURITIES, AND ADULTERATIONS. — The presence of accidental impurities (such as insects, dust, &c.) may be readily detected by alterations in the colour, odour, and flavour of the arrow-root.

Other cheaper feculas are sometimes substituted for the genuine arrow-root. I have myself met with one only of these substitutions, namely refined sago-meal (see *ante*, p. 145); and in this case the microscope readily detected the fraud. When squeezed in the hand, the sago-meal crackled like arrow-root; but when submitted to microscopic examination, the truncated extremity of many of the particles giving them either a mullar shape or dihedral summit, the irregular or tuberculated surface, and the size of the particles, readily served to distinguish it from arrow-root.

Potato-starch is said to have been sometimes sold for West Indian arrow-root. I have met with it in commerce under the name of English arrow-root. It is devoid of the dull or dead white appearance presented by West India arrow-root. The naked eye, or, still better, a pocket lens, readily distinguishes its large glistening particles from those of genuine arrow-root. The microscope instantly detects the difference. The particles of potato-starch are larger than those of arrow-root, and have coarser and more distinct rings. Moreover, the shape of the particles serves to distinguish them (see *Potato-starch*). Lampadius[3] observed that potato-starch evolves a peculiar odour when boiled with water and sulphuric acid, and that arrow-root does not evolve this odour when treated in a similar way. Arrow-root, moreover, " is destitute of that fetid unwholesome oil, extractable by alcohol from potato-starch."[4] Mixed with one and a half or twice its weight of concentrated hydrochloric acid, arrow-root yields an opaque paste, whereas that produced by potato-starch is transparent. Arrow-root takes a longer time than potato-starch to

[1] *Phil. Trans.* 1827.
[2] *Ann. des Scien. Nat.* 2de sér. Botanique, 1838, pp. 183–184.
[3] *Pharmaceutisches Central-Blatt für* 1832, S. 638.
[4] Ure, *Recent Improvements in Arts, Manufactures, and Mines*, p. 10, 1844.

become viscid, when mixed with equal parts of acid and water.[1]   Other kinds of feculas which are said to have been substituted (on account of their cheapness) for the genuine arrow-root, such as Tahiti arrow-root (see *ante*, Tacca oceanica, p. 221), East India arrow-root (see Curcuma angustifolia), Brazilian arrow (see Jatropha Manihot), rice-starch (see *ante*, p. 73), and are readily distinguishable by the microscope.

Physiological Effects.—By the Indians of South America, and even by some Europeans, the *roots* (tubers) have been supposed to possess alexipharmic properties.[2]   But their chief, if not their only real value, is that of yielding the starch called *arrow-root*, which is a much-esteemed non-nitrogenised alimentary principle, which, like some other agents of this kind (see Vol. i. p. 64), are useful in the animal economy for the production of fatty and saccharine matters, lactic acid, and heat.   Arrow-root is one of the most palatable and digestible of the starches.

Uses.—The *roots* (tubers) have been used by the South American Indians to counteract the effects of wounds inflicted by poisoned arrows.   Very recently[3] the expressed juice of the root has been lauded as an antidote to poisons taken into the stomach, and to the bites and stings of venomous insects and reptiles.

The starch or *arrow-root* is employed at the table as an article of food, in the form of puddings.   It forms an agreeable, non-irritating diet for invalids or infants.   In irritation of the alimentary canal, of the pulmonary organs, or of the urinary apparatus, it is especially valuable as a nutritive, emollient, and demulcent.

Administration.—To invalids and infants arrow-root (the starch) is exhibited when boiled in water or milk and flavoured.   Milk disagrees with some patients, and in such is of course to be avoided.   The addition of sugar improves the flavour and increases the nutritive qualities.   Spices, lemon-juice, or wine, may be employed according to circumstances.

74. Canna edulis, *Ker.*—Tous-les-Mois?

Sex. Syst. Monandria, Monogynia.

(Amylum dictum " Tous-les-Mois.")

The starch or fecula called Tous-les-Mois was introduced to the notice of the British public by the late Mr. Olpherts,[4] of St. Kitts, about 1836.   It was at first stated to be the produce of *C. coccinea* ; but as this species, like *C. indica*, has fibrous, and not tuberous roots, it is tolerably clear that this cannot be the source of the starch in question.

There is good reason for believing that *C. edulis* of Ker is a native of the West Indies, and that it is the species which yields tous-les-mois.   Descourtilz[5] and Lunan[6] speak of a species of Canna with fleshy tuberous roots, which grows in the West Indies, and which they call C. indica.   But the character of the roots just mentioned shows that the West Indian plant is not C. indica, Linn.   Ruiz and Pavon[7] speak of a South American plant, which they term Canna indica of Linnæus, whose fleshy tubers are eaten by the

---

[1] Scharling, *Pharmaceutical Journal*, vol. ii. p. 417, 1843.

[2] Sloane's *Jamaica*, vol. i. p. 254.

[3] Hamilton, *Pharmaceutical Journal*, vol. vi. pp. 23 and 25, 1847.

[4] Hamilton, *ibid.* vol. vii. p. 56, 1847 ; also the *Medico-Chirurg. Review* for Oct. 1, 1836; and Ryan's *Med. and Surg. Journal* for August 1836.

[5] *Fl. Méd. des Antilles*, p. 3, tab. 240.

[6] *Hortus Jamaicensis*, vol. ii. p. 417.

[7] *Flora Peruviana*.

Peruvians, who call the plant *Achira*. They considered it to be the C. indica of Linn. But when their herbarium came into Mr. Lambert's possession he raised plants from the seeds of the original specimens, and found the species to be a new one, which he named *C. edulis*.[1]

Mr. Lambert afterwards received seeds, from Dr. Gillies of Mendoza, of a Canna known in South America as "*Achira*." This has been described and figured[2] as a new species, under the name of *C. Achiras* (more properly "*C.* Achira"); but it is not improbable that it may prove to be identical with C. edulis.

C. glauca is also said to yield a valuable starch.[3]

My friend Mr. Wordsworth, assistant-surgeon to the London Hospital, and who resided some time at St. Kitts, tells me that he cultivated the tous-les-mois in his garden. Its height was about 4 feet; and its tubers three or four times the size of the fist. In order to extract the fecula, the tubers are rasped by means of a circular or wheel-rasp[4] worked by a treddle. The tuber is held against the edge of the rasp, at the point marked *a* in the accompanying figure. The starch is obtained from this pulp by the ordinary methods of washing, straining, decantation of the supernatant liquor, and desiccation of the deposited starch.

The quantity of starch procured from the roots of the tous-les-mois plant has not been satisfactorily ascertained. Ricord Madianna[5] obtained from a pound of the root two ounces of starch of a fine quality : this is equal to 12·5 per cent. It is probable, however, that on the large scale the product would be much greater.

FIG. 85.

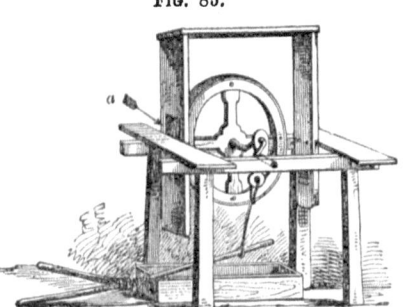

Wheel-rasp used for rasping the tubers of the Tous-les-Mois plant.

Tous-les-mois-starch is imported from St. Kitts. To the naked eye it greatly resembles potato-starch. On account of the large size of its particles it has a satiny or glistening appearance, and is devoid of that dead white or opaque appearance presented by the West Indian arrow-root. Examined by a pocket lens, the sparkling and glistening appearance of its particles is very obvious. When submitted to examination by means of the compound microscope, its particles are seen to be very large[6] (in this respect exceeding those of all other starches), somewhat egg-shaped, to have a very distinct nucleus, central cavity, or hilum, and concentric rings indicative of their laminated structure. Strictly speaking, their shape is oval or oblong; but generally more or less ovate. The circular hilum is usually placed at the narrow extremity; very rarely it is double; once I have seen it treble. The rings are numerous, regular, close, but somewhat unequally so. The hilum and the body of the particle are frequently cracked.

Potato-starch is the only amylaceous substance which can be confounded with tous-les-mois. The two starches may be distinguished by a careful attention to their relative sizes and shapes, to the appearance of their rings, the position of the hilum, and the action of polarised light on them.

First, the particles of potato-starch are, on the average, smaller than those of tous-les-

---

[1] *Botanical Register*, tab. 7.

[2] *Ibid.* tab. 1358.

[3] Bennett, *Ceylon and its Capabilities*, p. 127, 1843.

[4] Piso (*Hist. Nat. Brasiliæ*, p. 53, 1648) represents a somewhat similar machine as being used in the preparation of cassava or tapioca starch.

[5] *Journ. de Pharmacie*, t. xvi. p. 306, 1830.

[6] The following measurements, in parts of an English inch, of the particles of "tous-les-mois," were made for me by Mr. George Jackson :—

Particles.	Length.	Breadth.	Particles.	Length.	Breadth.
1	0·0042	0·0035	4*	0·0032	0·0020
2	0·0037	0·0026	5*	0·0025	0·0017
3*	0·0031	0·0027	6	0·0013	0·0010

The most prevalent-sized particles are those marked thus *.

mois, and are subject to greater irregularity of size (both as regards different sorts of potatoes and the different particles of the same potato). Secondly, the larger particles of potato starch are more irregular in shape than those of tous-les-mois: the latter are more constantly rounded, or oblong, or ovate-oblong: the former are oval, often approximating in shape to an oyster-shell, a mussel-shell, or a triangle with rounded corners, and being frequently gibbous or tumid at different parts of their surface. Thirdly, the rings seen on particles of tous-les-mois are fine, regular, uniform, concentric, and crowded: those of potato starch are coarser, irregular, often excentric, irregularly drawn out, distorted, or more and unequally distant from each other. In potato-starch a greater number of complete rings are visible, and we can trace the lines around the hilum, even in the case of many of the larger rings; but in tous-les-mois this can be done with a very few of the smaller rings only. Fourthly, in both the hilum is situated nearer to the end of the particle; but in potato-starch this character is less obvious, the hilum frequently being less distant from the centre of the particle than in the case of tous-les-mois. Lastly, when viewed by polarised light the cross is less frequently regular in potato-starch than in tous-les-mois: in the former the arms are often distorted.

Tous-les-mois of commerce contains about 16·74 per cent. of hygroscopic water. It is very soluble in boiling water; and, according to Dr. Shier's experiments, yields a jelly which is considerably more tenacious than the jelly of any other starch, but which, in clearness or translucency, is inferior to that of arrow-root and of some other substances.

The composition of tous-les-mois starch is assumed to be the same as that of other starches, viz. $C^{12}H^{10}O^{10}$

In its dietetical qualities tous-les-mois resembles other starches. It yields very agreeable articles of food for invalids and others, and appears to be very readily digested.

ORDER XVII. ZINGIBERACEÆ, Lindl.—GINGERWORTS.

DRYMYRHIZEÆ, Vent.—SCITAMINEÆ, R. Brown.

CHARACTERS.—Calyx superior, tubular, 3-lobed, short. Corolla tubular, irregular, with 6 segments in 2 whorls; the outer 3-parted, nearly equal, or with the odd segment sometimes differently shaped; the inner (sterile stamens) 3-parted, with the intermediate segment (labellum) larger than the rest, and often 3-lobed, the lateral segments sometimes nearly abortive. Stamens 3, distinct, of which the two lateral are abortive, and the intermediate one fertile; this placed opposite the labellum, and arising from the base of the intermediate segment of the outer series of the corolla. Filament not petaloid, often extended beyond the anther in the shape of a lobed or entire appendage. Anther 2-celled, opening longitudinally, its lobes often embracing the upper part of the style. Pollen globose, smooth. Ovary 3-celled, sometimes imperfectly so; ovules several, attached to a placenta in the axis; style filiform; stigma dilated, hollow. Fruit usually capsular, 3 celled, many-seeded [sometimes by abortion 1-celled]; occasionally berried (the dissepiments generally central, proceeding from the axis of the valves, at last usually separate from the latter, and of a different texture, R. Br.) Seeds roundish or angular, with or without an aril (albumen floury, its substance radiating, and deficient near the hilum, R. Br.); embryo enclosed within a peculiar membrane (vitellus, R. Br. Prodr. membrane of the amnios, ibid. in King's Voyage, 21) with which it does not cohere.—Aromatic, tropical, herbaceous plants. Rhizome creeping, often jointed. Stem formed of the cohering base of the leaves, never branching. Leaves simple, sheathing their lamina, often separated from the sheath by a taper neck, and having a single midrib, from which very numerous, simple, crowded veins diverge at an acute angle. Inflorescence either a dense spike, or a raceme, or a sort of panicle, terminal or radical. Flowers arising from among spathaceous membranous bracts, in which they usually lie in pairs (Lindley).

PROPERTIES.—The rhizomes contain a volatile oil and resin, which confer on them aromatic or acro-aromatic qualities. Many of them abound in starch, the particles of which (like those of plantain-starch, see ante, p. 223) are flattened discs. This is sometimes extracted and used as food. Some of them are remarkable for the yellow colouring matter which they yield.

The seeds also contain volatile oil and resin, and possess aromatic or acro-aromatic qualities.

75. ZINGIBER OFFICINALE, *Roscoe.*—THE NARROW-LEAVED GINGER.

Amomum Zingiber, *Linn.* D.
Sex. Syst. Monandria, Monogynia.
(Rhizoma, *L. E.*—Radix, *D.*)

HISTORY.—Dioscorides[1] and Pliny[2] speak of ginger: the former calls it ζιγγίβερις; the latter, *zingiberi* and *zimgiberi.*

BOTANY. **Gen. Char.**—*Corolla* with the outer limb 3-parted, inner 1-lipped. *Filament* lengthened beyond the anther into a simple incurved beak. *Capsule* 3-celled, 3-valved. *Seeds* numerous, arillate. — *Rhizocarpial* plants. *Rhizomes* tuberous, articulated, creeping. *Stems* annual, enclosed in the sheaths of distichous leaves. *Leaves* membranous. *Spikes* cone-shaped, radical or rarely terminal, solitary, consisting of 1-flowered imbricated bracts (Blume[3]).

Sp. Char.—*Leaves* sub-sessile, linear-lanceolate, smooth. *Spikes* elevated, oblong. *Bracts* acute. *Lip* 3-lobed (Roxburgh).

Rhizome biennial. *Stems* erect and oblique, and invested by the smooth sheaths of the leaves; generally 3 or 4 feet high, and annual. *Leaf-sheaths* smooth, crowned with a bifid ligula. *Scapes* solitary, 6 to 12 inches high. *Spikes* the size of a man's thumb. *Lip* dark purple. *Ovary* oval, with numerous *ovules ; style* filiform; *stigma* funnel-shaped, ciliate. *Capsule* roundish, unilocular. *Seeds* numerous; mostly abortive.[4]

Hab.—Cultivated in the tropical regions of Asia and America, and at Sierra Leone. Native soil doubtful, probably Asia.

PREPARATION.—*Green ginger* is sometimes imported from Jamaica. It consists of soft and juicy rhizomes with buds, and appears to have undergone but little preparation beyond picking and washing. The young shoots put forth every spring by the perennial rhizome are used in the manufacture of the delicious *preserved ginger (conditum zingiberis).* These shoots are carefully picked, washed, scalded, scraped, peeled, and then preserved in jars with syrup (Dr. P. Browne). The finest preserved ginger is imported from Jamaica usually in jars. Barbados preserved ginger is seldom brought over. The China preserved ginger is stringy. It is sometimes imported in the dried state.

The dried rhizomes, called in the shops *ginger (radix zingiberis)* are prepared when the stalks are wholly withered, and the rhizomes are about a year old. In Jamaica this happens in January or February. The rhizomes are dug up and separately picked, washed, and scraped ; and afterwards dried in the sun and open air (Dr. P. Browne). The product is the uncoated ginger of the shops, formerly called *white ginger (zingiber album).*

The coated ginger of the shops has obviously not undergone this careful preparation. In Barbados the rhizomes are dug up, scraped clean, and sun-dried.[5] The *black ginger (zingiber nigrum)* formerly prepared in Jamaica

---

[1] Lib. ii. cap. 190.
[2] *Hist. Nat.* lib. xii. cap. 14, ed. Valp.
[3] *Enumeratio Plantarum Java.*
[4] Roxburgh, *op. cit.* ; and Dr. P. Browne, *History of Jamaica.*
[5] Hughes, *Nat. Hist. of Barbados,* p. 233, 1750.

is obtained by picking and cleaning the rhizomes, scalding them gradually in boiling water, and afterwards sun-drying them.[1]

DESCRIPTION.—The *rhizome,* called in commerce *ginger root,* or simply *ginger (radix zingiberis),* occurs in flattish, jointed, branched, or lobed, palmate pieces, called *races* or *hands,* which rarely exceed four inches in length.

Barbados ginger, the old sorts brought from Malabar and Bengal, and African ginger, are covered by a dry shrivelled epidermis commonly called the " coat :" hence these sorts are usually said to be *coated* or *unscraped ;* whereas the ginger of Jamaica, and the new sorts which of late years have been brought from Malabar and Bengal, have been deprived of their epidermis, and are, therefore, said to be *uncoated* or *scraped.* The external colour varies in the different sorts from pale or bright yellow to dark or brown : the palest sort is the fine Jamaica ginger ; the darkest being the Bengal old sort, and the other sorts being intermediate. Ginger breaks moderately short, but the fractured surface presents numerous projecting pointed fibres, imbedded in a mealy or farinaceous tissue. A transverse section of the larger and more perfect pieces shows an outer, horny, resinous-looking zone, surrounding a farinaceous centre, which has a speckled appearance from the cut extremities of the fibres and ducts. The internal varies like the external colour : the best ginger is that which cuts pale but bright. The consistence of ginger, as ascertained by cutting, varies from soft to hard, or, as it is termed in trade, " flinty :" the soft being preferred. The taste of ginger is aromatic, hot, and biting : the odour of a fresh-broken piece is peculiar and pungent, though aromatic.

VARIETIES.—Seven kinds of ginger, distinguished partly by their place of growth and partly by their quality, are known in English commerce. Of these, two are from the West Indies, four from the East Indies, and one from Africa.

A. **West Indian Gingers.**—This division includes Jamaica and Barbados gingers.

1. *Jamaica ginger.*—Imported in barrels holding 1 cwt. each. It is an uncoated, pale sort, and when of fine quality occurs in large, bold, fleshy races, which cut soft, bright, and pale-coloured. Inferior samples are small in the race, darker-coloured, more or less flinty, and shrivelled.

2. *Barbados ginger.*—Imported in bags of about 60 or 70 lbs. It is a coated sort, in short flat races, which are darker-coloured than Jamaica ginger, and are covered with a corrugated epidermis.

B. **East Indian Gingers.**—This division includes two sorts from Malabar and two from Bengal, all of which are more liable to be wormy than either the West Indian or African sorts.

α. Malabar Gingers.

3. *Coated Malabar Ginger ; Unscraped Malabar Ginger ; Old sort of Malabar Ginger ; Common Malabar Ginger ; Bombay Ginger.*—Imported from Bombay in bags or packets. It is a coated, dark, small sort.

4. *Uncoated Malabar Ginger ; New sort of Malabar Ginger ; Telli-*

---

[1] Dr. P. Browne, *op. cit.*—According to Dr. Wright (*Lond. Med. Journ.* vol. viii. ; also *Memoir of the late Dr. Wright,* p. 185, 1828), two sorts of ginger are cultivated in Jamaica, viz. the white and the black : the latter has the most numerous and the largest roots.

cherry Ginger; Calicut Ginger; Cochin Ginger.—A pale uncoated sort, imported in chests, casks, or bags, sometimes from Tellicherry, but usually from Calicut or Cochin. It resembles Jamaica ginger both in external appearance and flavour, but has externally more of a brownish or reddish tint. It first appeared in English commerce about 1841.

β. Bengal Gingers.

5. *Coated Bengal Ginger; Common Bengal Ginger; Old sort of Bengal Ginger.*—Imported in bags. It is a coated or unscraped dark sort, which cuts flinty and brownish, but is plumper and less wormy than common Malabar ginger.

6. *Uncoated Bengal Ginger; Scraped Bengal Ginger; New sort of Bengal Ginger; Calicut sort of Bengal Ginger.*—Imported in chests of about 1½ cwt. It is an uncoated sort, darker than Jamaica ginger. It is not so large as the uncoated Malabar sort, and is harder and darker.

C. **African Ginger.**—Only one kind of African ginger is known, viz. that from Sierra Leone.

7. *Sierra Leone Ginger; African Ginger.*—Imported in casks or bags. It is a coated sort; the races being generally larger, less flat, and less plump than those of the Barbados sort, which in other respects they resemble.

Chinese Ginger.—[The Chinese ginger described by Bassermann[1] was stated in the preceding edition of this work to be unknown in English commerce; the only ginger imported into England from China being *preserved ginger.* We are informed, however, by Mr. Daniel Hanbury, that lately some dried Chinese ginger has been in the market. It is unscraped and coated, and cuts flinty and brownish. Each piece is perforated for suspension on a cord. This is probably the same described by Bassermann.—ED.]

ASSORTMENT.—The uncoated gingers—namely, the Jamaica, uncoated Malabar, and uncoated Bengal—are assorted for commercial purposes, according to their qualities, somewhat thus—

1. Bold, soft, and bright ginger.	3. Flinty and dark.
2. Smaller, but soft and bright.	4. Shrivelled, and only fit for grinding.

The Barbados, African, and coated Malabar and Bengal gingers, are usually sold unassorted.

[The following are the quantities of ginger imported into England for six years :—

	Cwts.			Cwts.
In 1849	27,767	In 1852		19,919
1850	33,996	1853		21,852
1851	35,399	1854		24,616—ED.]

WASHED GINGER; BLEACHED GINGER.—Ginger is sometimes washed in water, and then dried, by wholesale dealers, prior to its being offered for sale to the retailers.

Some of the darker sorts are bleached by washing them in a solution of chloride of lime, and sometimes by exposing them to the fumes of burning sulphur. By this treatment the ginger acquires a chalky-white character, and is then often termed *white-washed* ginger.

Ginger is said[2] to be sometimes washed in whiting and water (or whitewashed) under the pretence of preserving it from insects.

---

[1] *Pharmaceutisches Central-Blatt für* 1835.
[2] Brande, *Dict. of Mat. Med.*

Adulteration.—Powdered ginger is said to be sometimes admixed with flour and other amylaceous substances. The microscope would readily detect the adulteration, except in the case of East Indian arrow-root (*Curcuma angustifolia*), the particles of which are similar in appearance to those of ginger.

Composition.—Ginger was analysed in 1817 by Bucholz,[1] and in 1823 by Morin.[2]

Bucholz's Analysis.		*Morin's Analysis.*
Pale yellow volatile oil	1·56	Volatile oil.
Aromatic, acrid, soft resin	3·60	Acrid soft resin.
Extractive, soluble in alcohol	0·65	Resin insoluble in ether and oils.
Acidulous and acrid extractive, insoluble in alcohol	10·50	Gum. Starch.
Gum	12·05	Woody fibre.
Starch (analogous to bassorin)	19·75	Vegeto-animal matter.
Apotheme, extracted by potash (ulmin?)	26·00	Osmazome.
Bassorin	8·30	Acetic acid, acetate of potash, and sulphur.
Woody fibre	8·00	The ashes contained carbonate and sulphate of
Water	11·90	potash, chloride of potassium, phosphate of lime,
		alumina, silica, and oxides of iron and manganese.
White Ginger	102·31	Ginger.

1. Volatile Oil of Ginger.—Is pale yellow, very fluid, lighter than water, odour that of ginger; taste at first mild, afterwards acrid and hot.

2. Soft Resin.—Obtained by digesting the alcoholic extract of ginger first in water, then in ether, and evaporating the ethereal tincture. The residual resin is yellowish-brown, soft, combustible, has an aromatic odour and a burning aromatic taste. Is readily soluble in alcohol, ether, oil of turpentine, and hot almond oil.

3. Starch.—Ginger-starch consists of thin flat discs, which resemble those of East Indian arrow-root (see *Curcuma angustifolia*) and plantain-starch (see *ante*, p. 223).

Physiological Effects.— Ginger is one of the aromatic stimulants (see Vol. i. p. 227) which possess considerable pungency or acridity. Its dust applied to the mucous membrane of the nostrils acts as an irritant, and provokes sneezing. The rhizome chewed is a powerful sialogogue. The powder mixed with hot water, and applied to the skin, causes a sensation of intense heat and tingling, and slight redness. When taken into the stomach, ginger operates as a stimulant—first, to the alimentary canal; secondly, to the body generally, but especially to the organs of respiration. Like some other spices (the peppers for instance), it acts as an excitant to the genital organs. Furthermore, it has been said to increase the energy of the cerebral functions. It is less acrid than pepper.

Uses.—Its principal consumption is as a *condiment*. Its powers in this way are considerable, while its flavour is by no means disagreeable, and its acridity scarcely sufficient to enable it, when taken with food, to irritate or inflame.

As a *stomachic* and *internal stimulant*, it serves several important purposes. In enfeebled and relaxed habits, especially of old and gouty individuals, it promotes digestion, and relieves flatulency and spasm of the stomach and bowels. It checks or prevents nausea and griping, which are apt to be

---

[1] Gmelin's *Handb. d. Chem.*
[2] *Journ. de Pharm.* ix. 253.

produced by some drastic purgatives. It covers the nauseous flavour of many medicines, and communicates cordial and carminative qualities to tonic and other agents. As a *sialogogue* it is sometimes chewed to relieve tooth-ache, relaxed uvula, and paralytic affections of the tongue. As a *counter-irritant* I have frequently known a *ginger plaster* (prepared by mixing together powdered ginger and warm water, and spreading the paste on paper or cloth) relieve violent headache when applied to the forehead.

ADMINISTRATION.—*Powdered ginger* may be administered, in doses of from ten grains to a scruple or more, in the form of a pill. Made into a paste with hot water, it may be applied as a *plaster*, as already mentioned.

Preserved ginger (*conditum zingiberis*), though commonly used as a sweetmeat, may be taken with advantage as a medicine to stimulate the stomach. *Ginger lozenges, ginger pearls* (commonly termed *ginger seeds*), and *ginger pipe*, are useful articles of confectionary, which are frequently of benefit in dyspepsia accompanied with flatulence.

1. TINCTURA ZINGIBERIS, L. E. D.; *Tincture of Ginger.* (Ginger, bruised [in coarse powder, *E. D.*), ℥iss. [℥viij. *D.*] ; Rectified Spirit, Oij. Macerate for seven days [fourteen days, *D.*], and strain. "Proceed by per-colation or digestion, as directed for tincture of cinchona," *E.*)—A very valuable carminative. It is commonly employed as an adjunct to tonic, stimu-lant, and purgative mixtures. Its dose is f℥j. to f℥ij. The tincture, if made with proof spirit, becomes turbid by keeping, in consequence of the mucilage it contains.

Essence of Ginger is prepared as a tincture, except that the quantity of rhizome should be increased. Some preparers of it concentrate the tincture by distilling off part of the alcohol.

2. SYRUPUS ZINGIBERIS, L. E. D.; *Syrup of Ginger.* (Ginger, sliced, ℥iss.; Boiling Distilled Water, Oj.; Sugar, lb. iiss.; Rectified Spirit, a suf-ficiency. Macerate the ginger in the water for four hours, and strain, and proceed as ordered for the Syrupus Althææ. The Edinburgh College orders the same proportions as the London. The Dublin College makes this syrup by agitating together f℥j. of Tincture of Ginger with f℥vij. of simple Syrup.) —Used for flavouring. It is scarcely strong enough to be of much value. The *syrupus zingiberis* of the United States Pharmacopœia is made by adding f℥ij. of Tincture of Ginger (prepared with ℥viij. of Ginger and Oij. *wine measure*, of Alcohol) to a gallon of Syrup, and evaporating the alcohol by a water-bath.

3. INFUSUM ZINGIBERIS ; *Infusion of Ginger ; Ginger Tea.*—This is a very useful domestic remedy, and is prepared by digesting from ℈ij. to ℈iv. of Ginger in f℥vj. of Boiling Water, for two hours. When flavoured, it is employed as a carminative in flatulence, &c., in doses of one or two table-spoonfuls.

4. GINGER BEER.—For the following excellent formula for the preparation of this popular and agreeable beverage, I am indebted to Mr. Pollock, of Fenchurch Street:—"Take of White Sugar, lb. xx.; Lemon- (or Lime-) juice, f℥xviij.; Honey, lb. j.; Ginger, bruised, ℥xxij.; Water, Cong. xviij. Boil the ginger in three gallons of water for half an hour; then add the sugar, the juice, and the honey, with the remainder of the water, and strain through a cloth. When cold, add the White of one Egg and f℥ss. of Essence of Lemon: after standing four days, bottle. The bottles are to be laid on their sides in a cellar, and the beer is ready for use in about three weeks. If a little yeast be used, the beer is ready in a day or two; but in this case it does not keep well." This yields a very superior beverage, and one which will keep for many months. Lemon-juice may be purchased for sixpence a pint in Botolph Lane, Thames Street. A formula for the preparation of *Ginger-beer Powders* has already been given (see Vol. i. p. 568).

76. Zingiber Cassumunar, *Roxburgh.*

Sex. Syst. Monandria, Monogynia.

(Radix.)

The root of this plant is "perennial, tuberous, furnished with long, white, fleshy fibres, and jointed like ginger, but much larger; when fresh, of a deep yellow; possessing a strong, not very agreeable, camphoraceous smell, and warm, spicy, bitterish taste" (Roxburgh). Sir Joseph Banks and Dr. Comb (to whom specimens of it were given) thought that it was the true cassumunar of the shops.[1] But the great resemblance of cassumunar root to round zedoary leads me to think that it is obtained from a species of *Curcuma.*

About the year 1672, Dr. Pechey received from his brother, factor to the East India Company, a root which was called *cassumunar* (variously spelt casmunar, casumunar, &c.), *rysagone* (or risagon), and *bengale* (or bengalle).[2] These names were probably fictitious, and were merely given to conceal the secret of its nature.

This root is still found in the warehouses of some London druggists, who call it *cassumunar root (radix cassumunar)*, and consider it to be identical with *zerumber root* (see *Curcuma zedoaria*). It appears to me to be the *turmeric-coloured zedoary* of Ainslie, the *zedoaria radice lutea* of Breynius,[3] the *tommon besaar* or *tommon lawac* of Rumphius.[4] It occurs in segments (halves or quarters) of an ovate tuber (which in the dried state must have been about the size of a pigeon's egg), the external surface of which is marked with circular rings and the bases of the root-fibres, and is of a dirty turmeric-yellow colour. Internally it is reddish-brown, and has some resemblance, in its colour and pellucidity, to a fresh-fractured surface of Socotrine aloes. Its flavour is warm and aromatic; its odour is somewhat like that of turmeric. It has not been analysed. Its effects must be similar to those of zedoary and ginger. It was at one time used in convulsive and other cerebral diseases,[5] but has fallen into disuse.

77. CURCUMA LONGA, *Linn.*—THE LONG-ROOTED TURMERIC.

Sex. Syst. Monandria, Monogynia.

(Rhizoma, *L. E.*—Radix, *D.*)

HISTORY.—Turmeric is probably the κύπειρος ἰνδικός (*Cyperus indicus*) of Dioscorides.[6] Both he and Pliny[7] state that this Indian Cyperus has the

---

[1] Roxburgh, *Asiatic Researches*, vol. xi.

[2] Pechey, *Some Observations made on the Root Cassumuniar, called otherwise Rysagone, imported from the East Indies* [MS. without date, in the library of the Royal Medical and Chirurgical Society of London]; Sir Hans Sloane, *Phil. Trans.* No. 264, p. 580.

[3] *Prodromus*, ii. 105.

[4] *Herb. Amboyn.* pars 5ta, p. 168.

[5] *Some Observations made upon the Root called Casmunar imported from the East Indies*, published by a Doctor of Physick [Dr. Pechey?] in Gloucestershire. London, reprinted in the year 1693.

[6] Lib. i. cap. iv.

[7] *Hist. Nat.* lib. xxi. cap. lxx. ed. Valp.

form of ginger, and that, when chewed, it colours the saliva yellow like saffron. The word *curcuma* is derived from *kurkum*, the Persian name for saffron.[1]

BOTANY. **Gen. Char.**—Tube of the *corolla* gradually enlarged upwards; limb 2-lipped, each 3-parted. *Filament* broad. *Anther* incumbent, with 2 spurs at the base. *Style* capillary. *Capsule* 3-celled. *Seeds* numerous, arillate.—Stemless plants, with palmate tuberous roots. *Leaves* with sheathing petioles, bifarious, herbaceous. *Scape* simple, lateral or central. *Spike* simple, erect, comose, somewhat imbricated at the base with bracts or saccate spathes. *Flowers* dull yellow, 3 to 5 together, surrounded by bracteolæ.[2]

Sp. Char.—*Bulbs* small, and with the numerous, long, *palmate tubers*, inwardly of a deep orange-yellow. *Leaves* long-petioled, broad-lanceolate, of a uniform green (Roxburgh).

Hab.—Much cultivated about Calcutta, and in all parts of Bengal, also in China and Cochin-China. One acre yields about 2000 lbs. of the fresh root.

DESCRIPTION.—The *tubers*, called in the shops turmeric (*radix curcumæ, seu terra merita*), are of two kinds: one *round* (*Curcuma rotunda*), the other *long* (*Curcuma longa*), but both produced on the same plant. The first are round, oval, or ovate, about two inches long and one inch in diameter, pointed at one end, and marked externally with numerous annular wrinkles. The second are cylindrical, not exceeding the thickness of the little finger; 2 or 3 inches long, somewhat contorted, tuberculated. Both kinds are yellowish externally, internally more or less orange-yellow, passing into reddish-brown. The fractured surface has a waxy appearance. The odour is aromatic, somewhat analogous to ginger, but peculiar: the taste is aromatic. When chewed, it tinges the saliva yellow. Its powder is orange-yellow. The tubers are frequently worm-eaten.

If a thin slice of turmeric root be examined by the compound microscope, it is seen to consist chiefly of rounded or oblong, yellow, readily separable cells or vesicles, which appear to be filled with a minutely granular matter, and to be contained in an hexagonal cellular tissue. Intermixed with these cells are observed globules of a viscid, oleaginous, orange-coloured liquid. By boiling the slices in rectified spirit, the oleaginous liquid is dissolved, and the cells are deprived of their yellow colour. The colourless cells appear still to be filled with a granular matter. On the addition of iodine, the cells, but not the hexagonal tissue in which they are contained, acquire a dark blue colour, showing their amylaceous nature.

VARIETIES.—Five varieties of turmeric are known in the English market; namely, China, Bengal, Madras, Malabar or Bombay, and Java turmeric. These are readily distinguishable from each other by their external appearance; but if they were sorted according to their resemblance, the China and Java turmerics would be placed in one group, the Madras and Malabar in a second group, and the Bengal in a third.

1. *China turmeric.*—This sort consists of smooth, plump, round, and long tubers (*Curcuma rotunda et longa*, figs. 86 and 87) of a greenish-yellow hue externally. They yield a bright powder, and on that account are much preferred for medicinal purposes. Hence they fetch a higher price than any

---

[1] Royle, *Essay on the Antiquity of Hindoo Medicine*, p. 87.
[2] Blume, *op. cit.*

other sorts of turmeric. Probably if much of it were brought to market it would not fetch more than the Bengal sort.

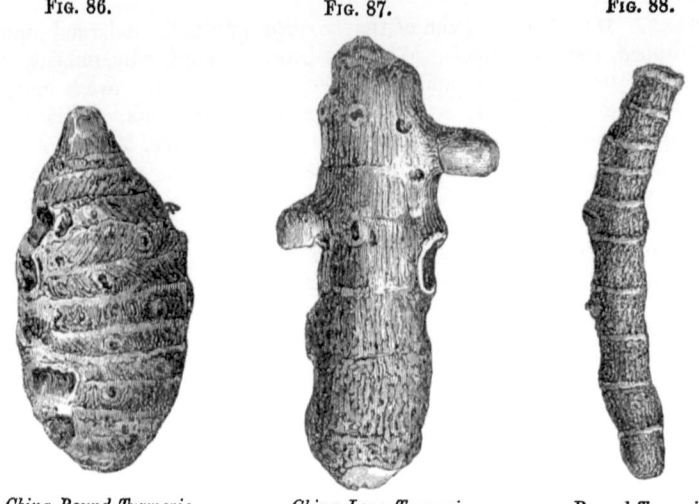

| Fig. 86. | Fig. 87. | Fig. 88. |

China Round Turmeric.　　　*China Long Turmeric.*　　　*Bengal Turmeric.*

2. *Bengal turmeric.*—This sort consists of thin or narrow long tubers (*Curcuma longa,* fig. 88) which are moderately smooth externally, and of a greyish dull yellow colour. They break with a deep reddish fracture. Although from the dull appearance of its narrow tubers it is not a very inviting sort to the inexperienced eye, yet it fetches a higher price than the Madras sort, on account of its being a much stronger dye.

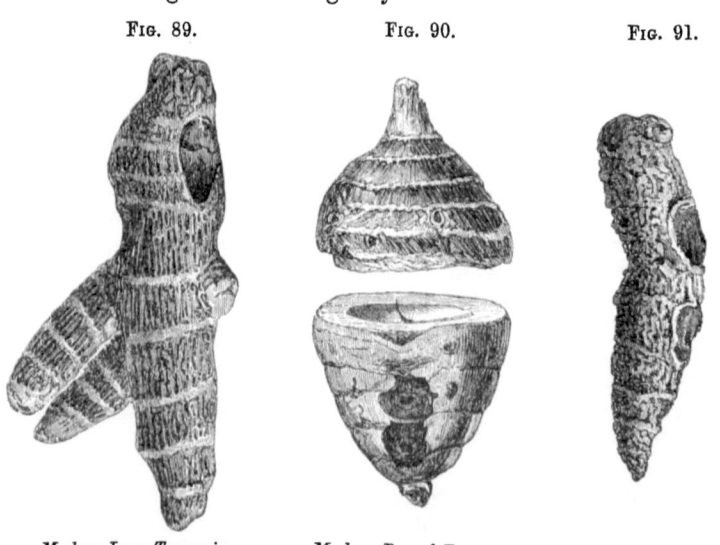

| Fig. 89. | Fig. 90. | Fig. 91. |

Madras Long Turmeric.　　*Madras Round Turmeric.*　　*Malabar Turmeric.*

3. *Madras turmeric.*—This is the most showy of all the kinds of turmeric. It consists principally of large long tubers (*Curcuma longa,* fig. 89),

but mixed with transverse segments of round tubers (*C. rotunda*, fig. 90). Externally the tubers are marked by longitudinal wrinkles, the surface of which is rubbed and bright yellow : internally the colour is that of a fresh-fractured surface of gamboge.

4. *Malabar turmeric ; Bombay turmeric.*—This sort is not constantly found in the market. It consists principally of long tubers (*C. longa*, fig. 91) :

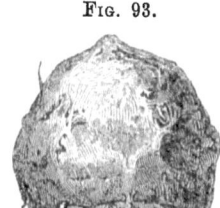

FIG. 92.

FIG. 93.

the round tubers (*C. rotunda*) being few and of very inferior quality. This sort of turmeric is smaller and more shrivelled than the Madras sort, but otherwise somewhat resembles it.

5. *Java turmeric.*—Not frequently found in the English market. In a general way it may be said to resemble the China sort. It consists of both round and long tubers (*C. rotunda et longa*, fig. 92), but chiefly the latter. They have a greenish-yellow hue.

Under the name of *bulbs of Batavian turmeric* I have received a sample of round tubers (fig. 93), said to be from Java. Dr. Th. Martius notices this sort as having been brought for many years from Batavia, and adds that it contains much colouring matter, and is probably the produce of *Curcuma viridiflora*.

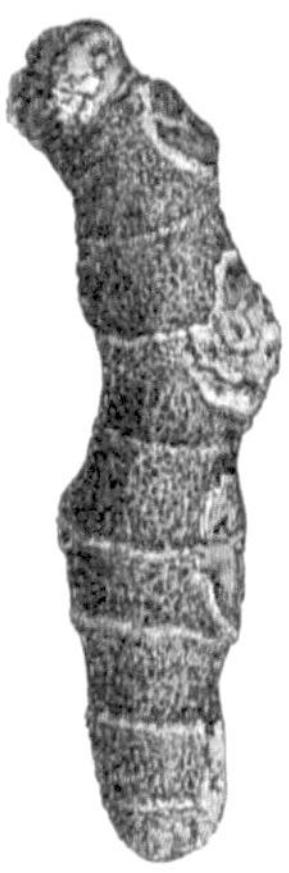

Java Turmeric.　　*Batavian Turmeric.*

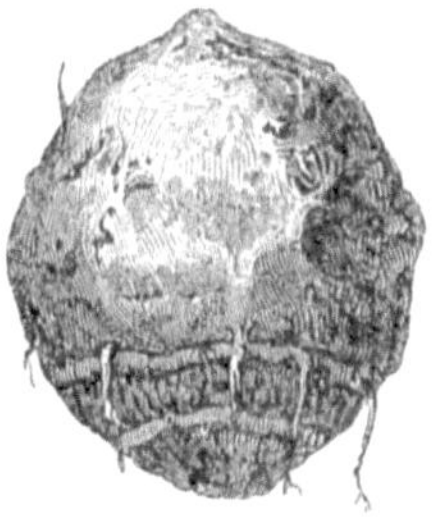

COMPOSITION.—Two analyses of turmeric have been made : one by John,[1] and a second by MM. Vogel and Pelletier.[2]

John's Analysis.		Vogel and Pelletier's Analysis.
Yellow volatile oil.......................	1	Acrid volatile oil.
Curcumin	10 to 11	*Curcumin.*
Yellow extractive	11 to 12	Brown colouring matter.
Gum	14	Gum (a little).
Woody fibre	57	Starch.
Water and loss	7 to 5	Woody fibre.
		Chloride of calcium.
Turmeric	100	Turmeric.

CURCUMIN ; *Yellow Colouring Matter.*—Is obtained, mixed with some volatile oil and chloride of calcium, by digesting the alcoholic extract of turmeric in ether, and evaporating the ethereal tincture to dryness. In the mass, *curcumin* is brownish-yellow, but when powdered it becomes full yellow. It is tasteless, odourless, almost insoluble in water, but readily soluble in alcohol and ether. These properties show that it is of a resinous nature. The alkalies colour it reddish-brown, and readily dissolve it. The alcoholic solution, evaporated with boracic acid, becomes red. Hydrochloric acid also reddens it. The alcoholic solution of curcumin produces coloured precipitates with several salts, as acetate of lead and nitrate of silver.

CHEMICAL CHARACTERISTICS.—The alkalies change an infusion of turmeric, or turmeric paper, to reddish-brown. A similar alteration of colour occurs when turmeric paper is exposed to the vapour of hydrochloric acid gas, or is touched with oil of vitriol. If to tincture of turmeric boracic acid be added,

[1] Gmelin's *Handb. d. Chem.*
[2] *Journ. de Pharm.* i. 289.

and the mixture be evaporated to dryness, an orange-red residue is obtained, whereas without the acid the residue is yellow. By this test the yellow colouring matter of turmeric can be distinguished from that of rhubarb (see *Rheum*). Sulphate of copper causes a yellowish precipitate with an infusion of turmeric. A similar effect is produced by sesquichloride of iron.

PHYSIOLOGICAL EFFECTS.—Are those of a mild aromatic stimulant (see Vol. i. p. 227). The colouring matter becomes absorbed, and communicates a yellow tinge to the urine.[1] According to Mr. Gibson,[2] the colouring matter of turmeric is somewhat changed by the digestive organs; for the stools of animals fed with this root were green, whilst both logwood and madder exhibited their respective hues after passing through the intestines.

USES.—Employed as a condiment, colouring ingredient, and test. It is a constituent of the well-known *curry powder* and *curry paste*, and of many other articles of Indian cookery. Formerly it had some reputation in hepatic and other visceral diseases, and especially in jaundice.

As a test, it is used to detect the presence of free alkalies, which change its yellow colour to a reddish-brown. But alkaline earths and the alkaline carbonates, borates, and sulphurets, as well as boracic, sulphuric, and hydrochloric acids, change the colour of turmeric from yellow to brown. Though not a very delicate test, it is often a very useful one.

1. TINCTURA CURCUMÆ; *Tincture of Turmeric.*—Prepared by digesting one part of bruised Turmeric in six parts of Proof Spirit. Employed for the preparation of turmeric paper. Diluted with water, it yields a slightly turbid yellow liquid, which is sometimes used in the class-room as a test for alkalies, &c.

2. CHARTA CURCUMÆ; *Charta exploratoria flava ; Turmeric Paper.*— Prepared with white, bibulous, or unsized paper, which is to be brushed over with, or soaked in, tincture of turmeric, and dried in the air, the access of alkaline and acid fumes being prevented. Mr. Faraday[3] directs it to be prepared with a *decoction of turmeric* (prepared by boiling one ounce of the coarsely-powdered turmeric in ten or twelve ounces of water, straining through a cloth, and allowing the fluid to settle for a minute or two). Turmeric paper is employed as a test for alkalies, &c., which render it reddish or brownish.

78. CURCUMA ANGUSTIFOLIA, *Roxburgh.*—THE NARROW-LEAVED TURMERIC.

Sex. Syst. Monandria, Monogynia.

(Fæcula tuberis. East Indian Arrow-root, *Offic*)

HISTORY.—This plant was found by H. T. Colebrook, Esq. in the forests extending from the banks of the Sona to Nagpore, and was by him introduced into the Botanic Garden at Calcutta.[4]

BOTANY. **Gen. Char.**—Vide *Curcuma longa.*

Sp. Char.—*Bulb* oblong, with pale, oblong, pendulous *tubers* only. *Leaves* stalked, narrow lanceolate. *Flowers* longer than the bracts.

---

[1] Lewis, *Mat. Med.*; and Reiger, quoted by Murray, *App. Med.* vol. v. p. 78.
[2] *Mem. of the Lit and Phil. Soc. of Manchester,* vol. i. 2d ser. p. 148.
[3] *Chemical Manipulation.*
[4] Roxburgh, *Fl. Indica,* vol. i. p. 31.

Hab.—East Indies : from the banks of the Sona to Nagpore (Roxburgh). Also in abundance on the Malabar coast (Ainslie).

EXTRACTION OF THE FECULA.—From the tubers of several species of Curcuma is obtained, in the East Indies, a fecula called *tikor*.

According to Dr. Roxburgh,[1] the biennial roots of the genus Curcuma consist of what he calls *bulbs, tubers,* and *fibres*. The *bulbs* are formed during the first year, and support the aërial parts of the plants : hence they may be termed *phyllophorous receptacles*. From these bulbs issue the *palmate tubers*, and chiefly the *fibres* or genuine roots; the latter issuing from the lower part of the bulbs. Some of the fibres end in a single oblong, pearl-coloured, solid *tuber*. From these tubers, and from no other parts, the natives of various parts of India obtain starch.

At Bhagulpore this is procured from *C. leucorrhiza*. "The root is dug up, and rubbed on a stone, or beat in a mortar, and afterwards rubbed in water with the hand, and strained through a cloth ; the fecula having subsided, the water is poured off, and the Tikor (fecula) dried for use."[2]

At Travancore, and also, according to Bennett,[3] at Bombay, from the *C. angustifolia*. "So much of it has been made of late years on the Malabar coast, where the plant grows in abundance, that it has become a considerable object in trade, and is much prized in England."[4]

C. rubescens is another species which also yields the fecula called tikor.

DESCRIPTION.—*Curcuma starch* (*amylum curcuma*) or *tikor* is imported from the East Indies under the name of *East India arrow-root*. But as this name is also applied to the starch of Maranta arundinacea cultivated in the East Indies, I have thought it advisable to distinguish it by the name of "Curcuma starch." Two kinds of Curcuma starch are imported from Calcutta ; one white, the other buff-coloured.

α. *White tikor*, or *curcuma starch*, or *white East Indian arrow-root*, is a fine white powder, readily distinguishable, both by the eye and the touch, from West Indian arrow-root. To the eye it somewhat resembles a finely-powdered salt (as bicarbonate of soda or Rochelle salt). When pinched or pressed by the fingers, it wants the firmness so characteristic of West Indian arrow-root, and it does not crepitate to the same extent when rubbed between the fingers.

Examined by the microscope, the particles of this starch are found to be transparent flattened discs of about the $\frac{1}{3333}$ of an inch in thickness.[5] Their shape is ovate, or oblong-ovate, with a very short neck or nipple-like projection at one extremity, where is situated the part called the hilum. The largest are about $\frac{1}{370}$th of an inch in length, and $\frac{1}{770}$th of an inch in breadth.[6] On

---

[1] Roxburgh, *Asiatic Researches*, vol. xi. p. 218 ; also, *Fl. Indica*, vol. i. p. 21.
[2] Roxburgh, *Fl. Indica*, vol. i. p. 30.
[3] *Ceylon and its Capabilities*, p. 151.
[4] Ainslie, *Mat. Indica*, vol. i. p. 19, 1826.
[5] The particles of plantain-starch, like those of curcuma-starch, are flat discs.
[6] The following measurements, in parts of an English inch, of the particles of East India arrow-root, were made for me by Mr. George Jackson :—

Particles.	Length.	Breadth.	Thickness.
1	0·0027	0·0013	
2	0·0029	0·0011	
3*	0·0022	0·0011	
4*	0·0017	0·0011	Average 0·0003
5*	0·0013	0·0008	
6	0·0012	0·0007	
7	0·0007	0·0004	

account of their flatness they have but little lateral shading, except when viewed edgeways. The hilum or nucleus is placed at the narrow extremity,—is circular, very small, and not very distinct. The rings (or rather portions of rings) are seen both on the flat surface and on the edges; they are numerous, close, and very fine.

β. *Buff-coloured tikor,* or *curcuma-starch; pale buff-coloured East Indian arrow-root.*—In the form of powder, or of pulverulent masses, which are dirty- or buffy-white. Paddy husks, woody fibre, and various impurities, are intermixed.

To the microscope both kinds present the same appearance, from which it is probable that they are obtained from the same plant, but with unequal degrees of care. The particles of East Indian arrow-root are very unequal in size, but on the average are larger than those of West Indian arrow-root.

COMPOSITION.—Not ascertained, but doubtless analogous to that of other starches, viz. $C^{12}H^{10}O^{10}$.

EFFECTS AND USES.—Analogous to those of the West Indian starch. Its commercial value, however, is much below that of the latter. At Travancore it forms a large portion of the diet of the inhabitants (Roxburgh).

79. Curcuma Zedoaria, *Roxburgh.*—Round Zedoary.

Sex. Syst. Monandria, Monogynia.

(Tubera.)

Dr. Roxburgh gave some of the dried roots of this plant to Sir Joseph Banks, who ascertained that they agreed well with the *Zedoaria rotunda* of the shops.[1]

1. ZEDOARIA ROTUNDA.—The *zedoary root* (*radix zedoariæ*) now found in the shops of English druggists is the *round zedoary* (*zedoaria rotunda*) of pharmacological writers. It occurs in segments (halves, quarters, or flat sections) of a roundish or ovate tuber. The external portion of the tuber is marked by the remains, membranes, and fibres, and is of a pale brownish-grey or whitish appearance. When cut, it presents a yellowish marbled appearance, not very dissimilar to the cut surface of rhubarb. It has a warm, aromatic, bitter taste, and an aromatic odour. It has been analysed by Bucholz[2] and by Morin.[3] Its constituents, according to the latter chemists, are—*Volatile oil, resin, gum, starch, woody fibre, vegeto-animal matter (?), osmazome (?), free acetic acid, acetate of potash, sulphur,* and in the ashes *carbonate* and *sulphate of potash, chloride of potassium, phosphate of lime, alumina, silica, oxides of iron* and *manganese.* It possesses aromatic and tonic properties. It is less heating than ginger and galangal, and is more analogous to turmeric.

2. ZEDOARIA LONGA.—The root called *long zedoary* (*Zedoaria longa*) is no longer found in the shops of English druggists. It is in pieces scarcely so long and wide as the little finger. Its chemical and medicinal properties resemble those of round zedoary. It is, perhaps, the *zerumbet root* (*radix zerumbet*), for a piece of which I am indebted to Dr. Royle. It is very similar in shape to a curved or arched piece of long turmeric. Its colour is yellowish-grey.

The plant which yields long zedoary has not been satisfactorily ascertained; but it is probably the *Curcuma Zerumbet* of Roxburgh, who states that the *zerumbet* or *kuchoora* of the native druggists of Calcutta are the roots of this species of Curcuma, and that they are principally obtained from Chittagong. He also adds that he sent the sliced and dried bulbous and palmate tuberous roots to Sir J. Banks, who ascertained that they were the real *zedoaria* of our Materia Medica, and that the root of *C. Zedoaria* was the *Zedoaria rotunda* of the shops.

---

[1] Roxburgh's *Flora Indica,* vol. i. pp. 23 and 24.
[2] Trommsdorff's *Journal,* xxv. 2, p. 3.
[3] *Journ. de Pharm.* t. ix. p. 257.

3. ZEDOARIA LUTEA.—The *turmeric coloured zedoary* of Ainslie,[1] the *yellow zedoary* (*zedoaire jaune*) of Guibourt, is probably the *cassumunar root* (*radix cassumunar*) of English druggists (see *ante*, p. 236).

80. AMOMUM CARDAMOMUM, *Linn.*—THE CLUSTER OR ROUND CARDAMOM.

Sex. Syst. Monandria, Monogynia.

(Semina.)

HISTORY.—The fruit of this plant is the ἄμωμον of Dioscorides,[2] the *Amomi uva* of Pliny.[3]

BOTANY. **Gen. Char.**—*Inner limb of the corolla* 1-lipped. *Filament* dilated beyond the anther, with an entire or lobed crest. *Capsule* often berried, 3-celled, 3-valved. *Seeds* numerous, arillate.—*Herbaceous perennials*, with articulated creeping *rhizomes*. *Leaves* in 2 rows, membranous, with their sheaths split. *Inflorescence* spiked, loosely imbricated, radical (Blume).[4]

Sp. Char.—*Leaves* with short petioles, lanceolate. *Spikes* half immersed in the earth, loosely imbricated with villous, lanceolate, acute, 1-flowered *bracts*. *Lip*, with the interior margin, 3-lobed. *Crest* 3-lobed (Roxburgh).

Hab.—Sumatra, Java, and other islands eastward to the Bay of Bengal.

DESCRIPTION.—The fruit of this plant is the *round cardamom* (*Cardamomum rotundum*) of the shops. It varies in size from that of a black currant to that of a cherry. It is roundish or roundish-ovate, with three convex rounded sides or lobes, more or less striated longitudinally, yellowish or brownish-white, sometimes with a red tint, and when examined by a pocket lens shows the remains of hairs, the greater part of which have probably been rubbed off. The seeds are brown, angular, cuneiform, shrivelled, with an aromatic, camphoraceous flavour. The fruits in their native clusters or spikes (constituting the *Amomum racemosum*) are rarely met with : a fine sample is in the Sloanian collection of the British Museum.

FIG. 94.

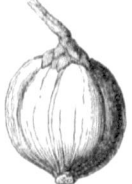

Round Cardamom.

COMPOSITION.—It has not been analysed. Its constituents are probably analogous to those of the Malabar cardamom (*Elettaria Cardamomum*).

EFFECTS AND USES.—Similar to those of the Malabar cardamom. Round cardamoms are not employed in this country. They are officinal in the French Codex, and said to be consumed in the Southern parts of Europe. [There is great doubt, however, that it is so, for though abundant in the markets of the East, they are (according to Mr. Daniel Hanbury) "seldom seen in Europe, except in cabinets of materia medica." They vary in price from 2s. 6d. to 5s. a pound in the market at Bangkok.[5]—ED.]

---

[1] *Materia Indica*, vol. i. pp. 491 and 493.
[2] Lib. i. cap. xiv.
[3] *Hist. Nat.* lib. xii. cap. xxviii. ed. Valp.
[4] *Op. cit.*
[5] *Pharm. Trans.* for Feb. and March 1855.

81. AMOMUM GRANUM PARADISI, *Hooker fil.*[1]

Sex. Syst. Monandria, Monogynia.

HISTORY.—[The species known under this name was long supposed to yield the officinal grains of paradise. The *A. Melegueta* is now ascertained, however, to be the only source of that officinal article.

BOTANY.—The botanical history of these seeds has been involved in much obscurity. Recent valuable communications to botanical science by Drs. Daniell and Hooker have done much, however, to throw light on this intricate subject. *Amomum Grana Paradisi* and *Amomum Melegueta* are now known as distinct species. The Amomum described by Smith as *A. Grana Paradisi* is identical with *Amomum exscapum* of Sims. The seeds of this species do not yield true grains of paradise.

FIG. 95.

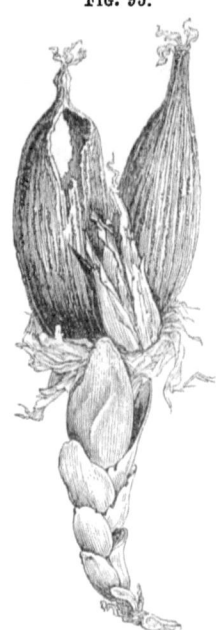

Amomum Granum Paradisi, Hooker fil.

(Natural size. From a specimen in Smith's herbarium in the collection of the Linnean Society.)

Gen. Char.—Vide *Amomum Cardamomum.*

Sp. Char. — Foliis elliptico-lanceolatis acuminatis, ligula obtusa v. biloba scapo multifloro bracteis laxe imbricatis puberulis obtusis mucronatis perianthio exteriore tubo brevi limbo obtuso interiore extus puberulo, lobis lateralibus obtusis, dorsali ovato-oblongo obtuso, labello amplo late obovato-rotundo marginibus undulato plicatis filamento basi utrinque processibus 2 subulatis, antheræ apice integro v. bifido lobulis lateralibus patulis subulatis loculis puberulis, staminodiis linearibus obtusis, ovario pubescente, fructu ampullaceo v. elliptico-ovato, v. lanceolato profunde sulcato pubescente, seminibus brunneis subquadrato-rotundatis, testa atro-brunnea nitida.

Hab.—Sierra Leone.

DESCRIPTION.—But little need be said of this drug. Unripe specimens of the fruit, which is remarkable for being deeply sulcated and covered with minute hairs, have the seeds invested with a very pale silvery epidermis; older ones are very dark brown, and highly polished. These seeds are highly aromatic, but do not possess the pungency of the real grains of paradise.

COMPOSITION.—These seeds do not appear to have been analysed. They are not found in the markets.

EFFECTS AND USES.—Probably much like those of the true grains of paradise.—ED.]

82. AMOMUM MELEGUETA, *Roscoe.*

Sex. Syst. Monandria, Monogynia.

(Semina.)

HISTORY.—The source of the officinal "Grains of Paradise." The term "*Malagueta*[2] *pepper*" has been applied to the fruit or seeds of several zin-

---

[1] [Hooker's *Journal of Botany and Kew Gardens Miscellany*, vol. vi. p. 295, 1854.]
[2] This word is variously spelt Malagueta, Malaguetta, Melegueta, Mellegetta, Meligetta, &c. Several etymologies of it have been given : some say the seeds have been so called in consequence of their resemblance to Turkey millet, termed by the Italians *melica* or *melega*. Savary says the

giberaceous plants,[1] as well as to the pimento or allspice.[2]   It is usually considered to be synonymous with the terms "*grains of paradise*" and "*Guinea grains.*"

Malagueta pepper is said to have been known in Italy before the discovery of the Guinea coast by the Portuguese in the 15th century.   It was brought by the Moors, who used to cross the great region of Madingha and the deserts of Lybia, and carry it to Mundi Barca (or Monte da Barca), a port in the Mediterranean.   The Italians, not knowing the place of its birth, as it is so precious a spice, called it *grana paradisi.*[3]

BOTANY.— [This Amomum has been much confounded in its pharmaceutical relations.   It is certainly the true producer of the grains of paradise of the shops.—ED.]

FIG. 96.

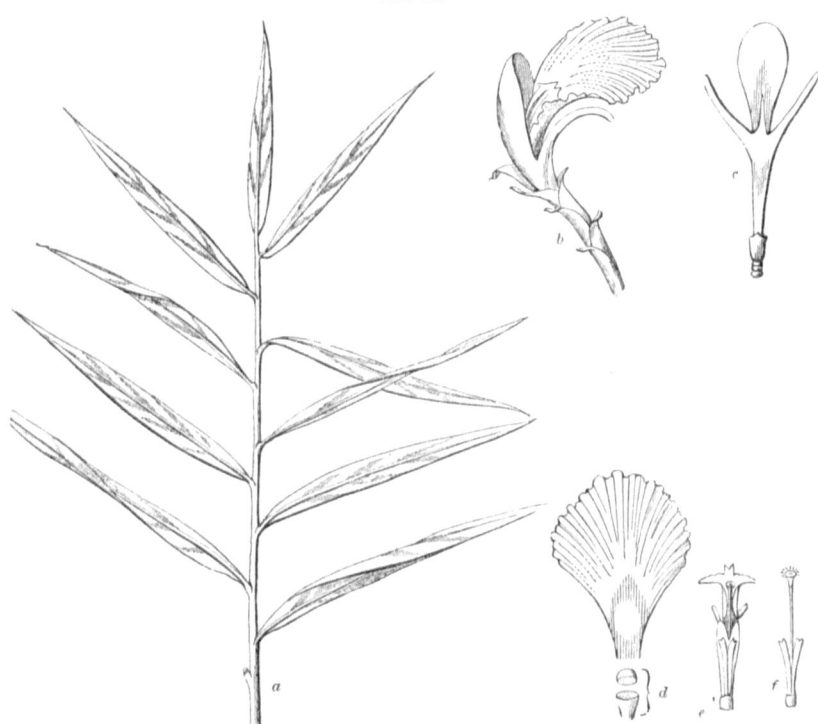

Leaves and Flower of Amomum Melegueta, Roscoe.

a. Stem and leaves.	*d.* Interior limb of corolla or lip.
b. Entire flower and floral bracts.	*e.* Filament, anther, stigma, style, and ovary.
c. Exterior limb of corolla.	*f.* Style and barren anthers (germinal processes).

term is derived from *mala gente,* the designation applied by the Portuguese to the people of the coast yielding the seeds.   Another derivation (suggested to me by Mr. R. Thomson, of the London Institution) is *Melli* (also written *Melle* and *Máli*), a kingdom of Nigritia; and *gitti* (or *gitter*), a Portuguese name for pepper.   Barbot says the Portuguese word malagueta is from the native name for the pepper, *emanegéta.*

[1] See a paper on "*Grains of Paradise,*" by the author, in *Pharm. Journ.* vol. ii. p. 443, 1843.
[2] See Ortega, *Historia natural de la Malagueta, ó Pimienta de Tavasco,* Madrid, 1780.
[3] De Barros, quoted in the *Encyclop. Metropol.* art. *Guinea.*

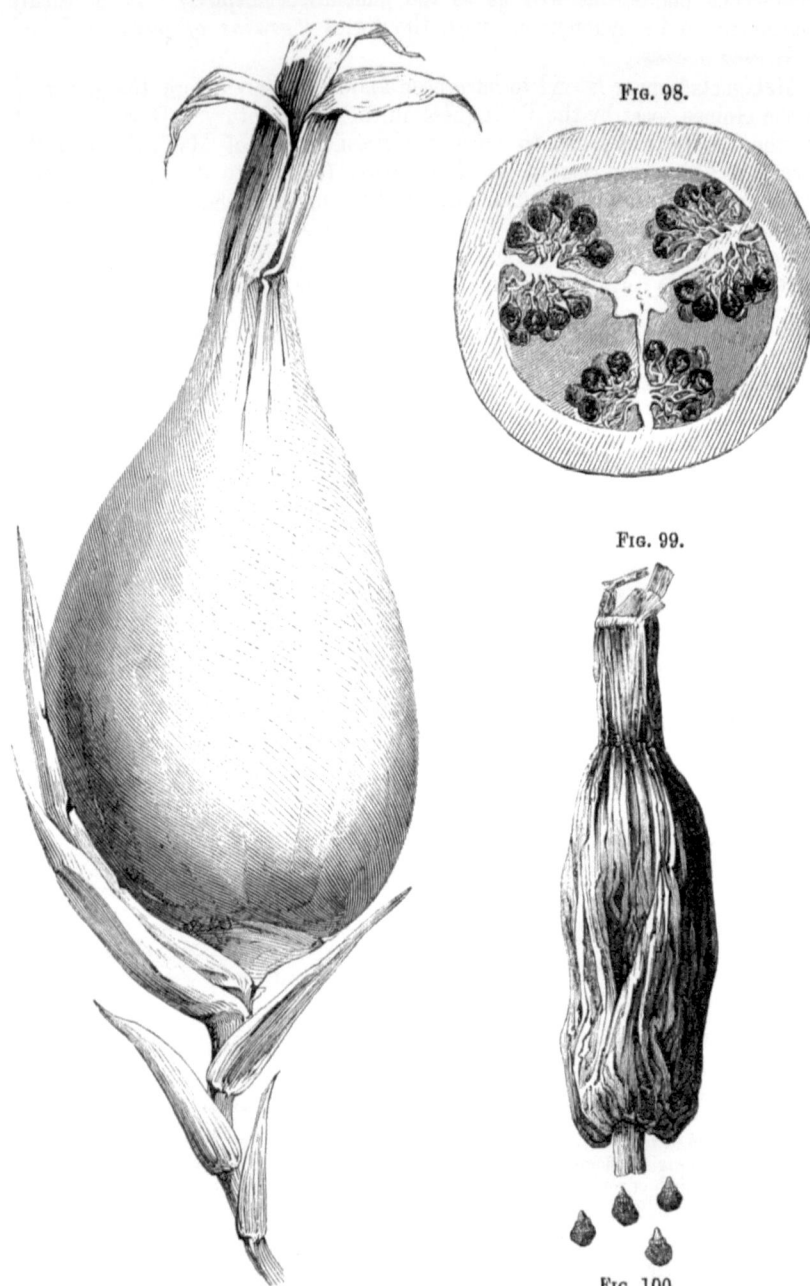

Fig. 97.

Fig. 98.

Fig. 99.

Fig. 100.

Fruit of Amomum Melegueta, Roscoe.

Fig. 97. Entire fruit preserved wet.   Fig. 99. Entire fruit dried.
Fig. 98. Transverse section of ditto.   Fig. 100. Seeds of ditto.

[**Gen. Char.**—Vide *A. Cardamomum.*

Sp. Char.—Foliis anguste lanceolatis, vaginis gracilibus, scapo unofloro, bracteis lineari oblongis cuspidatis perianthio exteriore spathaceo acuminato, interiore foliolo dorsali oblongo, lateralibus e basi lanceolata sensim acuminatis, labello late obovato quadrato, margine undulato crispato, filamenti processibus lateralibus subulatis, antheræ lobo terminali subtriangulari apice integro obtuso dentato v. bifido angulis lateralibus subelongatis sublatisve, ovario glabro, staminodiis liberis subulatis, fructu ampullaceo ovato v. ellipticooblongo glabro, perianthii tubo æquilongo coronato, seminibus angulato globosis pallide brunneis, testa nitida verruculata.

Hab.—Western coast of Africa; Demerara.—ED.]

DESCRIPTION. *a.* **Of the dried Fruits.**—I have met with two kinds of dried fruits whose seeds bear the name of grains of paradise or Guinea grains.

1. *Fruit* (fig. 101).—These are oval or oval-oblong capsules, somewhat reddish-brown, and wrinkled longitudinally. Their length (exclusive of stalk and beak) rarely exceeds 1½ inch; and their diameter is about ½ an inch. The seeds agree with the grains of paradise brought from Cape Palmas and Sierra Leone. I am indebted to Dr. Daniell for specimens gathered from the high lands on the right of the river Congo. Some of them are strung on a cord,—the usual form in which they are sold in Africa. [These fruits were thought by Dr. Pereira to agree with the Grain of Paradise Amomum described by Afzelius. The researches of Dr. Daniell, however, render it almost certain that they are merely the produce of stunted specimens of A. Melegueta, which must henceforth be regarded as the only source of the true grains of paradise of commerce.—ED.]

2. *Fruit* (fig. 102).—These fruits are larger than the preceding, and more ovate. Exclusive of beak and stalk they are two inches long and one inch in diameter. They are ovate or ovate-oblong, coriaceous, wrinkled as if shrivelled, yellowish-brown. The seeds are identical with those sold in the shops as grains of paradise or Guinea grains [and are, like the above, the produce of Roscoe's A. Melegueta.—ED.]

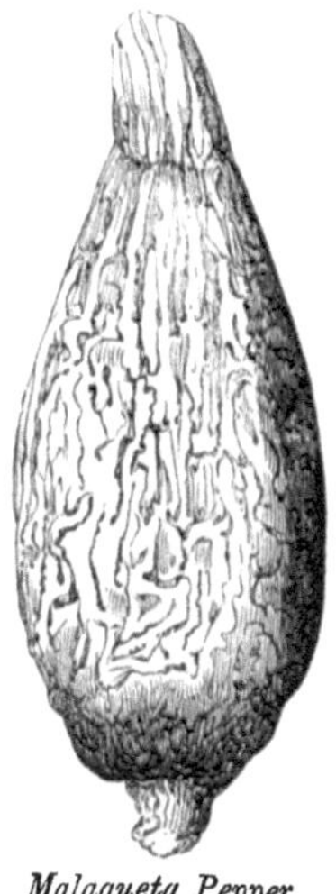

FIG. 101.　　　FIG. 102.

Malagueta Pepper Fruit.

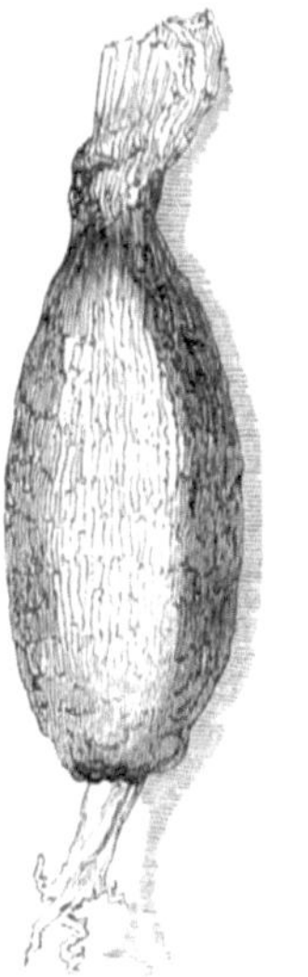

Capsule of Malagueta Pepper Fruit.

(From Dr. Burges's collection in the College of Physicians.)

(From a specimen in the Sloanian collection of the British Museum, where it is labelled "Melegetta,—a pod from Guinea.")

β. **Of the Seeds.**—The seeds, called in the shops *grains of paradise* (*grana paradisi*) or *Guinea grains* (*grana guineensia*), are roundish or ovate, frequently bluntly angular, and somewhat cuneiform; shining golden-brown; minutely rough, from small warts and wrinkles; internally white. Their taste is aromatic, and vehemently hot or peppery; when crushed and rubbed between the fingers, their odour is feebly aromatic. Their greatest diameter rarely exceeds 1¼ line. The acrid taste resides in the seed-coats.

Two sorts are distinguished by the importers :—

1. *Guinea grains from Acra.*—These are somewhat larger, plumper, and more warty than the ordinary sort. On the umbilicus of the seeds there is a short, conical, projecting tuft of pale-coloured fibres. This sort fetches a somewhat higher price than the next sort.

2. *Guinea grains from Cape Palmas and Sierra Leone.*—Smaller and smoother than the preceding. They are devoid of the projecting fibrous tuft on the umbilicus. Being somewhat cheaper than the foregoing sort, they form the ordinary grains of paradise of the shops.

Commerce.—Grains of paradise are imported, in casks, barrels, and puncheons, from the coast of Guinea. [The quantities of " grains of paradise and Guinea" imported during six years are, in cwts. as follows :—

	Cwts.		Cwts.
In 1849	1,247	In 1852	440
1850	1,316	1853	183
1851	96	1854	249.—Ed.]

"*Extract or preparation of Guinea grains*" was formerly imported.[1]

The heavy duty formerly imposed on grains of paradise was intended to act as a prohibition of their use.[2]

Composition.—[Grains of paradise have recently been elaborately examined by Sandrock, who finds them to contain—*Volatile oil, fatty oil, two resins,* which he distinguishes by the letters a and β, *peculiar astringent matter, albumen, gum* and *vegetable mucilage, pectine, extractive matter, starch, woody fibre, chloride of potassium, sulphate of potash, phosphate of lime, phosphate of magnesia,* and *silica.*[3]—Ed.]

Physiological Effects.—Analogous to those of pepper. A very erroneous notion prevails that these seeds are highly injurious.[4]

Uses.—Rarely employed as an aromatic. Esteemed in Africa as the most wholesome of spices, and generally used by the natives to season their food.[5]

Its principal consumption is in veterinary medicine, and to give an artificial strength to spirits, wine, beer, and vinegar.

By 56 *Geo.* III. c. 58, no brewer or dealer in beer shall have in his possession or use grains of paradise, under a penalty of £200 for each offence ; and no druggist shall sell it to a brewer, under a penalty of £500 for each offence.

83. Amomum maximum, *Roxburgh.*—The Great-winged Amomum.
(Fructus : Java Cardamom, *offic.*)

History.—This plant was first described by Roxburgh.[6]

Botany. **Gen. Char.**—Vide *Amomum Cardamomum.*

Sp. Char.—*Leaves* stalked, lanceolate, villous underneath. *Spikes* oval, even with the earth. *Bracts* lanceolate. *Lip* elliptical. *Coronet* of 1 semilunar lobe. *Capsules* round, 9-winged (Roxburgh).

The *capsule* is "almost globular, size of a gooseberry, 3-celled, 3-valved, ornamented with 9 [7 to 13, *Blume*] firm, short, ragged (when old and dry), membranaceous wings.

[1] Frewin, *Digested Abridgment of the Laws of the Customs,* 1819.
[2] *Fourth Report of the African Institution,* p. 16.
[3] [*Archiv der Pharmacie,* Jan. 1853, p. 18.]
[4] Roscoe, *op. cit.*
[5] *Fourth Report of the African Institution.*
[6] *Asiatic Researches,* xi. p. 344.

The *seeds* possess a warm, pungent, aromatic taste, not unlike that of cardamoms, but by no means so grateful" (Roxburgh). The *Nepal cardamom*, described by Dr. Hamilton,[1] appears to be identical with the Java cardamom. Dr. Hamilton says the plant yielding it " is a species of *Amomum*, as that genus is defined by Dr. Roxburgh, and differs very much from the cardamom of Malabar."

Hab.—The Malay Islands (Roxburgh); Java (Blume). Cultivated in the mountainous parts of Nepal, where it is propagated by cuttings of the root [rhizome]; the plants yield in three years, and afterwards give an annual crop (Hamilton).

DESCRIPTION.—The fruit of this plant is known in commerce by various names; such as *greater Java cardamoms* (*cardamomi majores javanenses*, Th. Martius; *Java cardamoms*, offic.; *Nepal cardamoms, desi elachi* [i. e. *country cardamoms*] of Hindustan, Hamilton; the *bura elachee* [i. e. *great cardamoms*] of Saharunpore,—the *Bengal cardamoms* of the Calcutta market, Royle; *cardamome ailé de Java* and *cardamome fausse maniguette*, Guibourt) are oval or oval-oblong, frequently somewhat ovate, 3-valved, from 8 to 15 lines long, and from 4 to 8 lines broad, usually flattened on one side, convex on the other, occasionally curved, sometimes imperfectly 3-lobed, and resembling in their form the pericarp of the cocoa-nut (fig. 103). Their colour is dirty greyish-brown. They have a coarse, fibrous, aged appearance, are strongly ribbed, and when soaked in hot water (fig. 104) become almost globular, and present from 9 to 13 ragged, membranous wings, which occupy the upper half or three-fourths of the capsule, and are scarcely perceptible in the dried state of the pericarp. By the possession of wings these cardamoms are distinguished from all others of commerce, and hence might be called the *winged cardamoms*. Occasionally the footstalk is attached, with, now and then, portions of brown, membranous, imbricated scales, as long as the fruit. At the opposite or winged extremity of the capsule are frequently the fibrous remains of the calyx. Seeds (fig. 105) somewhat larger than grains of paradise, dull, dirty brown, with a shallow groove on one side, internally white; taste and odour feebly aromatic. One hundred parts of the fruit consist, according to Th. Martius,[2] of seventy parts seeds, and thirty parts pericarpial coats. They are imported from Calcutta in bags.

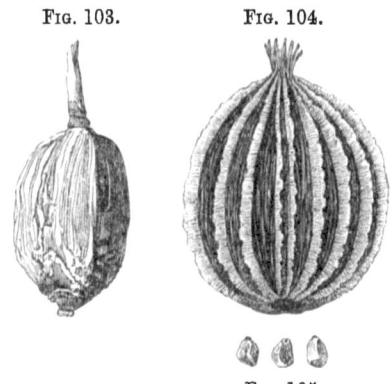

FIG. 103.   FIG. 104.

FIG. 105.

Java Cardamoms.

Fig. 103. The dried fruit of commerce.
Fig. 104. The fruit which has been soaked in water to expand the wings.
Fig. 105. Seeds.

COMPOSITION.—Analogous, probably, to that of the Malabar cardamom, except in the quantity of volatile oil which it yields; for Martius procured only four scruples of it from a pound of the fruit. The oil obtained was white and thickish.

EFFECTS AND USES.—Java cardamoms are not used here. They are of inferior quality, and when brought to this country are usually sold in bond for continental use. In 1839 a quantity of them was sold at sevenpence per lb.

84. Amomum Korarima.—The Korarima Cardamom.

The fruit of this plant is the *Cardamomum majus* of Valerius Cordus,[3] of Matthiolus,[4]

[1] *An Account of the Kingdom of Nepal,* ed. 1819.
[2] *Pharmakognosie.*
[3] *Hist. Stirpium,* lib. iv. p. 195, 1561.
[4] *Comment. in* vi. *lib. Diosc.* Venet. 1583.

Geoffroy,[1] Smith,[2] and Geiger.[3] In Dr. Burges's Collection of Materia Medica at the College of Physicians, there are several fine specimens marked "*Cardamomum maximum Matthioli*" (fig. 106).

FIG. 106.　　　　FIG. 107.

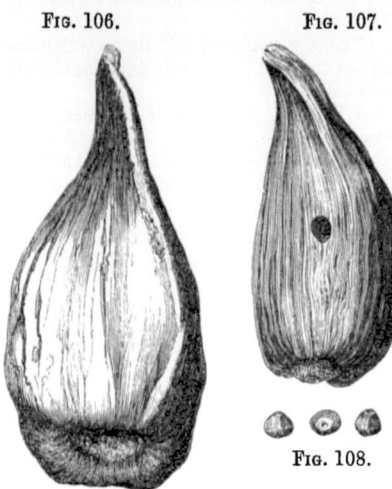

FIG. 108.

Korarima Cardamom.

Fig. 106. The "Cardamomum maximum Matthioli" of Dr. Burges's Collection in the College of Physicians.

Fig. 107. The "Korarima" of Dr. Beke.

Fig. 108. Seeds of ditto.

Under the name of *Korarima*, or *Gurágie spice*, I have received specimens of the same fruit, which had been brought from Abyssinia by Major Harris's embassy, by Dr. Beke, and by Mr. Charles Johnston[4] (fig. 107).

In former editions of this work I followed Sir J. E. Smith,[5] in considering this fruit to be identical with the *Amomum madagascariense* of Lamarck,[6] and the *A. angustifolium* of Sonnerat.[7] As there is some reason to doubt the propriety of this proceeding, I have considered it advisable to designate the plant provisionally the "*Amomum Korarima;*" the word Korarima (pronounced in English Korahrēēma) being the Galla name for the fruit which in Arabic is called *Heil*.[8]

The capsule is ovate, pointed, flattened on one side, striated, with a broad circular umbilicus or scar at the bottom, around which is an elevated, notched, and corrugated margin. Some authors, who have mistaken the base of the capsule for its summit, have compared the shape to that of a fig.

Some of the fruits which I received from Abyssinia had been perforated and strung upon a cord (fig. 107), probably for the purpose of hanging them to dry. Dr. Beke thinks that the pierced or perforated fruits are those which have been gathered before they were perfectly ripe.

The seeds (fig. 108) are rather larger than grains of paradise, roundish or somewhat angular, abrupt at the base, olive-brown, with an aromatic flavour analogous to that of the Malabar cardamom, but totally devoid of the vehemently hot acrid taste of the grains of paradise.

The Korarima is brought to the market of Báso, in southern Abyssinia, from Túmhe (known among the native merchants as the "*country of the Korarima*"), somewhere about 9° N. lat. and 35° E. long. It is carried to Massowáh, the port of northern Abyssinia on the Red Sea, and exported from thence to India. Dr. Rüppell was informed that the annual export is of the value of one thousand dollars (about £200 sterling). Although it is not impossible that the same fruit may grow in Madagascar, yet it is highly improbable that the Korarima of Abyssinia is the produce of Madagascar.[9]

At Báso, Dr. Beke purchased it at the rate of forty for one penny sterling. [At Musswah Mr. Vaughan found the capsules selling at one dollar per 1000.—Ed.]

---

[1] *Mat. Méd.* ii. 366.

[2] Rees' *Cyclop.* art. *Mellegetta*.

[3] *Handb. d. Pharm.* Bd. ii.

[4] *Pharmaceutical Journal*, vol. vi. p. 466, 1847.

[5] Rees' *Cyclop.* vol. xxxix. Addenda.

[6] *Encycl. Botan.* t. i. p. 133, Ill. tab. i.

[7] *Voyage aux Indes*, t. ii. p. 242.

[8] [In the former edition of this work the word was written *Kheil* or *Khil*. According to Mr. Vaughan, however (*Pharm. Journ.* vol. xii. p. 587), *Heil* is the correct name.—Ed.]

[9] Dr. Beke, *Pharmaceutical Journal*, vol. vi. p. 511.

85. Amomum citratum.

Cardamomum majus.—In Dr. Burges's Collection at the College of Physicians is a capsule (in a bad state of preservation) marked "*Cardamomum majus.*" It has a fibrous tuft at one extremity, and is much split at the other. The seeds are angular, oblong, larger than those of Malabar cardamoms, shining brownish-yellow, and have a large concave depression (hilum) at one extremity. They have a warm aromatic flavour, somewhat analogous to that of the oil of lemon-grass. When crushed, they evolve the odour of this oil. Hence I have given them the specific name "*citratum,*" as by this character they are readily distinguished from all other seeds of this order with which I am acquainted.

I have found the same fruits in the Sloanian collection of the British Museum. They are tied together in bunches. One sample is unnamed; another is marked in the catalogue "12057. *Grana Paradisi.*"

FIG. 109.

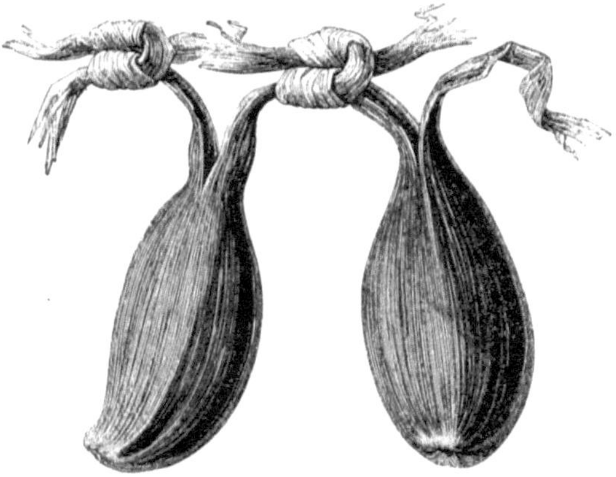

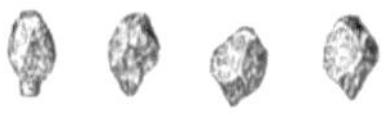

FIG. 110.

Amomum citratum.

Fig. 109. Fruits tied together in a bunch.—Fig. 110. Seeds.

I have met with the same fruits in a collection at Apothecaries' Hall; and I am indebted to Mr. Warrington for the specimen from which fig. 109 was taken. The capsules are tied together in bunches, as shown in the accompanying figure.

86. Amomum Clusii, *Smith.*—Clusius's Cardamom.

Fructus, xiv., Clusius, Exotic. lib. ii. cap. xv. pp. 37 and 38; *Granis paradysi sive Mellegetæ affinis fructus*, Bauhin, Pinax, p. 413; *Amomum Clusii*, or *Long-seeded Amomum*, Smith, Rees' Cyclop. vol. xxxix. Addenda.—Capsule ovate, pointed, slightly triangular, cartilaginous, striated, smooth, yellowish- [reddish-, *Smith*] brown. The seeds have scarcely any flavour, are oblong or ovate, inclining to cylindrical, dark-brown, highly polished, as if varnished; with a pale yellowish-brown, corrugated, and notched margin surrounding the scar.

On comparing my specimen (fig. 111), which was given to me by a druggist, with the one marked *A. Clusii* in Sir J. E. Smith's collection of fruits in the possession of the Linnean Society, I find the seeds of the latter are somewhat longer, and rather more cylindrical; in other respects the two specimens agree.

I have subsequently received from Dr. T. W. C. Martius specimens of a fruit marked "*Cardamomum maximum von Amomum Clusii?*" The capsules are somewhat plumper, but in other respects they agree with the preceding. I gave one of them to Professor Guibourt, who has published a figure of it.[1]

FIG. 111.

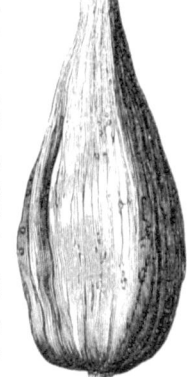

Amomum Clusii.

---

[1] *Hist. Nat. des Drog.* 4ème édit. t. ii. p. 220, fig. 120, 1849.

[87. Amomum Danielli, *Hooker fil.*—Bastard Melligetta.

HISTORY.—The above title has been given by Dr. Hooker to a species of Amomum noticed by Dr. Pereira, in the last edition of this work, as nearly resembling, if not identical with, the *A. Clusii.* He noticed, however, that the capsules differed. Dr. Daniell sent him the specimens from which the figures here given were taken (figs. 112, 113, 114).

FIG. 112.   FIG. 113.

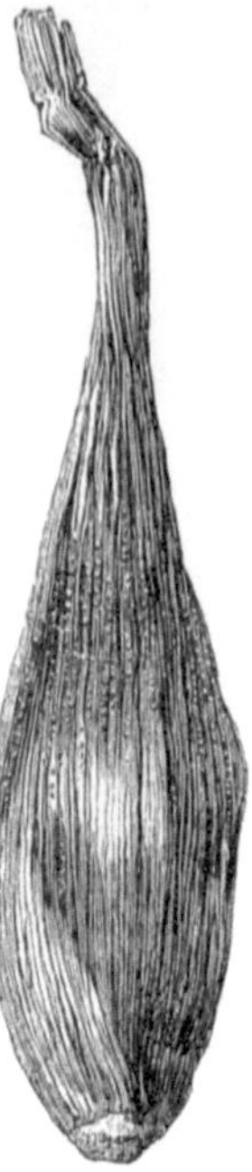

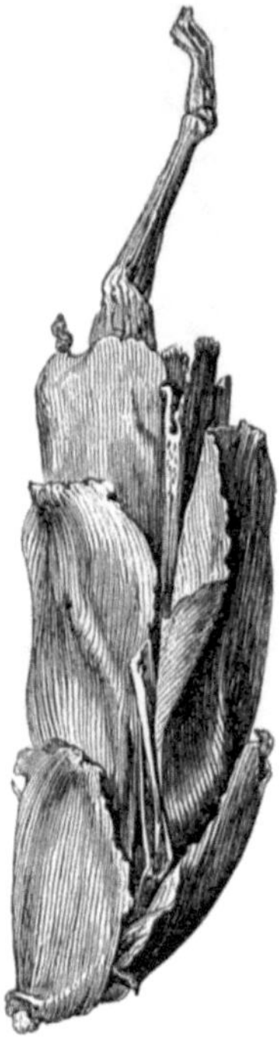

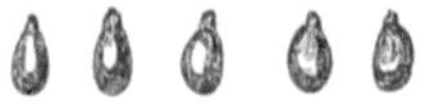

The following are the characters given by Dr. Hooker:—

A. Danielli.—Glaberrimum caule elongato folioso, foliis lineari-lanceolatis (1¼ ped. longis, 3 unc. latis), longe acuminatis striato venosis, scapis radicalibus floriferis 2 unc., fructiferis 4—6 unc. longis, 3—5 floris, bracteis oblongo-cymbiformibus obtusis, floribus flavis, corollæ lobis lateralibus patentibus, subulato acuminatis dorsali amplo obovato-oblongo cæteris longiore, labello late lineari-oblongo planiusculo rigido margine subundulato filamento basi utrinque appendicula subulata aucto fructu lineari ampullatio rostrato.

Hab.—Gold and slave coasts; Fernando Po; Clarence Town. Abundant. Flowers June and July.

A tall handsome species growing from 8 to 9 feet high; the stem an inch or more thick. The flowers are of a beautiful yellow colour,[1] thus differing from the true Melligetta, and, indeed, from all previously-described West African Amoma. The seeds are contained in a soft acidulous pulp of pleasant flavour, which the natives use to allay thirst, and also to prevent the irritating effects of cathartic medicines. The natives call it *Barsalo,* to distinguish it from a smaller Alpine variety named *Tokolo m'pomah,* which may, according to Dr. Daniell, be the same as, or closely allied to, the true Melligetta, which has very pungent seeds.[2]—ED.]

FIG. 114.

Fruits and Seeds of Amomum Danielli.

88. Amomum macrospermum, *Smith.*—Large-seeded Guinea Amomum.

(Semina.)

Zingiber Meleguetta, Gaertner de Fructib. vol. i. p. 34, pl. xii. fig. 1; *Fructus Cajuputi,* Trew, Commercium Litterarium, ann. 1737, Norimbergæ, p. 129, tab. 1, fig. 7-11; also. Herb. Blackwellianum emend. et auctum, vol. iii. cent. vi. tab. 584, fig. 9-13, Norimb. 1773.—Native of Sierra Leone.

The *capsule (fructus cajuputi,* Trew; *Cardamomum bandaense,* T. W. C. Martius; *grand*

---

[1] [*Pharmaceutical Journal,* vol. xii. p. 72.]
[2] [Dr. Hooker describes a variety, β (purpureum).—ED.]

cardamome de Gaertner, Guibourt; *mabooboo* of the natives of Sierra Leone,[1] is ovate, pointed, somewhat striated, about 2 inches long and 6 lines broad, with a corrugated beak.

The *seeds (semina cajuputi,* Trew) are ovate, or nearly globular, or somewhat oblong, variously angular, scarcely larger than grains of paradise, smooth, polished, greenish-grey or lead-coloured, with a strong umbilicated scar at their base, with a whitish or pale-yellow margin; flavour slightly aromatic. Smith says that Gaertner's figure represents them scarcely half large enough. This statement, however, does not apply to the seeds of my specimens.

The seeds yield, by distillation, a volatile oil. Cartheuser[2] obtained from half a pound of them a drachm and a half of a pale-yellowish, aromatic, camphoraceous oil, resembling, but less fragrant and penetrating than, cajuput oil. Trew erroneously supposed that these seeds were the source of the cajuput oil of commerce, and hence have arisen the erroneous denominations of " fructus et semina cajuputi" applied to the fruit and seeds of this species.

The seeds are aromatic, but are much inferior to those of the Malabar cardamom.

I have received from Dr. Daniell specimens of the fruit of this or some closely allied species growing at Gambia and Cape St. Mary. One of the specimens consists of a stalk five inches long, supporting two capsules, and clothed with bracts. The seeds are angular, and lead-coloured. Dr. Daniell tells me that the natives of Africa suck the acidulous pulp of the fruit.

FIG. 115.   FIG. 116.

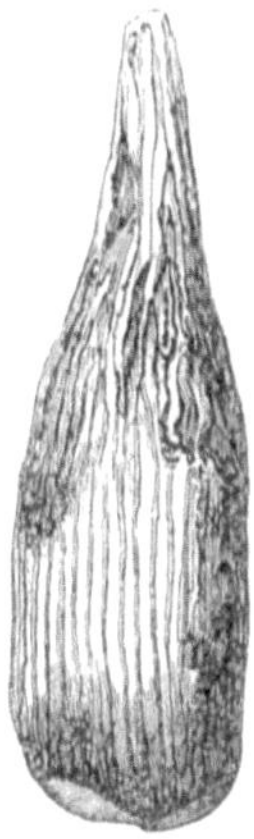

(From a specimen in the Sloanian Collection.) | (Banda cardamom of Martius,[3] and its seeds.)

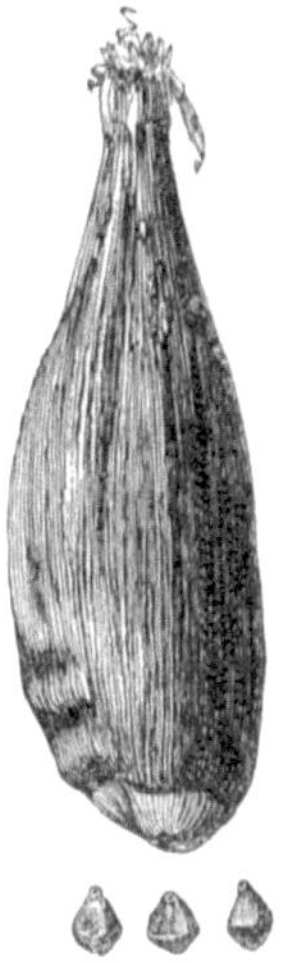

Amomum macrospermum.

89. Amomum globosum, *Loureiro ?*

(Semina.)

Mé tlé, Cochinch.; *Tsào keu,* Chin. Loureiro, Fl. Cochin.—Mountains of Cochinchina and China.

[Much valuable information has been collected on the subject of Chinese cardamoms by Mr. Daniel Hanbury, who has worked out the subject with great zeal and intelligence. In accordance with M. Guibourt's views, he divides this cardamom into the *large* round and the *small* round China cardamoms (see figs. 117—121).

Mr. Hanbury remarks as follows on these two commercial varieties, both of which, however, appear to be the product of the *Amomum globosum :—*

" Fine specimens of this fruit [large variety] were procured by my brother, Mr. Thomas Hanbury, at Singapore,—in the drug-shops of which place, he tells me, it appears by no means plentiful. Deprived of the husk (fig. 120), I have also received it from Canton and Shanghae; from the latter place under the above-mentioned character, *Tsaou-kow,*—the

---

[1] Sir J. E. Smith (Rees' *Cyclop. Suppl.*) states, on the authority of Afzelius, that the African name is " Mabooboo." But Nyberg (*Remedia Guineensia,* Upsal, 1813) says that the name " Mabubu" is applied to a species which he calls *Amomum latifolium,* whose seeds, in size, shape, and colour, agree with grape-seeds.

[2] *Dissert. nonnullæ select. physico-chem. ac medicæ,* Francof. 1775.

[3] Professor Guibourt (*Hist. Nat. des Drog.* 4ème édit. p. 218, fig. 119) has figured one of the specimens given to me by Dr. Martius; but he has erroneously stated that the figure was from a specimen in the Sloanian Collection of the British Museum.

same name, I presume, as that given by Loureiro, as applied to his *Amomum globosum*. In the Sloanian collection in the British Museum, there is a small specimen of this fruit.

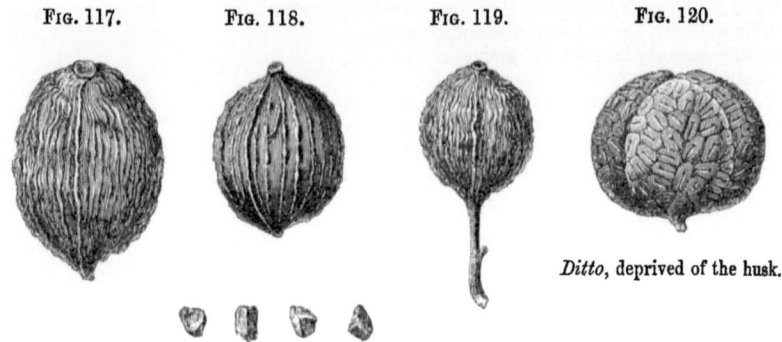

Fig. 117.   Fig. 118.   Fig. 119.   Fig. 120.

Ditto, deprived of the husk.

Large Round China Cardamom (fruits and seeds).

"The *large round China cardamom* varies considerably in size, my specimens being from $1\frac{2}{10}$ inches to $\frac{6}{10}$ of an inch in length. The capsules are somewhat oval or globular, pointed at either extremity, obscurely 3-sided (except at the base, where the triangular character is strongly marked); they are sometimes attached to a long pedicel. The pericarp closely invests the mass of seeds; it is brown, thin, and strongly marked externally with interrupted longitudinal ridges; it is hardly aromatic. The seeds are coherent into a 3-lobed mass (fig. 120); they are generally light greyish-brown, angular, with a deep furrow on one side; they have a slight aromatic odour and taste, the latter suggestive of thyme (*Thymus vulgaris*), though much weaker.

"This cardamom is a native of the South of China, and of Cochin China, whence it is exported. It appears to be much employed in Chinese medicine as a stomachic.

"Specimens of the *small round China cardamom* are preserved in the Musée d'Histoire Naturelle at Paris. M. Guibourt likewise possesses specimens, and has kindly presented me with one. I have never received this cardamom direct from China.

"The following description of the *small round China cardomom* is taken chiefly from M. Guibourt's work:—

Fig. 121.

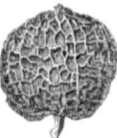

Small Round China Cardamom.

"Capsules pedicelled, nearly spherical, from 7 to 8 lines in diameter, slightly striated longitudinally, and much wrinkled in all directions by drying; it is probable, however, that the fruit was smooth when recent. The capsule is thin, light, easily torn, yellowish externally, white within. The seeds form a globular coherent mass. They are rather large and few in number, somewhat wedge-shaped, of an ashy-grey, a little granular on the surface, and present on the outer face a bifurcate furrow, shaped like a **Y**. They possess a strongly aromatic odour and taste.

"To this description I may add that, compared with the *large round China cardamom*, the capsules in question are more wrinkled in a network manner, more fragile and thin, and (from immaturity?) much less adherent to the mass of seeds; they are more globose, not triangular at the base, but flat, or even depressed like an apple. Their colour, in all the specimens I have seen, is a brownish-yellow. I cannot confirm M. Guibourt's remark as to the highly aromatic properties of the seeds.

"This cardamom, which appears to bear the same Chinese name as the foregoing, is attributed by M. Guibourt to the *Amomum globosum* of Loureiro."[2]—Ed.]

---

[1] *Flora Cochinchinensis*, Berolini, 1793, t. i. p. 6.
[2] *Pharm. Journal*, February and March 1855.

90. Amomum villosum, *Loureiro?*

(Semina.)

Sa nhon, Cochinch.; *Sŏ Xā mi,* Chin., Loureiro.—Mountains of Cochinchina.

I am indebted to Professor Guibourt for specimens of a fruit which he calls the *hairy China cardamom* (*cardamome poilu de la Chine*), and which, in the collection of the Muséum d'Histoire Naturelle, is termed (by mistake?) *tsao-keou.*

Capsules ovate, oblong, obtusely triangular. *Seeds* have no linear depression or groove, as those of the preceding variety, and by the absence of this they may be readily dis tinguished from it; coherent in masses, which are 3-lobed, not quite globular. In my specimens the pericarp is rugous, as if eroded; but when examined by a magnifier, it is seen to be covered by asperities and the remains of fine downy hairs. The flavour of the seeds is aromatic and terebinthi-nate, but not powerful.

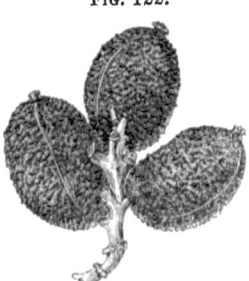

FIG. 122.

M. Guibourt thinks this fruit may perhaps be the pro-duce of *Amomum villosum* of Loureiro, the oriental names of which, however, are very different to that on the speci-men in the Paris Museum. Loureiro states that the seeds of A. villosum are subcalefacient and stomachic, and are exported from the provinces of Qúi-nhon and Phy-yeu, in Cochinchina (where they grow spontaneously) to China,

Hairy China Cardamom.

where they are largely used in medicine. [The woodcut here given is drawn from a specimen in the possession of one of the Editors, and for which he is indebted to Mr. Daniel Hanbury. Mr. H. has received specimens from Singapore and from China.—ED.]

BLACK CARDAMOM, *Guibourt.*—I am indebted to M. Guibourt for a fruit which he calls the *black cardamom of Gaertner* (*cardamome noir de Gaertner*), or the fruit of *Zingiber nigrum*, Gaertner. The *capsule* is larger than the short Malabar cardamoms, acuminate at its two extremities, and formed, as it were, of two obtusely-triangular pyramids joined base to base. The *pericarp* ash-brown, aromatic, but less so than the seeds. *Seeds* annular, brown, slightly aromatic, but devoid of the terebinthinate flavour.

FIG. 123.

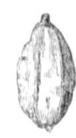

Gaertner states that his plant is the *Alughas* of the Ceylonese. But the black cardamom of Guibourt is certainly not Roxburgh's Alpinia Allughas.

Black Cardamom (Guibourt).

[Mr. Daniel Hanbury has given a description of this cardamom.[1] He received it from Mr. Lockhart, as met with in the drug-shops of China. He has called it the *bitter-seeded cardamom.* Fig. 124 (page 256) is copied from one of the woodcuts given by Mr. Hanbury.

91. Amomum xanthioides, *Wallich.*[2]

Amomum with small round brown-coloured fruits in clusters, No. 101 in W. Gomez's *Tavoy Catalogue,* 1827. MS. in the possession of the Linnean Society of London.

Amomum xanthioides, No. 1956.—Wallich, *Catalogus Plantarum quas in itinere Burma-nico a mense Augusti* 1826, *ad finem Maii* 1827, *observavit N.W.* MS. in the possession of the Linnean Society.

Amomum? xanthioides.—Wall., *Catal. of the East Indian Herbarium,* No. 6557.

Mr. Daniel Hanbury writes—"Among some specimens of drugs received from China through the kindness of my friend Mr. Lockhart, was a quantity of the capsules of a fruit resembling the hairy China cardamom, but differing from it in the much more spiny character of the pericarp.

"Upon comparison, it proved identical with a species collected at Tavoy, Gulf of

---

[1] [*Pharm. Journal,* Feb. and March 1855.]

[2] [The notice here given is abridged from Mr. Daniel Hanbury's account of the specimens in the *Pharm. Journ.* for Feb. and March 1855.—ED.]

Martaban, in 1827, by Mr. W. Gomez, in whose MS. collecting-book (above quoted) it is defined as 'Amomum (with small round brown-coloured fruits in clusters).'

FIG. 124.

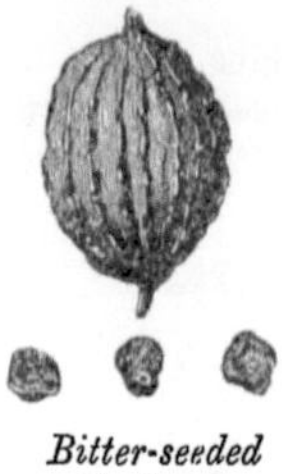

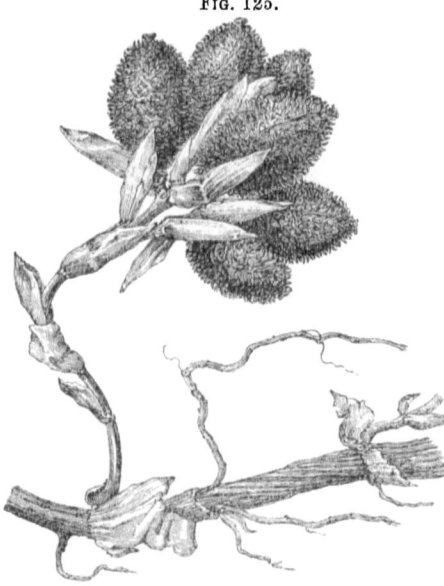

Bitter-seeded
Cardamom
(fruits and seeds).

"In Dr. Wallich's MS. Catalogue of Burmese Plants (entitled as above) occurs the following, in the doctor's own hand:—

"'1956. *Amomum xanthioides*, Wall.—Very like *A. aculeatum*, Roxb., but differing seemingly in the linear-lanceolate not cordate leaves, and the fruit, which consists in short, rounded clusters from the repent root; it is of an oblong obtuse form, thickly covered with prickles. Seems a tall species. Tavoy. ½ 27.'

"The next notice of *Amomum xanthioides* I find in the MS. Catalogue of the East Indian Herbarium of the Linnean Society, inserted thus:—

"'6557. Amomum? xanthioides, Wall. (A. aculeato Roxb. prox.) Tavoy, W. G.'

"From this last entry, it will be observed that a doubt seems to have been felt as to the genus of the plant in question,—a doubt, I confess, that appears to me groundless, if *Amomum aculeatum* is an admitted *Amomum*.

FIG. 125.

"The capsules of *Amomum xanthioides*, received by me under the name *Sha-jin-kŏ*,[1] had been deprived of seeds; indeed, the terminal syllable in the Chinese name signifies *husk* or *shell*. Yet from a few capsules which had escaped the shelling process, I had an opportunity of examining the seeds which, I suspected, were not unknown in the English market. I believed them to constitute the cardamom *seeds*[2] occasionally offered at the London drug sales, and which I had traced to Moulmein and Penang.

"This opinion has been unexpectedly confirmed. While this notice was in the hands of the printer, I received through the kindness of R. Padday, Esq., of Singapore, three samples of "bastard cardamoms" obtained from Bangkok in Siam. These *bastard cardamoms* have mostly been deprived of the husk: the seeds are either detached, or united with the partitions into 3-lobed masses. But the fruits retaining the husk are so evidently those of *Amomum xanthioides*, that I have no hesitation in referring the bastard cardamoms to that species. I also identify them with the cardamom *seeds* of the London market.

Fruit of Amomum xanthioides, Wallich.
(From a specimen in the herbarium of the Linnean Society.)

"The seeds of *A. xanthioides* much resemble those of the Malabar cardamom, but are not so rugose: they are, however, distinguishable by their peculiar aromatic taste and smell.

"I have received no information regarding the uses of these cardamom husks, which, it would appear, are exported to China, and there consumed.

"By a letter from Robert Hunter, Esq., of Bangkok, addressed to Mr. Padday, I learn that the so-called bastard cardamoms are the produce of the Laos Country and of Cambodia, where they grow wild in the more elevated regions of the mountain forests. Their commercial value is small, those of the first quality being worth, in Siam, about 3¼d. sterling per lb."—ED.]

---

[1] "I do not attach much value to this Chinese name, which I think is sometimes applied to the *Hairy China Cardamom*.

[2] "I mean the seeds *per se*. Malabar cardamoms deprived of pericarp are, I believe, never imported.

92. Alpinia Galanga, *Linn.*; A. chinensis, *Roscoe (?)*.

Sex. Syst. Monandria, Monogynia.

(Rhizoma.)

Two kinds of *galangal root (radix galangæ)*, a *lesser* and a *greater*, have long been known in medicine : to these Guibourt has added a third, which he calls *light galangal*. These three sorts are the produce of different parts of the East, and probably of different species of Alpinia.

1. *Radix galangæ majoris ; greater* or *Java galangal root.*—This is the root of the *Alpinia Galanga*, Linn. It is a coarser and larger root, with a feebler and somewhat different odour from that of the lesser galangal root. Although it occasionally comes to Europe, I cannot learn that it finds any use here.

1. *Radix galangæ minoris ; lesser* or *Chinese galangal root.*—This is the root of a plant growing in China, according to Guibourt,[1] the *Alpinia chinensis*, Roscoe (*Hellenia chinensis*, Willd.) It may perhaps be *Alpinia alba*, which Kœnig calls *Galanga alba*. It is brought to England from China either directly or by way of Singapore. It is the only sort usually kept by English druggists. It occurs in pieces which are as thick as the finger, seldom exceeding three inches in length, cylindrical or somewhat tuberous, often forked, sometimes slightly striated longitudinally, and marked with whitish circular rings. Externally its colour is dull reddish-brown ; internally pale, reddish-white. Its odour is agreeably aromatic ; its taste peppery and aromatic. It has been analysed by Bucholz[2] and by Morin.[3] The former obtained *volatile oil* 0·5, *acrid soft resin* 4·9, *extractive* 9·7, *gum* 8·2, *bassorin* 41·5, *woody fibre* 21·6, *water* 12·3, loss 1·3. It is a warm and agreeable aromatic, and is sometimes administered in the form of infusion in dyspepsia. Its effects, uses, and doses, are analogous to those of ginger. It is, however, rarely employed in England,—its principal consumption being on the continent.

3. *Radix galangæ levis ; galanga léger*, Guibourt ; *light galangal root.*—This variety, according to M. Guibourt, is characterised by its great lightness ; its weight being not more than a third of that of the previous sort. Its epidermis is smooth and shining. [By the late Dr. Pereira it was thought perhaps to be the root of *Alpinia nutans* (Roscoe), which Dr. Roxburgh[4] states is odorous, and is sometimes brought to England for Galanga major ; but Mr. Daniel Hanbury has obtained some of the root of *Alpinia nutans,* and it differs much from Guibourt's "light galangal." Mr. H. received the specimen from Mr. J. S. Stuchbury, of Demerara.—Ed.]

93. Alpinia alba, *Roscoe*.

(Semina.)

Hellenia alba, Willd.; *Heritiera alba*, Retz.; *Languas vulgare*, Kœnig ; *Amomum medium*, Loureiro, Fl. Cochinch.—The latter gives *Tsao quo* as the Cochinchina name, and *Thao qua* as the Chinese name of the plant.   Fig. 126.

Specimens of this fruit are in the Muséum d'Histoire Naturelle of Paris, where they are labelled *tsao-quo*. For my specimens I am indebted to Professor Guibourt, who calls the fruit the *ovoid China cardamom (cardamome ovoïde de la Chine)*. [Mr. Daniel Hanbury states that the ovoid cardamom exists in Dr. Burges's collection at the Royal College of Physicians, under the name of *Grana Paradisi in capsulis*. The seeds are very large, angular, and striated.—Ed.]

The dried fruit is about the size and shape of a large nutmeg ; it is ovoid, from 10 to 14 lines long, and from 6 to 8 lines broad, rather rigid, striated longitudinally, yellowish-brown with a reddish tint [scarlet when recent, *Kœnig*].

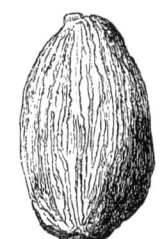

Ovoid China Cardamom.

---

[1] Guibourt, *Hist. Nat. des Drogues simples*, t. ii. p. 200, 4ème éd. 1849.
[2] Trommsdorff's *Journal*, xxv. 2, p. 3.
[3] *Journ. de Pharm.* ix. p. 257.
[4] *Asiatic Researches*, vol. xi. p. 318.

Grows in the province of Yu-nan. The seeds are aromatic, and are used by the natives as a condiment. They are said to be useful in intermittents. Kœnig terms the plant *Galanga alba,* and says it is much used among the Malays.

94. ELETTARIA CARDAMOMUM, *Maton.*—THE TRUE OR OFFICINAL CARDAMOM.

Alpinia Cardamomum, *Roxb. L.*—Renealmia Cardamomum, *Rosc.*—Amomum Cardamomum, *D.*

Sex. Syst. Monandria, Monogynia.

(Semina, *L. D.*—The fruit; Cardamoms, *Ed.*)

HISTORY.—A medicine, called Cardamom (καρδάμωμον), is mentioned by Hippocrates,[1] Theophrastus,[2] and Dioscorides,[3] the first of whom employed it in medicine. But it is now scarcely possible to determine what substance they referred to, as their notices of it are brief and imperfect; though I believe it to have been one of the fruits which we call cardamoms. Pliny[4] speaks of four kinds of cardamoms, but it is almost impossible to ascertain with any certainty what species he refers to.

BOTANY. **Gen. Char.**—The same as that of Amomum, but the *tube of the corolla* filiform, and the *anther* naked (Blume).

Sp. Char.—*Leaves* lanceolate, acuminate, pubescent above, silky beneath. *Spikes* lax. *Scape* elongated, horizontal. *Lip* indistinctly three-lobed (Blume).

Rhizome with numerous fleshy fibres. *Stems* perennial, erect, smooth, jointed, enveloped in the spongy sheaths of the leaves; from 6 to 9 feet high. *Leaves* subsessile on their sheaths, entire; length from 1 to 2 feet. *Sheaths* slightly villous, with a roundish ligula rising above the mouth *Scapes* several, (3 or 4) from the base of the stems, flexuose, jointed, branched, 1 to 2 feet long. *Branches* or *racemes* alternate, one from each joint of the scape, suberect, 2 or 3 inches long. *Bracts* solitary, oblong, smooth, membranaceous, striated, sheathing, one at each joint of the scape. *Flowers* alternate, short-stalked, solitary at each joint of the racemes, opening in succession as the racemes lengthen. *Calyx* funnel-shaped, 3-toothed at the mouth, about three-quarters of an inch long, finely striated, permanent. Tube of *corolla* slender, as long as the calyx; limb double, exterior of 3 oblong, concave, nearly equal, pale greenish-white divisions; inner lip obovate, much larger than the exterior divisions, somewhat curled at the margin, with the apex slightly 3-lobed, marked chiefly in the centre with purple violet stripes. *Filament* short, erect; *anther* double emarginate. *Ovary* oval, smooth; *style* slender, *stigma* funnel-shaped. *Capsule* oval, somewhat 3-sided, size of a small nutmeg [!], 3-celled, 3-valved. *Seeds* many, angular (Roxburgh).

Hab.—Mountainous parts of the coast of Malabar.

PRODUCTION. — Cardamoms are produced naturally or by cultivation. Between Travancore and Madura they grow without cultivation,[5] and also at

---

[1] Pages 265, 572, 603, 651, ed. Fœs.
[2] *Hist. Plant.* lib. xi. cap. vii.
[3] Lib. i. cap. 5.
[4] *Hist. Nat.* lib. xii. cap. xxix. ed. Valp.
[5] Hamilton [Buchanan], *Journey through Mysore, Canara, and Malabar,* vol. ii. p. 336.

certain places in the hills which form the lower part of the Ghaûts in Caduti-nada and other northern districts of Malayata.[1]   The cardamoms of the Wynaad, which are esteemed the best, are cultivated: the spots chosen for the cardamom farms are called *Ela-Kandy*, and are either level or gently sloping surfaces on the highest range of the Ghaûts after passing the first declivity from their base.[2]   " Before the commencement of the periodical rains, in June, the cultivators of the cardamom ascend the coldest and most shady sides of a woody mountain; a tree of uncommon size and weight is then sought after, the adjacent spot is cleared of weeds, and the tree felled close at its root.   The earth, shaken and loosened by the force of the fallen tree, shoots forth young cardamom plants in about a month's time."[3]

The quantity of cardamoms brought for sale at Malabar is about 120, or, according to another account, only 100 candies, from the following places:[4] —

	Candies of 640 *lbs.*	*Candies of* 640 *lbs.*
Coorg	40	30
Wynaad	57	65
Tamarachery	20	3
Cadutinada or Cartinaad	3	2
	120	100

The cardamoms of the Wynaad are shorter, fuller of seed, and whiter, than those of Malabar, and sell for 100 rupees a candy more.   Those of Coorg have fewer fine grains, but they have also fewer black or light ones.   The cardamoms of Sersi (western part of Soonda) are inferior to those of Coorg.[5]

[The quantities on which duty was paid in five years in this country was—

	lbs.
In 1840	6,246
1841	5,628
1842	6,501
1843	5,329
1844	7,694.—ED.]

DESCRIPTION.—The fruit of the *Elettaria Cardamomum* constitutes the *small, officinal, Malabar cardamom* (*cardamoms,* Ed.; *cardamomum minus,* Clusius, Matthiolus, Bontius, Geoffroy, Dale, Geiger, Th. Martius, and Guibourt: *cardamomum malabarense*).   It is an ovate oblong, obtusely triangular capsule, from three to ten lines long, rarely exceeding three lines in breadth; coriaceous, ribbed, greyish or brownish yellow.   It contains many angular blackish or reddish brown rugose seeds (*cardamomum,* L.; *carda-momum excorticatum,* Offic.), which are white internally, have a pleasant aromatic odour, and a warm, aromatic, agreeable taste.[6]   100 parts of the fruit yield 74 parts of seeds and 26 parts of pericarpial coats.[7]

---

[1] Hamilton, *op. cit.* vol. ii. p. 510.
[2] White, *Trans. of Linn. Soc.* vol. x. p. 237.
[3] Capt. Dickson, in Roxburgh's *Fl. Indica.*
[4] Hamilton, *op. cit.* vol. ii. p. 538.
[5] Hamilton, *op. cit.* vol. ii. p. 538, and vol. iii. p. 228.
[6] For some drawings of the minute structure of the seeds, vide Bischoff's *Handb. d. botanik. Terminal.* tab. xliii. fig. 1876 and 1954.
[7] Th. Martius, *Pharmakogn.*

Three varieties of Malabar cardamoms are distinguished in commerce; viz. *shorts, short-longs,* and *long-longs.* The two latter differ from each other in size merely.

Fig. 127.　Fig. 128.　Fig. 129.

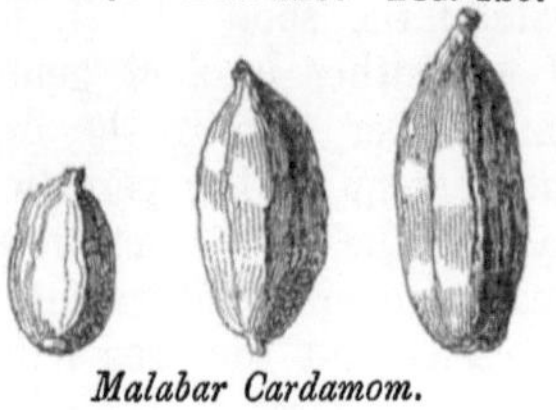

Malabar Cardamom.

Fig. 127. Shorts.
Fig. 128. Short-longs.
Fig. 129. Long-longs.

a. SHORTS.　*Malabar cardamoms properly so called; Petit cardamome* (Guibourt); *? Wynaad cardamom* (Hamilton); *Prima species Elettari planè rotunda et albicans* (Rheede).[1]—From 3 to 6 lines long, and from 2 to 3 lines broad; more coarsely ribbed, and of a browner colour, than the other varieties. This is the most esteemed variety.

β. SHORT-LONGS.　*Secunda species Elettari oblongior sed vilior* (Rheede).—Differs from the third variety in being somewhat shorter and less acuminate.

γ. LONG-LONGS.　*Moyen cardamome* (Guib.); *Tertia species Elettari vilissima et planè acuminata* (Rheede).—From 7 lines to an inch long, and from 2 to 3 lines broad: elongated, somewhat acuminate. This, as well as the last variety, is paler and more finely ribbed than var. *a. shorts.* The seeds also are frequently paler (in some cases resembling those of the Ceylon cardamom) and more shrivelled.

The three sorts are brought from Bombay in chests. The shorts are usually the dearest, and fetch from 3d. to 6d. per lb. more than the longs. The long-longs are seldom brought over. From Madras, only long cardamoms (usually short-longs, rarely long-longs) are brought: they are generally packed in bags, and are lighter by weight than the Bombay sort, and usually fetch 3d. per lb. less than the latter. [We are informed by a friend who has much experience in the drug trade, that the value of Madras cardamoms is usually 6d. to 9d. per lb. under the Malabar short-longs.—ED.]

COMPOSITION.—The small cardamom was analysed by Trommsdorff in 1834.[2] He obtained the following results:—*Essential oil* 4·6, *fixed oil* 10·4, *a salt of potash* (*malate?*) combined with *a colouring matter* 2·5, *fecula* 3·0, *nitrogenous mucilage* with *phosphate of lime* 1·8, *yellow colouring matter* 0·4, and *woody fibre* 77·3.

1. VOLATILE OR ESSENTIAL OIL OF CARDAMOM. — Is obtained from the seeds by distilling them with water.　50 lbs. of good short Malabar cardamoms yielded, at one operation, about f₃viss. of oil for every lb. of fruit.[3] It is colourless, has an agreeable odour, and a strong, aromatic, burning taste. Its sp. gr. is 0·943. It is very soluble in alcohol, ether, oils (both fixed and volatile), and acetic acid. It is insoluble in potash-ley. By keeping, it becomes yellow, viscid, and loses its peculiar taste and smell. It then detonates with iodine, and takes fire when placed in contact with concentrated nitric acid. On this oil depend the odour, flavour, and aromatic qualities of the seeds. Its composition is analogous to that of oil of turpentine, being $C^{10}H^8$.

2. FIXED OIL OF CARDAMOM.—Is insoluble in alcohol, ether, and the oils both fixed and volatile. Nitric acid, assisted by heat, reddens it. It has some analogy to castor oil.

3. STARCH.—Schleiden says that in these seeds he has discovered amorphous paste-like starch in the cells.

PHYSIOLOGICAL EFFECTS.—The effects of cardamoms are those of a very agreeable and grateful aromatic, devoid of all acridity.

USES.—Cardamoms are employed partly on account of their flavour, and partly for their cordial and stimulant properties. They are rarely administered

---

[1] Rheede, pars xi. tab. 4, 5, and 6.
[2] *Journ. de Chim. Méd.* t. i. p. 196, 2nde Sér.
[3] *Private information.*

alone, but generally either as adjuvants or correctives of other medicines, especially of stimulants, tonics, and purgatives. [The greater portion of the cardamoms brought to this country is re-exported to the north of Germany, where cardamoms are much used by confectioners, as also in every household, in order to flavour pastry. In England their use is confined to medicine. —ED.]

ADMINISTRATION.—Though cardamoms enter into a considerable number of pharmaceutical compounds, only two preparations derive their names from these seeds. They are the following :—

1. TINCTURA CARDAMOMI, E.; *Tincture of Cardamoms*. (Cardamom seeds, bruised, ℥ivss.; Proof Spirit, Oij. Macerate for seven days, and strain. "This tincture may be better prepared by the process of percolation in the same way with the tincture of capsicum, the seeds being first ground in a coffee-mill," *E.*)—This compound is agreeably aromatic. It is used as an adjunct to cordial, tonic, and purgative mixtures. Dose fȝj. to fȝij.

2. TINCTURA CARDAMOMI COMPOSITA, L. E. D.; *Compound Tincture of Cardamoms*. (Cardamom seeds, bruised; Caraway seeds, bruised, of each ȝiiss. [ȝss. *D.*]; Cochineal, powdered, ȝiiss. [ȝj. Ed. ȝij. *D.*]; Cinnamon, bruised, ȝv. [℥j. *D.*]; Raisins [stoned], ℥v.; Proof Spirit, Oij. [Oiij. *D.*] Macerate for seven days [fourteen days, *D.*], and filter. "This tincture may also be prepared by the method of percolation, if the solid materials be first beaten together, moistened with a little spirit, and left thus for twelve hours before being put into the percolator," *Ed.* The *Dublin College* omits the raisins.)—This tincture is used for the same purposes and in the same doses as the former preparation, over which it has the advantage of a more agreeable flavour. Moreover, its colour often renders it useful in prescribing.

95. ELETTARIA MAJOR, *Smith.*—THE GREATER OR CEYLON ELETTARIA.

Alpinia Granum Paradisi, *Moon.*

(Fructus ; Ceylon Cardamom, *offic.*)

HISTORY.—The fruit of this plant was known to Clusius,[1] who has noticed and figured it under the name of the *Cardamomum majus vulgare.*[2]

BOTANY.—The flower has not yet been described, but the other parts of the plant are so similar to the corresponding parts of Elettaria Cardamomum, that I have no difficulty in referring this plant to the genus Elettaria. Sir James Edward Smith,[3] who was acquainted with the fruit only, observes,

---

[1] *Exoticorum*, lib. i. pp. 186 and 187.
[2] For further details respecting the history of this cardamom, the reader is referred to a paper by the author, in the *Pharmaceutical Journal*, vol. ii. p. 384, 1842.
[3] Rees's *Cyclopædia*, vol. xxxix. art. *Elettaria*.

"we are persuaded they must belong to the same genus as the Malabar Cardamom."

Gen. Char.—See *Elettaria Cardamomum*, p. 258.

Sp. Char.—*Capsule* lanceolate oblong, acutely triangular, with flat sides. *Calyx* three-lobed (Smith).

Rhizome with numerous fibres. *Stem* erect, smooth, enveloped by leaf sheaths. *Leaves* sessile on their sheaths, silky beneath, acuminate ; the shorter ones lanceolate, the larger ones oblong-lanceolate : breadth 2 to 3 inches, length not exceeding 15¼ inches. *Sheaths* about half the length of the leaves, with a roundish ligula. *Scape* from the upper part of the rhizome, flexuose, jointed, 9 inches long, branched; the branches alternate, one from each joint of the scape, sub-erect, half an inch long, supporting two or three pedicels of about 3-10ths of an inch. *Bracts* solitary, sheathing at each joint of the scape, withered; partial ones, solitary, ovate, acute. *Flowers* not present. *Capsules* one or two on each branch of the scape, with the permanent calyx attached to them : their characters are described in the text.

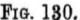

Fig. 130.

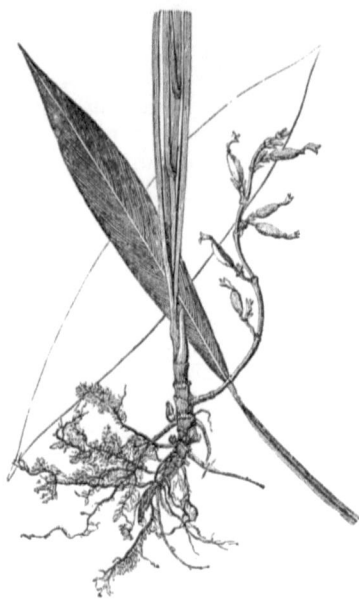

Elettaria major.

The plant from which the above description has been drawn formed part of a collection made for me in Ceylon by my much lamented friend and pupil, the late Mr. Frederick Saner, Assistant-Surgeon in Her Majesty's 61st regiment. He received it from Mr. Lear, Acting Superintendent of the Royal Botanic Gardens in Ceylon, whose letter, describing it as "*Alpinia* [Amomum] *Granum paradisi*," I have in my possession. I presume, therefore, that it is the plant which Mr. Moon,[1] the former superintendent of the Gardens, has described under the same name. The following facts favour this conclusion :—

1. Mr. Moon states that its Singalese name is *Ensal*, a term which both Hermann[2] and Burmann[3] gave as the native name for cardamom.

2. Mr. Moon states that it is cultivated at Candy. If the real grain of paradise plant were cultivated in Ceylon, it would be somewhat remarkable that its seeds are never exported. Now I have carefully examined the list of exports from that island for several years, but the words grain of paradise never once occur; and all the seeds imported into England under that name, I find, by the Customs House returns, come from the western coast of Africa. On the other hand, the Ceylon cardamom comes, as its name indicates, from that island.

[The above remarks were written by the author in the third edition of this work. We print them to show how the conclusion to which he arrived, from the above uncertain data, has been shown to be perfectly correct. It is now certain that the plant yielding the true grains of paradise does not grow in the east (see page 244 *et seq.*)—Ed.]

Hab.—Cultivated at Candy.

---

[1] *A Catalogue of the Indigenous and Exotic Plants growing in Ceylon,* Colombo, 1824.
[2] *Musæum Zeylanicum,* p. 66, Ed. 2nda, Lugd. Bat. 1726.
[3] *Thesaurus Zeylanicus,* p. 54, Amstelæd. 1737.

COMMERCE.—Bertolacci[1] says that the Ceylon cardamom is collected chiefly in the Candian territory, and that he was informed it was indigenous, but was introduced by the Dutch. The quantity exported from 1806 to 1813 inclusive varied from 4½ to 18 candies annually. Percival[2] states that cardamoms grow in the south-east part of Ceylon, particularly in the neighbourhood of Matura. I am informed that occasionally Ceylon cardamoms come from Quillon.

FIG. 131.

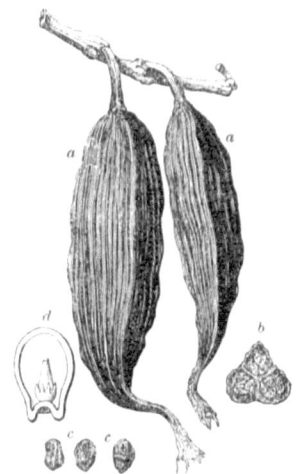

Ceylon Cardamoms.

a a, The dried capsules of commerce.
b, Transverse section of a capsule.
c c, Seeds.
d, Magnified view of a section of a seed, to show the embryo seated in vitellus (Lindley).

DESCRIPTION.—The *Ceylon cardamom*, or, as it is sometimes termed in English commerce, the *wild cardamom* (*cardamomum zeylanicum; cardamomum medium*, Matth. and Geoffr.; *cardamomum majus,* Bont. and Dale; *cardamomum majus vulgare,* Clusius; *cardamomum majus officinarum*, C. Bauhin; *cardamomum longum*, Th. Martius and Geiger; *grande cardamome*, Guib.) is a lanceolate-oblong capsule, acutely triangular, more or less curved, with flat and ribbed sides, about an inch and a half long and one-third of an inch broad. At one extremity we frequently find the long, cylindrical, permanent, three-lobed calyx; at the other the fruit stalk, which is sometimes branched. The pericarp is coriaceous, tough, brownish or yellowish ash-coloured, 3-celled. The seeds are angular, rugged, have a yellowish-red tinge, a fragrant and aromatic but peculiar odour, and a spicy flavour. The long diameter of the vitellus is parallel to that of the embryo. Th. Martius[3] says that 100 parts of these fruits yield 71 parts of seeds, and 29 parts of pericarpial coats.

COMPOSITION, EFFECTS, AND USES.—Ceylon cardamoms have not been analysed. Their constituents, as well as their effects and uses, are doubtless analogous to those of the Malabar cardamom. Their commercial value is about one-third that of the latter. They are chiefly used on the Continent.

ORDER XVIII. ORCHIDEÆ, *R. Brown.*—ORCHIDS.

ORCHIDES, *Jussieu.*—ORCHIDACEÆ, *Lindley.*

CHARACTERS.—*Flowers* irregular, gynandrous. *Perianth* adherent (superior), coloured, or rarely herbaceous; its parts arranged in 2 rows. *Column* consisting of the stamens and style consolidated into a central body. *Stamens* 3, the central only being perfect, except in Cypripedium, where the central is abortive and the two lateral perfect; *pollen* powdery, or cohering in waxy masses. *Ovary* adherent (inferior), 1-celled, composed of 6 carpels, of which 3 have parietal placentæ; *stigmas* usually confluent in a mucous disk.

---

[1] *Agricultural, Commercial, and Financial Interests of Ceylon*, p. 157, 1817.
[2] *Account of Ceylon*, 1805.
[3] *Pharmakognosie.*

Capsule membranous or coriaceous, rarely fleshy. *Seeds* innumerable, without albumen; *embryo* solid. *Roots* fasciculated and fibrous, sometimes with fleshy tubercles. *Leaves* never lobed; their veins usually parallel, very rarely somewhat reticulated. *Stem* sometimes swollen and jointed, forming *pseudo-bulbs*.

PROPERTIES.—See *Salep* and *Vanilla*.

96. Orchis, *Linn.*

Sex. Syst. Gynandria, Monaudria.

(Radix ; Salep.)

The term *salep*[1] (*radix salep*) is applied to the prepared tubercles of several orchideous plants.

1. ORIENTAL SALEP.—This is usually imported from the Levant, and is said to be the produce of Turkey, Natolia, and Persia. It consists of small ovoid tubercles, frequently strung on a cord. In 1825-6 salep of the value of 35,000 francs was imported into France from Persia.[2] Salep is the produce, probably, of different species of *Orchis*. Fraas[3] states that the σαλήπ or σαλέπι of Greece is collected from *O. Morio*, and also from *O. mascula, coriophora,* and *undulatifolia*. Dr. Royle thinks that the salep of Cashmere is obtained from a species of *Eulophia*. Caventou[4] states that the constituents of salep are gum (which does not become coloured by iodine), much bassorin, a little starch, common salt, and phosphate of lime. Others, however, have found an abundance of starch in salep;[5] and it is probable, therefore, that the quantity varies at different seasons, and is most abundant before the tubercle is exhausted by the nutrition of the stem.[6]

2. INDIGENOUS SALEP.—That prepared from *Orchis mascula* is most valued; but the roots of some of the palmated sorts, as *Orchis latifolia*, are found to answer almost equally well. Geoffroy,[7] Retzius,[8] and Moult,[9] have each pointed out the method of preparing it. The latter directs the roots to be washed and the brown skin removed by a brush or by dipping the root in hot water and rubbing it with a coarse linen cloth. The roots are then put on a tin plate and placed in an oven heated to the usual degree for six or ten minutes, in which time they will have lost their milky whiteness and acquired a transparency like horn. They are then removed and allowed to dry and harden in the air. The fresh roots of the orchis contain a peculiar odorous principle (which is almost entirely dissipated by drying), starch, mucilaginous matter, a small quantity of bitter extractive, ligneous matter, salts, and water.

Salep possesses the dietetical properties of the starchy and mucilaginous substances (see Vol. i. p. 64). Its medicinal properties are those of an emollient and demulcent. It was formerly in repute as an aphrodisiac and restorative, and as a preventive of miscarriage,[10] but it has no claim to these powers. The notion of its aphrodisiac properties seems to have been founded on the doctrine of signatures.

Indigenous salep was recommended by Dr. Thomas Percival[11] as a wholesome article of food; and in a medicinal point of view as a restorative, emollient, and demulcent.

Mucilage of salep (*mucilago radicis salep ; decoctum salep*) is prepared, according to the Hamburg *Codex*, with 5 grains of powdered salep and ʒj. of distilled water. Dissolve by boiling and constantly stirring, and strain.

---

[1] The term *saloop* is sometimes applied to sassafras tea.
[2] Chevalier, *Journ. de Pharm.* xv. 536, 1829.
[3] *Synopsis Plant. Fl. Classicæ,* p. 279, 1845.
[4] *Ann. Chim. Phys.* xxxi. 345.
[5] *Journ. de Pharm.* xii. 201, 1826 : Pfaff, *Syst. d. Mat. Méd.* i. 131 ; vi. 90.
[6] Raspail, *Chimie Organique.*
[7] *Hist. de l'Acad. Royale des Sciences,* 1740.
[8] *Swedish Transactions,* 1764.
[9] *Phil. Trans.* vol. lix.
[10] *Some Observations made upon the Root called Serapias or Salep, imported from Turkey, shewing its admirable Virtues in preventing Women's Miscarriages,* written by a Doctor of Physick in the Countrey to his Friend in London, 1694.
[11] *On the Preparation, Culture, and Use of the Orchis Root* (in the *Essays, Medical and Expemental,* 1773).

97. Vanilla, *Swartz.*

Sex. Syst. Gynandria, Monandria.

(Fructus.)

HISTORY.—Vanilla (so called from *vainilla* or *baynilla*, the diminutive of *vaina* or *bayna*, a sheath or pod) is said[1] to have been brought to the Continent, as a perfume, about the year 1510. It could not, however, have obtained much attention; for Clusius,[2] who received it from England in 1602, confesses that he had not seen it before; and he calls it *lobus oblongus aromaticus.* Hernandez[3] describes the vanilla plant under the name of *tlilxochitl* or *aracus aromaticus.* The pods were afterwards denominated *benzanelles* quasi *benzionelles*, on account of their benzoin-like odour.[4]

BOTANY. **Gen. Char.**—*Fruit* a long pulpy pod, with round seeds not inclosed in a loose membrane (Lindley).

Species.—Although, until recently, most authors have ascribed the vanilla of commerce to the *V. aromatiea* of Swartz, yet the assertion rested upon no certain or known fact, but chiefly upon the belief that *V. planifolia* bore no odoriferous fruit.[5] Morren,[6] however, by artificial impregnation, obtained fruit from the *V. planifolia*, which, in fragrance and other qualities, vied with the best vanilla of commerce; and it is probable, therefore, that this species yields part at least of the best or Mexican vanilla.

But Schiede[7] states that there are four forms of vanilla in Mexico, which he calls respectively *V. sativa, V. sylvestris, V. pompona*, and *V. inodora ;*[8] the first two of which he thinks have been confounded under the name of *V. planifolia.* He did not, however, see the flowers of any of these species; and, therefore, it is impossible to characterise them. He likewise mentions a *baynilla de mono* or *monkey vanilla*, which he did not examine; and also a *baynilla mestiza* or *hybrid vanilla*, a fruit intermediate between that of V. sativa and V. sylvestris.

But although the best vanilla comes from Mexico, there are other sorts which are the produce of other parts of tropical America, and which are certainly not the produce of *V. planifolia ;* I shall, therefore, also notice such other species as probably contribute some of the vanilla of commerce.

1. V. PLANIFOLIA, Andrews, Bot. Rep. t. 538.—Fruit very long; cylindrical, and very fragrant.—West Indies (Aiton), Mexico (?), and Guatemala (?).—Probably yields the best Mexican vanilla.—Schiede's *V. sativa* and *V. sylvestris* are perhaps referable to this species :—

a. V. sativa, Schiede; *Baynilla mansa* or *cultivated vanilla* of the Mexicans. Leaves oblong, succulent, the floral ones very small; fruits without furrows.—Grows wild; and is also cultivated in Papantla, Misantla, Nautla, and Colipa.—Yields the finest sort of vanilla. This, probably, is the *La Corrienté* or Current Vanilla of Desvaux.[9]

β. V. sylvestris, Schiede; *Baynilla cimarrona* or *wild vanilla* of the Mexicans. Leaves oblong-lanceolate, succulent, the floral ones very small; fruits with two furrows.—Grows in Papantla, Nautla, and Colipa.—Its fruit is collected in Papantla, and mixed with that of the preceding sort.—According to the information furnished to Desvaux, this form is

---

[1] Morren, *Annals of Natural History*, vol. iii. p. 1, 1839.

[2] *Exotic.* lib. iii. cap. xviii. p. 72, 1605.

[3] *Rerum Medic. Novæ Hisp. Thesaurus*, p. 38, Romæ, 1651.

[4] Mentzelius, *Index Nomin. Plant.* Berol. 1682.

[5] Plumier, who published a figure of *V. aromatica*, expressly states in his MS., published by Geoffroy (*Traité de Mat. Méd.* t. ii. p. 363, 1741), that his plant differs from the Mexican species in being inodorous.

[6] *Annals of Natural History*, vol. iii. p. 1, 1839.

[7] Schlechtendal's *Linnæa*, Bd. iv. S. 573, Oct. 1829; also, *Pharmaceutisches Central-Blatt für* 1830, S. 46.

[8] *V. inodora*, the *baynilla de puerco* or *hog vanilla* of the Mexicans, is, Schiede states, a distinct species, but, being deficient in volatile oil, is not used. Desvaux says that in drying it gives ont a disagreeable odour, and from this has obtained the name of "hog" vanilla.

[9] *Ann. Sciences Nat.* 3me Sér. Botanique, t. vi. p. 119, 1846.—Desvaux says that there are two varieties of *La Corrienté :* one which is well filled wiih seeds and pulp, and has a fine skin,—this is the most esteemed; the other, or *Cuéruda* (leathery) has a thick skin, and, though inferior, is *legitimate* in commerce : it is the *Lec, Leq,* or *Leg* of some parts of South America.

the same species as the preceding; but, growing wild in the woods, and deprived of the solar rays, it yields a smaller fruit.

2. V. AROMATICA, Swartz, in Act. Upsal. vi. 66.—Fruit cylindrical. very long.—South America : Brazil.—Said by Martius.to yield the *true vanilla* (*veræ siliquæ vanillæ*).

3. V. GUIANENSIS, Splitberger, Ann. Scien. Nat., 2de Sér., t. xv. Bot. p. 279, 1841.— Fruit fragrant, 6-8 inches long, 3-edged, straight or somewhat falcate; sides 11-15 lines broad, one somewhat convex, two flattish, angles obtuse.—Surinam. Probably yields *La Guayra vanilla*, and the *large vanilla* (*vanille grosse*) of Guiana.

4. V. PALMARUM, Lindley, Gen. and Sp. of Orchid. Plants, p. 437; Splitberger, Ann. Scien. Nat., 2de Sér., t. xv. p. 283.—Fruit fleshy, 2 inches long and ½ an inch diameter, cylindrical, or slightly 3-faced, obtuse at the extremities, bivalved.—Bahia. Yields a vanilla inferior in fragrance to the preceding.

5. V. POMPONA, Schiede; *Baynilla pompona* or *large vanilla* of the Mexicans.—Fruit with two furrows, rich in volatile oil, with an agreeable odour, yet will not dry, but always remains soft, and cannot be transmitted to Europe as an article of commerce. Humboldt[1] says that it has scarcely any sale on account of its odour. Desvaux observes that it is certainly the vanilla called by some authors *bova* (*vanille bouffie, tumid* or *swollen vanilla*), and which is found in French commerce under the name of *vanillon*.

CURING.—The preparation or curing of vanilla varies probably in different places. At Misantla the fruits are sun-dried, and afterwards sweated in blankets; or, when the weather is unfavourable, they are dried by artificial heat.[2] In some places they are dipped in boiling water, then suspended in the sun to dry, and afterwards oiled.[3] These different processes have for their object not merely the preservation of the fruits, but the development and preservation of their odour, which is supposed to be effected by a kind of fermentation; for in the fresh state, Aublet says, they have no aroma. The seat of the odour has been variously stated to be in the seeds, the pulp, and the fruit-coats: probably all these parts possess it in different degrees.

DESCRIPTION.—The dried fragrant fruits of several species of vanilla constitute the *vanilla* or *vanilloes* of the shops (*fructus* vel *capsula vanillæ; siliquæ vanigliæ* vel *banigliæ*).

Four sorts are known in the English market; viz. the Mexican or Vera Cruz, the Honduras, the La Guayra, and the Brazilian or Bahia. A fifth sort I have received by private hand.

1. *Mexican* or *Vera Cruz Vanilla*.—Imported from Vera Cruz tied in bundles of 50 pods, weighing, when of good quality, about 9½ or 10 oz. The heavier the bundle, the better the quality, and the greater the value per lb. The bundles come packed in tin cases, each holding 60 bundles. I have met with two varieties :—

α. —*Finest Mexican Vanilla*.—This consists of pods which are 7 or 8 inches long, ⅓ of an inch wide, tapering at the extremities, and curved at the base. They are longitudinally wrinkled, soft, clammy, and dark brown. Their odour is very fragrant, resembling, but being more delicious than, that of balsam of Peru. By keeping they become coated with brilliant acicular crystals, and are then called *crystallised vanilla*.

β. *Second Mexican Vanilla*.—The pods of this sort are shorter (being about 5 inches long), narrower, drier, paler, and less odorous than the preceding, with only a few isolated or no crystals on them. In other respects this sort agrees with the preceding.

Desvaux states that in Mexico five legitimate sorts of vanilla are distinguished: viz. the *primiera* (the *grande fina* of Humboldt), or the finest; *chica-fina* (the *mancuerna* of Humboldt), or small fine; *sacate*, or middlings; *resacate*, or middling-middlings; and *basura*, or the sweepings,

The *puerca* and *pompona* are not considered to be legitimate sorts.

Bourbon vanilla, according to Bourchardat,[4] differs from Mexican vanilla only in being somewhat smaller, redder, less brown, drier, and less unctuous.

2. *Honduras Vanilla*.—Imported from Honduras. Its value is from 2s. to 4s. per lb. The fruits are cylindrical, or slightly flattened, 3½ or 4 inches long, ⅓rd or ⅜ths of an inch in diameter, longitudinally wrinkled, brown, and dry. Their odour is vanilla-like, but feeble, and not of that fragrant kind which characterises the best vanilla.

---

[1] *Political Essay on the Kingdom of New Spain*, translated by J. Black, vo . iii. p. 26, 1822.
[2] Desvaux, *op. supra cit.*
[3] Aublet, *Hist. des Plantes de la Guiane Françoise*, t. ii. 1775.
[4] *Journ. de Pharm.* 3e Sér. t. xvi. p. 274, 1849.

3. *La Guayra Vanilla.*—Imported from La Guayra in Venezuela, in various packages (mostly tins in cases). It is an inferior sort, chiefly used by perfumers, and fetches from 2s. to 4s. per lb.

The fruits are large flattened, or somewhat plano-convex, or obscurely triangulated pods, from 5 to 7 inches long, $\frac{1}{2}$ to $\frac{3}{4}$ of an inch wide, somewhat narrowed at the extremities, a little twisted or curled, longitudinally wrinkled, here and there presenting a somewhat blistered appearance, brown, with a peculiar (sweetish fruity) vanilla odour. On the flattened side, at each edge, is a more or less distinct welt-like suture.

In the Museum of the Pharmaceurical Society are two pods, probably of the same sort, received from Mr. Stutchbery of Demerara. They are, however, $7\frac{1}{2}$ inches long, more distinctly triangular, blackish externally, and appear as if oiled. They were sent along with a pod of what I preserved to be *V. guianensis*, preserved wet.

La Guayra vanilla is probably the produce of *V. guianensis* of Splitberger. It is perhaps the *large vanilla (vanille grosse)* of Aublet; and is said by Dr. T. W. C. Martius to be sometimes met with under the name of *vanillon*.

4. *Brazilian* or *Bahia Vanilla.*—This consists of pods of about $7\frac{1}{2}$ inches long and $\frac{3}{4}$ of an inch wide. The samples which I have seen have been divided longitudinally, and, strictly speaking, therefore, are half pods. This sort is blackish, and damp and sticky to the touch, somewhat as if it had been covered with treacle or some glutinous substance. By digestion in spirit it is deprived of its glutinous coating. It is sometimes brought over quite wet. By some persons it is said to have been preserved in sugar, and that to this substance it owes its dampness. Its odour is not equal to that of the best vanilla. This sort of vanilla corresponds with the fruit neither of *V. aromatica* of Swartz, nor of *V. palmarum*, Lindley,—the only two species of vanilla which, according to Martius, are found in the Brazils. Is it *V. pompona* of Schiede?

5. *Panama Vanilla.*—I have received a single pod only of this. It is flat, $3\frac{1}{2}$ inches long, nearly $\frac{3}{4}$ths of an inch wide, dark brown, and fragrant.

Goodness.—The best vanilla is dark shining brown, plump, heavy, pliant, and soft, and has a fine fragrant smell. The crystallised variety is preferred.

Shrivelled, dull, dry, pale or yellowish brown, faintly smelling, or musty or mouldy pods are bad.

Sometimes dry shrivelled pods are freshened up with balsam of Peru, or are rolled in benzoic acid to give them a crystallised appearance.

Composition.—The crystallised vanilla was analysed by Bucholz,[1] who obtained the following results :—Odorous brownish yellow fixed oil, 10·8 ; soft resin, scarcely soluble in ether, 2·3 ; bitter extractive with some acetate of potash, 16·8 ; acidulous, bitterish, astringent extractive, 9·0 ; sweet extractive, 1·2 ; saccharine matter with benzoic acid, 6·1 ; gum, 11·2 ; starchy matter, 2·8 ; woody fibre, 20·0 ; oxydised extractive dissolved by potash, 7·1 ; gum extracted by potash, 5·9 ; benzoic acid, 1·1 ; water and loss, 5·7.— The ashes of the insoluble fibre consisted of the carbonates of soda, potash, lime and magnesia, sulphate of lime, sulphates, chlorides, alumina, oxide of iron, and oxide of copper.

The nature of the *odorous principle*[2] of vanilla has not been satisfactorily made out. It probably resembles that of the balsam of Peru, and belongs to the cinnameine series. By distillation with water, alcohol, or ether, vanilla yields no volatile oil : the liquid obtained by distillation with water being nearly inodorous. It is said that when the fruit is mature it yields from two to six drops of a liquid which has an exquisite odour, and bears the name of *balsam of vanilla*—none of which, however, reaches Europe, though it is stated to be used in Peru.

The *soft needle-like crystals* which incrust the finest kind of vanilla are usually regarded as benzoic acid. They are slightly soluble in hot water, and the solution, according to my experiments, reddens litmus. Bley,[3] who examined them, denies that their solution reddens litmus, and considers them to be a peculiar solid volatile oil. They require to be farther examined. [In the meantime it may be observed that many dealers, especially those of Paris, in which city there is a very large consumption of vanilla for the flavouring

---

[1] Buchner's *Repertorium*, Bd. ii. S. 253, 1828.
[2] An odour more or less allied to that of vanilla, and therefore called the *vanilla odour*, is common to many vegetable substances (see Virey, *Journ. de Pharm.* t. vi. p. 591 ; also Mérat and De Lens, *Dict. Mat. Méd.* t. vi. p. 843, and Suppl. p. 727.)
[3] *Pharmaceutisches Central-Blatt für* 1831, p. 579.

of ices and chocolate, have a method of bringing out the crystals of benzoic acid to the surface of the pod by artificial means. This is accomplished by wrapping the vanilla in flannel, and replacing it in its tin canister. This is put in a cold cellar for some weeks, and in the best qualities the crystals appear. If the vanilla does not acquire this crystalline character on its surface when thus treated, it is not considered to be in a healthy state. Hence dealers give the preference to the crystallised article.—ED.]

PHYSIOLOGICAL EFFECTS.—Vanilla is an aromatic stimulant. Its effects probably resemble those of balsam of Peru. It is considered to have an exhilarating effect on the mental functions, to prevent sleep, to increase the energy of the muscular system, and to act as an aphrodisiac.[1]

USES.—As a medicinal agent it is not employed in England. On the Continent it has been used in hysteria, melancholia, impotency, asthenic fevers, rheumatism, &c.

Its principal use in this country is to flavour chocolate and various articles of confectionary (ices, creams, &c.), liqueurs, &c. It is also employed in perfumery.

ADMINISTRATION.—It is exhibited in the form of powder or tincture.

1. *Pulvis Vanillæ; Powder of Vanilla.*—Vanilla is powdered by the intervention of sugar. The pods being cut in small pieces are pounded in an iron mortar with sugar, then sifted, the residue powdered with more sugar, and so on. The powders are then to be mixed. The quantity of sugar required varies according to the state of dryness or succulency of the pods; but in general four parts of sugar are required for one part of vanilla. This powder is used for aromatising various culinary and medicinal preparations. It may be administered medicinally in doses of a drachm; equal to about twelve grains of the pure vanilla.

2. *Tincture of Vanilla; Essence of Vanilla.*—This is prepared by digesting 1 part of good Mexican vanilla in 6 parts of rectified spirit. When inferior sorts of vanilla are used, the proportion of this substance is increased.—Vogler[2] states that a tincture of balsam of Peru is sometimes substituted for that of vanilla.

2. Leaves with netted (reticulated) veins. *Dictyogens; Retosæ.* Lindley.

† Flowers unisexual, with the perianth adherent to the ovary (*inferior ovary*).

ORDER XIX. DIOSCOREACEÆ, *Lindl.*—YAMS.

DIOSCOREÆ, *R. Brown.*

CHARACTERS.—Twining endogenous plants with reticulated *leaves*, unisexual regular *flowers*, a 6-parted superior *perianth*, 6 *stamens*, a 3-celled inferior *ovary* with 1- or 2-seeded cells, and capsular or berried *fruit*.

PROPERTIES.—See *Dioscorea* and *Tamus*.

98. Dioscorea, *Linn.*—The Yam.

Sex. Syst. Diœcia, Hexandria.

(Tuber.)

In tropical countries (East and West Indies, Africa, Polynesia) the tuberous roots of many species of *Dioscorea* or *Yam*[3] are used as food. Of seventeen species described by Roxburgh,[4] eleven are stated to be employed for food. The four following are cultivated in India, and are esteemed in the order in which they are enumerated:—*D. globosa,*

---

[1] Sundelin, *Heilmittellehre,* ii. 203, 3te Aufl.

[2] *Pharmaceutisches Central-Blatt fur* 1848, S. 448.

[3] The term *yam* is frequently, but erroneously, applied to the tubers of *Tacca* and *Arum* (see *ante*).

[4] *Fl. Indica,* vol. iii. p. 797.

D. alata, D. purpurea, and *D. rubella.* Roxburgh also says that *D. atropurpurea* is extensively cultivated at Malacca, Pegu, and the eastern islands; and that *D. fasciculata* is cultivated to a considerable extent in the vicinity of Calcutta, not only for food, but to make starch of the roots. In the West Indies several species are used as food; the chief are—*D. aculeata, D. alata, D. bulbifera,* and *D. sativa.* The tuberous roots sold in the London shops as West India yams are said to be those of *D. alata.*

Yams are large fleshy roots, sometimes weighing from thirty to forty pounds each. Some of them are highly acrid in the fresh state, but become agreeable articles of food when cooked, owing to the dissipation or decomposition of the acrid principle.

The fresh root of *Dioscorea sativa,* from the West Indies, was analysed by Süersen,[1] who obtained the following results:—resin, 0·05; uncrystallizable sugar, 0·26; mucilage, 2·94; starch, 22·66; ligneous fibre, 6·51; nitrogenised matter, quantity undetermined; and water, 67·58. The fresh roots yield 0·52 of ashes, containing carbonate of lime and silica.

The following are the per-centage quantities of *yam-starch* obtained by Dr. Sheir[2] from the fresh roots of several species of Dioscorea:—

Per-centage of Starch.		Per-centage of Starch.	
Common yam (*D. sativa*)	24·47	Buck yam (*D. triphylla*)	16·07
Barbados yam (*D——?*)	18·75	Another sample	15·63
Guinea yam (*D. aculeata*)	17·03	A third	14·83 (From a dark-coloured variety.)

I am indebted to Dr. Sheir for specimens of the starches of three species; viz. *D. sativa, D. aculeata,* and *D. triphylla.* They were prepared in the Colonial Laboratory at Demerara. They are beautifully white, inodorous, and tasteless. Examined by the microscope, the particles of the three starches present a general similarity of character. They are large, somewhat compressed, elliptical or ovate, or somewhat obtusely triangular. They may be compared in shape to the seed of the common scarlet runner bean (*Phaseolus multiflorus*), and are surrounded by rings, which, when viewed on the middle of the flat side of the particle, appear to be but slightly curved. In the latter character they approximate to curcuma starch. Some of the particles present one or two slight nipple-like projections analogous to those of maranta starch. In polarised light they present the usual crosses observed with most other starches. Their size[3] is about $\frac{1}{500}$th of an inch in length, and about $\frac{1}{1000}$th of an inch in breadth.

Yams are roasted and boiled, and eaten like potatoes. "They are dressed in various forms, being boiled in soups or broths, &c., made into pudding, or roasted in the fire."[4] Some of them, however, are violently acrid, causing vomiting and diarrhœa, even after being carefully cooked. This is said to be the case with *D. triphylla* and *dæmona.* Yet Dr. Wright and Dr. Sheir declare that the roots of *D. triphylla* are nearly equal to potatoes.

---

[1] Quoted by L. Gmelin, *Handb. d. Chemie,* Bd. ii. S. 1334.

[2] *Report on the Starch-producing Plants of the Colony of British Guiana,* by John Sheir, LL.D. Demerara, 1847.—Dr. James Clark (*Medical Facts and Observations,* vol. vii. 1797) obtained from 4 lbs. of the roots of *D. triphylla* 5 oz. 2 dr. of starch, and from the same quantity of the roots of *D. bulbifera,* 8 oz. of starch.

[3] The following measurements, in parts of an English inch, of the particles of yam starch, were made for me by Mr. George Jackson:—

	Guinea Yam.		Common Yam.		Buck Yam.	
Particles.	Length.	Breadth.	Length.	Breadth.	Length.	Breadth.
1	0·0025	0·0020	0·0019	0·0012	0·0030	0·0015
2	0·0018	0·0014	*0·0019	0·0009	*0·0022	0·0014
3	*0·0015	0·0011	*0·0016	0·0010	*0·0017	0·0010
4	*0·0012	0·0010	0·0012	0·0008	*0·0016	0·0008
5	*0·0012	0 0007	0·0009	0·0006	0·0010	0·0007
6	0·0010	0·0006				
7	0·0013	0·0005				

The most prevalent sized particles are those marked thus.*

[4] Dr. Wright, *Medicinal Plants growing in Jamaica,* in the *Memoir* of his life, p. 208, 1828.

99. Tamus communis, *Linn.*—Common Black Bryony.

Sex. Syst. Diœcia, Hexandria.

(Radix.)

Ἄμπελος μέλαινα, Dioscor. lib. iv. cap. 185 ? ; *Chironia, Gynæcanthe* aut *Apronia*, Pliny, lib. xxiii. cap. 17, ed. Valp.? ; *Bryonia nigra*, Gerard, 871.—Indigenous. The root (*radix bryoniæ nigræ*) is large and fleshy, black externally, white internally. When fresh, it possesses some acridity. No analysis of it has been made. Taken internally, it acts as a diuretic, and has been esteemed as a lithic. It is kept in the herb shops, and sold, like Solomon's seal, as a topical application for removing bruise marks. In France, it is called the *herbe aux femmes battues,* or the *herb for bruised women.*

†† Flowers with the perianth free from the ovary (*superior ovary.*)

Order XX. SMILACEÆ, *Lindl.*—SARSAPARILLAS.

CHARACTERS.—*Flowers* biennial or polygamous. *Calyx* and *corolla* both alike, free, 6-parted. *Stamens* 6, inserted into the perianth near the base; seldom hypogynous. *Ovary* 3-celled, the cells 1- or many-seeded : *style* usually trifid; *stigmas* 3. *Fruit* a roundish berry. *Albumen* between fleshy and cartilaginous; *embryo* usually distant from the hilum.—*Herbaceous* plants or *under shrubs*, with a tendency to climb. *Stems* scarcely woody. *Leaves* reticulated. (*Lindley.*)

PROPERTIES. See *Smilax.*—The *Ripogonum parviflorum*[1] of R. Brown, a native of New Zealand, where it is called *kareao*, is said to possess virtues similar to those of sarsaparilla, and may be termed the *New Zealand sarsaparilla.* The stems yield 12 per cent. of extract, which is bitter, and contains starch-gum and traces of astringent matter.[2]

100. SMILAX, *Linn.*—several Species of, yielding Sarsaparilla.

Sex. Syst. Diœcia, Hexandria.

(Radix dicta Zarza seu Sarsaparilla.)

HISTORY.—The root of sarsaparilla was brought into Europe from the West Indies, about the year 1530, with the character of being a medicine singularly efficacious in the cure of lues venerea.[3] Monardes[4] says that, when the Spaniards first saw it, they called it, *çarça-parilla,* on account of its resemblance to the çarça-parilla of Europe (*Smilax aspera*).[5] The Spanish term *zarzaparilla* (from *zarza,* a bramble ; and *parilla,* a vine) signifies a thorny vine.

BOTANY. **Gen. Char.**—*Diœcious.* *Perianth* 6-parted, nearly equal, spreading. MALE FLOWERS : *stamens* 6; *anthers* erect. FEMALE FLOWERS : *perianth* permanent; *ovary* 3-celled, the cells 1-seeded; *style* very short;

---

[1] Allan Cunningham, in *Hooker's Companion to the Botanical Magazine*, vol. ii.

[2] See a paper by the author, in the *Pharmaceutical Journal*, vol. v. p. 73.

[3] Pearson, *Observations on the Effects of various Articles of the Materia Medica in the Cure of Lues Venerea*, 1800.

[4] Clusii, *Exotic.* lib. x. cap. xxii. p. 317.

[5] [According to Dr. X. Landerer the stalks and fruit of this European species are sold in the Mizir bazaars of Constautinople as excelling in efficacy the genuine sarsaparilla.—ED.]

stigmas 3. *Berry* 1- to 3-seeded. *Seeds* roundish; *albumen* cartilaginous; *embryo* remote from the hilum. (R. Brown, *Prodrom.* p. 293.)

Species.—Considerable uncertainty prevails as to the botanical origin of the various sorts of sarsaparilla of commerce. From four species of Smilax, a great part, at least, of this drug is obtained.

1. S. OFFICINALIS, HBK.—*Stem* twining, shrubby, prickly, quadrangular, smooth; the young shoots are unarmed, and almost round. *Leaves* ovate-oblong, acute, cordate, netted, 5- to 7-nerved, coriaceous, smooth, a foot long, and 4-5 inches broad; the young ones are narrow, oblong, acuminate, and 3-nerved. *Petioles* smooth, an inch long, bearing two tendrils above the base. *Flowers* and *fruit* unknown.—Grows in New Granada, on the banks of the Magdalena, near Bajorque. It is called *zarzaparilla* by the natives, who transmit large quantities of it to Carthagena and Mompox; whence it is shipped for Jamaica and Spain (Humboldt).[1] According to Pohl, it is collected near the river Abaité, in the western part of the province of Minas Geraes (Martius).

This species probably yields the sarsaparilla exported from Colombia (Savanilla, Santa Marta, Caraccas and its port La Guayra, St. Margarita and its port Porta Arenas,) and Guatemala (Costa Rica).

2. S. MEDICA, Schlechtendal, in Linnæa, vi. 47.—*Stem* angular, armed at the joints with straight prickles, with a few hooked ones in the intervals. *Leaves* shortly acuminate, smooth, 5- to 7-nerved; inferior ones cordate, auriculate-hastate; upper ones ovate-cordate. *Peduncle* axillary, smooth, about an inch long. *Inflorescence* an 8- to 12-flowered umbel. *Fruit* red, size of a small cherry; contains 1—3 reddish-brown *seeds*. *Embryo* cylindrical, lodged in horny albumen (T. F. L. Nees).[2]

Schiede[3] says that of the numerous species of Smilax which grow on the eastern slope of the Mexican Andes, this is the only species which is collected in the villages of Papantla, Tuspan, Nautla, Misantla, &c., and carried to Vera Cruz, from whence it is sent into European commerce under the name of *zarzaparilla*. We may, therefore, safely state that Mexican sarsaparilla (Vera Cruz and Tampico) is the produce of this species.

3. S. PAPYRACEA, Poiret; *S. syphilitica*, Mart. (non Humb.) Reise, iii. 1280; *Sipó êm* of the natives.—*Stem* 4-cornered or plane-angular, polished, prickly. *Leaves* somewhat membranous, oval-oblong, obtuse at both ends, or usually pointletted at the apex, quite entire, unarmed, 5-ribbed with 3 more prominent ribs. *Cirrhi* inserted beneath the middle of the petiole.—Province of Rio Negro, in marshy spots on the Japura, near Porto dos Miranhos (Martius); near Ega (Pœppig); and near Borba, in the province of Rio Negro (Riedel).—Yields Brazilian (also called Maranham, Para, or Lisbon) sarsaparilla. This species has also been found at Guatemala. Specimens were forwarded to the late Dr. Pereira from that locality, and have been described by Mr. Robert Bentley.[4]

The " Rio Negro Sarsa" of Dr. Hancock[5] is perhaps the produce of this species.

[1] *Nov. Gen. et Spec.* i. p. 215.
[2] Nees, *Pl. Med. Suppl.*
[3] *Linnæa*, Bd. iv. S. 576, 1829.
[4] *Pharm. Journ.* vol. xii. p. 470.
[5] *Trans. Med.-Bot. Soc.* 1829.

The preceding are the species of Smilax from which probably the greater part, if not all, of the sarsaparilla of commerce is obtained. Other species, however, which have been mentioned in connection with this drug require to be noticed.

4. S. sarsaparilla, Linn.—It is common in the hedges and swamps of the United States of America; but, notwithstanding its name, it does not yield any of the sarsaparilla of commerce; and there is no evidence that it ever did yield any. Dr. Wood[1] remarks, that its root would certainly have been dug up and brought into the market, had it been found to possess the same properties with the imported medicine.

5. S. syphilitica, HBK.—Humboldt and Bonpland discovered it in New Granada, on the river Cassiquiare, between Mandavala and San Francisco Solano.[2] In the former edition of this work, I stated, on the authority of Martius,[3] that this species yielded Brazilian sarsaparilla. But this botanist has subsequently[4] ascertained that he had mistaken *S. papyracea* for this species.

Poeppig[5] states that *S. syphilitica*, HBK., is collected at Maynas (in Colombia), and forms the *sarsa fina* which is mixed with *sarsa gruésa* (*S. cordato-ovata*, Pers.) and sent to Para.

6. S. cordato-ovato, Persoon.—Cayenne; Maynas. Yields *sarsa gruésa* (see supra).

7. S. Purhampy, Ruiz, Memoria sobre las virtudes, &c. &c., Purhampy, p. 65.—Peru.[6] Yields one of the best sorts of sarsaparilla, which Ruiz calls *China peruviana*. Lindley thinks this may be the same species as S. officinalis.

8. S. obliquata, Poiret.—Peru. Guibourt[7] ascribes to this species the *Peruvian sarsaparilla* of commerce, but I know not on what authority.

[Dr. Bertold Leeman has lately declared his belief that the greater portion of the sarsaparilla imported under the commercial names of "Jamaica," "Lisbon, or Brazilian," and "Guatemala, or red Paraguay" sarsaparilla, is the produce of one and the same species, the *Smilax officinalis* of Humboldt and Bonpland. He further states that the *S. medica* and *S. papyracea* are identical with *S. officinalis*. We shall treat of the subject irrespective of these views, which appear to require confirmation.[8]—Ed.]

General Description.—The *sarsaparilla* or *sarza* (more properly *zárza*) of commerce (*radix sarsaparillæ* vel *sarzæ*) consists essentially of the *roots* of the before-mentioned and perhaps also of other species of Smilax. In some sorts of sarsaparilla the roots are attached to a portion of the *rhizome*.

a. The *rhizome* or *rootstock* (*rhizoma*), called by druggists the *chump*, is a tuberous subterranean stem, which in the living plant is placed horizontally or obliquely in the earth. It grows throwing out aerial stems and roots at the more pointed extremity, and gradually dies off at the thicker and older end. One or more *aerial stems* are frequently found attached to the rhizome of the shops; these are rounded or square, with *nodes* and usually with *aculei* or prickles. If a transverse section be made of either the rhizome or aerial stem no distinction of bark, wood, and pith is perceptible.

β. The *roots* (*radices*) are called by Schleiden[9] adventitious (*r. adventitiæ*): they are usually several feet long, and of variable thickness; on the average about that of a writing quill. The thin shrivelled roots are more or less wrinkled or furrowed longitudinally, and in trade are usually said to be *lean*; while the thick, plump, swollen ones are described as being *gouty*.

---

[1] *United States Dispensatory.*
[2] *Nova Gen. et Sp. Plant.* t. i. 271.
[3] *Reise in Brasilien*, Bd. iii.
[4] *Systema Materiæ Medicæ Veg. Brasil.*, 1843.
[5] *Reise in Chile, Peru und auf dem Amazonstrome wahrend der Jahre* 1827-32, Bd. i. S. 459, *Pharm. Central Blatt. für* 1832, S. 57; and *für* 1835, S. 908.
[6] *Flora Medica.*
[7] *Hist. Nat. des Drog.* t. ii. p. 182. 4ème édit. 1849.
[8] *Pharm. Journal*, vol. xiii. p. 385.
[9] *Jahresbericht über die Fortschritte in der Pharmacie im Jahre*, 1847, p. 81.

The latter usually abound in starch, and are said to be *mealy*. Frequently, especially in some sorts of sarsaparilla, the roots are said to be *bearded*; that is, they give off, more or less abundantly, fibres, which are themselves often divided into fibrils.

The colour of the roots varies, being more or less red or brown, frequently with a grayish tint. The washed or unwashed condition, the greater or less care taken of them in drying, the time of year when they were collected, the colour and nature of the soil in which they grew, as well as the species or sort of plant from which they are obtained, and many other circumstances, doubtless modify the colour. The taste of the root is mucilaginous and slightly acrid. The acridity is only perceived after chewing the root for a few minutes. The odour is somewhat earthy.

By a transverse section the roots are seen to consist of a cortex or rind, and a ligneous cord or meditullium inclosing the pith, somewhat in the manner of an exogenous stem.

The *cortex* or *rind* consists, 1st, of the *cuticle* or *epidermis*, composed of compact cells; 2ndly, of the *outer cortical layers*, composed of coloured (from golden yellow to deep orange red), elongated, thick, flattened cells (some of which are porous), which form a *subcuticular tissue* (*epiphlœum* or *periderm?*); and 3rdly, of the *inner cortical layers*, consisting of shorter, thinner, cylindrical, often porous cells with large intercellular spaces. In some sorts of sarsaparilla most of these cells abound in starch, while a few contain bundles of acicular crystals (oxalate of lime?) called *raphides*. The mealy cortex is frequently colourless, but sometimes has a roseate tint.

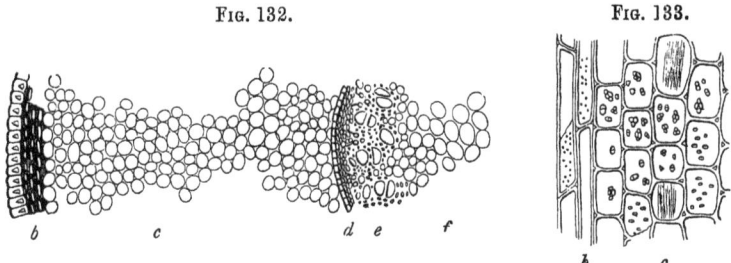

FIG. 132. FIG. 133.

Fig. 132. Transverse section of the cortex and half of the diameter of the meditullium.
Fig. 133. Longitudinal section of the cortex.

Magnified Sections of Sarsaparilla.

a. Cuticle or epidermis.
b. Outer cortical layers (subcuticular tissue).
c. Inner cortical layers. Most of the cells abound in starch; some few contain raphides.

d. Cellular layer or nucleus sheath.
e. Woody zone (vascular-bundle-circle).
f. Medulla or pith.

The *ligneous cord* or *meditullium* consists of, 1st, a *cellular layer* (*liber?*), called by Schleiden the *Kernscheide* or *nucleus-sheath*, whose cells are empty, thick, and strongly coloured (like those of the outer cortical layers); 2ndly, a *woody zone*, called by Schleiden the *Gefässbündelkreis* or *vascular-bundle-circle*, usually of a pale yellowish colour, and composed of woody tissue, vessels,[1] and cambial cells; and 3rdly, *medulla* or *pith*,

---

[1] The apertures in the woody zone, seen with the naked eye in a transverse section of the root, are those of large vessels. Occasionally we perceive an isolated bundle of vessels whose interior is filled up with a yellowish-red colouring matter.

generally colourless, composed of cylindrical cells (like those of the inner cortical layers) which often abound in starch. Sometimes an isolated vessel, or a small group of vessels surrounded by a thin layer of ligneous cells, is seen in the pith.

The chief anatomical characters, which vary in the different species of sarsaparilla, are the relative breadths of the cortical, ligneous, and medullary layers, the characters of the cells of the nucleus sheath, and the number of layers composing the subcuticular tissue. Schleiden pretends that he can, by these characters, distinguish the South American, Central American, and Mexican sarsaparillas from each other. The following is the way in which he applies them :—*South American sarsaparillas*, he says, have, almost without an exception, a mealy cortex and a vascular-bundle-circle whose breadth, from the nucleus sheath to the pith, is one-fourth, or at most one-third, the diameter of the pith. They have, therefore, a large white pith. The *Central American* and *Mexican sarsaparillas* have, on the other hand, a vascular-bundle-circle whose breadth is commonly equal to, and sometimes exceeds, the diameter of the pith. Sometimes, but rarely, the pith is half as thick again as the vascular-bundle-circle. The Central American and Mexican sarsaparillas are, according to Schleiden, readily distinguished from each other by the nucleus sheath, whose cells, in the *Central American* sorts, are either quadrangular or somewhat elongated transversely (tangentially), and are nearly equally thick on all sides (fig. 134); whereas in the *Mexican* sort these cells are elongated in the direction from within outwards (radially), and have walls which are thicker on the inner than on the outer side (fig. 135).

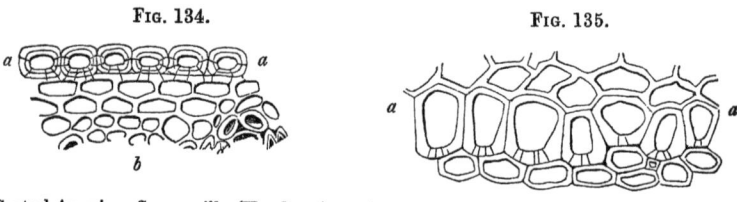

FIG. 134.   FIG. 135.

Central American Sarsaparilla (Honduras). | South American Sarsaparilla (Vera Cruz).

Magnified Views of the Cells composing the Nucleus-sheath (according to Schleiden).

a, a, a, a, The cells of the sheath. | *b,* A portion of the woody zone.

The Central American and Mexican sorts are less strikingly distinguished, according to Schleiden, by the external cortex (subcuticular tissue), which, in the Central American, consists of only one, rarely two, layers of very thick cells, and altogether has fewer cellular layers; while the Mexican has from 2 to 4 layers of very thick cells, and altogether sometimes 6 or 7 layers.

COMMERCIAL SORTS.—Several sorts of sarsaparilla are met with in commerce, and are well known to our dealers; but I find that, with some exceptions, there is a great want of precision in the names applied to some of the varieties. The terms *Jamaica, Lima, Honduras,* and *Lisbon* or *Brazilian,* are, by English dealers, applied to sorts which are well known to them either by the characters of the roots or the mode of packing. There is another kind, called by English druggists *gouty* or *Vera Cruz* sarsaparilla, which appears to me to be identical with that called by Continental and American writers *Caraccas sarsaparilla;* under which name I shall describe it.

α. **Geographical Classification.**—Sarsaparilla is exclusively the produce of America, and grows in the southern part of North America and the northern part of South America. The exact limits are not known.

1. *Mexican sarsaparilla.*—This is the produce of *Smilax medica*, and is the growth of Papantla, Tuspan, Nantla, Misantla, &c. It is usually shipped at Vera Cruz, and is, therefore, usually known in commerce by the name of *Vera Cruz sarsaparilla.* From Tampico, another Mexican port, a similar sort of sarsaparilla is also exported, which is known in Europe as *Tampico sarsaparilla.* According to Monardes, the first sarsaparilla which came to Europe was brought from New Spain (Mexico). He describes it as being whiter, somewhat yellowish, and smaller than the Honduras sort.

2. *Central American sarsaparilla.*—Guatemala produces sarsaparilla, which is sometimes exported to Jamaica, but which has only lately been distinguished in European commerce as the produce of Guatemala. *Honduras sarsaparilla* is a well-known and distinct sort in the London market. Monardes says it was the second kind known in Europe. He describes it as darker and thicker than the Mexican sort ; and says that it was more esteemed. *Costa Rica sarsaparilla* is usually sold as *Lima sarsaparilla*, with which it agrees in quality. Much sarsaparilla is collected on the Mosquito coast by the Seco Indians, who sell it to the Sambos. The latter carry it in their doreys to Truxillo, where they barter it for goods.[1] I have been informed that sarsaparilla, the produce of the Mosquito Shore of St. Juan de Nicaragua, is sometimes sent to England by way of Jamaica.

3. *Colombian sarsaparilla.*—Since 1831 Colombia has been divided into three independent states, viz. New Granada, Venezuela, and Ecuador, from all of which sarsaparilla is exported to Europe, either directly or indirectly, by way of Jamaica or New York.

a. New Granada.—According to Humboldt and Bonpland, sarsaparilla (*Smilax officinalis*) is collected on the banks of the Magdalena, and transmitted to Carthagena and Mompox, whence it is shipped for Jamaica and Spain. Occasionally sarsaparilla is imported into England from Santa Marta and Savanilla.

β. Venezuela.—From la Guayra (the sea-port of the Caraccas) is shipped to the United States of America and Europe *Caraccas sarsaparilla.* Sarsaparilla is sometimes imported into England from Porta Arenas.

γ. Ecuador.—Occasionally sarsaparilla is imported into London from Guayaquil ; but whether it is the produce of Maynas or of Central America I know not.

4. *Brazilian sarsaparilla.*—This is a well-known sort, and is imported from Para ; and according to Martius is the produce of *Smilax papyracea.* Poeppig, however, says that two sorts of sarsaparilla, *sarsa fina* and *sarsa gruésa*, are collected in Maynas and transmitted to Peru : the first is the produce of *Smilax syphilitica*, the second of *S. cordato-ovata.*

5. *Peruvian sarsaparilla.*—Sarsaparilla is sometimes imported from Lima ; but whether it is the produce of Peru or of Maynas, or of Central America, I know not. Under the name of *Lima sarsaparilla* is sold, not only the sarsaparilla from Lima, but also that from Costa Rica. It is probable

---

[1] Young, *Narrative of a Residence on the Mosquito Shore during the Years* 1839, 1840, and 1841, Lond. 1842.

that no sarsaparilla grows on the western declivity of the Andes, and that the sarsaparilla exported from Lima is either the produce of Maynas or has been carried to Lima from some other ports on the Pacific.

A considerable portion of sarsaparilla is imported into London from Jamaica (*Jamaica sarsaparilla*), from Valparaiso, and from New York; and formerly also from Lisbon (*Brazilian sarsaparilla*). But it is not the produce of these places.

β. **Qualitative Classification.**—The various commercial sorts of sarsaparilla differ from each other in the anatomical and other characters of the roots, in the manner in which they are folded and packed, and in the absence or presence and character of the attached rhizomes and stalks. I have already given a sketch of Schleiden's anatomical arrangement of the commercial sorts of sarsaparilla roots. I shall not adopt it, because I do not consider it accurate or easily applied. His classification would associate Costa Rica sarsaparilla with that of Honduras, and the Lima with the Caraccas and Brazilian sorts. I shall arrange the sarsaparillas of commerce in two divisions: the first including those commonly termed mealy; the second, those which are not mealy.

Div. 1. *Mealy Sarsaparillas.*

(Sarsaparillæ farinosæ seu amylaceæ.)

These are characterised by the mealy character of the inner cortical layers, which are white or pale-coloured. The meal or starch is sometimes so abundant, that a shower of it, in the form of white dust, falls when we fracture the roots. The thickest mealy coat which I have measured was barely $\frac{1}{10}$th of an inch in thickness. Compared with the diameter of the meditullium or ligneous cord, the thickness of the mealy coat is sometimes nearly equal to it, but usually does not exceed the $\frac{1}{3}$ or $\frac{1}{2}$ of it. The thick mealy roots have a swollen appearance, and are technically called *gouty* by the dealers: the cortex being brittle is frequently cracked transversely in rings, and readily falls off. The colour of the mealy coat varies from white to yellowish or pinkish.

FIG. 136.

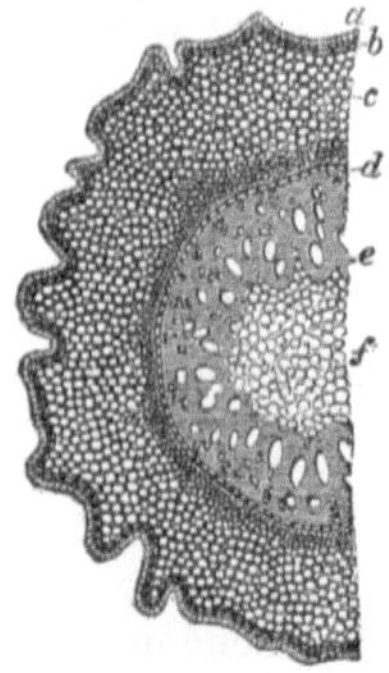

Magnified view of a section of mealy (Honduras) *sarsaparilla.*

a. Cuticle or epidermis.
b. Outer cortical layers.
c. Mealy coat, or inner cortical layers.
d. Cellular sheath.
e. Woody zone.
f. Medulla or pith.

The medulla or pith is frequently very amylaceous.

If a drop of oil of vitriol be applied to a transverse section of the root of mealy sarsaparilla, the mealy coat is *but little altered in colour;* while the woody zone becomes dark purplish or almost black. Sometimes the pith also acquires a darkish tint.

A decoction of mealy sarsaparilla, when cold, becomes dark blue on the addition of tincture of iodine.

The aqueous extract of mealy sarsaparilla, when rubbed down with distilled water in a mortar, does not completely dissolve, but yields a turbid liquid, which becomes blue on the addition of iodine.

This division includes three commercial sorts of sarsaparilla; namely, the *Brazilian,* the *Honduras,* and a third kind, which by English dealers is commonly called *gouty* or *Vera Cruz* sort, but which, by Continental and American writers, is usually denominated *Caraccas.*

[To these we must now add the *Guatemala sarsaparilla,* obtained from the Smilax papyracea. The four commercial sorts will then bear arrangement according to the late author's plan, as follows :—]

A. Pith 2- to 4-times the breadth of the woody layer; cells of the nucleus sheath elongated radially, [and having walls which are thicker on the inner than on the outer side.—ED.]

    a. Pale, folded, often swollen (or gouty) roots with the rhizomes or stems attached . . . . 1. *Caraccas.*

    β. Reddish brown, unfolded roots with rhizome or stems attached, packed in rolls or cylindrical bundles . . . . 2. *Brazilian.*

B. Pith 1- to 1½ times the breadth of the woody layer.

    [*a.* Folded roots; cells of the nucleus sheath square, or elongated transversely, and nearly equally thick on all sides . 3. *Honduras.*

    β. Unfolded roots without rhizome, packed in rolls or cylindrical bundles; cells of the nucleus sheath elongated radially, and having walls which are thicker on the inner than the outer side . . . . 4. *Guatemala.*[1]
                                                  ED.]

1. CARACCAS SARSAPARILLA (*Radix Sarsaparillæ de Caraccas*).—This is the *gouty* or *Vera Cruz sarsaparilla* of most English dealers. It would appear to come to this country by various routes. One sample which I have received, came, as I was informed, by Mr. Price (of the firm of Price and Gifford, drug-brokers), from the Pacific side of South America by way of Valparaiso. Mr. Luckombe, of the firm of Hodgkinson and Co., informs me that some of this sort of sarsaparilla has come by way of New Orleans. Dr. Wood[2] states that it is imported in large quantities into the United States from La Guayra (the port of the Caraccas). He says it comes in oblong packages of about one hundred pounds, surrounded with broad strips of hide, which are connected laterally with thongs of the same material, and leaves much of the root exposed. The roots, he adds, are separately, closely, and carefully packed, and are often very amylaceous internally.

FIG. 137.

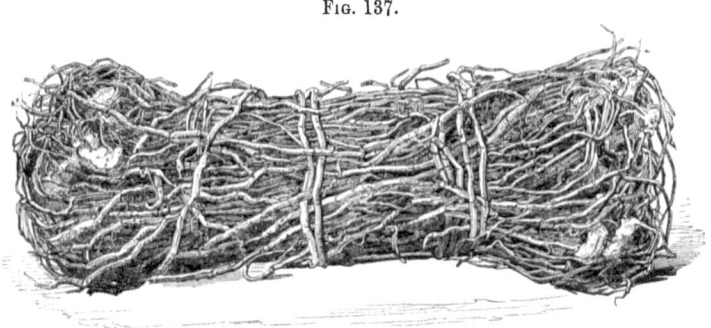

Bundle of Caraccas Sarsaparilla.

I have a bundle (fig. 137) of this sarsaparilla (called by English druggists *gouty* or *Vera Cruz sarsaparilla*) which was imported into Liverpool from

---

[1] [Mr. Bentley's paper on this subject is of great interest. The above arrangement is in accordance with his description. See *Pharm. Journ.* vol. xii. p. 470.—ED.]
[2] *United States Dispensatory.*

Valparaiso. It weighs 5½ lbs. It is flattened, about 2½ feet long, scarcely 1 foot broad at its widest parts, and is 3 or 4 inches thick. At each extremity are two rhizomes, with portions of rounded or obscurely square stems bearing a few small prickles. The roots are pale yellowish or reddish grey, and are very amylaceous. The cells of the nucleus sheath are elongated radially, and their walls are thicker on the inner side (fig. 135).

This sort is probably the produce of *Smilax officinalis* and *S. syphilitica*, HBK.

Guibourt's *Maracaibo sarsaparilla* is perhaps only a variety of Caraccas sarsaparilla.

2. Brazilian Sarsaparilla; *Lisbon, Portugal,* or *Rio Negro Sarsaparilla* (*Radix Sarsaparillæ brasiliensis,* seu *lisbonensis; S. de Maranon; S. de Para; S. insipida*).—Prior to the introduction of the Jamaica sort of sarsaparilla into the London Market, the Lisbon sort commanded the highest price.[1] This is usually imported from Para and Maranham. It is brought over unfolded, tied in rolls or cylindrical bundles (*sarsaparilla longa*) of from three to five feet long, and about a foot in diameter.

In the museum of the Pharmaceutical Society is a roll (fig. 138) weighing 14¼ lbs.: its length is 3 feet 1 inch, and its diameter 7 inches.

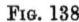

Fig. 138.

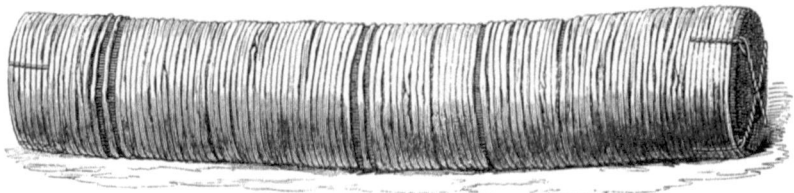

A Roll of Brazilian Sarsaparilla.

It is free from the rhizome or chump. But as it is not easy to get at the interior of the rolls, this sort of sarsaparilla is more liable to false packing than any other sort. It has fewer longitudinal wrinkles than the Jamaica kind, fewer radicles, especially at one end; has a reddish-brown colour, and abounds in amylaceous matter, both in the cortex and pith. Its decoction is much paler coloured than the Jamaica variety.

This sort of sarsaparilla is collected on the branches of the Amazon: according to Poeppig, at Huallaga, Intay, Jurua, Rio de los Enganos; according to Martius, at Ucayala, Ica, Jupura, and Rio Negro.

Martius[2] says that the Indians gather it all the year round, according to the state of the weather and of the rivers. After being dried over a fire, the roots are tied up in bundles with a flexible stem called *Timbotitica;* and to prevent them being worm-eaten, they are preserved in the gables of the houses, where they are exposed to smoke.

The same writer[3] also states that this sarsaparilla is the produce of *Smilax papyracea* and *S. officinalis.* Poeppig tells us that there are two sorts of sarsaparilla which the dealers mix together; these are *sarsa fina,* a thin lean

[1] Pope, *Med.-Chir. Trans.* vol. xii. p. 344, 1823.
[2] *Reise,* Bd. iii. S. 1280.
[3] *Systema Mat. Med. Brasil.*

sort, less active, but also less liable to be worm-eaten,— and *sarsa gruésa,* a thicker, more active sort, but more liable to be attacked by insects : the first, he says, is the produce of *S. syphilitica,* the second of *S. cordato-ovata.* Schleiden suggests that *S. Purhampuy* of Ruiz may perhaps yield some Brazilian sarsaparilla.

3. HONDURAS SARSAPARILLA ; *Mealy Sarsaparilla* (*Radix Sarsaparillæ de Honduras ; S. acris* vel *gutturalis*).—It is imported from Belize, and other parts of the Bay of Honduras. It comes in large and smaller bundles two or three feet long, folded lengthwise (in a kind of hank), and secured in a compact form by a few transverse circular turns. A large bundle (fig. 139) in the museum of the Pharmaceutical Society is $2\frac{1}{2}$ feet long, from 10 to 12 inches in diameter, and weighs about 17 lbs. A smaller bundle (fig. 140) is 2 feet 2 inches long, $3\frac{1}{2}$ inches in diameter, and weighs about 2 lbs.

FIG. 139.

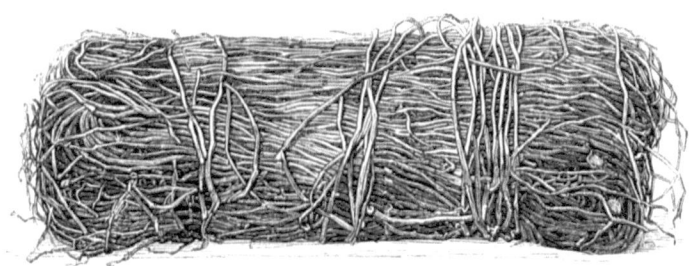

FIG. 140.

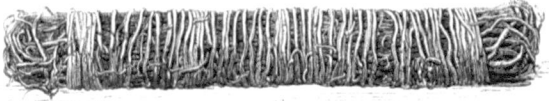

Figs. 139 and 140. *Large and Smaller Bundles of Honduras Sarsaparilla.*

The bundles are packed in bales, weighing from 80 to 110 lbs. or more, and imperfectly covered by skins. In the interior of the bundles are found roots of inferior quality, rhizomes with adherent stems, stones, chumps of wood, &c. The roots are furnished with a few rootlets. The general colour of the roots is dirty greyish- or reddish-brown. The cortex is very mealy, and the meditullium or central cord is thinner than in the Jamaica sort. The cells of the nucleus sheath are square, or are elongated tangentially, and are equally thick on all four sides (see fig. 134).

The taste of the root is amylaceous, and ultimately somewhat acrid. Its decoction becomes intensely blue by the addition of a solution of iodine. Its powder is fawn-coloured, and, when rubbed with water and tincture of iodine, becomes intensely bluish black. From five pounds of the root of fine quality about one pound of extract may be produced (Hennell). A sample, examined by Mr. Battley, yielded six and a half ounces of extract from three pounds of root, which is about ten and a half ounces from five pounds : 874 grains of the cortical portion of the root yielded 230 grains of extract (Battley). In one operation, in the laboratory of a friend of mine, 170 lbs. of root yielded 45 lbs. of extract. According to Mr. Pope, the cortex yields twice as much extract as the meditullium.

Nothing whatever is known respecting the botanical origin of this sort of sarsaparilla; [but Mr. Bentley inclines to believe it produced by the *Smilax papyracea*, inasmuch as the distinctive characters between it and the next described article are by no means remarkable.—Ed.]

[4. Guatemala Sarsaparilla (*Smilax papyracea*).—Newly described as a commercial article by Mr. Robert Bentley (Pharm. Journ. vol. xii. p. 470). This sarsaparilla was given to the late Dr. Pereira by the importers. The roots are unfolded and tied together in the middle by a flexible monocotyledonous stem into a loose and somewhat cylindrical bundle (see fig. 141). It

Fig. 141.

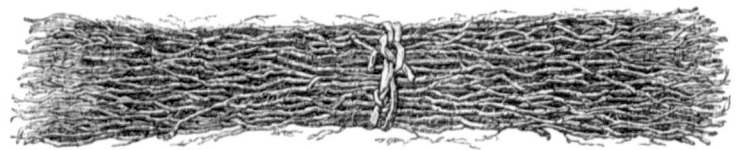

Guatemala Sarsaparilla.

is free from rhizome or chump. The roots are much furrowed longitudinally, and are frequently swollen or gouty, like the Caraccas and Vera Cruz sarsaparillas. There are branched rootlets, or beard. The taste is amylaceous, and perhaps slightly acrid, but there is no perceptible odour. A transverse section exposes a thick cortical portion, colourless, or of pale roseate hue. In thickness this cortex is from one-half to one-third that of the meditullium. A decoction is paler than that of the Jamaica sarsaparilla. Solution of iodine produces in it an immediate dark blue precipitate. According to the experiments of Mr. Daniel Hanbury, this sarsaparilla yields 22 per cent. of extract, which is an extremely favourable result.—Ed.]

Div. 2. *Non-mealy Sarsaparillas.*

(Sarsaparillæ non-farinosæ vel non-amylaceæ.)

The sarsaparillas of this division are characterised by a deeply coloured (red or brown) usually non-mealy cortex. The cortex is red, and much thinner than in the mealy sorts. Although by the microscope starch grains can be detected in the inner cortical layers, yet their number is comparatively small, and is quite insufficient to give the mealiness which characterises the sarsaparillas of the first division. The diameter of the meditullium or ligneous cord is much greater than in the mealy sarsaparillas, and is frequently six or more times greater than the thickness of the cortex. The roots have never that swollen appearance called by dealers gouty, and which is frequently observed in the mealy sorts.

Starch grains are usually recognisable in the pith by the microscope.

If a drop of oil of vitriol be applied to a transverse section of the root of the non-mealy sarsaparillas, both cortex and wood acquire a dark red or purplish tint.

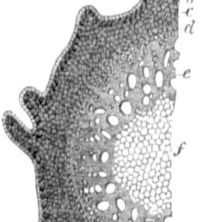

FIG. 142.

A decoction of non-mealy sarsaparilla, when cold, does not yield a blue colour when a solution of iodine is added to it.

This division includes the sorts known in commerce by the names of *Jamaica* and *Lima* sarsaparillas, as well as a sort which I have received as a *lean Vera Cruz* sarsaparilla.

They differ from the Caraccas, Brazilian, and Honduras sarsaparillas, in having a red or brown usually non-mealy cortex. In the relative thickness of the pith and woody layer they agree with the Honduras sarsaparilla ; but they differ from it in having the cells somewhat elongated radially, in this respect approaching the Caraccas and Brazilian sorts.

I have been unable to detect any anatomical difference between the roots of the Jamaica, the so-called Lima, and the lean Vera Cruz sorts. The Jamaica and Lima sorts are, I believe, not essentially different from each other. Both are probably the produce of Central America. They differ in colour somewhat, in the mode of packing, and in the route by which they reach England. What I have received as lean Vera Cruz sarsaparilla might pass for a lean, thin, pale-coloured Lima sort whose roots are unfolded.

Magnified view of a section of Non-mealy (Jamaica) Sarsaparilla.

a. Cuticle or epidermis.
b. Outer cortical layers.
c. Red inner cortical layers.
d. Cellular sheath.
e. Woody zone.
f. Medulla or pith.

5. JAMAICA SARSAPARILLA, offic.; *Red-bearded Sarsaparilla* (*Radix Sarsaparillæ jamaicensis* vel *rubræ*).—This sort first appeared in the London market about 1819 or 1820.[1]

The roots are folded and made up in bundles (*sarsaparilla rotunda*) of about a foot or half a yard long, and four or five or more inches broad. These bundles are neither trimmed nor closely packed.

The bundle from which fig. 143 was taken, was about 17 inches long, from 5 to 7 inches wide, and 3 inches

FIG. 143.

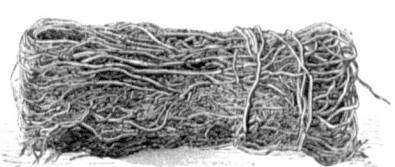

Bundle of Jamaica Sarsaparilla.

thick : its weight was 21½ oz. In the museum of the Pharmaceutical Society are some plaits of Jamaica sarsaparilla. One of these (fig. 144) weighs 5½ ounces, and is 4½ feet long, and 1¾ inches wide.

FIG. 144.

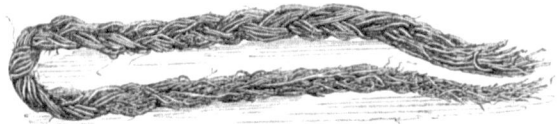

A Plait of Jamaica Sarsaparilla.

[1] Pope, *Med.-Chir Trans.* vol. xii. p. 344, 1823.

The bundles of Jamaica sarsaparilla are packed in circular bales of from 60 to 80 lbs. each. The roots of this sort are long, slender, furnished with numerous small fibrous rootlets (called the *beard*). Its cortex is brownish, but with an orange-red tint, which distinguishes it from other kinds of *red* sarsaparilla. The cortex is reddish, and when examined by the microscope is found to contain some starch globules. The meditullium has frequently a reddish tint. When chewed, Jamaica sarsaparilla tinges the saliva. Its taste is not remarkably mucilaginous, but slightly bitter, and after a few minutes slightly acrimonious. Its decoction is deepened in colour by a solution of iodine, but no blue is perceptible. Its powder is pale reddish brown, and when rubbed with water and tincture of iodine becomes blue, but less intensely so than the powder of the Honduras variety. It yields a larger quantity of extract than the other varieties: its extract is perfectly soluble in cold water. From three pounds of average quality about one pound of extract may be obtained (Hennell, also Battley); but from the same quantity of root of very fine quality nearly one pound and a quarter of extract may be procured (Hennell). 874 grains of the cortical portion of the root yielded 484 grains of extract (Battley). According to Mr. Pope, the cortex yields five times as much as the meditullium.

Jamaica sarsaparilla is not the produce of the island whose name it bears, but, as I have been informed by wholesale dealers, of the Mosquito shore on the eastern coast of Honduras and of St. Juan, from whence it is brought to England by way of Jamaica; and occasionally it is said to be brought from Guatemala. [We have official information as to the sources of Jamaica sarsaparilla, which we give in the following table.—Ed.]

Account of the Quantities of Sarsaparilla imported into Jamaica in each year from 1846 to 1853 inclusive, distinguishing the Countries from which imported.

	1846.	1847.	1848.	1849.	1850.	1851.	1852.	1853.
	lbs.	lbs.	lbs.	lbs.	lbs.	lbs.	lbs.	lbs.
Guatemala	—	59,42	—	—	—	—	—	—
Columbia	76,907	26,871	—	—	—	—	—	—
United States	—	—	—	203	16	—	495	140
New Granada	—	44,290	78,975	70,243	58,588	53,345	90,171	74,459
Total	76,907	77,103	78,975	70,446	58,604	53,345	90,666	74,599

[*The Quantities of Sarsaparilla exported from Jamaica to Great Britain were—*

In 1846	90,696 *lbs.*	In 1850	67,105 *lbs.*
1847	63,529	1851	46,968
1848	68,367	1852	71,400
1849	30,165	1853	62,339—Ed.]

This accords with Humboldt's statement before mentioned, that sarsaparilla is exported from Colombia (he says from Carthagena and Mompox) into Jamaica.

But although this table may be relied on for showing the countries from which sarsaparilla is imported into Jamaica, it does not establish the place of growth.

It is probable that Jamaica sarsaparilla is the produce of *Smilax officinalis*.

In the collection of Materia Medica at Apothecaries' Hall, London, is a sample of sarsaparilla said to have been grown in Jamaica ; but it does not resemble the Jamaica sarsaparilla of commerce. Its colour is pale cinnamon brown. Internally it is mealy.

6. LIMA SARSAPARILLA (*Radix Sarsaparillæ de Lima*).—This name is of course strictly applicable to sarsaparilla brought from Lima only, from whence, in fact, the first parcels came. But of late years sarsaparilla of the same quality has been brought from various other places ; and the dealers, to distinguish it from other kinds, have called it the *Lima sort ;* and gradually the term Lima sarsaparilla has been applied, rather to indicate the quality than the place of shipment. The true Lima sort is brought round Cape Horn ; whereas much of the so-called Lima sort is the produce of Costa Rica, and is brought from the Caribbean Sea. I know of one importation of 99,000 lbs. from Costa Rica. The Lima sort is also brought from Guajaquil and Valparaiso.

Although some druggists prefer good parcels of Costa Rica to Lima sarsaparilla, still the general run of the Lima parcels comes nearer to Jamaica than the Costa Rica sort. On the whole, however, it is difficult to say whether any dealer can with certainty distinguish the Lima and Costa Rica sorts.

I am informed that the Costa Rica sort sometimes comes from St. Marta, Savanilla, and Caraccas ; though that from Costa Rica is usually of a better description.

Lima (including Costa Rica) sarsaparilla is imported folded in bundles or hanks of about 2 or 3 feet long, and 6 or 9 inches in diameter, with the attached rhizome (chump) contained in the interior of the bundle. The bundle of which a cut (fig. 145) is subjoined came *viâ* Jamaica : it weighed 2 lbs. 13 oz. ; was two feet long, and 6 inches in diameter.

FIG. 145.

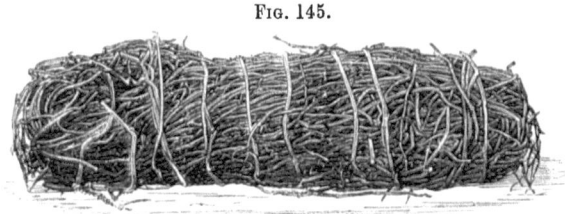

Bundle of Lima Sarsaparilla.

The bundles are usually packed in bales of from 60 to 80 lbs. each.

In quality Lima sarsaparilla closely resembles the Jamaica sort; but it yields a smaller quantity of extract. Its colour is brown or greyish-brown. Occasionally a few roots are found in a bale of good Lima sarsaparilla, which, as well as their rhizome and stem, are light clay-coloured. The stems are square and prickly : the prickles are few and small, except in the clay-coloured variety.

Lima sarsaparilla is probably the produce of *Smilax officinalis.*

Occasionally a knobby root or rhizome, like the *radix Chinæ*, with a round stem, and long, smooth, wiry, brown root-fibres, is found in a bale of Lima sarsaparilla. A transverse section of the stem presents, to the naked eye, a structure somewhat similar to that of the common cane. I have received the same root (under the name of *Salsepareille-Squine de Macaraïbo*) from Professor Guibourt, who found it in Caraccas sarsaparilla.

7. VERA CRUZ SARSAPARILLA (*Radix Sarsaparillæ de Vera Cruce*).—Much confusion exists about the sarsaparilla called the Vera Cruz sort; this name being usually applied to the gouty Caraccas sort before described. The sort which I received some years ago under the name of "lean Vera Cruz sarsaparilla," I was informed came from Vera Cruz; but it is now seldom met with. It is the sort which Mr. Pope[1] described as "lean, dark, and fibrous." The bundle (fig. 146) is 2 feet long, and, at the widest part, 2 inches broad: its weight is 7 ounces. The roots are unfolded (*sarsaparilla longa*), and have the *chump* attached at one end.

FIG. 146.

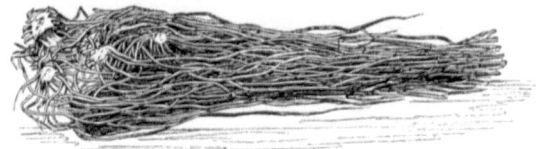

Bundle of Vera Cruz Sarsaparilla.

They are thin, tough, of a greyish-brown colour, with a shrivelled, thin, non-mealy cortex. They give off very few rootlets. This sort yields a deep-coloured decoction, which is unchanged by a solution of iodine.

Vera Cruz sarsaparilla is the produce of *Smilax medica*.

Tampico sarsaparilla is probably identical with the Vera Cruz sort.

THERAPEUTICAL VALUE AND QUALITY.—The relative therapeutical values of the different sorts of sarsaparilla are not easily determined. There are only two ways by which we can attempt to arrive at them,—one chemical, the other clinical or empirical. But, while on the one hand we have neither comparative analyses of the various commercial sorts of this root, nor an accurate knowledge of its active principle; so, on the other, we have no clinical observations of the relative effects of the different sorts, and great difficulty exists in the way of making them, on account of the immediate and obvious effects of this root being very slight. To this absence of actual precise information must be ascribed the different relative values assigned to the various sorts in different countries.

In the southern parts of Europe, where sarsaparilla has been the longest in use, the *thickest* and most *mealy* roots, irrespective of the country producing them, are preferred. It is, however, quite certain that starch is not the active principle of the root, but is regarded as being contemporaneous with it. I believe this opinion to be erroneous; for 1stly, the mealy sarsaparillas give to the test of oil of vitriol slighter indications of the presence of smilacin than the non-mealy sorts; 2ndly, the mealy sorts are the least acrid to the taste; and 3rdly, the largest quantity of extract is obtained from a non-mealy sort, viz. that brought *viâ* Jamaica.

In England the non-mealy sarsaparillas are almost universally, and, as I believe, properly preferred; and of these the Jamaica sort is most esteemed, and next to this, that called the Lima.

The *colour* of the root is not to be absolutely depended on, but roots having a deep orange-red tint are preferred. *Taste*, perhaps, is the best

---

[1] *Med.-Chir. Trans.* vol. xii. p. 344, 1823.

criterion : the more acrid and nauseous the taste, the better is the quality of the root. This test has been much insisted upon by Dr. Hancock.[1] The *quantity of extract* yielded by a given weight of the root has been much insisted upon by Mr. Battley and Mr. Pope as a test of goodness; both these writers have asserted the superiority of Jamaica sarsaparilla, because it yields a larger quantity of extract. But though a sarsaparilla which yields very little extract cannot be regarded as good, yet it does not follow, especially in the absence of comparative trials, that a sarsaparilla which yields the most abundant extract is necessarily the best, since the quantity may arise from the presence of mucilage and other inert matters. The *beard* is another criterion of goodness : the greater the quantity of root-fibres (technically callled *beard*), the better the sarsaparilla.

COMMERCE.—[The following table is from an official source.—ED.]

ACCOUNT *showing the Quantities of Sarsaparilla imported into the United Kingdom, and distinguishing the Countries from which imported, in each Year from 1849 to 1854.*

Countries from which imported.	1849.	1850.	1851.	1852.	1853.	1854.
	lbs.	*lbs.*	*lbs.*	*lbs.*	*lbs.*	*lbs.*
Russia, Northern Ports.............	822	360	671	—	—	—
Hanseatic Towns	—	—	—	6,049	11,910	9,946
Holland...............:	—	—	137	433	127	—
Belgium...........................	—	—	—	1,346	—	—
The Channel Islands	—	—	—	3,949	—	—
France	—	20,032	314	62	214	16
Portugal	—	6,242	1,479	7,550	—	—
Duchy of Tuscany	—	—	273	910	—	1,155
Sardinian Territories..............	—	—	—	—	136	—
Naples and Sicily	—	—	343	—	—	—
Sierra Leone	—	—	—	3	—	—
Turkey	—	—	73	—	2,582	—
Mauritius	—	—	70	—	—	—
British India	—	56	14,788	22,756	20,785	2,333
Hudson's Bay Company, Settlements of.........................	—	—	—	—	—	109
Newfoundland	—	8,131	309	—	349	—
Canada	5	113	—	—	—	14
New Brunswick...................	—	40	—	—	—	—
Jamaica..........................	82,437	49,702	63,885	66,467	87,628	9,113
St. Vincent	—	—	—	—	—	5,431
Bahamas	272	—	—	—	—	—
Honduras	47	49,988	60,316	95,752	45,915	46,060
St. Thomas	—	—	—	—	408	23,958
United States of America	11,317	44,719	3,537	34,795	61,957	18,067
Mexico	3,968	32,335	6,516	1,419	2,470	4,693
Central America	3,958	2,699	3,1265	20,293	15,463	17,320
New Granada....................	340	12,201	864	2,661	27,758	72,909
Venezuela	100	—	—	—	1,061	1,288
Ecuador..........................	59	—	—	—	9,085	17,879
Brazil............................	6,220	12,247	17,810	16,517	24,662	17,582
Oriental Republic of the Uruguay	—	—	—	—	—	3,669
Chili	7,636	—	—	—	16,498	8,014
Peru	1,753	6,559	988	—	5,849	733
Total...............	118,934	245,424	203,997	280,962	334,857	260,289

[1] *Transactions of the Medico-Botanical Society,* 1829.

COMPOSITION.—Sarsaparilla was analysed by Cannobio;[1] by Pfaff;[2] by Batka;[3] and by Thubeuf.[4]

Cannobio's Analysis.	Pfaff's Analysis.	Batka's Analysis.	Thubeuf's Analysis.
Bitter acrid resin.. 2·8	Balsamic resin .... 2·0	1. A crystalline matter (parallinic acid).	1. A crystalline substance (salseparine).
Gummy extractive . 5·5	Acrid extractive .. 2·5	2. A colouring (crystal-line) matter.	2. A colouring matter.
Starch .... 54·2	Extractive similar to cinchona .... 3·7	3. An essential oil.	3. A resinous matter.
Woody fibre ...... 27·8	Common extractive 9·4	4. Gum.	4. Ligneous matter.
Loss .... 9·7	Gummy extractive . 1·4	5. Bassorin.	5. Starch.
	Starch .... trace	6. Starch.	6. Chloride potassium.
Sarsaparilla [Hon-duras?] ....100·0	Albumen.......... 2·2	7. Albumen.	7. Nitrate potash.
	Woody fibre ...... 75·0.	8. Extractiform matter.	8. Fixed aromatic thick oil.
	Moisture.......... 3·0	9. Gluten and gliadine.	9. Waxy substance.
	Loss .... 0·8	10. Fibrous and cellular tissue.	
		11. Pectic acid.	Sarsaparilla.
	Sarsaparilla [Vera Cruz] ....100·0	12. Acetic acid.	
		13. Salts—namely, chlo-rides of calcium, po-tassium, and mag-nesium; carbonate of lime, oxide of iron, and alumina.	
		Sarsaparilla.	

Batka[5] separately analysed the bark, wood, and pith of Jamaica sarsaparilla, and obtained the following results :—

Epidermis.[6]	Cortical Pith.[7]	Woody Nucleus and Pith.
Volatile oil (with some acrid Colouring matter. [resin.	Starch.	Yellow soft resin.
Acetates.	Gum.	Starch.
Frothing resin (parill-resin, parillinic acid ?).	Vegetable gluten.	Gum.
Extractive matter.	Extractive matter.	Pectates.
Albumen and bassorin.	Albumen.	Vegetable gluten.
Chlorides.	Resinous colouring matter.	Frothing resin.
Starch and gum.	Amylaceous fibre and tegument.	Creosote (a trace).
		Woody fibre.

1. ESSENTIAL OIL OF SARSAPARILLA.—Sarsaparilla contains a small quantity of vola-tile oil.

The following experiments were made by a friend, a manufacturing chemist, who gave me the products for examination. 140 lbs. of Jamaica sarsaparilla were distilled, by steam heat, at twice, with 220 gallons of water. 50 gallons of a milky liquid were obtained, which were again submitted to distillation until 20 gallons had passed over. 20 lbs. of common salt were added to the distilled product, and heat being applied, 3 gallons were drawn over. The liquor was milky, held in solution carbonate of ammonia, and contained a few drops of a volatile oil, which was heavier than water, was soluble in rectified spirit, and had the odour and acrid taste of sarsaparilla. 100 lbs. of Jamaica sarsaparilla were distilled with 100 gallons of water. The distilled liquor was acid, and formed a white precipitate with solutions of acetate of lead. It was re-distilled: the liquor that first passed over was not ammoniacal, but towards the end of the process became so.

2. SMILACIN.—Discovered in 1824 by Palotta,[8] who termed it pariglin. Folchi, about the same time, also procured it, and gave it the name of smilacin. Thubeuf, in 1831,

[1] Brugnatelli, Giornale de Fisica, Dec. 2, p. 421, 1818.
[2] Syst. de Mat. Med. Bd. vii. S. 90, 1824.
[3] Journ. de Pharm. t. xx. p. 43, 1834.
[4] Ibid. xx. 682, 1834.
[5] Pharmaceutisches Central-Blatt für 1834, S. 902.
[6] By epidermis, I presume the author means both epidermis properly so called and the outer cortical layers.
[7] By cortical pith (Rindemark), the author obviously means the inner cortical layers.
[8] Journ. de Pharm. x. 543.

called it *salseparin*. In 1833, Batka announced that the active principle of this root was an acid, which he termed *parallinic acid*. Lastly, in 1834, Poggiale[1] showed the identity of these different substances.

It is procured by decolorising a concentrated hot alcoholic tincture of sarsaparilla by animal charcoal. The tincture deposits, on cooling, impure smilacin, which may be purified by repeated solution and crystallisation. Soubeiran[2] has proposed a more economical process.

It resides both in the cortical portion and in the woody zone.

Smilacin is a white, crystallisable, odourless, and, in the anhydrous state, almost tasteless substance; very slightly soluble in cold water, more so in boiling water, and depositing from the latter by cooling. Its solution has the bitter acrid taste of sarsaparilla, and froths on agitation. It is soluble in alcohol, ether, and oils. It does not combine with acids to form salts. Strong sulphuric acid colours it red, then violet, and lastly yellow. It dissolves in cold and pure hydrochloric acid: the solution becomes red and afterwards gelatinous when heated. It is soluble in strong nitric acid: if the solution be heated, nitrous gas escapes; and by evaporation a solid residuum is obtained, which is soluble in boiling water, from which it precipitates in white flocks as the liquid cools.

Smilacin is closely allied to, if it be not identical with, saponin. Now, as the latter is readily converted into an acid (*esculic acid*), so probably is the former: hence, perhaps, the parallinic acid of Batka may not be absolutely identical with smilacin, but bear the same relation to it that esculic acid does to saponin.

Smilacin has the following composition :—

	Poggiale. (Mean of 12 analyses.)	*Henry.*	*Petersen.*
Carbon	65·23	62·84	62·80
Hydrogen	8·67	9·76	9·14
Oxygen	28·80	27·40	28·06
Anhydrous smilacin	100·00	100·00	[Parillina] 100·00

Poggiale gives the following formula for its atomic constitution, $C^8H^7\frac{1}{2}O^3$; while O. Henry assumes $C^9H^9O^3$, and Petersen[4] $C^9H^8O^3$. As no definite compound of smilacin has been obtained, these formulæ are of little value. Thubeuf says that hydrated [crystallised] smilacin contains 8·56 water.

Cullerier[5] gave it to nine syphilitic patients. In doses of six grains the stomach readily supported it; but nine grains caused weight at the stomach and nausea. It appeared to relieve the patients' symptoms, and, in one case, seemed to effect a cure.

According to Palotta, pariglin, in doses of from two to thirteen grains, acts as a debilitant, reducing the circulation, sometimes producing constriction of the œsophagus, and exciting nausea and diaphoresis. He thinks it might be useful in chronic rheumatism, skin diseases, &c.

3. STARCH.—This is found in both the cortical and medullary cells. It is most abundant in the Caraccas, Brazilian, and Honduras sarsaparillas, to which it gives their mealy character. According to Schleiden, it exists in two forms,— as grains, and as paste.

The *starch-grains* are arranged in groups of 2, 3, 4, or 6; their shapes being modified by their mutual compression; the prevailing form being that of a muller. Their average length is about $\frac{1}{2000}$th of an inch.[6] The nucleus (central cavity or hilum) is scarcely perceptible by ordinary light (Schleiden says that the grains are without evident central

---

[1] *Journ. de Chim. Méd.* x. 577.
[2] *Nouv. Traité de Pharm.* ii. 166.
[3] *Journ. de Pharm.* xx. 682.
[4] Thomson, *Organic Chemistry*, 279.
[5] *Journ. de Chim. Méd.* t. i. p. 45, 2de sér.
[6] The following measurements, in parts of an English inch, of the grains of starch of sarsaparilla were made for me by Mr. George Jackson :—

1	0·0006
2	*0·0005
3	*0·0004
4	0·0003
5	0·0002

The bulk of this specimen consisted of particles of the size of those distinguished by an asterisk. One of the hemispherical or muller-shaped particles measures 0·0007 by 0·0005. A compound grain, consisting of three grains, was found to be 0·0005 in diameter.

cavity); but by the aid of polarised light its position may be determined, as it is at the junction of the arms of the cross. In some grains it can be detected by common light. Towards the circumference of some of the grains a series of faint parallel curved lines are observed.

Starch-paste, or *amorphous starch*, is found in some of the cortical cells. It is more abundant in Vera Cruz sarsaparilla, which is sun-dried, than in the Brazilian sort, which has been dried by exposure to the smoke of fires: hence, probably, its formation depends on the season, and not on the action of heat on the grain starch. Iodine colours it blue. This so-called starch-paste, or amorphous state, is, perhaps, only imperfectly formed and closely aggregated starch-grains.

4. RESIN AND EXTRACTIVE.—These principles require further examination. On them probably depends a part, at least, of the medicinal properties of sarsaparilla.

CHEMICAL CHARACTERISTICS.—A decoction of sarsaparilla froths greatly when shaken. It scarcely, if at all, reddens litmus. Diacetate of lead and protonitrate of mercury cause precipitates. Alkalies deepen the colour of the decoction. If a strong decoction be added to oil of vitriol, a red colour is produced (owing to the action of the acid on the smilacin?).

Decoctions of mealy sarsaparilla become dark blue (*iodide of starch*) on the addition of a solution of iodine. Decoctions of non-mealy sorts are usually somewhat darkened by iodine, but the effect frequently disappears after a few minutes. If a solution of persalt of iron be added to the decoction, more or less darkening is usually produced. The greatest effect is produced with decoctions of either Jamaica or Lima sarsaparilla: with those of the Honduras and Brazilian sorts the effect is much feebler. In some cases a flocculent precipitate slowly subsides.[1] If oil of vitriol be applied to a section of sarsaparilla, a greater or less portion of the woody surface (the woody zone, and, in the case of Jamaica and Lima sarsaparilla, the cortex also) becomes dark red, and then violet (owing to the action of the acid on the smilacin?). The same colour is also produced by the action of the acid on a fresh cut surface of the rhizome (*chump*). If a strong decoction of mealy sarsaparilla be poured into alcohol, a copious precipitate (*starch*) is produced.

PHYSIOLOGICAL EFFECTS. *α. On Vegetables.*—Not ascertained.

β. On Animals.—Not ascertained.

γ. On Man.—Imperfectly determined; no experiments having been made to ascertain its physiological effects.

To the taste, sarsaparilla is slightly acrid, and somewhat nauseous. Diaphoresis is by far the most common effect of its internal use. When the skin is kept cool, diuresis is not unusual. But in estimating the diaphoretic or diuretic power of sarsaparilla, we must take into consideration the amount of liquid in which the medicine is usually taken, and the other medicines which are frequently conjoined with it: for in many instances the diaphoresis or diuresis is referable rather to these than to sarsaparilla.

In several cases I have given the powder of this root in very large doses, in order to ascertain its effects. Nausea, vomiting, and temporary loss of appetite, were alone observed.

Dr. Hancock[2] says, that on one patient, an African, an infusion of four ounces of Rio Negro sarsa acted as a narcotic, producing nausea, great prostration of strength, torpor, and unwillingness to move. The pulse was scarcely altered, unless it were a little retarded. Though the effects here

---

[1] See also Marquart's comparative examinations of several kinds of sarsaparilla, in the *Pharmaceutical Journal*, vol. viii. p. 126, 1843.

[2] *Trans. Med.-Bot. Soc.* 1829.

stated agree, to a certain extent, with those ascribed to smilacin, they cannot be regarded as the ordinary effects of this root.

In some conditions of system, especially those of a cachectic kind, sarsaparilla acts as a powerful and valuable alterative tonic. Its continued use is often attended with improvement of appetite and digestion, augmentation of strength, increase of flesh, the production of a more healthy tone of mind, and the palliation, or, in some cases, complete disappearance, of various morbid symptoms,—as eruptions, ulcerations, and pains of a rheumatic character. Sarsaparilla differs in several respects from the bitter vegetable tonics. Though it is not devoid of, yet it does not, as they do, abound in a bitter principle. It is not adapted for the cure of intermittents, or of simple debility. But its best effects are seen in those depraved conditions of system which the public, and even some medical men, ascribe to the presence of a morbid poison, or to a deranged condition of the fluids. Hence it is frequently denominated *a purifier of the blood.* Those who do not adopt the pathological notion here referred to, call it an *alterative.* The varieties of sarsaparilla which abound in starch (as the *Caraccas* and *Honduras* sorts) possess demulcent and nutritive properties.

USES.—By many practitioners sarsaparilla is considered to possess no remedial properties; by others it is regarded as a medicine of great efficacy. Considering that more than 100,000 lbs. of it are annually consumed in this country, the number of those who entertain the latter opinion cannot be small. It has been justly remarked by Mr. Lawrence,[1] that physicians have no confidence in it, and surgeons a great deal. I think that this fact is readily explained by the circumstance that physicians are much less frequently called in to prescribe for those forms of disease in the treatment of which surgeons have found sarsaparilla so efficacious. Many practitioners have doubted or denied its remedial activity on what, it must be admitted, are very plausible grounds; viz. that the root possesses very little taste and no smell; that by the ordinary mode of using it, it produces very slight, if any, obvious effects on the animal economy; and that it has failed in their hands to relieve or cure diseases in which others have asserted they found it effectual. They are, therefore, disposed to refer any improvement of a patient's health, under the long-continued use of sarsaparilla, either to natural changes in the constitution, or to the influence of the remedial means with which the sarsaparilla was conjoined. But I would observe, that hitherto no experiments have been made to ascertain what effects the long-continued employment of sarsaparilla may give rise to in the system of a healthy man; and we are not warranted in assuming that none would result, because none are observable from the employment of a few doses. Moreover, it is to be remembered that some of our most powerful poisons prove the most efficacious remedies when given in such small doses that they excite no other obvious effect on the system than the removal of morbid symptoms. Witness the beneficial influence of the minute doses of arsenious acid in lepra. Furthermore, no one has ascribed to sarsaparilla the power of a specific, and its warmest advocates admit its occasional failure. But so often has it been found, that various diseases, which had resisted all other tried remedial means, and were gradually increasing, became stationary, and afterwards subsided, under the use of sarsaparilla,

---

[1] *Lectures on Surgery,* in the *Lond. Med. Gaz.* vol. v. p. 770.

that a large majority of British surgeons, including the most eminent of the present day, have been compelled to admit its therapeutic power.

As no obvious relationship exists between its known physiological effects and its apparent therapeutic agency, an argument has been raised against its medicinal activity, on the ground that we cannot explain its *methodus medendi;* but, for the same reason, we might refuse to admit the power of cinchona to cure ague. Mr. Lawrence[1] justly observes, that, although we cannot point out the manner in which a remedy "operates, we are not, on that account, to withhold our confidence in its power. It is enough for us, in medical science, to know that certain effects take place. In point of fact, we are in many cases unable to distinguish the *modus operandi* of medicines—the manner in which their influence is produced." The most plausible explanation of the agency of alterative medicines is that offered by Müller,[2] and which I have before had occasion to notice (see *ante*, p. 90). It assumes that these remedies cause changes in the composition of the nutritive fluids (the chyle and blood), and thereby produce slight chemical alterations in organs morbidly changed in composition, by which already existing affinities are annulled, new ones induced, and the vital principle enabled to effect the further restoration and cure. This hypothesis may be used to explain the remedial influence of sarsaparilla.

Sarsaparilla has been found especially serviceable in the following maladies:—

1. *In inveterate venereal disease.*—It is beneficial principally when the malady is of long continuance, and the constitution is enfeebled and emaciated, either by the repeated attacks of the disease, or by the use of mercury. In such cases it is, as Sir William Fordyce[3] correctly observed, "the great restorer of appetite, flesh, colour, strength, and vigour." When the disease resists, or is aggravated by, the use of mercury, sarsaparilla evinces its most salutary powers. It is given to relieve venereal pains of a rheumatic character; to remove venereal eruptions; to promote the healing of ulcers of the throat; and to assist in the cure when the bones are affected. In recent chancre, or bubo, it is of little use; nor does it appear to possess the least power of preventing secondary symptoms. We cannot ascribe to it "the same anti-syphilitic properties—that is, the same power of arresting or curing the venereal disease—that experience warrants us in attributing to mercury."[4] Sarsaparilla is sometimes given alone, but more frequently with other remedies : as with stimulating diaphoretics (mezereon, sassafras, and guaiacum), or with mercurials in small or alterative doses, or with acids (especially the nitric), or with alkaline substances (as potash or lime), or with iodine or with the bitter tonics. It is difficult to lay down concise rules to guide us in the selection of these adjuncts. In venereal pains and eruptions, sudorifics, the copious use of warm diluents, and warm clothing, are especially applicable, and should be conjoined with sarsaparilla. In scrofulous constitutions, with enlarged glands, it will be for the most part advisable to avoid the use of mercury. In such I have seen the alkalies most serviceable. When extreme debility is present, the bitter tonics and nitric acid are often added to sarsa-

[1] *Op. cit.* p. 769.
[2] *Physiology*, vol i. pp. 59 and 363.
[3] *Medical Observations and Inquiries*, vol. i. p. 169.
[4] Lawrence, *op. cit.* p. 769; see also Mr. Pearson's *Observations on the Effects of various Articles of the Materia Medica in the Cure of Lues Venerea*, p. 39, 1800.

parilla with benefit. When the periosteum is affected iodide of potassium should be conjoined.

2. *In chronic rheumatism* sarsaparilla is often advantageously conjoined with powerful sudorifics and anodynes (as opium or hyoscyamus), especially when any suspicion exists as to the venereal origin of the disease.

3. *In obstinate skin diseases* benefit is frequently obtained by the use of sarsaparilla. Its employment is not confined to cutaneous affections of one particular elementary form, since it is given with good effect in papular, vesicular, pustular, and tubercular skin diseases, of a chronic kind, when they occur in enfeebled and emaciated constitutions. Though, in these cases, its value principally depends on its tonic and alterative effects, its diaphoretic operation is to be encouraged by the use of diluents and warm clothing.

4. *In cachectic conditions of the system generally,* sarsaparilla may be given, often with the best effects, and never with any ill consequences, save that of producing slight nausea. Indeed, one of the great advantages of sarsaparilla over many other alteratives and tonics is, that although it may fail in doing good, it never does any harm beyond that of now and then causing slight disorder of stomach. In chronic abscesses, attended with profuse discharge, diseases of the bones, obstinate ulcers, chronic pulmonary affections accompanied with great wasting of the body, enlarged glands, and various other maladies connected with a depraved state of the system, sarsaparilla is often a very useful medicine.

ADMINISTRATION.—Sarsaparilla is administered in substance, and in the form of infusion, decoction, extract, and syrup.

1. **PULVIS SARZÆ;** *Powdered Sarsaparilla.*—The ordinary dose of this is from half a drachm to one or two drachms. Half an ounce frequently nauseates, and in some cases gives rise to vomiting. Powder of Jamaica sarsaparilla is to be preferred to that of other varieties. It is redder than that of the Honduras kind, and produces a much less intense blue colour when rubbed with water and tincture of iodine. I have been informed that some druggists employ, in the preparation of the powder, the roots from which the extract has been prepared. This fraud may be detected by the powder being almost devoid of taste, macerating it in water, and carefully comparing the infusion with one prepared from an unadulterated sample. The microscope might sometimes be carefully employed to detect adulterations of powdered sarsaparilla. The presence of foreign starch grains would indicate the presence of some other vegetable in the suspected powder.

[2. **INFUSUM SARSAPARILLÆ,** U. S. (Take Sarsaparilla, bruised, ℥j.; Boiling Water, Oj. Digest it for two hours in a covered vessel, or strain, or by displacement.)—ED.]

3. **INFUSUM SARSAPARILLÆ COMPOSITUM;** *Compound Infusion of Sarsaparilla.* Formerly ordered by the Dublin College. (Sarsaparilla root previously cleared with cold water, and sliced, ℥j.; Lime Water, Oj. Macerate for twelve hours in a covered vessel, with occasional agitation, and strain.) —According to Mr. Battley,[1] lime water is not so good a solvent for the constituents of sarsaparilla root as distilled water; for 874 grains of the root

---

[1] *Lond. Med. Rep.* xix. 169.

lost only 140 grains by maceration in lime water, whereas the same quantity of root lost 175 grains in distilled water. The dose of this infusion is from f℥iv. to f℥vj. two or three times a day.

4. DECOCTUM SARZÆ, L. E.; *Decoctum Sarsaparillæ,* D.; *Decoction of Sarsaparilla.* (Sarza, sliced [in chips, *E.*; and cleansed with cold water, *D.*], ℥v. [℥ij. *D.*]; Distilled Water, Oiv. [Boiling Water, Oiss. *D.*] Boil down to two pints, and strain.) The Edinburgh College orders maceration for four hours, and then the removal of the root for bruising. It is then replaced, and the liquor boiled down. The Dublin College orders digestion in water for an hour, boiling for ten minutes. The product should measure a little more than a pint.—An objection has been taken to this, as well as to all preparations of sarsaparilla made by boiling, that the heat employed volatilizes or decomposes the active principle of the root. "An infusion of sarsaparilla," says Soubeiran,[1] "which is odorous and sapid, loses both its odour and taste by boiling for a few minutes : these changes speak but little in favour of the decoction. On the other hand, it is known that the fibrous parts of vegetables always give less soluble matters to water, when treated by decoction ; and if it be added that sarsaparilla is completely exhausted by hot water, I cannot see what advantages the decoction can possess over preparations made by other methods." Without denying the injurious effects of long boiling, and, therefore, the superiority of preparations made without it, I cannot admit that either the decoction or extract of sarsaparilla is inert. No objection, however, exists to the substitution of an *infusion* for a decoction. But it is advisable to employ a somewhat larger quantity of the root, and to have it crushed before macerating it. The proportions of root and water, in the above preparation, are such that one ounce of the decoction contains the extractive of one drachm only of the root. Hence the extract or syrup is usually conjoined.

Mr. Jacob Bell[2] objects to taking out the roots after maceration, in order to bruise them, on the ground that by this process the wood may absorb a larger portion of the virtues of the bark in return for the inert starch which it gives out. An infusion or decoction of Jamaica sarsaparilla usually produces little or no blue colour with tincture of iodine; whereas the corresponding preparations of Honduras sarsaparilla (the kind usually met with, cut in small split lengths, in the shops) becomes bluish black on the addition of a solution of iodine. The dose of *Decoctum Sarzæ* is f℥iv. to f℥viij. three or four times daily.

5. DECOCTUM SARZÆ COMPOSITUM, L. E; *Decoctum Sarsaparillæ compositum,* D.; *Compound Decoction of Sarsaparilla.* (Decoction of Sarsaparilla, boiling hot, Oiv.; Sassafras, sliced and bruised ; Guaiacum-wood shavings; Liquorice-root, bruised, of each ʒx.; Mezereon [bark of the root], ʒiij. [℥ss. *E.*] Boil for a quarter of an hour, and strain.) The Dublin College orders of the Sliced Root, ℥ij.; Sassafras Root in chips, Guaiacum Wood, and Liquorice Root, of each, ℥ij.; Mezereon Root Bark, ʒj ; Boiling Water, Oiss. Digest one hour, boil ten minutes, cool, and strain. The

---

[1] *Nouv. Traité de Pharm.* t. ii. p. 168.
[2] *Pharmaceutical Journal,* vol. i. p. 55, 1841.

product should measure about Oj.—This preparation is an imitation of the celebrated *Lisbon Diet Drink.* The objections made to the use of ebullition in preparing the simple decoction apply equally to the present preparation. The additions are for the most part valueless. The guaiacum-wood is useless, water not being able to dissolve the resin. The volatile oil contained in the sassafras-wood is in part dissipated by the boiling. The mezereum, an active agent, is used in such small quantity that it can confer but little medicinal power. The liquorice is employed merely to communicate flavour. An improvement in the present formula would be to omit the guaiacum, to increase the quantity of sarsaparilla and mezereum, to substitute maceration for decoction, and to add oil of sassafras. The dose of the officinal preparation is from fʒiv. to fʒvj. three or four times a day. The syrup or extract is usually conjoined with it. During its use the skin should be kept warm.

A *Liquor Sarzæ compositus concentratus* is usually kept in the shops for the extemporaneous preparation of the compound decoction of Sarsaparilla.

6. SYRUPUS SARZÆ, L. E.; *Syrup of Sarsaparilla.*—(Sarza, lb. iiiss.; Distilled Water, *Cong.* iij.; Sugar, ʒxviij.; Rectified Spirit, fʒij. Boil down the sarza in C. ij. of the water to a gallon, pour off the liquor and strain while yet warm; boil down the sarza again in the remaining water to half, and strain, evaporate the mixed liquors to two pints, and dissolve the sugar in them; lastly, when cold, mix in the spirit. The Edinburgh College somewhat modifies the above process, and omits the spirit. Their preparation is weaker than the above. The Dublin College substitutes a Syrupus Hemidesmi, or Syrup of Indian Sarza, the formula for which is as follows :—Of Indian Sarsaparilla, bruised, ʒiv.; Boiling Distilled Water, Oj.; Refined Sugar, in powder, as much as is sufficient. Infuse in the water for four hours, strain, allow subsidence to take place. Decant the clear liquor, add twice the weight of sugar, and dissolve it by a steam or water heat.)—Simonin[1] has successfully prepared the syrup by the percolation method.

This I conceive to be a very unnecessary preparation; for, as the late Dr. A. T. Thomson[2] justly observes, " it can be much better and more easily supplied by rubbing up a few grains of the extract with some simple syrup." It is, however, frequently prescribed as an adjunct to the decoction. Prepared with Jamaica sarsaparilla it is not liable to ferment, and its flavour is somewhat agreeable, being very analogous to that of West Indian molasses. A few drops of solution of potassa sometimes prevent its disagreement with the stomach.

The *Syrup of Sarsaparilla* of the United States Pharmacopœia is intended to represent the famous French *Sirop de Cuisinier.* It is prepared with proof spirit, which extracts the acrid principle of the root without taking up the inert fecula; and the tincture being evaporated, to get rid of the alcohol, is made into syrup. By this means the long-continued boiling is avoided. As the editors of the *United States Dispensatory* speak most confidently of the remedial value of this preparation, I subjoin the formula for its preparation, taken from the American Pharmacopœia :—

Syrup of Sarsaparilla, U.S.—" Sarsaparilla, bruised, lb. ij.; Guaiacum wood, rasped, ʒiij.; Red Roses, Senna, Liquorice root, bruised, each, ʒij.; Oil of Sassafras, Oil of Anise,

---

[1] *Journ. de Pharm.* xx. 110.
[2] *London Dispensatory*, 9th edit.

each ℳv.; Oil of Partridge-berry [*Gualtheria procumbens*, an astringent aromatic] ℳiij.; Sugar, lb. viij.; Diluted Alcohol, Ox. [*wine measure*]. Macerate the Sarsaparilla, Guaiacum wood, Roses, Senna, and Liquorice root, in the diluted Alcohol for fourteen days; then express and filter through paper. Evaporate the tincture, by means of a water-bath, to four pints and a half; then add the Sugar, and dissolve it, so as to form a syrup. With this, when cold, mix the Oils previously triturated with a small quantity of syrup." The dose is fℨss. (equivalent to somewhat less than ℨj. of the root), taken three or four times a day.

A *Syrupus Sarzæ Compositus* is usually kept in the shops.

7. EXTRACTUM SARZÆ LIQUIDUM, L.; *Extractum Sarsaparillæ fluidum*, E. and D.; *Fluid Extract of Sarsaparilla*, Offic. (Sarsaparilla, lb. iiiss. [in chips, lb. j. *E.*]; Distilled Water, C. v.; [Boiling Water, Ovj. *E.*]; Rectified Spirit, ℨij. *L.* The Dublin College orders of Sarsaparilla, lb. j.; Boiling Water, Oviij.; Rectified Spirit, a sufficiency. Digest the root for two hours in Ov. of water, at 212°, and decant. Add the remaining water, digest again for two hours, decant. Evaporate the mixed liquors, by steam or water heat, to a syrupy consistence: when cold, add as much spirit as will make up the entire twenty ounces. The London College gives the following directions:—Boil the sarza in Oiij. of water down to Oxij., decant, and strain while hot. Boil the sarza again in the remaining water to half, and strain. Evaporate the mixed liquors to ℨxviij., and when the extract is cold, mix in the spirit. The Edinburgh College directs as follows:—"Digest the root for two hours in four pints of the water; take it out, bruise it, replace it in the water, and boil for two hours; filter and squeeze out the liquid; boil the residuum in the remaining two pints of water, and filter and squeeze out this liquor also; evaporate the united liquors to the consistence of thin syrup; add, when the product is cool, as much rectified spirit as will make in all sixteen fluid-ounces: filter. This fluid extract may be aromatised at will with various volatile oils or warm aromatics.")

[The solid extract of sarza, of former London and Dublin Pharmacopœias, is now little prized, and we have recourse in pharmacy to the more convenient form of a liquid. There are a variety of preparations of sarza sold by dealers prepared by secret methods, and greatly vaunted by the inventors. One of these, known as De Vere's fluid extract of sarza, deserves special notice: it is prepared with great care, and, according to Dr. Scott, (who has written an interesting little history of it,) it is made from the Smilax papyracea. The root has a remarkably red cortex. The figure appended to Dr. Scott's book does not agree with that lately given by Mr. Bentley as the Smilax papyracea. The botanical history, however, of this subject is far from satisfactorily made out. Whatever we may think respecting the preservation of the secret of its manufacture, it must be allowed that the extract of Dr. Scott is a remarkably fine preparation, and he deserves much credit for the great pains he has taken in working out the subject of sarsaparilla as he has done.—Ed.]

In this country Jamaica sarsaparilla is preferred for the preparation of the extract; and next to this the Lima sort. If Honduras, or any other mealy sarsaparilla, be employed, the product contains a large quantity of starch-gum. Extract of Jamaica sarsaparilla, when rubbed on white paper or porcelain, exhibits a reddish tint not observable in the extract of the Honduras kind. The flavour and odour are characters which assist in distinguishing well-prepared extract. Rubbed up with water it is almost completely soluble, and the solution, which should be clear, scarcely deposits anything by stand-ing. The dilute solution should not remain blue on the addition of a solution of iodine. But extract prepared from a mealy sarsaparilla does not completely dissolve in water, and yields a turbid liquor, which becomes dark blue on the addition of a solution of iodine.

In England the fibrils or *beard* of Jamaica sarsaparilla are preferred to both root and rhizome (*chump*); they contain less starch and woody fibre than the latter, and I am informed that they yield a greater portion of extract.

The quantity of extract obtained from Jamaica sarsaparilla has already been alluded to (see p. 282). The following table is from the papers of Thubeuf.[1]

6 *lbs. of Sarsaparilla.*		*yielded of Extract.*
	Red Jamaica sarsaparilla	℥xxj. ℨij.
	Red sarsaparilla of the Coast [Costa Rica?]......	℥xxj. ℨij.
Roots cleaned and de-prived of rhizome...	Vera Cruz sarsaparilla	℥xvij. ℨvij.
	Caraccas sarsaparilla.............................	℥xv. ℨiij.
	Honduras sarsaparilla	℥xiv.
	Lisbon sarsaparilla	℥xiij. ℨjss.
Rhizome cut thin and bruised		℥ix. ℨiijss.

Extract made by the evaporation of an infusion prepared by the displace-ment process is devoid of starch, and is consequently richer in the active principles. By the avoidance of ebullition, the destruction or dissipation of volatile matters is less likely to be effected. In effecting the evaporation of the decoction or infusion, steam heat should be employed; and the tempera-ture of the liquid should not be allowed to exceed 212° F. When the con-centrated decoction (especially of the Honduras kind) is allowed to cool, as at night, a kind of fermentation is readily set up, and gas is copiously evolved. Extract of sarsaparilla, when it has been kept for some time, frequently becomes covered by cubical crystals of chloride of potassium.

It deserves notice that though smilacin is said to be soluble in boiling alcohol and ether, yet I find that the extract of Jamaica sarsaparilla yields but little to these liquids.

Extract of sarsaparilla is declared by many writers to be an inert and useless preparation; but the assertions are, for the most part, founded rather on theoretical than practical considerations. I have extensively used it, and believe that when properly prepared from Jamaica sarsaparilla it is a most valuable and efficient remedy; and the enormous quantity of it which is consumed by the profession generally (including some of the most eminent of its members), is a proof that many others entertain a similar opinion. It is given in doses of from half a drachm to two or three drachms three or four times a day. It should be rubbed down with water, and flavoured by the tincture of orange-peel, or by some volatile oil (as the oil of cloves, allspice, lemon, or cinnamon). Alkalies render its flavour somewhat dis-agreeable, though they frequently increase greatly its remedial powers.

7. EXTRACTUM SARZÆ COMPOSITUM; *Compound Extract of Sarsa-parilla.*—Not in any Pharmacopœia, though kept in the shops. It is made

---

[1] *Journ. de Pharmacie,* t. xvi. p. 701; and t. xviii. p. 157.

by mixing, with extract of sarsaparilla, an extract prepared by evaporating a decoction of mezereon bark, liquorice root, and guaiacum shavings, and a small quantity of oil of sassafras. This preparation is employed as a convenient substitute for the compound decoction of sarsaparilla. The dose of it, and the mode of exhibition, are the same as of the simple extract. Three quarters of an ounce of the compound extract are equal to a pint of the compound decoction.

101. Smilax China, *Linn.*

(Radix.)

SMILAX CHINA, Kaempf. Amoen. Exot., p. 783; Loureiro, Fl. Cochinchinensis, p. 622.—A native of Japan, China, and Cochin China.—The *China root* of the shops (*radix Chinæ orientalis* seu *veræ* vel *ponderosæ*) is said to be the produce of this species. But, according to Roxburgh,[1] the roots of *S. glabra* and *S. lanceæfolia*, which are used in the East in medicine, are not to be distinguished by the eye from the roots of *S. China*, brought from China.

China root is imported into England, usually in baskets, from Calcutta and Singapore. Dr. O'Shaughnessy[2] states that it is largely imported into Calcutta from the eastward. It is said to be the produce of the province of Quansi, in China. It occurs in large, ligneous, knotty pieces, of from three to eight inches long, and an inch or two thick. Externally it has a greyish-brown colour, and internally a light flesh or yellowish-white colour. It is inodorous, and has a slightly astringent taste. It has been analysed by Reinsch,[3] who found it to consist of wax 0·3, balsamic resin 0·4, crystalline matter (smilacin) 2·8, with sugar, tannic acid, salts, and resinous colouring matter (quantity not stated), tannic acid with salts, reddish gummy colouring matter, and smilacin 4·8, starch-gum, vegetable gluten, and salts 2·6, starch 23·5 with salts, starch with tannic acid 34·0, woody fibre 20·0, and water 12·0 (=100·4). It was introduced into Europe in 1535 as an infallible remedy for the venereal disease, and obtained great celebrity in consequence of the benefit which the Emperor Charles the Fifth is said to have derived from it in gout. Its effects are not very obvious, but it is said to be diaphoretic. It tinges the sweat. It has been used in the same maladies as sarsaparilla; viz. venereal diseases, rheumatism, gout, obstinate skin diseases, &c. It is given in the form of decoction.

SPURIOUS CHINA ROOTS.—Several smilaceous roots, the produce of the New World, but resembling the oriental China root, have been described under the name of *American* or *occidental China root* (*radix Chinæ Americanæ* vel *occidentalis*). Their origin is by no means well ascertained, though they are usually said to be the produce of *Smilax Pseudo-China*, Linn. Hernandez[4] notices three sorts; one of which he calls *Olcacatzan* or Mexican China root; a second termed *Phaco;* and a third called *Cozolmecatl.*

One or more sorts of *occidental China root* are frequently found in the middle of the bundles of Lima and some other kinds of sarsaparilla.

Brazilian China root, known by the various names of *Juapecanga, Inhapecanga, Japicanga, Jupicanga*, and *Raiz de China branca* vel *rubra*, is obtained from several species of *Smilax:* viz. *S. Japicanga*, Grisebach; *S. syringoides*, Grisebach (*Jupicanga*, Piso, Med. Braz. i. 99); *S. brasiliensis*, Grisebach (*S. glauca*, Martius, Reise, i. 283); and *S. syphilitica*, Humboldt. It has not been analysed. Its uses resemble those of oriental China root.[5]

---

[1] *Fl. Indica*, vol. iii. p. 792.

[2] *Bengal Dispensatory.*

[3] Buchner's Repertorium, 2ter Beihe, Bd. xxxii. S. 145, 1843.

[4] *Rerum. Med. Nov. Hispan. Thesaurus*, pp. 212-213, Romæ, 1651.

[5] For a figure and description of Brazilian China root, see Goebel and Kunze's *Pharmaceutische Waarenkunde*, Bd. ii. S. 129, Taf. xviii. fig. 2.

102. Smilax aspera, *Linn.*
(Radix.)

Σμῖλαξ τραχεῖα, Dioscorides, lib. iv. cap. 144. *Smilax*, Pliny, lib. xvi. cap. 63.—A native of the South of Europe. Its roots constitute *Italian sarsaparilla* (*Sarsaparilla italica*). They have not been analysed. Their effects, uses, and mode of administration resemble those of the ordinary sarsaparilla brought from America.[1]

The roots of *Hemidesmus indicus*, or Indian sarsaparilla, are frequently sold in London under the name of Smilax aspera. They will be noticed hereafter.

Class IV. Exogenæ, *DC.*—Exogens.
DICOTYLEDONES, *Jussieu.*

CHARACTERS.—*Trunk*, consisting of bark, wood, and pith, placed one within the other; the pith being innermost. *Bark*, composed of strata (the younger and inner being called *endophlæum* or *liber*), each usually increasing by the deposit of new matter on its inner side. *Wood*, consisting of ligneous strata, traversed by *medullary rays*, and increasing by the deposit of new woody matter on its outer side (*exogenous growth*): the older and inner strata are called *duramen*, or *heart wood;* the younger and outer strata are termed *alburnum*, or *sap wood*. *Leaves* usually articulated with the stems; their veins commonly branching and anastomosing (*netted, reticulated*). *Flowers*, if with a distinct calyx, often having a quinary, sometimes a quaternary, rarely a ternary, arrangement. *Embryo* with 2 or more cotyledons (*dicotyledonous*); if 2, they are opposite; if more than 2 (*poly-cotyledonous*), they are verticillate, radicle naked, *i. e.* elongating, without penetrating any external case (*exorrhizous*).

This class includes two sub-classes :—1. *Gymnospermæ*, or naked-seeded exogens ; 1. *Angiospermæ*, or covered-seeded exogens.

Sub-class I. *Gymnospermæ—Gymnosperms.*
GYMNOGENS, *Lindl.*

CHARACTERS.—*Ovules* naked, in an open carpellary leaf or pervious disk, fertilised by direct application of the pollen to the foramen (*micropyle*) without the intervention of stigma, style, and ovary. *Ligneous tissue* porous at the sides, the pores being apparently surrounded each by one or two circles.

This sub-class includes two orders :—1. *Cycadeæ*, or Cycads ; 2. *Pinaceæ*, or Conifers.

ORDER XXI. CYCADACEÆ, *Lindl.*—CYCADS.
CYCADEÆ, *Richard* and *R. Brown.*

CHARACTERS.—Gymnosperms with a simple continuous *stem*, parallel-veined pinnate *leaves*, and *scales* of the cone antheriferous.

PROPERTIES.—Mucilage and starch are the useful products of this order. They are found in the stems and seeds (see *Cycas* and *Zamia*). The seeds of *Dion edule* yield a starch which is used in Mexico as arrow-root. (*Lindley.*)

---

[1] For further details respecting the medicinal properties of Smilax aspera, see Mérat and De Lens, *Dict. Univ. de Mat. Méd.* t. vi. p. 374, 1834; and Dierbach's *Neuest. Entdeck. in d. Mat. Med.* Bd. iii. Abt. ii. S. 1088. 1847.

103. Cycas, *Linn.*

Sex. Syst. Diœcia, Polyandria.

No product of this genus is employed in Europe, either as medicine or as food. From the stems of *C. circinalis* and *C. revoluta* a starch is obtained, of which a kind of *sago* is said to be made in the East. I have prepared starch from both of these species, and find that its microscopic characters are entirely different from those of the sago starch of European commerce. The starch of *C. circinalis* consists of grains united in masses of from 2 to 6: the single grains are rendered more or less irregular or polygonal by their mutual compression, but hemispherical and mullar-shaped particles predominate. Their size[1] varies, but is on the average smaller than that of the starch-grains of genuine sago. The so-called hilum frequently appears split and surrounded by rings. In polarised light the grains show a distinct cross.—The starch of *C. revoluta*, of which *Japan sago* is said to be made, resembles that of the preceding species. None of it comes to England.—A clear mucilage, which concretes into a gum like tragacanth, exudes from fresh-wounded parts of several species of Cycas.[2]

104. Zamia, *Linn.*

Sex. Syst. Diœcia, Polyandria.

In the Bahamas, and some other of the West India Islands, a starch is obtained from the trunk of some species of this genus which is employed as an excellent sort of arrow-root. None of it, to my knowledge, comes to Europe as an article of commerce. In the Museum of Œconomic Botany, at the Botanic Garden, Kew, there is a specimen of a starch, sent from Jamaica by Mr. Purdie, and stated to be " A nutritious powder made from the trunk of *Zamia integrifolia*, and sold in the West India markets." In external appearance it resembles West Indian arrow-root (Maranta arundinacea); but when examined by the microscope it is found to consist of rather large-sized grains,[3] some of which are spheroidal; but most of them are the separated parts of compound grains, and, therefore, are variously shaped owing to their mutual compression; some being hemispheres, others mullar-shaped grains, &c. The nucleus and rings are scarcely discernible. Most

---

[1] The following measurements, in parts of an English inch, of the starch of *C. circinalis*, were made for me by Mr. George Jackson:—

	Single Grains.	*Compound Grains.*
	0·0015	0·0015 by 0·0018.
	0·0013	0·0013 by 0·0010.
	0·0010	
Round..........	0·0008 by 0·0007	
	0·0005	
	0·0004	
	0·0003	
Hemispherical {	0·0011 by 0·0009	
	0·0007 by 0·0006	

Those particles of which one diameter only is given had a circular outline, and were probably mullar-shaped grains seen endwise.

[2] Roxburgh, *Fl. Indica*, vol. iii. p. 749.

[3] The following measurements of 12 grains were made for me by Mr. George Jackson:—

MEASUREMENTS OF STARCH FROM ZAMIA INTEGRIFOLIA.

	Parts of an English Inch.			*Parts of an English Inch.*
1.	0·0022 × 0·0021		7.	0·0011 × 0·0009
2.	0·0022 × 0·0018		8.	0·0013 × 0·0010
3.	0·0020 × 0·0019		9.	0·0009 × 0·0007
4.	0·0019 × 0·0016		10.	0·0007 × 0·0006
5.	0·0017 × 0·0014		11.	0·0004 × 0·0004
6.	0·0014 × 0·0013		12.	0·0003 × 0·0003

of the grains present a superficial protuberant scar (like the hilum of some seeds), the situation of which is remote from the nucleus (as ascertained by polarised light).

[*Zamia media* (*Florida arrow-root*).—This is an intermediate species between *Z. integri-folia* and *Z. angustifolia*. It differs from the former in having more numerous, longer, and narrower leaflets, which are perfectly entire, or nearly destitute of serratures at the apex. The footstalk is hairy at the base, and the female cone is obtuse, not pointed. The root is a large spheroidal or somewhat tapering coated tuber, rough and dark-coloured externally, fleshy, internally white and succulent, and when incised pouring forth a fluid of gummy consistence, which hardens in small tears at the point of exit. This root is called *Coonti root* in Florida by the Indians and white settlers, and the farina prepared from it is also called *Coonti*. As a nutriment, it is found in the shops of the northern cities of the United States under the name of *Florida arrow-root*. When carefully prepared it has a mealy appearance and feel, is of a pure white colour, and somewhat lustrous appearance : it is apt to be lumpy. The mode of preparation is the same as that of Bermuda arrow-root. The form of the granule is that of the half, third, or fourth of a solid sphere. Some of the granules are completely mullar-shaped : in fact, the form is exactly that given by Raspail for the granule of the Maranta arundinacea, which is invariably round. *Florida arrow-root* is employed for the same purposes, and in the same manner, as the other species of farina in use.—ED. From the American edition.]

ORDER XXII. PINACEÆ, *Lindley.*—CONIFERS.

CHARACTERS.—*Flowers* monœcious or diœcious, naked. *Males* monandrous or monadelphous ; each floret consisting of a single *stamen*, or of a few united, collected in a deciduous amentum ; about a common rachis ; *anthers* 2-lobed or many-lobed, bursting longitudinally ; often terminated by a crest, which is an unconverted portion of the scale out of which each stamen is formed. *Females* in cones. *Ovary* spread open, and having the appearance of a flat scale destitute of style or stigma, and arising from the axil of a membranous bract. *Ovule* naked ; in pairs or several, on the face of the ovary, inverted, and consisting of one or two membranes, open at the apex, together with a nucleus. *Fruit* consisting of a cone formed of the scale-shaped ovaries, become enlarged and indurated, and occasionally of the bracts also, which are sometimes obliterated, and sometimes extend beyond the scales in the form of a lobed appendage. *Seed* with a hard crustaceous integument. *Embryo* in the midst of fleshy oily albumen, with 2 or many opposite *cotyledons ;* the *radicle* next the apex of the seed, and having an organic connection with the albumen. *Trees* or *shrubs*, with a branched trunk abounding in resin. *Wood* with the ligneous tissue marked with circular disks. *Leaves* linear, acerose or lanceolate, entire at the margins ; sometimes fascicled in consequence of the non-development of the branch to which they belong ; when fascicled, the primordial leaf to which they are then axillary is membranous, and enwraps them like a sheath. (*Lindley.*)

PROPERTIES.—Every part of coniferous plants contains an oleo-resinous juice, which, by distillation, is resolved into volatile oil and resin. The medicinal properties of this juice have been before noticed (see Vol. i. pp. 228-9).

Sub-order I. ABIETEÆ.

Ovules inverted; pollen oval, curved.

105. PINUS, *DC.*—THE PINE.

Sex. Syst. Monœcia, Monadelphia.

(Oleo-resinæ.)

BOTANY. **Gen. Char.**—*Flowers* monœcious. MALES :—*catkins* racemose, compact and terminal ; squamose ; the *scales* staminiferous at the apex. *Stamens* 2; the *anthers* 1-celled. Females: *catkins* or *cones* simple, imbricated with acuminate scales. *Ovaries* 2. *Stigmas* glandular. Scales of the *cone* oblong, club-shaped, woody; umbilicato-angular at the apex. *Seeds* [nuts, *DC.*] in pairs, covered with a sharp-pointed membrane. *Cotyledons* digitato-partite. *Leaves* 2 or many, in the same sheath (DC. and Dubuy, *Bot. Gall.*)—Hardy, evergreen trees.

Species.—1. Pinus sylvestris, Linn.; *Wild Pine* or *Scotch Fir.*— *Leaves* in pairs, rigid. *Cones* ovato-conical, acute; young ones stalked, recurved, as long as the leaves; generally in pairs. Crest of the *anthers* very small. *Embryo* 5-lobed. (*Bot. Gall.*)—Highlands of Scotland, Denmark, Norway, and other northern countries of Europe. Flowers in May and June. A tall, straight, hardy, long-lived tree, determinately-branched. Its *wood* is the red or yellow deal. It yields *common turpentine, tar,* and *pitch.*

2. Pinus Pinaster, Aiton, Lambert; *P. maritima,* DC.; *the Pinaster* or *Cluster Pine.*—*Leaves* twin, very long, rigid, pungent, furnished at the base with a reflexed scale. *Cones* oblong-conical, obtuse, very smooth, bright, shorter than the leaves. *Scales* bristly (*Bot. Gall.*)—Southern maritime parts of Europe. Very abundant in the neighbourhood of Bordeaux, and between this town and Bayonne. It is a much larger tree than the Scotch Fir. Flowers in May. It yields *Bordeaux turpentine, galipot, tar,* and *pitch.*

3. Pinus palustris, Lambert; *the Swamp Pine. Leaves* 3, very long. *Cones* subcylindrical, armed with sharp prickles. *Stipules* pinnatifid, ragged, persistent (Lambert).—A very large tree, growing in dry sandy soils, from the southern parts of Virginia to the Gulf of Mexico. " Its mean elevation is 60 or 70 feet, and the diameter of its trunk about 15 or 18 inches for two-thirds of this height. The *leaves* are about a foot in length, of a brilliant green colour, and united in bunches at the end of the branches. The names by which the tree is known in the Southern States are *long-leaved pine, yellow pine,* and *pitch pine ;* but the first is the most appropriate, as the last two are applied also to other species. This tree furnishes by far the greater proportion of *turpentine, tar,* &c. consumed in the United States, or sent from this to other countries."[1]

4. Pinus Tæda, Lambert; *the Frankincense Pine.* — Abundant in Virginia. Yields *common turpentine,* but of a less fluid quality than that which flows from the preceding species.

5. Pinus Pinea, Lambert, DC.; *the Stone Pine.* — Grows in the south of Europe and northern part of Africa. Yields the cones called, in the shops, *pignoli pines,* the seeds of which, termed *pine nuts* (πιτυίδες, Diosc.; *pityida,* Pliny; *nuclei pineæ pineoli*) are used as a dessert.

6. Pinus Pumilio, Lambert; *the Mugho* or *Mountain Pine.*—A native of the mountains of the South of Europe. An oleo-resin, called *Hungarian balsam (balsamum hungaricum),* exudes spontaneously from the extremities of the branches, and from other parts of the tree. By distillation of the young branches with water, there is obtained in Hungary an essential oil, called *Krummholzöl,* or *oleum templinum.*

---

[1] *United States Dispensatory.*

7. PINUS CEMBRA, Lambert, DC.; *the Siberian Stone Pine.* — The seeds, like those of Pinus Pinea, are eaten. By distillation the young shoots yield *Carpathian balsam* (*balsamum carpathicum; b. Libani*).

106. ABIES, *DC.*—THE FIR.

Sex. Syst. Monœcia, Monadelphia.
(Oleo-resinæ.)

BOTANY. **Gen. Char.**—*Flowers* monœcious. MALES : *catkins* solitary, not racemose; the *scales* staminiferous at the apex. *Stamens* two; the *anthers* 1-celled. FEMALES : *catkins* simple. *Ovaries* 2. *Stigmas* glandular. Scales of the *cone* imbricated; thin at the apex, rounded, (neither thickened, angular, nor umbilicated on the back). *Cotyledons digitato-partite. Leaves* solitary in each sheath (*Bot. Gall.*)

Species.—1. ABIES EXCELSA, DC.; *A. communis*, Hort.; *Pinus Abies*, Linn.; *the Norway Spruce Fir.—Leaves* tetragonal. *Cones* cylindrical; the scales rhomboid, flattened, jagged, and bent backwards at the margin (*Bot. Gall.*)—A native of Germany, Russia, Norway, and other parts of Europe; also of the northern parts of Asia. Commonly cultivated in England. Flowers in May and June. A very lofty tree, growing sometimes to the height of 150 feet. It yields by spontaneous exudation *common frankincense* (*abietis resina*, L.; *thus*, D.), from which is prepared *Burgundy pitch* (*pix abietina*, L., *pix burgundica*, E. D.)

The leaf-buds (*gemmæ* seu *turiones abietis*) of this species of Abies, as well as of the Silver Fir (*Abies Picea*), are used on the Continent, in the form of decoction or beer; or, with the woods of guaiacum and sassafras, and juniper berries, in the form of tincture (*tinctura pini composita*, Ph. Bor.) They are employed in scorbutic, rheumatic, and gouty complaints.

2. ABIES BALSAMEA, Lindley; *Pinus balsamea*, Linn., Lambert; *the Canadian balsam Fir; Balm of Gilead Fir.—Leaves* solitary, flat, emarginate, subpectinate, suberect above. Scales of the flowering *cone* acuminate, reflexed.—An elegant *tree*, seldom rising more than 40 feet. Inhabits Canada, Nova Scotia, Maine, Virginia, and Carolina. Yields *Canada balsam* (*Terebinthina canadensis*, L.; *Balsamum canadense*, E. D.)

3. ABIES CANADENSIS, Lindley;[1] *Pinus canadensis*, Linn., Lambert; *the Hemlock Spruce Fir.*—Said to yield an oleo-resin analogous to Canada balsam.

4. ABIES PICEA, Lindley; *Abies pectinata*, DC.; *Pinus Picea*, Linnæus; *the Silver Fir.*—Mountains of Siberia, Germany, and Switzerland. Yields *Strasburgh turpentine.*

5. ABIES NIGRA, Michaux; *Pinus nigra*, Lambert; *the Black Spruce Fir.*—The concentrated aqueous decoction of the young branches is *essence of spruce*, used in the preparation of *spruce beer.*[2]

Essence of spruce (*essentia abietis*) is prepared by boiling the young tops of some coniferous plant (in America, those of *Abies nigra*, or *black spruce*, are used) in water,

---

[1] Loudon's *Encyclopædia of Plants.*
[2] *United States Dispensatory.*

and concentrating the decoction by evaporation. "It is a thick liquid, having the colour and consistence of molasses, with a bitterish, acidulous, astringent taste."[1] It is used in the preparation of spruce beer.

Spruce beer (*cerevisia abietis*) is thus prepared:—Take of Essence of Spruce, *half a pint*; Pimento (bruised), Ginger (bruised), Hops, of each, *four ounces*; Water, *three gallons*. Boil for five or ten minutes; then strain, and add, of warm Water, *eleven gallons*; Yeast, *a pint*; Molasses, *six pints*. Mix, and allow the mixture to ferment for twenty hours."[2] It is sometimes taken as an agreeable and wholesome drink in summer. It is diuretic and anti-scorbutic, and is, in consequence, employed in long sea-voyages as a preventive of scurvy.

107. LARIX EUROPŒA, DC.—THE COMMON LARCH.

Sex. Syst. Monœcia, Monadelphia.

(Terebinthina Veneta, *L. D.*)

Botany.   **Gen. Char.**—*Flowers* monœcious.   *Character* as in Abies; but the *cotyledons* are simple, and never lobed.   *Cones* lateral.   *Leaves,* when first expanding, in tufted fascicles, becoming somewhat solitary by the elongation of the new branch (*Bot. Gall.*)

Sp. Char.—*Leaves* fascicled, deciduous.   *Cones* ovate-oblong.   Edges of *scales* reflexed, lacerated.   *Bracts* panduriform (Lambert).

Hab.—Alps of Italy, Switzerland, Germany, Siberia, &c.   Cultivated in woods.

Products.—This species yields *larch* or *Venice turpentine*.   When the larch forests of Russia take fire, a gum issues forth from the medullary part of the trunks, during combustion, which is called *Orenburgh gum* (*gummi orenburgense*).   A saccharine matter exudes from the larch, about June, which is called *manna of the larch*, or *manna de Briançon*.   Lastly, a fungus, called *Polyporus officinalis*, is nourished on this tree.

Medicinal Substances obtained from the preceding Coniferous Plants.

The term *turpentine* (*terebinthina*) is ordinarily applied to a liquid, or soft solid oleo-resinous juice of certain coniferous plants, as well as of the *Pistachia Terebinthus*, a plant of the order *Terebintaceæ*, Juss. Indeed, this last-mentioned plant, *Pistachia Terebinthus*, is probably the true *Terebinthus* of the ancients (Τερμίνθος, Theoph. and Dioscorides). When submitted to distillation, these juices are resolved into *volatile oil* and *resin*.   The roots, and other hard parts of coniferous trees, yield, by a kind of *distillatio per descensum*, the thick liquid called *tar*, from which *pitch* is procured.   Hence it will be convenient to speak of the coniferous terebinthinates under four heads:—1st, the *oleo-resinous juices*; 2dly, the *volatile oil* obtained therefrom by distillation; 3dly, the *resinous residuum*; 4thly, *tar* and *pitch*.

---

[1] *United States Dispensatory.*
[2] *Ibid.*

1. Oleo-Resinæ Terebinthinæ.—Terebinthinate Oleo-Resins.

At first these oleo-resins are liquid, but by age and exposure to the air they become, more or less speedily in the different varieties, solid, partly by the volatilization, and partly by the resinification, of the volatile oil. They have a certain general similarity in taste and odour. They soften and become very fluid by heat, readily take fire in the air, and burn with a white flame, and, if the supply of air be limited, with the copious deposition of finely-divided carbon (*lamp black*). They are almost completely soluble in alcohol and ether; and yield, by distillation, a volatile oil and a resinous residuum. It must not be inferred that the identical volatile oil and resin, into which these oleo-resins are resolved by distillation, pre-exist in the juices which yield them; for in some cases it is certain they do not, but are products, not educts, as I have elsewhere[1] shown. Thus balsam of Canada possesses the property of *right*-handed circular polarisation; and, by distillation, yields a volatile oil and a residual resin, both of which enjoy the power of *left*-handed circular polarisation. It is obvious, therefore, that during distillation some molecular change must have been effected in the proximate principles of the balsam. American turpentine, on the other hand, possesses the power of *left*-handed circular polarisation : but by distillation, yields a volatile oil (oil of turpentine of English commerce) which produces *right*-handed polarisation. Water acquires a terebinthinate flavour when digested with them; and by the aid of the yolk or the white of an egg, or still better by that of vegetable mucilage, forms an emulsion with them.

1. COMMON TURPENTINE (*Terebinthina vulgaris*, L. D.)—Under this name we find oleo-resins brought from various parts of the world, obtained from different species of *Pinus*, and, though agreeing in the main in their properties, possessing certain distinctive characters. At the present time the London market is almost exclusively supplied from the United States of America, a small quantity only being occasionally imported from Bordeaux.

a. American or *White Turpentine* (the *Térébinthinate de Boston* of the French) "is procured chiefly from the *Pinus palustris*, partly also from the *Pinus Tæda*, and perhaps some other species inhabiting the Southern States. In former times large quantities were collected in New England; but the turpentine trees of that section of the Union are said to be nearly exhausted; and our commerce is almost exclusively supplied from North Carolina and the south-eastern parts of Virginia."[2]

The method of procuring this turpentine is as follows :—A hollow is cut in the tree, a few inches from the ground, and the bark removed for the space of about 18 inches above it. The turpentine runs into this excavation from about March to October; more rapidly, of course, during the warmer months. It is transferred from these hollows into casks.[3]

It is imported from New York in casks; those from North Carolina holding 2 cwts., while those from South Carolina contain 2½ cwts. It is yellowish-white, with an aromatic odour, and a warm, pungent, bitterish taste. It is translucent or opaque. Its consistence varies, being semifluid, or, in cold weather, that of a soft solid. It contains various impurities (leaves,

Pharmaceutical Journal, vol. v. p. 67, 1845.
United States Dispensatory.
Michaux, *N. Am. Sylv.* iii. ; Way, *Trans. of the Society of Arts*, vol. xxviii. p. 89 ; Duhamel, *Traité des Arbres*, t. ii. p. 146, Paris, 1755.

twigs, chips, &c.)   That got from the first tappings is the best, and is called *virgin turpentine.*   Recent American turpentine is said[1] to yield 17 per cent. of essential oil.

This sort of turpentine possesses the property of left-handed circular polarization; but it yields by distillation a volatile oil having right-handed polarization.

American turpentine is melted and strained, and in this state it is some-times called *refined turpentine.*

Old and concrete American turpentine is sometimes sold for *frankincense* (*thus* vel *abietis resina.*)

β. *Bordeaux turpentine* is obtained by making incisions in the *Pinus Pinaster,* Lambert (*P. maritima,* DC.), and collecting the turpentine in hollows at the foot of the tree.   Every month these hollows are emptied, and the oleo-resin conveyed in pails to a reservoir.   In this state it is called *soft gum* (*gumme molle*).   It is purified either by heating it in large boilers, and filtering through straw (*térébenthine galipot*), or by exposing it in a barrel, the bottom of which is perforated by holes, to the sun; the liquid which drains through is called *térebinthine au soleil.*   The last method yields the best product, since less volatile oil is dissipated by it.[2]   The turpentine which flows during the winter is called *galipot* in Provence, *barras* in Guienne.   It is in the form of semi-opaque, solid, dry crusts of a yellowish-white colour, a terebinthinate odour, and a bitter taste.[3]

Bordeaux turpentine is whitish, thickish, and turbid.   It has a disagreea-ble odour, and an acrid, bitter, nauseous taste.   On standing it separates into two parts: one thinner, yellow, and almost transparent; another thicker, whitish, and of the consistence of thick honey, having a granular consistence. Bordeaux turpentine readily becomes hard and dry by exposure to the air. It possesses the property of left-handed circular. polarization; and yields by distillation an oil which also has left-handed polarization.   It enjoys, with balsam of copaiva, the property of solidifying with magnesia, and in this respect is distinguished from Strasburgh turpentine.

Common turpentine has been analysed by MM. Moringlane, Duponchel, and Bonastre,[4] and by Unverdorben.[5]   The last-mentioned chemist found it to consist of *two volatile oils* (*oil of turpentine*), *pinic acid,* a little *sylvic acid,* a trace of an *indifferent resin* not soluble in oil of petroleum, and a small quantity of *bitter extractive.*   The quantity of volatile oil varies from 5 to 25 per cent. of the weight of the turpentine.   Laurent has dis-covered in Bordeaux turpentine a resinous acid, *pimaric acid,* isomeric with pinic acid.

2. LARCH OR VENICE TURPENTINE (*Terebinthina veneta,* L. D.; *Tere-binthina laricea*).—Obtained from *Larix europœa,* DC., by boring the trunks of the trees, and adapting to each hole a wooden gutter, which con-veys the juice into a tub or trough, from which it is afterwards withdrawn for filtration.[6]   Through the kindness of Professor Guibourt I have received an authentic sample of larch turpentine.   It was collected in the wood of the

---

[1] *United States Dispensatory.*
[2] Guibourt, *Hist. des Drog.* t. ii. p. 578 ; Duhamel, *Traité des Arbres,* t. ii. p. 147.
[3] Guibourt, *op. cit.*
[4] *Journ. de Pharm.* t. viii. p. 329.
[5] Berzelius, *Traité de Chim.* ; and Gmelin, *Handb. d. Chem.*
[6] Duhamel, *Traité des Arbres,* t. i. p. 335.

Bishop of Maurienne, in Savoy, by order of the bishop, and at the urgent solicitation of M. Bonjean, pharmacien, naturalist of Chambery. The same kind of turpentine, collected in Switzerland (*Swiss turpentine*)[1] is sold in Paris as *Strasburgh turpentine* (*Térébenthe de Strasbourg*),[2] and was formerly called *Venice turpentine*. It is a thick and consistent fluid, flowing with difficulty; is sometimes transparent, but more frequently cloudy; has a yellow or greenish-yellow tint; an odour which is peculiar, not very agreeable, weaker than that of either Strasburgh or common turpentine, but less disagreeable than the latter; and an acrid, very bitter taste. It has little or no tendency to concrete by keeping,—a property known to Pliny,[3] and which distinguishes it from common turpentine.

A factitious substance (*terebinthina veneta factitia*) is sold by London druggists for Venice turpentine. It is prepared by melting together oil of turpentine and black rosin. A similar preparation is found in the shops of the United States of America,[4] and is probably identical with that imported from America under the name of Venice turpentine.[5]

Berzelius and Unverdorben[6] have submitted Venice turpentine to examination, and with the following results :—

Berzelius's Analysis.	*Unverdorben's Analysis.*
1. Oil of turpentine, probably composed of two oils.	1. Volatile oil, which readily distils.
2. Resin insoluble in cold oil of petroleum.	2. Volatile oil, which distils less readily, and has a tendency to resinify.
3. Resin soluble in cold oil of petroleum.	3. Succinic acid (small quantity).
	4. Much pinic acid.
	5. A little sylvic acid.
	6. Indifferent resin, insoluble in oil of petroleum.
	7. Bitter extractive.
Old Venice Turpentine.	Fresh Venice Turpentine.

Larch resin yields, according to Berzelius,[7] from 18 to 25 per cent. (according to Guibourt, only 15 to 24 per cent.) of volatile oil, which possesses the power of left-handed circular polarisation. Its odour is citron-like, and on this account the oil might be substituted for essence of lemons in the preparation of *scouring drops*. Its sp. gr. is 0·863.

3. STRASBURGH TURPENTINE (*Terebinthina argentoratensis*; *Térébenthine au citron, ou Térébenthine d'Alsace*, Guib.)—This is obtained from *Abies Picea*. The peasantry in the vicinity of the Alps collect it by puncturing the vesicles adhering to the bark with sharp-pointed hooks, and receiving the juice in a bottle. It is afterwards filtered through a rude kind of bark funnel.[8] Strasburgh turpentine is very fluid, transparent, of a yellowish colour, has a very agreeable odour of citron, and a taste moderately acrid and bitter. It consists, according to Caillot,[9] of *volatile oil* 33·5, *resin* insoluble

---

[1] Guib. MSS.
[2] Idem, *Hist. des Drog.* 3me éd. t. ii. p. 577.
[3] *Hist. Nat.* lib. xvi. cap. 19, ed. Valp.
[4] *United States Dispensatory.*
[5] Dr. Maton, in Lambert's *Description of the Genus Pinus*; and Dr. A. T. Thomson, *London Dispensatory.*
[6] Berzelius, *Traité de Chim.* t. v. p. 477 ; and Gmelin, *Handb. d. Chem.*
[7] Berzelius, *op. cit.*
[8] Duhamel, *Traité des Arbres*, t. i. p. 9.
[9] *Journ. de Pharm.* xvi. p. 436.

in alcohol 6·20, *abietin* (a crystallisable resin) 10·85, *abietic acid* (? pinic and sylvic acids) 46·39, *extractive* and *succinic acid* 0·85, *loss* (principally volatile oil) 2·21.

4. CANADIAN TURPENTINE or *Canada Balsam* (*Terebinthina canadensis; Balsamum canadense*) is obtained from *Abies balsamea* in Canada and the state of Maine. [It is imported in barrels of 1½ to ¾ cwt.—ED.] Between the bark and the wood of the trunk and branches of these trees are vesicles containing this oleo-resin, which exudes when they are broken, and is received in a bottle. It is imported in casks containing each about one cwt. When fresh it has the consistence of thin honey, but by age gradually solidifies : it is yellow, transparent, very tenacious, of a peculiar and agreeable terebinthinate odour, and of a slightly bitter, somewhat acrid, taste. Like Bordeaux turpentine, it solidifies when mixed with a sixth of its weight of calcined magnesia. It is imperfectly soluble in alcohol.

Canada balsam has been analysed by Bonastre,[1] who obtained the following results :—*volatile oil* 18·6, *resin* easily soluble in alcohol 40·0, *subresin* difficultly soluble 33·4, *fibrous caoutchouc like subresin* 4·0, *acetic acid* traces, *bitter extractive* and *salts* 4·0.

Balsam of Canada possesses the property of right-handed circular polarisation : but both the oil and resin, into which it is resolved by distillation, have left-handed polarisation.[2] It is used by varnish-makers, by opticians as a cement, and by microscopists as a medium for mounting objects.

The great value of Canada balsam for optical purposes depends on its transparency and its refractive power, which is nearly equal to that of glass. When used to connect the pieces of an achromatic lens, it prevents the loss of light by reflection, and excludes moisture and other foreign bodies from the space between the surfaces of the glasses. In Nicol's prisms (single image prisms of Iceland spar), it serves the important purpose of transmitting the ordinary ray, and of interrupting the passage of the extraordinary one; its index of refraction being intermediate between that of Iceland spar for the ordinary ray, and that of the same substance for the extraordinary ray. The following table of indices of refraction serves to illustrate the preceding statements :—

Indices of Refraction.		*Indices of Refraction.*	
Canada balsam	1·528 to 1·549	Flint glass	1·576 to 1·642
Plate glass	1·500 to 1·550	Iceland spar, ordinary ray	1·654
Crown glass	1·525 to 1·544	Iceland spar, extraordinary ray	1·483

5. COMMON FRANKINCENSE (*Abietis resina*, L.; *Thus*, D.)—This is the spontaneous exudation of *Abies excelsa*. I am indebted for an authentic sample of this oleo-resin to Mr. Daniel Hanbury, who collected it, in the autumn of 1849, from the *A. excelsa*, in Switzerland. It is a soft solid, glistening in places, as if covered with a film of water. Its colour is not uniform : it is whitish, yellowish, pinkish, or pale violet red, and dark in different portions. The pinkish or violet red or peach-blossom hue seems to have been produced by exposure of the resin to the air and light, and in this circumstance resembles the peach-blossom red colour which assafœtida acquires under similar circumstances. It is probable, however, that this tint is not permanent. Its odour is not disagreeable, but is somewhat like that of Strasburgh turpentine. Guibourt says it is analogous to that of castoreum. The taste is balsamic, and without any bitterness. When melted in water,

---

[1] *Journ. de Pharm.* viii. 337.
[2] See a paper by the author, in the *Pharmaceutical Journal*, vol. v. p. 67, 1845.

and strained through a coarse cloth, it forms *Burgundy pitch* (*pix abietina* vel *burgundica; poix jaune* ou *blanche*). An authentic sample, prepared by Mr. D. Hanbury from *thus* collected by himself, is of an opaque whitish-yellow colour, somewhat resembling emplastrum plumbi.

The substance sold as common frankincense in the London shops is usually concrete American turpentine; and most of the so-called Burgundy pitch found in commerce is a fictitious article. Common frankincense or Thus has been analysed by Caillot,[1] who obtained the following results :—*volatile oil* 32·00, *resin* insoluble in alcohol 7·40, *abietin* (a crystallisable resin) 11·47, *abietic acid* (? pinic and sylvic acids) 45·37, *extractive* and *succinic acid* 1·22, *loss* (principally volatile oil) 2·54.

PHYSIOLOGICAL EFFECTS.—The effects of terebinthinate substances have been before noticed (see Vol. i. p. 229). Locally they operate as irritants. Applied to the skin they cause rubefaction, and sometimes a vesicular eruption. Swallowed they give rise to a sensation of warmth at the stomach, in large doses occasion sickness, and promote the peristaltic movement of the intestines. After their absorption they operate on the general system as stimulants, and excite the vascular system, especially of the abdominal and pelvic viscera. Their influence is principally directed to the secreting organs, more especially to the mucous membranes and the urinary apparatus. They act as diuretics, and communicate a violet odour to the urine. This odour depends on a portion of the oil having undergone a slight change in its nature during its passage through the system. Part of the oil, however, is thrown off unchanged; for Moiroud[2] has observed, that at the same time that the turpentines cause a violet odour, they flow in part with the urine. " I have verified," says he, " this double phenomenon on many horses, to whom turpentine has been given, for some days, in the enormous dose of ten or twelve ounces." But the kidneys are not the only parts engaged in getting rid of the absorbed turpentine. All the secreting organs, but more especially the bronchial surfaces and the skin, are occupied in the same way. By these the oil is exhaled apparently unchanged, or at least with its usual odour. During the circulation of the terebinthinate particles in the system, they exercise a local influence over the capillaries and secerning vessels, in the vital activity of which they effect a change. In certain morbid conditions, this change is of a most salutary nature. In catarrhal affections of the mucous membranes the secerning vessels become constringed under the use of terebinthinates, and the discharge is, in consequence, checked.

The most important, because by far the most active, constituent of the terebinthinate oleo-resins is volatile oil. Hence their effects are almost identical with those of the latter, and will be noticed hereafter (see p. 313). Some slight differences, however, are to be noticed. They are less rapidly absorbed, are more permanent in their operation, confine their influence principally to the apparatus of organic life, not affecting, at least to the same extent, the brain, and act less powerfully on the cutaneous system. We have few data on which to rely in judging of the comparative influence of the different terebinthinates; but as their most active constituent is volatile oil, we may fairly infer that those which possess the greatest liquidity, and which, in

---

[1] *Journ. de Pharm.* t. xvi. p. 436.
[2] *Pharmacol. Vétérin.* p. 312.

consequence, contain the largest quantity of oil, are the most powerful prepa-rations. *Venice* and *Strasburgh turpentines* stand in this respect pre-emi-nent. *Canada balsam* is valuable on account of its purity and agreeable flavour. In activity, purity, and flavour, *common turpentine* holds the lowest rank.

Uses.—The terebinthinate oleo-resins are, with some exceptions, applicable for the same purposes as the volatile oil. The following are the principal cases in which they are employed :—

1. *In mucous discharges from the urino-genital organs ;* as gonorrhœa, gleet, leucorrhœa, and chronic cystirrhœa.

2. *In chronic catarrh, both mucous and pituitous,* occurring in old persons of a lax fibre and lymphatic temperament.

3. *In chronic mucous diarrhœa, especially when accompanied with ulceration of the mucous follicles.*

4. *In colic and other cases of obstinate constipation,* Cullen[1] found a turpentine emulsion used as a clyster "one of the most certain laxatives."

5. *In chronic rheumatism,* especially sciatica and lumbago, the turpen-tines are occasionally used.

6. *As detergents and digestives* they have been sometimes applied to indolent and ill-conditioned ulcers.

Administration.—The dose of the terebinthinate oleo-resins is from a scruple to a drachm. They are given in the form of *pill, emulsion,* or *elec-tuary.* To communicate to the softer kinds a consistence fit for making pills, liquorice powder may be added to them. Bordeaux turpentine and balsam of Canada, mixed with about one-twenty-eighth part of their own weight of calcined magnesia, solidify in about twelve hours : the acid resins combine with the magnesia, and form solid resinates, which absorb the volatile oil. A turpentine emulsion is made with the yolk of egg, or mucilage of gum Arabic, sugar, and some aromatic water. To form an electuary the turpentine is mixed with sugar or honey. An emulsion, containing from half an ounce to an ounce of turpentine, may be used as a clyster in obstinate constipation, ascarides, &c.

The terebinthinate oleo-resins yield several officinal substances, and enter into several preparations :—

1. Terebinthina vulgaris, L. D. yields *Oleum Terebinthinæ,* L. E. D., and *Resina,* L. E. D.; and enters into the composition of *Emplastrum Galbani,* L., and *Unguentum Elemi,* L.

2. Terebinthina veneta, E. D. is a constituent of *Emplastrum Cantharidis compo-situm,* E., and *Unguentum Infusi Cantharidis,* E.

3. Abietis Resina, L., Thus, D., yields *Pix Abietina,* L. (*Pix Burgundica,* E. D.); and enters into the composition of *Emplastrum Galbani,* L., *Emplastrum Opii,* L., *Emplastrum Picis,* L., *Emplastrum aromaticum,* D., and *Emplastrum Thuris,* D.

2. Oleum Terebinthinæ, *L. E. D.*—Oil of Turpentine.

This essential oil is frequently, though erroneously, called *spirits* or *essence of turpentine.*

Preparation.—It is obtained by submitting to distillation a mixture of

---

[1] *Treat. of the Mat. Med.*

American turpentine (which has been melted and strained) and water in due proportions, in the ordinary copper still, with a naked fire. The distilled product is found to consist of oil of turpentine swimming on water; the residue in the still is resin. If no water be employed, a much higher temperature is required to effect the distillation, and danger is thereby incurred of causing empyreuma. Mr. Flockton, a large distiller of turpentine in this metropolis, informs me that the average quantity of oil yielded by American turpentine is from 14 to 16 per cent. He also tells me that Bordeaux turpentine yields an oil having a more disagreeable odour, and a rosin of inferior quality.

The *Dublin College* formerly ordered oil of turpentine to be prepared as follows :—Take of common Turpentine, *by weight*, lb. v. ; Water, Oiv. [*wine measure*]. Distil the oil from a copper alembic; yellow resin will remain after the distillation.

To deprive it of all traces of resinous and acid matters, oil of turpentine should be re-distilled from a solution of potash; and this is actually done, as Mr. Flockton informs me. The British Colleges, with the exception of Edinburgh, now give no formula for its preparation : the directions formerly given are as follow :—

Take of Oil of Turpentine, Oj. [Oij. *wine measure*, D.] ; Water, Oiv. [*wine measure*, D.] Let the oil cautiously distil.—The Dublin College directs a pint and a half only of the oil to be distilled.

PROPERTIES.—Pure oil of turpentine is a colourless, limpid, very inflammable fluid. It has a peculiar, and, to most persons, disagreeable odour, and a hot taste. When pure, it is neutral to test paper. Its sp. gr. is 0·86 at about 70° F. It boils at about 314° F. ; the density of its vapour is 4·76 (Dumas). It is very slightly soluble in hydrated alcohol; but 100 parts of alcohol, of sp. gr. 0·840, dissolve 13 or 14 parts of it, and absolute alcohol takes up a still larger proportion. The oil is also soluble in ether. Exposed to the air, it absorbs oxygen, becomes yellowish and somewhat denser, owing to the formation of resin (*pinic* and *sylvic acids*). This resinification is accompanied with the production of a small quantity of formic acid.

Fig. 147.

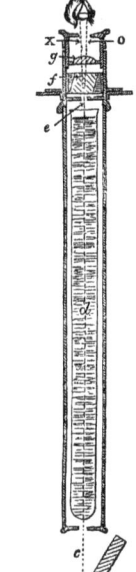

Oil of turpentine enjoys the power of rotating the ray of plane-polarised light; but the direction of rotation is different in the English and French oils,—in the former being right-handed, in the latter left-handed.

Plan of the apparatus for showing the circular polarisation of oil of turpentine.

a, A ray of common or unpolarised light.
b, A glass reflector, placed at an angle of 56°·45, for effecting the plane-polarisation of the light.
c, The reflected plane-polarised ray.
d, The oil of turpentine, which effects the double refraction and rotation of the plane-polarised light.
e, The emergent circularly polarised light.
f, The analyser (a double refracting rhomb of calcareous spar), which produces two coloured images : one caused by ordinary refraction, and called the *ordinary image* (o) ; the other by extraordinary refraction, and termed the *extraordinary image* (x).
g, A lens employed to produce well-defined images.

FIG. 148.

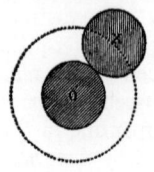

*Ordinary and extra-
ordinary images.*

When the eye is applied to the aperture above or in front of the lens *g*, two circular discs of coloured light (fig. 148) are perceived; one (*o*) the ordinary, the other (*x*) the extraordinary image. The colours of these images are complementary to each other. By rotating the analyser (*f*) on its axis, the extraordinary image (*x*) revolves around the ordinary image (*o*); each image undergoing a succession of changes of colour; the sequence of colours being different for the English and French oils of turpentine.

SEQUENCE OF COLOURS FOR OIL OF TURPENTINE AS OBTAINED BY THE RIGHT-HANDED
ROTATION OF THE ANALYSER.

English Oil of Turpentine. (Obtained from American turpentine, the produce of *Pinus palustris* and *P. tæda.*		*French Oil of Turpentine.* (Obtained from Bordeaux turpentine, the produce of *Pinus Pinaster.*)	
Ordinary Image.	*Extraordinary Image.*	*Ordinary Image.*	*Extraordinary Image.*
Red	Green.	Red	Green.
Orange	Blue.	Violet ⎱	Yellow.
Yellow	⎰ Indigo. ⎱ Violet.	Indigo ⎰	
		Blue	Orange.
Green	Red.	Green	Red.
Blue	Orange.	Yellow	⎰ Violet. ⎱ Indigo.
Indigo ⎱ Violet ⎰	Yellow.	Orange	Blue.
Red	Green.	Red	Green.

Moreover, the degree of rotatory power is not uniform.

English oil of turpentine (obtained by distillation with water from American turpentine) is remarkable for its comparatively feeble odour. A sample of oil whose sp. gr. was 0·863 had a molecular power of right-handed rotation of 18·5 to 18·7.

French oil of turpentine (obtained by distillation from Bordeaux turpentine) enjoys the power of left-handed rotation ; the intensity of which, however, is subject to some variation, as the following table shows :—

	Sp. Gr.	Left-handed Rotatory Power.
Unrectified oil	0·8806	28·83
First product of the rectification with water	0·8736	31·657
Latter product of the rectification with water	0·889	22·327
Oil rectified without water	0·873	32·23
Oil rectified without water preserved 10 years with potash	0·87	33·95

It is obvious, therefore, that the molecular constitution of oil of turpentine is not constant.

Bouchardat found that the unrectified oil was an imperfect solvent of caoutchouc ; and the oil rectified without water a better one. But the same oil distilled from bricks was pyrogenous, had a slight lemon-yellow colour, a sp. gr. of 0·8422, a rotatory power of only 8°·68, and a much increased power of dissolving caoutchouc. Rectified oil of turpentine is sold in the shops under the name of *camphene*, for burning in lamps. When it has become resinified by exposure to the air, it is unfit for the purposes of illumination, and requires to be rectified from carbonate of potash, or some similarly active substance, to deprive it of resin.

The *sweet oil of turpentine* or *sweet spirits of turpentine,*—sold in the shops for " painting without smell,"—does not appear to differ from the rectified oil of turpentine of English commerce.

The common or unrectified oil of turpentine, sold in the shops under the name of *turps*, contains resin, and is, in consequence, denser and more viscid than camphene. Its sp. gr. varies from 0·87 to 0·884.
Oil of turpentine is composed of

	Atoms.	Eq. Wt.	Per Cent.
Carbon	20	120	88·23
Hydrogen	16	16	11·76
Oil of Turpentine	1	136	99·99

[In 1853 the duty on foreign oil of turpentine was abolished, since which time American oil comes largely into this market, its value being generally 1s. per cwt. more than that of the English, because for the latter the packages are charged separately, while in the price of the former the original casks are included, the value being 35s. to 45s. per 112 lbs.—ED.]

Hydrates of oil of turpentine.—Four hydrates of oil of turpentine are known. When the commercial oil is exposed to an intense cold, crystals either of the binhydrate $C^{20}H^{16},2HO$, or of the hexahydrate $C^{20}H^{16},6HO$, are deposited. The latter forms large prismatic crystals, which, at a temperature of about 217½° F., became converted into the quadhydrate, $C^{20}H^{16},4HO$. The monohydrate, $C^{20}H^{16},HO$, is a liquid which List calls *terpinol*.

Hydrochlorate of oil of turpentine; Artificial Camphor.—When hydrochloric acid is passed into oil of turpentine, surrounded by ice, two compounds are obtained,—one solid, called *solid* or *Kind's artificial camphor*; the other fluid, and termed *liquid artificial camphor, terebene*, or *terebylene*.

Solid artificial camphor, $C^{20}H^{16},HCl$, is white, transparent, lighter than water, and has a camphoraceous taste. It is neutral to test-paper, fuses at a temperature above the boiling point of water, and is volatilisable usually with the evolution of hydrochloric acid. It burns in the air with a greenish sooty flame; and when the flame is blown out, evolves a vapour which has a terebinthinate odour. Distilled with lime, it yields chloride of calcium, water, and a volatile oil called *camphilene*, which is isomeric with oil of turpentine, but has no rotatory power in relation to polarised light. The quantity of solid artificial camphor yielded by oil of turpentine depends on the sort of oil employed. From Thénard's experiments, it would appear that French oil of turpentine yields the largest produce. Artificial camphor does not produce the lesion of the nervous system which is caused by ordinary camphor. Orfila found that half an ounce of it, dissolved in olive oil, and given to a dog, caused merely a few small ulcers in the mucous membrane of the stomach.

CHARACTERISTICS OF OIL OF TURPENTINE.—As a volatile oil, it is recognised by its combustibility, its burning with a very sooty flame, its almost insolubility in water, its solubility in alcohol and ether, its volatility, and its evaporating without leaving any greasy stain on paper. It is sometimes used to adulterate other more costly volatile oils; and it may then be detected by one or more of the following characters:—1st, its remarkable odour; 2dly, its rotatory power in relation to polarised light; 3dly, its being only very slightly soluble in diluted spirit; 4thly, its ready admixture with, and solubility in, the fixed oils; 5thly, its not being able to dissolve, in the cold, santaline (the colouring principle of the wood of *Pterocarpus santalinus*), whereas some of the other volatile oils (as oil of lavender) do dissolve it; 6thly, by the violent action of both chlorine and iodine on it.

PHYSIOLOGICAL EFFECTS.   *a. On Vegetables.*—Plants exposed to the vapour of this oil are rapidly destroyed.[1]

β. On Animals.—On both vertebrated and invertebrated animals it operates as a poison. Injected into the veins of horses and dogs it excites pneumonia.[2] Two drachms thrown into the veins of a horse caused trembling, reeling, falling, inclination to pass urine and stools, and frequent micturition. Inflammatory fever, with cough, continued to the eighth day; then putrid fever appeared. On the ninth day death took place. The body presented all the signs of putrid fever and pneumonia (Hertwich). Schubarth[3] found that two drachms of the rectified oil, given to a dog, caused tetanus, failure of the pulse and breathing, and death in three minutes. The skin of the horse is very sensible to the influence of oil of turpentine, which produces acute pain. "It is a remarkable circumstance," says Moiroud,[4] "that this pain is not accompanied with any considerable hyperæmia. It is quickly produced, but is of short duration." Oil of turpentine is sometimes employed by veterinarians as a blister, but it is inferior to cantharides, and, if frequently applied, is apt to blemish (*i. e.* to cause the hair of the part to fall off). In doses of three ounces it is a most valuable antispasmodic in the colic of horses.[5] In small doses it acts as a diuretic. Tiedemann and Gmelin[6] detected oil of turpentine in the chyle of a dog and a horse to whom this agent had been given.

γ. On Man.—In *small doses* (as six or eight drops to f℥j.) it creates a sensation of warmth in the stomach and bowels, becomes absorbed, circulates with the blood, and in this way affects the capillary vessels, and is thrown out of the system by the different excretories, on the secerning vessels of which it acts in its passage through them. The exhalations of the skin and bronchial membranes acquire a marked terebinthinate odour, while the urine obtains the smell of violets. By its influence on the renal vessels it proves diuretic. By the same kind of local influence on the cutaneous vessels it proves sudorific. It appears to have a constringing effect on the capillary vessels of the mucous membranes, for, under its use, catarrhal affections of, and hemorrhages from, these parts are frequently checked, and often are completely stopped. Its continued use sometimes brings on irritation of the urinary organs, or, when this state pre-existed, it is often aggravated by the use of turpentine.

In a *medium dose* (f℥j. or f℥ij.) its effects are not constant. Dr. Ed. Percival[7] saw two drachms given without any unpleasant effect being produced either on the digestive or urinary organs; they acted as an agreeable stomachic, and promoted the catamenia. Mr. Stedman,[8] on the other hand, has seen this dose produce strangury, bloody urine, suppression of this secretion, fever,

---

[1] De Candolle, *Phys. Vég.* p. 1347.
[2] Hertwich and Gaspard, quoted by Wibmer, *Wirk. d. Arzn. u. Gifte*, Bd. iv. p. 212.
[3] Wibmer, *op. cit.*
[4] *Pharm. Vétér.* p. 314.
[5] Youatt, *The Horse*, in *Library of Useful Knowledge.*
[6] *Versuch üb. d. Wege auf welch. Subst. ins Blut gelang.*
[7] *Ed. Med. and Surg. Journ.* vol. ix.
[8] *Edinb. Med. Essays*, vol. ii. p. 42.

thirst, and vomiting. These two cases, however, may be regarded as the opposite extremes; and, in general, we may expect, from a medium dose, a feeling of heat in the stomach and bowels, accelerated peristaltic motion, increased frequency of pulse, diaphoresis, diuresis, and sometimes irritation of the urinary organs. Occasionally it provokes the catamenia.

In *a large* or *maximum dose* (f₃iv. to f₃ij.) its effects are not constant. It usually causes a sensation of abdominal heat, sometimes nauseates, and in general operates as a tolerably active purgative, without causing any unpleasant effects. I have administered from one to two fluidounces in a considerable number of cases of tape-worm, and have rarely seen any ill consequences therefrom. " It has been given," says Dr. Duncan,[1] " even to the extent of four ounces in one dose, without any perceptible bad effects, and scarcely more inconvenience than would follow from an equal quantity of gin." Cases are reported, however, in which it has failed to produce purging, and in such it has acted most violently on the system, accelerating the pulse, depressing the muscular power, and giving rise to a disordered state of the intellectual functions, which several persons have compared to intoxication. A remarkable and well-detailed instance of this occurred in the person of Dr. Copland,[2] who refers the disorder of the cerebral functions, in his case, to diminished circulation of blood in the brain; while the gastric heat, &c. he ascribes to increased vascular activity in the abdominal region. The oil passed off most rapidly by the skin and lungs (principally by the latter), and the air of the apartment became strongly impregnated with its effluvia. In some cases it causes sleepiness. Purkinje[3] experienced this effect from one drachm of the oil. Dr. Duncan has sometimes seen it produce " a kind of trance, lasting twenty-four hours, without, however, any subsequent bad effect." The same writer adds, "the largest dose I have known given has been three ounces, and without injury." A scarlet eruption is mentioned by Wibmer as being produced in one case by an ounce of the oil.

Uses.—The following are the principal uses of the oil of turpentine :—

1. *As an anthelmintic.*—It is the most effectual remedy for *tape-worm* we possess. It both causes the death of, and expels the parasite from the body. To adults it should be given in doses of an ounce at least. I have frequently administered an ounce and a half, and sometimes two ounces. Occasionally, as in Dr. Copland's case, it fails to purge, but becoming absorbed, operates most severely on the system, causing disorder of the cerebral functions. It is said to be more apt to act thus in persons of a full and plethoric habit. To prevent these ill consequences an oleaginous purgative should be either conjoined with it, or given at an interval of four or five hours after it. An excellent and safe method of employing it is to combine it with a castor-oil emulsion. *Chabert's empyreumatic oil* (described Vol. i. p. 238) used by Bremser[4] against tape-worm, consists principally of oil of turpentine. A very effectual remedy for the *small thread-worm* (*Ascaris vermicularis*) is the turpentine enema.

2. *In blennorrhœa.*—Oil of turpentine sometimes checks or stops profuse

---

[1] *Edinb. Dispensatory.*
[2] *Lond. Med. and Phys. Journ.* vol. xlvi. p. 107.
[3] Quoted by Wibmer, *Wirk. d. Arzn.*
[4] *Traité sur les Vers Intest.* p. 488.

chronic discharges from the mucous membranes.   It appears to effect this by
a topical influence over the capillary and secerning vessels, in its passage
through them out of the system.   In many cases it would appear to confine
its operation to the production of an increase of tonicity in the vessels which
pour out mucus; but in other instances, especially in blennorrhœa of the
urinary apparatus, it seems to set up a new kind of irritation in the affected
membrane, which supersedes the previously existing disease.   Hence its use
is not admissible in acute or recent affections of these tissues.   In gonorrhœa
and gleet I have frequently employed it as a substitute for balsam of copaiva
with success.   In leucorrhœa it has occasionally proved serviceable.   In
catarrhus vesicæ or cystirrhœa it now and then acts beneficially; but it
requires to be used in small doses and with great caution.   In chronic pulmonary catarrh, either mucous or pituitous, it is said to have been employed
with advantage.   In chronic diarrhœa and dysentery it has proved advantageous : in these cases it has a direct local action on the affected part, besides
exerting its influence over this in common with other mucous membranes
after its absorption.

3. *In hemorrhages.*—In sanguineous exhalations, called hemorrhages,
from the mucous surfaces, oil of turpentine may, under some circumstances,
act efficaciously.   On the same principle that it checks excessive secretion of
mucus in catarrhal conditions of these tissues, so we can readily conceive it
may stop the exhalation of blood.   But it is only admissible in cases of a
passive or atonic character, in the absence of plethora and a phlogistic diathesis.[1]
In purpura hæmorrhagica it has been recommended as a purgative by Dr.
Whitlock Nichol,[2] Dr. Magee,[3] and others.   I have seen it act injuriously
in this disease, while blood-letting has seemed to relieve.

4. *In puerperal fever.*—The use of the oil of turpentine as a specific in
this disease was introduced by Dr. Brenan, of Dublin ;[4] and strong testimony
was subsequently borne to its efficacy by several highly respectable practitioners.[5]
Dr. Brenan gave one or two table-spoonfuls of the oil, every three or four
hours, in cold water, sweetened; and applied flannel soaked in the oil to the
abdomen.   But the apparent improbability of a stimulant like turpentine
curing an inflammatory disease, has prevented many practitioners placing any
faith in it, or even giving it a trial.   In other instances, the unconquerable
aversion which patients have manifested to it has precluded its repetition.
Lastly, it has failed, in the hands of some of our most accurate observers, to
produce the good effects which Dr. Brenan and others have ascribed to it, and
in some instances has appeared to aggravate the malady.   These reasons have
been conclusive against its employment,—at least, in the way advised by Dr.
Brenan.   But there are two valuable uses which may be made of turpentine,
in puerperal fever : it may be given in the form of clyster, to relieve a tympanitic condition of the intestines, and for this purpose no remedy perhaps is
superior to it; secondly, flannel soaked in the hot oil may be applied to the

---

[1] Adair, *Med. Facts and Observ.* vol. iv. p. 25; Copland, *Lond. and Med. Phys. Journ.* vol. xlvi.
p. 194.
[2] *Ed. Med. and Surg. Journ.* vol. xviii. p. 540.
[3] *Ibid.* vol. xxiv. p. 307.
[4] *Thoughts on Puerperal Fever, and its Cure by Spirits of Turpentine,* Lond. 1814.
[5] *Vide* Bayle, *Bibl. Thérap.* t. iv.

abdomen, to cause rubefaction, as a substitute for a blister, to the employment of which several objections exist.

5. *In ordinary fever.*—As a powerful stimulant in some forms of low fever, oil of turpentine has been well spoken of by Dr. Holst,[1] Dr. Chapman,[2] Dr. Douglas,[3] and more recently by Dr. Wood.[4] When the skin is dry, the bowels flatulent, and ulceration of the mucous membrane suspected, it often proves most serviceable.

5. *In rheumatism.*—In chronic rheumatism oil of turpentine has long been celebrated. Its beneficial influence depends on its stimulant and diaphoretic operation, and is more likely to be evinced in old and debilitated persons. I have found medium doses occasionally succeed when small ones have failed. But for the most part I have not met with that success with it in chronic rheumatism, to induce me to place much confidence in it. In the form of liniment it has often proved serviceable.

7. *In sciatica and other neuralgic affections.*—Oil of turpentine was proposed as a remedy for sciatica by Drs. Pitcairn and G. Cheyne. Its efficacy was subsequently confirmed by Dr. Home.[5] More recently it has been extensively employed, and with great success, in France, in sciatica as well as in various other neuralgias.[6] But it has proved more successful in those which affect the lower extremities. My own experience does not lead me to speak very favourably of it. In a disease the pathology of which is so imperfectly understood as is that of neuralgia, it is vain to attempt any explanation of the *methodus medendi* of an occasional remedy for it. I have known oil of turpentine now and then act most beneficially in sciatica, without giving rise to any remarkable evacuation by the bowels, skin, or kidneys, so that the relief could not be ascribed to a cathartic, a diaphoretic, or a diuretic operation.

8. *In suppression of urine.*—I have seen oil of turpentine succeed in reproducing the urinary secretions when other powerful diuretics had failed.

9. *In infantile diabetes.*—Dr. Dewees[7] has cured three cases of diabetes [?] in infants under fifteen months old "by keeping the bowels freely open, and putting a quantity of spirits of turpentine upon the clothes of the children, so as to keep them in a terebinthinate atmosphere."

10. *In nephritic diseases.*—In some diseases of the kidneys, as ulceration, the use of oil of turpentine has been much extolled. It has proved successful in renal hydatids.[8] [?]

11. *In dropsy.*—Oil of turpentine has occasionally proved serviceable in the chronic forms of this disease.[9] Its efficacy depends, in part, on its derivative operation as a stimulating diuretic; and in part, as I conceive, on its powerful influence over the capillary and secerning vessels, by which it exercises a direct power of checking effusion. It is inadmissible, or is contra-

[1] *Hufeland's Journ.* Bd. xx. St. 2, S. 146.
[2] *Elem. of Therap.* 4th edit. vol. ii. p. 129.
[3] *Dubl. Hosp. Rep.* vol. iii.
[4] *North Amer. Med. and Surg. Journ.* April 1826.
[5] *Clin. Experiments.*
[6] Martinet, *Lond. Med. and Phys. Journ.* March 1829 ; Bayle, *Bibl. Thérap.* t. iv.
[7] *Treatise on the Physical and Moral Treatment of Children.*
[8] Bayle, *op. cit.*
[9] See the authorities quoted by Dr. Copland, *Lond. Med. and Phys. Journ.* vol. xlvi. p. 201.

indicated, in dropsies accompanied with arterial excitement, or with irritation of the stomach or the urinary organs. When the effusion depends on obstruction to the return of venous blood, caused by the pressure of enlarged or indurated viscera, tumours, &c. turpentine can be of no avail. But in the atonic forms of dropsy, especially in leucophlegmatic subjects, attended with deficient secretion of the skin and kidneys, this oil is calculated to be of benefit. Dr. Copland[1] has used it in the stage of turgescence, or invasion of acute hydrocephalus, as a drastic and derivative.

12. *In spasmodic diseases.*—Oil of turpentine has been employed successfully in the treatment of epilepsy by Drs. Latham, Young, Ed. Percival, Lithgow, Copland, and Pritchard.[2] No benefit can be expected from this or any other medicine when the disease depends on organic lesion within the osseous envelopes of the nervous centres. But when the disease is what Dr. Marshall Hall terms *centripetal* or *eccentric* (as the convulsion of infants frequently is)—that is, takes its origin in parts distant from the cerebro-spinal axis, which becomes affected only through the incident or excitor nerves—we can easily understand that benefit may be obtained by the use of au agents like this, which, while it stimulates the abdominal viscera, operates as a cathartic and anthelmintic, and produces a derivative action on the head. A more extended experience of its use in chorea, hysteria, and tetanus, is requisite to enable us to speak with confidence of its efficacy in these diseases, though a few successful cases have been published.[3]

13. *In inflammation of the eye.*—Mr. Guthrie[4] has employed oil of turpentine in inflammation of the iris and choroid coat, on the plan recommended by Mr. Hugh Carmichael.[5] In some cases, especially those of an arthritic nature, it succeeded admirably; in others it was of little or no service. It was given in doses of a drachm three times a day.

14. *In tympanites.*—To relieve flatulent distension of the stomach and bowels, and the colic thereby induced, both in infants and adults, oil of turpentine is a most valuable remedy. It should be given in full doses, so as to act as a purgative; or when, from any circumstance, it cannot be exhibited by the mouth, it may be employed in the form of clyster. Dr. Ramsbotham[6] speaks in the highest terms of the efficacy of the oil of turpentine in the acute tympanites of the puerperal state, and thinks that most of the cases of the so-called puerperal fever, which yielded to this oil, were in fact cases of acute tympanites; and in this opinion he is supported by Dr. Marshall Hall.

15. *In obstinate constipation.*—Dr. Kinglake,[7] in a case of obstinate constipation, with a tympanitic condition of the intestines, found oil of turpentine a successful cathartic, after the ordinary means of treating these cases had been assiduously tried in vain. Dr. Paris[8] also speaks highly of it in obstinate constipation depending on affections of the brain.

---

[1] *Op. cit.* p. 202.
[2] Copland's *Dict. of Pract. Med.* p. 806.
[3] Copland, *Lond. Med. and Phys. Journ.* vol. xlvi. p. 199 ; Phillips, *Med.-Chir. Trans.* vol. vi. ; Elliotson, *Lancet*, May 1830 ; Gibbon, *Lond. Med. Gaz.* vol. vii. p. 428.
[4] *Lond. Med. Gaz.* vol. iv. p. 509.
[5] *Loc. cit.* vol. v. p. 836.
[6] *Lond. Med. Gaz.* vol. xvi. p. 118.
[7] *Lond. Med. and Phys. Journ.* vol. xlvi. p. 272.
[8] *Pharmacologia.*

16. *To assist the passage of biliary calculi.*—A mixture of three parts sulphuric ether and two parts oil of turpentine has been recommended as a solvent for biliary calculi.[1] But there is no foundation for the supposition that the relief which may be obtained by the use of this mixture in icterus, and during the passage of a biliary calculus, depends on the dissolution of the latter.

17. *As an external remedy.*—Oil of turpentine is employed externally, as a *rubefacient*, in numerous diseases, on the principle of counter-irritation, before explained (Vol. i. p. 127). Thus, in the form of liniment, it is used, either hot or cold, in chronic rheumatism, sprains, sore-throat, neuralgic affections of the extremities, &c. In the form of fomentation the hot oil is applied to produce redness of the skin in puerperal peritonitis, as I have already mentioned. As a powerful local *stimulant*, it was recommended by Dr. Kentish[2] as an application to burns and scalds, his object being to restore the part gradually, not suddenly, to its natural state, as in the treatment of a case of frostbite. The practice is most successful when the local injury is accompanied with great constitutional depression. I can bear testimony to its efficacy in such cases, having employed it in several most severe and dangerous burns with the happiest results. In that form of gangrene which is not preceded by inflammation, and is called *dry* or *chronic*, oil of turpentine may occasionally prove serviceable, especially when the disease affects the toes and feet of old people. There are many other topical uses to which it has been applied; but as they are for the most part obsolete, at least in this country, I omit any further mention of them. They are fully noticed in the works of Voigtels[3] and Richter.[4] Oil of turpentine is the principal ingredient in *Whitehead's Essence of Mustard*, which contains also camphor and a portion of the spirits of rosemary. *St. John Long's liniment* consisted of oil of turpentine and acetic acid, held in suspension by yolk of egg.[5]

ADMINISTRATION.—When given as a diuretic, and to affect the capillary and secerning vessels (in catarrhal affections of the mucous membranes, dropsy, suppression of urine, hemorrhage, &c.), the dose is from six or eight minims to f3j.; as a general stimulant (in chronic rheumatism, chorea, &c.), or to produce a change in the condition of the intestinal coats (in chronic dysentery), from f3j. to f3ij.; as an anthelmintic (in tape-worm) or as a revulsive (in apoplexy, in epilepsy previous to an expected paroxysm, &c.) from f3ss. to f3ij. It may be taken floating on some aromatic water to which some hot aromatic tincture, as *tinctura capsici*, has been added; or it may be diffused through water by the aid of mucilage or an emulsion; or it may be made into a linctus with honey or some aromatic syrup.

1. ENEMA TEREBINTHINÆ, L. E. D.; *Clyster of Turpentine.* (Oil of Turpentine, f3j.; Yolk of one Egg. Rub them together, and add Decoction of Barley, f3xix., L.—The *Edinburgh College* substitutes plain Water for Barley Water.—The *Dublin College* directs f3j. of Oil of Turpentine to be

---

[1] Durande, *Observ. sur l'Efficacité du Mélange d'Ether sulph. et d'Huile volatile de Téréb. dans Coliques hépat. produites par des Pierres Biliaires,* 1790.
[2] *Essay on Burns.*
[3] *Arzneimittell.* Bd. ii. S. 260.
[4] *Ibid.* Bd. ii. S. 74.
[5] Dr. Macreight, *Lancet* for 1837-8, vol. ii. p. 485.

rubbed with f℥xvj. of mucilage of barley.)—Used as an anthelmintic in ascarides ; as an antispasmodic and purgative in colic, obstinate constipation, and
tympanites. Dr. Montgomery[1] says "it is much used in cases of peritoneal
inflammation."

2. LINIMENTUM TEREBINTHINÆ, L. D.; *Linimentum Terebinthinatum,*
E.; Turpentine Liniment. (Soft Soap, ℥ij.; Camphor, ℥j.; Oil of Turpentine,
f℥xvj. "Shake them together until they are mixed," *L.*—Resinous Ointment,
℥iv.; Oil of Turpentine, f℥v.; Camphor, ℥ss. Melt the ointment, and gradually mix with it the camphor and oil till a uniform liniment be obtained,"
E.—Ointment of Resin, ℥viij.; Oil of Turpentine, f℥v. "Having melted the
ointment, gradually mix the oil of turpentine with it," *D.*)—Introduced by
Dr. Kentish[2] as a dressing for burns and scalds. The parts being first bathed
with warm oil of turpentine, alcohol, or camphorated spirit, are to be covered
with pledgets of lint thickly spread with this liniment. When the peculiar
inflammation, excited by the fire, has subsided, milder applications are then to
be resorted to. This liniment may also be used in any other cases requiring
the employment of a more stimulant application than the ordinary soap
liniment.

3. Resinæ Terebinthinæ.—Terebinthinate Resins.

1. *Resina*, L. E. D.—*Rosin or Common Resin.*

PREPARATION.—This is the residue of the process for obtaining oil of
turpentine. It is run, while liquid, into metallic receivers coated with whiting
to prevent adhesion, and from these is ladled into wooden moulds or casks.
When the distillation is not carried too far, the product contains a little water,
and is termed *yellow rosin (resina flava).* A more continued heat expels
the water and produces *transparent rosin ;* and if the process be pushed as
far as it can be without producing a complete alteration of properties, the
residue acquires a deep colour, and is termed *brown* or *black rosin,* or *colo-*
phony (resina nigra seu *colophonium).* If melted rosin be run into cold
water contained in shallow tanks, and a supply of cold water be kept up until
the rosin has solidified, a pale yellow product is obtained, called *Flockton's*
patent rosin.
[Since the abolition of the duty in 1853, a good deal of American rosin is
brought to this market. It is very much purer than the English, and the
difference, independently of colour, is distinguishable by the naked eye : on
looking through moderately sized pieces, the English rosin shows little specks
(impurities), while the American is free from them. The latter fetches from
25 to 100 per cent. more than the former, the qualities being classed, according
to their colour, into amber, red, and brown, and the intermediate varieties.
There is also an English article called "elastic" rosin, which is manufactured by Mr. Flockton on a large scale.—ED.]
PROPERTIES.—Rosin is compact, solid, brittle, almost odourless and tasteless, with a smooth shining fracture, becomes electric by friction, is fusible at
a moderate heat, decomposable at a higher temperature, and burning in the air

---

[1] *Observations on the Dublin Pharmacopœia.*
[2] *Essay on Burns.*

with a yellow smoky flame.   It is insoluble in water, but soluble in alcohol, ether, and the volatile oils.   With wax and the fixed oils it unites by fusion; with the caustic alkalies it unites to form a *resinous soap* (the *alkaline resinates*, principally the *pinates*).   Heated with concentrated sulphuric or nitric acid, mutual decomposition takes place.

By distillation rosin yields *rosin oil* and *tar*.   *Rosin oil* is a mixture of four carburets of hydrogen : *retinaphte*, $C^{14}H^8$; *retinyle*, $C^{10}H^{12}$; *retinole*, $C^{32}H^{16}$; and *metanaphthaline*, $C^{20}H^8$.   The rosin oil which distils over at from $226\frac{1}{2}°$ F. to $302°$ F. is a mixture of retinaphte and retinyle.   It is sometimes used in the arts as a substitute for oil of turpentine.   The part which boils at about $464°$ F. is retinole : it enters into the composition of some printing inks.   Mixed with lime, it forms a sort of grease for wheels, machinery, &c.   Rosin oil has been used in the preparation of *rosin gas*.[1]

Yellow rosin is opaque and yellow, or yellowish-white.   Its opacity is owing to water, with which it is incorporated.   By continued fusion this is got rid of, and the rosin then becomes transparent (*transparent rosin*).   *Brown rosin*, or *colophony*, is more or less brown and transparent.

Composition.—Rosin is a compound or mixture of *pinic acid* (principally), *colophonic acid* (variable in quantity), *sylvic acid* (a small quantity), and traces of *an indifferent resin*.[2]

Pinic and sylvic acids are isomeric : according to Laurent, their equivalent is expressed by the formula $C^{40}H^{29}O^3,HO$; and their salts by the formula $MO,C^{40}H^{29}O^3$.

1. Pinic Acid.—It is soluble in cold alcohol of sp. gr. 0·883.   The solution forms a precipitate (*pinate of copper*) on the addition of an alcoholic solution of acetate of copper.   *Pinate of magnesia* dissolves with difficulty in water.

2. Colophonic Acid (*Colopholic Acid*).—Formed by the action of heat on pinic acid; and therefore the quantity of it contained in rosin varies according to the heat employed.   Rosin owes its brown colour to it.   It is distinguished from pinic acid by its greater affinity for salifiable bases, and its slight solubility in alcohol.[3]

3. Sylvic Acid.—Is distinguished from pinic acid by its insolubility in cold alcohol of sp. gr. 0·883.

4. Indifferent Resin.—Is soluble in cold alcohol, oil of petroleum, and oil of turpentine.   It forms with magnesia a compound readily soluble in water.

Physiological Effects.—Not being used internally, its effects when swallowed are scarcely known.   It is probable, however, that they are of the same kind as those of common turpentine, though very considerably slighter.   In the horse it acts as a useful diuretic, in doses of five or six drachms.[4]   Its local influence is mild,   " It may be considered," says Dr. Maton,[5] " as possessing astringency without pungency."

Use.—Powdered resin has been applied to wounds to check hemorrhage, and is occasionally used for this purpose in veterinary practice.   But the principal value of rosin is in the formation of plasters and ointments, to which it communicates great adhesiveness and some slightly stimulant properties.

---

[1] Pelouze and Frémy, *Cours de Chimie générale*, t. iii. p. 543, 1850.
[2] Unverdorben, in Gmelin, *Hand. d. Chem.* ii. 520.
[3] Berzelius, *Traité de Chim.* t. v. p. 489.
[4] Youatt, *The Horse*, in the *Library of Useful Knowledge*.
[5] Lambert's *Pinus*.

1. CERATUM RESINÆ, L.; *Unguentum Resinosum,* E.; *Unguentum Resinæ,* D.; *Yellow Basilicon* or *Basilicon Ointment,* offic. (Resin, Wax, of each ℥xv.; Olive Oil, Oj. Melt the Resin and the Wax together with a slow fire; then add the Oil, and press the Cerate, while hot, through a linen cloth, *L.*—The *Edinburgh College* orders of Resin, ℥v.; Axunge, ℥viij.; Bees' Wax, ℥ij. Melt them together with a gentle heat, and then stir the mixture briskly while it cools and concretes.—The *Dublin College* directs of Yellow Wax, ℥iv.; Resin, lb. ss.; Prepared Lard, lb. j. Melt by a gentle heat, strain through flannel, and stir till it concretes.)—A mildly stimulant, digestive, and detergent application to ulcers which follow burns, or which are of a foul and indolent character, and to blistered surfaces to promote a discharge.

2. EMPLASTRUM RESINÆ, L. D.; *Emplastrum Resinosum,* E.—Has been already described, Vol. i. p. 812.

2. *Pix Burgundica,* E. D.—*Burgundy Pitch.*

(Pix abietina, *L.*)

PREPARATION.—True Burgundy pitch is prepared by melting common frankincense (*Abietis resina,* L.; *Thus,* D.) in hot water, and straining through a coarse cloth. By this process part of the volatile oil and the impurities are got rid of. The substance sold as Burgundy pitch in the shops is rarely prepared in this way, but is fictitious. Its principal constituent is rosin, rendered opaque by the incorporation of water, and coloured by palm oil. One maker of it informed me that he prepared it from old and concrete American turpentine. A sample of genuine Burgundy pitch was prepared by Mr. D. Hanbury from Thus collected by himself in Switzerland. In colour it somewhat resembled *emplastrum plumbi.* Its odour resembled the Burgundy pitch imported from Hamburgh, and which, when strained, constitutes the best commercial Burgundy pitch.

Hamburgh Burgundy pitch is of a dark colour, and contains many impurities. It would appear to be melted but unstrained Thus. It yields, when re-melted and strained, a Burgundy pitch which is darker coloured, but which otherwise agrees with the genuine sample prepared by Mr. Hanbury.

PROPERTIES.—Genuine Burgundy pitch is hard, brittle when cold, but readily taking the form of the vessel in which it is kept. It softens by the heat of the hand, and strongly adheres to the skin. Its colour is yellowish-white; its odour is not disagreeable; its taste slightly bitter. Fictitious Burgundy pitch is usually of a fuller yellow colour than the genuine, and has a somewhat less agreeable odour.

COMPOSITION.—Consists of *resin* principally, and a small quantity of *volatile oil.*

PHYSIOLOGICAL EFFECTS.—Its effects are similar to those of the other terebinthinate resins. In activity it holds an intermediate station between common turpentine and rosin; being considerably less active than the first, and somewhat more so than the last of these substances. Its local action is that of a mild irritant. In some persons it excites a troublesome vesiculo-pustular inflammation.[1]

---

[1] Rayer, *Treatise on Diseases of the Skin,* by Dr. Willis, p. 366.

USES.— It is employed as an external agent only, spread on leather, forming the well-known *Burgundy pitch plaster* (*emplastrum picis burgundicæ*), which is applied to the chest in chronic pulmonary complaints, to the loins in lumbago, to the joints in chronic articular affections, and to other parts to relieve local pains of a rheumatic character. It acts as a counter-irritant or revulsive.

EMPLASTRUM PICIS, L. E.; *Plaster of Pitch*. (Burgundy Pitch, lb. ij.; Resin of the Spruce Fir [Thus], lb. j. Resin, Wax, of each ʒiv.; Expressed Oil of Nutmeg, ʒj.; Olive Oil, Water, of each fʒij. Add first the Resin of the Spruce Fir, then the Oil of Nutmegs, the Olive Oil, and the Water, to the Pitch, Resin, and Wax, melted together. Lastly, mix them all, and boil down to a proper consistence. *L.*—The formula of the *Edinburgh College* is as follows: Burgundy Pitch, lb. iss.; Resin and Bees' Wax, of each, ʒij.; Oil of Mace, ʒss.; Olive Oil, fʒj.; Water, fʒj. Liquify the Pitch, Resin, and Wax, with a gentle heat; add the other articles; mix them well together, and boil till the mixture acquires a proper consistence.)—Stimulant and rubefacient; used in the same cases as the simple Burgundy pitch.

4. Pix liquida and Pix solida.—Tar and Pitch.

1. *Pix Liquida*, L. E. D.—*Vegetable Tar*.

HISTORY.—This is the πίττα of Theophrastus,[1] the πίσσα ὑγρά (*liquid pitch*) or κῶνος of Dioscorides,[2] and the *pix liquida* of Pliny.[3]

PREPARATION. —Two kinds of *tar* are known in commerce; namely, *coal tar* and *wood tar*. They are obtained in the destructive distillation,—the first of coal, the second of wood.

Of wood tar there are two sorts: one procured in the northern parts of Europe and in America from the waste of fir timber, and known in commerce as *Stockholm tar, Archangel tar, American tar*, &c.; the other obtained as a secondary product in the manufacture of pyroligneous acid and gunpowder charcoal. The former is the kind used in medicine. That which is procured from *Pinus sylvestris* in the northern parts of Europe is considered to be much superior to American tar.

The process now followed seems to be identical with that practised by the Macedonians, as described by Theophrastus. It is a kind of *distillatio per descensum* of the roots and other woody parts of old pines. As now carried on in Bothnia, it is thus described by Dr. Clarke:[4]— "The situation most favourable to the process is in a forest near to a marsh or bog, because the roots of the fir, from which tar is principally extracted, are always most productive in such places. A conical cavity is then made in the ground (generally in the side of a bank or sloping hill); and the roots of the fir, together with logs and billets of the same, being neatly trussed in a stack of the same conical shape, are let into this cavity. The whole is then covered with turf, to prevent the volatile parts from being dissipated, which, by

---

[1] *Hist. Plant.* lib. ix. cap. ii. and iii.
[2] Lib. i. cap. xciv.
[3] *Hist. Nat.* lib. xxiv. cap. 24, ed. Valp.
[4] *Travels in Scandinavia*, part iii. p. 251 ; see also Duhamel, *Traité des Arbres*.

means of a heavy wooden mallet and wooden stamper, worked separately by two men, is beaten down, and rendered as firm as possible about the wood. The stack of billets is then kindled, and a slow combustion of the fir takes place, without flame, as in working charcoal. During this combustion the tar exudes, and a cast-iron pan being at the bottom of the funnel, with a spout which projects through the side of the bank, barrels are placed beneath this spout to collect the fluid as it comes away. As fast as the barrels are filled, they are bunged, and ready for immediate exportation." Wood-tar is also obtained as a secondary product, in the manufacture of acetic acid, by the dry distillation of wood.

Fig. 149.

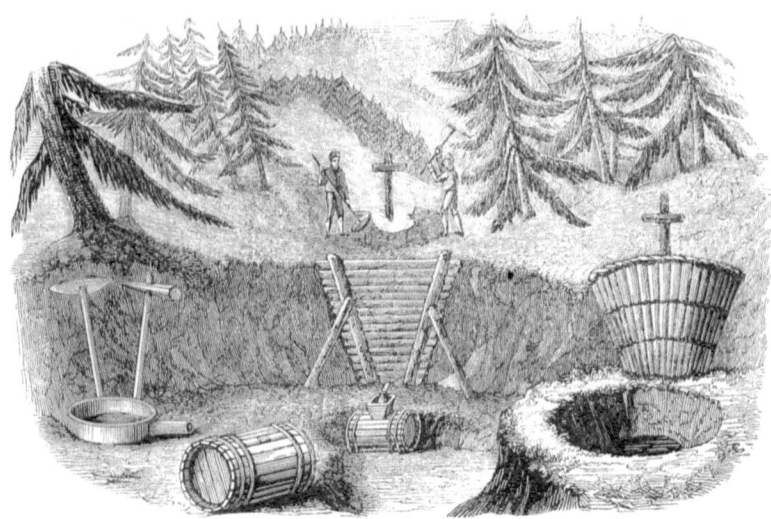

Preparation of Tar.

COMMERCE.—Wood-tar is imported into this country chiefly from the northern parts of Europe (Russia, Sweden, Norway, Denmark, and North Germany),—partly from the United States of America. It usually comes in barrels, each holding 31½ gallons; twelve barrels constituting a *last*. Tar is also produced in this country.

PROPERTIES.—It is a dark-brown, viscid, semi-liquid substance, which preserves during a long period its softness. [Its viscidity is destroyed by heat. It then becomes so liquid that it easily permeates hempen fibres; and it is in this state that it is largely employed for impregnating hemp previously to this being worked into ropes and cables.—ED.] It is soluble in alcohol, ether, and the oils both fixed and volatile. Submitted to distillation, it yields an aqueous acid liquor (*pyroligneous acid*), and a volatile oily matter (*oil of tar*); the residue in the still is *pitch*. [The vapour of tar is highly inflammable.—ED.]

COMPOSITION.—Wood-tar is a very complex substance. It consists principally of *pyretine* (pyrogenous or empyreumatic resin), *pyroleine* (pyrogenous oil), *acetic acid*, and *water*.—Reichenbach has obtained from it *kreosote, paraffin, eupion, picamar, kapnomor, pittacal,* and *cedriret.*—*Pyren* and *chrysen* have likewise been found in it. The tar obtained from coniferous woods contains in addition *colophony* and *oil of turpentine*.

PHYSIOLOGICAL EFFECTS.—The effects of tar are analogous to those of turpentine, but modified by the presence of acetic acid and the pyrogenous products. Locally it acts as a stimulant; and when applied to chronic skin diseases and indolent ulcers, it frequently induces a salutary change in the action of the capillary and secerning vessels, evinced by the improved quality of the secretions and the rapid healing of the sores. In such cases it is termed detergent, digestive, or cicatrisant. Swallowed, it acts as a local irritant and stimulant, becomes absorbed, and stimulates the secreting organs, especially the kidneys, on which it operates as a diuretic. Slight[1] states that a sailor swallowed a considerable quantity of liquid tar, which caused vomiting, great lassitude, and violent pain in bowels and kidneys. The urine was red, and, as well as the other evacuations, had the odour of tar. The head and the pulse were unaffected. The *vapour of tar*, inhaled, acts as a stimulant and irritant to the bronchial membrane, the secretion of which it promotes.

USES.—Tar is rarely employed *internally*. It has, however, been administered in chronic bronchial affections, and in obstinate skin diseases.

The *inhalation of tar vapour* was recommended by Sir Alex. Crichton[2] in phthisis; but at best it proves only a palliative, and it frequently, perhaps generally, fails to act even thus, and in some cases occasions a temporary increase of cough and irritation.[3] In chronic laryngeal and bronchial affections it has more chance of doing good.[4] Sir A. Crichton's directions for using it in phthisis are as follows :—The tar employed should be that used in the cordage of ships; to every pound of which, half an ounce of carbonate of potash must be added, in order to neutralise the pyroligneous acid generally found mixed with it, the presence of which will necessarily excite coughing. The tar thus prepared is to be placed in a suitable vessel over a lamp, and to be kept slowly boiling in the chamber during the night as well as the day. The vessel, however, ought to be cleansed and replenished every twenty-four hours, otherwise the residuum may be burned and decomposed,—a circumstance which will occasion increased cough and oppression on the chest.

Applied *externally*, tar is used in various forms of obstinate skin diseases, especially those which affect the scalp, lepra, &c.

ADMINISTRATION.—Internally, tar is administered either in substance, in the form of pills made up with wheat flour, of electuary with sugar, or in the form of tar water. In substance it may be taken to the extent of several drachms daily.

1. AQUA PICIS LIQUIDÆ; *Tar Water*. (Tar, Oij.; Water, Cong. j. Mix, stirring with a stick for a quarter of an hour; then, as soon as the tar subsides, strain the liquor, and keep it in well-stoppered jars.)—Tar water has the colour of Madeira wine, and a sharp empyreumatic taste. It reddens litmus, but does not effervesce on the addition of a solution of carbonate of

---

[1] Wibmer, *Wirk. d. Arzneim.* Bd. iv. S. 215.
[2] *Practical Observations on the Treatment and Cure of several varieties of Pulmonary Consumption, and on the Effects of the Vapour of boiling Tar in that disease,* 1823.
[3] Dr. Forbes, Translation of Laennec's *Treatise on Diseases of the Chest*, p. 365.
[4] Trousseau and Pidoux, *Traité de Thérap.* t. i. p. 459.

potash, though its colour becomes deepened. With a solution of bicarbonate of potash a very slight effervescence takes place. By persulphate of iron tar water is rendered very dark, or even blackish. The volatile oil contained in tar water is partly held in solution by acetic acid, which, as is well known, dissolves kreosote. It consists of water holding in solution acetic acid, and pyrogenous oil and resin. Notwithstanding the high eulogies passed on it by Bishop Berkeley,[1] tar water is now rarely employed. It is occasionally administered in chronic catarrhal and nephritic complaints, to the extent of one or two pints daily. As a wash in chronic skin diseases, especially those affecting the scalps of children, I have frequently seen it used, and sometimes with apparent benefit.

2. UNGUENTUM PICIS LIQUIDÆ, L. E. D.; *Tar Ointment.* (Tar, Mutton Suet, of each lb. j. Melt them together, and press through a linen cloth. The *Edinburgh College* takes of Tar, ℥v., and Bees' Wax, ℥ij. Melt the wax with a gentle heat, add the tar, and stir the mixture briskly, while it concretes on cooling, *E.* [Take of Tar, Oss.; Yellow Wax, ℥iv. Melt the wax with a gentle heat, then add the tar, and stir the mixture until it concretes, *D.* Ed.]—Its principal use is as an application to ring-worm of the scalp, and scalled head, in which it sometimes succeeds, but more frequently fails to cure. It is now and then applied to foul ulcers.

3. OLEUM PICIS LIQUIDÆ; *Oleum Pini rubrum; Oil of Tar.*—This is obtained by distillation from tar. It is a reddish, limpid fluid, having the odour of tar. It is a mixture of various volatile constituents of tar. By redistillation it may be rendered colourless, and then becomes very similar to oil of turpentine. It is occasionally used as an application to ring-worm of the scalp, and scalled head. Swallowed in a large dose it has proved fatal.[2]

2. Pix, L.—Black Pitch.

(Pix arida, *E.*—Bitumen aridum e Pice liquidâ præparatum, *L.*)

HISTORY.—This is the πίσσα ξηρά (*dry pitch*) of Dioscorides,[3] which, he says, some call παλίμπισσα (*pitch reboiled*).

PREPARATION.—The residuum in the still after the distillation of wood-tar is *pitch* (*pix*, L.)

PROPERTIES.—At ordinary temperatures it is a black solid, having a brilliant fracture. It softens at 99° F., and melts in boiling water. It dissolves in alcohol, and in solutions of the alkalies and of the alkaline carbonates.

COMPOSITION.—Pitch is composed of *pyrogenous resin* and *colophony*.

PHYSIOLOGICAL EFFECTS.—Made into pills with flour or any farinaceous substance, pitch may be taken to a great extent, not only without injury, but with advantage to the general health. It affords one of the most effectual means of controlling a languid circulation, and an inert and arid condition of the skin.[4] As a local remedy it possesses great adhesiveness, and when applied to wounds and ulcers acts as a stimulant and digestive.

---

[1] *Siris, a Chain of Phil. Reflex. and Inq. concerning Tar Water*, new edit. Lond. 1744.
[2] *Lancet* for 1832–3, vol. ii. p. 598; also March 8th, 1834.
[3] Lib. i. cap. 97.
[4] Bateman, *Synopsis of Cutaneous Diseases*, p. 53, 6th ed.

Uses.—Bateman[1] speaks favourably of the internal use of pitch in *ichthyosis*. It has been employed also in other obstinate skin diseases. But the principal use of pitch is in the form of ointment, as an application to cutaneous affections of the scalp.

ADMINISTRATION.—Dose from grs. x. to ʒj. made into pills with flour. The unpleasant pitchy flavour of the pills is materially diminished by keeping them for some time.

UNGUENTUM PICIS, L.; *Unguentum Basilicum nigrum* vel *Tetrapharmacum*. (Black Pitch, Wax, Resin, of each ʒxj.; Olive Oil, Oj. Melt them together, and press through a linen cloth.)—Stimulant and digestive; used in the obstinate cutaneous eruptions of the scalp.[2]

Sub-order II. CUPRESSEÆ.

Ovules erect; pollen spheroidal.

108. JUNIPERUS COMMUNIS, *Linn.*—COMMON JUNIPER.

Sex. Syst. Diœcia, Monadelphia.

(Fructus, *L. E. D.*—Cacumina, *E. D.*—Oleum e fructu destillatum, *L. E. D.*)

HISTORY.—The tree which in our translation of the Bible[3] is called the *juniper*, is supposed to have been a leguminous plant, either broom or furse (*genista* vel *ulex*).

Juniperus communis is a native of Greece, and must, therefore, have been known to the ancient Greeks. Sibthorp[4] thinks that it may perhaps be the ἄρκευθος μικρά of Dioscorides,[5]—a name which Fraas[6] considers to have been applied to *Juniperus oxycedrus*. The last-mentioned authority is of opinion that the κέδρος μικρά of Dioscorides[7] is our juniper. The fruit mentioned in the Hippocratic writings under the name of ἀρκευθίς, and which was used in some disorders of females, was the produce of a species of *Juniperus*,—perhaps of the *J. phœnicia*, which is very common in Greece and the islands of the Archipelago, and whose fruit is yellowish, but has the size, form, and powers of that of the common juniper.

BOTANY. **Gen. Char.**—*Diœcious*, rarely *monœcious*. MALES :—*Catkins* ovate; the *scales* verticillate, peltato-pedicellate. *Anthers* 4 to 8, unilocular. FEMALES :—*Catkins* globose; the 3 concave scales united. *Stigma* gaping. *Galbulus* composed of the united and fleshy scales, and containing 3 triquetrous osseous *seeds*.

[1] *Op. cit.*
[2] Vide *Unguentum Picis liquidæ.*
[3] *Job*, xxx. 4; 1 *Kings*, xix. 4.
[4] *Prod. Fl. Græcæ.*
[5] Lib. i. cap. 103.
[6] *Synopsis Plant. Fl. Classicæ*, p. 259, 1845.
[7] Lib. i. cap. 105.

Sp. Char.—*Leaves* 3 in each whorl, spreading, linear-subulate, keeled, mucronate, longer than the galbulus.

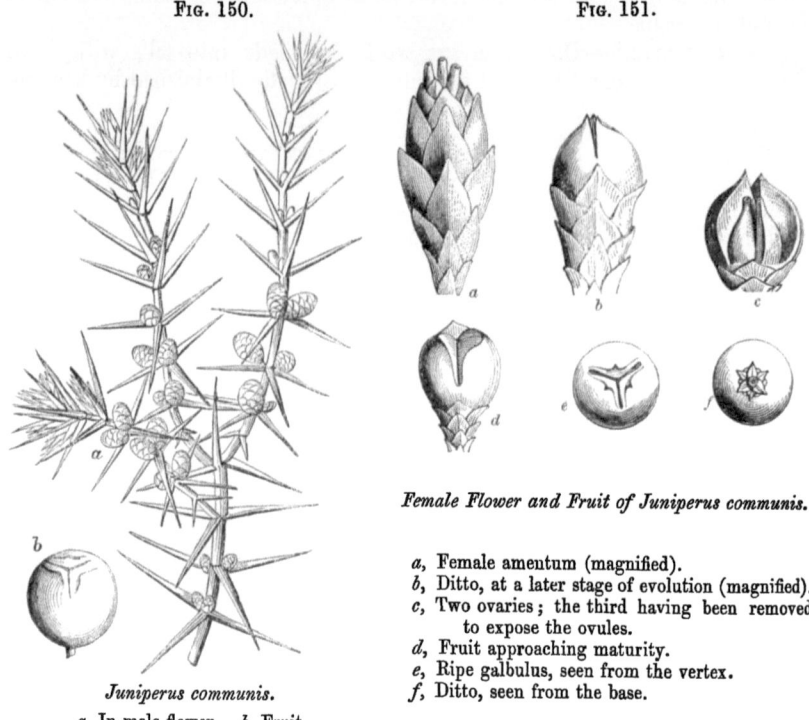

FIG. 150.   FIG. 151.

Juniperus communis.

a, In male flower. *b*, Fruit.

Female Flower and Fruit of Juniperus communis.

a, Female amentum (magnified).
b, Ditto, at a later stage of evolution (magnified).
c, Two ovaries; the third having been removed
    to expose the ovules.
d, Fruit approaching maturity.
e, Ripe galbulus, seen from the vertex.
f, Ditto, seen from the base.

A bushy *shrub*. *Leaves* evergreen, numerous, with a broad flat shallow channel above, the keel beneath with a slender furrow, pungent, glaucous on the upper side, dark green beneath. *Flowers* axillary, sessile, small; the *males* discharging a copious cloud of yellow pollen: *females* green, on scaly stalks. *Fruit* commonly called *a berry*, but is in reality that kind of cone called by botanists a *galbulus*, which has fleshy coalescent carpella, whose heads are much enlarged. It requires two seasons to arrive at maturity. The galbulus is black tinged with blue, and is scarcely more than half the length of the leaves.

Loudon[1] mentions no fewer than seven varieties; but some of these are probably distinct species.

Juniperus nana (Smith), Dwarf Alpine Juniper, has a procumbent stem; imbricated, incurved, linear-lanceolate leaves; and fruit nearly as long as the leaves.—Indigenous. On mountains.

Hab.—North of Europe. Indigenous, growing on hills and healthy downs, especially where the soil is chalky. It flowers in May.

DESCRIPTION.—In this country the *fruit* and *tops*, and, on the continent, the *wood*, are officinal.

---

[1] *Arboretum*, vol. iv. p. 2489.

Juniper berries (*baccæ juniperi*), as the dried fruit of the shops is commonly termed, are about the size of a pea, of a blackish-purple colour, covered by a glaucous bloom. They are marked superiorly with a triradiate groove, indicating the adhesion of the succulent carpella; inferiorly with the bracteal scales, which assume a stellate form (see fig. 151, *e* and *f*). They contain three seeds. Their taste is sweetish, with a terebinthinate flavour; their odour is agreeable and balsamic.

Juniper tops (*cacumina* seu *summitates juniperi*) have a bitter terebinthinate flavour and a balsamic odour.

Juniper wood (*lignum juniperi*) is obtained either from the stem or root; it evolves a balsamic odour in burning, and, by distillation with water, yields volatile oil. On old stems there is sometimes found a resinous substance (*resina juniperi; sandaraca germanica*).

Sandarach or Juniper Resin.—The resin called *sandarach* (*sandaraca*), or *gum juniper* (*gummi juniperi*), is imported from Mogadore. It is the produce of *Callitris quadrivalvis*, Vent. (*Thuja articulata*, Desf.) Though sold by chemists and apothecaries, it is not employed in medicine. It is used in the manufacture of varnishes. Its powder is commonly known under the name of *pounce*.

Commerce.—Juniper berries are imported in bags and barrels from Rotterdam, Hamburgh, Leghorn, Trieste, and other European ports. In 1838, duty was paid on 5896 cwts.

Composition.—Juniper berries were analysed in 1822 by Trommsdorff,[1] and in 1831 by Nicolet.[2] Trommsdorff obtained *volatile oil* 1·0, *wax* 4·0, *resin* 10·0, *a peculiar species of sugar with acetate and malate of lime* 33·8, *gum with salts of potash and lime* 7·0, *lignin* 35·0, *water* 12·9 (= 103·7, *excess* 3·7).

1. Oil of Juniper (see below).
2. Resin.—Is green, according to Trommsdorff. Nicolet obtained it in the crystalline state, and found it to consist of C^5,H^2,O^1.
3. Wax.—Is brittle. Consists, according to Nicolet, of $C^{13},H^{8\frac{1}{2}},O^4$.
4. Sugar.—Is crystallisable, and analogous to grape sugar, according to Trommsdorff. But Nicolet describes it as being like molasses.

Physiological Effects.—Juniper berries and tops are analogous in their operation to the terebinthinate substances. Three ounces of the berries act on the larger herbivorous animals as a diuretic.[3] On man, also, these fruits operate on the urinary organs, promoting the secretion of urine, to which they communicate a violet odour.[4] In large doses they occasion irritation of the bladder and heat in the urinary passages. Piso[5] says their continued use causes bloody urine. They promote sweat, relieve flatulency, and provoke the catamenia. Their activity is principally dependent on the volatile oil which they contain, and which, according to Mr. Alexander's experiments,[6] is, in doses of four drops, the most powerful of all the diuretics.[7]

Uses.—Juniper berries or oil are but little used in medicine. They may be employed, either alone or as adjuncts to other diuretic medicines, *in drop-*

---

[1] Gmelin's *Handb. d. Chem* ii. 1380.
[2] Thomson's *Organic Chemistry*, p. 899.
[3] Moiroud, *Pharm. Vétér.*
[4] Cargillus, in Ray, *Hist. Plant.* t. ii. p. 1412.
[5] Murray, *App. Med.*
[6] *Experimental Essays*, p. 149, 1768.
[7] See his *Table*, at p. 251.

sical disorders, indicating the employment of renal stimuli. Van Swieten[1] speaks favourably of their use in mild cases of ascites and anasarca. *In some affections of the urino-genital apparatus* juniper may be employed with advantage. Thus, in mucous discharges (as gonorrhœa, gleet, leucorrhœa, and cystirrhœa) it may be used under the same regulations that govern the employment of copaiva and the terebinthinates. Hecker[2] praised it in the first stage of gonorrhœa. Juniper has been employed in some other diseases.[3]

Administration.—The dose of the *berries* is one or two drachms, triturated with sugar. The *infusion* (prepared with an ounce of the berries and a pint of boiling water) is a more convenient mode of exhibition: the dose is f℥iv. every four hours.

1. JUNIPERI OLEUM, L. E. D.; (*Anglicum*, L.); *Oil of Juniper; English Oil of Juniper.*

—Is obtained by submitting the fruit, tops, or wood, to distillation with water. The full-grown green fruit yields more than the ripe fruit, for in the act of ripening a portion of the oil becomes converted into resin. It is limpid, transparent, nearly colourless, and lighter than water, and causes the left-handed rotation of polarised light,—in this respect agreeing with French oil of turpentine. It has the odour of the fruit, and an aromatic balsamic taste. It dissolves with difficulty in alcohol. According to Blanchet, it consists of two isomeric oils, carburets of hydrogen, $C^{20}H^{16}$: one colourless, and more volatile; a second coloured, and less volatile. Both, when agitated with a solution of salt, form crystalline hydrates. The more volatile oil almost entirely constitutes the oil obtained from the ripe fruit. It is soluble in alcohol and in hydrochloric acid, with which it forms a liquid artificial camphor. Its density is 0·839.

The oil is, perhaps, the best form for exhibiting juniper. The dose is two to six drops, either in the form of pill, or diffused through water by the aid of sugar and mucilage.

Oleum empyreumaticum Juniperi.—By the dry distillation of the wood of *Juniperus Oxycedrus* there is obtained, in France, a tarry oil called *huile de cade* (*oleum cadinum*). It is a brownish, inflammable liquid, having a strong empyreumatic and resinous odour, and an acrid caustic taste. It is employed in veterinary medicine,—to cure ulcers in horses, and, formerly, to cure the itch in sheep. Oil of tar, which is often substituted for it, is considered to be inferior. It has also been used in the human subject, both externally and internally,—in obstinate skin diseases, worms, and toothache. Dose, a few drops.

2. SPIRITUS JUNIPERI COMPOSITUS, L. E. D.

[Take of Oil of Juniper, ʒiss.; Oil of Caraway, Oil of Fennel, each ♏xij.; Proof Spirit, Cong. j. Dissolve, *L.*—Juniper Berries, bruised, lb. j.; Caraway, bruised; Fennel, bruised, aa. ℥iss.; Proof Spirit, Ovij.; Water, Oij. Macerate the fruits in the spirit for two days, add the water, and distil off seven pints, *E.*—Juniper Berries, bruised, ℥viij.; Caraway Seed, bruised; Fennel Seed, bruised, of each ʒj.; Proof Spirit, Cong. ss.; Water, Oj. Macerate the berries and seeds in the spirit for twenty-four hours; then add the water, and with a slow fire distil half a gallon, *D.*—Ed.]—This preparation, when sweetened, may be regarded as an officinal substitute for *genuine Hollands* and *English gin*, both of which

---

[1] *Commentaries*, English edit. 12mo. vol. xii. p. 431.
[2] *Anweisung d. vener. Krankh.* quoted by Voigtels, *Arzneim.* Bd. ii. Abt. 2, S. 510.
[3] Consult on this subject Vogt, *Lehrb. d. Pharmakodyn.*; Richter, *Arzneimittell.*; and Sundelin, *Spec. Heilmittell.*

compounds are flavoured with juniper. It is used as an adjunct to diuretic mixtures. The dose is fʒij. to fʒiv.

[3. **INFUSUM JUNIPERI**, D. (Take of Juniper Berries, bruised, ℥j. ; Boiling Water, Oss. Infuse for one hour in a covered vessel, and strain. The product should measure about eight ounces, *D.*)—ED.]

109. JUNIPERUS SABINA, *Linn.*—COMMON SAVIN.

Sex. Syst. Diœcia, Monadelphia.

(Cacumen recens et exsiccatum ; Oleum e cacumine destillatum, *L.*—Tops, *E. D.*)

HISTORY.—This is the βράθυ of Dioscorides,[1] the *sabina* of Pliny [2] Each of these writers notices both the cypress-leaved and the tamarisk-leaved varieties of savin.

BOTANY.   **Gen. Char.** — Vide *Juniperus communis.*

Sp. Char.—*Leaves* ovate, convex, densely imbricated, erect, decurrent, opposite ; the oppositions pyxidate (*Bot. Gall.*)

A small bushy *shrub. Branches* closely invested by the very small glandular *leaves. Galbulus* round, purple, somewhat smaller than that of Juniper communis.

Loudon[3] mentions five varieties. Of these the most interesting are the two following :—

α. *J. S. cupressifolia*, Aiton.—The Cypress-leaved Savin. La Sabine mâle. Leaves acute, more spreading, 3 lines long.

β. *J. S. tamariscifolia*, Aiton.— The Tamarisk-leaved or Berry-bearing Savin. La Sabin femelle. Leaves shorter, almost appressed and obtuse.

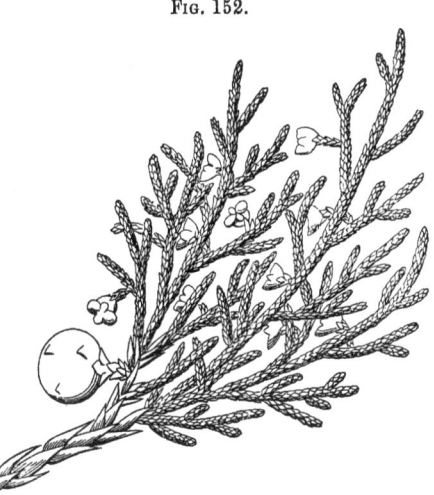

FIG. 152.

Juniperus Sabina in Fruit.

Another variety, *J. S. foliis variegatis*, has variegated leaves. A fourth, *J. S. prostrata*, is a low trailing plant. The fifth, *J. S. alpina*, is procumbent, and more slender than the fourth.

HAB.—Midland and southern parts of Europe, Asiatic Russia. Cultivated in gardens in this country. Flowers in April.

JUNIPERUS VIRGINIANA, Linn., the *Red Cedar* (the wood of which is used for black-lead pencils), is used in the United States as a substitute for savin.

DESCRIPTION.—The officinal parts of the plant are the *tops* (*cacumina summitates*), which consist of the young branches with their attached leaves. They have, in the fresh state (*cacumen recens*), a strong, peculiar, heavy odour, especially when rubbed ; and a nauseous, resinous, bitter taste. The dried tops (*cacumina exsiccata*) are yellowish-green, and less odorous than the fresh ones.

---

[1] Lib. i. cap. 104.
[2] *Hist. Nat.* lib. xxiv. cap. 61, ed. Valp.
[3] *Arboretum*, vol. iv. p. 2499.

Composition.—Some experiments on the composition of savin were made by Berlisky.[1]   In 1837, an analysis of this plant was made by a young chemist of the name of Gardes.[2]   The constituents are *volatile oil, resin, gallic acid, chlorophylle, extractive, lignin,* and *calcareous salts.*

Oil of Savin (see *post*).

Chemical Characteristics.—An aqueous infusion of savin is yellowish, has the odour and bitter taste of the herb, and forms a soluble green compound (*gallate? of iron*) on the addition of sesquichloride of iron, but is unchanged by a solution of gelatin.   Oxalate of ammonia causes, in the infusion, a white precipitate (*oxalate of lime*).   Alcohol acquires a green colour when digested with the tops : on the addition of water to the alcoholic tincture, some *resin* is separated.   By distillation with water or ether, both the fresh and dried tops (but especially the first) yield *volatile oil.*

Detection.—Savin is sometimes employed for criminal purposes, and, therefore, occasionally becomes the subject of medico-legal inquiries. Powdered savin in the stomach and bowels might, on account of its green colour, be mistaken for bile : but when mixed with distilled water it entirely subsides ; and, provided no bile be intermixed, the supernatant liquor will be devoid of a green colour.   The powder, when dry, may be detected to be that of savin by the peculiar odour of this herb.   The odorous principle (volatile oil) might, if the quantity of powder be sufficient, be separated by submitting this to distillation with water or ether.   Moreover, savin powder yields a green colour to alcohol, and its aqueous infusion strikes a green colour with the tincture of the sesquichloride of iron.   If the powder be coarse, the microscope may give us important aid in detecting savin.   A careful examination of the woody fibres will detect their circular pores (fig. 153, A B), characteristic of the Gymnosperms ; and by the shape of the apex of the leaves (when these can be obtained), savin (fig. 153, C D) may be distinguished from another poisonous gymnospermous plant (fig. 153, E), namely the Yew (*Taxus baccata*).[3]

Fig. 153.

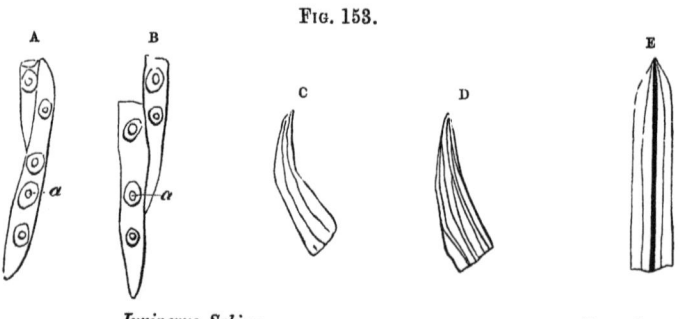

Juniperus Sabina.   *Taxus baccata.*

A B, Woody fibres (magnified) of Savin ; showing *a a,* the pores.
C D, Magnified extremity of the leaf of Savin, showing the subulate linear leaves.
E, Magnified extremity of the leaf of Yew (*Taxus baccata*), showing the linear acute leaves.

---

[1] Trommsdorff's *Journ.* viii. 1, 94.
[2] *Journ. de Chim. Méd.* t. iii. p. 331, 2de sér.
[3] See an interesting report of a case of poisoning by savin, in which the above characters were successfully made use of to detect the poison, by Dr. A. Taylor and Mr. Charles Johnson, in the *Lond. Med. Gaz.* for Aug. 8th, 1845, p. 646. [See also Taylor *On Poisons,* p. 521.]

PHYSIOLOGICAL EFFECTS. α. *On Animals.*—Savin acts on animals as an acrid poison. Orfila[1] applied two drachms of the powder to an incised wound in the leg of a dog; inflammation and infiltration of the limb took place, and death occurred in about thirty-six hours. Four drachms introduced into the stomach of a dog, and the œsophagus tied, caused death in thirteen hours; the stomach was bright red, and the rectum a little inflamed. Orfila infers that its effects depend principally on its absorption, and its action on the nervous system, the rectum, and the stomach. A drachm of *oil of savin* was given by Hillefield[2] to a cat. It caused a flow of saliva, anxiety, frequent discharge of urine, dulness, trembling, and, in an hour and a quarter, bloody urine. The animal having been strangled, the bladder was found contracted, with some coagulated blood contained in its cavity.

β. *On Man.*—Oil of savin, the active principle of the herb, is a powerful local irritant. When applied to the skin, it acts as a rubefacient and vesicant. On wounds and ulcers its operation is that of an acrid (not chemical) caustic. Swallowed in large doses, it occasions vomiting, purging, and other symptoms of gastro-intestinal inflammation. In its operation on the system generally, it is powerfully stimulant. " Savin," says Sundelin,[3] " operates not merely as irritants generally do, as a stimulant to the arterial system, but it also eminently heightens the vitality of the venous system, the circulation in which it quickens. It next powerfully stimulates the absorbing vessels and glands, the serous, the fibrous, and the mucous membranes, and the skin. It operates as a specific excitant and irritant on the kidneys, and yet more obviously on the uterus. The increased secretion of bile, and the augmented volume of the liver, both of which conditions have sometimes been observed after the copious and long-continued use of savin, appear to be connected with its action on the venous system." Mohrenheim[4] mentions the case of a woman, 30 years of age, who swallowed an infusion of savin to occasion abortion. Violent and incessant vomiting was induced. After some days she experienced excruciating pains, which were followed by abortion, dreadful hemorrhage from the uterus, and death. On examination, the gall-bladder was found ruptured, the bile effused in the abdomen, and the intestines inflamed. The popular notion of its tendency to cause abortion leads, on many occasions, to the improper use of savin; and the above is not a solitary instance of the fatal consequences thereof. A fatal case of its use as an emmenagogue is recorded by Dr. Dewees.[5] That it may frequently fail to provoke premature labour is shown by the case, related by Fodéré,[6] of a woman who, in order to produce abortion, took every morning, for twenty days, one hundred drops of this oil, and yet went her full time and brought forth a living child. It ought to be well known that in those cases in which it may succeed in causing miscarriage, it can only do so at the risk of the woman's life. Vogt[7] says that it has a tendency to induce an apoplectic state in the fœtus. The emmenagogue power of savin is fully established. Perhaps the observations of Home[8] are

[1] *Toxicol. Gén.*
[2] Wibmer, *Wirk. d Arzneim. u. Gifte*, Bd. iii. H. 1, p. 191.
[3] *Heilmittellehre*, Bd. ii. S. 180, Auf. 3te.
[4] Murray, *App. Med.* vol. i. p. 59.
[5] *Compend. Syst. of Midwifery*, pp. 133–4.
[6] *Méd. Lég.*
[7] *Pharmakodyn.*
[8] *Clinical Experiments*, p. 419.

the most satisfactory of any on this subject, confirmed as they are by the reports of many other accurate observers.

Uses.—Savin is not much used internally; but in cases of amenorrhœa and chlorosis depending on or accompanied by a torpid condition or deficient action of the uterine vessels, it may be given as a powerful uterine stimulant. In such cases it proves a most efficient remedy. According to my own observation, it is the most certain and powerful emmenagogue of the whole materia medica. My experience of it, therefore, confirms the statements of Home.[1] Though I have employed it in numerous cases, I never saw any ill effects result from its administration. Of course its use is contraindicated where irritation of the uterus, or indeed of any of the pelvic viscera, exists, [or when the female is in a pregnant state.—Ed.] In chronic rheumatism, with a languid circulation in the extreme vessels, Chapman[2] speaks in very high terms of it. It has been used as an anthelmintic.

As a topical agent, savin is frequently employed, mostly in the form of the cerate, to make *perpetual blisters*. Equal parts of savin and verdigris, in powder, form one of the most efficacious applications for the removal of venereal warts. The powder, an infusion, or the expressed juice of the plant, is occasionally applied to warts, to old and indolent ulcers, and in cases of psora and tinea.

Administration.—By drying, savin loses part of its volatile oil, and hence the *powder* is not the best preparation of it. It is, however, sometimes given in doses of from five to fifteen grains. A *decoction* and *extract* are also objectionable preparations, on account of the heat employed in making them. An *infusion* may be prepared by digesting ʒj. of the fresh herb in fʒviij. of boiling water : the dose is one or two table-spoonfuls. The *oil* is by far the most convenient and certain preparation of savin. A *conserve* of the fresh leaves is sometimes used.

1. OLEUM SABINÆ, E. D.; *Oil of Savin*.—This is obtained by submitting the fresh tops to distillation with water. [The tops yield about three per cent. of the oil.—Ed.] It is a limpid liquid of a light yellow colour, having the unpleasant odour of the plant, and a bitter acrid taste. Its sp. gr. is 0·915. [Its boiling point is 315°.—Ed.] Its composition is analogous to that of oil of turpentine, being $C^{20}H^{16}$, [or according to Dumas, $C^{10}H^8$.—Ed.] It agrees with English oil of turpentine in its power of effecting the right-handed rotation of plane polarised light. [This oil is very soluble in ether, and may be removed by this liquid from watery decoctions or infusions in which it is diffused. It forms a turbid mixture with rectified spirit. When treated with its volume of concentrated sulphuric acid, it acquires a dark red-brown colour, and when this mixture is added to distilled water, a dense white precipitate is separated. The odour is the best and the most characteristic test.— Ed.] Winckler[3] states that he dissolved one ounce of savin oil in the same quantity of concentrated sulphuric acid, and then distilled it from milk of lime (to remove the sulphurous acid), and obtained two drachms of an oil which was undistinguishable from the volatile oil of thyme. The dose of oil of savin, as

---

[1] *Clinical Experiments*, p. 419.
[2] *Elem. of Therap.*
[3] Buchner's *Repertorium*, 2te Reihe, Bd. xlii. S. 330, 1846.

an emmenagogue, is from two to six drops, diffused in a mucilaginous or oleaginous mixture.[1]

2. UNGUENTUM SABINÆ, L. D. ; *Ceratum Sabinæ,* E. ; *Savin Ointment.* (Fresh Savin, bruised, lb. ss. ; White Wax, ℥iij. ; Lard, lb. j. Mix the savin in the lard and wax melted together, then press through a linen cloth. [The *Edinburgh College* orders of Fresh Savin, 2 parts ; Bees'-wax, 1 part ; Axunge, 4 parts. Melt the wax and axunge together, add the savin, and boil them together until the leaves are friable, then strain, *E.*] Savin Tops, dried, and in fine powder, ℨj. ; Ointment of White Wax, ℥vij. Mix the powder intimately with the ointment by trituration, *D.* [The U.S. Pharmacopœia directs Savin in powder, ℨij. ; Resin Cerate, lb. j. Mix the savin with the cerate previously melted.]—The boiling directed by the Edinburgh College is considered objectionable on account of the loss of a portion of the oil. The colour of this cerate should be a fine green, and its odour that of the plant : the former property depends on chlorophylle, and the latter on the presence of oil of savin. Savin cerate is used as a dressing to blistered surfaces, to produce what is termed a *perpetual blister*. It is preferred to the Ceratum cantharidis as being less acrid, and not liable to cause strangury. It is sometimes applied to seton tapes, to increase the discharge from setons.

ANTIDOTES.—In a case of poisoning by savin herb or its oil, the first indication is to remove the poison from the stomach and bowels, by the stomach-pump, and castor oil. Opiates and demulcent drinks should then be given. The warm bath may be advantageously employed. Blood-letting should be resorted to if the inflammatory symptoms indicate, and the condition of the system permit it.

---

[1] [The dose and medicinal properties of this oil have given rise to some discussion since the former edition of this work was published. In a case tried at the Cornwall Lent Assizes, 1852, the accused, a medical man, was convicted and sentenced to transportation for administering *oil of savin* to a female with intent to procure miscarriage. The proof of intent rested partly on medical and partly on moral circumstances. It appeared that the prisoner had given fourteen drops of the oil, in three doses, daily,—a quantity which, according to the medical evidence at the trial, was greater than should have been prescribed for any lawful purpose. The medicinal dose, as an emmenagogue, on the authority of Christison, is from two to five *minims*, and according to Pereira, from two to six *drops*. The quantity given by the prisoner, although a full dose, was not, therefore, greater than these authorities recommend ; and his criminality appears to have rested not so much on the dose given, as on the question whether he knew, or as a medical man had reason to *suspect*, that the female for whom he prescribed it was pregnant. No medical authority would recommend oil of savin in full doses for *pregnant* females ; and with regard to the existence or non-existence of pregnancy in a special case, medical men are reasonably presumed to have better means of satisfying themselves than non-professional persons. The prisoner's innocence, therefore, rested on the presumption that he implicitly believed what a young woman told him regarding her condition —that he had no reason to *suspect* her pregnancy, and therefore did not hesitate to select and prescribe a medicine which is very rarely used by practitioners, and certainly has an evil reputation. If the prosecutrix is to be believed, she told the prisoner that she had disease of the heart and liver, and that nothing more was the matter with her. It is absurd to suppose that oil of savin should be prescribed for diseases of this kind. The prisoner, on the hypothesis of innocence, must have intended the medicine to act on the uterus, and must have inferred the existence of an obstruction of menstruation from natural causes irrespective of pregnancy. The jury do not appear to have given him credit for such ignorance of his profession, and this probably led to his conviction : there can be no doubt, from the evidence, that the oil was administered with guilty intention. Every competent practitioner would undoubtedly satisfy himself that a young female, whose menses were obstructed, was *not pregnant*, before he prescribed full doses of this oil three times a day, or he would fairly lay himself open to a suspicion of criminality. If pregnancy were only *suspected*, this would be sufficient to deter a practitioner of common prudence from prescribing, in any dose, a drug which may exert a serious action on the system. A report of this case will be found in the *Med. Times and Gazette*, April 17, 1852, p. 404.—ED.]

ORDER XXIII. TAXACEÆ, *Lindl.*—TAXADS.

TAXINEÆ, *Endl.*

CHARACTERS.— Naked-seeded exogens, with repeatedly branched, continuous *stems*, simple *leaves* often fork-veined, solitary female *flowers*, 2-celled *anthers* opening longitudinally, membrane next the nucleus of the *ovule* inclosed, *seed* usually supported or surrounded by a succulent imperfect cap-shaped pericarp, *embryo* straightened, dicotyledonous, and *albumen* fleshy.

PROPERTIES.—The Taxaceæ agree with the Pinaceæ in the resinous quality of their juices, but abound more in bitter astringent, and some of them in narcotico acrid principles.

110. Taxus baccata, *Linn.*—Common Yew.

Sex. Syst. Diœcia, Monadelphia.

(Folia et semina.)

Σμῖλαξ, by some called ϑύμαλος, by the Romans termed τάξος, Dioscorides, lib. iv. cap. 80; *Taxus*, Pliny, lib. xvi. cap. 20 et 33, and lib. xxiv. cap. 72.—A tree often attaining a considerable bulk. Leaves scattered, nearly sessile, 2-ranked, crowded, linear, acute, entire, very slightly revolute, about 1 inch long, dark green, smooth and shining above, paler with a prominent midrib beneath, terminating in a small harmless point. Flowers axillary sessile. Fruit drooping, consisting of a succulent, sweet, internally glutinous, scarlet cup, enclosing an oval, brown, nuciform seed, unconnected with the fleshy part. — In 1828, Peretti[1] analysed yew (the *leaves ?*), and obtained a bitter volatile oil, a bitter non-crystallisable substance, a yellow colouring matter, resin, tannin, gallic acid, chlorophylle, mucilage, sugar, and malate of lime. In 1818, Chevallier and Lassaigne[2] examined the pulpy cup of the *fruit*, and found in it a non-crystallisable fermentable sugar, gum, malic and phosphoric acids, and a carmine-red fatty matter. In 1843, Martin[3] analysed the seeds, and obtained from them a volatile oil having a terebinthinate odour, fixed oil, a green very bitter resin, sugar, albumen (in small quantity), sulphate of lime, and vegetable fibre. The poisonous properties of yew were known to the ancient Greeks and Romans, and have been fully established by modern experience, although some few writers have expressed doubts concerning them. Percival[4] states that three children were poisoned by the fresh leaves. Dr. Mollan[5] has mentioned the case of a lunatic who died in fourteen hours after taking yew-leaves: the symptoms were giddiness, sudden prostration of strength, vomiting, coldness of the surface, spasms, and irregular action of the heart. Mr. Hurt[6] has reported an interesting case of a child, three years and a half old, who died in less than four hours after eating the fruit: the symptoms were vomiting, convul-

FIG. 154.

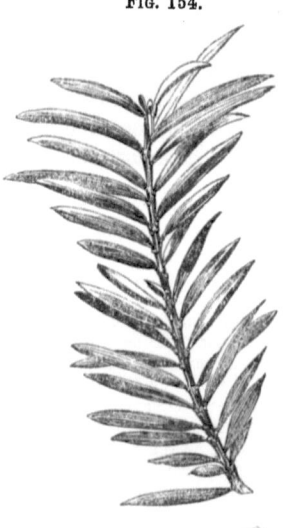

Taxus baccata.

a, Young. *b*, Older fruit.

[1] *Journ. de Pharm.* t. xiv. p. 537, 1828.
[2] *Ibid.* t. iv. p. 558, 1818.
[3] *Jahresbericht über d. Fortschritte d. Pharm. in Jahre* 1843, S. 18.
[4] *Essays, Med. Phil. and Exper.* vol. iii. p. 257.
[5] *Dublin Hospital Gazette,* May 15, 1845, p. 109.
[6] *Lancet,* Dec. 10, 1836.

sions, purple lips, and dilated pupil. [The symptoms produced by yew-leaves and berries are pretty uniform in character : convulsions, insensibility, coma, dilated pupils, pale countenance, small pulse, and cold extremities, are the most prominent. Vomiting and purging are also observed. In two cases of recent occurrence, the subject of one, a girl of about five years of age, died in a comatose state in four hours after she had eaten the berries; and the other, a boy aged four years, died nineteen days after taking the berries, obviously from severe inflammation of the bowels.[1] There is a vulgar but erroneous notion that the yew-leaves are not poisonous when fresh, and that in any case they act only mechanically. A case related above shows the fallacy of this opinion, and the other cases prove that there is a specific poison in the yew, since it exists in the berries as well as in the leaves. If cattle recover from the primary effects on the nervous system, they are liable to die, after several days, from inflammation of the bowels. On one occasion the intestines of an ox which had obviously died from the effects of yew-leaves, were found in a highly inflamed and gangrenous state.—ED.] Considered both in a toxicological and therapeutical point of view, the yew appears to hold an intermediate position between savin and foxglove. To savin it is allied by its botanical affinities and chemical composition, as well as by its acrid, evacuant, diuretic, and emmenagogue properties. But, on the other hand, its relation to the neurotics, especially to sedatives, is marked by the giddiness, irregular and depressed action of the heart, convulsions, and insensibility which it produces. It is said that when used for medicinal purposes it is unlike digitalis in not being apt to accumulate in the system. As a poison, it belongs to the class of acro-narcotics ; as a medicine, it is used as a sedative, antispasmodic, emmenagogue, lithic, and resolvent. As a sedative it has been proposed by Rempinelli and Martin to be used as a substitute for, and under the same indications as, digitalis. As an emmenagogue it has been given in cases similar to those for which savin is sometimes administered. Dr. A. Taylor[2] says that "infusion of yew-leaves, which is popularly called yew-tree tea, is sometimes used for the purpose of procuring abortion by ignorant midwives." As a lithic it has been employed in calculous complaints ; as an antispasmodic in epilepsy and convulsions ; as a resolvent in hepatic and gouty complaints. In pulmonary and vesical catarrh it has likewise been used. The *powder* of the leaves or seeds is given in doses of from half a grain to two or three grains. The *extract of the leaves* (*extractum taxi*, Cod. Hamb.), prepared by evaporating the expressed juice of the leaves, is administered in doses of one or two grains, and gradually increased. The *alcoholic and ethereal extract* of the seeds is employed in doses of from ⅛th to ⅓rd of a grain. In cases of poisoning by yew, the first indication is to expel the poison from the stomach by the means already pointed out. The sedative and narcotic effects are to be counteracted by stimulants, such as ammonia (see the treatment for poisoning by foxglove).

Sub-class II. *Angiospermæ.— Angiosperms.*

EXOGENS, *Lindl.*

CHARACTERS.—*Ovules* enclosed in an ovary, and fertilised by the application of the pollen to the stigma.

In accordance with the classification followed by De Candolle, the natural orders of this sub-class will be arranged in the four following sub-divisions :—1st, *Monochlamydeæ;* 2dly, *Corollifloræ ;* 3dly, *Calycifloræ ;* and 4thly, *Thalamifloræ.*

SUB-DIVISION I. MONOCHLAMYDEÆ, *De Cand.*

APETALÆ, *Endlicher.*

Flowers frequently unisexual. Perianth absent, rudimentary or simple, calycine or coloured, free or connate with the ovary.

---

[1] [*Prov. Journal*, Nov. 29, 1848, p. 662; and Dec. 27, p. 708.]
[2] *On Poisons*, p. 790.

Order XXIV. LIQUIDAMBARACEÆ, *Richard.*— LIQUIDAMBARS.

Balsamifluæ, *Blume, Endl.*—Altingiaceæ, et olim Balsamaceæ, *Lindley.*

Characters.—Tall *trees*, with amentaceous unisexual *flowers;* a 2-celled, 2-lobed, many-seeded *capsule;* and winged *seeds*, with the embryo inverted in fleshy albumen.
Properties.—Balsamic, fragrant.

111. Liquidambar, *Linn.*

Altingia, *Noronha.*

As this is the only genus of the Order, its characters are necessarily those of the latter.[1] It consists of a very small number of species, of which none probably are officinal. But as their balsamic products have been confounded with storax and balsam of Peru (two officinal substances), a short notice of them is requisite.

1. L. styraciflua, Linn.; *Sweet Gum; White Gum (American Liquidambar Tree).*— A native of the United States and Mexico, attaining, in the southern districts, an immense size. In Louisiana and Mexico there is obtained, by making incisions into the stem, a fluid balsamic juice called *liquidambar* or *copalm balsam.* In this fluid state it constitutes the *liquid liquidambar*, or *oil of liquidambar* of Guibourt. It is transparent, amber-yellow, has the consistence of a thick oil, a balsamic odour, and an aromatic, acrid, bitter taste. By time it concretes, and becomes darker coloured. The soft solid called by Guibourt *soft* or *white liquidambar* is perhaps a mixture of the opaque deposit of the fluid balsam and of the latter rendered concrete by keeping. It is a soft, almost opaque solid, very similar in appearance to concrete turpentine. Its odour is similar to, though weaker than, the liquid balsam. Its taste is balsamic and sweetish. Bonastre[2] analysed a very fluid sample, recently received from America, and found it to consist of—*volatile oil*, 7·0 ; *semi-concrete matter*, 11·1 ; *benzoic acid*, 1·0 ; *crystalline matter soluble in water and alcohol*, 5·3 ; *yellow colouring matter*, 2·05 ; *oleo-resin*, 49·0 ; *styracin*, 24.0 ; loss, 0·55. The volatile oil consists, according to Henry, of $C^{10}H^7$. Styracin is a fusible, crystalline substance, soluble in boiling alcohol, and composed, according to Henry, of $C^{11}H^5O^2$. The proportion of benzoic [cinnamic?] acid is increased by time. Mr. Hodgson[3] obtained from a sample which he examined 4·2 per cent.

Liquidambar has been confounded with both *white balsam of Peru* and *liquid storax.* The liquidambar which I have received from M. Guibourt is quite different from a genuine sample of the *white balsam of Peru* received by me from Guatemala, and it is equally different from the liquid storax of the shops. Dr. Wood[4] observes that some of the genuine juice of *liquidambar styraciflua* brought from New Orleans, which he examined, had an odour entirely distinct from that of liquid storax. A thick, dark-coloured, opaque, impure substance is obtained from the young branches of this species by boiling them in water and skimming off the fluid balsam which rises to the surface. This also has been confounded with liquid storax, but none of it comes to this country. The *effects* and *uses* of liquidambar are similar to those of storax and other balsamic substances. The dose of it is from ten to twenty grains.

2. L. Altingia, Blume; *Altingia excelsa*, Noronha.—A native of Java, where it is called *Ras-sama-la (Rasamalla* or *Rosa-mallas* auct.) It yields a fragrant balsam, which by some writers has been regarded as the liquid storax of the shops. But the latter

---

[1] [The *L. Altingia* is found in the woods of Java. It differs from the *L. styraciflua* and *orientale* in having ovate instead of palmate leaves. They are also lanceolate acuminate, and serrated. This tree, according to Lindley, yields the fragrant stimulating liquid storax or Rasamala of the Malay Archipelago.—Ed.]
[2] *Journ. de Pharm.* t. xvii. p. 338, 1831.
[3] *Journal of the Philadelphia College of Pharmacy*, vi. 190.
[4] *United States Dispensatory.*

substance comes to England by way of Trieste, and, according to Landerer,[1] is the produce of *Styrax officinale;* and as such I shall describe it hereafter (see *Styrax officinale*). Petiver[2] says that the *Rosa-mallas* grows in Cobross, an island at the upper end of the Red Sea, near Cadess, which is three days' journey from Suez. Its bark is removed annually, and boiled in salt water until it comes to a consistence like birdlime: it is then separated, put in barrels (each holding 420 lbs.), and sent to Mocha, by way of Judda. The Arabs and Turks call it *Cotter Mija.* Dr. Marquart[3] analysed some of the genuine resin of *L. Altingia,* and by distillation with carbonate of soda obtained a volatile oil resembling styrol, and a substance resembling styracin, but which had a different composition.

3. L. ORIENTALE, Miller; *L. imberbe,* Aiton; *Platanus orientalis,* Pocock.—This tree grows in Cyprus, where it is called *Xylon Effendi* (the wood of our Lord). By incisions made in the bark, it yields a kind of white turpentine, and a very fragrant oil. Dr. Lindley thinks it is probable that the liquid storax of the shops is collected from this tree; but I do not agree with him in this opinion.

ORDER XXV. SALICACEÆ, *Lindl.*—WILLOWWORTS.

SALICINEÆ, *Richard.*

CHARACTERS.—*Flowers* unisexual, amentaceous. *Stamens* distinct or monadelphous; *anthers* 2-celled. *Ovary* superior, 1-celled; *ovules* numerous, erect, at the base of the cell, or adhering to the lower part of the sides; *style* 1 or 0; *stigmas* 2 or 4. *Fruit* coriaceous, 1-celled, 2-valved, many-seeded. *Seeds* either adhering to the lower part of the axis of each valve, or to the base of the cell; comose; *albumen* 0; *embryo* erect; *radicle* inferior.—*Trees* or *shrubs.* *Leaves* alternate, simple, with deliquescent primary veins, and frequently with glands; *stipules* deciduous or persistent (*Lindley*).

PROPERTIES.—The barks of the species of this Order are astringent and tonic; the astringency being due to tannic acid, and the tonic property to salicine or some other bitter principle. An oleo-resinous or balsamic substance, of a stimulant nature, is secreted by the buds of some of the species.

112. SALIX, *Linn.*—WILLOW.

Sex. Syst. Diœcia, Diandria.

(Cortex e speciebus salicis diversis; Salicis cortex, *E.*)

HISTORY.—Dioscorides[4] speaks of the astringent qualities of the ἰτέα, or *willow* (*Salix alba?*), which was employed in medicine by the ancients. For a long series of years it fell into disuse, but was again brought into notice in 1763 by the Rev. Mr. Stone,[5] who published a paper on the efficacy of the bark of *Salix alba,* as a remedy for agues. The broad-leaved willow bark (*Salix Caprea*) was subsequently introduced into practice by Mr. James,[6] whose observations on its efficacy were afterwards confirmed by Mr. White[7] and Mr. G. Wilkinson.[8]

BOTANY. **Gen. Char.**—*Flowers* diœcious, or rarely monœcious, amentaceous; *scales* imbricated; a *gland* surrounding the stamens or ovary.

---

[1] *Pharmaceutisches Central-Blatt für* 1840, p. 11.
[2] *Phil. Trans.* vol. xxvi. p. 44.
[3] *Jahrb. für prakt. Pharmacie,* Bd. v. p. 486 (quoted by Dierbach, in the *Ergänzungsheft* to Geiger's *Handb. d. Pharm.* 2te Aufl. 1843).
[4] *Lib.* i. cap. 136.
[5] *Phil. Trans.* vol. liii. p. 195.
[6] *Observations on a particular Species of Willow,* 1792.
[7] *Observations and Experiments on the Broad-leaved Willow Bark,* 8vo. Bath, 1798.
[8] *Experiments and Observ. on the Cortex Salicis latifoliæ,* 8vo. Newcastle-upon-Tyne [1803].

Males:—*Stamens* 2 to 5, usually 2, sometimes the 2 united into 1, and then the anther is 4-celled. Females:—*Seeds* comose; the *radicle* inferior (*Bot. Gall.*)

Species.—Sir J. E. Smith[1] mentions sixty-four indigenous species of Salix; but pharmacological and botanical writers are not agreed as to which species possesses the most medicinal power. The best practical rule to follow is this:—Select those whose barks possess great bitterness, combined with astringency. The following are those which are in the greatest repute:—

1. Salix Russelliana, Smith; *The Bedford Willow.*—*Leaves* lanceolate, tapering at each end, serrated throughout, very smooth. *Footstalks* glandular or leafy. *Germen* tapering, stalked, longer than the scales. *Style* as long as the stigmas (Smith).—A *tree.* In marshy woods and wet meadows, in various parts of Britain. Flowers in April and May. Its bark abounds in tannic acid. On account of its astringency, Sir J. E. Smith regards it as the most valuable officinal species; and he observes, that if it has occasionally disappointed medical practitioners, they probably chanced in such cases to give the *S. fragilis.*

2. Salix alba, Linn.; *The Common White Willow.*—*Leaves* elliptic-lanceolate, pointed, serrated, silky on both sides; the lowest serratures glandular. *Stamens* hairy. *Germen* smooth, almost sessile. *Stigmas* deeply cloven. *Scales* rounded (Smith).—A tall *tree.* River-sides and moist woods, in various parts of Britain. Flowers in May. Its bark, called *cortex salignum,* or *cortex anglicanum* of some writers, is astringent, but less so than that of the preceding species.

3. Salix Caprea, Linn., E.; *Salix latifolia rotunda,* Bauhin; *Great Round-leaved Willow.*—*Stem* erect. *Leaves* roundish-ovate, pointed, serrated, waved, pale and downy beneath. *Stipules* somewhat crescent-shaped. *Catkins* oval. *Germen* stalked, ovate, silky. *Stigmas* nearly sessile, undivided. *Capsules* swelling (Smith).—A *tree.* Indigenous, very common; growing in woods and hedges. Flowers in April. Its bark is the *broad-leaved willow bark (cortex salicis latifoliæ)* recommended by James, White, and Wilkinson (see *ante,* p. 337).

4. Salix fragilis, Linn.; *The Crack Willow.*—*Leaves* ovate-lanceolate, pointed, serrated throughout, very smooth. *Footstalks* glandular. *Germen* ovate, abrupt, nearly sessile, smooth. *Scales* oblong, about equal to the stamens and pistils. *Stigmas* cloven, longer than the style (Smith).—A *tree.* Indigenous: about the banks of rivers. Flowers in April and May.

5. Salix pentandra, Linn.; *Sweet Bay-leaved Willow.*—This species is officinal in the Prussian Pharmacopœia, and is preferred by Nees von Esenbeck to all other species. Its bark is the *cortex salicis laureæ* of some pharmacologists.

6. Salix purpurea, Linn.; *Bitter Purple Willow.*—This species deserves notice on account of the intense bitterness of its bark.

Description.—Willow bark (*cortex salicis*) varies in its appearance and qualities according to the species and the age of the tree from which it is procured. In the dried state it is usually quilled and odourless. It should have a bitter and astringent taste.

---

[1] *Engl. Flora,* iv.

COMPOSITION.—The bark of *Salix alba* was analysed by MM. Pelletier and Caventou,[1] who obtained the following results :—*Bitter yellow colouring matter, green fatty matter* similar to that found in cinchona, *tannin, resinous extract, gum, wax, woody fibre,* and a *magnesian salt* containing an organic acid.

These celebrated chemists failed to isolate *salicine,* which must have been contained in their bitter yellow colouring matter, either mixed or combined with some other matter. Their resinous extract is probably identical with what Braconnot calls *corticin.*

1. TANNIC ACID.—This is the astringent principle of willow bark. Sir H. Davy[2] gives the following as the quantities of tannin [impure tannic acid] in the bark of two willows :—

		480 lbs. of bark.	lbs. of tannin.
Leicestershire Willow	[*Salix Russelliana*]	large size	33
Common Willow......	[*Salix ——?*]......	large	11

2. SALICINE.—See *post.*

CHEMICAL CHARACTERISTICS.—A decoction of the bark, made with distilled water, is coloured dark green (*tannate of iron*) by sesquichloride of iron ; but, made with spring water, dark purple. Solution of gelatin produces a precipitate (*tannate of gelatin*) in the decoction, but tincture of nutgalls causes no turbidity. A strong decoction of willow bark, containing much salicine, is reddened by concentrated sulphuric acid.

PHYSIOLOGICAL EFFECTS.—Willow bark possesses both bitterness and astringency. It belongs, therefore, to the *astringent bitters,* the effects of which have been elsewhere noticed. It is not so apt to disturb the stomach as cinchona, but its tonic and febrifuge powers are less than those of the latter. Vogt[3] ascribes to it balsamic properties.

USES.—It has been employed as an indigenous substitute for cinchona. The indications for its use, therefore, are the same as those for the latter. It is given in intermittents, dyspeptic complaints accompanied with, or dependent on, a debilitated condition of the digestive organs, passive hemorrhages, chronic mucous discharges, in the stage of convalescence after fever, and as an anthelmintic. As a local astringent, the powder or infusion is sometimes employed, but there are many more efficient remedies of this kind.

ADMINISTRATION.—The dose of the *powder* is ʒss. to ʒj. The *infusion* or *decoction* (prepared with ʒj. of the bark and Oj. of water) may be given in doses of from fʒj. to fʒiij.

SALICINUM ; *Salicine.*—Obtained in a more or less impure state by Brugnatelli, Fontana,[4] in 1825, and by Leroux and Buchner[5] in 1828, and in a pure state by Leroux[6] in 1829. Has been found in about fourteen species of *Salix* and eight species of *Populus.*[7] It has been detected in the bark, leaves, and flowers. Herberger obtained 250 grains, Merck 251 grains, from 16 ounces of the bark and young twigs of *Salix Helix :* Erdmann,

---

[1] *Journ. de Pharm.* t. vii. p. 123.
[2] *Elements of Agricultural Chemistry*, 4th edit. p. 83.
[3] *Pharmakodynamik*, Bd. i. S. 658.
[4] *Journ. de Chim. Méd.* t. i. p. 216, 1825.
[5] *Repert. für d. Pharm.* Bd. xxix. S. 411, 1828 ; also *Journ. de Pharm.* xvi. 242.
[6] *Ann. de Chim. et de Phys.* t. xliii. p. 440, also *Journ. de Chim. Méd.* t. vi. p. 340, 1830.
[7] Herberger, *Pharmaceutisches Central-Blatt für* 1838, S. 848.

however, procured, by another process, 300 grains from a pound of the bark of *Salix pentandra*.[1]　Merck's process for obtaining it, as stated by Liebig,[2] is as follows :—

"Dried or fresh willow bark is cut small, and exhausted by repeated boiling with water. The decoctions are concentrated, and while boiling treated with litharge till the liquor appears nearly colourless. The dissolved oxide of lead is removed, first by sulphuric acid, afterwards by sulphuret of barium, and, after the separation of sulphuret of lead, evaporated, when salicine crystallises, and is purified by repeated solution and crystallisation (Merck). From willow bark, which is fresh and rich in salicine, it may be obtained by cautious evaporation of the cold aqueous infusion (Merck). The oxide of lead removes from the solution gum, tannin, and extractive matter, which would impede the crystallisation of the salicine. It also combines with the salicine, forming a kind of salt, which is decomposed by the sulphuric acid and sulphuret of barium. If the latter be carefully added, neither sulphuric acid nor baryta remain in the solution; and the sulphuret of lead which separates, acts as a decolorising agent."

Salicine crystallises in silky colourless needles and laminæ. It is white, very bitter, inodorous, neutral to vegetable colours, fusible at 230° F., and combustible at a higher temperature. It rotates to the left a ray of plane polarised light. It is much more soluble in boiling than in cold water, 100 parts of which dissolve only 5·6 parts of salicine. It is also soluble in alcohol, but not so in ether or the volatile oils. It is not precipitated by any agent. Cold oil of vitriol colours it blood-red.[3] By this test the presence of salicine is detected in its solutions, and in decoctions of willow and poplar barks, or in the barks themselves. Chromic acid (or a mixture of bichromate of potash and sulphuric acid) converts salicine ($C^{26}H^{18}O^{14}$) into hydruret of salicyle (also called salicylous acid), $C^{14}H^{5}O^{4}$,H (*oil of meadow-sweet*), carbonic acid, and formic acid. Hence this acid may be employed as a test for salicine. For this purpose 3 parts of salicine, 3 of bichromate of potash, and 24 of water, are to be dissolved in water, and to the solution 4½ parts of oil of vitriol diluted with 12 parts of water are to be added. On the application of heat the well-known odour of the flowers of meadow-sweet (*Spiræa ulmaria*) is evolved. If diluted hydrochloric or sulphuric acid be boiled with a solution of salicine, the fluid becomes suddenly turbid, and deposits a precipitate of saliretine, glucose[4] being at the same time formed.

$$C^{26}H^{18}O^{14} \quad + \quad 4HO \quad = \quad C^{14}H^{8}O^{4} \quad + \quad C^{12}H^{14}O^{14}$$

Salicine.　　　Water.　　　Saligenine.　　　Glucose.

By the prolonged action of heat, saligenine loses the elements of water (2HO) and becomes saliretine ($C^{14}H^{6}O^{2}$). [This is the formula of the hydruret of benzoyle and of benzoine.—ED.]

---

[1] *Pharmaceutisches Central-Blatt für* 1838, S. 852.

[2] *Turner's Chemistry*, 7th edit. p. 816.

[3] Phloridzin, veratria, piperin, oil of bitter almonds, and other bodies, are also coloured red by oil of vitriol. [The colour produced by sulphuric acid in salicine is rather a carmine red. When bichromate of potash is added, the colour is deepened, and oxide of chrome is set free. Strong nitric acid gives a pale yellowish colour, deutoxide of nitrogen being evolved.—ED.]

[4] [There are two varieties of *glucose* found in fruit :—A crystallisable body represented as above by the formula $C^{12}H^{14}O^{14}$. This turns the plane of polarised light to the right, like cane-sugar and dextrine. The second variety is uncrystallisable. It is represented by the formula $C^{12}H^{12}O^{12}$. This turns the plane of polarised light to the left, like gum (see Regnault, *Cours de Chimie*, tom. iv. p. 141).—ED.]

[Salicine yields different products with nitric acid, according to its degree of concentration. One part of salicine digested for one or two days with ten parts of nitric acid (1·161) produces a yellow liquid, from which white crystalline needles of a substance called *helicine* are deposited. Its formula is $C^{26}H^{16}O^{14}+3HO$. It loses 3 eq. of water at 212° without undergoing decomposition, and it melts at 347°. Like salicine, it is not very soluble in cold, but is easily dissolved by boiling water. *Helicine* undergoes some remarkable transformations. Thus alkaline solutions (potash or ammonia), yeast (fermentum cerevisiæ), and synaptase, convert it to glucose and the oil of Spiræa ulmaris, or meadow-sweet, $C^{14}H^6O^4$. Thus—

$$C^{26}H^{16}O^{14} \quad + \quad 2HO \quad = \quad C^{12}H^{12}O^{12} \quad + \quad C^{14}H^6O^4$$

Salicine.　　Water.　　Glucose.　　Oil of Spiræa.

When the nitric acid is more concentrated, salicine is converted by it to oxalic and carbazotic acids.

Yeast and albuminous substances generally exert no action on salicine, but synaptase (the albuminous principle of the sweet and bitter almond, which acts as a ferment to amygdaline) resolves salicine at a temperature of 104° into sugar and saligenine.

$$C^{26}H^{18}O^{14} \quad + \quad 2HO \quad = \quad C^{12}H^{12}O^{12} \quad + \quad C^{14}H^8O^4$$

Salicine.　　Water.　　Glucose.　　Saligenine.

If the solution be heated, the sugar is obtained by evaporation as grape-sugar, $C^{12}H^{14}O^{14}$.

Saligenine ($C^{14}H^8O^4$).—This compound is obtained by the above process from the fermented mixture of synaptase and salicine, in rhomboidal crystals of a pearly lustre. It is very soluble in water, alcohol, and ether. Fifteen parts of cold water dissolve one part, and its solubility is greatly increased by boiling. It exerts no rotatory power on polarised light. It melts at 179°, and, as already explained by the author, it is converted by diluted acids and heat into *saliretine* and sugar. In the conversion of salicine to sugar this is no doubt a transition-product. The solution of saligenine gives with the persalts of iron a deep indigo-blue colour. It is unchanged in air; but if oxidised by platinum black it loses 2 eq. of hydrogen, and is converted to hydruret of salicyle and water.

$$C^{14}H^8O^4 \quad + \quad O^2 \quad = \quad C^{14}H^6O^4 \quad + \quad 2HO$$

Saligenine.　　Oxygen.　　Hydruret of salicyle.　　Water.—ED.]

Salicine has been repeatedly subjected to analysis. [It contains no nitrogen.—ED.]

	Atoms.		Eq. Wt.		Per Ct.		Piria.[1]							
							I.		II.		III.		IV.	
Carbon	26	...	156	...	54·54	...	54·87	...	54·24	...	54·73	...	54·48	
Hydrogen	18	...	18	...	6·29	...	6·36	...	6·39	...	6·43	...	6·31	
Oxygen	14	...	112	...	39·17	...	38·77	...	39·37	...	38·84	...	39·21	
Salicine	1	...	286	...	100·00	...	100·00	...	100·00	...	100·00	...	100·00	

[According to Piria, salicine is constituted of sugar and saligenine: thus—

$$C^{26}H^{18}O^{14} \quad = \quad C^{12}H^{10}O^{10} \quad + \quad C^{14}H^8O^4$$

Salicine.　　Sugar.　　Saligenine.

It appears to be easily converted to *salicylous acid*, or hydruret of salicyle, by diluted sulphuric acid and bichromate of potash, as described by the author. This acid is represented by the formula $C^{14}H^6O^4$, or $C^{14}H^5O^3+HO$. It is isomeric with benzoic acid, and is identical in composition and properties with the oil of Spiræa ulmaria. It is a colourless oily liquid, boiling at about

---

[1] *Ann. de Chim. et de Phys.* 3me sér. t. xiv. p. 257, 1845.

380°. It exerts no rotatory power on the plane of polarised light. It is almost insoluble in water, but is very soluble in alcohol and ether. It reddens and afterwards bleaches litmus. It has a hot taste and an aromatic odour resembling that of bitter almonds. A persalt of iron produces with it a rich violet colour. Salicine, as mentioned by the author (*infra*), appears to be invariably changed in the animal organism into salicylous acid. It has been noticed that insects which feed on the willow-bark (and especially one variety of beetle) produce this transformation. If the insect be placed on a sheet of white paper impregnated with a solution of a persalt of iron, and it be irritated while passing over the paper, it will emit salicylous acid, indicated by the track of the insect assuming an intense violet colour.—ED.]

PROPERTIES.—Salicine possesses tonic properties analogous to disulphate of quina, than which it is less liable to irritate the stomach. In its passage through the system salicine undergoes oxidation, and is converted into hydruret of salicyle (*salicylous acid*), which is found in the urine. Its presence is detected by a persalt of iron, which strikes an intense violet colour with urine containing it.[1] It is employed in dyspepsia, intermittents, and other diseases for which cinchona and disulphate of quina are usually exhibited. In the event of the latter becoming scarce, salicine would prove an exceedingly valuable substitute. The dose of it is from 10 to 30 grains. It may be given in powder mixed with sugar, or dissolved in some aromatic water.[2] Its quickest action in intermittents is said to be obtained when it is given in powder.[3] [Buchner states that 12 grains in divided doses will generally arrest ague.—ED.]

ORDER XXVI. CUPULIFERÆ, *Richard.*

CORYLACEÆ, *Mirbel.*

CHARACTERS.—*Flowers* unisexual: males amentaceous; females aggregate or amentaceous. *Males:*—Stamens 5 to 20, inserted into the base of the scales, or of a membranous valvate calyx, generally distinct. *Females:*—Ovaries crowned by the rudiments of an adherent (superior) calyx, seated within a coriaceous involucre (*cupule*) of various figure, and with several cells and several ovules, the greater part of which are abortive; *ovules* twin or solitary, pendulous or peltate; *stigmas* several, subsessile, distinct. *Fruit* a bony or coriaceous 1-celled nut, more or less enclosed in the involucre. *Seeds* solitary, 1, 2, or 3: *embryo* large, with plano-convex, fleshy cotyledons, and a minute superior radicle.—*Trees* or *shrubs*. *Leaves* with stipules, alternate, simple, often with veins proceeding straight from the midrib to the margin (*Lindley*).

PROPERTIES.—The prevailing quality of this Order is astringency, owing to the presence of tannic acid in the wood as well as in the bark.

Besides the species presently to be described, the following may be here briefly referred to:—*Quercus tinctoria*, or the *Black Oak*, is a native of America. Its bark, called *quercitron*, is used by dyers. In the United States it is employed medicinally, but it is said to be disposed to irritate the bowels.—The large capsules or acorn-cups of *Quercus Ægilops* are imported from the Levant, under the name of *Velonia*. They are astringent, and are employed by dyers.—A saccharine substance exudes from the leaves of *Quercus mannifera* in Kurdistan.[4]

---

[1] Laveran and Millon, *Comptes rendus*, t. xix. p. 347; and *Annuaire de Chimie*, p. 585, 1845. These writers state that salicylic acid was also produced; but Wöhler and Frerichs found that hydruret of salicyle did not become changed into salicylic acid in its passage through the system.
[2] Blom, *Beobacht. u. Beitr. üb. die Salicine*, Potsdam, 1835.
[3] *Lond. Med. Gaz.* Feb. 28, 1840.
[4] Lindley, *Botanical Register*, May and June, 1840.

113. QUERCUS PEDUNCULATA, *Willd.*—THE COMMON BRITISH OAK.

Quercus Robur, *Linn.*
Sex. Syst. Monœcia, Polyandria.
(Cortex, *L. D.*—The Bark, *E.*)

HISTORY.—The oaks (*Quercus* of botanists) were held sacred by the Greeks, Romans, Gauls, and Britons. They are mentioned in the Old Testament.[1] Both Dioscorides and Galen were acquainted with their astringent qualities. " Every part of the oak" (δρῦς ; *Q. sessiliflora* and *pedunculata*, according to Fraas, but according to Sibthorp *Q. Ægilops*), says Dioscorides,[2] " but especially the liber, possesses an astringent property."

BOTANY.   **Gen. Char.**—Monœcious.   MALE FLOWERS :—*Catkins* lax and pendulous.   *Perianth* lacerated.   *Stamens* 5 to 10.
FEMALE FLOWERS : — *Invo-
lucre* scaly ; the *scales* numerous, imbricated ; combined
with a coriaceous, hemispherical
cup.   *Perianth* 6-lobed, adnate to the ovary.   *Ovary*
3-celled ; 2 of the cells abortive.   *Stigmas* 3.   *Nut* 1-
celled, 1-seeded, surrounded
at the base by the cupule
(*acorn-cup*).   (*Bot. Gall.*)

Sp. Char.—*Leaves* deciduous, shortly-stalked, oblong-
obovate, deeply sinuate ; their
sinuses rather acute, lobes
obtuse.   *Fruits* 2 or 3 upon
a long peduncle (*Hooker*).

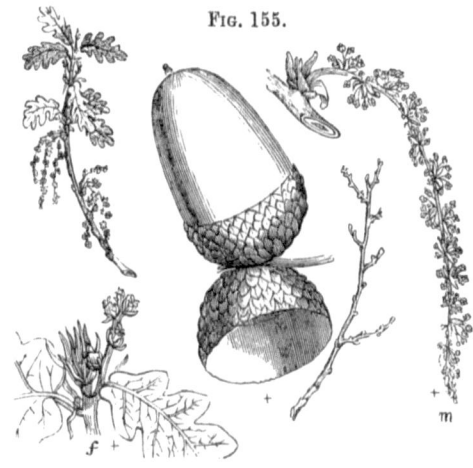

FIG. 155.

Quercus pedunculata.

A large and handsome *tree*, remarkable for its longevity.   *Twigs* round, smooth, greyish-brown.   *Leaves* bright green, furnished with a single midrib sending off veins into the lobes.   *Male flowers* yellowish ; *females* greenish, tinged with brown.

Hab.—Indigenous, growing in woods and hedges.   Flowers in April. It is found in most European countries.

BARKING.—In the spring the barks of trees contain more astringent matter, and are more readily separated from the wood.   The usual time for barking the oak is from the beginning of May to the middle of July.   The barkers make a longitudinal incision with a mallet furnished with a sharp edge, and a circular incision by means of a barking bill.   The bark is then removed by the peeling-irons ; the separation being promoted, when necessary, by beating the bark with the square end of the mallet.   It is then carefully dried in the air, by setting it on what are called lofts or ranges, and it is afterwards stacked.[3]

---

[1] *Isaiah*, i. 29, 30.
[2] Lib. i. cap. 142.
[3] Loudon's *Encyclopædia of Agriculture*, 3d edit. p. 658-9.

DESCRIPTION.—Oak bark (*cortex quercûs*) consists of pieces of from one to two feet long, which vary in their appearance according to the age of the stem or branch from which they have been taken. The bark of young stems is thin, moderately smooth, covered externally with a silvery or ash-grey cuticle, and is frequently beset with lichens. Internally it is, in the fresh state, whitish; but, when dried, brownish, red, fibrous. The bark of old stems is thick, very rough externally, cracked, and wrinkled, and is usually of inferior quality.

COMPOSITION.—According to Braconnot,[1] oak bark contains — *tannic acid, tannates of lime, magnesia, potash, gallic acid, uncrystallizable sugar, pectin,* and *lignin.*

The quantity of TANNIN [impure tannic acid] obtained by Davy[2] from oak bark is as follows :—

	Tannin afforded.
480 *lbs. of*	
Entire bark of middle-sized oak, cut in spring	29 lbs.
„ coppice oak	32
„ oak, cut in autumn	21
White interior cortical layers of oak bark.........................	72

Biggins[3] obtained 30 parts of tannin from the bark of an oak felled in winter, while the same weight of the bark of an oak felled in spring yielded him 108 parts.

CHEMICAL CHARACTERISTICS.—Decoction of oak bark reddens litmus, and becomes dark blue or purple (*tannate of iron*) on the addition of sesqui-chloride of iron. A solution of gelatin causes a precipitate (*tannate of gelatin*) with it. A solution of emetic tartar causes no precipitate with the decoction. [If alcohol be added to the decoction, concentrated to the consistence of a syrup, it causes the precipitation of *pectin*. A decoction, rendered alkaline by a fixed alkali, deposits a gelatinous matter (*pectic acid*) on the addition of acetic acid.—*Braconnot.*]

PHYSIOLOGICAL EFFECTS.—The effects of oak bark are similar to those of other vegetable astringents containing tannic acid, and have been already described.

USES.—The principal value of oak bark in medicine arises from its astringent property. Thus we employ a decoction of it as a gargle in relaxed conditions of the uvula, and in chronic inflammatory affections of the throat;[4] as a wash in flabby, ill-conditioned, or bleeding ulcers; as an injection in leucorrhœa, in piles, or in prolapsus of the uterus or rectum; as an internal astringent in old diarrhœas, in the last stage of dysentery, and in alvine hemorrhages. Poultices made of powdered oak bark have been applied with benefit to mortified parts.[5] Mr. Lizars[6] states that he has obtained "wonderful success" in the cure of reducible herniæ by bathing the groin (the hernia having been previously reduced) three or four times daily with a warm inspissated decoction of oak bark, and then applying a truss. The practice, however, is not a new one.[7]

The inhalation of finely-powdered oak bark is said to have proved very

---

[1] *Ann. de Chim. et de Phys.* t. i. p. 381.
[2] *Elem. of Agricult. Chem.* 4th edit. p. 83.
[3] Pfaff, *Syst. d. Mat. Med.* Bd. ii. S. 207.
[4] Cullen, *Mat. Med.* vol. ii. p. 45.
[5] Barton, *Collection towards a Mat. Med. of the United States.*
[6] *Ed. Med. and Surg. Journal,* July 1822.
[7] See the references in Ploucquet's *Literatura Medica,* t. ii. p. 297.

beneficial in supposed cases of pulmonary consumption.[1] The inspiration of impalpable powders of other astringents has been already noticed as a remedy for phthisis.   Connected with this, the popular opinion of the exemption of operative tanners from phthisis pulmonalis deserves to be mentioned.   Dr. Dods,[2] who has paid some attention to this subject, concludes that the popular notion is correct; and he ascribes the exemption to " the inhalation of that peculiar aroma, or volatile matter, which is constantly arising from tan-pits during the process of tanning with bark."   Hitherto, however, no suffi-cient evidence has been advanced to prove that tanners are exempt from the disease.

As a tonic, oak bark has been employed in medicine, but it is much inferior to cinchona.   Baths made of a decoction of this substance have been used by Dr. Eberle in the intermittents of very young children with benefit; and Dr. Fletcher (of Virginia) has recommended the same remedy in tabes mesenterica.[3]   The decoction, powder, and extract have been taken internally in intermittents, but they are very apt to irritate the stomach.   Dr. Cullen[4] says that both by itself, and joined with chamomile flowers, he has prevented the paroxysms of intermittents.

ADMINISTRATION.—Dose of the *powder* from half a drachm to one or two drachms.

DECOCTUM QUERCUS, L. E. D.; *Decoction of Oak Bark.* (Oak Bark, bruised, ʒx. [ʒiss. *D.*] ; Water [distilled, *L.*], Oij. [Oiss. D.]   Boil down to a pint, and strain, *L. E.*   Boil for ten minutes in a covered vessel, and strain, *D.*)—Used as a local astringent for various purposes, in the form of gargle, injection, or lotion.   Administered in doses of fʒij. to fʒvj.   Some-times employed as a bath, especially for children.

114. QUERCUS INFECTORIA, *Olivier.*—THE GALL, OR DYER'S OAK.

Sex. Syst. Monœcia, Polyandria.

(Galla ; Tumor ramuli a cynipe Gallæ tinctoriæ excitatus, *L.*—Gallæ; Excrescences, *E.*—Galls ; The Excrescences formed by Diplolepis gallæ tinctorum, *D.*)

HISTORY.—Hippocrates employed the nutgall (κηκίς) as an astringent, both internally and externally.[5]   Dioscorides[6] describes it as the fruit of the oak; and the same error is found in the works of comparatively recent writers, as of Pomet.[7]

BOTANY.   **Gen. Char.**—Vide *Quercus pedunculata.*

Sp. Char.—*Leaves* ovate-oblong, sinuate-dentate, very smooth, deciduous. *Fruit* sessile, very long.[8]

Small tree or *shrub*, from 4 to 6 feet high.   *Stem* crooked.   *Leaves* on short petioles, with a few short mucronate teeth on each side.   *Acorn* 2 or 3 times as long as the cupules.

---

[1] Eberle, *Treatise on Mat. Med.* 2d edit. vol. i. p. 268.
[2] *Lond. Med. Gaz.* vol. iii. p. 497.
[3] Eberle, *op. cit.* vol. i. pp. 267-8.
[4] *Mat. Med.* vol. i. p. 45.
[5] Ed. Fœs. pp. 609, 267, &c.
[6] Lib. i. cap. 146.
[7] *Hist. of Drugs*, Engl. translation, 1712.
[8] Olivier, *Voy. dans l'Empire Ottom.* t. ii. p. 64.

Hab.—Asia Minor, from the Bosphorus to Syria, and from the Archipelago to the frontiers of Persia.

FORMATION OF GALLS.—The term *gall* (*galla*) is applied to an excrescence or tumour formed on any part of a vegetable in consequence of the puncture of an insect. In general, the insects which give rise to galls are the gall-flies, constituting the genus *Cynips*, and forming the tribe *Gallicolæ* (*Diphlolepariæ*, Lat.) of the order *Hymenoptera*. But sometimes they are plant-lice, or *Aphidii* of the order *Hemiptera*. Thus the very astringent *Chinese galls* called *Woo-pei-tsze* (fig. 156), of which I have elsewhere[1] given a description, are produced, as the late Mr. Doubleday[2] has shown, by an Aphidian.

FIG. 156.

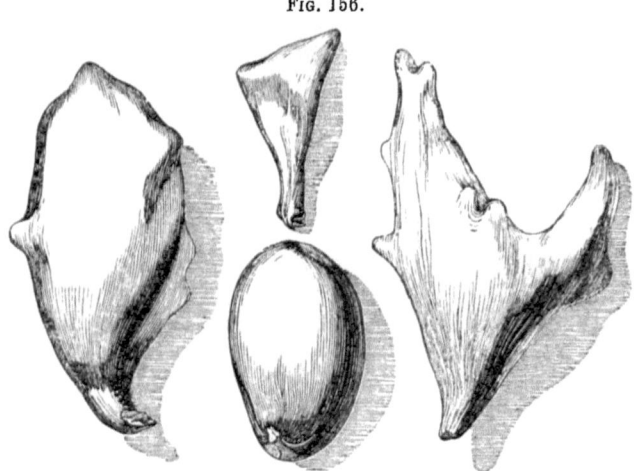

Chinese Galls, or Woo-pei-tsze.

The gall-flies (*Cynips*) are those insects by whose puncture the officinal galls are produced, and to which, therefore, our attention must be principally directed. The females of these insects are supplied with an ovipositor, called by Latreille the *borer* (*terebra*), channelled with lateral teeth. By means of this instrument they are enabled to perforate the foliaceous or cortical parts of plants for the purpose of depositing their eggs, along with an acrid liquor, in the wound thus made. The irritation thereby produced gives rise to an influx of the juices of the plant to the wounded part, and an excrescence is formed, which is termed *a gall* (*galla*). Here the insect usually undergoes its transformations: the egg produces the larva (or maggot), which feeds on the juices of the plant, and is changed into the pupa. This afterwards becomes the perfect insect (*imago*), and, perforating the gall, produces a small, round hole, through which it escapes from its prison-house.

The external form and appearance of galls are very constant when formed by the same insect on the same part of the same plant; but the galls of different species of vegetables, and of different parts of the same plants, as well as those of the same vegetable species, produced by a different insect, vary considerably. There is reason for believing that the form and appearance

---

[1] *Pharmaceutical Journal*, vol. iii. p. 384, 1844.
[2] *Ibid.* vol. vii. p. 310, 1848.

of the gall is determined more by the insect than by the plant; for we sometimes have on the same oak two kinds of galls, of very dissimilar appearance, produced by different insects.

OAK GALLS.—Most, if not all plants, but especially the oaks, are liable to the production of galls. The *oak galls* vary considerably in size, shape, texture, and other properties, according to the species and part of the oak in which they grow, and the insect by whose puncture they are produced. From their fancied resemblance to nuts, apples, currants, and other fruit, they have been respectively called *nut-galls, apple-galls, currant-galls, grape-galls, cherry-galls, artichoke-galls.*[1]

The largest species of British oak galls is the *oak apple* or *oak sponge*, produced by *Cynips Quercûs terminalis.* They are astringent, like nutgalls.

The small round *currant-galls* are produced by *C. Q. pedunculi.* They are scattered over the rachis of the amentum, giving it the appearance of a bunch of currants.

The *artichoke-gall* or *oak-strobile* is a beautiful foliose gall, produced by *C. Q. gemmæ.*

Galls of various species are produced on oak-leaves. One of the larger sorts is red and succulent, and has been called the *cherry-gall.* A smaller one is called by Reaumur the *currant-gall.* Mr. Westwood states that the large ones (as large as a boy's marble) are formed by *C. Q. folii.*

The large *Mecca* or *Bussorah galls,*[2] sometimes called *Dead-sea apples, mad-apples (mala insana),* or *apples of Sodom (poma sodomitica),* are produced on the *Quercus infectoria* by a species of *Cynips* which Mr. Westwood calls *C. insana.*

FIG. 157.   *b*

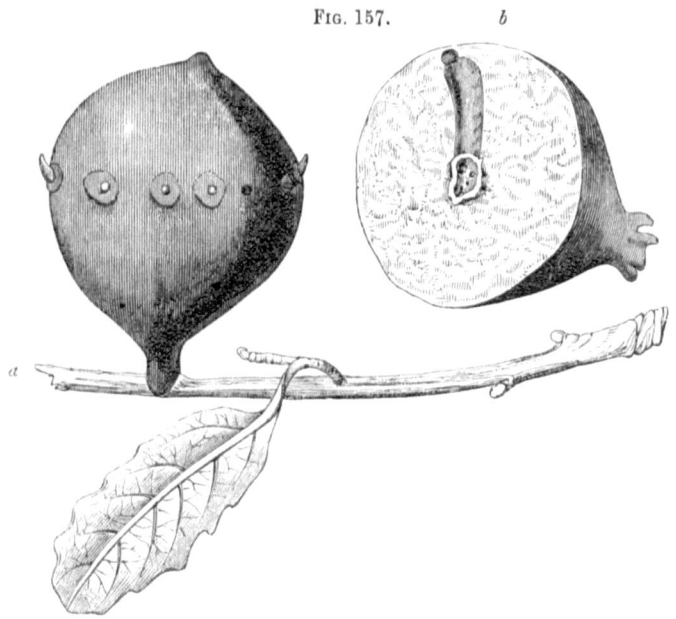

Mecca or Bussorah Galls.

a, Branch bearing a gall.   *b*, Section of a gall.

---

[1] For further details respecting galls, the reader is referred to Reaumur's article on this subject, in his *Mémoires pour servir à l'Histoire des Insectes,* 4to. vol. iii. 1737; also to Westwood's *Introduction to the Modern Classification of Insects,* 2 vols. 8vo. 1838–40.

[2] See a notice of this gall, by the author, in the *Pharmaceutical Journal,* vol. viii. p. 422.

A very irregular, deeply-furrowed, angular gall is formed on the capsule of the *Quercus pedunculata* by the *Cynips Quercûs calycis.* This is the *acorn-gall.* It is sometimes used in Germany by dyers, as a substitute for nutgalls, under the name of *Knoppern* or *Knobben.* These galls appear to me to be identical with some which I have received from M. Guibourt under the name of *gallon de Hongrie ou du Piémont.* The acorn, with its capsule, is usually attached to it. A very similar-shaped gall, attached by its middle to a young branch, is frequently found intermixed: this M. Guibourt calls the *horned gall* (*galle. corniculée*).

NUTGALLS.—The *nutgalls* (*gallæ* officinarum) of commerce are produced by the *Cynips gallæ tinctoriæ* on the *Quercus infectoria.* Ollivier[1] says that this insect lives on this species of Quercus only. On the sides and at the ends of the branches and shoots of this tree, the female makes a puncture and deposits her egg. An excrescence is soon formed, within which the larva is developed, which is changed first into the pupa and then into the imago. As soon as the perfect insect is produced, it eats its way out. If we examine those galls from which the animal has escaped, we observe externally a circular hole, of about a line in diameter, leading to a canal of from $2\frac{1}{2}$ to $3\frac{1}{2}$ lines long, which passes to the centre of the gall. But in those galls in which the insect has not put off its pupa state, we find neither an external hole nor an internal canal. In the imperforated gall, the part sometimes called "the kernel" is the cocoon of the insect in the pupa state (Kirby and Spence). Guibourt[2] states that in the immediate envelope of the central cavity of the gall he detected starch grains, and, in the exterior covering, chlorophylle and volatile oil. Guibourt has also observed, around the spherical amylaceous mass, cells serving for the respiration of the insect. Those galls from which the insect has escaped are commonly larger, lighter-coloured, and less astringent: they are termed *white galls.*

The nutgalls of different countries vary in their size, shape, weight, and quality of surface.

1. *Levant Nutgalls (Gallæ levanticæ).*—These are the ordinary nutgalls of the shops. They are in general about the size of a nut, somewhat round, tuberculated or warty; whence they were formerly called spiny or prickly galls (*galles à l'épine, gallæ spinosæ*), to distinguish them from the smooth French and other galls. They are imported from Syria, Smyrna, and Constantinople. The most esteemed *Syrian galls (gallæ syricæ)* are the produce of Mosul on the Tigris: these are the *Mosul galls (gallæ mossulicæ).* The *Aleppo galls (gallæ haleppenses)* usually pass for Mosul galls. *Tripoli galls (gallæ tripolitanæ)* come from Tripoli (also called Taraplus or Tarabulus, whence the corrupt name of "Tarablous galls"), and are inferior to the Aleppo galls. The *Turkey galls (gallæ turcicæ)* usually come from Constantinople or Smyrna [they are the produce of Anatolia.] *Smyrna galls (gallæ smyrnenses)* are not so heavy, are lighter-coloured [and may be ranked with Tripoli galls, which are now rarely met with], and contain a larger admixture of white galls than those brought from Aleppo. The galls brought from Bombay (*East India galls*) are probably the produce of Persia or neighbouring parts.[3] [They are heavy, but less sightly than those from the

---

[1] *Op. cit.*
[2] *Hist. Nat. des Drogues simples,* 4me édit. t. ii. 1849.
[3] *Mat. Indica,* vol. i. p. 145.

Levant. The latter possess a bloom which improves their appearance. The Bombay galls lose this during their transit from Persia to Bombay, and thence to England.—ED.]

In commerce three kinds of Levant galls are distinguished—viz. *black* or *blue, green,* and *white ;* but there is no essential distinction between the two first.

α. *Black* or *blue nutgalls (gallæ nigræ* seu *cæruleæ) ; green nutgalls (gallæ virides).*—These are gathered before the insect has escaped, and are called by the natives *yerli.* They vary from the size of a pea to that of a hazel-nut, and have a greyish colour. The smallest have a blackish-blue tint, and are distinguished by the name of *black* or *blue galls ;* while the larger and greener varieties are called *green galls.* Externally they are frequently tuberculated, but the surface of the tubercles and of the intervening spaces is usually smooth. Their texture is compact but fragile. They have no odour, but a styptic and powerfully astringent taste.

β. *White galls (gallæ albæ).*—These are for the most part gathered after the insect has escaped ; and hence they are perforated with a circular hole. They are larger, lighter-coloured (being yellowish or whitish), less compact, less heavy, and less astringent. They are of inferior value. [These galls vary in colour from white to pink. The whitest and heaviest are most esteemed, and are used for tanning valuable skins or furs. Those that approach a reddish pink are less heavy, and but little esteemed.—ED.]

γ. *Small Aleppo nutgalls.*—Occasionally there is imported from Aleppo a small sort of nutgall, called the *coriander gall.* Somewhat larger than these is another sort of small Aleppo gall, called the *small crowned Aleppo galls (gallæ haleppenses coronatæ).* They are about the size of a pea, or a little larger, and crowned superiorly by a circle of points or tubercles like the fruit of the myrtle or Eugenia. Although very small, they are often perforated by a large hole, so that they must have attained their maximum size ; and, there-fore, are a distinct sort from the usual Aleppo kind. Rather larger than these, and having a speckled surface, is a sort which has received the name of *Turkish diamonds.*

2. *European Nutgalls.*—Various sorts of nutgalls are produced in Europe. The *Istria* and *Abruzzi nutgalls* are intermediate in size between the usual Levant galls and the small Aleppo sort. They are somewhat turbinate or pear-shaped, wrinkled, and usually have a short peduncle. [These are mostly used by the silk-dyers of France.—ED.] The *Morea nutgalls* are about the size of the preceding, but they are " crowned." They are chiefly used on the Rhine. *French nutgalls* are spherical, very light, usually very smooth or even polished, but sometimes very slightly wrinkled. *Hungarian, Italian,* and *Bohemian nutgalls* are but little known in England.

[One variety, described in former editions of this work as a sort of Levant gall, is now known to be the produce of the Capitanata in the kingdom of Naples. They are known under the name of *marmorine nutgalls (galles marmorines,* Guibourt) of the French writers, and are about the size of the black or blue galls, but without tubercles or warts. The surface, however, is dull and roughish, something like orange berries. Their shape is round, with some-times a little elongation where the peduncle is attached. Trieste is the chief market for these galls. They are thence transmitted into Germany.—ED.]

[The following table represents the quantity of galls on which duty was paid during five years :—

	Cwt.			Cwt.
1840	1787		1843	2175
1841	2029		1844	3135.—Ed.]
1842	2783			

Composition.—Nutgalls were analysed by Sir H. Davy,[1] who obtained the following results :—

Matter soluble in water = 37 ; viz. {	Tannin .... 26·0
	Gallic acid, with a little extractive .... 6·2
	Mucilage and matters rendered insoluble by evaporation 2·4
	Carbonate of lime and saline matter .... 2·4
Matter insoluble in water (*lignin*) .... 63·0

Good Aleppo Nutgalls.. 100·0

Pelouze[2] found in 100 parts of nutgalls the following constituents : *tannic acid* 40·0, *gallic acid* 3·5, *ellagic acid* and *insoluble matter* 50, *extractive colouring matter* 6·5 = 100·0.

1. Tannic Acid (see *post*).
2. Gallic Acid (see *post*).
3. Ellagic or Bezoardic Acid (*Acidum ellagicum* vel *bezoardicum*), $C^{14}H^2O^7,3HO$.—Discovered by Braconnot, who called it *ellagic* acid, from the French word *galle* spelt backwards. It is probably produced by the slow decomposition of the tannic acid contained in the nutgall [under exposure to the air. The ellagic acid remains as a sediment mixed with gallic acid at the bottom of the vessel in which the strong infusion, decoction, or paste of galls, has been allowed to become mouldy. The mould is removed, the liquid portion drained off, and the sediment treated with boiling water, which dissolves and removes the gallic acid. The undissolved residue is then boiled with a solution of potash, which removes the ellagic acid under the form of ellagate of potash. This salt is obtained by evaporation in crystalline scales, scarcely soluble in pure water, but easily dissolved in water which is at all alkaline. From the salt of potash, the ellagic acid may be readily separated by other acids, under the form of a yellowish powder.—Ed.] It is a yellowish-grey insipid powder, scarcely soluble in cold water, a little more so in alcohol, but insoluble in ether. Like the tannic and gallic acids it forms a bluish-black precipitate with the persalts of iron. Hot nitric acid, according to Braconnot, gives it a blood-red colour. The acid has recently acquired additional interest in consequence of the discovery by Mr. Thomas Taylor[3] (subsequently confirmed by Merklein and Wöhler[4]), that the *Oriental Bezoar* is an ellagic acid calculus formed in the intestines of animals (usually a species of wild goat, termed by the Persians *Pasen*), which feed on vegetable substances containing tannin, from which the ellagic acid is produced [by changes in the system of the animal analogous to those of oxidation in the air.] Ellagic acid, therefore, must be regarded as identical with *bezoarine* (*Bezoarstoff* of John). [This acid loses 2 eq. of water when heated to 248°. Its formula is then $C^{14}H^2O^7,HO$. In combination with bases its formula is found to be $C^{14}H^2O^7$.—Ed.]

Chemical Characteristics.—Infusion of nutgalls reddens litmus paper, forms an inky compound (*tanno-gallate of iron*)[5] on the addition of a ses-

---

[1] *Phil. Trans.* for 1830.
[2] *Ann. de Chimie et de Physique*, t. liv. p. 337.
[3] *Lond. and Edin. Philosoph. Magazine* for May 1844, and also for January 1846 ; and *Catalogue of the Museum of the Royal College of Surgeons*, published in July 1845.
[4] *Ann. der Chem. u. Pharm.* Bd. lv. S. 129, 1845.
[5] [This compound is familiarly known under the name of *Ink*. It is chiefly a tannate of iron, and this resists chemical change better than gallate of iron. For the preparation of good and durable

quisalt of iron, and a yellowish-white precipitate (*tannate of gelatin*) with a solution of gelatin. If a piece of skin, depilated by lime, be immersed in the infusion, and agitated with it from time to time, all the tannic acid is absorbed, the filtered liquor striking a blue colour (*gallate of iron*) with the sesquisalts of iron, but giving no precipitate with a solution of gelatin. Infusion of galls forms precipitates (*metallic tannates* or *tanno-gallates*) in many metallic solutions; it also produces a precipitate (*a tannate*) in aqueous solutions of the vegetable alkaloids [unless too much diluted.]

TABLE OF METALLIC PRECIPITATES BY A STRONG INFUSION OF GALLS.[1]

Metal.	Solution employed.	Precipitate according to	
		Brande.	Dumas.
Manganese............	Neutral protochloride	Dirty yellow	0
Iron	Neutral protosulphate	Purple tint.........	0
Iron	Persulphate	Black..............	Blue-black.
Zinc	Chloride...................	Dirty yellow	0
Tin	Acid protochloride..............	Straw-yellow	Yellowish.
Tin	Acid perchloride	Fawn-yellow	Yellowish.
Cadmium	Chloride...................	(?)	0
Copper	Protochloride..................	Yellow brown......	?
Copper	Nitrate	Green..............	Grey.
Lead	Nitrate	Dingy yellow......	White.
Antimony	Emetic tartar..................	Straw-yellow	White.
Bismuth............	Tartrate of bismuth and potassa	Yellow and copious	Orange.
Cobalt	Chloride...................	0	Yellow-white.

PHYSIOLOGICAL EFFECTS.—As nutgalls contain a larger portion of tannic acid than any other known vegetable production, they possess in the highest degree the properties of an astringent.

USES.—The following are the principal uses of nutgalls:—

1. *As a tonic in intermittents.*—Notwithstanding Poupart's favourable report of the use of galls in these cases, they scarcely deserve notice, as we have in arsenic, cinchona, and sulphate of quina, much more effective and certain febrifuges.

---

ink, it is proper that the salt of iron should not be in the form of persalt, but in that mixed condition of proto- and persalt which is found in the common green sulphate of iron. The salt of iron should not be in excess, or the ink will speedily turn brown. If the infusion of galls be disproportionately large, the ink, under moderate exposure to air and light, will rapidly become mouldy. We subjoin a formula for good ink which we have employed for some years, and have found effectual:—Take of Powdered Galls, ʒiss.; Gum Senegal, ʒiss.; Green Sulphate of Iron, ʒj.; Water, ʒxx. Boil the galls for three hours in ʒxv. of the water, making up the loss by evaporation. After cooling, strain the liquid from the sediment, and dissolve in it the gum. When the gum is thoroughly mixed with the decoction of galls, add to it in a wide basin, by degrees, a filtered solution of the green vitriol in five ounces of the water. Mix thoroughly by agitation, and expose the liquid to the air for three or four days, occasionally stirring it. It slowly changes from a purple-brown to a blue-black colour. It should be closely bottled before it has become perfectly black. Some lumps of camphor should be placed in the bottle, as this tends to prevent mouldiness; and the ink should be kept in a dark place, as light favours the decomposition of tannic acid and the production of mould. When first used, the ink may appear pale, but by exposure it deepens in colour, the protoxide being converted to peroxide of iron.—ED.]

[1] Brande's *Manual of Chemistry*, 1848.

[2] Discrepancies arise from the strength of the solutions as well as from their acid or basic characters, so that neutral solutions should as far as possible be used.

2. *As an astringent in hemorrhages,* especially passive alvine hemorrhages.

3. *In chronic mucous discharges,* as old diarrhœas.

4. *As a chemical antidote.*—Nutgalls may be given in poisoning by ipecacuanha, emetina, the organic alkaloids generally, and those vegetable productions whose activity depends on an organic alkaloid; as opium, white hellebore, colchicum or nux vomica. Their efficacy arises from the tannic acid, which combines with the vegetable alkali to form a tannate possessing less activity than the other salts of these bases; perhaps because of its slight solubility. Nutgalls are recommended as an antidote in cases of poisoning by emetic tartar, but I very much doubt their efficacy.

5. *As a topical astringent.*—Nutgalls are applicable in any cases requiring the topical use of a powerful vegetable astringent. Thus, in the form of gargle, in relaxation of the uvula; as an injection, in gleet and leucorrhœa; as a wash, in flabby ulcers, with profuse discharge; *prolapsus ani* seu *vaginæ;* and in the form of ointment, in piles.

ADMINISTRATION.—The dose of the *powder* is from ten to twenty grains. Nutgalls are also used in the form of *infusion* and *tincture.*

Roasted nutgalls (*gallæ torrefactæ*) are used in the manufacture of copying-ink (see *Pyrogallic Acid,* post).

Besides the following officinal formulæ for the use of galls, others have been published by Mouchon.[1]

1. INFUSUM GALLÆ; *Infusion of Galls.*—Prepared by digesting ℨiv. of coarsely powdered nutgalls in f℥vj. of boiling water. Employed as a chemical antidote, and as a reagent or test. The dose is from f℥ss. to f℥ij.; or, in cases of poisoning by the vegetable alkalies, f℥iv.

2. TINCTURA GALLÆ, L. D.; *Tinctura Gallarum,* E.; *Tincture of Galls.* (Galls, bruised, ℨv.; Proof Spirit, Oij. Macerate for fourteen days [strain, express, *D.*], and filter. "This tincture may be prepared either by digestion or percolation, as directed for tincture of capsicum," *E.*) [The proportions of galls and spirit used in the three Pharmacopœias are now precisely similar. —ED.])—A powerful astringent. Dose from f℥ss. to f℥ij. Diluted with water, it forms a very useful and convenient astringent gargle and wash. Its principal use is as a chemical test, especially for the persalts of iron, [chalybeate waters], gelatin, and the vegetable alkaloids. After it has been kept for some time its tannic acid becomes converted into gallic acid, and it then ceases to occasion precipitates in solutions of gelatin and of the vegetable alkaloids, [although it still serves to detect iron. Paper impregnated with it serves as a portable test for solutions of iron.—ED.]

3. UNGUENTUM GALLÆ, D.; *Ointment of Galls.* (Galls, in very fine powder, ℨj.; Ointment of White Wax, ℨvij. Rub the powdered galls with the ointment until a uniform mixture is obtained.)—Astringent. Mixed with zinc ointment, it is applied to piles after the inflammatory stage is passed. Mr. B. Bell[2] recommends an ointment composed of equal parts of powdered galls and hog's lard or butter, in external hemorrhoidal swellings.

---

[1] *Gaz. des Hôp. Civ. et Milit.* 13 Avril, 1837.
[2] *Syst. of Surgery.*

4. UNGUENTUM GALLÆ COMPOSITUM, L.; *Unguentum Gallæ et Opii,* E.; *Compound Ointment of Galls.* (Galls, in very fine powder, ʒvj.; Opium, powdered, ʒiss. [ʒj. *E.*]; Lard, ʒvj. [ʒj. *E.*] Mix.)—An excellent astringent application to *blind piles* (*i. e.* piles without hemorrhage) and prolapsus ani. The opium diminishes the pain which the galls might otherwise occasion, when the hemorrhoidal tumours are very sensible. From ʒss. to ʒj. of camphor is frequently added to this ointment. [The *Unguentum Gallæ* of the *United States* Pharmacopœia is prepared according to the following formula:—(Galls, in powder, ʒj.; Lard, ʒvij. Mix them, *U.S.*) Dr. Carson remarks that a smoother ointment, and one which leaves no gritty or rough deposit on irritable surfaces, is prepared by adding ʒj. of aqueous extract of galls to ʒj. of simple ointment.—ED.]

5. ACIDUM TANNICUM, D.; *Acidum Quercitannicum*; *Tannic Acid*: in the impure state called *Tannin*, the *Tanning Principle*, or *Materia Scytodephica* (σκυτοδεψικός, belonging to curriers).—Extracted from nutgalls by ether in the percolation or displacement apparatus.[1] The ether employed is that of commerce (which contains about 10 per cent. of water). The tannic acid is at first dissolved by the ether, but is afterwards precipitated, in the form of a thick syrup, by the water contained in the ether. The syrupy stratum, consisting chiefly of the water holding tannic acid dissolved, is to be repeatedly washed with pure ether *in vacuo,* or at a temperature not exceeding 100° F. The residue is almost pure tannic acid. [The process introduced into the last *Dublin* Pharmacopœia is based on a principle similar to this.—ED.] Galls, in tolerably fine powder, ʒviij.; Sulphuric Ether, Oiij.; Distilled Water, ʒv. Incorporate the water and ether by agitation, and pour the resulting solution, in successive portions, upon the galls, previously introduced into a glass or porcelain percolator. The liquid which accumulates in the lower bottle will consist of two distinct strata, the heavier of which is to be separated and evaporated to dryness, finally applying an oven heat,— which, however, should not exceed 212°. From the lighter liquid the ether may be removed by distilling it by means of a water-bath, and with the aid of a Liebig's condenser.[2]

Tannic acid is a spongy, brilliant, light, odourless, white, or commonly yellowish, uncrystalline solid. It dissolves in water, alcohol, and ether; but less so in ether than in alcohol. [Water is its best solvent.] In the solid state it is unalterable in the air; but dissolved in water it absorbs oxygen, and is transformed into carbonic acid, which escapes, and gallic acid, which remains in solution : hence it should be dissolved only at the time we are about to use it.

[The aqueous solution, when boiled, becomes turbid. Provided it be not exposed to air, but kept in a bottle quite full, the aqueous solution may be preserved for a long time without undergoing chemical change. If exposed to air, it becomes dark-coloured, mouldy, and loses its property of precipitating gelatin; but it does not appear that there is any production of gallic acid when the tannic acid is pure. The conversion alluded to by the author appears to depend on a species of fermentation, from the presence of some nitrogenous matter, of the same nature as ordinary ferment, contained in the crude gall nut. The conversion to gallic acid is prevented by all those substances which destroy the fermenting properties of yeast. It has been hitherto considered that the access of oxygen is necessary to this change; but, according to Regnault, oxygen or air is not

---

[1] Pelouze, *Ann. de Chim. et de Physique,* t. liv.
[2] [*Pharmaceutical Journal,* June 1853, p. 597.—ED.]

required; and in this respect the gallic resembles the alcoholic fermentation. Regnault states that gallic acid is a result of the decomposition of an extract of galls even in a vessel hermetically sealed. It is not improbable, therefore, that the production of gallic acid may be in some cases increased by the addition of ordinary ferment (yeast), as it is often procured with difficulty and only in small quantity from common galls.—Ed.]

The following are the *characteristics* of this substance:—It has an intensely astringent taste, and a slightly acid reaction. It produces with a solution of gelatin a white precipitate (*tannate of gelatin*); with a solution of a sesquisalt of iron, a deep blue compound (*tannate of iron*); and with solutions of the vegetable alkalies, white precipitates (*tannates*), slightly soluble in water, but very soluble in acetic acid. The mineral acids also cause precipitates with concentrated solutions of tannic acid, as do the alkalies and their carbonates. [The carbonates are decomposed by a strong solution of it. The diluted sulphuric or hydrochloric acid, on boiling, converts it to gallic acid.—Ed.] Gelatinous alumina rapidly absorbs tannic acid from its solution, and forms an insoluble compound with it. [When a few drops of a solution of this acid are added to a glass of lime-water, a dense white precipitate is formed (*tannate of lime*), acquiring rapidly a grey and a dingy green colour. It thence passes through various shades to a dark purple-brown colour. Tannic acid is dissolved by strong sulphuric acid, forming a dingy purple-brown solution, almost black. It does not produce the red or crimson colour of gallic acid under the same circumstances, and there is a black deposit when it is added to water.—Ed.]

Tannic acid is composed of $C^{18}H^8O^{12} = C^{18}H^5O^9, 3HO$; consequently its equivalent or atomic weight in the hydrated state is 212. [In combination, the 3 eq. of water are replaced by 3 eq. of metallic oxide. Thus, on boiling for some time a solution of tannic acid with a solution of acetate of lead, a yellow precipitate is formed, the formula of which is $3PbO, C^{18}H^5O^9$.—Ed.] Its symbol is $\overline{Tan}, 3HO$; or $\overline{Qt}, 3HO$.

Tannic acid is employed in medicine, in chemistry, and in the arts. Considered as a medicine, tannic acid is a powerful agent of the astringent class. As a *topical* remedy, it is probably the most powerful of all vegetable astringents or styptics. Its chemical action on fibrin, albumen, and gelatin explains this. It is the active principle of a very large proportion of vegetable astringents. Given to a dog in doses of from 7½ to about 93 grains, it did not affect the health of the animal: it caused constipation, but its appetite remained the same. The urine gradually became darker-coloured and opaque, and was found to contain both gallic and pyrogallic acids, and a humus-like substance. The tannic acid had become converted into these bodies during its passage through the animal system.[1] The gallic acid was detected in the urine by the blackish-blue precipitate produced by the persalts of iron, and by no precipitate being produced with gelatin. Pyrogallic acid was detected by the bluish-black precipitate produced by the protosalts of iron. On the human subject tannic acid operates as a constipating agent, when given in a sufficient dose and frequently repeated. Cavarra[2] states that 2½ grains taken three days successively produced this effect on himself. The *remote* effects of tannic acid are not so obvious, but they appear to be astringent, though in

---

[1] Wöhler and Frerichs, *Chemical Gazette*, vol. vi. p. 231, 1848.
[2] Cavarra, *Lond. Med. Gaz.* vol. xx. p. 171, 1837.

a much feebler degree. As the tannic acid becomes changed into gallic acid during its passage through the system, it is probably the latter agent which operates on remote parts as an astringent when tannic acid is administered. If this opinion be correct, tannic acid would act, as Dr. Garrod[1] has suggested, less powerfully as a remote astringent than an equal weight of gallic acid. But, as a topical astringent, tannic is far more powerful than gallic acid; because its chemical reaction on albumen, gelatin, and fibrin is energetic, while gallic acid exerts no action on these principles.

Tannic acid is used as an astringent chiefly in hemorrhages and profuse secretions; and also to constringe relaxed fibres. In hemorrhages it has been used both topically as a styptic (in bleeding gums, piles, and uterine hemorrhage), and remotely as an astringent (in hemorrhage from the lungs, stomach, bowels, kidneys, and uterus). In chronic fluxes it has likewise been employed both as a topical and a remote remedy: topically in gonorrhœa, gleet, leucorrhœa, and ophthalmia; remotely in pulmonary catarrh, diarrhœa, dysentery, leucorrhœa, gonorrhœa, and cystirrhœa. To restrain the phthisical sweating it has been recommended by Charvet and others, and Giadorow[2] states that, given in combination with opium, he cured (?) two cases of diabetes by it. To constringe fibres, it is applied to spongy gums and prolapsed bowel. As an application to sores, it has been employed by Ricord in chancres, and by Mr. Druitt[3] in sore nipples. Dr. Scott Alison[4] has recently recommended its use in various other cases:—as a tonic or peptic in dyspepsia; as a "histogenetic" to promote the genesis and improve the quality of the blood, in rickets; as a nervine in nervous debility and languor; and to arrest or retard the growth of heterologous formations (tubercle and malignant disease). It has likewise been given as an antidote to check excessive vomiting from ipecacuanha or emetina.—Tannic acid may be administered in doses of from 3 to 10 or more grains, in powder, pill, or solution. When we employ it as a remote agent, the pill-form seems to be the most appropriate mode of exhibition.—As a lotion or injection, it may be used in the form of aqueous solution, containing from 4 to 6 or more grains in the fluidounce. It has also been employed in the form of ointment, composed of ʒij. of the acid dissolved in fʒij. of distilled water, and mixed with ʒxij. of lard.

In chemistry, tannic acid is employed as a reagent or test. Its solution should be fresh made when used, and preserved in a bottle kept full.

In the arts it serves various useful purposes. It is the active principle of the tanning substances. In the manufacture of white wines it is used to coagulate the substance called *glaïadine*, which is apt to excite the viscous fermentation in these wines.

6. ACIDUM GALLICUM, D.; *Gallic Acid*.—It is usually prepared by exposing for a long time an infusion of nutgalls to the air at a moderate temperature, removing now and then a mouldy skin which forms on the surface of the liquid. A sediment of impure gallic acid is obtained, which requires to be purified by solution in boiling water, decolorised by animal charcoal, and crystallised. In this process the tannic acid of the nutgalls is

---

[1] *Lancet*, Dec 30, 1848.
[2] *Annali universali di Medicina*, quoted by Dr. Dunglison, in his *New Remedies*, 5th edit. 1846.
[3] *Provincial Med. Journal*, Oct. 9th, 1844.
[4] *London Journal of Medicine*, 1850.

assumed to absorb atmospheric oxygen, and to be converted into gallic acid, carbonic acid, and water.

$$C^{18}H^8O^{12} \quad + \quad O^8 \quad = \quad 2(C^7H^3O^5) \quad + \quad 4CO^2 \quad + \quad 2HO$$

| Hydrated tannic acid. | | Gallic acid. | Carbonic acid. | Water. |

This process is favoured by the presence of a nitrogenised matter, which acts as a ferment; and the decomposition is termed the *gallic fermentation*.[1] The mouldy skin which forms on the surface is called *mycoderma,* and resembles mother of vinegar.

[Two processes are given in the last *Dublin* Pharmacopœia,—one similar to that described by the author. We here subjoin them.

Galls, in coarse powder, lb. j.; Distilled Water, as much as may be necessary. Having placed the galls in a porcelain dish, pour on as much water as will convert them into a thick paste, and keep them in this moistened condition for six weeks, at a temperature of between 60° and 70°, adding water from time to time, so as to supply what is lost by evaporation. Let the residue be boiled for twenty minutes with forty-five ounces of water, and then placed on a calico filter. The filtered solution, on cooling, will afford a copious precipitate. Let this be drained on a calico filter, then subjected to strong expression, after having been first enveloped in blotting-paper, and again dissolved in ten ounces of boiling water. When, upon ceasing to apply heat, the solution has cooled down to 80°, pour it off from the crystals which have formed, and, having washed these with three ounces of ice-cold water, dry them,—first in blotting paper, and finally by a steam or water heat.

By boiling the undissolved portion of the galls with forty-five additional ounces of water, filtering into a capsule containing the liquor decanted from the crystals formed in the preceding process, evaporating down to the bulk of ten ounces, and cooling to 80°, an additional quantity of the crystallised acid will be obtained.

Or : Galls, lb. j.; Oil of Vitriol of commerce, f℥xxvj.; Water, Ov. ℥xiv. Steep the galls for twenty-four hours in one pint of the water, then transfer them to a glass or porcelain percolator, and pour on a pint and a half of the water in successive portions. Dilute five ounces of the oil of vitriol with an equal bulk of water, and, when the mixture has cooled, add it to the infusion obtained by percolation, stirring well, so as to bring them into perfect contact. Let the viscid precipitate which forms be separated by a filter, and to the solution which passes through add five ounces more of the oil of vitriol, which will yield an additional precipitate. This being added to that previously obtained, let both be enveloped in calico, and subjected to powerful pressure. Dissolve the residue in the rest of the oil of vitriol, this latter being first diluted with what remains of the water; boil the solution for twenty minutes, then allow it to cool, and set it by for a week. Let the deposit which has formed at the end of this period be pressed, dried, and then dissolved in three times its weight of boiling water; clearing the solution, if necessary, by filtration; and when it has cooled down to 80° decant the liquid from the crystalline sediment which has formed, and wash the latter with three ounces of

---

[1] [It has been already stated (*ante*, p. 354) that air is not absolutely necessary to the gallic fermentation (see *Pharmaceutical Journal*, Oct. 1854, p. 182; March 1853, p. 444).—Ed.]

ice-cold water. Finally, let it be transferred to blotting-paper, and, when deprived by this of adhering liquid, let it be dried perfectly, at a temperature not exceeding 212°.

The gallic acid obtained by either of the preceding processes may be rendered nearly white by dissolving it in twenty times its weight of boiling distilled water, and causing the solution to traverse a stratum of prepared animal charcoal spread upon a calico filter. When the liquid passes through colourless, it should be evaporated to one-sixth of its volume, and then suffered to cool, in order to the separation of the crystallised acid, *D*. [By redissolving the crystals in alcohol, and evaporating slowly the alcoholic solution, it may be obtained in a state of great purity.—ED.]

PROPERTIES.—Pure gallic acid is a colourless, crystallisable acid, with an acidulous and styptic taste. It is soluble in water, alcohol, and slightly so in ether, and its solutions have a strongly acid reaction. It produces a deep blue colour with the salts of the sesquioxide of iron, in which circumstance it agrees with tannic acid; but it differs from the latter acid in not precipitating solutions of gelatin, albumen, or the salts of the alkaloids. To detect gallic acid mixed with tannic acid, the latter may be previously removed from its solution by precipitation with a solution of gelatin. The gallic acid may then be detected by the salts of the sesquioxide of iron. It does not occasion any precipitate with the salts of the pure protoxide of iron.

[Among other properties of this acid may be mentioned the following :—Its aqueous solution is not decomposed by keeping, except when exposed to air. It then becomes brown, a vegetable mould is formed on the surface, and we have found this liquid to possess the property of precipitating gelatin. Gallic acid, when in excess, forms stable salts with alkaline bases; but when the alkali predominates, oxygen is absorbed, and the liquid undergoes various changes of colour. Potash and ammonia poured on crystals of gallic acid produce a rich red-coloured solution. A small quantity of a solution of gallic acid added to a glass of lime water, produces at first a white precipitate (gallate of lime). This rapidly becomes blue, and passes through a violet tint to a dark purple colour. The crystals, dissolved in boiling concentrated sulphuric acid, produce a rich crimson-red solution. When poured into cold water, a red crystalline precipitate is formed, having the formula $C^7H^2O^4$. The gallic acid merely loses an equivalent of water. It deoxidises nitric acid, producing a red colour like that caused by morphia. When a solution of gallic acid is added to a solution of nitrate of silver, there is no precipitate, but the silver is slowly reduced. If the mixture be warmed, the reduction of the metal is instantaneous. On account of this property, gallic acid is much used in photography. Gallic acid equally reduces the solutions of gold.—ED.]

Free from colour. Destroyed by heat. Soluble in water and rectified spirit. To the preparations of sesquioxide of iron dissolved in water it imparts a bluish-black colour: but it throws down nothing from a solution of isinglass.—*Ph. Lond.*

Gallic acid consists of $C^7H^3O^5$,HO : hence its equivalent or atomic weight is 94. [It loses 1 eq. of water at 212°, and becomes $C^7H^3O^5 = 85$.—ED.] When heated by an oil-bath to 365° or 400° F., it gives out carbonic acid, and is resolved into *pyrogallic acid* ($C^6H^3O^3$). If, however, it is rapidly heated to 480° F., it gives out water, carbonic acid, and becomes *metagallic acid* ($C^{12}H^3O^3$).

Uses.—Gallic acid is employed in medicine as an astringent; but as a topical agent it is greatly inferior to tannic acid. [The powdered acid placed in a deep cut has been found to arrest the hemorrhage without causing pain; and a lotion formed of ʒij. of acid in a pint of warm water has subdued the inflammation in erysipelas of the face.—Ed.] Unlike the tannic acid, it causes precipitates neither in gelatinous nor in albuminous solutions: and a piece of skin does not absorb gallic acid from its aqueous solution, as it does tannic acid from its solution. Its chemical action on the constituents of the animal tissues is thus much weaker than that of tannic acid. No obvious effects result from the introduction of a few grains into the stomach. Twenty-four grains have produced a sweetish taste and a slight feeling of internal heat; but no other effect.[1] It has been administered in doses of from fifteen to thirty grains against the Tænia Solium, but without any benefit. For reasons already stated it is probable that, in equal doses, it is more powerful, as a remote astringent, than tannic acid. Dr. Todd[2] says that in all cases of hemorrhage—whether hæmoptysis, hæmatemesis, hæmaturia, or any other form dependent on hemorrhagic tendency—he considers it to be the best styptic we possess. The dose of it is from three to ten grains or more three or four times a day. It may be used in the same forms as tannic acid.

[The experience of Dr. Todd regarding the efficacy of gallic acid as an internal astringent, has been lately confirmed by Dr. Richard Neale, of University College Hospital. This gentleman has found it serviceable in five-grain doses in hæmoptysis, hæmaturia, hæmatemesis, menorrhagia, and in the discharge of blood from the bowels. Under its use in ten-grain doses he found that the œdema attending albuminuria nearly disappeared; and although the case ultimately proved fatal, the symptoms were greatly ameliorated.

In cases of acute tonsillitis and scarlatinal sore-throat, he has found great benefit arising from the use of the under-mentioned gargle :—℞ Acidi Gallici, Ʒij.; Liq. Sodæ Chlorinatæ (Beauf.), ʒij.; Aquæ destillatæ calidæ, ℥viij. M. Ft. gargarisma sæpe utend.

This gargle assumes a dark olive-brown colour, owing to the action of the excess of alkali in the chloride of lime upon the gallic acid, but the taste is said not to be unpleasant.[3]—Ed.]

7. ACIDUM PYROGALLICUM ; *Pyrogallic Acid.*—[This acid has within the last few years been brought into very extensive use in one branch of photography; namely, in the collodion process on glass. It is procured, as stated by the author, as a result of the effect of heat on gallic acid or powdered galls. Crystallised gallic acid is gradually heated by an oil-bath to about from 365° to 400°, and the vessel is maintained at this temperature for a long time. The gallic acid at first loses an equivalent of water; it then melts, carbonic acid is evolved, and pyrogallic acid slowly sublimes in small white crystalline scales, leaving a brown residue in the retort. The change may be thus expressed :—

$$C^7H^3O^5 \quad = \quad C^6H^3O^3 \quad + \quad CO^2$$

| Gallic acid. | Pyrogallic acid. | Carbonic acid. |

It will be perceived, therefore, that in constitution it resembles the neutral organic compounds, gum, starch, and sugar, in the fact that the oxygen and hydrogen are in the

---

[1] Chevallier, *Dict. des Drogues,* t. i. p. 93, Paris, 1827.
[2] *London Medical Gazette,* N.S. vol. viii. p. 101, January 19, 1849.
[3] [*Med. Times and Gazette,* May 12, 1855, p. 458.]

proportions to form water. Powdered galls, or the dry evaporated extract of galls, will also yield this acid. For this purpose the substance may be cautiously heated to the temperature above mentioned in an earthen vessel, and a paper cone placed over the vessel to receive the sublimed crystals.

Properties.—Pyrogallic acid is a crystallisable volatile acid. It is readily soluble in water, alcohol, and ether. It differs remarkably from gallic acid by reason of its very great solubility in cold water. It is usually seen in white crystalline scales. It melts at $257°$, and is sublimed at about $400°$ without change. If heated rapidly above this temperature it is converted into water and metagallic acid. It strikes a rich blue colour with the protosalts of iron, and a blue green with the persalts. It produces, when added to lime water, a beautiful crimson colour, which becomes rapidly altered by oxidation. It reduces silver in the *cold* instantly; and by the aid of heat it reduces the salts of gold and mercury. It is dissolved by concentrated sulphuric acid, but when the mixture is heated it is carbonised and decomposed, thus differing strikingly from gallic acid in this respect. When combined with an excess of potash, it absorbs oxygen perfectly, and with great rapidity, acquiring a brown colour. It has thus been used in the analysis of gases for the removal of free oxygen in neutral mixtures. The crystals moistened with strong ammonia acquire at first a yellow, and then a dingy brown colour. Gallic acid produces with ammonia a bright crimson-red colour, passing slowly to brown. The aqueous solution of pyrogallic acid, when exposed to air, undergoes rapid changes by oxidation, and is speedily decomposed.[1]—Ed.]

Pyrogallic acid, in an impure form, is employed in the preparation of a hair-dye and of copying ink. By the dry distillation of galls, it is obtained partly in the form of a sublimate, partly in the fluid form. The sublimate and fluid are to be dissolved in distilled water, the solution deodorised by animal charcoal, concentrated by evaporation, and then mixed with spirit of wine and some agreeable volatile oil. The resulting compound is a *hair dye*, which stains the hair dark brown; and the tint is not removed by sweat or moisture. It must be cautiously applied, as it stains the hands.[2] Roasted nutgalls are used in the manufacture of copying ink on account of the dark colour which the pyrogallic acid produces with the sulphate of the protoxide of iron.

[8. ACIDUM METAGALLICUM ; *Metagallic Acid.*—When gallic or pyrogallic acid is suddenly heated to a temperature of $480°$, a small quantity of pyrogallic acid is sublimed; but the greater part is converted into water, carbonic acid, and metagallic acid. This remains in the retort as a brownish-coloured substance, resembling in appearance and chemical properties humic and ulmic acids. Its formula is $C^6H^2O^2$. Its production from gallic acid is represented in the subjoined equation:—

---

[1] [Notwithstanding the well-marked chemical distinctions between gallic and pyrogallic acids, an attempt was lately made to include pyrogallic acid under the Talbotype patent, as being *ejusdem generis* with gallic acid. A patent for paper was assumed to include collodion, and a patent for gallic acid was assumed to include pyrogallic acid, although neither substance was known to science when the patent was taken out! In the case of *Talbot* v. *Laroche*, tried at Guildhall in December 1854, the plaintiff, a scientific man, on being asked the distinction between the two acids, said that by sublimation gallic acid " did not *change its distinctive nature*, but became more soluble in water." Several chemical gentlemen gave some support to this opinion, although it involved the postulate that a product of decomposition by heat was of the same nature as the substance which produced it. The reduction of a salt of silver is no proof of identity, or otherwise tannic and formic acids and the protosalts of iron might be included under the gallic acid patent. The learned judge who tried this case showed a masterly power of analysing scientific subtleties; and he so placed the matter before the jury, that they gave a verdict to the effect that gallic acid and pyrogallic acid were in substance not the same; thus extinguishing the claim of the patentee.

Pyrogallic differs from gallic acid photographically in its immediate, uniform, and complete reduction of the salt of silver which has only for one moment received the impression of the solar rays. The acid could not be used in mixture with nitrate of silver, as gallic acid is directed to be used under the patent (gallo-nitrate of silver), on account of its immediate decomposition of the salts of silver, while gallic acid alone would operate too slowly on the collodion-film. That the altered condition of the collodion-film is revealed by the chemical action of a solution of pyrogallic acid, furnishes a wonderful instance of the molecular change produced instantaneously by the solar rays. But for this, it might have been supposed that the light had produced no change.—Ed.]

[2] *Pharmaceutical Journal*, vol. iii. p. 585, 1844.

$$C^7H^3O^5 \quad = \quad C^6H^2O^2 \quad + \quad CO^2 \quad + \quad HO$$

Gallic acid.   Metagallic acid.   Carbonic acid.   Water.

Metagallic acid is also the result of the decomposition by heat of tannic acid.

It is insoluble in water, but soluble in alkaline liquids, forming brown-coloured solutions, from which acids precipitate the original substance unchanged.—Ed.]

[115. Quercus tinctoria, *Bartram.*—Black or Dyer's Oak.

Sex. Syst. Monœcia, Polyandria.

Gen. Char.—See *ante*, p. 342.

Sp. Char.—The *leaves* are obovate or oblong, sinuate, lobed, pubescent beneath. *Male flowers* in slender, long, filiform aments. *Cup* turbinate. *Acorn* small, ovoid, flattened at top.

This is one of the largest forest-trees of the United States, attaining in favourable situations the height of ninety or one hundred feet, with spreading branches, and a rough, dark-coloured bark.

The bark when separated is thick and rugged, full of fissures, and black externally; internally, it is fibrous and of a red colour, increased by drying. It breaks with a rough fracture. That obtained from the young shoots and smaller branches is smoother externally, and the inner fibres are finer. The odour is strong, and the taste is bitter and styptic, tinging the saliva yellow when chewed. The cellular integument contains a yellowish-brown colouring principle. The interior layer when separated constitutes *Quercitron Bark,* used for the purpose of dyeing; it is shipped to Europe.

In consequence of the colour imparted to leather, it is not much used for tanning. As it soils the clothes an objection is urged against it in medicine.

The medicinal properties and uses are the same as those enumerated under *Q. pedunculata.*—Ed.]

[116. Quercus alba, *Linn.*—White Oak.

Sex. Syst.—Monœcia, Polyandria.

Gen. Char.—See *ante*, p. 342.

Sp. Char.—*Leaves* obovate, oblong; obliquely divided into obtuse lobes; *segments* oblong, entire; *cup* hemispherical, tuberculated; *acorn* ovoid, oblong; *fruit* in pairs.

This tree is less elevated than the *Q. tinctoria.* It forms, however, a larger and more regularly-expanded head with numerous horizontal branches. The trunk and branches have a whitish hue: hence the name *White Oak.* The leaves are of a silvery appearance, with a hoary under surface. The young leaves are covered with a fine silky down.

The bark is rough externally, of a light colour; the effete epidermis being arranged in flat layers. On drying, the internal layer becomes brown. It breaks with a stringy fracture. The odour is decided and tan-like; taste astringent and bitter. This bark is used in tanning. For medicinal purposes it is preferred to the black oak.

DECOCTUM QUERCUS ALBÆ, U.S.; *Decoction of White Oak Bark.* (Take of White Oak Bark, bruised, an ounce; Water, a pint and a half. Boil down to a pint, and strain.)—Used as the *Decoctum Quercûs,* p. 345.—Ed.]

117. Quercus Suber, *Linn.*—The Cork Tree.

Sex. Syst. Monœcia, Polyandria.

(Cortex.)

Φελλός, Theophrast., Hist. Plant. lib. iii. cap. 16 ; *Suber*, Pliny, Hist. Nat. lib. xvi. cap. 13, and lib. xxiv. cap. 8.—This species of Quercus has a cracked fungous bark, and ovate-oblong, bluntish, coriaceous, entire or sharply serrated leaves, which are downy beneath. It is a native of northern parts of Africa and of the southern parts of Europe, especially of Spain, Portugal, and France. It grows to the height of 20 or 30 feet.—According to Mohl,[1] the bark of a young branch of Quercus Suber consists of four distinct parts : 1st, an exterior layer or *epidermis* ; 2dly, *colourless cellular tissue*, the *epiphlœum* of Link, the *phlœum* (φλοιός, the bark of trees) or *peridermis* of Mohl, the *suberous envelope* of some writers; 3dly, *green parenchyma*, the *mesophlœum* of Link, the *herbaceous* or *cellular integument* of others; 4thly, a *fibrous layer* called *endophlœum* or *liber*. Of these four layers, two (namely, the 2nd and 4th) are useful in pharmacy and medicine.

1. SUBER; *Cork ; Cortex exterior Quercûs Suberis ; Exterior Bark of the Cork Tree.*— The substance known in commerce as *cork* is the *epiphlœum* or *suberous envelope* above mentioned. When the branches are from three to five years old, the epidermis cracks by distension, and the second layer enlarges on the inner side by the deposition of new layers. These constitute *cork*.[2] It falls naturally every eight or nine years, but for commercial purposes is usually removed one or two years before this period. That season of the year is selected when the bark adheres the most firmly to the wood, in order that the cork may be raised without endangering the separation of the liber from the alburnum. By this precaution the trees are not at all injured by the corking process ; nay, they are said to be more healthy and vigorous than when the cork is allowed to accumulate on their stems. The trees yield these crops from the age of 15 to 150 years.

To remove the cork, an incision is made from the top to the bottom of the tree, and a transverse circular incision at each extremity ; the cork is then stripped off. To flatten it, a number of layers are piled up in a pit of water, and loaded with weights to keep them down. Subsequently they are dried, and in that state exported. Our supply is principally derived from Spain and Portugal. To close the transverse pores, cork is charred.

The physical properties of cork are too well known to need description. Its leading character is elasticity. In this respect it is similar to the wood of *Anona palustris*, called *cork wood*, and which is used in Jamaica by the country people, instead of corks, to stop up their jugs and calabashes.[3] When thin slices of cork are examined by the microscope, they present a cellular appearance, the cells being four-cornered and tabular.

The most important chemical examinations of cork are those of Chevreul[4] and Doepping.[5] According to Chevreul, cork contains traces of a *volatile oil, wax* (cerin), *soft resin, red and yellow colouring principles, tannic acid, a nitrogenous brown substance, gallic acid, acetic acid, calcareous salts,* and *suberin*. The substance to which the name of *suberin* has been given is the body which remains after cork has been successively treated with alcohol, ether, water, and diluted hydrochloric acid. In its form and physical characters it differs but little from ordinary cork. According to Doepping, it cannot be obtained pure, but always contains *cork-cellulose* ($C^{24}H^{5}O^{20}$), some *cork wax* ($C^{25}H^{5}O^{3}$), and a small quantity of a *nitrogenous body*. He found it to consist of carbon 67·8, hydrogen 8·7, nitrogen 2·3, and oxygen 21·12. When cork is treated with nitric acid, the suberin yields suberic acid ($C^{8}H^{6}O^{3}$), which imparts a peculiar character to cork and to all barks containing cork.[6]

The uses of cork for making floats for fishermen's nets, anchor-buoys, stoppers to vessels (*obturamenta cadorum*), and women's winter shoes, are mentioned by Pliny. On account of the tannic acid which it contains, cork is an improper substance for closing vessels containing chalybeate liquids (especially such as are intended for analysis), as the iron is

---

[1] *Lond. and Edinb. Phil. Mag.* vol. xii. p. 53, 1838.
[2] See also Dutrochet, *Comptes rendus*, t. iv. p. 48, Paris, 1838.
[3] *The Civil and Natural History of Jamaica*, by P. Browne, M.D., p. 256, Lond. 1789.
[4] *Ann. Chimie*, t. xcvi. p. 155.
[5] *Annalen d. Chem. u. Pharm.* Bd. xlv. S. 286, 1843 ; also, *The Chemical Gazette*, July 1, 1843.
[6] Mulder, *The Chemistry of Vegetable and Animal Physiology*, p. 478, 1849.

in part absorbed by the cork [and blackens it by forming in its substance tannate of iron. The whole of the water may thus become discoloured.—ED.]

Cork was formerly employed in medicine. Reduced to powder, it was applied as a styptic: hung about the necks of nurses, it was thought to possess the power of stopping the secretion of milk; lastly, burnt cork, mixed with sugar of lead and lard, has been used as an application to piles.

2. CORTEX ALCORNOCÆ EUROPÆÆ; *European Alcornoque[1] Bark; Cork Tree Bark.*—The bark of the cork-oak which I received from Spain under the name of *alcornoque bark* bears considerable resemblance to oak-bark, and was probably obtained from the younger branches of the cork tree. It is ash-grey externally, and wrinkled or grooved internally. The bark imported from Italy, Spain, and Barbary, under the name of *cork-tree bark*, and which is used by tanners, appears to be the inner bark of older stems. It consists apparently of the third and fourth layers above mentioned. It is in fibrous or stringy pieces, externally rusty red, internally deeply grooved or furrowed. It has very little odour, and an astringent taste. For tanning purposes the Italian bark is considered inferior to the Spanish and Barbary barks. In its medicinal properties European alcornoque bark resembles oak bark. It owes its astringency to tannic acid. Its powder, in the dose of a drachm, has been used in hemorrhages and diarrhœa.[2]

3. CORTEX ALCORNOCÆ AMERICANÆ; *American Alcornoque Bark.*—This is the genuine alcornoque bark of French and German pharmacologists. The Spanish colonists have applied the name of alcornoque bark to one or more American barks which possess some real or fancied resemblance to the alcornoque bark of their mother-country. Humboldt[3] says that the *Bowdichia virgilioides* (HBK.) is called by the inhabitants of the districts where it grows, in South America, the alcornoque. In another place,[4] he states that the same name is given to a *Malpighia* (Byrsonima) on account of the suberous bark of the trunk. Nees von Esenbeck[5] considered *Byrsonima crassifolia* (Malpighia crassifolia auct.) to be the source of the American alcornoque bark. The bark which comes from South America, and is considered to be genuine alcornoque bark, occurs in large flat, occasionally arched, pieces, having some resemblance to coarse flat cinchona bark. The epidermis is usually wanting. Externally the bark is reddish, or dark cinnamon-brown; internally it is pale. The taste is slightly bitter. It has been repeatedly subjected to analysis. Biltz[6] gives as the constituents—*peculiar crystalline matter* (alkornin), 1·15; *matter soluble in alcohol, not in ether* (oxydised tannin?), 1·67; *tannin* with a *lime salt*, 14·27; *gummy extractive*, with *starch*, a *nitrogenous substance*, and a *supersalt of lime*, 33·74; *woody fibre* and *loss*, 47·71; *ashes* of the woody fibre, 1·46 = 100·0.

American alcornoque bark possesses astringent properties. It was introduced into European practice in 1811 as a remedy for phthisis, but, after a short trial, it soon fell into disuse, and there are no grounds for supposing that it has any curative powers whatever in this disease.—Dose, in powder, ℈j. to ℨj. It may also be used in the form of infusion or decoction (prepared with ℥ss. of bark and f℥viij. of water) in doses of f℥j. or f℥ij. The dose of the extract is from gr. x. to ℈j.[7]

ORDER XXVII. ULMACEÆ, *Mirbel.*—ELMWORTS.

CHARACTERS.—*Flowers* hermaphrodite or by abortion unisexual, in loose clusters, never in catkins. *Calyx* membranous, imbricated, campanulate, inferior, irregular. *Petals* 0. *Stamens* definite; inserted into the base of the calyx; erect in æstivation. *Ovary*

---

[1] *Alcornoque* is the Spanish name for the cork-oak. It is of Arabic origin, being derived from *dorque*, signifying "denuded or badly clothed," adding the article *al*, changing *d* into *c*, and introducing the syllable *no* into the middle of the word (*Diccionario de la Lengua Castellana*, compuesto por la Real Academia Española, 1726–39).

[2] Chomel, *Abrégé de l'Hist. des Plantes usuelles*, t. ii. p. 332, 1761.

[3] *Nova Genera et Species Plantarum*, t. vi. p. 295.

[4] *Personal Narrative*, vol. vi. part i. p. 6.

[5] Geiger's *Hand. d. Pharm.* 2te Aufl. 2te Abth. 2te Halfte, S. 1651.

[6] Brande's *Archiv*, xii.; also L. Gmelin's *Handb. d. Chemie*, Bd. ii. p. 1322.

[7] For further details respecting alcornoque bark the reader is referred to a paper by the author in the *Pharmaceutical Journal*, vol. vi. p. 362, 1847.

superior, 1- or 2-celled; *ovules* solitary, pendulous; *stigmas* 2, distinct. *Fruit* 1- or 2-celled, indehiscent, membranous, or drupaceous. *Seed* solitary, pendulous; *albumen* none, or in very small quantity; *embryo* straight or curved, with foliaceous cotyledons; *radicle* superior.—*Trees* or *shrubs*, with rough, alternate, deciduous leaves, and stipules.

PROPERTIES.—The plants of this Order bear some analogy to those of Cupuliferæ in their chemical and medicinal properties. Their bark contains tannic acid,—combined, however, with mucilaginous and bitter matters. Hence it is reputed astringent and tonic.

Dr. M'Dowall, of Virginia, has proposed the bark of *Ulmus fulva* for bougies, tents, and catheters.[1]

118. ULMUS CAMPESTRIS, *Linn.*—THE COMMON SMALL-LEAVED ELM.

Sex. Syst. Pentandria, Digynia.

(Cortex interior, *L.*)

HISTORY.—Dioscorides[2] speaks of the astringent property of the bark of the elm (πτελέα), as does also Pliny.[3]

BOTANY.   **Gen. Char.**—*Flowers* hermaphrodite. *Calyx* campanulate, 4- to 5-toothed, coloured, persistent. *Stamens* 3 to 6. *Ovary* compressed. *Stigmas* 2. *Fruit* (a samara) suborbicular, with a broad membranous margin (*Bot. Gall.*)

Sp. Char.—*Leaves* doubly serrated, rough. *Flowers* nearly sessile, 4-cleft. *Fruit* oblong, deeply cloven, naked (Sir J. E. Smith).

A large *tree*, with rugged *bark*. By the latter character it is readily distinguished from *Ulmus glabra*, which has a smooth, dark, lead-coloured bark.

Hab.—Southern parts of England. Flowers in March or April.

DESCRIPTION.—The officinal part of the elm is the inner cortical portion, or *liber*. To obtain it, the *bark* should be separated from the tree in spring; and, after the epidermis and a portion of the external cortex have been removed, the *liber* should be quickly dried. As met with in the shops, the *inner elm bark* (*cortex ulmi*) consists of thin tough pieces, which are inodorous, and have a brownish-yellow colour, and a mucilaginous, bitter, very slightly astringent taste.

COMPOSITION.—According to Rink,[4] 100 parts of elm bark contain— *resin* 0·63, *gum* and *mucus* 20·3, *impure gallic acid* (tannin?) 6·5, *oxalate of lime* 6·3 (?), *chloride of sodium* (?) 4·6.

1. TANNIC ACID.—Davy[5] states that 480 grs. of elm bark yielded 13 grs. of tannin.

2. ULMIC ACID; *Ulmin.*—On many trees, especially the elm, there is not unfrequently observed a substance which was supposed to be a morbid production. When dried, it consists of a mucilaginous matter, and carbonate or acetate of potash. By the combined agency of the air and the carbonate, the organic matter is altered in its properties, and is converted into a brown substance, which combines with the potash. This brown matter has been termed *ulmin*, or *ulmic acid*. It may be formed, artificially, by a variety of processes; as by heating a mixture of wood and potash, by the action of sulphuric acid on vegetable matters, and by other methods.

CHEMICAL CHARACTERISTICS.—Infusion of elm bark becomes green (*tan-*

---

[1] *Brit. and For. Med. Review*, July 1838, art. *Elm Bark Surgery*, p. 259.
[2] Lib. i. cap. 111.
[3] *Hist. Nat.* lib. xxiv. cap. 33.
[4] Geiger, *Hand. d. Pharm.*; and Wittstein's *Handwörterbuch*.
[5] *Phil. Trans.* 1803, p. 233.

nate of iron) on the addition of a salt of the sesquioxide of iron, and forms a precipitate (*tannate of gelatin*) with a solution of gelatin.

PHYSIOLOGICAL EFFECTS.—The effects of elm bark are those of a mild astringent tonic, containing a considerable quantity of mucilage, which gives it a demulcent property. Hence, in the classification of Richter,[1] it is arranged as a *mucilaginous astringent.* The decoction, taken in full doses, accelerates the pulse, and acts as a diaphoretic and diuretic.

USES.—Lysons[2] recommended the decoction of this bark in cutaneous eruptions, and Dr. Lettsom[3] found it successful in ichthyosis. It has now fallen almost into disuse. It has been employed as a cheap substitute for sarsaparilla.[4]

ADMINISTRATION.—Used only in the form of decoction.

DECOCTUM ULMI, L. ; *Decoction of Elm Bark.* (Fresh Elm Bark, bruised, ℥iss. ; Distilled Water, Oij. Boil down to a pint, and strain.)— Formerly given in skin diseases ; now fallen into disuse. Dose, f℥iv. to f℥vj. three or four times a day.

[119. ULMUS FULVA, *Mich.*—SLIPPERY ELM.

(Slippery Elm Bark, *U.S.*)

Sp. Char.—*Leaves* very scabrous above, rather unequal, and somewhat cordate at base. *Buds* clothed with a fulvous tomentum. *Flowers* in dense subsessile fascicles. *Samara* orbicular, naked on the margin (*Beck. Bot.*)

This is sometimes called also Red Elm. It is from 20 to 40 feet high, with rugate branches. The leaves are from 4 to 6 inches long, and 2 or 3 inches broad, lanceolate oval, or obovate oblong, conspicuously acuminate, doubly serrate, the upper surface scabrous, beneath tomentose pubescent. *Stipules* pilose. *Flowers* on short pedicels, numerous, in dense lateral clusters. *Calyx* about 7-cleft ; segments obtuse, clothed and ciliate, with a reddish tawny pubescence. *Stamens* often 7, much exserted ; anthers dark purple. *Styles* granular pubescent, purple. *Samara* orbicular, about half an inch in diameter, radiately veined, pubescent in the centre, on a slender pedicel as long as the calyx ; margin smooth, cleft at apex between the styles ; segments acuminate by the pubescent adnate styles, and so incurved and overlapped as to give the margin the appearance of being entire at the apex (*Darlington*).

This plant is common in the United States, growing in low grounds and along fences.

The inner bark is fibrous, and is removed from the trunk and large branches of the tree in long pieces. It is found in the shops in this form, or ground into powder. It is bland and demulcent, and is used as a substitute for flaxseed and other demulcent articles. From the powder can be made an excellent poultice by mixing it with the requisite quantity of hot water.

INFUSUM ULMI, U.S. ; *Infusion of Slippery Elm Bark.*—Made by mace-

---

[1] *Arzneimitt.* Bd. i.
[2] *Medical Transactions*, vol. ii. p. 203.
[3] *Medical Memoirs*, p. 152.
[4] Jeffreys, *Cases in Surgery*, Lond. 1820.

rating an ounce of Slippery Elm Bark in a pint of boiling water. Used for the ordinary purposes of a demulcent solution.—ED.]

ORDER XXVIII. URTICACEÆ, *Endl.*—NETTLEWORTS.

URTICEÆ, *Jussieu.*

CHARACTERS.—*Flowers* herbaceous, inconspicuous, polygamous. *Calyx* membranous, lobed, persistent. *Stamens* definite, distinct, inserted in the base of the calyx, and opposite its lobes. *Ovary* superior, simple. *Ovule* solitary, erect. *Fruit* a simple indehiscent nut, naked or surrounded by the persistent calyx. *Embryo* straight, with fleshy albumen; cotyledons flat; radicle superior.—*Trees, shrubs,* or *herbs.* *Leaves* frequently covered with asperities or stinging hairs. *Stipules* mostly persistent, rarely deciduous or absent.

PROPERTIES.—The Order is now very circumscribed, and contains but few properties interesting to the physician. The most remarkable property of the Order is the acridity (sometimes very extreme) of the liquid contained in the epidermoid gland at the base of the stinging hair. Endlicher[1] says that it is bicarbonate of ammonia; but this is an obvious error, as ammonia in any known form is incompetent to produce the violent effect ascribed to some of the East Indian Urticaceæ.

Urtication, or flagellation by a bunch of nettles (*Urtica dioica*), is an old method of treating palsy.[2]

120. Parietaria officinalis, *Linn.*—Common Wall-Pellitory.

Sex. Syst. Tetrandria, Monogynia.

(Herba.)

This is a common indigenous plant, which was formerly in great repute as a diuretic and lithontriptic. By some practitioners it is still highly esteemed. It is used in calculous and other urinary affections, and also in dropsies. The *expressed juice* may be taken in doses of one or two fluidounces. Or the *decoction* (prepared by boiling ʒj. of the herb in a pint of water) may be substituted. The *extract* has also been used. On account of a nitrate which the plant contains, the extract is said to have taken fire in making it.[3]

ORDER XXIX. CANNABINACEÆ, *Lindl.*—HEMPWORTS.

CANNABINEÆ, *Endl.*

CHARACTERS.—*Flowers* diœcious. MALES : in racemes or panicles. *Calyx* herbaceous, scaly, imbricated. *Stamens* 5, opposite the sepals; *filaments* filiform; *anthers* terminal, 2-celled, opening longitudinally. FEMALES : in spikes or cones. *Sepal* 1, enwrapping the ovary. *Ovary* free, 1-celled. *Ovule* solitary, pendulous. *Stigmas* 2, subulate. *Fruit* 1-celled, indehiscent. *Embryo* without albumen, hooked, or spirally coiled ; radicle superior, lying against the back of the cotyledon.

PROPERTIES.—There are only two species in this family, and each of these will be separately noticed. One of these (*Cannabis sativa*) is remarkable for the tenacity of its fibre, and the narcotic intoxicating quality of its juices; the other (*Humulus Lupulus*) for its bitter principle, and its fragrant oil, whose vapour is soporific.

---

[1] *Enchiridion Botanicon.*
[2] Celsus, lib. iii. cap. 27.
[3] Withering, *Arrangement of British Plants,* 7th edit. vol. ii. p. 237.

121. CANNABIS SATIVA.—COMMON HEMP.

Sex. Syst. Diœcia, Pentandria.

(Herba et resina. The extract, *D.*)

HISTORY.—This plant was well known to the ancient Greeks and Romans, but they do not appear to have been acquainted with its narcotic properties. Dioscorides[1] merely mentions that the expressed juice of the seeds of κάνναβις allays ear-ache, and the same statement is made by Galen.[2] Herodotus[3] mentions it, and states that the Scythians cultivated it and made themselves garments of it. He also adds that they threw the seeds on red-hot stones, and used the perfumed vapour thereby obtained as a bath, which excited from them cries of exultation. This I presume refers to the intoxicating properties of its smoke. The hemp may have been, as Dr Royle[4] suggests, the "assuager of grief" or the *nepenthes* (νηπενθές) of which Homer[5] speaks as having been given by Helen to Telemachus in the house of Menelaus. Helen is stated to have received the plant from a woman of Egyptian Thebes. It is known in India as the "increaser of pleasure," the "exciter of desire," the "cementer of friendship," the "cause of a reeling gait," and the "laughter-mover."[6]

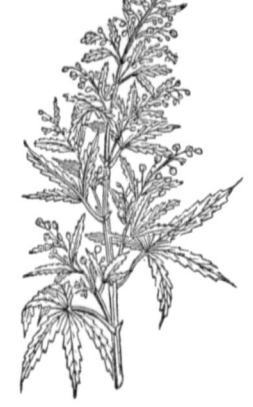

FIG. 158.

Cannabis sativa.

Pliny[7] mentions it under the name of *Cannabis.*

BOTANY. **Gen. Char.**—*Flowers* diœcious. MALES: —*Flowers* racemose. *Calyx* 5-parted, imbricated. *Stamens* 5. FEMALES:—*Flowers* in spikes. *Calyx* (bract?) 1-leaved, acuminate, rolled round the ovary. *Ovary* roundish. *Style* short. *Stigmas* 2, filiform, pubescent. *Fruit* 1-celled, 2-valved.

Sp. Char.—The only species.

Annual. Stem 3 to 5 or 6 feet high, erect, branched, angular. Leaves on long weak petioles, digitate, serrated, roughish. Stipules subulate. Flowers in clusters, axillary. The whole plant has a clammy feel.

CANNABIS SATIVA var. INDICA; *Indian Hemp.*—The plant which grows in India and has been described by some botanists[8] under the name of *Cannabis indica*, or *Indian Hemp*,[9] does not appear to possess any specific differences from the common hemp. Roxburgh[10] and most other distinguished botanists have accordingly considered it identical with the *Cannabis sativa* of Linnæus and Willdenow.

---

[1] Lib. iii. cap. 165. The κάνναβις ἀγρία of this author (lib. iii. cap. 106) is the *Althæa cannabina* of modern botanists.

[2] *De Simpl. Med. Facult.* lib. vii. cap. 5.

[3] Lib. iv. *Melpomene,* lxxiv. and lxxv.

[4] *Illustrations of the Botany of the Himalayan Mountains,* p. 334.

[5] *Odyssey,* iv. 220.

[6] Royle, *op. supra cit.;* also Dr. O'Shaughnessy, *On the Preparation of the Indian Hemp or Gunjah,* Calcutta, 1839.

[7] *Hist. Nat.* lib. xix. cap. 56; and lib. xx. cap. 97.

[8] Rumphius, *Herbarium Amboinense,* vol. v. t. 77.

[9] In the United States of America, the denomination of *Indian hemp* is applied, both in the Pharmacopœia and Dispensatory, to the *Apocynum cannabinum;* and it has been imported and sold in London for the real Indian hemp (*Cannabis sativa* var. *indica*), according to the statement of Dr. Fred. J. Farre (*Lond. Med. Gaz.* May 5, 1843, p. 209).

[10] *Flora Indica,* vol. iii. p. 772.

C. indica branches from the ground up to within two feet of the top; whereas common hemp grows three or four feet before it branches. The fruit also of *C. indica* is smaller and rounder. I have carefully compared *C. indica* (both that grown in the Chelsea Garden and that contained in Dr. Wallich's Herbarium in the possession of the Linnean Society) with the *C. sativa* in Linnæus's collection, and I cannot discover any essential distinction between them. The male plants appear to me to be in every respect the same.[1] In the female plants, the flowers of *C. indica* were more crowded than those of common hemp.

Hab.—Persia, Caucasus, hills in the north of India. Cultivated in various other countries.

DESCRIPTION.—The parts employed in Asia for the purposes of intoxication, and in Europe for medicine, are the herb (leaves) and the resin.

1. *Herba cannabis sativæ.*—This is used in India in two forms; one called *gunjah*, the other *bang*. The *hashish* of the Arabs differs somewhat from gunjah.

α. *Gunjah.*—This is the dried hemp plant which has flowered, and from which the resin has not been removed. It is sold in the Calcutta bazaars, for smoking chiefly, in bundles of about two feet long and three inches in diameter, each containing twenty-four plants. That which I have received from Dr. O'Shaughnessy, and also found in commerce, consists of cylindrical or fusiform masses (about the size and shape of the fingers) of a greyish or greenish-brown colour, and composed of stems, leaves, and petioles pressed together. It has a faint odour and feeble bitterish taste.

β. *Bang, Subjee,* or *Sidhee.*—This consists of the larger leaves and capsules without the stalks. I have not met with this in commerce.

γ. *Háshish* or *Hashish.*—This, according to Steeze,[2] consists of the tops and tender parts of the plant collected after inflorescence.

2. *Resina Cannabis sativæ.*—The concreted resinous exudation from the leaves, slender stems, and flowers, is called *Churrus*. The mode of collecting it is somewhat analogous to that adopted in Crete for the collection of ladanum. "In Central India and the Saugor territory, and in Nipal, Churrus is collected during the hot season in the following singular manner:—Men clad in leathern dresses run through the hemp-fields, brushing through the plant with all possible violence; the soft resin adheres to the leather, and is subsequently scraped off and kneaded into balls, which sell from five to six rupees the seer. A still finer kind—the *Momeea* or *waxen Churrus*—is collected by the hand in Nipal, and sells for nearly double the price of the ordinary kind. In Nipal, Dr. M'Kinnon informs me, the leathern attire is dispensed with, and the resin is gathered on the skins of the naked coolies! In Persia, it is stated by Mirza Abdul Razes that the Churrus is prepared by pressing the resinous plant on coarse cloths, and then scraping it from these and melting it in a pot with a little warm water. He considers the Churrus of Herat as the best and most powerful of all the varieties of the drug.[3] Churrus, such as I have received it from Dr. O'Shaughnessy, is in masses having the shape and size of a hen's egg, or of a small lemon, and formed by the adhesion of superimposed elongated pieces.

---

[1] This agrees with a remark in the *Hortus Cliffortianus*—"Quod mas in Horto Malabarico exhibitus nostra sit planta nullum dubium detur; fœmina autem parum recedit foliis ternatis, tamen et ejusmodi plantas in sole macro apud nos observamus non infrequenter."

[2] *Pharm. Journal,* vol. v. p. 83, 1845, [See also the same journal, Oct. 1854, p. 165.—ED.]

[3] O'Shaughnessy, *op. supra cit.* p. 6.

It has a dull greyish-brown colour, and not much odour. It consists of resinous and various foreign matters (fragments of flowers, leaves, and seeds).

3. *Fructus Cannabis sativæ.*—The fruits, called usually *hemp seed* (*semen cannabis*), are small ash-coloured, shining, nut-like or seed-like bodies. They are demulcent and oleaginous, but not narcotic. They are employed for feeding cage-birds. They are said by Burnett[1] to possess the singular property of changing the colour of the plumage of bullfinches and goldfinches from red and yellow to black, if the birds are fed on the seeds for too long a time or in too large a quantity (?).

Composition.—The *leaves* of common hemp have been submitted to analysis by Tscheepe,[2] by Schlesinger,[3] and by Bohlig.[4] The results of the two former of these are as follows :—

TSCHEEPE.		SCHLESINGER.	
Chlorophylle.		Bitter matter...............................	1·25
Gluten.	} Green fecula.	Chlorophylle soluble in ether............	4·75
Phosphate of lime.		Chlorophylle soluble in alcohol	9·375
Brown extractive.		Green resinous extractive	5·0
Sweetish bitter extractive.		Colouring matter	10·15
Brown gum.		Gummy extract	19·45
Lignin.		Malate of lime with extractive	6·775
Soluble albumen.		Extractive	6·875
Salts of ammonia, potash, lime, and magnesia.		Vegetable albumen........................	8·0
Alumina.		Lime, magnesia, and iron	9·5
Silica.		Lignin	12·0
		Loss	6·875
Leaves of Cannabis sativa.		Leaves dried at 200° F...................	100·000

Bohlig found a great agreement between the constituents of common hemp and those of the stinging nettle (*Urtica dioica*).

Dr. Kane[5] has made an ultimate analysis of the leaves and herb of hemp, as well as of their ashes; but the results have no medical interest.

Hemp seeds have been analysed by Bucholz,[6] who obtained—*fixed oil* 19·1, *resin* 1·6, *sugar* with extractive 1·6, *gummy extract* 9·0, soluble *albumen* 24·7, *woody fibre* 5·0, *husk* 38·3, loss 0·7 = 100·0.

1. Volatile Oil of Hemp.—This has hitherto been procured in such small quantities that its properties are but imperfectly known. When the dried plant is distilled with a large quantity of water, traces of the oil pass over, and the distilled liquor has the odour of the plant.

2. Cannabin; *Resin of Hemp.*—This appears to be the active principle of hemp. It is a soft, neutral resin, soluble in alcohol and in ether, and separable, by the addition of water, from its alcoholic solution, in the form of a white precipitate. It has a warm, bitterish, acrid, somewhat balsamic taste, and a fragrant odour, especially when heated. Messrs. T. and H. Smith[7] say that it very much resembles jalap-resin or jalapine, except in remaining soft even after continued drying, and in its odour and taste.

3. Fixed Oil of Hempseed; *Hempseed Oil; Oleum Cannabis.*—This is a drying oil obtained in Russia, by expression, from hempseeds, which yield about 25 per cent. of it. At first it is greenish-yellow, subsequently yellow. It has an acrid odour, but a mild taste. Its sp. gr. is 0·9276 at 52°. It dissolves readily in boiling alcohol, in 30 parts

---

[1] *Outlines of Botany*, p. 560, 1835.
[2] Gmelin, *Hand. d. Chemie*, Bd. ii. S. 1324.
[3] *Pharmaceutisches Central-Blatt für* 1840, S. 490.
[4] *Ibid.* S. 519.
[5] *Lond. Edinb. and Dubl. Phil. Mag.* for February 1844 ; also, *Industrial Resources of Ireland.*
[6] Quoted by L. Gmelin, *Handb. d. Chemie.*
Pharmaceutical Journal, vol. vi. p. 127, 1846.

of cold alcohol. At —17° F. it freezes. It is used in the preparation of a soft soap, in paint, and in lamps for the purpose of illumination ; but it is apt to clog the wick by the formation of a viscid adherent varnish. When boiled it makes a good varnish.

PHYSIOLOGICAL EFFECTS.—A general statement of the effects of Indian hemp has already been made (see Vol. i.) Its action as a neurotic is essentially that of a cerebro-spinal. It operates as a *phrenic :* in moderate doses producing exhilaration, inebriation with phantasms, and more or less confusion of intellect, followed by sleep ; in large doses causing stupor. Hence it may be called an exhilarant, inebriant, phantasmatic, hypnotic or soporific, and stupefacient or narcotic.

On Orientals the inebriation or delirium produced by it is usually of an agreeable or cheerful character, exciting the individual to laugh, dance, and sing, and to commit various extravagances,—acting as an aphrodisiac, and augmenting the appetite for food. In some it occasions a kind of reverie. It renders others excitable and quarrelsome, and disposes to acts of violence.[1] The singular form of insanity said to be brought on by it has already been noticed in the first volume of this work.

It acts as an *anæsthetic.* It relieves pain, and is, therefore, employed as an anodyne or paregoric. Moreover, Mr. Donovan[2] found that under its influence his sense of touch and feeling gradually became obtuse, until at length he lost all feeling unless he pinched himself severely ; and Dr. Christison[3] states he felt a pleasant numbness of his limbs after its use.

Its influence as a *cinetic,* or agent affecting the action of the muscles, is remarkable. It relieves spasm, and is, therefore, frequently used as an antispasmodic. On Orientals large doses produce a cataleptic condition (in which the muscles are moderately contracted, but flexible and pliant, and the limbs retain any position or attitude in which they may be placed).

The following illustrative cases are taken from Dr. O'Shaughnessy's paper on Indian hemp :—

At two P.M. a grain of the resin of hemp was given to a rheumatic patient. At four P.M. he was very talkative, sang, called loudly for an extra supply of food, and declared himself in perfect health. At six P.M. he was asleep. At eight P.M. he was found insensible, but breathing with perfect regularity, his pulse and skin natural, and the pupils freely contractile on the approach of light. Happening by chance to lift up the patient's arm, the "professional reader will judge of my astonishment," observes Dr. O'Shaughnessy, "when I found that it remained in the posture in which I placed it. It required but a very brief examination of the limbs to find that the patient had by the influence of this narcotic been thrown into that strange and most extraordinary of all nervous conditions,— into that state which so few have seen, and the existence of which so many still discredit,— the genuine *catalepsy* of the nosologist. We raised him to a sitting posture, and placed his arms and limbs in every imaginable attitude. A waxen figure could not be more pliant or more stationary in each position, no matter how contrary to the natural influence of gravity on the part. To all impressions he was meanwhile almost insensible." He continued in this state till one A.M., when consciousness and voluntary motion quickly returned. Another patient who had taken the same dose fell asleep, but was aroused by the noise in the ward. He seemed vastly amused at the strange aspects of the statue-like attitudes in which the first patient had been placed. "On a sudden he uttered a loud peal of laughter, and exclaimed that four spirits were springing with his bed into the air. In vain we attempted to pacify him ; his laughter became momentarily more and

---

[1] It has been stated that the men who attempted the assassination of Lord Cornwallis in India were intoxicated by Indian hemp (Thornton, *History of the British Empire in India,* vol. ii. p. 486, 1842).

[2] *Dublin Journal of Medical Science,* Jan. 1845.

[3] *Dispensatory.*

2 B

more uncontrollable. We now observed that the limbs were rather rigid, and in a few minutes more his legs and arms could be bent, and would remain, in any desired position. He was moved to a separate room, where he soon became tranquil; his limbs in less than an hour gained their natural condition, and in two hours he expressed himself perfectly well and excessively hungry."

On Europeans I have never heard of a cataleptic state being produced by this drug. In a case of tetanus under my care in the London Hospital, and which was carefully watched by Dr. O'Shaughnessy and myself, the resinous extract of Indian hemp was given in increasing doses up to twenty grains. It caused stupor and cessation of spasms, but no perfect cataleptic state. The only tendency to this condition which was observed was when the arm of the patient was lifted and then cautiously let go: it fell slowly and gradually, not quickly, as it would have done under ordinary conditions: the patient was at this time quite insensible.

[Mr. B. Taylor, who tried the effects of the extract upon himself, thus describes his feelings and sensations. The dose taken was a teaspoonful and a half:—

"The sense of limitation,—of the confinement of our senses within the bounds of our own flesh and blood,—instantly fell away. The walls of my frame were burst outward, and tumbled into ruin; and without thinking what form I wore—losing sight even of all idea of form—I felt that I existed throughout a vast extent of space. * * * * It is difficult to describe this sensation, or the rapidity with which it mastered me. In the state of mental exaltation in which I was then plunged, all sensations as they rose suggested more or less coherent images. They presented themselves to me in a double form: one physical, and therefore to a certain extent tangible; the other spiritual, and therefore revealing itself in a succession of splendid metaphors. * * * * My curiosity was now in a way of being satisfied: the spirit (demon, shall I not rather say?) of Hasheesh had entire possession of me. The thrills which ran through my nervous system became more rapid and fierce, accompanied with sensations that steeped my whole being in unutterable rapture. I was encompassed by a sea of light, through which played the pure harmonious colours that are born of light. While endeavouring in broken expressions to describe my feelings to my friends, who sat looking upon me incredulously—not yet having been affected by the drug—I suddenly found myself at the foot of the great pyramid of Cheops. The tapering courses of yellow limestone gleamed like gold in the sun, and the pile rose so high that it seemed to lean for support on the blue arch of the sky. I wished to ascend it, and the wish alone placed me immediately upon its apex, lifted thousands of feet above the wheat-fields and palm-groves of Egypt. I cast my eyes downwards, and, to my astonishment, saw that it was built, not of limestone, but of huge square plugs of Cavendish tobacco. * * * * The most remarkable feature of these illusions was, that at the time I was most completely under their influence I knew myself to be seated in the tower of Antonio's hotel in Damascus, knew that I had taken hasheesh, and that the strange gorgeous and ludicrous fancies which possessed me were the effect of it."[1]—ED.]

By internal use it acts as a *mydriatic*, causing preternatural dilatation of the pupil. But Dr. Lawrie[2] states that when applied around the eye it does not cause dilatation of the pupil. Indian hemp does not appear much to affect the secretions. It neither excites nausea nor lessens the appetite. It neither causes dryness of the tongue nor constipation of the bowels. It does not appear to check or otherwise affect the bronchial secretions. I am disposed to think that it is somewhat sudorific. Drs. Ballard and Garrod[3] state that in large doses it communicates an odour to the urine like that evolved when the tincture is mixed with water, and in part like that of the Tonquin bean.

Compared with opium, Indian hemp differs in its operation on the system in several remarkable circumstances: as by its inebriating, phantasmatic, and aphrodisiac effects; by its causing catalepsy and dilatation of pupil; and by

[1] *Pictures of Palestine*, by Bayard Taylor, 1853.
[2] *Lond. and Edinb. Monthly Journal of Medical Science*, Nov. 1844, p. 947.
[3] *Elements of Materia Medica*.

its not causing nausea, loss of appetite, dry tongue, constipation, or diminution of the secretions.

Dr. Hooke, in his account of Indian hemp (Bangue) read to the Royal Society, Dec. 18, 1689, notices the various odd tricks shown by persons while in the ecstasy caused by this plant; and adds that when this condition subsides the patient finds himself mightily refreshed and exceedingly hungry. The general effects of Indian hemp on man, as stated by Dr. O'Shaughnessy from his own observations, are alleviation of pain (mostly), remarkable increase of appetite, unequivocal aphrodisia, and great mental cheerfulness. Its more violent effects were delirium of a peculiar kind, and a cataleptic state.

Its effects on *animals* were analogous: he gave ten grains of Nipalese Churrus dissolved in spirit to a middling-sized dog:—" In half an hour he became stupid and sleepy, dozing at intervals, starting up, wagging his tail as if extremely contented; he ate some food greedily; on being called to, he staggered to and fro, and his face assumed a look of utter and helpless drunkenness. These symptoms lasted about two hours, and then gradually passed away. In six hours he was perfectly well and lively." It would appear that Indian hemp acts more powerfully in India than in Europe. My experiments (detailed in the second edition of this work, pp. 1097-8) fully bear out this statement. Dr. O'Shaughnessy, when in England, satisfied himself of the difference of the effect of Indian hemp in this country and in Bengal; and he observes,[1] that while in India he had seen marked effects from half a grain of the extract, or even less, and had been accustomed to consider one grain and a half a large dose, in England he had given ten or twelve or more grains to produce the desired effect.

Uses.—Indian hemp is chiefly employed as a medicine, for its hypnotic, anodyne, and antispasmodic properties; occasionally, also, for its mental influence (*i. e.* as a phrenic and nervine). Compared with opium, it is less certain than the latter agent,—over which, however, it has several advantages. Thus it does not constipate the bowels, lessen the appetite or create nausea, produce dryness of the tongue, or check the pulmonary secretion, as opium is well known to do. Moreover, in some patients in whom opium causes headache and various distressing feelings, Indian hemp occasionally acts without any of these inconveniences; but I have heard others object to its continuance on the ground of its very unpleasant effects.

As a *hypnotic,* I have used it with advantage in spirit-drinkers, and have succeeded in one or two cases in producing sleep with it where large doses of morphia had failed. In some hysterical patients, and in cases of chorea, I have occasionally employed it to induce sleep where the use of opium was from some cause objectionable. Dr. Clendinning[2] speaks favourably of its soporific influence in pulmonary affections and low fever. It has the great advantage over opium of neither repressing the secretions nor lessening the appetite for food.

As an *anodyne* it is, I think, in general, decidedly inferior to opium; but there are occasions where its use is to be preferred to the latter agent. In acute and subacute rheumatism, in gout, and in neuralgia, it frequently alleviates the pain.

As an *antispasmodic* it has been employed in tetanus, hydrophobia, malignant cholera, chorea, and infantile convulsions. In the cases of tetanus (both traumatic and idiopathic) and of hydrophobia which I have seen treated with it, it completely failed to give permanent relief. In one case of traumatic tetanus it alleviated the pain and spasms, but the patient, notwithstanding,

---

[1] *Pharmaceutical Journal,* vol. ii. p. 594, 1843.
[2] *Medico-Chirurg. Transactions,* vol. xxvi.

died. In a case under the care of Professor Miller[1] it was given, and the
patient recovered. [Mr. Hodson, of Bishop Stortford, also found it successful
in the treatment of a case of traumatic tetanus in a child seven years of
age. The dose given was from a grain to a grain and a half every three or
four hours, continued several days.[2]—ED.] It has failed, however, in the
hands of Mr. Potter[3] and others. And in a case of idiopathic tetanus in
Guy's Hospital, under the care of Dr. Babington,[4] it proved useless. In
chorea I have found it serviceable, sometimes as an antispasmodic, at others
as a hypnotic ; and the same may be said of its use in hysteria.

As a *phrenic*, or medicinal agent affecting the mental functions, Indian
hemp has also been employed. Dr. Clendinning speaks favourably of its use
as a nervine stimulant, in removing languor and anxiety, and raising the
pulse and spirits; and Dr. Conolly thinks that it may be useful in some
chronic forms of mania.[5] Dr. Sutherland has not obtained any good effect
from it.[6]

ADMINISTRATION.—In England, Indian hemp is usually administered in
the form of resinous or alcoholic extract, and of tincture.

1. EXTRACTUM CANNABIS INDICÆ ALCOHOLICUM ; *Resinous* or *Alcoholic Extract of Indian Hemp.*

—This is the preparation usually sold in the shops
under the name of *resin of Indian hemp* or *cannabin* (see *ante*, p. 368).
Dr. O'Shaughnessy directs it to be prepared by boiling the rich adhesive
tops of the dried gunjah in rectified spirits until all the resin is dissolved.
"The tincture thus obtained is evaporated to dryness in a vessel placed over
a pot of boiling water. The extract softens at a gentle heat, and can be made
into pills without any addition." Mr. Robertson,[7] of Calcutta, prepared it by
a kind of percolation process ; the vapour of alcohol
being transmitted through the dry herb. At first
a thin tarry matter containing much resin, latterly
a brown liquor containing little resin but much
extractive, passed over. At this point water was
substituted for the spirit in the still, and as much
as possible of the spirit retained by the plant thus
expelled from it. Part of the alcohol was removed
from the fluid by distillation; but the rest was
dissipated by evaporation at a temperature not
exceeding 150° F. From 1 cwt. of the plant about
8 lbs. of extract were obtained at one operation,
which was so slowly conducted as in all its stages
to last a fortnight.

The following is the process given by the Messrs.
Smith, of Edinburgh,[8] for the preparation of this
extract :—Digest bruised gunjah in successive

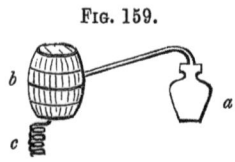

FIG. 159.

*Apparatus for the percolation
of alcohol vapour through
the dried herb of Indian
hemp.*

a, The still, charged with strong
   spirits.
b, The cask, containing the
   plant, and into the side
   of which the nose of the
   still was introduced.
c, Common condensing worm.

---

[1] *Lond. and Edinb. Monthly Journal of Medical Science*, Jan. 1845.
[2] [*Med. Times and Gazette*, May 1, 1852.]
[3] *Lancet*, vol. i. p. 36, Jan. 11, 1845.
[4] *Ibid.* vol. ii. p. 351, Dec. 14, 1844.
[5] See also Moreau, *Du Haschisch et de l' Aliénation Mentale, Etudes Psychologiques*, Paris, 1845.
[6] *Further Report of the Commissioners in Lunacy*, p. 392, 1847.
[7] *Pharmaceutical Journal*, vol. vi. p. 71, 1846.
[8] *Ibid.* p. 171, 1846.

quantities of warm water till the expressed water comes away colourless; and again for two days, at a moderate heat, in a solution of carbonate of soda, in the proportion of one part of the salt to two of gunjah. Colouring matter, chlorophylle, and inert concrete oil being thus removed, express and wash the residuum, dry it, and exhaust it by percolation with rectified spirit. Agitate with the tincture, milk of lime containing an ounce of lime for every pound of gunjah, and, after filtration, throw down the excess of lime by a little sulphuric acid. Agitate with the filtered liquor a little animal charcoal, which is afterwards to be removed by filtration. Distil off most of the spirit, add to the residual tincture twice its weight of water in a porcelain basin, and let the remaining spirit evaporate gradually. Lastly, wash the resin with fresh water till it comes away neither acid nor bitter, and dry the resin in thin layers. This resin contains the peculiar taste and odour of the gunjah. A temperature of 180° F. acting for eight hours on thin layers of it exposed to the air does not impair its activity. 100 lbs. of dry gunjah yield about 6 or 7 lbs. of this extract.

DOSE.—The dose of the alcoholic extract of Indian hemp is generally from gr. j. to grs. v. I have usually found one grain of the extract kept in the London shops to act as a narcotic. The Messrs. Smith state that two-thirds of a grain of the pure resin produced on themselves and others powerful narcotic effects. In a case of tetanus under my care in the London Hospital, the dose of the extract (supplied by Dr. O'Shaughnessy, who watched the case with me) was gradually increased to grs. xx. It may be administered in the form of pill; or better, by diffusion through an emulsion (prepared by rubbing the extract with olive oil, in a warm mortar, and gradually adding mucilage, and afterwards water), or by solution in rectified spirit, and dropping the tincture into water immediately before its administration.

2. EXTRACTUM CANNABIS INDICÆ PURIFICATUM, D. (Extract of Indian Hemp of commerce, ʒj.; Rectified Spirit, fʒiv. Dissolve the extract in the spirit, and when the dregs have subsided decant the clear liquid, and evaporate, by means of a water-bath, to the consistence of a soft extract, D.)

3. TINCTURA CANNABIS INDICÆ, D.; *Tincture of Indian Hemp.*— This is usually prepared by dissolving ʒj. of the alcoholic extract of Indian hemp in fʒxx. of rectified spirit. These are the proportions directed to be used by Dr. O'Shaughnessy; but, probably by a typographical error, he has ordered *proof* spirit instead of rectified spirit. Dose from ♏x. to fʒj. Dr. O'Shaughnessy gives in tetanus ʒj. every half hour until the paroxysms cease or catalepsy is induced; in cholera, ten drops every half hour. It may be administered in an emulsion or mucilaginous mixture, or in water sweetened with sugar. It should be swallowed soon after it has been added to the aqueous liquid, as the resin is precipitated, and is apt to adhere to the side of the vessel. The *Dublin College* gives the subjoined formula:—Purified Extract of Indian Hemp, ʒss.; Rectified Spirit, Oss. Dissolve the extract in the spirit, D.

OTHER PREPARATIONS OF INDIAN HEMP.—By the Asiatics, Egyptians, and others who employ Indian hemp for the purposes of intoxication, various preparations of this drug are in use. In some of these the plant itself is employed, either rubbed up with water and made into a draught, or formed into an electuary. But a favourite mode of using it is to extract the active principle by some fatty matter (generally butter or oil), by which an oleaginous solution or fatty extract is obtained. For this purpose the hemp is boiled in butter or oil, with a little water,—usually until the water is boiled away. It is said that the fatty extract thus obtained will preserve its intoxicating powers for years. It is usually mixed up with other ingredients, and taken in the form of an electuary, confection, or pastile. The *majoon* used at Calcutta,[1] the *mapouchari* employed at Cairo,[2] and the *dawames* of the Arabs,[3] are preparations of this kind. Lastly, hemp is also used for smoking in pipes.

ANTIDOTES.—In a case of poisoning by Indian hemp, the treatment should be the same as that for poisoning by opium (which see).

122. HUMULUS LUPULUS, *Linn.*—THE COMMON HOP.

Sex. Syst. Diœcia, Pentandria.

(Amentum, *L.*—Catkin, *E.*—The dried Strobiles, *D.*)

HISTORY.—This plant is probably the *Lupus salictarius* of Pliny.[4] Its culture was introduced into this country from Flanders, in the reign of Henry VIII.[5]

BOTANY. **Gen. Char.**—*Diœcious.* MALES :—*Calyx* 5-partite. *Stamens* 5. FEMALES :—*Strobiles* consisting of large, persistent, concave scales

FIG. 160.

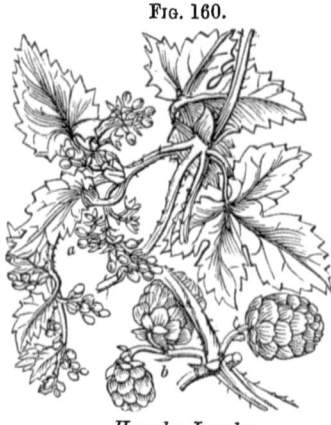

Humulus Lupulus.

a, The male plant.   *b*, The female ditto.

[bracts], having a single flower in the axilla of each. *Ovary* 1. *Styles* 2. *Seed* 1, with an arillus. *Embryo* spirally contorted (*Bot. Gall.*)

Sp. Char.—The only species.

Perennial. Stems annual, long, weak, and climbing, scabrous. *Leaves* petiolate, 3- to 5-lobed, serrated, veiny, rough. *Flowers greenish-yellow.*

Hab.—Thickets and hedges in many parts of Europe. Indigenous [?]. Flowers in July.

CULTIVATION.—The female plant is cultivated in several counties in England, especially Kent, Sussex, Surrey, Worcestershire, and Herefordshire. The third year after planting it generally comes into full bearing. *Stacking* or *setting the poles* is performed in April or May. The *gathering* or *picking* takes place in September. The cones are dried in kilns, and are then packed in hempen sacks, called *bags* or *pockets*. This operation is called *bagging*.[6]

DESCRIPTION.—The aggregate fruits of the Humulus Lupulus are strobiles or catkins (*strobili* seu *amenta lupuli*), in commerce termed *hops*. They consist of scales, nuts, and lupulinic glands or grains. The *scales* are the enlarged and persistent bracts, which enclose the nuts : they are ovate, membranous, and at their base glandular. The *nuts* (achenia) are small, hard,

---

[1] O'Shaughnessy, *op. supra cit.*

[2] Buchner's *Repertorium*, 2te Reihe, Bd. xlix. S. 359, 1848 ; also 3tte Reihe, Bd. i. S. 94, 1848.

[3] Moreau, *op. supra cit.*

[4] *Hist. Nat.* lib. xxi. cap. 50, ed. Valp.

[5] Beckmann, *Hist. of Invent.* vol. iv. p. 340.

[6] Loudon's *Encyclopædia of Agriculture.*

nearly globular, and covered with aromatic, superficial, globose glands. The *lupulinic glands* or *grains* (commonly termed *yellow powder* or *lupulin*) are the most important parts of the strobiles. By thrashing, rubbing, and sifting, Dr. Ives[1] procured 14 ounces from six pounds of hops ; and he therefore concluded that dry hops would yield about a sixth part of their weight of these grains. They are usually intermixed with sand. They are rounded, of a cellular texture, golden yellow, and somewhat transparent. They are sessile, or nearly so. The common centre, around which the cells are arranged, has been called the *hilum*. By drying they lose their spherical form. Placed in water they give out an immense number of minute globules. Under other circumstances they become ruptured, and allow an inner envelope to escape. According to Turpin[2] they consist of *two vesicles,* one enclosing the other. The inner one contains *globules, an aromatic oil,* and *a gas.* He also states, that in the bubbles of the disengaged gas an immense number of crystals are formed.

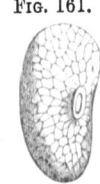

Fig. 161.

*Dried Lupulinic grain, with its hilum (mag-
nified).*

COMPOSITION.—Payen, Chevallier, and Pelletan,[3] analysed the scales and lupulinic grains. Dr. Ives[4] also examined the latter.

LUPULINIC GRAINS.		SCALES.
Payen, Chevallier, and Pelletan's Analysis.	Ives's Analysis.	Payen, Chevallier, and Pelletan's Analysis.
Volatile oil .... 2·00	Tannin...... 4·16	Astringent matter.
Bitter principle (Lupulite) ...... 10·30		Inert colouring matter.
Resin ....50 to 55·00	Extractive . 8·33	Chlorophylle.
Lignin .... 32·00		Gum.
Fatty, astringent, and gummy	Bitter prin-	Lignin.
matters, osmazome, malic	ciple...... 9·16	Salts (of potash, lime, and ammonia,
and carbonic acid, several	Wax.........10·00	containing acetic, hydrochloric,
salts (malate of lime, acetate } traces.		sulphuric, nitric, &c. acids).
of ammonia, chloride of	Resin ......30·00	The scales usually contain a portion
potassium, sulphate of pot-		of lupulinic matter, from which it
ash), &c. ..../	Lignin ......38·33	is almost impossible to free them.
99·30	100·00	

1. VOLATILE OIL OF HOPS.—Resides in the lupulinic grains. Obtained by submitting these, or hops which contain them, to distillation with water. Its colour is yellowish, its odour that of hops, its taste acrid. It is soluble in water, but still more so in alcohol and ether. Its sp. gr. is 0·910. By keeping, it becomes resinified. It is said to act on the system as a narcotic. The water which comes over, in distillation, with the oil, contains acetate of ammonia, and blackens silver ; from which circumstance the presence of sulphur is inferred.

2. BITTER PRINCIPLE OF HOPS ; *Lupulite ; Lupuline.*—Is procured by treating the aqueous extract of the lupulinic grains, united with a little lime, with alcohol. The alco-
holic tincture is to be evaporated to dryness, the residue treated with water, and the solution evaporated. The residue, when washed with ether, is lupulite. It is neutral, uncrystallisable, yellowish white, very bitter, soluble in 20 parts of water, very soluble in alcohol, and slightly so in ether. The aqueous solution froths by agitation ; it forms no precipitate with either tincture of nutgalls or acetate of lead. Lupulite contains no nitrogen. It is devoid of the narcotic property of the oil. In small doses it is said to

---

[1] *Journal of Science,* vol. xi. p. 205.
[2] *Mémoires de l'Acad. Royale des Sciences,* t. xvii. p. 104, 1840 ; see also Raspail, *Chim. Org.*
[3] *Journ. de Pharm.* t. viii. p. 209 ; and *Journ. de Chim. Méd.* t. ii. p. 527.
[4] *Journal of Science,* vol. xi. p. 205.

have caused loss of appetite and diminished digestive power; but a repetition of the experiment is very desirable.

3. Tannic Acid; *Tannin.*—In the manufacture of beer, this principle serves to precipitate the nitrogenised or albuminous matter of the barley, and, therefore, for clarification. [All genuine beer, however, contains tannic acid.—Ed.]

4. Resin.—Is of a golden yellow colour, and becomes orange-yellow by exposure to the air. It is soluble in both alcohol and ether. It appears to be the oil changed into resin, partly by oxidisement.

Chemical Characteristics.—A decoction of hops reddens litmus, owing to the presence of free acid. Sesquichloride of iron strikes an olive-green colour (*tannate of iron*). A solution of gelatin renders the filtered decoction turbid (*tannate of gelatin*). Chloride of barium occasions with it a white precipitate (*sulphate of baryta*).[1] Oxalate of ammonia also causes a white precipitate (*oxalate of lime*).

Physiological Effects.—The odorous emanations (vapour of the volatile oil) of hops possess narcotic properties. Hence a pillow of these cones promotes sleep, as I have several times witnessed. Moreover, we are told that stupor has occasionally been induced in persons who have remained for a considerable time in hop warehouses.

The lupulinic grains are aromatic and tonic. They appear also to possess soothing, tranquillising, and, in a slight degree, sedative and soporific properties. But the existence of any narcotic quality has been strongly denied by Dr. Bigsby,[2] Magendie,[3] and others. "I have tried, at different times," says Magendie, "both the lupuline [lupulinic grains] in substance, and its different preparations, on animals, but I have never observed that it is a narcotic, although this property is one which is most strikingly displayed in experiments on animals. Dr. Maton[4] found that it allayed pain, produced sleep, and reduced the frequency of the pulse from 96 to 60 in twenty-four hours. Both infusion and tincture of hops are mild but agreeable aromatic tonics. They sometimes prove diuretic, or, when the skin is kept warm, sudorific. Their sedative, soporific, and anodyne properties are very uncertain.

Uses.—A pillow of hops (*cervicale* seu *pulvinus, pulvinar lupuli*) is occasionally employed in mania, and other cases in which inquietude and restlessness prevail, and in which the use of opium is considered objectionable. In hop countries it is a popular remedy for want of sleep. The benefit said to have been obtained from it by George III., for whom it was prescribed by Dr. Willis, in 1787, brought it into more general use. Hops are given internally to relieve restlessness consequent upon exhaustion and fatigue, and to induce sleep in the watchfulness of mania and of other maladies; to calm nervous irritation; and to relieve pain in gout, arthritic rheumatism, and after accouchement. Though they sometimes produce the desired effect, they frequently fail to give relief. Dr. Maton used it, with good effect, as an anodyne in rheumatism. As a tonic, hops are applicable in dyspepsia, cachectic conditions of the system, or any other maladies characterised by debility.

Hops have been applied, topically, in the form of fomentation or poultice,

---

[1] [Sulphuric acid, sometimes sulphurous acid, may be detected in hops, owing to the common practice of drying them with the vapour of burning sulphur mixed with coke or charcoal. Bad foreign hops are said to be much improved by this process; but this of course is only in external appearance.—Ed.]

[2] *Lond. Med. Rep.* vol. iv. p. 287.

[3] *Formulaire.*

[4] *Observations on Humulus Lupulus,* by A. Freake, 2d edit.

as a resolvent or discutient, in painful swellings and tumors. Freake employed an ointment composed of lard and the powder of the hop, as an anodyne application to cancerous sores.[1]

[Dr. Sigmund has frequently, since 1844, borne testimony to the narcotic and sedative power of this substance in affections of the male organs of generation, and especially when erections impede the healing of wounds or ulcers, the chordee of gonorrhœa, and in pollution. One great advantage it possesses over opium and other narcotics is, that it does not interfere with digestion or any other function. He cautions us against mistaking it for *lupulin*, which consists of the yellow glands or grains of the scales of the female flower, *lupulit*, a chemical preparation of the bitter principle, called also by some lupulin, but which does not possess the power of lupulinic grains. An efficacious tincture is prepared from ʒj. of the powder and ʒiij. of spirit, of which 20 to 50 drops form a dose.[2]—ED.]

But the principal consumption of hops is in the manufacture of beer and ale, to which they communicate a pleasant bitter and aromatic flavour, and tonic properties; while, by their chemical influence, they check the acetous fermentation. Part of the soporific quality of beer and ale is usually ascribed to the hops used in the manufacture of these beverages.

ADMINISTRATION.—The best preparation of hops for internal use is the yellow powder (*lupulinic grains* or *lupulin*). The *infusion* and *tincture* are less eligible modes of exhibition. The *extract* is still more objectionable. *Well-hopped beer* is a convenient mode of administering hops, when fermented liquors are not contraindicated.

1. INFUSUM LUPULI, L.; *Infusion of Hops.* (Hops, ʒvj.; Boiling Distilled Water, Oj. Macerate for four hours in a vessel lightly covered, and strain). (Hops, ʒss.; Boiling Water, Oj. Macerate for two hours, *U. S.*)— Dose, fʒj. to fʒij.

2. TINCTURA LUPULI, L.; *Tinctura Humuli; Tincture of Hops.* (Hops, ʒvj. [ʒv. *U. S.*]; Proof Spirit, Oij. Macerate for fourteen days, and strain.)—Dose, fʒss. to fʒij.

3. EXTRACTUM LUPULI, L. E.; *Extract of Hops.* (Hops, lb. iiss. [lb. j. *E.*]; Boiling Distilled Water, *Cong.* ij. [*Cong.* j. *E.*] Macerate for twenty-four hours, then boil down to a gallon [Oiv. *E.*], and strain the liquor while hot; lastly, evaporate [in the vapour bath, *E.*] to a proper consistence.— Dose, gr. v. to ℈j. Whatever virtue this preparation possesses is owing to the bitter principle or lupulite.

4. LUPULINA; *Yellow Powder; Lupulinic Grains* or *Glands.* (Separated from the strobiles by rubbing and sifting.)—Dose, grs. vj. to grs. xij. taken in the form of powder or pills.

5. TINCTURA LUPINÆ, D.; *Tinctura Lupuli,* E. (Take any convenient quantity of Hops, recently dried; separate by friction and sifting the yellowish-brown powder attached to the scales. Then take of this powder, ʒv.; and of Rectified Spirit, Oij.; and prepare the tincture by percolation or digestion, as directed for tincture of capsicum. *Ph. Ed.*) (Take of Lupulin, ʒv.; Rectified Spirit, Oij. Macerate for fourteen days, strain, express, and filter, *D.*)— Dose, ʒss. to ʒij.

---

[1] *Op. cit.* p. 13; see also *Annals of Medicine*, vol. ii. p. 403.
[2] *Med. Times and Gazette*, June 16, 1855.

ORDER XXX. MORACEÆ.

MOREÆ, *Endlicher.*

CHARACTERS.—*Flowers* unisexual. MALES :—*Calyx* 0, or 3—4-parted. *Stamens* 3—4, inserted into the base of the calyx and opposite its segments. FEMALES :—*Calyx* 0, or 4—5-parted. *Ovary* 1-celled, rarely 2-celled. *Ovules* solitary, pendulous, or amphitropal, with the foramen uppermost. *Fruit* small nuts or utricles, 1-seeded, inclosed within the succulent receptacle, or collected in a fleshy head formed by the consolidated succulent calyx. *Seed* solitary, with a thin brittle testa; embryo lying in fleshy albumen, hooked, with the radicle long, superior, folded down towards the cotyledons.—*Trees* or *shrubs*, with a milky juice. *Leaves* furnished with stipules.

PROPERTIES.—Various. The milky juice of some species is bland and potable; of others acrid and poisonous. In India *Ficus elastica* yields caoutchouc. *Maclura tinctoria* furnishes the dye wood called *Fustic*, whose colouring principle is termed *morine.*

123. MORUS NIGRA, *Linn.*—THE COMMON MULBERRY.

Sex. Syst. Monœcia, Tetraudria.

(Fructûs Succus, *L.*)

HISTORY.—The mulberry (μορέα) is mentioned by Hippocrates[1]—" Mora calefaciunt et humectant ac alvo secedunt," says the Father of Physic. Dioscorides[2] also speaks of the mulberry.

BOTANY. **Gen. Char.**—Monœcious. *Catkins* unisexual. *Calyx* 4-lobed; the lobes concave. *Stamens* 4, alternate with the segments of the calyx. *Ovary* free. *Stigmas* 2. *Seeds* 1-2, covered by the pulpy calyx (*Bott. Gall.*)

Sp. Char.—*Leaves* cordate, ovate, lobed, or unequally dentate ; rough and thickish. *Fruit* dark purple (*Bot. Gall.*)

FIG. 162.

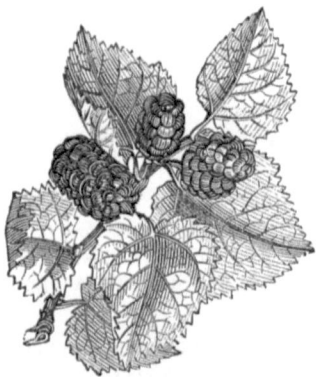

Morus nigra.

A small *tree,* with rugged bark. *Flowers* greenish. " *Fruit,* consisting of the female flowers, become fleshy and grown together, inclosing a dry membranous pericarp" (Lindley).

Hab.—Native of Persia and China. Cultivated for its fruit. Flowers in May.

DESCRIPTION.—The fruit is usually called *a berry (bacca mori nigræ),* but is, in fact, that kind called by botanists *a sorosis.* Its odour is peculiar and agreeable ; its taste is peculiar, pleasant, acidulous, and sweet. The juice is dark violet red.

COMPOSITION.—The fruit has not been analysed. Its principal constituents are —*violet-red colouring matter, tartaric acid, sugar,* and *woody fibre.* The root has been analysed by Wackenroder.[3]

PHYSIOLOGICAL EFFECTS.—Mulberries are alimentary in a slight degree; they allay thirst, diminish febrile heat, and, in large quantities, prove laxative.

[1] *De victûs ratione,* lib. ii. cap. 360, ed. Fœs.
[2] Lib. i. cap. 180.
[3] Gmelin's *Handb. d. Chem.* ii. 1324.

USE.—They are employed as an agreeable aliment, and are well adapted to check preternatural heat and relieve thirst in fevers, but are objectionable when a tendency to diarrhœa exists. They owe their retention in the Pharmacopœia to their colour and flavour.

SYRUPUS MORI, L.; *Syrup of Mulberry*. (Juice of Mulberries, strained, Oj.; Sugar, lb. ijss. Dissolve the sugar in the mulberry juice with a gentle heat, and proceed in the same manner as directed for Syrup of Lemons.)—Used as a colouring and flavouring substance. Its acidity prevents its being used with alkalies, earths, or their carbonates.

124. FICUS CARICA, *Linn.*—THE COMMON FIG.

Sex. Syst. Polygamia, Triœcia, *Linn.*—Polygamia, Diœcia, *Willd.*—Diœcia, Triandria, *Pers.*
(Fici: fructus præparatus, *L.*—Fici: the dried fruit, *E. D.*)

HISTORY.—In the Old Testament we are informed that Hezekiah (who lived 600 years before Christ) used figs as a topical application to a boil.[1] The fig-tree is the συκῆ of Dioscorides,[2] the *Ficus* of Pliny.[3]

BOTANY. **Gen. Char·** — Monœcious. *Flowers* numerous, pedicellated, inclosed within a fleshy receptacle, which is umbilicated, and nearly closed at the apex, hollow within. *Calyx* 3—5-lobed: lobes acuminate. *Male-flowers* near the umbilicus. *Stamens* 3—5. *Ovary* free (Desf.); semi-adnate (Gaertn.) *Style* 1. *Stigmas* 2. *Drupe* or *utricle* 1-seeded, sunk into the pulpy receptacle. *Coat* of the nut fragile, crustaceous (*Bott. Gall.*)

Sp· Char.—*Leaves* cordate, palmate, scabrous above, pubescent beneath (*Bot. Gall.*) —A small *tree*. Flowers in June. *Receptacle* green. At the base of each receptacle are two or three bracteal scales.

FIG. 163.

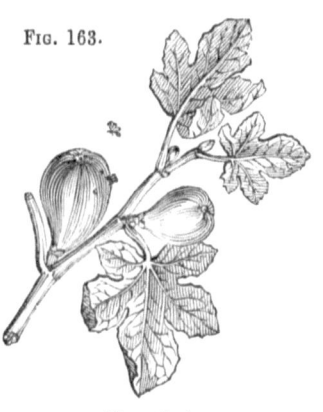

Ficus Carica.

FIG. 164.

A, Receptacle:—*a a*, bracteal scales; *b*, umbilicus.
B, Longitudinal section of receptacle:—*a*, flowers seated on *b*, the inner side of the receptacle.
C, Female flower.
D, Section of ditto.
E, Male ditto.

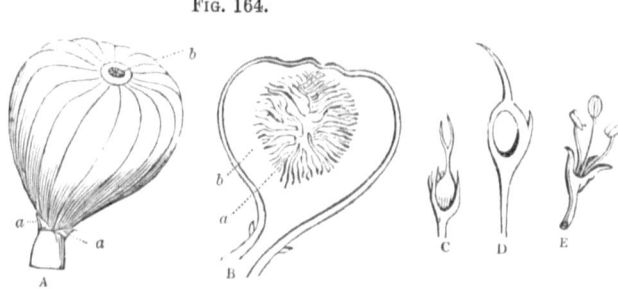

Ficus Carica.

[1] *Isaiah*, xxxviii. 21.
[2] Lib. i. cap. 183.
[3] *Hist. Nat.* lib. xx. iii. cap. 63.

HAB.—Native of Asia and South of Europe.   [Carica a Cariâ regione dicta.—ED.]

DESCRIPTION.—Figs (*fici* seu *caricæ*) constitute that kind of collective fruit called, by Mirbel, a *syconus*. They consist of fleshy, hollow, pyriform receptacles, within which are numerous, small, seed-like bodies (*achenia*, Lindley; *utricles*, Auctor). In the unripe state they contain an acrid and bitter juice, but which, when they are ripe, is replaced by sugar. Ripe figs are dried in the sun, or in ovens, and are afterwards packed in drums and baskets, in which they are imported. As met with in the shops, they are more or less compressed, are covered with a whitish, saccharine efflorescence,[1] have a brownish or yellowish colour, and are somewhat translucent. They have a peculiar and agreeable odour, and contain a sweet viscid pulp, in which are the achenia. *Turkey* or *Smyrna figs* are the largest, most juicy, and sweetest; hence they are sometimes termed *fat figs* (*caricæ pingues*): they are distinguished into *pulled* and *flat*. Of 20,406 *cwts.* of figs imported in 1830, no fewer than 18,801 came from Turkey (*Parliam. Return*).

COMPOSITION.—Bley[2] analysed Smyrna figs, and obtained the following result:—*Sugar of figs* 62·5, *fatty matter* 0·9, *extractive with chloride of calcium* 0·4, *gum with phosphoric acid* 5·2, *woody fibre* and *seeds* [achenia] 15·0, and *water* 16·0 = 100·0.

PHYSIOLOGICAL EFFECTS.—Figs are nutritive, emollient, demulcent, and laxative. In the fresh state they are both agreeable and wholesome: when dried, as we receive them, they readily disorder the stomach and bowels, and occasion flatulence, griping, and mild diarrhœa.

USES.—In those countries where they are plentiful, figs are used as food. Here they are chiefly employed as a dessert. Internally they are given in the form of demulcent decoctions (as the *Decoctum Hordei compositum*, L., and *Mistura Hordei*, E.) in pulmonary and nephritic affections. As laxatives they are sometimes taken with the food to relieve habitual constipation, and enter into the composition of *Confectio Sennæ*, L. (*Electuarium Sennæ*, E.) Roasted or boiled, and split open, they are employed as suppurative cataplasms in gum-boils.

125. DORSTENIA CONTRAJERVA, *Linn.*; and D. BRASILIENSIS, *Lam.*

Sex. Syst. Tetrandria, Monogynia.
(Radix.)

HISTORY.—The earliest notice of this plant is that by Monardes,[3] who states that the word *contrayerva* is the Indo-Spanish term for alexipharmic or counter-poison. In 1581, Clusius[4] received from Sir Francis Drake a root which he called, after the donor, *Drakena radix*, and which has been supposed to be contrayerva root.

---

[1] [This efflorescence is crystallised grape sugar. It only appears on the imported figs soon after cold weather sets in.—ED.]
[3] *Pharm. Central-Blatt für* 1831, S. 27.
[4] Clusius, *Exoticorum*, lib. x. p. 311.
[5] *Ibid.* p. 83.

BOTANY. **Gen. Char.**—Monœcious. *Flowers* arranged upon a fleshy receptacle, usually flat and expanded, and extremely variable in form : *males* on the surface of the receptacle, 2-lobed, fleshy, diandrous ; *females* immersed in the receptacle, also 2-lobed in most species. *Ovary* 1—2-celled, with a single suspended ovule in each cell. *Style* 1. *Stigma* 2-lobed. *Achenia* lenticular, imbedded in the fleshy receptacle, from which they are projected with elasticity when ripe.—Dwarf *herbaceous* plants with scaly rhizomata (Lindley).

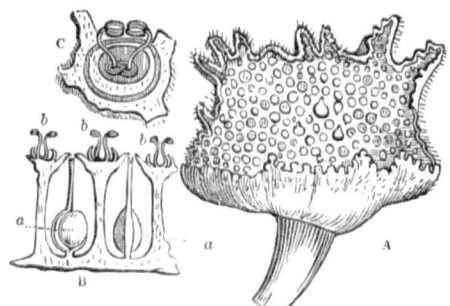

FIG. 165.

Dorstenia Contrajerva.

A. Entire receptacle.
B. Section of ditto :—*a.* Female flowers ; *b.* Male ditto.
C. Male flower in its superficial hollow.

Species.—1. *D. Contrajerva*, Linn.—Caulescent ; *stem* covered with spreading green scaly stipules. *Leaves* palmate ; the lobes lanceolate, acuminate, coarsely serrated and gashed, occasionally almost pinnatifid. *Receptacle* on a very long stalk, quadrangular, wavy, or plated (Lindley). A native of New Spain, Mexico, Peru, Tobago, St. Vincent's (Willd.) The root of this is not met with in commerce.

2. *D. brasiliensis*, Lam.—A native of Jamaica, Brazil, and Trinidad. This yields the contrayerva root usually met with in the shops.

DESCRIPTION.—The contrayerva root (*radix contrajervæ*) usually found in the shops is imported from the Brazils. It consists of an ovoid or oblong rootstock, terminating inferiorly in one or several long, tapering, more or less curved root-fibres. From the sides of the root-stock also arise numerous slender fibres. Externally the colour is yellowish-brown. The odour of the root is peculiar but aromatic. The taste is warm, bitterish, slightly acrid.

I have also found another kind of contrayerva root in the shops. The rootstalk is smaller, cylindrical, blackish-brown, with fewer fibres. The receptacle and leaves are attached ; the latter are reniform. This may be the *Drakena radix* of Clusius.

COMPOSITION.—The root has not been analysed. It contains, according to Geiger,[1] *volatile oil, bitter extractive*, and *starch*. To which may be added *resin, free acid*, and *woody fibre*.

PHYSIOLOGICAL EFFECTS.—Stimulant, tonic, and diaphoretic. Its operation is very analogous to that of serpentary root, between which and the rhizome of the sweet flag it deserves to be arranged. The root of the *Dorstenia brasiliensis* often proves emetic.[2]

USES.—Obsolete, or nearly so. It has been employed in fevers of a low type, and in other diseases requiring a mild, stimulant, and diaphoretic treatment.

---

[1] *Hand. d. Pharm.*
[2] De Candolle, *Essai sur les Propriétés Méd.*

ADMINISTRATION.—The dose of the root in *powder* is Əj. or ʒss. The *infusion* (prepared by digesting from ʒiv. in fʒvj. of boiling water) may be given in doses of fʒj. or fʒij. The *Pulvis contrajervæ compositus* (composed of powdered contrayerva root, ʒv. and prepared shells, lb. jss.) is no longer officinal.

ORDER XXXI. ARTOCARPACEÆ, *Lindley*.

ARTOCARPEÆ, *R. Brown ; Endl.*

CHARACTERS.—*Flowers* unisexual, in dense heads. MALES.—*Calyx* 0, or consisting of 2—4 sepals. *Stamens* opposite the sepals. FEMALES :—*Flowers* arranged over a fleshy receptacle. *Calyx* tubular, with a 2—4-cleft or entire limb. *Ovary* free, 1-celled. *Ovules* suspended. *Fruit* surrounded by a dry or fleshy receptacle, or composed of consolidated fleshy calyxes, within which lies a multitude of nuts. *Seeds* erect, parietal, or pendulous. *Embryo* more or less albuminous, straight, with the radicle directed towards the vertex of the ovary.—*Trees* or *shrubs*, with a milky juice. *Leaves* alternate. *Stipules* large, convolute.

PROPERTIES.—The milky juice is variable in quality : in some species being poisonous, in some edible, in others neither. It usually, if not invariably, contains caoutchouc.— The *Artocarpus incisa*, or *Bread fruit tree*, and the *A. integrifolia* or *Jak fruit*, deserve notice on account of their important alimentary uses. *Artocarpus incisa* is a native of the islands of the Pacific and of the Moluccas. Its fruit is to the inhabitants of Polynesia what corn is to the people of other parts of the world. *Artocarpus integrifolia* is cultivated throughout southern India, and all the warmer parts of Asia. Its fruit forms a very considerable article of food in Ceylon.[1]

126. Antiaris toxicaria, *Leschinault.*—Antsjar or Upas.

This is the celebrated *Antsjar* or *Upas* poison tree of Java, rendered notorious principally in consequence of certain gross falsehoods concerning it, about the year 1780, by a person of the name of Foersch, said to have been a surgeon in the service of the Dutch East India Company. Malefactors, says this person, when they receive sentence of death, are offered the chance of life, if they will go to the Upas-tree for a box of poison; and although every precaution is taken to avoid the injurious influence of the emanations of the tree, yet of 700 criminals who went to collect the poison, scarcely two out of twenty returned. Foersch further adds, that for fifteen or eighteen miles around this tree no living animal of any kind has ever been discovered.[2] Dr. Horsfield[3] and M. Leschinault[4] have shown that the above statements are for the most part fabulous. From their observations it appears that the *true poison tree* of Java is the *Antiaris toxicaria*[5] (fig. 166). It is one of the largest forest trees of Java, being from 60 to 100 feet high. The milky juice is collected by incision, and is then inspissated by boiling along with the juice of arum, galanga, and onions. The poison, when brought to this country, is found to be a thick fluid of a grayish-brown or fawn-colour, and an unpleasant odour. It consists, according to Pelletier and Caventou,[6] of *a peculiar elastic resin, slightly soluble*

---

[1] Hooker, *Bot. Mag.* vol. ii. N.S.

[2] See the translation of Foersch's paper, in Burnett's *Outlines of Botany*, 552; also *Penny Magaz.* vol. ii. p. 321.

[3] *Quarterly Journal*, vol. ii. p. 331.

[4] *Ann. du Mus. d'Hist. Nat.* t. xvi. p. 476.

[5] For a very elaborate account of this tree, by M. I. J. Bennett, see Dr. Horsfield's *Plantæ Javanicæ rariores*, p. 52.

[6] *Ann. Chim. et Phys.* t. xxvi. p. 44.

gummy matter analogous to bassorin, and *a bitter matter soluble in water.* This bitter matter is composed of *a colouring matter* absorbable by charcoal, *an undetermined acid,* and *antiarin,* the active principle of the plant, and which is precipitable by tincture of galls.

FIG. 166.

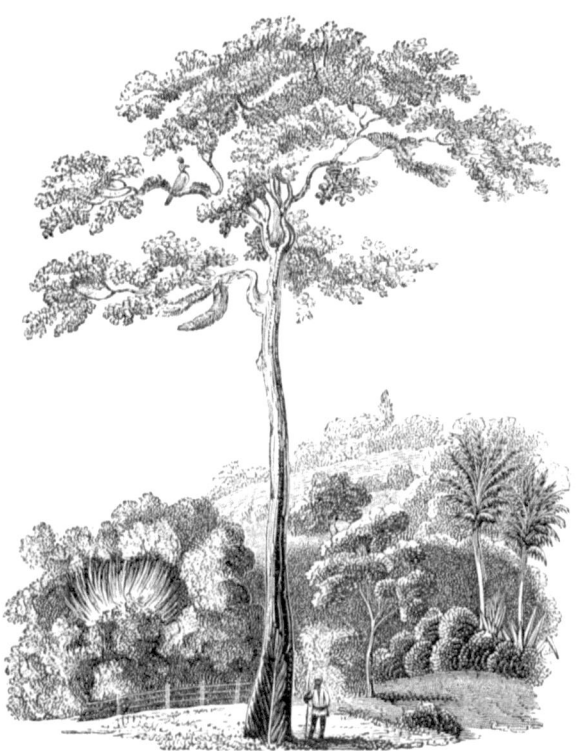

Arbor toxicaria, Ipo., Rumph; *Antiaris toxicaria,* Leschinault.
(From Blume's *Rumphia.*)

More recently, Mulder[1] has submitted this juice to analysis, and found it to consist of *vegetable albumen* 16·14, *gum* 12·34, *antiar-resin* 20·93, *myricin* 7·02, *antiarin* 3·56, *sugar* 6·31, and *extractive* 33·70. The antiar-resin was composed of $C^{16}H^{12}O$. Antiarin consisted of $C^{14}H^{10}O^5$. Sir B. Brodie[2] says the poison renders the heart insensible to the stimulus of the blood. Magendie and Delile[3] found that, besides acting on the brain and spinal marrow, it proved emetic. According to Andral, it causes convulsions with alternations of relaxation.

ORDER XXXII. PIPERACEÆ, *Richard.*—PEPPERWORTS.

CHARACTERS.—*Flowers* naked, hermaphrodite, with a bract on the outside. *Stamens* 2 or more, arranged on one side, or all round the ovary; to which they adhere more or

---

[1] *Pharmaceutisches Central-Blatt für* 1838, S. 511.
  Phil. Trans. for 1811.
[3] Orfila, *Toxicol. Gén.*

less; *anthers* 1—2-celled, with or without a fleshy connective; *pollen* roundish, smooth. *Ovary* superior, simple, 1-celled, containing a single erect, orthotropal *ovule; stigma* sessile, simple, rather oblique. *Fruit* superior, somewhat fleshy, indehiscent, 1-celled, 1-seeded. *Seed* erect, with the embryo lying in a fleshy sac, placed at the apex of the seed on the outside of the albumen.—*Shrubs* or *herbaceous plants.* *Stems* articulated. *Leaves* opposite, verticillate, or alternate, in consequence of the abortion of one of the pair of leaves. *Stipules* 0, or in pairs, or single and opposite the leaf. *Flowers* usually sessile, sometimes pedicellate, in spikes which are either terminal or axillary; or opposite the leaves (*Lindley*).

PROPERTIES.—Fruits remarkable for their hot taste, and acrid and stimulant properties. These qualities they owe to the presence of an acrid oil and resin.

127. PIPER NIGRUM, *Linn.*—THE BLACK PEPPER.

Sex. Syst. Diandria, Trigynia.

(Fructus immaturus, *L.*—Dried unripe Berries, *E. D.*)

HISTORY.—The ancient Greeks were acquainted with pepper (πέπερι), their knowledge of which must have been derived, directly or indirectly, from the Hindoos. Hippocrates[1] employed it in several diseases. Pliny[2] notices its uses as a condiment, and expresses his astonishment that it should have come into general use, since it has neither flavour nor appearance to recommend it.

BOTANY. **Gen. Char.**—*Spadix* covered with flowers on all sides. *Flowers* hermaphrodite, rarely dioecious, each supported by a scale. *Stamina* 2 or

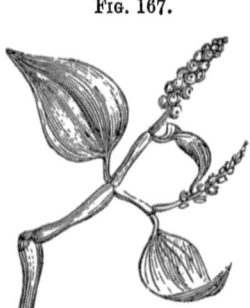

FIG. 167.

Piper nigrum.

more. *Ovarium* with 1 solitary erect *ovule.* *Stigma* punctiform, obtuse, or split. *Berry* 1-seeded. *Embryo* dicotyledonous [monocotyledonous, *Blume*], inverted (Blume).

Sp. Char.—*Stem* shrubby, radicant, climbing, terete. *Leaves* ovate or elliptical, acuminate, occasionally somewhat oblique, subcordate, 5—7-nerved, coriaceous, smooth, recurved at the margin, glauco-greenish beneath. *Spadices* shortly pedunculated, pendulous. *Fruits* distinct (Blume).[4]

Stem 8—12 feet long, jointed, dichotomous. *Fruit* at first green, then red, afterwards black.

According to Dr. Roxburgh,[5] *Piper trioicum* is cultivated, and yields excellent pepper.

Hab.—Cultivated in various parts of India and its islands (Roxburgh), also in the West Indies.

PREPARATION.—When any of the berries on a spadix change from green to red, the whole are considered fit for gathering; for if they are allowed to become fully ripe, they are somewhat less acrid, and, moreover, easily drop off. When collected, they are spread out and dried in the sun, and the stalks separated by hand-rubbing. They are afterwards winnowed.[6] The dried and shrivelled berries constitute *black pepper* (*piper nigrum*).

---

[1] *De morb. mul.* &c.

[2] *Hist. Nat.* lib. xii. cap. 14, ed. Valp.

[3] *Enum. Plant. Javæ*, p. 64.

[4] *Op. cit.*

[5] *Fl. Indica*, vol. i. p. 153.

[6] Marsden, *History of Sumatra*, 3d edit. p. 137.

White pepper (*piper album*) is prepared from the best and soundest grains, taken at their most perfect age of maturity. These being soaked in water, swell and burst their tegument, which is afterwards carefully separated by drying in the sun, hand-rubbing, and winnowing.[1]

COMMERCE.—The pepper countries extend from about the longitude of 90° to that of 115° E., beyond which no pepper is to be found; and they reach from about 5° S. latitude to about 12° N., where it again ceases. The following estimate of the production of pepper is drawn up by Mr. Crawford :[2]—

PRODUCTION OF PEPPER.

Sumatra (west coast)	20,000,000 lbs.
Sumatra (east coast)	8,000,000
Islands in the Straits of Malacca	3,600,000
Malay Peninsula	3,733,333
Borneo	2,666,667
Siam	8,000,000
Malabar	4,000,000
Total	50,000,000

DESCRIPTION.—*Black pepper* (*piper nigrum*) is round, covered externally with a brownish-black corrugated layer (the remains of the succulent portion of the berry), which may be readily removed by softening it in water. Internally we have a hard, whitish, spherical, smooth seed, which is horny externally but farinaceous internally. The taste of both nucleus and covering is acrid and hot. Amongst wholesale dealers three sorts are distinguished :—

1. *Malabar pepper.*—This is the most valuable : it is *brownish-black*, free from stalks, and nearly free from dust.

2. *Sumatra pepper.*—This is the cheapest sort. It is *black*, mixed occasionally with a few stalks, and contains from one to five per cent. of dust. (Under the name of Sumatra pepper some dealers include the Penang or brownish-black sort, and the black Sumatra sort.)

[3. *Penang pepper; Batavia pepper.*—This is the cheapest sort. It is sometimes blackish, but usually earthy-coloured. It generally contains from two to ten per cent. of dust. The grains are large.—ED.]

The heavier the pepper is, the more it is esteemed in the market. The heaviest of all, being hard and smooth, is called *shot pepper*, which is always Malabar, Sumatra, or Penang sort. Most dealers sift their black pepper before offering it for sale, and use the dust (called P. D.) for pickling or grinding.

Fulton's decorticated pepper is black pepper deprived of its husk by mechanical trituration.

Bleached pepper, or *English bleached pepper*, is Penang pepper bleached by chlorine. In this state it ought perhaps to be classed among the white peppers.

White pepper (*piper album*) is the fruit deprived of the external fleshy portion of the pericarp. The grains are larger than those of black pepper, spherical, whitish, and smooth, horny externally ; internally they are farinaceous or hollow in the centre. They are less acrid and pungent than black pepper. In commerce three sorts are distinguished :—

---

[1] Marsden, *op. cit.*
[2] M'Culloch, *Dict. of Commerce.*

2 c

1. *Tellicherry pepper*, which is of two kinds.   The *fine Tellicherry pepper* is not larger, but it is whiter and brighter than any other description of white pepper, and fetches a higher price.

2. *The Penang.*—[This is the boldest white pepper made, but it is inferior in colour to the *Tellicherry* sort.—Ed.]

3. *Batavia.*—This sort resembles *Tellicherry* in shape, and is preferred to the Singapore kind.   There is another description, called *Limed Batavia*, but this is *limed* for the Dutch market.

4. *Singapore.*—[This is the lowest of the four sorts.   It is usually more or less mixed with shrivelled grains.   The production is greater than that of the others.—Ed.]

5. *English bleached white pepper.*—When the two preceding sorts are scarce, brown Penang pepper is bleached.   The yellowest and largest grains are chosen for this purpose, for neither an expensive nor small sort would pay.

[An attempt has been made to convert black to white pepper by depriving it of the outer coating ; but the loss in weight is so great, and the article when made is so inferior in quality, that the process is not carried on.   It is to be observed, that the three first peppers are bleached before they go into consumption : hence we are hardly justified in making a distinct variety under the head of *English bleached pepper.*—Ed.]

Composition.—In 1819, Oersted discovered *piperin* in pepper.   In 1821 black pepper was analysed by Pelletier.[1]   In 1822 white pepper was analysed by Lucä.[2]

BLACK PEPPER (*Pelletier*).	WHITE PEPPER (*Lucä*).	
Acrid soft resin.	Acrid resin	16·60
Volatile oil.	Volatile oil	1·61
Piperin.	Extractive, gum, and salts	12·50
Extractive.	Starch	18·50
Gum.	Albumen	2·50
Bassorin.	Woody fibre	29·00
Starch.	Water and loss	19·29
Malic acid.		
Tartaric acid.		
Potash, calcareous and magnesian salts.		
Woody fibre.		
Black pepper.	White pepper	100·00

Dr. Ure[3] obtained, from 100 parts of white peppercorns, a trace of volatile oil, 8½ grs. of a pungent resin containing a small fraction of piperin, about 60 grs. of starch with a little gum, and nearly 30 grains of matter (lignin) insoluble in hot or cold water.

Lucä found no *piperin* in white pepper, but Poutet[4] subsequently detected it.   Probably, therefore, in Lucä's analysis the piperin was contained in the resin.

1. Resin of Pepper (*Resina Piperis*).—This is a very acrid substance, soluble in alcohol and ether, but not so in volatile oils.   It possesses in high perfection the acrid properties of pepper.   Dissolved in ether, it was employed by Dr. Lucas in intermittents, and in two out of three cases with success.[5]   In the museum of the Pharmaceutical

[1] *Ann. de Chim. et de Phys.* xvi. 344.
[2] Schwartze, *Pharm. Tabellen.*
[3] *Supplement* to Ure's *Dict. of Arts*, p. 200, 1844.
[4] *Journ. de Pharm.* t. vii.
[5] Dierbach, *Neuest. Entd. in d. Mat. Med.* Bd. i. S. 252, 1837.

Society are two kinds of pepper resin: one called the "green resin," the other the "red resin."

2. VOLATILE OIL OF PEPPER (*Oleum Piperis*).—When pure this is colourless; it has the odour and taste of pepper. Its sp. gr. is 9·9932 (Lucä). Its composition is $C^{10}H^8$. It absorbs hydrochloric acid in large quantity, but does not form a crystalline compound with it. According to Meli,[1] it possesses the same febrifuge properties as piperin,— perhaps because it retains some of the latter principle. It has been used in some forms of dyspepsia depending on general debility.

3. PIPERIN.—This substance was discovered by Oersted in 1819, but was more accurately examined by Pelletier in 1821. It exists in black, white, and long pepper, and also in cubebs. It is a crystalline substance, the crystals being rhombic prisms, with inclined bases. It fuses at 212° F., is insoluble in cold water, and is only very slightly soluble in boiling water. Its best solvent is alcohol: the solution throws down piperin when water is added to it. Ether dissolves it, but not so readily as alcohol. Acetic acid is likewise a solvent for it.

Piperin when pure, is white; but as met with in commerce it is usually straw-yellow. It is tasteless and inodorous. It was at first supposed to be an alkali; but Pelletier has shown that it possesses no analogy with vegetable alkalies, and that it is related to the resins. With strong sulphuric acid it forms a blood-red liquid. Nitric acid colours it first greenish-yellow, then orange, and afterwards red. The action of hydrochloric acid is similar. Its formula, according to Regnault, is $C^{34}H^{19}NO^6$.

Piperin has been recommended and employed by Meli and several other physicians[2] as a febrifuge in intermittent fevers. It is said to be more certain and speedy, and also milder in its action, than the cinchona alkalies. Moreover, we are told that it might be procured at a cheaper rate than sulphate of quina. Its dose is about six or eight grains in powder or pills. Sixty grains have been taken in twenty-four hours, without causing any injurious effects. Meli considers two or three scruples sufficient to cure an intermittent. Magendie[3] proposes it in blenorrhagia, instead of cubebs.

4. STARCH. — Both black and white peppercorns contain abundance of very minute starch-grains.

ADULTERATION.—Sago is said to have been used to adulterate ground white pepper. The microscope would readily detect the fraud ; the starch-grains of sago being very much larger than those of pepper, from which they also differ in shape.

PHYSIOLOGICAL EFFECTS.—Pepper is one of the acrid species whose general effects have been already noticed. Its great acridity is recognised when we apply it to the tongue. On the skin it acts as a rubefacient and vesicant.[4] Swallowed, it stimulates the stomach, creates a sensation of warmth in this viscus, and, when used in small doses, assists the digestive functions, but if given in large quantities induces an inflammatory condition. Thirty white peppercorns, taken for a stomach complaint, induced violent burning pain, thirst, and accelerated pulse, which continued for three days, until the fruits were evacuated.[5] Wendt, Lange, and Jager[6] have also reported cases in which inflammatory symptoms supervened after the use of pepper. On the vascular and secerning systems pepper acts as a stimulant. It accelerates the frequency of the pulse, promotes diaphoresis, and acts as an excitant to the mucous surfaces. On one of my patients (a lady) the copious use of pepper induces burning heat of skin, and a few spots of *Urticaria evanida* usually on the face. "I have seen," says Van Swieten,[7] "a most ardent and danger-

[1] Dierbach, *op. cit.*
[2] Dierbach, *op. cit.* Bd. i. S. 176, 1828.
[3] *Formulaire.*
[4] Richard, *Dict. de Méd.* t. xvii. p. 307.
[5] Wibmer, *Arzneim. u. Gifte*, Bd. iv. S. 220.
[6] Quoted by Wibmer, *op. cit.* S. 119.
[7] *Commentaries*, English transl. vol. v. p. 57.

ous fever raised in a person who had swallowed a great quantity of beaten pepper." It has long been regarded as a stimulant for the urino-genital apparatus. The opinion is supported by the well-known influence of the peppers over certain morbid conditions of these organs. Moreover, the beneficial effect of pepper in some affections of the rectum leads us to suspect that this viscus is also influenced by these fruits.

USES.—It is employed as a condiment, partly for its flavour, partly for its stimulant influence over the stomach, by which it assists digestion. As a gastric stimulant it is a useful addition to difficultly-digestible foods, as fatty and mucilaginous matters, especially persons subject to stomach complaints from a torpid or atonic condition of this viscus. Infused in ardent spirit it is a popular remedy for preventing the return of the paroxysms of intermittent fevers, given shortly before the expected attack. The practice is not recent, for Celsus[1] advises warm water with pepper to relieve the cold fit. The febrifuge power of this spice has been fully proved, in numerous cases, by L. Frank,[2] Meli,[3] Riedmüller (Dierbach), and others; though Schmitz[4] denies it. Barbier[5] says that in some instances where large doses were exhibited death occurred in consequence of the aggravation of a pre-existent gastritis. It has been employed in gonorrhœa as a substitute for cubebs. In relaxed uvula, paralysis of the tongue, and other affections of the mouth or throat requiring the use of a powerful acrid, pepper may be employed as a masticatory. In the form of ointment it is used as an application to tinea capitis. Mixed with mustard it is employed to increase the acridity of sinapisms.

ADMINISTRATION.—The dose of black pepper (either of corns or powder) is from five to fifteen grains; the powder may be given in the form of pills.

1. CONFECTIO PIPERIS, L.; *Electuarium Piperis*, E.; *Confectio Piperis Nigri*, D.; *Confection of Black Pepper*. (Black Pepper, Elecampane-root [Liquorice-root in powder, *E.*], of each lb. j.; Fennel Seeds, lb. iij.; Honey, Sugar, of each lb. ij. Rub the dry ingredients together to a very fine powder, L. Black Pepper in fine powder, Liquorice Root in powder, of each ℥ss.; Refined Sugar, ℥j.; Oil of Fennel, f℥ss.; Clarified Honey, by weight, ℥ij. Rub the dry substances together into a very fine powder, then add the honey and oil, and beat them into a uniform mass, D. The *London College* keeps this in a covered vessel, and directs the honey to be added when the confection is to be used. But the *Edinburgh* and *Dublin Colleges* order the honey to be added immediately after the ingredients have been mixed.)—This preparation is intended to be a substitute for a quack medicine, called "*Ward's Paste*," which has obtained some celebrity as a remedy for fistulæ, piles, and ulcers about the rectum. Its efficacy doubtless depends on the gentle stimulus it gives to the affected parts. Sir B. Brodie[6] observes, that severe cases of piles are sometimes cured by it; and he thinks that it acts on them topically, the greater part of the paste passing into the colon, becoming blended with the fæces, and in this way coming in contact with

[1] Lib. iii. cap. 12.
[2] *Journ. Complém. du Dict. des Scienc. Méd.* t. viii. p. 371.
[3] *Ibid.* t. xiii. p. 124.
[4] Rust's *Magaz.* Bd. xvi.
[5] *Traité Élém. de Mat. Méd.* 2de édit. t. ii. p. 57.
[6] *Lectures* in *Lond. Med. Gaz.* vol. xv. p. 746.

the piles, on which it operates as a local application, much as *vinum opii* acts on the vessels of the conjunctiva in chronic ophthalmia. In confirmation of this view, he mentions the case of a patient attended by Sir Everard Home, who was cured by the introduction of the paste into the rectum. Confection of black pepper is adapted for weak and leucophlegmatic habits, and is objectionable where much irritation or inflammation is present. The dose of it is from one to two or three drachms twice or thrice a day. " It is of no use," says Sir B. Brodie, " to take this remedy for a week, a fortnight, or a month: it must be persevered in for two, three, or four months." As it is apt to accumulate in and distend the colon, gentle aperients should be exhibited occasionally during the time the patient is taking the confection.

2. **UNGUENTUM PIPERIS NIGRI**; *Ointment of Black Pepper.* (Prepared Hogs' Lard, lb. j.; Black Pepper, reduced to powder, ʒiv. Make an ointment.)—Formerly in vogue for the cure of tinea capitis. [It is no longer officinal.—ED.]

[3. **EXTRACTUM PIPERIS FLUIDUM**, U.S.; *Fluid Extract of Black Pepper.* (Take of Black Pepper, lb. j.; Ether, a sufficient quantity. Put the powder into a percolator, and pour ether gradually upon it, until two pints of filtered liquor are obtained. From this, distil off, by means of a water-bath at a gentle heat, a pint and a half of ether, and expose the residue in a shallow vessel until the whole of the ether has evaporated, and the deposit of piperin and crystals has ceased. Lastly, separate the piperin by expression through a cloth, and keep the liquid portion.

This preparation is of semifluid consistence, of a dark colour, and possessed strongly of the odour and taste of black pepper. It may be used in those cases in which this article is usually employed. Dose, grs. xx. to ʒss.—ED.]

---

128. CHAVICA[1] ROXBURGHII, *Miquel.*[2]—COMMON LONG PEPPER.

Sex. Syst. Diandria, Trigynia.
(Fructus immaturus, *L.*—Dried Spikes, *E.*)

SYNONYMES.—*Piper longum*, Linn. in part; figure in Nees' Plant. Medic. tab. 23.·

HISTORY.—Long pepper (πέπερι μακρόν) is mentioned both by Dioscorides[3] and Galen.[4]

BOTANY. **Gen. Char.**—Woody. *Spikes* solitary, opposite to the leaves. *Flowers* sessile, diœcious. *Bracts* with short stalks, nearly quadrangular, peltate. *Style* very short or 0. *Berries* sessile, united with the permanent bracts and the thickened rachis of the spike. *Seeds* oblong, or almost lenticular, with a crustaceous finely scrobiculate testa and a mealy albumen.

---

[1] Chavica is the Sanscrit name for plants of this kind.
[2] *Systema Piperacearum*, Rotterdam, 1843. See also *Pharmaceutisches Central-Blatt für* 1839, pp. 415 and 431; and *für* 1845, p. 9;—and *Buchner's Repertorium*, Bd. xxxvi. S. 229, 1844; and Bd. xxxix. S. 14, 1845.
[3] Lib. ii. cap. 189.
[4] *De Simpl. Med. Facult.* lib. viii. cap. 16, 11.

Sp. Char.—Rather hairy; lower leaves roundish-ovate, 7-nerved; female spikes cylindrical, about as long as their stalk.

Hab.—India. Found wild among bushes on the banks of watercourses up towards the Circa mountains. It flowers and bears fruit during the wet and cold seasons (Roxburgh). It is cultivated in Bengal, and in the valleys amongst the Circar mountains. The roots and thickest parts of the stems, when cut into small pieces and dried, form a considerable article of commerce all over India, under the name of *Pippula moola.*

DESCRIPTION.—When fully grown, but yet unripe, the spadices are gathered and dried by exposure to the sun. They are then packed in bags for sale. As met with in commerce, *long pepper* (*piper longum*) is greyish-brown, cylindrical, an inch or more in length, having a mild aromatic odour but a violent pungent taste. [In its natural state its colour is brown, but it usually receives a slight coating of lime. The best comes from Singapore and Batavia.—ED.]

The long pepper imported from our possessions in India is the produce of *Chavica Roxburghii,* Miq. But that which is brought to Europe from the Dutch colonies is the produce of *Chavica officinarum,* Miq.

COMPOSITION.—This pepper was analysed by Dulong in 1825.[1] The following are the substances he obtained from it :—*Acrid fatty matter* (resin?), *volatile oil, piperin, nitrogenous extractive, gum, bassorin, starch, malates and other salts.*

The VOLATILE OIL OF LONG PEPPER is colourless, and has a disagreeable odour and an acrid taste.

PHYSIOLOGICAL EFFECTS.—The effects of long pepper are analogous to those of black pepper. Cullen[2] and Bergius[3] consider it less powerful; but most other pharmacologists are agreed on its being more acrid. Medicinally it may be employed in similar cases. It is used principally in pickling, and for culinary purposes. It is a constituent of several pharmacopœial preparations.

129. Chavica Betle, *Miquel.*—Betle Pepper.

PIPER BETLE, *Linnæus.*—The leaf of this plant (as well as of *Chavica Siriboa,* Miq.) is extensively used by the Malays and other nations of the East, who consider it a necessary of life. The mode of taking it in Sumatra consists simply in spreading on the *sirih* (the leaf of the Chavica Betle) a small quantity of *chunam* (quick-lime prepared from calcined shells), and folding it up with a slice of *pinang* or Areca nut. As a result of mastication there exudes a juice which tinges the saliva of a bright red colour, and which the leaf and nut, without the lime, will not yield. This hue being communicated to the mouth and lips, is esteemed ornamental, and an agreeable flavour is imparted to the breath. The juice is usually, but not always, swallowed. To persons who are not habituated to this composition it causes giddiness, astringes and excoriates the mouth and fauces, and deadens for a time the faculty of taste. Individuals, when toothless, have the ingredients previously reduced to a paste, that they may dissolve without further effort.[4]

[1] *Journ. de Pharm.* t. xi. p. 52.
[2] *Mat. Med.* vol. ii. p. 209.
[3] *Mat. Med.* ed. 2nda, t. i. p. 29.
[4] Marsden, *Hist. of Sumatra,* 3d edit. p. 281.

130. CUBEBA OFFICINALIS, *Miq.*—THE CUBEB PEPPER.

Sex. Syst. Diandria, Trigynia.

(Fructus immaturus, *L.*—Fruit, *E.*—The Berries, *D.*)

SYNONYME.—*Piper Cubeba*, Linn. fil., Blume, L.

HISTORY.—It is somewhat doubtful when cubebs were first employed in medicine, and by whom they were first noticed. I am inclined to believe, however, that they are mentioned in the Hippocratic writings[1] under the name of μυρτίδανον : for 1st, the remedy termed μυρτίδανον is distinguished from pepper (πέπερι), and is said to be *a round Indian fruit which the Persians call pepper.* 2ndly, the modern Greek name for cubebs is μυρτίδανον.[2] The word cubebs is derived from the Arabic name for these fruits, which first occurs in the writings of Serapion,[3] Rhazes, and Avicenna. From the same source Actuarius[4] derived the name κομβέβας, by which he has designated cubebs. Cubebs were in use in England more than 500 years ago, for in 1305 Edward I. granted to the Corporation of London the power of levying a toll of one farthing a pound on this article in its passage over London Bridge.[5]

BOTANY. **Gen. Char.**—Woody. *Spike* solitary, opposite the leaves. *Flowers* diœcious. *Ovary* sessile. *Stigmas* 3—5, sessile. *Berries,* by the contracted basis, apparently stalked (pseudo-pedicellate). *Seed* roundish, with leathery or horny testa and mealy albumen. (Condensed from Miquel).

Sp. Char.—*Leaves* smooth; the lower ones unequal, somewhat cordate at the base, ovate, acute ; the upper ones more oblong-ovate, with rounded base, and smaller ; those of the male plant 5-nerved, of the female plant 5—9-nerved. *Fruit* globose, shorter than their stalks.—A climbing shrub.

Hab.—Grows wild in Bantam, the western part of Java; also on some of the neighbouring islands.—Cultivated in the lower parts of Java.

The above is, according to Miquel, the mother-plant of the genuine cubebs. But a neighbouring species,—*Cubeba canina*, Miquel,—yields a fruit which, according to Blume, also forms part of the cubebs of commerce. This plant grows on the Sunda and Molucca islands. The fruits and seeds of the two species are thus distinguished.

C. OFFICINALIS, *Miq.*	C. CANINA, *Miq.*
Berries far more numerous, crowded, almost globose, scarcely acuminate ; when dry, rugous, blackish-brown, having a very acrid, aromatic, almost bitter taste.	Fewer, more remote, ovate ; when dry, remarkably beaked (rostrate), black, smaller, scarcely rugous, having a weaker, almost anise-like taste.
Seed-coat (spermoderm), greyish-brown, traversed by eight longitudinal nerves, oblong-globular.	Reddish, almost shining, lined (*striolata*) longitudinally, spherical.
Fruit-stalks (formed of the thin lower portion of the berry) longer than the berries.	Nearly of the same length as the berries.

---

[1] *De Morbis Mulierum*, lib. ii. p. 672, ed. Fœsii.—The term μυρτίδανον was also used to signify a myrtle-like plant, and likewise a rough excrescence growing on the μυρσίνη (*Ruscus aculeatus*). See Dioscorides, lib. i. cap. 156.

[2] *Pharmacopœia Græca*, Athenis, 1837.

[3] In his account of cubebs, Serapion has translated what Dioscorides has said of μυρσίνη (*Ruscus aculeatus*), and added everything which Galen has stated respecting καρπήσιον. But Galen expressly states that καρπήσιον resembles φοῦ (the root of *Valeriana Dioscoridis*) ; and it is improbable, therefore, that cubebs and carpesium should be identical.

[4] C. Bauhini *Pinax*.—No Greek edition of Actuarius has been published, and I am, therefore, obliged to quote his writings at second-hand. In my copy of the Latin translation (*De Medicamentorum compositione*, J. Ruellio interprete, p. 69 *b*, 1546), the phrase runs thus—" carpesii (cubebe barbari vocant)."

[5] *Liber Niger Scaccarii*, vol. i. p. *478 ; also *The Chronicles of London Bridge*, p. 155.

DESCRIPTION.—The dried unripe fruit of this plant constitutes the *cubebs* *cubebæ* vel *piper caudatum*) of the shops.[1] In appearance, cubebs resemble black pepper, except that they are lighter coloured, and are each furnished with a stalk two or three inches long, and from which circumstance they have received their name *caudatum*. The cortical portion of cubebs (that which constituted the fleshy portion of the fruit) appears to have been thinner and less succulent than in black pepper. Within it is a hard spherical seed, which is whitish and oily. The taste of cubebs is acrid, peppery, and camphoraceous; the odour is peculiar and aromatic.

[Besides the well-known commercial cubebs, there are also to be met with in the market "wild cubebs." They are both imported from Batavia and Singapore. We have been favoured by Mr. A. Faber with good samples of the two kinds.

The importation of cubebs in the ten years from 1835 to 1844 amounted to 8260 bags, and the consumption to 5717 bags of about 70 lbs. each, making the average annual consumption of those years 40,019 pounds.—ED.]

COMPOSITION.—Three analyses of cubebs have been made: one by Trommsdorff, in 1811;[2] a second by Vauquelin, in 1820;[3] and a third by Monheim, in 1835.[4]

Vauquelin.	*Manheim.*	
1. Volatile oil, nearly solid.	1. Green volatile oil	2·5
2. Resin, like that of copaiva.	2. Yellow volatile oil	1·0
3. Another coloured resin.	3. Cubebin	4·5
4. A coloured gummy matter.	4. Balsamic resin	1·5
5. Extractive.	5. Wax	3·0
6. Saline matter.	6. Chloride of sodium	1·0
	7. Extractive	6·0
	8. Lignin	65·0
	Loss	15·5
Cubebs.	Cubebs	100·0

1. ESSENTIAL OIL OF CUBEBS.—(See *post.*)

2. RESIN OF CUBEBS.—Vauquelin has described two resins of cubebs: one is green, liquid, acrid, and analogous, both in odour and taste, to balsam of copaiva; the other is brown, solid, acrid, and insoluble in ether.

3. CUBEBIN.—From cubebs is obtained a principle to which the term *cubebin* has been applied. It is very analogous to piperin. Cassola, a Neapolitan chemist,[5] says, it is distinguished from the latter principle by the fine crimson colour which it produces with sulphuric acid, and which remains unaltered for twenty or twenty four hours; more-

---

[1] [CUBEBA CLUSII; *African Cubebs.*—The article known under this name, called also *Piper caudatum*, or tail pepper, has been recently examined by Mr. Stenhouse. By the action of potash on an alcoholic extract of these cubebs, he obtained a crop of large and nearly colourless crystals, in the form of oblique four-sided prisms, resembling *piperine.* The crystals are very soluble in hot spirit of wine, pretty soluble in ether, but insoluble in water. When distilled with potash, they yield a volatile base, which has the characteristic odour of *piperidine.* Ultimate analysis showed their composition to be $C^{68}H^{38}N^2O^{12}$. Mr. Stenhouse concludes that, whatever may be their botanical characters, the chemical properties of African cubebs prove that they are really a species of pepper, containing, as they do, *piperine*, and not *cubebine*, the non-nitrogenous crystallisable principle of the Cubeb tribe, which possesses no basic properties. It is curious, that while the *smell* of the African cubebs is very similar to that of ordinary cubebs, the *taste* closely approaches that of common pepper (*Pharmaceutical Journal*, Feb. 1855, p. 363; for a further account of the history of the plant, see a paper by Dr. Daniell, *Pharmaceutical Journal*, Nov. 1854, p. 198).—ED.]

[2] Schwartz, *Pharm. Tabell.*
[3] *Ann. Phil.* 2d series, vol. iii. p. 202.
[4] *Journ de Pharm.* xx. 403.
[5] *Journ. de Chim. Méd.* t. x. p. 685.

over, cubebin is not crystallisable. [Engelhardt found a large deposit of cubebin from an ethereal infusion of cubebs which had been kept for some months. As this substance is almost insoluble in ether at the ordinary temperature, it was probably dissolved by the oils extracted by the ether. In the preparation of this substance, according to the general method, there would consequently be a considerable loss resulting from the extraction with ether previous to dissolving the cubebin in alcohol.[1]—ED.]

According to Monheim,[2] cubebin is identical with piperin, and he asserts that it is combined with a soft acrid resin. In this state it is soluble in ether, alcohol, the fixed oils, and acetic acid; but it is insoluble in oil of turpentine and dilute sulphuric acid. It fuses at 68° F.

Dr. Görres[3] gave cubebin, in both acute and chronic gonorrhœa, to the extent of one drachm, four times daily. But he premised the use of phosphoric acid.

4. EXTRACTIVE MATTER OF CUBEBS.—Vauquelin says, the extractive matter of cubebs is analogous to that found in leguminous plants. It is precipitable by galls, but not by acetate of lead.

PHYSIOLOGICAL EFFECTS.—Cubebs belong to the class of acrid substances already noticed in the first volume of this work. Their sensible operation is very analogous to that of black pepper. Taken in moderate doses, they stimulate the stomach, augment the appetite, and promote the digestive process. In larger quantities, or taken when the stomach is in an irritated or inflammatory condition, they cause nausea, vomiting, burning pain, griping, and even purging. These are their local effects. The constitutional effects are those resulting from the operation of an excitant,—namely, increased frequency and fulness of pulse, thirst, and augmented heat. They probably stimulate all the mucous surfaces, but unequally so   In some instances cubebs give rise to an eruption on the skin like urticaria. Not unfrequently they cause headache; and occasionally disorder of the cerebro-spinal functions, manifested by convulsive movements or partial paralysis, as in a case related by Mr. Broughton.[4]

Cubebs appear to exercise a specific influence over the urino-genital apparatus. Thus, they frequently act as diuretics, and at the same time deepen the colour of, and communicate a peculiar aromatic odour to the urine. Their stimulant operation on the bladder is well illustrated by a case related by Sir Benjamin Brodie.[5]   A gentleman, labouring under chronic inflammation of the bladder, took fifteen grains of cubebs, every eight hours, with much relief. Being anxious to expedite his cure, he, of his own accord, increased the dose to a drachm. This was followed by an aggravation of the symptoms: the irritation of the bladder was much increased, the mucus was secreted in much larger quantity than before, and ultimately the patient died,—" his death being, I will not say occasioned," adds Sir Benjamin, " but certainly very much hastened, by his imprudence in overdosing himself with cubebs." Three drachms of cubebs caused in Pül[6] nausea, acid eructations, heat at the pit of the stomach, headache, uneasiness, and fever.

USES.—The principal use of cubebs is in the treatment of *gonorrhœa.* They should be given in as large doses as the stomach can bear, in the early part of the disease; for experience has fully proved that in proportion to the length of time gonorrhœa has existed, the less amenable is it to the influence

[1] *Pharmaceutical Journal*, July 1854, p. 37.
[2] *Journ. de Chim. Méd.* t. x. p. 685.
[3] Dierbach, *Neusten Entd. in d. Mat. Méd.* S. 253, 1837.
[4] *Lond. Med. Gaz.* vol. i. p. 405.
[5] *Ibid.* vol. i. p. 300.
[6] *Arzneim. u. Giften*, Bd. iv. S. 217.

of cubebs. In some instances an immediate stop is put to the progress of the malady. In others the violent symptoms only are palliated; while in many (according to my experience in most) cases no obvious influence over the disease is manifested. The presence of active inflammation of the urethra does not positively preclude the use of cubebs, though I have more than once seen them aggravate the symptoms. Mr. Jeffreys[1] thinks the greatest success is met with in the more inflammatory forms of the disease. Cubebs have been charged with inducing swelled testicle; but I have not observed this affection to be more frequent after the use of cubebs than when they were not employed. Mr. Broughton[2] gave them to fifty patients, and in forty-five they proved successful. Of these only two had swelled testicle. The explanation of the *methodus medendi* is unsatisfactory. Sir A. Cooper[3] thinks that cubebs produce a specific inflammation of their own on the urethra, which has the effect of superseding the gonorrhœal inflammation. The occasional occurrence of a cutaneous eruption from the use of cubebs deserves especial attention, as I have known it create a suspicion of secondary symptoms.

Cubebs have been recommended in gleet and leucorrhœa.[4] In abscess of the prostate gland, twenty or thirty grains of cubebs, taken three times a day, have in many cases appeared to do good.[5] They seemed to give a gentle stimulus to the parts, and to influence the disease much in the same way that Ward's Paste operates on abscesses and fistulæ, and ulcers of the rectum. In cystirrhœa also they have occasionally proved serviceable in small doses.[6] In piles, likewise, they are given with advantage.[7] The efficacy of cubebs in mucous discharges is not confined to the urino-genital mucous membrane. In catarrhal affections of the membrane lining the aerian passages, it proves exceedingly useful, especially when the secretion is copious and the system relaxed. Formerly cubebs were employed as gastric stimulants and carminatives in dyspepsia, arising from an atonic condition of the stomach. They have also been used in rheumatism. The Indians macerate them in wine, and take them to excite the sexual feelings.

ADMINISTRATION.—Cubebs, in the form of *powder*, are given in doses varying from ten grains to three drachms. In affections of the bladder and prostate gland the dose is from ten grains to thirty grains. In gonorrhœa, on the other hand, they should be administered in large doses. Mr. Crawford[8] says, that in Malay countries they are given in doses of three drachms, six or eight times during the day.

1. OLEUM CUBEBÆ, E.; *Volatile Oil of Cubebs.* (Prepared by grinding the fruit, and distilling with water.)—By distillation, cubebs yield about 10·5 per cent. of a transparent, slightly-coloured (when pure, colourless), volatile oil, which is lighter than water (sp. gr. 0·929), and has the cubeb odour, and a hot, aromatic, bitter taste. Its formula is $C^{10}H^8$.

---

[1] *Observations on the Use of Cubebs, or Java Pepper, in the Cure of Gonorrhœa,* 1821.
[2] *Med.-Chir. Trans.* vol. xii. p. 99.
[3] *Lancet,* vol. iii. p. 201, 1824.
[4] Dr. Orr, *Ed. Med. Journ.* vol. xviii. p. 318.
[5] Sir B. Brodie, *Lond. Med. Gaz.* vol. i. p. 396.
[6] *Ibid.* p. 300.
[7] *Ibid.* xv. 747.
[8] *History of the Indian Archipelago,* vol. i. p. 465.

By keeping, it sometimes deposits crystals (*cubeb stearoptene* or *cubeb camphor*), the primary form of which is the rhombic octohedron.[1] They form a hydrate whose composition is $C^{10}H^8,HO$. Their odour is that of cubebs; their taste, at first, that of cubebs and camphor, afterwards cooling. They are fusible at 133° F., soluble in alcohol, ether, and oils, but are insoluble in water. Oil of cubebs is an excellent and a most convenient substitute for the powder. The dose of it, at the commencement of its use, is ten or twelve drops. This quantity is to be gradually increased as long as the stomach will bear it. In some instances I have given it to the extent of a fluidrachm for a dose. It may be taken suspended in water by means of mucilage, or dropped on sugar; or, in the form of *gelatinous capsules of cubebs*. A combination of oil of cubebs and oil of copaiva forms a very useful medicine in some cases of gonorrhœa.

2. EXTRACTUM OLEO-RESINOSUM CUBEBÆ; *Oleo-resinous Extract of Cubebs.*—Dublanc directs this to be prepared by adding the oil to the resinous extract of cubebs, which is prepared by digesting the cake, left after the distillation of the oil, in alcohol, and distilling off the spirit.[2] The process of Mr. Procter, Jun.,[3] appears to be a better one. It consists in exhausting cubebs by ether in the displacement apparatus, and submitting the ethereal tincture to distillation in a water-bath. The residual *ethereal extract of cubebs* has a dark olive brown colour, and contains all the volatile oil, cubebin, and resin (the active principles of the fruit), as well as most of the waxy matter, but none of the extractive. 1 lb. avoirdupoise of cubebs yields 2 oz. of ethereal extract. One drachm of it, therefore, is equal to one ounce of cubebs. It may be administered in the form of emulsion, pills, or capsules. Dose from grs. v. to ʒss.

3. TINCTURA CUBEBÆ, L. D.; *Tincture of Cubebs.* (Cubebs, ʒv.; Rectified Spirit, Oij. Macerate for fourteen days, and filter.)—Dr. Montgomery[4] says, " I have found this tincture cure gonorrhœa both speedily and satisfactorily." The dose of it is one or two drachms, three times a day.

Some druggists keep a more concentrated tincture.

[**4. EXTRACTUM CUBEBÆ FLUIDUM**, U.S.; *Fluid Extract of Cubebs.* Take of Cubebs, lb. j.; Ether, a sufficient quantity. Put the cubebs into a percolator, and having packed it carefully, pour ether gradually upon it until two pints of filtered liquor are obtained; then distil off by means of a water bath, at a gentle heat, a pint and a half of the ether, and expose the residue in a shallow vessel until the whole of the ether has evaporated. The dose is from grs. v. to ʒss.—Ed.]

131. ARTANTHE ELONGATA, *Miquel.*—MATICO-PLANT.

Sex. Syst. Diandria, Monogynia.

(The leaves, D.)

SYNONYMES.—*Piper angustifolium*, Ruiz and Pavon, Fl. Peruv.; *Piper elongatum*, Vahl.; *Stephensia elongata*, Kunth.; *Moho Moho* id est

---

[1] Brooke, *Ann. Phil.* N.S. vol. v. p. 450.
[2] *Journ. de Pharm.* t. xiv. p. 40.
[3] *Pharmaceutical Journal*, vol. vi. p. 319, 1846.
[4] *Observations on the Dubl. Pharm.* p. 439, Lond.

Nodus Nodus, vernacul. name.—This plant has long been in use among the natives of Peru in venereal diseases; and having been employed on some oc-

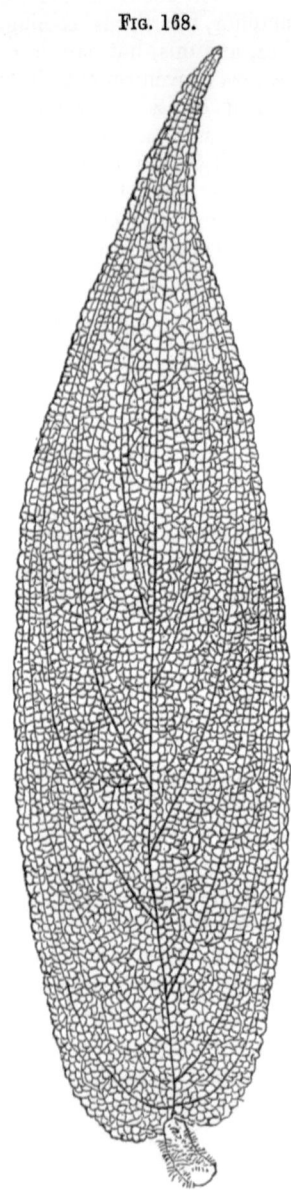

Artanthe elongata.

Fig. 168.

casion by a soldier as a mechanical agent to staunch blood, it got the name of the *Soldier's herb,* and, in 1839, was introduced into this country as an internal or chemical styptic. The term *matico* (*matecô* or *matica*) is not exclusively applied to the leaves of this plant; but to those of others also. Dr. Lindley has given to the Museum of the Pharmaceutical Society some leaves of the *Eupatorium glutinosum,* Kunth. They are marked *Matico,* and are said to be excellent in powder for staunching blood and healing wounds. In appearance and texture they closely resemble the leaves of Artanthe elongata; and would, I doubt not, be equally valuable as a mechanical styptic.

DESCRIPTION.—Artanthe elongata is a shrub of about 12 feet high, with jointed stem and branches. Its leaves are harsh, short-stalked, oblong-lanceolate, acuminate; pubescent beneath, tessellated or rough on the upper side on account of the sunken veins. The spikes are solitary, cylindrical, and opposite the leaves; the bracts lanceolate; and the flowers hermaphrodite.—It grows at Huanuco, Cuchero, Panao, Chaclea and Muna in Peru; and flowers from July to September.

Matico (*herba maticæ*) is imported in serons, and consists of the dried leaves, stalks, and spikes (some unripe, others ripe), and more or less compressed into a lump. The colour of the dried plant is greenish; and the leaves, which are from 2 to 8 inches long, in structure somewhat resemble those of sage, and are easily reducible to powder. The plant has an aromatic odour, somewhat similar to that of cubebs.

COMPOSITION.—Matico has been analysed by Dr. J. F. Hodges,[1] who found the following substances in it :—*an aromatic volatile oil, a bitter principle* (maticine), *a soft dark green resin, a brown colouring matter, a yellow colouring matter, chlorophylle, gum and nitrate of potash, salts,* and *lignin.*— The oil of matico has a light green colour, and, when recent, the consistence of good castor oil, but becomes thick and

---

[1] *Memoirs and Proceedings of the Chemical Society,* vol. ii. p. 123, 1844.

crystalline on keeping.   The bitter principle, called maticine, is soluble in alcohol and water, but not in ether.   Infusion of matico yields a dark greenish colouring and precipitate with the sesquichloride of iron;[1] but undergoes no change on the addition of gelatin, emetic tartar, or perchloride of mercury.   It therefore contains little or no tannin.   Acetate of lead and infusion of nutgalls each occasion copious coloured precipitates.

Physiological Effects and Uses.—Matico is an aromatic bitter stimu-lant, which agrees with cubebs and the pepper in the character of its effects. Its active principles are volatile oil, resin, and the bitter principle.   Matico may be used (like lint, felt, or cobweb,) as a topical application for staunching blood, or from slight cuts and other wounds of the nose and gums, or leech-bites. It acts mechanically as a styptic by the structure of its leaf, which divides the blood and promotes its coagulation.   As an *internal* remedy it is appli-cable as a substitute for cubebs, in discharges from the mucous surfaces, as leucorrhœa and gonorrhœa.   It might, perhaps, be useful in diseases of the rectum, in similar cases to those in which the confection of pepper has been serviceable.   The Indians use the infusion as an aphrodisiac.[2]   Matico has been greatly lauded[3] as an internal styptic or astringent in internal hemorrhages (from the lungs, stomach, bowels, and uterus).   But the botanical, chemical, and sensible qualities of matico are opposed to the idea of its astringent properties ; and with regard to the supposed therapeutic evidence, it may be observed that, from the often temporary character and uncertain duration of internal hemorrhages generally, it is very difficult to determine the therapeutical influence of the agents called astringents, and to distinguish *post hoc* from *propter hoc* phenomena.   If matico have any styptic power, it is derived not from tannic or gallic acids, but from the volatile oil which the plant contains; and in that case the oils of pepper, cubebs, or turpentine, would be much more energetic and preferable.   [Dr. Ruschenberger, who became acquainted with matico during a visit to Peru in 1834, and introduced it into the United States, has used it locally in chronic ophthalmia with advantage.   With regard to its anti-hemorrhagic power, this gentleman informed the American editor of this work, that he applied it to arrest hemorrhage after an operation on the side of the neck below the angle of the jaw, in which there was considerable bleeding and difficulty in taking up the divided vessels, owing to the induration of the part from chronic inflammation ; and the application was successful.   The same arrest of the discharge of blood followed its use in hematemesis.[4]—Ed.]

Matico is administered in the form of powder, infusion, and tincture.   The dose of the *powder* is from ℈ss. to ʒij.

1. INFUSUM MATICO, D. ;   Matico Leaves, cut small, ℥ss. ;   Boiling Water, Oss.   Infuse for one hour in a covered vessel, and strain.   The product should measure about eight ounces.   *D.*—Dose from ℥j. to ℥ij.

2. TINCTURA MATICO, D. ;   Matico Leaves, in coarse powder, ℥viij. ;   Proof Spirit, Oij.   Macerate for fourteen days, strain, express, and filter.—Dose from ʒj. to ℥ij.

---

[1] Peppermint and other labiate plants yield infusions which produce a dark green colour with the sesquichloride of iron.

[2] Martius, *Pharmaceutical Journal*, 1843, vol. ii. p. 660.

[3] See Jeffrey's *Remarks on Matico*, 1843.

[4] Dr. Carson, in American edition.

Order XXXIII. EUPHORBIACEÆ, *Juss.*—SPURGEWORTS.

Euphorbiæ, *Juss.*

CHARACTERS. — *Flowers* unisexual. *Calyx* free (inferior), with various glandular or scaly internal appendages; sometimes wanting. *Corolla* usually absent, sometimes poly-petalous or monopetalous. *Stamens* definite or indefinite, distinct or monadelphous; *anthers* 2-celled. *Ovary* free (superior). *Ovules* solitary or twin, suspended from the inner angle of the cell. *Fruit* generally tricoccous, consisting of 3 carpels splitting and separating with elasticity from their common axis, occasionally fleshy and indehiscent. *Seeds* solitary or twin, suspended often with an aril; embryo enclosed in fleshy albumen; cotyledons flat; radicle superior.—*Trees, shrubs,* or *herbs,* often abounding in a milky juice. *Leaves* opposite or alternate, simple, rarely compound, often with stipules. *Flowers* axillary or terminal, sometimes enclosed within an involucre resembling a calyx. Some of the Euphorbiaceæ are succulent or fleshy, and have a considerable resemblance to Cacteaceæ; from which they may in general be distinguished by the presence of an acrid milky juice.

PROPERTIES.—Mostly acrids; operating, toxicologically, as acrid, narcotic-acrid, or acro-narcotic poisons; and medicinally, as rubefacients, suppurants, emetics, diuretics, and cathartics. The acrid or poisonous principle or principles reside in the roots, stems, leaves, and seeds. It is a constituent of the acrid milky juice found in many of the species. "M. Berthollet has recorded a remarkable instance of the harmless quality of the sap in the interior of a plant, whose bark is filled with a milky proper juice of a poisonous nature. He described the natives of Teneriffe as being in the habit of removing the bark from the *Euphorbia canariensis*, and then sucking the inner portion of the stem in order to quench their thirst, this part containing a considerable quantity of limpid and non-elaborated sap."[1] In some cases an acrid principle is found in the embryo, but not in the albumen of the seed. Thus Aublet[2] states that the kernels of *Omphalea diandra* are edible if the embryo be extracted; but if this be left in, they prove cathartic. In some cases, however, as those of *Croton* and *Ricinus*, the albumen also possesses acrid and poisonous properties. The chemical nature of the acrid principle or principles has not been determined. In some cases it appears to be volatile, in others fixed. If it be true that persons have been poisoned by sleeping under the Manchineel tree (*Hippomane Mancinella*), this species must give out a poisonous vapour. In some cases, however, resin appears to be the active principle; as in the officinal substance called gum euphor-bium.

The expressed oils of the seeds of several of the Euphorbiaceæ (as *Croton, Ricinus, Jatropha, Euphorbia,* and *Anda*) are purgative; in some cases violently so. They probably owe this to some active principle dissolved in the fixed oil; for the residual oil-cake acts as a drastic purgative, in some cases more so than the expressed oil. Sou-beiran[3] thinks that some of the euphorbiaceous seeds owe their purgative qualities to resin. The fixed oil of some of the seeds is remarkable for its more ready miscibility with, or solubility in, alcohol, than most other fixed oils. Some euphorbiaceous plants are devoid of acridity, or possess it in a very slight degree only. Some of these are aromatic, resiniferous, and tonic. Von Buch[4] says, the branches of *Euphorbia balsamifera* contain a mild sweet juice, which is eaten by the inhabitants of the Canary Isles. The aromatic tonic bark of the *Croton Eleutheria* is another exception to the very general acridity of these plants. Some of the roots are harmless and nutritious. Others of neighbouring species abound in nutritive starch (e. g. *tapioca-starch*), which resides in a poisonous juice.

---

[1] Henslow, *Botany,* in Lardner's *Cyclop.* p. 217.
[2] *Histoire des Plantes de la Guiane,* t. ii. p. 844.
[3] *Journ. de Pharm.* t. xv. p. 501, 1829.
[4] Nees and Ebermaier, *Med. Pharm. Bot.* Bd. i. S. 355.

TRIBE. EUPHORBIEÆ, *Bartling*.

Ovules solitary. *Seeds* albuminous. *Flowers* monœcious, apetalous: male and females mixed in a cup-shaped involucre.

132. EUPHORBIA CANARIENSIS, *Linn.*—THE CANARY EUPHORBIUM.

Sex. Syst. Dodecandria, Trigynia, *Linn.*—Monœcia, Monandria, *Smith.*
(Concrete resinous juice, *E.*)

HISTORY.—The plant which yields the saline waxy-resin called in the shops *gum euphorbium*, is said both by Dioscorides[1] (who calls it εὐφόρβιον) and Pliny[2] to have been first discovered in the time of Juba, king of Mauritania; that is, about, or a few years before, the commencement of the Christian era. Pliny says that Juba called it after his physician, Euphorbus; and that he wrote a volume concerning it, which was extant in Pliny's time. Salmasius, however, states that this word occurs in the writings of Meleager the poet, who lived some time before Juba. But in the passage in question the commonly received reading in the present day is not εὐφόρβης, but ἐκ φορβῆς.[3]

BOTANY. **Gen. Char.** — *Flowers* collected in monœcious heads, surrounded by an involucrum consisting of 1 leaf with 5 divisions, which have externally 5 glands alternating with them. *Males* naked, monandrous, articulated with their pedicel, surrounding the female, which is in the centre. *Females* naked, solitary. *Ovarium* stalked. *Stigmas* 3, forked. *Fruit* hanging out of the involucrum, consisting of 3 cells, bursting at the back with elasticity, and each containing 1 suspended seed (Lindley).

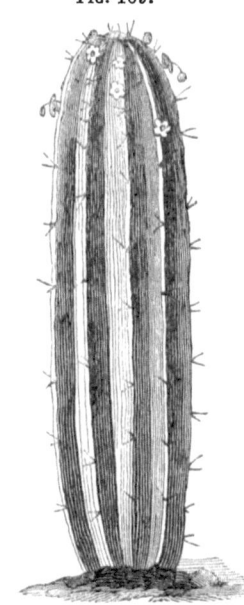

FIG. 169.

Euphorbia officinarum.

Sp. Char.—*Branches* channelled, with 4, rarely 5, angles, armed with double, straight, spreading, dark, shining *spines*.

These specific characters apply to the branches found mixed with the euphorbium of commerce. They agree with the description and figure of *Tithymalus aizoides lactifluus* seu *Euphorbia canariensis* of Plukenet.[4] This agrees with the statement of Miller,[5] who states that by looking over some euphorbium in a shop, he " found several spines amongst it, which exactly agreed with those of that plant." I feel very little hesitation, therefore, in referring the euphorbium of English commerce to *E. canariensis.*

From the *E. canariensis* of Willdenow and of some other botanists, this plant is distinguished by its straight spines; but on examining the *E. canariensis* at the Kew Garden, I

¹ *Lib.* iii. cap. 96.
² *Hist. Nat.* lib. xxv. cap. 38, ed. Valp. Pliny calls the plant *euphorbia*, and the resin *euphorbium* (lib. xxvi. cap. 34).
³ Dr. Greenhill, *Dict. of Greek and Roman Biography*, art. *Euphorbus*, vol. ii. p. 97.
⁴ *Almagest. Bot.* vol. ii. p. 370.
⁵ *Gardener's Dictionary*, vol. i. art. *Euphorbium*.

found as many of the spines straight as uncinate. The diameter of the stems, however, and even of the young shoots, is greater than that of stems found in the euphorbium of commerce. The species which most closely agrees with the latter in the sizes of the stems, the number of angles, and the number and directions of the spines, is *Euphorbia tetragona*. This species has mostly square stems; though some of the larger stems are somewhat channelled. The dried stems found in the euphorbium of commerce, however, appear to be uniformly channelled. The *E. officinarum* has many angles: the *Dergmuse* of Jackson[1] has many scolloped angles. *Euphorbia antiquorum* has been said to yield euphorbium, but the statement is denied by both Hamilton[2] and Royle.[3]

Hab.—The Canary Islands; Africa, in the neighbourhood of Mogadore?

Extraction.—Euphorbium is thus procured :—The inhabitants of the lower regions of the Atlas range make incisions in the branches of the plant, and from these a milky juice exudes, which is so acrid that it excoriates the fingers when applied to them. This exuded juice hardens by the heat of the sun, and forms a whitish-yellow solid, which drops off in the month of September, and forms the euphorbium of commerce, "The plants," says Mr. Jackson,[4] "produce abundantly once only in four years; but this fourth year's produce is more than all Europe can consume." The people who collect it, he adds, are obliged "to tie a cloth over their mouth and nostrils to prevent the small dusty particles from annoying them, as they produce incessant sneezing." The acrid resinous juice resides in the outer or cortical portion of the stem.

Properties.—Euphorbium consists of irregular yellowish, slightly friable tears, usually pierced with one or two holes, united at the base, and in which we find the remains of a double aculeus. These tears are almost odourless; but their dust, applied to the olfactory membrane, acts as a powerful sternutatory. Their taste is at first slight, afterwards acrid and burning. When heated, euphorbium melts, swells up imperfectly, evolves an odour somewhat like that of benzoic acid vapour, takes fire, and burns with a pale flame. Alcohol, ether, and oil of turpentine, are its best solvents; water dissolves only a small portion of it.

Composition.—Euphorbium has been the subject of several analyses—namely, in 1800, by Laudet;[5] in 1809, by Braconnot;[6] in 1818, by Pelletier[7] and by Mühlmann;[8] in 1819, by Brandes;[9] and more recently by Drs. Buchner and Herberger.[10]

Pelletier's Analysis.		*Brandes' Analysis.*	
Resin	60·8	Resin	43·77
Wax	14·4	Wax	14·93
Bassorin	2·0	Caoutchouc	4·84
Malate of lime	12·2	Malate of lime	18·82
Malate of potash	1·8	Malate of potash	4·90
Water and loss	8·8	Sulphates of potash and lime, and phosphate of lime	0·70
		Water and loss	6·44
		Woody fibre	5·60
Euphorbium	100·0	Euphorbium	100·00

[1] *Account of Morocco*, 3d edit. p. 134.
[2] *Trans. of the Linn. Soc.* vol. xiv.
[3] *Bot. of the Himalaya Mountains*, p. 328.
[4] *Op. cit.*
[5] Gmelin, *Hand. d. Chem.*
[6] *Ann. Chim.* lxviii. 44.
[7] *Bull. d. Pharm.* iv. 502.
[8] Gmelin, *op. cit.*
[9] *Ibid.*
[10] Christison, *Treatise on Poisons*.

RESIN is the active ingredient of euphorbium. It coincides in many of its properties with ordinary resins: thus, it is reddish-brown, hard, brittle, fusible, soluble in alcohol, ether, and oil of turpentine, and somewhat less so in oil of almonds. Its leading and characteristic property is intense acridity. It differs from some resins in being slightly soluble only in alkalies. It is a compound of two resinous substances.

a. One resinous substance is soluble in cold alcohol. Its formula, according to Mr. Johnston,[1] is $C^{40}H^{31}O^6$.

β. The other resinous substance is insoluble in cold alcohol. The mean of Rose's analyses[2] of it gives as the composition of this resin, *carbon* 81·58, *hydrogen* 11·35, and *oxygen* 7·07.

PHYSIOLOGICAL EFFECTS. *a. On Animals generally.*—Euphorbium acts on horses and dogs as a powerful acrid substance, irritating and inflaming parts with which it is placed in contact, and affecting the nervous system. When swallowed in large quantities, it causes gastro-enteritis (two ounces are sufficient to kill a horse); when applied to the skin, it acts as a rubefacient and epispastic. Farriers sometimes employ it, as a substitute for cantharides, for blistering horses; but cautious and well-informed veterinarians are opposed to its use.

β. *On Man.*—The leading effect of euphorbium on man is that of a most violent acrid; but under certain circumstances a narcotic operation has been observed. When *euphorbium dust is inhaled, and also applied to the face,* as in grinding this drug, it causes sneezing, redness and swelling of the face, and great irritation about the eyes and nose. To prevent as much as possible these effects, various contrivances are adopted by different drug-grinders; some employ masks with glass eyes, others apply wet sponge to the nose and face, while some cover the face with crape. The pain and irritation are sometimes very great. Individuals who have been exposed for some time to the influence of this dust, suffer from headache and giddiness, and ultimately become delirious. All the workmen of whom I have inquired (and they comprise those of three large firms, including the one alluded to by Dr. Christison) agree that these are the effects of euphorbium. An old labourer assured me that this substance produced in him a feeling of intoxication; and I was informed at one drug-mill of an Irish labourer who was made temporarily insane by it, and who, during the fit, insisted on saying his prayers at the tail of the mill-horse.

Insensibility and convulsions have been produced by euphorbium. The only instance I am acquainted with is the following:—A man was engaged at a mill where euphorbium was being ground, and remained in the room longer than was considered prudent. Suddenly he darted from the mill-room, and ran with great velocity down two pairs of stairs. On arriving at the ground-floor or yard he became insensible, and fell. Within five minutes I saw him: he was lying on his back, insensible and convulsed; his face was red and swollen, his pulse frequent and full, and his skin very hot. I bled him, and within half an hour he became quite sensible, but complained of great headache. He had no recollection of his flight down stairs, which seems to have been performed in a fit of delirium.

When *powdered euphorbium is applied to the skin*, it causes itching, pain, and inflammation, succeeded by vesication. When *swallowed*, it causes

---

[1] *Phil. Trans.* 1840, p. 365.
[2] Poggendorff's *Annalen*, xxxiii. 52.

2 D

vomiting and purging, and, in large doses, gastro-enteritis, with irregular hurried pulse and cold perspirations.

USES.—Notwithstanding that it is still retained in the Edinburgh Pharmacopœia, it is rarely employed in medicine. It was formerly used as an *emetic* and *drastic purgative* in dropsies; but the violence and danger of its operation have led to its disuse. Sometimes it is employed as an *errhine* in chronic affections of the eyes, ears, or brain; but its local action is so violent that we can only apply it when largely diluted with some mild powder, as starch or flour.

Mixed with turpentine or Burgundy pitch (or rosin), it is employed in the form of plaster, as a *rubefacient*, in chronic affections of the joints. As a *vesicant*, it is rarely employed. As a *caustic*, either the powder or alcoholic tincture (*Tinctura Euphorbii*, Cod. Hamb., prepared by digesting euphorbium, ℥j. in rectified spirit, lb. j.) is sometimes employed in carious ulcers.

ANTIDOTE.—In a case of poisoning by euphorbium, emollient and demulcent drinks, clysters (of mucilaginous, amylaceous, or oleaginous liquids), and opium, should be exhibited, and blood-letting and warm baths employed. In fact, as we have no chemical antidote, our object is to involve the poison in demulcents, to diminish the sensibility of the living part by opium, and to obviate the inflammation by blood-letting and the warm bath. If the circulation fail, ammonia and brandy will be required.

133. Euphorbia Lathyris, *Linn.*—Caper Spurge.

(Semina.)

This is an indigenous or naturalised biennial plant, which is cultivated in gardens. *Stem* solitary, erect, 2 or 3 feet high, purplish, round, smooth, like every other part. *Leaves* numerous, spreading in 4 rows, opposite, sessile, oblong, acute, entire, of a dark glaucous green; their base heart-shaped; the lower ones gradually diminishing. *Umbel* solitary, terminal large, or 4 repeatedly forked branches. *Bracts* heart-shaped, entire, tapering to a point. *Flowers* sessile in each fork, solitary, variegated with yellow and dark purple. *Nectaries* rounded with blunt horns. *Capsules* large, smooth (Smith).— The seeds (*sem. euphorbiæ lathyris; sem. cataputiæ minoris; grana regia minora*) are about the size of peppercorns. They yielded Soubeiran[1] *a yellow fixed oil, stearine, a brown acrid oil, a crystalline matter, a brown resin, an extractive colouring matter,* and *vegetable albumen.* The yellow fixed oil is purgative, but it owes this property to matters which it holds in solution. The brown acrid oil is the active principle: it has a disagreeable odour, approaching that of croton oil, and readily dissolves in alcohol and ether. Oil of caper spurge (*oleum euphorbiæ lathyris*) may be obtained by expression, by alcohol, or by ether. The expressed oil, unlike that of croton oil, is insoluble in alcohol. It is less active than the oil prepared by alcohol (as 3 is to 2). Both the milky juice of the plant and the seeds are acrid, and violently purgative. In a case of poisoning by the seeds, narcotic symptoms also were present.[2] The oil may be employed as an indigenous substitute for croton oil. The dose of it is from three to ten drops.[3] The capsules are pickled and used as a substitute for capers, which they resemble in size, appearance, and pungency. When recent, they are certainly acrid and poisonous; and it is probable, therefore, that the pickling process lessens or destroys their virulence; but the free use of the pickled fruits is dangerous.

[1] *Journ. de Pharm.* t. xv. p. 507, 1829 ; also, *Nouveau Traité de Pharmacie,* t. ii.
[2] Christison, *Treatise on Poisons.*
[3] Dierbach, *Neuesten Entd. in d. Mat. Med.* S. 76, 1837; Bailly, *Lancet,* June 10th, 1826.

134. Euphorbia Ipecacuanha, *Linn.*—Ipecacuanha Spurge.

(Radix.)

This plant (also called *American Ipecacuanha*) is a native of the United States of America. The dried root (*radix euphorbiæ ipecacuanhæ*; vel *rad. ipecacuanhæ spuriæ albæ*) is cylindrical, greyish-yellow, inodorous, and has a sweetish, not unpleasant, taste. According to Dr. Bigelow, it contains caoutchouc, resin, gum, and probably starch. Its active principle is perhaps resin. This root is "an energetic, tolerably certain emetic, rather milder than *E. corollata*, but, like that, disposed to act upon the bowels, and liable, if given in over-doses, to produce excessive nausea and vomiting, general prostration, and alarming hypercatharsis. It is, therefore, wholly unfit to supersede ipecacuanha."[1] The dose of the powdered root is from ten to fifteen grains. In small doses it is diaphoretic.

TRIBE. CROTONEÆ, *Blume.*

Ovule solitary. *Flowers* usually having petals, in clusters, spikes, racemes, or panicles.

135. CROTON TIGLIUM, *Lam.*—THE PURGING CROTON.

Croton Jamalgota, *Hamilton.*

Sex. Syst. Monœcia, Monadelphia.

(Oleum e semine expressum, *L.*—Expressed oil of the seeds, *E. D.*)

HISTORY.—Croton seeds are mentioned by Avicenna[2] and by Serapion[3] under the name of *Dend* or *Dende.* The earliest European describer of them is Christopher d'Acosta, in 1578,[4] who terms them *pini nuclei malucani.* When Commeline wrote, they were known in the shops by the name of *cataputia minor,* although they were sold by itinerants as *grana dilla* or *grana tilli.* They were much employed by medical men in the 17th century, and were known by various names, but principally by that of *grana tiglia.* They, however, went out of use,—probably in consequence of the violence and uncertainty of their operation. Their re-employment in modern practice is owing partly to the notices of them by Dr. White and Mr. Marshall, in the first edition of Dr. Ainslie's work;[5] but principally to the introduction of the oil, in 1820, by Dr. Conwell.[6]

BOTANY. **Gen. Char.** — *Flowers* monœcious, or very rarely diœcious. *Calyx* 5-parted. MALES :—*petals* 5 ; *stamens* 10 or more, distinct. FEMALES :—*petals* 0 ; *styles* 3, divided into two or more partitions. *Capsule* tricoccous [with 1 seed in each cell] (*Adr. de Jussieu*).

---

[1] *United States Dispensatory.*
[2] Lib. ii. cap. 219.
[3] *De Simplicibus*, cccxlviii.
[4] Clusius, *Exoticor.* p. 292.
[5] *Materia Medica of Hindostan*, 1813.
[6] See his *Récherch. sur les Propr. Méd. et l'Emploi en Méd. de l'Huile de Croton Tiglium*, 1824. For further historical details, consult Professor H. H. Wilson's paper in the *Transactions of the Med. and Phys. Society of Calcutta*, vol. i. p. 249.

Sp. Char.—Arboreous.   *Leaves* oblong-ovate, acuminate, 3—5-nerved, slightly serrate, smooth.   *Stamina* 15, distinct.   Each cell of the fruit filled by the seed.

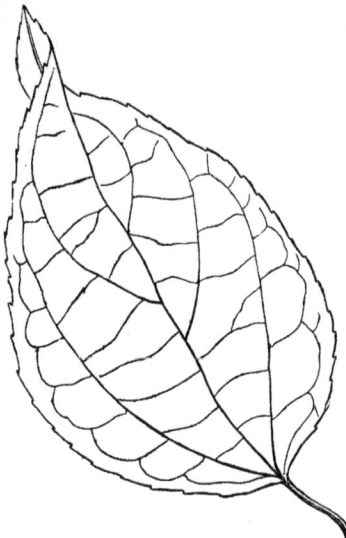

FIG. 170.

Leaf of Croton Tiglium.

A middle-sized *tree*, from 15 to 20 feet high.   *Bark* smooth, ash-coloured.   *Leaves* thin and membranous, sometimes cordate, and with two flat round glands at their base; when young, covered on both surfaces, but especially the lower one, with minute stellate hairs.   At the base of the leaves are two flat round glands.   *Raceme* terminal, erect, simple.   *Petals* of male flower white.

Hab.—Continent of India, islands forming the Indian Archipelago, and Ceylon.

The CROTON PAVANA[1] is said also to yield tiglium or croton seeds.   It is distinguished from C. Tiglium by having only ten stamina, and by the seeds being much smaller than the cells in which they are placed.   C. Pavana is a native of Ava, north-eastern parts of Bengal? Amboyna? Dr. Hamilton thinks it is the *Granum Moluccum* of Rumphius.

DESCRIPTION.—*Croton seeds* (*semina tiglii* seu *semina crotonis, grana tiglii, purging nuts* of some authors) in size and shape are very similar to castor seeds.   Viewed laterally, their shape is oval or oval-oblong; seen from either extremity, they have a rounded or imperfectly quadrangular form. Their length does not exceed 6 lines, their thickness is $2\frac{1}{2}$ to 3 lines, their breadth 3 or 4 lines.   Sometimes the surface of the seeds is yellowish, owing to the presence of an investing lamina (epidermis?).   The testa is dark brown or blackish, and is marked with the ramifications of the raphé.   The endocarp, or internal seed-coat, is thin, brittle, and of a light colour.   It encloses a yellowish oily albumen, which envelopes the embryo, whose cotyledons are foliaceous or membranous.   The seeds are without odour; their taste is at first mild and oleaginous, afterwards acrid and burning.   When heated, they evolve an acrid vapour.   The proportion of shell and kernel in 100 parts by weight of the seeds is thus stated by two authorities :—

	Nimmo.	*Caventou.*
Shell or seed-coats	36	33·3
Kernel or nucleus	64	66·6
	100	99·9

---

[1] Hamilton, *Trans. Linn. Soc.* vol. xiv. 257.

COMPOSITION.—Croton seeds were analysed in 1818 by MM. Pelletier and Caventou,[1] in 1822 by Dr. Nimmo,[2] and in 1823 by Brandes.[3]   The following are their results :—

Pelletier & Caventou.	Nimmo.	Brandes.	
Fixed oil and cro- tonic acid } 50	Acrid purga- tive principle } 27	Volatile oil.	traces
		Fixed oil, with *crotonic acid*, and an alkaloid (*crotonin*)	17·00
Gum	Fixed oil 33	*Crotonates* and colouring matter	0·32
Albumen(emulsin) } 50	Farinaceous } 40	Brownish-yellow resin, insoluble in ether	1·00
Lignin	matter	Stearine and wax.	0·65
		Extractive, sugar, and malates of potash and lime.	2·05
		Starchy matter, with phosphate of lime and magnesia	5·71
		Gum and gummoin	10·17
		Albumen	1·01
		Gluten.	2·00
		Seed-coats and woody fibre of the nucleus	39·00
		Water	22·50
Kernel.... 100	Kernel.... 100	Croton Seeds.	101·41

1. VOLATILE OIL OF CROTON SEEDS.—This is but imperfectly known, traces only of it having been obtained. Brandes regards it as extremely acrid, and thinks that by the united agencies of air and water it is converted into crotonic acid ; for the distilled water of the seeds becomes more acid by keeping.

2. FIXED OIL OF CROTON SEEDS.—This also is but imperfectly known. It must not be confounded with croton oil of the shops, which is a mixture of this and other constituents of the seeds. Fixed oil of croton seeds is, probably, a combination of crotonic and other fatty acids with glycerine.

3. CROTONIC ACID (*Jatrophic Acid*).—Discovered by Pelletier and Caventou. Though this acid exists in the free state in the seed, yet an additional quantity of it is obtained when the oil is saponified. For this purpose the oil is saponified by potash, the resulting soap decomposed by tartaric acid, and the watery fluid, from the surface of which the separated common fatty acids have been removed, is to be submitted to distillation. In this way is obtained an aqueous solution of a solid, very volatile, fatty acid, which congeals at 23° F., and, when heated a few degrees above 32° F., is converted into vapour, having a strong nauseous odour, which irritates the eyes and nose, and has an acrid taste.

At first Pelletier and Caventou regarded this acid as the active principle of the oil ; but Caventou subsequently expressed doubts on the subject, and stated that fresh experiments induced him to think that the irritating and volatile principle of the oil, which so strongly irritated the nose and eyes, was not of an acid nature. My colleague, Mr. Redwood, informs me that he has ascertained that crotonic acid and the crotonates are inert, or nearly so ; and my experiments with crotonic acid prepared by him support his statements.

Crotonic acid unites with bases forming a class of salts called *crotonates*, which are inodorous. The *crotonate of ammonia* precipitates the salts of lead, copper, and silver, white ; and the sulphate of iron, yellow. *Crotonate of potash* is crystalline, and dissolves, with difficulty, in alcohol. *Crotonate of barytes* is soluble in water ; but *crotonate of magnesia* is very slightly soluble only in this liquid.

4. CROTONIN.—The crystallisable substance considered by Brandes to be a peculiar alkaloid, which he called *crotonin*, and which appeared to be identical with the *tiglin* of Adr. de Jussieu, has been found by Weppen[4] to be (as formerly suggested by Soubeiran[5]) a magnesian soap with an alkaline reaction.

---

[1] *Journ. de Pharm.* t. iv. p. 289, 1818 ; and t. xi. p. 10, 1825. In the first paper croton seeds were, by mistake, said to be the seeds of *Jatropha Curcas.* Caventou corrected this statement in the second paper. In the *Journ. de Pharm. et de Chim.* for March 1850, M. Guibourt states that he has recently ascertained that the seeds of *J. Curcas* are sold by respectable dealers in Paris for croton seeds. It is stated by Mr. Frost (*Lond. Medic. Reposit.* vol. xvii. p. 464, 1822 ; and vol. xviii. p. 474, 1822) that in England the former seeds have been mistaken for the latter.

[2] *Quarterly Journal of Science,* vol. xiii. p. 62, 1822. Soubeiran (*Journ. de Pharm.* t. xv. 514, 1829) states, though I know not on what authority, that the oil which Dr. Nimmo analysed under the name of croton oil, was extracted from the Jatropha.

[3] *Archiv des Apothekervereins im nördl. Teutschland,* Bd. iv. (quoted by L. Gmelin, *Handb. d. Chem.* ii. 1320). See also *Berlin. Jahrb. für d. Pharm.* Bd. xxvi. Abt. i. S. 222, 1824.

[4] *Ann. d. Chem. u. Pharm.* Bd. lxx. S. 254, 1849 ; also *Chemical Gazette,* vol. vii. p. 355, 1849.

[5] *Nouv. Traité de Pharm.* t. ii. p. 103.

5. RESIN.—Is brown and soft, and has a disagreeable odour,—on account, doubtless, of the oil which it retains. It is soluble in alcohol, but insoluble in ether and in water. The alkalies dissolve it by separating a whitish matter. It contributes to the purgative properties of croton oil.

PHYSIOLOGICAL EFFECTS. 1. **Of the Seeds.** α. *On Animals generally.*— Croton seeds are powerful local irritants or acrids, causing inflammation in those living parts with which they are placed in contact. Orfila[1] found that three drachms being introduced into the stomach of a dog, and the œsophagus tied to prevent vomiting, caused death in three hours; and on examination of the body, the alimentary canal was found to be in a state of inflammation. In another experiment, a drachm caused death under the same circumstances. A drachm, also, applied to the cellular tissue of the thigh, was equally fatal. A dose of from twenty to thirty grains of the powder of the kernel given to the horse causes, in six or eight hours, profuse watery stools, and is recommended by some veterinarians as a purgative; but the uncertainty of its operation, and the griping and debility which it occasions, are objections to its use.[2] Lansberg[3] found that twenty of the seeds killed a horse, by causing gastro-enteritis. The pulse was frequent, small, and soft.

β. *On Man.*—In the human subject a grain of croton seed will frequently produce full purgation. Mr. Marshall[4] says that this quantity, made into two pills, is about equal in power to half a drachm of jalap, or to six grains of calomel. The operation, he adds, is attended with much rumbling of the bowels; the stools are invariably watery and copious. Dr. White recommends the seeds to be torrefied, and deprived of their seed-coats, before employing them.[5] Dr. Wallich informed me that the labourers in the Calcutta Botanic Garden were in the habit of taking one of these seeds as a purgative, but that on one occasion this dose proved fatal.

The seed-coats, the embryo, and the albumen, have each in their turn been declared to be the seat of the acrid principle; I believe the remarks which I shall have to make with respect to the seat of the acridity of castor-oil seeds, will apply equally to that of croton seeds.

The following is a case of poisoning by the inhalation of the dust of the seeds :—

Thomas Young, aged 31, a labourer in the East India warehouses, was brought into the London Hospital on the 8th of December, 1841, labouring under symptoms of poisoning by the inhalation of the dust of croton seeds. He had been occupied about eight hours in emptying packages of these seeds, by which he was exposed to their dust. The first ill effects observed were loss of appetite, then a burning sensation in the nose and mouth, tightness at his chest, and copious lachrymation, followed by epigastric pain. Feeling himself getting worse, he left the warehouse, but became very giddy, and fell down insensible. Medical assistance was procured, an emetic was administered, stimulants were exhibited, and he was wrapped in warm blankets. When he became sensible he complained of his mouth being parched, and that his throat was swelling. He was then removed to the hospital. On his admission he appeared in a state of collapse, complained of burning pain at the stomach, in the throat, and in the head, and of swelling and numbness of his tongue. The epigastrium felt hot and tense, the pupils were dilated, the breathing short and hurried, the countenance distressed, pulse 85, surface cold. He

---

[1] *Toxicol. Gén.*
[2] Youatt, *The Horse,* in *Library of Useful Knowledge.*
[3] Wibmer, *Arzneim. u. Gifte,* Bd. ii. S. 222.
[4] Ainslie, *Mat. Indica,* vol. i. p. 104.
[5] *Ibid.*

stated that his tongue felt too large for his mouth, and appeared to be without feeling, and he had bitten it two or three times to ascertain whether there was any sensation in it. On examination, however, no change could be observed in the size or appearance of the tongue or parts about the mouth. Hot brandy and water were given to him, and he was put into the hot bath with evident relief. He continued in the hospital for several days, during which time he continued to improve, but still complained of epigastric pain. It deserves notice that his bowels were not acted on, and on the day following his admission several doses of castor oil were given to him.

It would be interesting to know whether the seeds of Croton Pavana are equally active with those of Croton Tiglium ; and, also, whether the seeds of both species are found in commerce.

2. **Of the Oil.**   α. *On Animals generally.*—On vertebrated animals (horses, dogs, rabbits, and birds) it acts as a powerful local irritant or acrid. When taken internally, in moderate doses, it operates as a drastic purgative ; in large doses, as an acrid poison, causing gastro-enteritis. Moiroud[1] says that from twenty to thirty drops of the oil are, for the horse, equal to two drops for a man ; and that twelve drops injected into the veins cause alvine evacuations in a few minutes. Thirty drops administered in the same manner have caused, according to this veterinarian, violent intestinal inflammation and speedy death. A much less quantity (three or four drops) has, according to Hertwich,[2] terminated fatally when thrown into the veins. After death the large intestines have been found to be more inflamed than the small ones. Flies which had eaten some sugar moistened with the oil of croton died in three or four hours,— the wings being paralysed or immoveable before death.

β. *On Man.*—*Rubbed on the skin,* it causes rubefaction and a pustular or vesicular eruption, with sometimes an erysipelatous swelling of the surrounding parts. When rubbed into the abdomen, it sometimes, but not invariably, purges. Rayer[3] mentions a case in which thirty-two drops rubbed upon the abdomen produced purging, large vesicles, swelling and redness of the face, with small prominent, white, crowded vesicles on the cheeks, lips, chin, and nose. *Applied to the eye,* it gives rise to violent burning pain, and inflammation of the eye and face. In one case it produced giddiness.[4] Ebeling obtained relief by the application of a solution of carbonate of potash. *Swallowed in small doses,* as of one or two drops, it usually causes an acrid burning taste in the mouth and throat, and acts as a drastic purgative, giving rise to watery stools, and frequently increasing urinary secretion. Its operation is very speedy. Frequently it causes evacuations in half an hour: yet it is somewhat uncertain. Sometimes six, eight, or even ten drops may be given at a dose without affecting the bowels. In moderate doses it is less disposed to cause vomiting or purging than some other cathartics of equal power. Mr. Iliff,[5] however, observes that it produces nausea and griping more frequently than has been supposed.

The following is a case of poisoning by an *excessive dose* of croton oil :— A young man, aged 25, affected with severe typhoid fever, swallowed by mistake two and a half drachms of croton oil. At the end of three-quarters

---

[1] *Pharm. Vétér.* p. 272.
[2] Wibmer, *Arzneim. u. Gifte*, Bd. ii. S. 218.
[3] *Treatise on Diseases of the Skin*, by Dr. Willis, p. 367.
[4] Dierbach, *Neuesten Entd. in d. Mat. Med.* 1837, p. 201.
[5] *Lond. Med. Rep.* vol. xvii.

of an hour the skin was cold and covered with cold sweats, the pulse and action of the heart scarcely perceptible, respiration difficult; the points of the toes and fingers, the parts around the eyes and the lips, blue, as in malignant cholera; abdomen sensible to the touch; but no vomiting. In an hour and a half there were excessive and involuntary alvine evacuations, sensation of burning in the œsophagus, acute sensibility of the abdomen, skin colder, respiration and circulation difficult; the cyanosis extended over the whole body, the skin became insensible; and death occurred, with some of the symptoms of asphyxia, four hours after the poison was swallowed. No lesion was found in the gastric membrane. The intestines presented ulcerations such as are characteristic of typhus fever.[1] [A case is reported in which a female advanced in life took by mistake a tea-spoonful of an embrocation containing croton oil. She immediately complained of a hot burning sensation in the throat. She was seized with convulsions, and died in three days.[2]—Ed.]

In comparing croton oil with other violently acrid purgatives, we find it distinguished by its speedy operation, the great depression of the vascular system as well as the general feeling of debility which it produces, and by the uncertainty of its operation.

Uses.—The value of croton oil as an internal remedial agent depends principally on two circumstances—first, its powerful and speedy action as a drastic cathartic, by which it is adapted for obviating constipation, or for operating on the bowels as a counter-irritant; and secondly, on the smallness of the dose, which in practice presents many advantages. These circumstances render it peculiarly applicable in cases requiring powerful and speedy catharsis, and in which the patient cannot swallow, or does so with extreme difficulty, as in *trismus, coma,* and *some affections of the throat*; or where he will not swallow, as in *mania*. In all such cases the oil may be dropped on the tongue. *In obstinate constipation,* whether from the poison of lead or from other causes, it has sometimes succeeded where other powerful cathartics had been tried in vain. It is especially serviceable where the stomach is irritable, and rejects more voluminous purgatives; and it is of course objectionable in all inflammatory conditions of the digestive tube. In stercoraceous vomiting, with other constitutional symptoms of hernia, but without local evidence of displacement, and where the stomach rejected the ordinary senna draught, I have known oil of croton prove most effectual. *In torpid conditions of the intestinal canal, in tendency to apoplexy, in dropsy* unconnected with inflammation, *in paralysis,*—in a word, in any cases in which a powerful and speedy intestinal irritant is required, either for the purpose of evacuating the canal merely, or for acting as a revulsive or counter-irritant, and thereby relieving distant parts, croton oil is a very useful, and, on many occasions, most valuable cathartic. In employing it, two cautions are necessary: it must be avoided, or at least used with great caution, in extreme debility; and it is improper in inflammatory affections of the digestive organs. The great drawback to its use is its uncertainty. In one case it acts with extreme violence, in another it scarcely produces any effect. *In the diseases of children,* when a powerful purgative is required, croton oil has been

---

[1] *Journ. de Chim. Méd.* 2nde sér. t. v. p. 509.
[2] *Medical Gazette,* vol. xliii. p. 41.

administered, on account of the minuteness of the dose and the facility of its exhibition. In hydrocephalus, and other head-affections of children, I have several times used it where other cathartics had failed, or where extreme difficulty was experienced in inducing the patients to swallow the more ordinary remedies of this class. In some of these it has disappointed me. In the case of a child of four years of age, affected with incipient hydrocephalus, I gave six doses, of one drop each, of the oil without any effect. *In uterine obstructions* (chlorosis and amenorrhœa) it has occasionally proved serviceable. *In tape-worm* it has been recommended, but I have no experience of its efficacy.

Rubbed on the skin, croton oil has been employed to produce rubefaction and a pustular eruption, and thereby to relieve diseases of internal organs, on the principle of counter-irritation, before explained.[1] *Inflammation of the mucous membrane lining the air-passages, peripneumonia, glandular swellings, rheumatism, gout,* and *neuralgia,* are some of the diseases against which it has been applied in this way; and doubtless frequently with benefit. It is sometimes used in the undiluted form, but more commonly with twice or thrice its volume of olive oil, oil of turpentine, soap liniment, alcohol, ether, or some other convenient vehicle. But in all the cases just enumerated it has never appeared to me to present any advantage over many other counter-irritants in common use,—as emetic tartar; while the chance of causing purging is, in some cases, an objection to its use, and its greater cost sometimes precludes its employment on a large scale in pauper establishments. Frictions with it on the abdomen have been used to promote alvine evacuations, but it frequently fails to produce the desired effect. To promote the absorption of the oil in these cases, it should be dissolved in ether or alcohol, and the frictions are to be assiduously made.

ADMINISTRATION.—*Croton seeds* are rarely or never used in this country. Their farina may, however, be given in doses of a grain or two.

CROTONIS OLEUM, E.; *Tiglii Oleum,* L.; *Croton Oil.*—This is the expressed oil of the seeds. It is imported from the East Indies, principally from Madras and Ceylon, but in part from Bombay. I have been informed by an oil-presser at Calcutta that it is prepared like castor oil, except that it is strained instead of being boiled. In shelling the seeds, the women often suffer severely from swelling of the face. Croton oil is also expressed in England. The operation is usually effected by a Bramah's press in a room heated to about 75° F. The men engaged in the process are usually much affected by it; they suffer redness of the face, irritation of the eyes and air-passages, and purging. The following are the results obtained at two operations: the weights are avoirdupoise :—

	Seeds.			Oil obtained.
	cwts.	qrs.	lbs.	lbs.
Croton seeds	2	0	17	51
Ditto	5	3	10	150
Total	7	3	27	201

This gives a per-centage produce of about 22·46. The colour of the oil thus

---

[1] Bamberger, *De olei crotonis externe adhibiti efficacia,* Berol. 1833.

obtained, when viewed by transmitted light, was that of dark sherry. No use is made of the cake.

In France, the croton cake is subjected to the action of alcohol, and the oil thus obtained mixed with the previously expressed oil. Guibourt[1] obtained by expression 41·6 per cent. of oil from the kernels of the seeds, and subsequently 10·4 per cent. by the action of alcohol : making together 52 per cent. Calculating the shells at one-third the weight of the entire seeds, this product would be equal to nearly 35 per cent. for the entire seeds.

Genuine croton oil varies in colour from very pale yellow (like that of Canada balsam) to dark reddish-brown (like the deepest-coloured sherry). Its consistence is unctuous, and increases with age. It has an unpleasant but marked odour, and an acrid taste, and leaves behind an acrid sensation in the fauces. It reddens litmus, and is soluble in ether and in the fixed and volatile oils. The following are the characteristics of the goodness of the oil, according to the Edinburgh College :—

When agitated with its own volume of pure alcohol, and gently heated, it separates on standing, without having undergone any apparent diminution.

This statement is not correct, according to my observations. Pure croton oil expressed in London dissolves in alcohol (sp. gr. 0·796) without requiring to be "gently heated." The oil imported from the East Indies does, however, require to be heated with the alcohol to effect its solution. In the second place, separation does not take place, at ordinary temperatures, in the case of a mixture of English croton oil and alcohol. But by a low temperature, separation takes place on standing; but in that case the volume of oil is found to be slightly augmented. East India croton oil mixed with alcohol separates by repose : the volume of the oil, however, is increased, and that of the alcohol proportionately lessened.

In one experiment, 8 vols. of E. I. croton oil were mixed with 8 vols. of alcohol, sp. gr. 0·796, and gently heated. In two days separation had taken place : the oil now measured $8\frac{3}{4}$ vols., and the alcohol $7\frac{1}{4}$ vols. In a second experiment, 7 vols. of another E. I. croton oil were mixed with 7 vols. of alcohol : in four days separation had taken place : the oil measured $7\frac{1}{3}$ vols., and the alcohol $6\frac{7}{8}$ vols.

According to Dr. Maclagan, only 96 per cent. of the oil separates. It is obvious, therefore, that commercial croton oils, believed to be genuine, are not uniform in their relation to alcohol.

According to Mr. Twining,[2] there are two kinds of croton oil met with in commerce. One is dark yellow and thickish, the other is straw-coloured. The first is the more energetic. These oils, he thinks, may perhaps be obtained from different plants; the one from Croton Tiglium, the other from Croton Pavana. The croton oils found in the London market are of two kinds ; one exotic, imported from India and Ceylon,—the other expressed in London. These differ both in their appearance and relation to alcohol.

a. Oleum Crotonis exoticum; *Foreign* or *East Indian Croton Oil ; Pale Croton Oil.*—This is imported from Ceylon and the continent of India. It is paler than London expressed oil. Some samples are very transparent and pale yellow, like Canada balsam. Others (the more usual sort) are of a pale amber colour. If equal volumes of East India oil and alcohol (sp. gr. 0·796) be shaken together, an opaque milky mixture is obtained; but if the heat of a spirit-lamp be applied, the mixture becomes transparent and uniform.

[1] *Journ. de Pharm. et de Chim.* 3ème sér. t. xvii. p. 183, 1850.
[2] Dierbach, *op. cit.*

By standing, however, for twenty-four hours it separates into two strata; the lower one consisting of the oil which has taken up a small quantity of alcohol, and has, in consequence, become somewhat augmented in bulk; and the upper one, the alcohol, which has suffered a corresponding diminution in volume.

β. OLEUM CROTONIS ANGLICUM; *English Croton Oil; Dark Croton Oil.*—The oil expressed from croton seeds in London is darker-coloured than that usually imported from India. By transmitted light it is of a reddish-brown colour, like that of the deepest sherry, almost approaching to chesnut brown. By reflected light it has a greenish tinge. The dark colour of the oil may perhaps depend on some change which the seeds have suffered by keeping. After the oil has stood for a few months it is found to have deposited some white fat (margarine?). If equal volumes of alcohol (sp. gr. 0·796) and this oil be shaken together at ordinary temperatures, they form an uniform transparent mixture, and no separation takes place on standing for many weeks, unless the mixture be exposed to a low temperature. This fact, which was mentioned to me by Mr. Redwood, he has verified with various samples of croton oil expressed respectively by himself, by Mr. Morson, by Messrs. Herrings, and by Messrs. May and Co. I have verified it with a sample expressed by Messrs. Herrings. Exposure to artificial cold (as a freezing mixture), or to the atmosphere during a very cold night, will cause a separation: the oil is then found to have slightly increased in bulk, and the alcohol to have suffered a corresponding diminution of volume.

On what, it may be asked, does this difference in the properties of the East Indian and English croton oils depend? Does it arise from some difference in the mode of preparation? Or is the East Indian oil contaminated with jatropha oil? Dr. Christison observes that croton oil " is not easily adulterated with the common fixed oils, with the exception of castor oil, because this is the only common oil which possesses sufficient thickness to impart due unctuosity. Castor oil may be detected by the test mentioned in the Edinburgh Pharmacopœia. Absolute alcohol shaken with the adulterated oil will dissolve out the impurity, and thus lessen its volume; but no visible diminution is produced on pure croton oil. Five per cent. of castor oil may be thus detected; but the application of heat, as recommended by the College, is unnecessary." It is obvious, however, that this test is not applicable to English croton oil adulterated with castor oil, both of which oils are soluble in cold alcohol. If any fraud be practised in respect to croton oil, the adulterating ingredient is probably jatropha oil, which is less soluble in alcohol than croton oil.

Croton oil is exhibited in doses of one, two, or three drops. In some instances it is simply placed on the tongue,—as in coma, tetanus, and mania; or it may be taken in a tea-spoonful of syrup. These methods of administering it are objectionable, on account of the acrid taste produced. The usual mode of employing it is in the form of pill, made with conserve of roses or bread-crumb. Some have employed it in the form of emulsion, flavoured with a carminative oil or a balsamic substance; but the burning of the mouth and throat to which it gives rise is an objection to its use.

α. *Tinctura Crotonis; Tincture of Croton.*—This is prepared by digesting the seeds, or dissolving the oil in rectified spirit. Soubeiran's formula is one drop of croton oil and half a drachm of rectified spirit.

β. *Sapo Crotonis; Croton Soap.*—This is prepared with two parts of croton oil and one part of soap-boiler's lye. It is, in fact, a crotonate of soda. A croton soap is sold by Mr. Morson, of Southampton Row, Russell Square. It may be used as a purgative, in doses of from one to three grains. It has been said that the alkali diminishes the acrimonious property of the oil without affecting its cathartic powers,—a statement, however, which is highly improbable.

LINIMENTUM CROTONIS, D.; *Croton Liniment.* [(Croton Oil, f℥j.; Oil of Turpentine, f℥vij. Mix them with agitation, *D.* Another formula for this liniment is suggested by the author. It consists in mixing one part of croton oil with five parts of olive oil.)]—Rubbed repeatedly on the skin, it occasions redness and a pustular eruption. It is used as a counter-irritant.

ANTIDOTES.—In a case of poisoning by the seeds or oil, the first object is to remove the oil from the stomach. Mild, demulcent, and emollient drinks are then to be given. Alkaline substances have been recommended as chemical antidotes, but their efficacy is not proved. Full doses of opium will be requisite to check the diarrhœa. To relieve a failing circulation, ammonia and brandy may be given, and the warm bath employed.

136. CROTON ELEUTERIA, *Swartz* (Cascarilla Bush).—THE SEA-SIDE BALSAM OR SWEET-WOOD.

Sex. Syst. Monœcia, Monadelphia.

(Cortex, *L.* Bark probably of Croton Eleuteria, and possibly of other species of the same genus, *E.* The Bark, *D.*)

HISTORY.—Great confusion has existed with regard both to Cascarilla or Eleutheria bark, and the plant yielding it. The bark is said to have been first noticed by Vincent-Garcias Salat,[1] a Spaniard, in 1692. In the following year, Stisser,[2] a German professor, gave a more extended notice of it, and states that he had some of it given him by a person of distinction, at that time just returned from England, who told him that it was then the custom in England to mix it with tobacco, in order to render it more agreeable for smoking. By Dale[3] and some other pharmacologists it was thought to be *cortex thuris* or frankincense bark, and by Geoffroy[4] and others to be a species of cinchona bark. Its name *cascarilla* (the diminutive of *cascara,* the Spanish name for the rind or bark of trees) is also a Spanish name for Peruvian bark.

In 1754 Catesby[5] noticed and figured a plant which, he said, grew plentifully on most of the Bahama Islands, and yielded Cascarilla bark, or, as he called it, "*The Ilatheria bark, La Chacrilla.*" This plant is generally supposed to be the *Croton Cuscarilla,* Linn. (*C. lineare,* Jacq.); and several reasons led me, at one time,[6] to think that it might be the source of the cascarilla bark of the shops,—an opinion also entertained by Dr. Wood;[7] but Dr. Lindley[8] adduced several reasons for believing that the *Croton Eleuteria* was the true species, as Drs. Wright and Woodville had already asserted; and the subsequent receipt, by Dr. Lindley, of specimens of the

[1] *Unica quæsticuncula in quâ examinatur pulvis de quarango vulgò cascarilla in curatione tertianæ,* in 4to. Valentiæ, 1692. (Duval, *Journ. de Pharm. et de Chimie,* 3me sér. t. viii. p. 91, 1845 : see also Alibert, *Nouv. Elém. de Thérap.* t. i. p. 74, 5me édit. 1826.)

[2] *Acta laboratorii chymici,* specimen ii. Helmstadä, 1693 (quoted by Geoffroy). Stisser was the author of a letter to the Fellows of the Royal Society, entitled *De machinis fumiductoriis,* and published at Hamburgh in 1686.

[3] *Pharmacologia,* 3tia ed. p. 346, 1737. Many of the synonymes for this bark given in Dale's work are erroneous.

[4] *Treat. on Foreign Vegetables,* by R. Thicknesse, M.D. (chiefly taken from Geoffroy), Lond. 1749.

[5] *Nat. Hist. of Carolina, Florida, and the Bahama Islands.*

[6] See *Lond. Med. Gaz.* vol. xx. p. 489.

[7] *United States Dispensatory.*

[8] *Fl. Med.* p. 179.

plant from the Hon. J. C. Lees, Chief Judge in the Bahamas, has fully confirmed the accuracy of Dr. Lindley's opinion.[1] "The plant," says Mr. Lees, "is scarcely known here by the name of Cascarilla, but is commonly called Sweet-wood Bark, and often Eleuthera Bark, because it is chiefly gathered on the island of Eleuthera. It is the only bark receiving the name of Cascarilla exported from the Bahamas, where the tree grows in abundance."

The *Croton Cascarilla*, Don, *L.* (*C. pseudo-China*, Schiede) yields Copalchi (not Cascarilla) bark.

BOTANY. **Gen. Char.**—See *Croton Tiglium.*

FIG. 171.

Sp. Char.—A small tree; leaves ovate, obtuse, entire, beneath silvery and densely downy; racemes axillary and terminal, compound; flowers subsessile, monœcious (*Lindley*).

Branches and *twigs* angular, somewhat compressed. *Leaves* stalked, alternate, with a short but obtuse point. *Flowers* monœcious, sub-sessile. MALES:—*petals* whitish; *stamens* 10—12. *Ovary* roundish; *styles* 3, bifid; *stigmas* obtuse. *Capsule* roundish, minutely warted, not much bigger than a pea, with 3 furrows, 3 cells, and 6 valves.[2]

Hab.—The Bahama Islands, Jamaica.

DESCRIPTION. — *Eleutheria* or *cascarilla bark* (*cortex eleuteriæ* seu *cascarillæ*, *chaquerille* vel *schacharilla*) is in the form of fragments, or quills, of about one or two, more rarely three or four, inches long; the fragments being thin, and

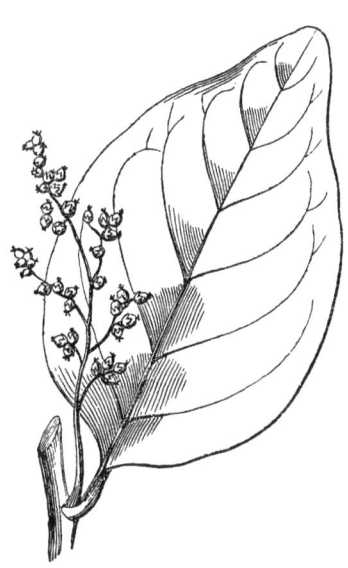

Croton Eleuteria.

usually curved both longitudinally and transversely, the quills varying in size from that of a writing pen to that of the little finger. The bark is compact, hard, moderately heavy, and has a short resinous fracture, not fibrous or splintery, as in cinchona barks. Some of the pieces are partially or wholly covered with a whitish rugous epidermis, cracked both longitudinally and transversely. If a longitudinal section of the bark be examined by the microscope, cells are observed filled with an orange-red matter (oleo-resin?). The cortical layers are of a dull brown colour. The taste of this bark is warm, spicy, and bitter; its odour is peculiar, but agreeable. When burned, it evolves a pleasant odour (which has been compared by Pfaff to that of vanilla or amber when heated), on which account it is a constituent of *fumigating*

---

[1] Specimens of the stems and bark accompanied the specimens of the plant. The former were kindly presented to me by Dr. Lindley.

Swartz, *Fl. Ind. occ.*

pastiles. Fée[1] has enumerated no fewer than forty-three species of lichens found on this bark. With one exception (*Parmelia perlata,* which I have never seen on cascarilla), every one of these lichens has an adherent, crustaceous, amorphous thallus. A very common species is *Lecidea Arthonioides,* Fée; the thallus of which is very white, and the apothecia minute, round, and black.

COMMERCE.—It is imported from Nassau, in New Providence (one of the Bahama Islands).

COMPOSITION.—Cascarilla bark was analysed by Trommsdorff,[2] who obtained from it the following substances :—*Volatile oil* 1·6, *bitter resin* 15·1, *gum* and *bitter matter with trace of chloride of potassium* 18·7, *woody fibre* 65·6. Meissner[3] detected in the ashes of the bark the *oxide of copper.* Brandes[4] has announced the existence of a peculiar alkaline substance (*cascarillina*).

1. VOLATILE OIL OF CASCARILLA (*Oleum Cascarillæ*).—It possesses the odour and taste of the bark. Its sp. gr. is 0·938. Its colour is variable, sometimes being greenish, at others yellow or blue. It consists of two oils, one boiling at 344°, which contains no oxygen (its formula probably being $C^{10}H^8$); the other less volatile and oxygenated. Nitric acid converts it into a yellow, pleasant-smelling resin. By distillation with water the bark yields about 1-120th of its weight of this oil.

2. RESIN.—Separated from the alcoholic tincture of the cascarilla by the addition of water. It is reddish-brown; has a balsamic, slightly bitter, not astringent taste; and, when thrown on hot coals, evolves an agreeable odour.

3. EXTRACTIVE.—Has a bitter, but not balsamic taste. Its watery solution reddens litmus, and is unchanged by either ferruginous solutions or tincture of nutgalls.

CHEMICAL CHARACTERISTICS. — The sesquichloride of iron deepens the colour of the infusion of cascarilla. The tincture of nutgalls causes turbidness, and at the end of twenty-four hours a very slight precipitate. A very concentrated alcoholic tincture deposits some resin on the addition of water.

PHYSIOLOGICAL EFFECTS.—Cascarilla bark belongs to the *aromatic bitters* before noticed; that is, it produces the combined effect of an aromatic and of a moderately powerful tonic; but it does not possess any astringency. Some pharmacologists place it with aromatics, others with tonics. Cullen,[5] though at one time uncertain as to which of these classes it belonged, ultimately classed it with the tonics. Krauss[6] states that moderate doses give rise, in very susceptible, especially in sanguine subjects, to narcotic effects; but though I have frequently employed it, I never observed an effect of this kind. Mixed with tobacco, and used for smoking, it is said to cause giddiness and intoxication.[7]

USES.—Cascarilla has been employed as a substitute for cinchona; and although it is inferior to the latter in tonic and febrifuge properties, its aromatic quality frequently enables it to sit easily on the stomach, without causing either vomiting or purging, which, in irritable affections of the alimentary canal, cinchona is apt to produce. In this country it is principally employed

---

[1] *Essai sur Cryptogames,* 1824.
[2] Gmelin, *Handb. d. Chem.* ii. 1319.
[3] *Ibid.*
[4] *Berl. Jahrb.* xxiii.
[5] *Mat. Med.*
[6] *Heilmittellehre,* S. 401.
[7] *United States Dispensatory.*

in those forms of dyspepsia requiring an aromatic stimulant and tonic. It is also used in cases of debility generally; and in chronic bronchial affections, to check excessive secretion of mucus. In Germany, where it is a favourite remedy, it is used in many other cases; such as low nervous fevers, intermittents, the latter stages of diarrhœa, and dysentery.

ADMINISTRATION.—The *powder* may be given in doses of from ten grains to half a drachm; but it is a less agreeable form than the infusion.

1. INFUSUM CASCARILLÆ, L. E. D.; *Infusion of Cascarilla.* (Cascarilla Bark, bruised, ʒiss.; Boiling distilled Water, Oj. Macerate for two hours in a vessel lightly covered, and strain [through linen or calico, *E.*] Cascarilla Bark, in coarse powder, ʒj.; Boiling Water, Oss. Infuse for one hour in a covered vessel, and strain. The product should measure about eight ounces, *D.*)—A light and aromatic bitter tonic. It is a good vehicle for acids and alkalies. The tincture of cascarilla is usually joined with it. Dose, from fʒj. to fʒij.

2. TINCTURA CASCARILLÆ, L. E. D.; *Tincture of Cascarilla.* (Cascarilla Bark, bruised [in moderately fine powder, *E.*], ʒv.; Proof Spirit, Oij. Macerate for fourteen days, and filter, *L.* " Proceed by percolation or digestion, as afterwards directed for tincture of cinchona," *E.* Cascarilla Bark, in coarse powder, ʒv.; Proof Spirit, Oij. Macerate for fourteen days, strain, express, and filter, *D.*)—Generally employed as an adjunct to tonic and stomachic infusions. Dose, from fʒj. to fʒij.

137. Croton pseudo-China, *Schlectendal.*—Copalche Bush.
(Cortex Copalche vel Copalchi.)

CROTON PSEUDO-CHINA, Schlectendal, Berlin. Jahrb. f. d. Pharmacie, 1829, p. 1 (with a figure); Linnæa, Bd. v. S. 84, 1830; and Bd. vi. S. 359, 1831; *Croton Cascarilla*, Don, Ed. New Phil. Journ. vol. xvi. p. 368.

This species of Croton was discovered by Schiede (Linnæa, Bd. iv. S. 211 and 579, 1829) between Plan del Rio and Puente, in Mexico. A small variety (*C. pseudo-China* var. *minor*) was found between Laguna Verde and Actopan. Both plants yield a bark very similar to that of cascarilla, and which is called in the apothecaries' shops of Jalapa *quina blanca* or *copalche.*

According to v. Bergen and v. Santen, four serons of this bark were imported in 1817 into Hamburgh from Cuba, under the name of *cascarilla de Trinidad.* In 1827 more than 30,000 lbs. of it came along with cinchona bark from Peru to Hamburgh, by way of Liverpool. Of this, 32 serons were shipped at Payta, and 300 serons at Guayaquil. It was said to be a *cinchona called copalchi* (*quina dit copalchi*). The Prussian minister, v. Altenstein, received it from Mexico under the name of *copalcke.*[1] In 1825 Mercadieu[2] published an analysis of it; and stated that it was known in Mexico as *copalchi* or *cortex amarus.* He showed a sample of it to Humboldt, who suggested that it might be the produce of *Croton suberosum*, HBK.

I have met with two sorts of copalche bark in English commerce:

1. *Quilled Copalche.*—Under the name of a *new kind of cinchona bark* I received copalche bark in the form of small thin quills, which in shape, size, and general appearance, resemble that kind of cinchona bark called by druggists "ash cinchona." In flavour it closely resembles cascarilla bark; and in burning evolves a similar odour. It is the kind

---

[1] Martiny, *Encycklop. d. med.-pharm. Naturalien- und Rohrwaarenkunde*, Bd. i. 1843; also, Göbel and Kunze, *Pharmaceut. Waarenkunde.*
[2] *Journ. de Chimie Méd.* t. i. p. 236 *bis*, 1825.

figured by Göbel and Kunze, and is doubtless the sort which the late Mr. Don mistook for genuine cascarilla bark. It might with propriety be called *Mexican cascarilla*. From genuine or Bahama cascarilla it is distinguished by the length of the quills, their colour, and the absence of transverse cracks. [According to Mr. Howard, about sixty bales of this bark have been lately imported from Puntas Arenas in the gulf of Nicoya; probably the produce of some part of Costa Rica. The appearance of the singularly indented resinous-looking derm, where denuded, is a highly characteristic feature of the species. Mr. Howard found that it contained a bitter alkaloid (*copalchin*) soluble in ether and precipitable as a white hydrate from its solution in acids. The bark contains in addition about six per cent. of fragrant wax, as well as some fatty matter. It is worthy of note that this alkaloid yields a deep green colour with chlorine and ammonia, in which respect it resembles quinine. The proportion contained in the bark is very small, being about 0·05 in 100 parts. The taste is not unlike that of quinine. It differs from this alkaloid in being apparently crystalline, and in not affording under the microscope the appearance which Herapath has assigned as the test for quinine. It also differs from quinidine.[1]—Ed.]

2. *Corky Copalche Bark.*—Under the name of *copalche* or *chiquique bark,* I have received a bark in coarser larger quills and twisted pieces covered with a very thick and much cracked corky coat. Its taste is very bitter. In burning, it evolves an aromatic odour. Is this the produce of *Croton suberosum?* Dr. Stark[2] states that he received it from Chili under the name of *natri;* and that at Santa Cruz it is known as *chiquique.*

Copalche bark has been analysed both by Mercadieu and Brandes. According to the latter chemist, 100 parts of the bark yield a *yellow bitter extractive with malates* 13·3, *brown tasteless extractive* obtained by potash 3·3, *acrid aromatic soft resin* 6·3, *green resin* 1·0, *semi-resin* 8·3, *fat with green resin* 1·1, *wax with malate of lime* 0·7, *glutinous nitrogenous matter* 33·3, *albumen* 8·7, *malate of lime* 3·3, *oxalate of lime* 4·1, *phosphate of lime* 1·4, *sulphates* and *muriates* 0·7, *ligneous fibre* 18·0, loss in *water and volatile oil* 6·2.

The medicinal properties of copalche resemble those of cascarilla bark. In Mexico it is used as a substitute for cinchona in the treatment of intermittents. It may be exhibited in powder, infusion, decoction, tincture, or spirituous extract, in the same doses as cascarilla. Dr. Stark says the infusion or decoction is best made by half an ounce of bark to a pint of water : the dose being a table-spoonful or small wine-glassful. The tincture he prepares with an ounce of bark to one pint of proof spirit; the dose being one or two tea-spoonfuls.

138. RICINUS COMMUNIS, *Linn.*—THE CASTOR-OIL PLANT, OR PALMA CHRISTI.

Sex. Syst. Monœcia, Monadelphia.

(Oleum e semine calore aut vi compressum, *L.*—Expressed oil of the seeds, *E.*—The seeds from which the oil is expressed, *D.*)

History.—The castor-oil plant was known in the most ancient times. Caillaud found the seeds of it in some Egyptian sarcophagi supposed to have been at least 4000 years old.[3] Whether this is, as some persons imagine,[4] the plant called *kikayon* in the Bible,[5] and which, in our translation, is termed the *gourd,* I cannot pretend to decide. The pious fathers Jerome and Augustin differed so much in their opinions as to what was the particular plant meant in the passage just referred to, that from words, we are told, they proceeded to blows![6] The ancient Greeks were acquainted with the *ricinus,*

---

[1] [*Pharmaceutical Journal*, Jan. 1855, p. 319.]
[2] *Ibid.* vol. ix. p. 463, April 1850.
[3] *Dict. Univ. de Mat. Méd.* t. vi.
[4] See Dr. Canvane's *Dissertation on the Oleum Palmæ Christi*, 2nd edit. Lond. 1769.
[5] *Jonah,* iv. 6.
[6] Harris, *Nat. Hist. of the Bible;* also, Kitto's *Cyclopædia of Biblical Literature*, vol. ii. p. 203, art. *Kikayon.*

for both Herodotus[1] and Hippocrates[2] mention it: the latter employed the root in medicine. Dioscorides[3] calls it the κίκι or κρότων. It was termed κρότων by the Greeks, and *ricinus* by the Romans,[4] on account of the resemblance of its seeds to a little insect bearing these names, which infests dogs and other animals, and whose common name in English is the *tick*.

BOTANY. **Gen. Char.**—*Flowers* monœcious. *Calyx* 3—5-parted, valvate. *Petals* 0. *Filaments* numerous, unequally polyadelphous; cells of the *anther* distinct, below the apex of the filament. *Style* short; *stigmas* 3, deeply bipartite, oblong, coloured, feathery; *ovary* globose, 3-celled, with an ovule in each cell. *Fruit* generally prickly, capsular, 3-coccous, with 1 seed in each cell.—*Trees, shrubs,* or *herbaceous* plants, sometimes becoming arborescent.

Leaves alternate, palmate, peltate, with glands at the apex of the petiole. *Flowers* in terminal panicles; the lower male, the upper female; all articulated with their peduncles, and sometimes augmented by biglandular bracts (*Lindley,* from *Endlicher*).

Sp. Char.—*Stem* herbaceous, pruinose. *Leaves* peltato-palmate, in 7 lobes; the lobes ovate acuminate, serrated. *Flowers* in long glaucous racemes. *Stigmas* 3, bifid at the apex. *Capsule* covered with spines.

The *stems* of plants growing in this country are round, greenish or reddish-brown, and blue pruinose, and branched. *Leaves* on long round petioles, 8- or 10-lobed. A large scutelliform gland on the petiole, near its junction with the lamina. *Filaments* capillary, branched. *Stigmas* reddish. *Capsules* supported on stalks, which are somewhat longer than the capsules themselves.

Hab. — India. When cultivated in Great Britain,

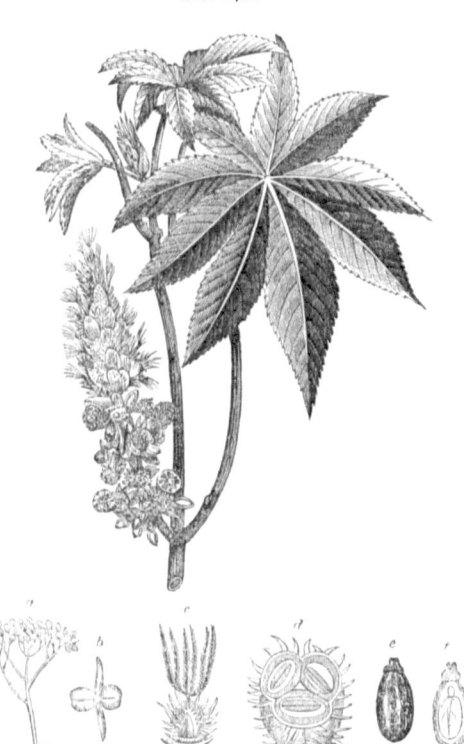

FIG. 172.

Ricinus communis.

a, Stamens. *b*, Anther. *c*, Stigmas. *d*, Capsule. *e*, Seed. *f*, Embryo.

---

[1] Lib. ii. *Euterpe,* 94.
[2] *De Nat. Mulieb.* p. 573, ed. Fœs.
[3] Lib. iv. cap. 164.
[4] Pliny, *Hist. Nat.* lib. xv. cap. 7.

Ricinus communis is an annual, seldom exceeding three or four feet high; but in other parts of the world it is said to be perennial, arborescent, and to attain a height of fifteen or twenty feet. Dr. Roxburgh[1] says that in India several varieties are cultivated, "some of them growing to the size of a pretty large tree, and of many years' duration." Clusius[2] saw it in Spain with a branched trunk as thick as a man's body, and of the height of three men. Belon[3] also tells us that in Crete it endures for many years, and requires the use of ladders to mount it. Ray[4] found it in Sicily as large as our common alder trees, woody, and long-lived; but it has been a question with botanists whether these arborescent and other kinds are mere varieties of, or distinct species from, the ordinary Ricinus communis.

The following (varieties or distinct species) are enumerated by Nees and Ebermaier[5] as common in gardens, and as distinguished principally by the colour and pruinose condition of the stem,—characters which, however uncertain in other cases, appear here to be constant.

1. RICINUS AFRICANUS (Willd.)—Stem not pruinose, green, or on one side reddish. The fruit-racemes abbreviated, the fruit-stalk longer than the capsule. Seeds attenuated on one side, marbled grey and yellowish-brown. [Arborescent. Cultivated in Bengal.[6]]

2. RICINUS MACROPHYLLUS (H. Berol.)—Nearly allied to the foregoing; stem quite green, not pruinose. Fruit-racemes elongated, fruit-stalk shorter than the fruit.

3. RICINUS LEUCOCARPUS (H. Berol.)—Stem pale green, white pruinose. Fruit-stalk as long as the fruit. The unripe fruit and prickles almost quite white.

4. RICINUS LIVIDUS (Willd.)—Stem, petiole, and midrib purple-red, not pruinose. Nearly allied to R. africanus, and, like this, more woody and perennial. [Arborescent. Cultivated in Bengal (Hamilton).]

5. RICINUS VIRIDIS (Willd.)—Stem pale green, blue pruinose, by which it is distinguished from R. macrophyllus. Seeds somewhat smaller, more oval, marked with white and fine brown. [Herbaceous. Cultivated in Bengal (Hamilton).]

DESCRIPTION.—*Castor seeds* (*semina ricini* seu *sem. cataputiæ majoris*) are oval, somewhat compressed, about four lines long, three lines broad, and a line and a half thick; externally they are pale grey, but marbled with yellowish-brown spots and stripes. The seed-coats consist, according to Bischoff,[7] of a smooth external coat (*epidermis seminalis*). 2dly, a difform, hard *testa*, consisting of two layers,—an external thick and dark brown one, and an internal one, thinner and paler. 3dly, a *cuticula nuclei* or *membrana interna*. The fleshy tumid *cicatricula stomatis* (also termed *strophiola*) is very evident at the upper end of the seed; beneath it is a small *hilum*, from which passes downwards the longitudinal *raphé*.[8] The *chalaza* is colourless.[9] The *nucleus* of the seed consists of oily *albumen* and an *embryo* the cotyledons of which are membranous or foliaceous.

COMPOSITION.—The only analysis of these seeds as yet published is that of Geiger.[10] The following are his results:—

---

[1] *Fl. Indica*, vol. iii. p. 689.
[2] *Exoticorum*, p. 299.
[3] *Observ.* lib. i. cap. 18.
[4] *Hist. Plant.* vol. i. p. 166.
[5] *Handb. d. med.-pharm. Botan.*
[6] Hamilton, *Linn. Trans.* vol. xiv.
[7] *Handb. d. bot. Term.* pp. 508, 510, and 512, tab. xl. fig. 1875.
[8] Bischoff, *ibid.* p. 515, &c. tab. xli. fig. 1747.
[9] *Ibid.* p. 518, tab. xliii. fig. 1901.
[10] *Handb. d. Pharm.* Bd. ii. S. 1671.

a. Seed-coats...........	Tasteless resin and extractive.............................	1·91	}	23·82
	Brown gum	1·91		
	Ligneous fibre..	20·00		
b. Nucleus of the seeds	Fatty oil..	46·19	}	69·09
	Gum	2·40		
	Casein (albumen)	0·50		
	Ligneous fibre with starch? (hardened albumen?) ...	20·00		
Loss (moisture)...		7·09		

Castor seeds... 100·00

1. VOLATILE ACRID PRINCIPLE (? *ricinoleic acid*).—This principle is not mentioned by Geiger, and its existence has been doubted or denied by others. But the following as well as other facts establish, in my opinion, its presence:—First, Guibourt[1] experienced a peculiar feeling of dryness of the eyes and throat, in consequence of having been exposed to the vapour arising from a vessel in which bruised castor seeds and water were boiling. Secondly, Planche obtained a permanent odorous principle by distilling a mixture of water and castor oil. Bussy and Lecanu[2] ascribe the occasional acridity of the oil to the production of fatty acids, by the action of the air on it.

2. FIXED OIL.—See *Olèum Ricini*, post.

3. ACRID RESIN?—Castor seeds appear to contain a fixed acrid principle, probably of a resinous nature, as suggested by Soubeiran.[3] The acrid principle (whatever its nature may be) appears to reside in both the *albumen* and *embryo* of the seeds. Jussieu[4] and some others have asserted that it resided exclusively in the embryo; while Boutron-Charlard and Henry, jun.[5] declared the albumen to be the exclusive seat of it. But any unprejudiced person may soon satisfy himself, by tasting separately the embryo and albumen, that both parts possess acridity. Dierbach[6] states that in fresh seeds the innermost seed-coat contains the acrid principle. If this be correct, it is most remarkable that the same coat, when dry, contains none. Calloud[7] found that castor cake (the residual cake left after the expression of the oil from the seeds), after having been deprived of all its principles soluble in alcohol, still contains an acrid principle, and excites vomiting when given in doses of about 7¼ grains.

PHYSIOLOGICAL EFFECTS.—Castor seeds possess considerable acridity. Bergius[8] states that a man masticated a single seed at bed-time: the following morning he was attacked with violent vomiting and purging, which continued the whole day. Lanzoni also states that the life of a woman was endangered by eating three grains of the seeds.[9] More recently, a girl, 18 years of age, was killed by eating " about twenty" seeds : the cause of death was gastro-enteritis.[10] [" The emmenagogue effects ascribed to the application of the *leaves* of the ricinus communis, by Drs. M'William and Tyler Smith, can easily be understood, when we remember their irritative character, and the consequences which we have found to be induced by irritation of the mammæ caused by other stimulants. ' When the breasts,' says Dr. M'William, ' are small and shrivelled, the plant is said to act more upon the uterine system, bringing on the menses if their period be distant, or causing their immoderate flow if their advent be near.'

" In the subjoined case, related by Dr. Tyler Smith, the effect produced may

[1] *Journ. de Chim. Méd.* t. i. p. 111.
[2] *Journ. de Pharm.* t. xiii. p. 80.
[3] *Ibid.* t. xv. p. 507, 1829.
[4] Quoted by De Candolle, *Essai sur les Propr. des Plantes*, p. 263.
[5] *Journ. de Pharm.* t. x. p. 466.
[6] Quoted by Nees and Ebermaier, *Handb. d. med.-pharm. Botan.*
[7] *Journ. de Pharm.* 3me sér. t. xiv. p. 189, 1848.
[8] *Mat. Med.* t. ii. p. 823, ed. 2nda.
[9] Marx, *Die Lehre von. d. Giften*, i. 128.
[10] *Lond. Med. Gaz.* vol. xix. p. 944 ; also Taylor *On Poisons*, p. 525.

have been owing partly to the application to the genitals. 'I have used,' says Dr. Tyler Smith, 'the remedy in a case of scanty menstruation of a remarkable kind. Owing to exposure to marsh malaria some years ago, the patient had scarcely a sign of coloured discharge at the usual catamenial periods. She used the infusion of the leaves of the red bofarcira at the date of her period, applying the infusion and leaves to the breasts, and the vapour to the genitals, with the effect of producing, in two days, a considerable flow of the catamenia.' "[1]—Ed.]

OLEUM RICINI, L. E. D.; *Castor Oil.*—This may be obtained from the seeds by expression, by decoction, or by the agency of alcohol. The chief part, if not the whole of the oil consumed in England, whether imported or extracted in England, is procured by expression.

Soubeiran[2] considers all processes in which heat is employed as objectionable, as a quantity of fatty acids is produced which renders the oil acrid. In America, on the contrary, heat is considered useful by expelling a volatile acrid principle.[3] It cannot be doubted that too high a temperature developes acrid matter. In England the oil is expressed, either by Bramah's hydraulic press or by the common screw-press, in a room artificially heated. It is purified by rest, decantation, and filtration. It is bleached by exposure to light on the tops of houses. In Calcutta it is prepared as follows:—The fruit is shelled by women; the seeds are crushed between rollers, then placed in hempen cloths, and pressed in the ordinary screw or hydraulic press. The oil thus procured is afterwards heated with water in a tin boiler until the water boils, by which the mucilage or albumen is separated as a scum. The oil is then strained through flannel and put into canisters. The castor seeds are distinguished according to the country yielding them. Two principal kinds are known, the large and the small nut; the latter yields the most oil.[4] The best East Indian castor oil is sold in London as cold drawn. In the southern provinces of India, according to Ainslie,[5] castor oil is obtained by decoction.

Much of the American castor oil is prepared by mere expression, rest, and decantation; but the following are the outlines of the process usually employed in the United States by those who prepare it on the large scale. The seeds, cleansed from the dust and fragments of the capsules, are placed in a shallow iron reservoir, where they are submitted to a gentle heat insufficient to scorch or decompose them, and not greater than can be readily borne by the hand. The object of this step is to render the oil sufficiently liquid for easy expression. The seeds are then introduced into a powerful screw-press, and submitted to pressure, by which a whitish oily liquid is obtained, which is mixed with a considerable quantity of water in clean iron boilers, and the impurities skimmed off as they rise to the surface. The water dissolves the mucilage and starch, and the heat coagulates the albumen, which forms a whitish layer between the oil and water. The clear oil is now removed, and boiled with a minute portion of water until aqueous vapour ceases to arise, and till a small portion of the liquid taken up in a phial preserves a perfect transparency when it cools. The effect of this operation is to clarify the oil, and to render it less irritating by driving off the volatile acrid matter. But much care is requisite not to push the heat too far, lest the oil acquire a brownish hue, and an acrid peppery taste similar to the West India medicine. One basket of the seeds yields five or six quarts, or about twenty-five per cent., of the best oil.[6]

In the West Indies the oil is obtained by decoction; but none of it comes to this country in the way of commerce. In Jamaica the bruised seeds are boiled with water in an iron pot, and the liquid kept constantly stirred. The oil, which separates, swims

---

[1] [Dr. Cormack, in *Assoc. Journ.* March 25, 1853.]
[2] *Nouveau Traité de Pharmacie.*
[3] *United States Dispensatory.*
[4] Private information from an oil-presser of Calcutta.
[5] *Materia Indica*, vol. i. p. 256.
[6] *United States Dispensatory.*

on the top, mixed with a white froth, and is skimmed off. The skimmings are heated in a small iron pot, and strained through a cloth. When cold, it is put in jars or bottles for use.[1] The object of the second heating is to dissipate the volatile acrid principle; but if the process be not suspended immediately after the water is driven off, the oil acquires a reddish-brown colour, an acrid flavour, and irritating qualities. It is said that the seeds are sometimes roasted to increase the product. By this process also the oil is coloured and rendered acrid. In Armenia the oil is obtained by decoction; in Russia by expression.[2] On the continent of Europe castor oil is sometimes obtained by the agency of alcohol. The process is more expensive, and the product is inferior.

The *oleum ricini alcoholicum*, in use in Italy, is apparently an alcoholic extract, composed of 72 per cent. of oil and 28 per cent. of alcohol and water. The dose is from half an ounce to an ounce.[3]

Properties.—Castor oil is a viscid oil, usually of a pale yellow colour, with a slightly nauseous odour and a mild taste. It is lighter than water, its sp. gr. being, according to Saussure, 0·969 at 55° F. When cooled down to about 0°, it congeals into a transparent yellow mass. By exposure to the air it becomes rancid, thick, and ultimately congeals, without becoming opaque; and hence it is called a *drying oil*. When heated to a little more than 500° F. it begins to decompose.

Solubility.—Castor oil is remarkable for its ready solubility in alcohol. Strictly speaking, castor oil and alcohol exercise a mutual solvent action on each other. When they are shaken together, an homogeneous transparent mixture is obtained. Rectified spirit of wine[4] may be substituted frequently with a similar result; but with some samples of genuine oil the mixture does not become clear until heat is applied; and, moreover, by standing a separation takes place into two strata,—an upper spirituous one, holding oil in solution; and an inferior oleaginous one, containing spirit. In one experiment 65 vols. of oil and 65 vols. of rectified spirit were mixed, and by shaking a transparent uniform mixture was obtained: after several weeks a separation had taken place: the upper stratum measured 12 vols., the lower one 118 vols. Of three samples of genuine oil, one English, a second West Indian, and the third East Indian, I find the English to be the most, and the East Indian the least soluble in rectified spirit.—I find that castor oil enables other fixed oils (olive, nut, lard, and other oils) to dissolve in alcohol. Thus, if 1 vol. of olive oil, 2 vols. of castor oil, and 2 vols. of rectified spirit, be mixed and heated, a transparent homogeneous solution is obtained.—Ether readily dissolves castor oil.

Varieties.—In the London market there are chiefly three sorts of castor oil; namely, the oil expressed in London from imported seeds, East Indian oil, and the American. West Indian and Australian oils are rarely to be met with.

1. *English Castor Oil.*—By this is meant castor oil drawn in England from imported seeds. It differs somewhat from the imported oil. I am informed that it is not bleached so completely by exposure to light as the East Indian oil. This is usually ascribed to the seeds having suffered some change before they are pressed. But something is probably due to the mode of preparation: in England the oil is not heated in boiling water, as it is in Calcutta.

[1] Wright, *Med. Plants of Jamaica*, in *Lond. Med. Journ.* vol. viii.
[2] *Chemical Gazette*, vol. i. p. 210, 1843.
[3] *Pharmaceutical Journal*, vol. vii. p. 354, 1848.
[4] According to Stoltze, benzoic acid augments the solubility of castor oil in spirit containing 75 per cent. of alcohol; that is, in spirit whose sp. gr. is 0·860. Camphor has a similar influence.

2. *East Indian Castor Oil* is the principal kind employed in this country. It is imported from Bombay and Calcutta. It is an oil of exceedingly good quality (both with respect to colour and taste), and is obtained at a very low price. It is procured from *Ricinus communis* and *R. lividus*. I am informed that occasionally it solidifies by keeping.

3. *American* or *United States Castor Oil* is, for the most part, imported from New York. All the samples which I have examined have been of very fine quality; and, in my opinion, had a less unpleasant flavour than the East Indian variety. Our druggists object to it, on the ground of its depositing a white substance (*margaritine*) in cold weather,—a circumstance which has led some persons to imagine that it had been mixed with some other fixed oil (lard oleine ?).

4. *West Indian Castor Oil.*—For a genuine specimen of this oil I am indebted to Mr. Spencer, of Lamb's Conduit Street, who received it some years since from the wife of the Governor of the Island of Tobago, on whose estate it was procured. Its colour is that of golden brown sherry.

5. *Australian Castor Oil.*—Of this I have seen but one sample, which was dark coloured. [The loss from breakage and leakage as a result of importation from India is immense. On account of the former, the package in duppers has been given up, and is now confined to tin canisters packed into cases containing about 160 lbs. The Americans pack their oil invariably in barrels or hogsheads; but it is never imported into England, except when the prices rule from 50 to 60 per cent. above the average of 5d. per lb. for East Indian oil. The American oil tastes less acrid than the latter, but it congeals quickly in cold weather, and becomes opaque. On this account it fetches much less in the English market than the oil from Calcutta.—Ed.]

Commerce.—Castor oil is imported in casks, barrels, hogsheads, and duppers. The latter are made, as I am informed, of gelatine (prepared by boiling the cuttings of skin) moulded in earthen moulds. In this country the oil is purified by decantation and filtration, and is bleached by exposure to solar light on the tops of houses. [The quantity of this oil imported annually during a period of seven years was as follows :—

	lbs.		lbs.
1843	1,051,792	1847	451,584
1844	1,223,264	1848	513,856
1845	1,801,632	1849	1,084,272—Ed.]
1846	1,477,168		

Composition.—The following is the *ultimate* composition of castor oil, according to the analyses of Saussure and Ure :—

	Saussure.	Ure.
Carbon	74·178	74·00
Hydrogen	11·034	10·29
Oxygen	14·788	15·71
Castor oil	100·000	100·00

The *proximate* principles have not been accurately determined. From Bussy and Lecanu's[1] researches we may infer that castor oil contains three fats, each composed of oxide of glyceryle and a fatty acid. But according to the more recent investigations of Saalmuller,[2] there can be but two fats in this oil. In addition to these fats there is probably a small proportion of an acrid resin. The following table, therefore, represents the

PRESUMED COMPOSITION OF CASTOR OIL.

Ricinoleine.
Margaritine.
Acrid resin ?

1. *Ricinoleine.*—This has not been isolated. It is the constituent of castor oil which by saponification yields oxide of glyceryle and a liquid acid, *ricinoleic acid*, $C^{38}H^{35}O^5$.

---

[1] *Journ. de Pharm.* t. xiii. p. 57, 1827.
[2] *Annal. d. Chem. u. Pharm.* Bd. lxiv. S. 108, 1848 ; also *The Chem. Gaz.* vol. vi. p. 74, 1848.

Bussy and Lecanu regard this acid as a mixture of two acids, which they term *ricinic* and *elaïodic* acids.

2. *Margaritine ;* or *Ricino-stearine.*—This is a solid white crystalline fat, which separates from castor oil in cold weather. By saponification it yields oxide of glyceryle and a solid crystallisable fatty acid called *margaritic acid*, which in its melting point (165° F.) and composition exhibits a great resemblance to stearic acid, $C^{68}H^{68}O^7$. But with a margaritic acid obtained from another sample of castor oil, he found the composition to approach more to that of palmitic acid, $C^{32}H^{32}O^4$.

According to Lecanu and Bussy, margaritic acid constitutes only 0·002 of the products of saponification of castor oil: it follows, therefore, that the proportion of margaritine in the oil must be small. But it is probable that the quantity is variable, and that the differences observed in the action of alcohol in the different specimens of castor oil depend on variations in the relative proportions of the margaritine and ricinoleine.

3. *Acrid Resin?*—Some years since Soubeiran[1] obtained from castor oil by a complicated process what he supposed to be a soft resinous oil, but which was evidently a complex product. To this he in part ascribed the purgative qualities of castor oil.

Products of Decomposition.—By saponification and distillation castor oil yields certain peculiar products by which it is characterised.

PRODUCTS OF SAPONIFICATION.		PRODUCTS OF DISTILLATION.	
100 *Parts of Castor Oil yielded:*		(*Average of Two Experiments :*)	
1. Fatty acids (viz. *ricinic, elaïodic,* and margaritic acids)	94	1. Distilled liquid	33·5
		(*a.*) Water.	
2. Glycerine	8	(*b.*) Acetic acid.	
		(*c.*) Acroleine (a small quantity).	
		(*d.*) Œnanthol. [acids.	
		(*e.*) Ricinic, elaïodic, and œnanthylic	
		2. Solid residuum	63·0
		3. Loss (inflammable gas)	3·5
Total	102	Castor oil	100·0

1. *Œnanthol.*—Described by Bussy and Lecanu as *volatile oil;* but more recently by Bussy[2] as œnanthol. It is a colourless limpid aromatic liquid, whose formula is $C^{14}H^{14}O^2$. It is scarcely soluble in water, but dissolves in alcohol and ether. It is rapidly oxidised in the air, and becomes *œnanthylic acid* ($C^{14}H^{13}O^3$,HO). It combines with water, forming a crystalline hydrate, $C^{14}H^{14}O^2$,HO. By the action of nitric acid it yields at a low temperature an isomeric compound called *metœnanthol ;* and at a high temperature, besides œnanthylic and other volatile fatty acids, a volatile oil resembling oil of cassia.

2. *Solid residuum of distillation.*—Pale yellow, elastic, spongy, having the consistence of soft new bread, gelatiniform, odourless, tasteless, combustible, solid. It is insoluble in alcohol, ether, and the oils (both fixed and volatile).

By the action of hyponitric acid on castor oil Boudet obtained a solid odorous fat called *palmine,* which by saponification yielded palmic acid, $C^{34}H^{32}O^5$,HO, and glycerine; and by the action of nitric acid on castor oil Mr. Tilley[3] obtained œnanthylic acid.

Adulteration.—Two kinds of frauds have been practised with regard to castor oil. One consists in the admixture of a small quantity of croton oil to it, with the view of increasing its activity. This mixture is introduced into gelatine capsules, and sold as *concentrated castor oil.* This fraud is a very dangerous one. I have heard of several cases in which very violent and dangerous effects were produced by these capsules on pregnant females.

The other fraud consists in the adulteration of the castor oil with some bland viscid cheaper oil. I have been informed that the oleine of lard, called *lard oil,* has been used for this purpose, but I have not been enabled to

[1] *Journ. d. Pharm.* t. xv. p. 507, 1829.
[2] *Ibid.* 3me sér. t. viii. p. 321, 1845 ; also, *Chemical Gazette,* vol. iii. p. 381, 1845.
[3] *Memoirs of the Chemical Society,* vol. i. p. 1, 1843.

procure evidence of it. This kind of fraud is said to be detected by alcohol, which dissolves the genuine castor oil, but not the admixed oil; and accordingly, in the Edinburgh Pharmacopœia the test of the purity of the oil is that "it is entirely dissolved by its own volume of alcohol." Unfortunately, however, for this test, castor oil may be adulterated with 33 per cent. of another fixed oil, and yet be soluble in its own volume of alcohol.

Physiological Effects.—α. *On Animals generally* castor oil acts as a laxative or mild purgative. Large animals, as the horse, require a pint or more for a dose; smaller ones need only a few ounces.[1] Mr. Youatt, however, declares this oil to be both uncertain and dangerous in the horse.[2]

β. *On Man.*—*Injected into the veins*, castor oil gripes and purges, and causes a nauseous oily taste in the mouth :[3] hence it would appear to have a specific influence over the mucous lining of the alimentary canal. *Swallowed* to the extent of one or two ounces, it usually acts as a mild but tolerably certain purgative or laxative, without producing any uneasiness in the bowels. "It has this particular advantage," says Dr. Cullen,[4] "that it operates sooner after its exhibition than any other purgative I know of, as it commonly operates in two or three hours. It seldom gives any griping, and its operation is generally moderate—to one, two, or three stools only." It not unfrequently occasions nausea, or even vomiting, especially if somewhat rancid; in many cases, I believe, rather from its disgusting flavour than from any positively emetic qualities. It has been stated by continental writers that castor oil is most unequal in its action, at one time operating with considerable violence, at another with great mildness; but I have never found it so, nor is it usually considered to be so in this country. I can, however, readily believe that a difference in the mode of its preparation, especially with reference to the heat employed, may materially affect its purgative property.

When castor oil has been taken by the mouth, it may be frequently recognised in the alvine evacuations ; but it presents itself under various forms, "sometimes resembling caseous flakes, or a soap-like scum, floating on the more fluid part of the dejection : occasionally it has been arranged in a form not unlike bunches of grapes, or more nearly of hydatids of a white colour; more generally, however, it is found mixed up with the fæces as a kind of emulsion ; and in some few instances it has been discharged under the form of solid tallow-like masses."[5] Mr. Brande[6] says in one case it was discharged from the bowels in the form of indurated nodules, which were at first regarded as biliary concretions. A remarkable case is mentioned by Dr. Ward, of a woman on whom this oil did not act as a purgative, but exuded from every part of her body.[7]

Uses.—Castor oil is used to evacuate the contents of the bowels in all cases where we are particularly desirous of avoiding the production of abdominal irritation (especially of the bowels and urino-genital organs). The principal, or I might say the only objection to its use in these cases, is its nauseous taste. The following are the leading cases in which we employ it :—

---

[1] Moiroud, *Pharm. Vétér.* p. 280.
[2] *The Horse*, in *Library of Useful Knowledge*, pp. 212 and 387.
[3] Dr. E. Hale, in Begin's *Traité de Thérapeutique*, p. 114.
[4] *Mat. Med.*
[5] Dr. Golding Bird, *Lond. Med. Gaz.* vol. xv. p. 225.
[6] *Dict. of Mat. Med.*
[7] *Lond. Med. Gaz.* vol. x. p. 377.

1. *In inflammatory affections of the alimentary canal,* as enteritis, peritonitis, and dysentery, a mild but certain purgative is oftentimes indicated. No substance, I believe, answers the indication better, and few so well, as castor oil.

2. *In obstructions and spasmodic affections of the bowels,* as intus-susception, ileus, and colic, especially lead colic, this oil is the most effectual evacuant we can employ.

3. *After surgical operations about the pelvis or abdomen* (for example, lithotomy, and the operation for strangulated hernia), as well as after *parturition,* it is the best and safest purgative.

4. *In inflammatory or spasmodic diseases of the urino-genital organs,* inflammation of the kidneys or bladder, calculous affections, gonorrhœa, or stricture, castor oil is a most valuable purgative.

5. *In affections of the rectum,* especially piles, prolapsus, and stricture, no better evacuant can be employed.

6. *As an anthelmintic* for tape-worms, castor oil was first employed by Odier. Arnemann, however, has shown that it possesses no peculiar or specific vermifuge properties.

7. *As a purgative for children* it has been used on account of its mildness, but its unpleasant taste [?] is a strong objection to its use.

8. *In habitual costiveness,* also, it has been recommended. Dr. Cullen observed that if castor oil be frequently repeated the dose might be gradually diminished ; so that persons who, in the first instance, required half an ounce or more, afterwards needed only two drachms.

[9. *In Asiatic or malignant cholera.*—During the epidemic cholera which prevailed in this metropolis in the summer of 1854, and to which no fewer than 13,297 persons fell victims, the use of castor oil as an *eliminant* was strongly recommended by Dr. Johnson, of King's College Hospital. It was extensively tried in hospital and private practice, and with very variable results. In some instances it appeared to aggravate the symptoms and exhaust the patient, while in others the apparent benefit which followed its use was ascribed to other causes. The Report of the "Treatment Committee" of the Board of Health, lately published, has enabled us, since the disappearance of the disease, to arrive at some estimate of the merits of the castor-oil treatment of cholera. The Committee, including the names of some eminent physicians of this metropolis, base their report on 2,749 cases of developed cholera, and taking the cases of collapse, treated by different methods, they find that the per-centage of mortality was as it is stated below :—

	Deaths.
Calomel and opium	59·2 per cent.
Calomel (larger doses)	60·9 ,,
Salines	62·9 ,,
Chalk and opium	63·2 ,,
Calomel (small doses)	73·9 ,,
Castor oil	77·6 ,,
Sulphuric acid	78·9 ,,

Assuming that these cases have been carefully compared, it is clear that castor oil has no claim to be considered as a remedy for cholera.

"In consequence of the very strong manner in which castor oil was recommended by Dr. Johnson in the treatment of Asiatic cholera, the physicians to the Dreadnought Hospital-ship considered it their duty, both in justice to Dr. Johnson and also to their patients, to give the reported remedy a fair trial in a series of cases. These cases were not selected, but taken indiscriminately for several days together.

" Immediately on admission, each patient had a salt-and-water emetic administered, in order to clear the stomach of any medicines or other liquid they might previously have taken. After copious vomiting had taken place, the castor oil was used. The medicine was given regularly under proper superintendence, and in no case was there any neglect or mismanagement on the part of the nurses. Constant friction to the extremities, by means of flesh-brushes or coarse towels, was also employed, and an abundant supply of iced water was given to all of the patients.

" The following is a brief but correct account of the cases so treated :—

" Out of 19 cases, 12 terminated fatally, and 7 recovered.

" Of the 12 fatal cases, 8 died during the stage of collapse, and 4 during the consecutive fever. The case (No. 16) was, at the commencement, but slightly collapsed, but afterwards became the worst case of consecutive fever that we had to treat.

" Of the 7 that recovered, in 1 the reaction was so great as to require a full bleeding; 3 had the consecutive fever slightly; and 3 recovered without any febrile symptoms at all.

" In 4 cases, calomel was given after the oil appeared to have produced no beneficial effect, and the patients were getting worse.

" Of the 4 thus treated, 2 recovered, and 2 died; the two that recovered had consecutive fever slightly; the 3rd died of consecutive fever; and the 4th died during the stage of collapse.

" Judging from the result, we are not justified in giving any credit to castor oil as a remedy in the treatment of Asiatic cholera."[1]—ED.]

Administration.—The dose of castor oil for children is one or two tea-spoonfuls; for adults, from one to two or three table-spoonfuls. To cover its unpleasant flavour, some take it floating on spirit (especially gin), but which is frequently contraindicated; others on coffee, or on peppermint or some other aromatic water [infusion of cloves]; or it may be made into an emulsion by the aid of the yolk of egg or mucilage of tragacanth.

139. Curcas purgans, *Adanson;* and C. multifidus, *Endlicher.* Physic Nuts.

(Semina.)

The seeds of both these species of Curcas are met with under the name of *physic nuts;* and as their effects and uses are similar, I include them under a common head.

Gen. Char.—*Flowers* monœcious. *Calyx* very short, 5-parted. MALES: *Corolla* globose-campanulate, 5-cleft. *Stamens* 10, united at the base, the 5 exterior alternating with the same number of conoid glands; filaments filiform; anthers turned inwards, 2-celled. FEMALES: *Corolla* much larger than the calyx, convolute; consisting of 5 petals. *Ovary* on a 5-lobed disc, 3-celled, with 1 ovule in each cell. *Styles* 3, filiform, distinct. *Stigmas* thick, 2-lobed. *Capsule* 3-coccous, with 1 seed in each cell.—Tropical *shrubs* of America. *Leaves* alternate, petiolated, angulate 5-lobed, quite entire, truncated at the base, reticulate 7-nerved, quite smooth. *Corymbs* with long peduncles; the males terminal; the females axillary (*Endlicher*).

Species.—1. CURCAS PURGANS, Adanson; *Jatropha Curcas*, Linn.; *English Physic Nut,*

---

[1] [*Medical Times and Gazette*, Oct. 7, 1854.]

Wright; *Physic-nut Tree*, Hughes, Browne; *Angular-leaved Physic Nut*, Miller; *Pinheiro de purga, Pinhaô paraguay*, Mart., Syst. Mat. Med. Brasil.—Leaves long-stalked, broadly cordate, angular, roundish; panicles terminal or axillary, in cymes.—West Indies; Brazils; coast of Coromandel; Ceylon.

The fruit is a tricoccous capsule about the size and shape of a walnut.

The seeds (*semina curcadis*), sometimes called *American* or *English physic nuts*, or simply *physic nuts* (*nuces catharticæ americanæ*), *Barbadoes seeds* or *nuts* (*nuces barbadenses*), *semina ricini majoris* or *gros pignon d'Inde*, have the shape of castor seeds, but are somewhat rough to the touch, and black, but marked with numerous minute cracks. The kernels are covered with a fine white pellicle (*cuticula nuclei*). The seeds have been analysed by Cadet de Gassicourt[1] and by Soubeiran.[2] The latter chemist found in them *a fixed oil, a peculiar fixed acrid resin, saccharine matter, gum*, a small quantity of *fatty acid, glutine* (emulsin?), a *free acid* (malic?), and some *salts*.

The expressed oil, commonly called *jatropha oil* (*oleum jatrophæ curcadis* vel *oleum infernale*), was imported a few years ago under the name of *oil of wild castor seeds*. It is sometimes expressed in England. As commonly met with, it has a yellowish colour, with a feeble odour, and during the cold weather deposits a white solid fat (margarine or stearine). When fresh and pure, it is described as being odourless, colourless, and quite limpid. 1000 parts of the seeds yielded to Guibourt 656 parts of kernels, from which he obtained 265 parts of a colourless very fluid oil, which in the cold deposited a considerable quantity of stearine. Jatropha oil differs from castor and croton oils in its slight solubility in alcohol; but mixture with castor oil augments its solubility. According to Mr. Quekett,[3] it is well adapted for burning in lamps; for which purpose it is employed in India.

Properties.—Jatropha *seeds* and *oil* resemble the seeds and oil of croton in their effects. Mr. Bennett[4] swallowed four seeds, and experienced a very unpleasant sensation in the stomach and bowels, with nausea, which, after an interval of nearly two hours, terminated in vomiting: their purgative effects followed soon afterwards, and were mild; the sickness had then passed away, but the burning sensation continued for some time longer. The kernels of five seeds caused in a labourer vomiting, purging, perspiration, debility, giddiness, and delirium. Four hours after taking the poison he walked to the London Hospital: the pupils were natural, the countenance pale, the hands cold, and the pulse 140. An opiate and a mild cordial were given to him, and he soon recovered.[5] Jatropha oil is occasionally used as a drastic purgative. It is less powerful than croton oil. Dr. Christison states that twelve or fifteen drops of it are about equal to one ounce of castor oil. The residual cake from which the oil has been expressed is very active. The last-mentioned authority found that a few grains of it caused violent vomiting and purging. The juice of the plant[6] has been successfully applied externally as a remedy for piles. Dr. McWilliam[7] says that a decoction of the leaves is used by the natives of the Cape Verd Islands to excite a secretion of milk in women who have borne a child, and who are not past child-bearing.[8]

2. CURCAS MULTIFIDUS, Endlicher, Enchir. Botan.; *Jatropha multifida*, Linn.; *Adenorhopium multifidum*, Pohl; *French Physic Nut; Spanish Physic Nut.*—Leaves large, stalked, palmate or digitate, many-lobed, smooth; lobes pinnatifid, cuneate. — West Indies; Brazils.—The capsule is yellowish, about the size of a walnut, obtusely 3-cornered, somewhat tapering above, 3-celled; each cell containing 1 seed. The seeds, called *French physic nuts* (*semina curcadis multifidi; nuces purgantes; avellanæ purgatrices; ben magnum*), are about the size of those of a common nut, rounded externally, with two flattened surfaces separated by an ovule internally. The seed-coat is marbled and smooth: the kernel is white.—The composition of these seeds is, according to Soubeiran,[9] similar to that of the seeds of the *Curcas purgans.*—The expressed oil (*oleum*

---

[1] *Journ. de Pharm.* t. x. p. 176, 1824.

[2] *Ibid.* t. xv. p. 503, 1829.

[3] *Practical Treatise on the Use of the Microscope*, p. 138, 1848.

[4] *Lond. Med. Gaz.* vol. ix. p. 8.

[5] Letheby, *Lond. Med. Gaz.* N.S. vol. vii p. 116, 1848.

[6] Lunan, *Hort. Jamaicensis*, vol. ii. p. 62; quoted by Dr. Hamilton in the *Pharmaceutical Journal*, vol. v. p. 26, 1845.

[7] *Report on the Boa Vista Fever*, 1847.

[8] See page 419, *ante.*

[9] *Journ. de Pharm.* t. xv. p. 506, 1829.

curcadis multifidi ; oleum pinhoen), as well as the seeds, are drastic cathartics. In their operation they resemble the preceding oil and seeds. Death is said to have been produced by them.[1]

3. The seeds of the Jatropha gossypifolia, Linn.; *Bastard French Physic Nut, Belly-ach,* or *Wild Cassada,* have also been used as purgatives in dropsies.[2]

140. Anda brasiliensis, *Raddi.*

(Semina.)

Anda, Piso, I. 72; II. 148; *Anda brasiliensis,* Raddi, Quarante piante, &c. 1821; *Anda Gomesii,* Ad. Jussieu, De Euphorb. Generib. 1824; *Anda-açu, Indayaçu, Purga de Gentio; Cocco de Purga, Purga dos Paulistas, Frutta d'Arara,* Brazil.—Brazil.— The fruit is about the size of an orange, with 2 large and 2 smaller angles. It contains two roundish nut-like seeds (*semina andæ brasiliensis*) about the size of small chesnuts. By pressure they yield a fixed oil (*oleum andæ brasiliensis; oil of anda-açu*). Both seeds and oil are purgative. One seed, according to Von Martius,[3] is a dose for a man. The expressed oil is clear and pale yellowish. Like jatropha oil, it is not very soluble in alcohol; but its solubility is increased by the addition of castor oil. Mr. Ure[4] found that in doses of 20 drops it operated moderately as a purgative.

141. MANIHOT UTILISSIMA, *Pohl.*[5]—BITTER CASSAVA.

Sex. Syst. Monœcia, Monadelphia.
(Fecula of the Root ; Tapioca, *E.*)

Synonymes.—*Jatropha Manihot,* Linn.; *Janipha Manihot,* HBK. ii. 85; Hooker, Bot. Mag. t. 3071. D.

History.—Monardes[6] describes the Indian method of making cassava bread; and Piso[7] notices the mode of preparing the farina called cream of *Tipioca [Tapioca].*

Botany. **Gen. Char.**—*Flores* monœcious. *Calyx* corolline, campanulate, 5-cleft, convolute. *Corolla* 0. *Stamens* 10, inserted on the margin of a fleshy disc, free, the alternate ones shorter: *filaments* filiform; *anthers* turned inwards, 2-celled. *Ovary* placed on the fleshy disc, 3-celled, with 1 ovule in each cell. *Style* short. *Stigmas* 3, many-lobed, the lobes consolidated into a conical sinuated-sulcated mass. *Capsule* 3-coccous; the cocci 2-valved and 1-seeded (*Endlicher*).

Sp. Char.—*Leaves* with very long petioles, deeply 7-parted, palmate; the segments lanceolate, acuminate, attenuated at the base, quite entire, the outer ones smaller, unequal, diverging, straggling. *Root* whitish-yellow (*Pohl*).

Root large, thick, tuberous, fleshy; containing an acrid, milky, highly poisonous juice. *Flowers* axillary, racemose.[8]

Hab.—Native of the Brazils; where, as well as in other parts of South America, it is cultivated.

---

[1] Sloane's *Jamaica,* vol. i. p. 36.
[2] Hamilton, *Pharmaceutical Journal,* vol. v. p. 27, 1845.
[3] *Systema Mat. Med. Veget. Brasil.*
[4] *Pharmaceutical Journal,* vol. ix. p. 9, 1849.
[5] *Plant. Brasil. Icones et Descript.,* fol. Vindob. 1827–31.
[6] Clusii *Exoticor.* lib. x. cap. 53, p. 330.
[7] *De Medicina Brasil.* p. 52.
[8] Hooker, *Bot. Mag.* t. 3071.

MANIHOT AIPI, Pohl; *Sweet Cassava*, Bancroft, Nat. Hist. of Guiana, 1769.—This is usually regarded as a variety of the above, but Pohl considers it to be a distinct species; characterised by the leaves, which are 5-parted, and by the root, which is reddish, and contains a milky non-poisonous juice. It is cultivated in the Brazils, and in Spanish America.

MANIHOT JANIPHA, Pohl; *Jatropha Janipha*, Linn.; *Janipha Loeflingii*, HBK.— This species is said to yield the *sweet* or *white cassava* of the West Indies. Dr. Hamilton[1] says it so closely resembles the *Janipha Manihot*, Linn. (*Manihot utilissima*, Pohl), that an experienced eye can hardly distinguish it with certainty. Is not the sweet cassava of the West Indies the *Manihot Aipi* of Pohl? Like the latter, it is devoid of poisonous properties.

DESCRIPTION.—1. *Bitter cassava root* is a large tuberous root[2] which abounds in a poisonous milky juice. It is difficult to distinguish it by its appearance from the sweet cassava root; but it is devoid of the tough, fibrous, or woody filaments found in the heart of the sweet cassava root; and it does not become soft, like the latter root, by boiling or roasting. The rasped root mixed with water, boiled, and then fermented, yields a spirituous liquor called *cassiri*.[3] *Cassava meal* is obtained by subjecting the grated root to pressure to express the juice, and then drying and pounding the residual cake. Of this meal *cassava bread* is made. The expressed juice by repose deposits the farina called *cassava starch*, of which *tapioca* is made. A sauce called *casareep* or *cassireepe* is made from the juice.[4]

2. *Sweet cassava root* resembles the bitter cassava root in external appearance; but, unlike the latter, it is not poisonous. It has a bundle of tough, fibrous, or woody filaments at the heart, running longitudinally through the root. By boiling or roasting it becomes soft, and is used at table.

A few pounds of *dried sweet cassava root* were sent to England from Jamaica on speculation, to ascertain whether it was likely to prove a profitable article of commerce. It consisted of transverse and longitudinal segments, which were beautifully white, had a very faint agreeable odour, and were mucilaginous or farinaceous to the taste. The circular discs were from one to two or more inches in diameter, and had in the centre the ligneous cord above alluded to. Some of the pieces were worm-eaten: a few were slightly scorched or burnt, apparently by over-heating in the drying process.

Cassava meal and *bread, cassava starch*, and *tapioca*, are prepared from the sweet as well as from the bitter cassava root.

COMPOSITION.—The bitter cassava root has been analysed by MM. O. Henry and Boutron-Chalard,[5] who inferred that it contained *free* [?] *hydrocyanic acid, starch*, a small quantity of *sugar*, an *organic salt of magnesia*,

[1] Hamilton, *Pharmaceutical Journal*, vol. v. p. 27, 1845.
[2] A figure of the root is given in the *Journ. de Pharm.* t. xxii. 1836.
[3] Dr. Hamilton, *Pharmaceutical Journal*, vol. v. p. 29, 1849.
[4] *Casareep* is the concentrated juice of the roots of the bitter cassava flavoured by aromatics. During the evaporation, the poisonous principle of the juice [prussic acid] is either dissipated or destroyed. Casareep is used to flavour soups and other dishes, and is the basis of the West Indian dish *pepper-pot*. It is a powerful antiseptic (Shier, *Report on the Starch-producing Plants of the Colony of British Guiana*, Demerara, 1847; Hamilton, *Pharmaceutical Journal*, vol. v. p. 30, 1845).—In French Guiana the term *cabiou* or *cabion* is applied to a similar condiment (Henry and Boutron-Chalard, *Journ. de Pharm.* t. xxii. p. 123). The inspissated juice flavoured with capsicum pods is used in the Brazils as a sauce, under the name of *Tycupí* or *Tucupí* (Martius, *Syst. Mat. Med. Veg. Brasil.* p. 94).
[5] *Journ. de Pharm.* t. xxii. p. 118, 1836.

a *bitter principle*, a *crystallisable fatty matter*, an *azotised matter* (vegetable osmazome), *phosphate of lime*, and *woody fibre*.

1. HYDROCYANIC ACID.—According to O. Henry and Boutron-Chalard, the active principle of the root is hydrocyanic acid. Their statement is confirmed by Dr. Christison, who examined some well-preserved juice from Demerara.[1]

2. VOLATILE ACRID PRINCIPLE ?—The vomiting and purging, and other abdominal symptoms ascribed to bitter cassava, would lead us to suspect that, like other euphorbiaceous plants, it contains an acrid principle.

PHYSIOLOGICAL EFFECTS.—The fresh roots, as well as the expressed juice, are virulent poisons, destroying life in a very short period of time. O. Henry and Boutron-Chalard describe the effects on guinea-pigs as resembling those caused by hydrocyanic acid; but death did not occur until from 40 to 55 minutes after the use of the poison. Ricord Madianna[2] has killed dogs in ten minutes with a poison obtained from this root. The symptoms described by Barham[3] are pain and swelling of the abdomen, vomiting and purging, dimness of sight, syncope, rapid diminution of the powers of life, and death in a few hours. Half a pint of the juice has produced death in an hour.[4]

USES.—Dr. Wright[5] says that the scrapings of the fresh root are successfully applied to ill-disposed ulcers; and Dr. Hamilton[6] speaks of the instantaneous relief which he experienced on himself from the application of a cataplasm of the rasped roots, with all their juices unexpressed, to the spot where a nest of chigres (*Pulex penetrans*) had been dislodged. The root is used to catch birds, which, by eating it, lose the power of flying.[7] It yields cassava meal and cassava starch.

1. FARINA MANDIOCÆ; *Cassava* or *Cassada Meal; Furinha de Pao,* or simply *Farinha; Farine de Manioc.*—This is obtained by washing and scraping the roots, then rasping or grating them, and subjecting the pulp to pressure, by which the poisonous juice is expressed. The residual compressed pulp is then dried over a fire, being stirred during the whole time. In this way is obtained *cassava meal.*[8]

Cassava meal is a mixture of *cassava starch, vegetable fibre,* and *proteine* or *albuminous* matters. Dr. Shier[9] found that in the sliced and dry roots the per-centage of nitrogen is 0·78, but in the cassava meal (the juice expressed) only 0·36. If these numbers be multiplied by 6·5, the per-centage quantity of proteine or albuminous matters in the dried root will be 5·0, and in cassava meal 2·34. I received from Dr. Shier two kinds of cassava meal; one called cassava meal, the other termed cassava flour. They may be distinguished as coarse and fine meal.

---

[1] [Prussian blue may be obtained from the expressed juice by the process usually adopted in liquids containing hydrocyanic acid.—ED.]
[2] Quoted by Sloane, *Jamaica,* vol. ii. p. 363.
[3] *Hortus Americanus,* p. 34, 1794.
[4] *Journ. de Pharm.* t. xvi. p. 310, 1830.
[5] *Med. Plants of Jamaica.*
[6] Martius, in Wibmer, *Arzneim. u. Gifte,* Bd. iii. S. 273.
[7] *Pharmaceutical Journal,* vol. v. p. 28, 1848.
[8] The details of the process for making cassava meal vary somewhat in different localities. According to Piso (*De Medicina Brasil.* lib. iv. p. 53), the roots are grated by a hand-mill somewhat similar to that used in the preparation of Tous-les-mois. Edwards (*Voyage up the River Amazon,* p. 24, Lond. 1847) says they are grated upon stones, and the pulp compressed in a slender bag of rattan six feet in length.
[9] *Report,* p. 15.

α. **Coarse Cassava Meal;** *Cassava Meal,* Shier ; *Couaque* or *Couac,* Guibourt.—This is meal which in coarseness is about equal to sawdust or small dried crumbs of bread. I have found a similar preparation in English commerce under the name of *" Tapioca Flour from Bahia."* Coarse cassava meal has a slight yellowish or brownish tint, varying in different samples.

β. **Fine Cassava Meal;** *Cassava Flour,* Shier ; *Farine de Manioc,* Guibourt.—This is a finer and whiter meal than the preceding. In fineness it resembles wheat flour.

Cassava bread or *cassava cakes* are made by baking the compressed cassava pulp on a hot plate, in the manner muffins and crumpets are baked in England. Cassava meal and cassava bread are important and valuable articles of food to the inhabitants of tropical America. The flavour of cassava cakes resembles that of Scotch oat-cakes.

2. AMYLUM MANDIOCÆ ; *Mandioca* or *Cassava Starch; Tapioca.*— The juice which is expressed from the rasped root deposits, on standing, an amylum or starch (*cassava starch*), of which *tapioca* is made.

a. **Cassava Starch;** *Tapioca Meal ; Brazilian Arrow-root ; Moussache* or *Cipipa.*—The fecula or starch deposited from the expressed juice of the cassava root, after being washed and dried in the air without heat, constitutes the *tapioca meal* or *Brazilian arrow-root* of commerce. It is usually imported into this country from Rio Janeiro. For some years past it has been imported into France from Martinique, and is sold as arrow-root (Guibourt). It is white and pulverulent, and resembles in external appearance genuine arrow-root (maranta starch). When examined by the microscope, however, it is readily distinguished. Cassava starch, when examined by this instrument, is found to consist of small single grains,[1] which, in the living plant, were united in groups or compound grains, each composed of 2, 3, or 4 grains. Most of the grains are mullar-shaped, and, therefore, have been united in groups of two each : when seen endwise, they appear circular or globular. Some of them are truncated egg-shaped grains, with one or two facets at the truncation. The nucleus, central cavity, or hilum, is circular, surrounded with rings, and bursts in a stellate manner. These statements apply equally to *bitter cassava starch* and *sweet cassava starch* sent to me from Demerara by Dr. Shier, as well as to starch obtained by myself from sweet cassava root received from Jamaica.

Cassava starch has not been analysed; but there can be no doubt that its composition is similar to that of other starches, and that its formula is $C^{12}H^{10}O^{10}$. Its effects and uses are also like those of other starches.

β. **Tapioca.**—This is imported from Bahia and Rio Janeiro. [The tapioca imported from Rio Janeiro is without exception much whiter, and has a more pearl-like appearance, than that from Bahia, which is coarse and has a

---

[1] The following are the measurements, in parts of an English inch, of ten grains of cassava starch. They were made by Mr. George Jackson :—

	Lengths.	Breadths.		Lengths.	Breadths.
1	0·0012	× 0·0012	6	0·0005	× 0·0004
2	0·0008	× 0·0008	7	0·0004	× 0·0004
3	0·0008	× 0·0007	8	0·0003	× 0·0003
4	0·0007	× 0·0006	9	0·00025	× 0·0002·5
5	0·0005	× 0·0004	10	0·0002	× 0·0002

yellowish tint. Both sorts are imported in barrels of about 140 lbs. The Rio tapioca is worth at least one-half more than the Bahia.—ED.] Tapioca is nothing more than cassava meal which while moist or damp has been heated, for the purpose of drying it, on hot plates. By this treatment the starch grains swell, many of them burst, and the whole agglomerate in small irregular masses or lumps. In consequence of the change thus effected in the starch grains, tapioca is partially soluble in cold water; and the filtered cold infusion strikes a blue colour with tincture of iodine. The drying to which it has been subjected renders it difficult of solution. In boiling water it swells up, and forms a transparent viscous jelly-like mass. Submitted to prolonged ebullition in a large quantity of water, it leaves an insoluble residue, which precipitates. This, when diluted with water and coloured by iodine, appears to consist of mucous flocks.

Made into puddings, tapioca is employed as a dietetical substance. Boiled in water or milk, and flavoured with sugar, spices, or wine, according to circumstances, it is used as an agreeable, nutritious, light, easily digestible article of food for the sick and convalescent. It is devoid of all irritating and stimulating properties.

142. Crozophora tinctoria, *Necker.*—**Turnsole.**

(Succus.)

Heliotropium tricoccum, Pliny, lib. xxii. cap. 29; *Croton tinctorium*, Linn.—South of France: Mediterranean coast. Cultivated since 1833 in the neighbourhood of Grand Gallargues, in the department of Gard, in France. The expressed juice is green; but under the combined influence of the air and ammonia it becomes purplish. Coarse sacking stained purple by this juice is termed *turnsole rags* (*tournesol en drapeaux*), or *bezetta*[1] *cærulea*. These rags are exclusively employed by the Dutch; but for what purpose is not well known, though it has been supposed for colouring cheese, confectionary, and liqueurs.[2]

ORDER XXXIV. ARISTOLOCHIACEÆ, *Lindley.* BIRTHWORTS.

ARISTOLOCHIEÆ, *Jussieu;* ASARINÆ, *Bartling.*

CHARACTERS.—*Flowers* hermaphrodite, axillary, solitary. *Calyx* adherent (superior), tubular, monosepalous, with the segments valvate or induplicate in æstivation, sometimes regular, sometimes very unequal. *Stamens* 6 to 12, epigynous, distinct, or adhering to the style and stigmas. *Ovary* inferior, 6-celled, very rarely 3—4-celled; *ovules* numerous, anatropal, horizontally attached to the axis. *Style* simple. *Stigmas* radiating, as numerous as the cells of the ovary. *Fruit* dry or succulent, 3—4—6-celled, many-seeded. *Seeds* thin, with a very minute embryo placed at the base of fleshy albumen.— *Herbs* or *shrubs*, the latter often climbing. *Wood* without concentric zones and insepa-rable wedges. *Leaves* alternate, simple, stalked.

PROPERTIES.—Not important. The roots possess stimulant properties, owing to the presence of volatile oil. Some of them are acrids. Bitter extractive renders them somewhat tonic.

---

[1] *Bezetta*, the diminutive of the Spanish word *bézo*, a lip, a term originally applied to pigments used to colour the lips.

[2] See an interesting notice of Turnsole by Mr. D. Hanbury, jun. in the *Pharmaceutical Journal*, vol. ix. p. 308, 1850.

143. ARISTOLOCHIA SERPENTARIA, *Linn.*—THE VIRGINIAN SNAKE-ROOT.

Aristolochia officinalis, *Nees* and *Ebermaier*.

Sex. Syst. Gynandria, Hexandria.

(Radix, *L.*—The Root, *E. D.*)

HISTORY.—The first writer who distinctly mentions *Virginian snake-root*, or *snake-weed*, is Thomas Johnson, an apothecary of London, in his edition of Gerarde's Herbal, published in 1633.

BOTANY.   Gen. Char.—*Calyx* tubular, ventricose at the base, dilated at the apex, and extended into a ligula. *Anthers* 6, subsessile, inserted on the style. *Stigma* 6-lobed. *Capsule* 6-angled, 6-celled (*Bot. Gall.*)

Sp. Char.—*Stem* flexuous, ascending. *Leaves* cordate, acuminate, on both sides pubescent. *Peduncles* nearly radical, unifloral. Lip of the *calyx* lanceolate (*Nees v. Esenbeck*).

Hab.—North America.

COLLECTION AND PROPERTIES.—The root (*radix serpentariæ*) is collected in Western Pennsylvania and Virginia, in Ohio, Indiana, and Kentucky.[1] It is imported in bales, usually containing about 100 lbs. As met with in the shops, it consists of a tuft of long, slender, yellowish or brownish fibres, attached to a long contorted head or caudex. The odour is aromatic, the taste warm and bitter.

COMPOSITION.—It was analysed by Bucholz in 1807;[2] by Chevallier in 1820;[3] and by Peschier in 1823.[4]

Bucholz's Analysis.		*Chevallier's Analysis.*
Volatile oil	0·50	Volatile oil.
Greenish-yellow soft resin	2·85	Resin.
Extractive matter..............	1·70	Extractive.
Gummy extractive	18·10	Starch.
Lignin	62·40	Ligneous fibre.
Water	14·45	Albumen.
		Malate and phosphate of lime.
		Oxide of iron and silica.
Serpentary root	100·00	Serpentary root.

1. VOLATILE OIL.—Grassmann[5] obtained only half an ounce from 100 lbs. of the root. Its colour is yellowish, its odour considerable, its taste not very strong.[6] Grassmann compares the odour and taste to those of valerian and camphor combined.

2. BITTER PRINCIPLE; *Extractive*, Bucholz and Chevallier.—This is very bitter, and slightly acrid. It is soluble in both water and spirit. Its solution, which is yellow, is rendered brown by alkalies, but is unchanged by the ferruginous salts.

PHYSIOLOGICAL EFFECTS.—These have been examined by Jörg and his pupils.[7] In *small doses* serpentary promotes the appetite. In *large doses* it causes nausea, flatulence, uneasy sensation at the stomach, and frequent but not liquid stools. After its absorption, it increases the frequency and

---

[1] *United States Dispensatory.*
[2] Gmelin, *Hand. d. Chem.*
[3] *Journ. de Pharm.* vi. 365.
[4] Gmelin, *op. cit.*
[5] Quoted by Dr. W. C. Martius, *Pharmacogn.*
[6] Lewis, *Mat. Med.*
[7] Wibmer, *Arzneim. u. Gifte*, Bd. i. S. 221; also, *Journ. de Chim. Méd.* t. vii. p. 493.

fulness of the pulse, augments the heat of the skin, and promotes secretion and exhalation. Furthermore, it would appear, from the experiments before referred to, that it causes disturbance of the cerebral functions, and produces headache, sense of oppression within the skull, and disturbed sleep. In these properties serpentary bears some analogy to, but is much weaker than, camphor. It is more powerful than contrayerva.

USES.—Its employment is indicated in cases of torpor and atony. It was formerly termed *alexipharmic*, on account of its fancied power of curing the bite of a rattlesnake and of a mad dog.[1] At the present time it is rarely employed. It has been much esteemed as a stimulant in *fevers*, both continued and intermittent. A scruple of serpentary, taken in three ounces of wine, is mentioned by Sydenham[2] as a cheap remedy for tertians in poor people. Dr. Cullen[3] considered it as suited for the low and advanced stage of typhus only. In an epidemical affection of the throat (called the *throat-distemper*), it was given internally as a diaphoretic, and used with sumach berries, in the form of a decoction, as a gargle, with benefit.[4]

ADMINISTRATION.—The dose of it in substance is from ten to thirty grains. The infusion is the best form for the administration of serpentary.

1. **INFUSUM SERPENTARIÆ**, L. E.; *Infusion of Serpentary or Snakeroot*. (Serpentary, ʒss.; Boiling Water, Oj. Infuse for four hours in a covered vessel, and strain [through linen or calico, *E.*])—Dose, fʒj. or fʒij. every two or three hours, according to circumstances.

2. **TINCTURA SERPENTARIÆ**, L. E. D.; *Tincture of Serpentary or Snake-root*. (Serpentary, bruised [in moderately fine powder, *E.*], ʒiiiss. Proof Spirit, Oij.; [and Cochineal, bruised, ʒj. *E.*] Macerate for seven days, and filter, *L. D.* "Proceed by percolation or digestion, as for the tincture of cinchona," *E.* Take of Virginia Snake-root, bruised, ʒiij.; Diluted Alcohol, Oij. Macerate for fourteen days, express and filter through paper, *U.S.*)— Used as an adjunct to tonic infusions. Dose, from fʒj. to fʒij.

144. ASARUM EUROPÆUM, *Linn.*—COMMON ASARABACCA.

Sex. Syst. Dodecandria, Monogynia.

(Folia.)

HISTORY.—This plant was used in medicine by the ancients.[5] Dioscorides[6] calls it ἄσαρον.

BOTANY. **Gen. Char.**—*Calyx* campanulate, 3-lobed. *Stamens* 12, inserted on the ovary; *anthers* adnate to the middle of the filaments. *Style* short. *Stigma* stellate, 6-lobed. *Capsule* 6-celled (*Bot. Gall.*)

---

[1] Dale, *Pharmacologia.*
[2] *Works*, translated by Dr. Pechey, 4th ed. p. 233.
[3] *Mat. Med.*
[4] *Med. Observ. and Inquir.* vol. i. p. 211.
[5] [It was introduced into the former editions of the London and Dublin Pharmacopœias. It is now removed from the Materia Medica.—ED.]
[6] Lib. i. cap. 9.

Sp. Char.—*Leaves* 2 on each stem, kidney-shaped, obtuse [somewhat hairy] (Smith[1]).

The branching *root-fibres* arise from an underground stem or *rhizome*. The aerial *stems* are several from each rhizome. *Leaves* petiolated. From the axil of the two leaves springs a solitary, rather large, drooping *flower*, upon a short peduncle, of a greenish-brown colour and coriaceous substance. Segment of the *calyx* incurved. *Capsule* coriaceous. *Seeds* ovate, with horny albumen.

Hab.—Indigenous. Perennial. Flowers in May.

Description.—The whole plant (root-fibres, rhizome, and aerial stems, with leaves and flowers) is kept in the shops under the name of *asarabacca* (*radix cum herbâ asari*), but the leaves only are directed to be used in the Pharmacopœia. Dr. Batty[2] states that the plant is gathered for medicinal uses in the woods near Kirby Lonsdale, Westmoreland. The *rhizome* is about as thick as a goose-quill, greyish, quadrangular, knotted. It has a pepper-like odour and an acrid taste. The *leaves* are almost inodorous, but have an acrid, aromatic, and bitter taste.

Composition.—Goerz[3] published an analysis of the root in 1784 ; Lassaigne and Feneulle another in 1820 ;[4] Regimbeau a third in 1827 ;[5] and Gräger a fourth in 1830.[6]

Gräger's Analyses.

Root.		Herb.	
Volatile oil		Asarin	0·10
Asarum-camphor }	0·630	Tannin	0·04
Asarin [? Asarite] }		Extractive	5·49
Asarin	1·172	Chlorophylle	1·52
Tannin	1·072	Albumen	2·12
Extractive	3·972	Citric acid	0·54
Resin	0·156	Ligneous fibre	15·00
Starch	2·048	Water	74·84
Gluten and albumen	1·010	Loss	0·35
Citric acid	0·316		
Ligneous fibre	12·800		
Salts (citrates, chloride, sulphate, and phosphates)	3·042		
Water	74·600		
Fresh root of asarabacca	100·818	Fresh herb of asarabacca	100·00

1. Volatile Oily Matters.—By submitting asarabacca root to distillation with water, three volatile oily matters are obtained; one liquid and two solid, at ordinary temperatures.

a. Liquid Volatile Oil (Oleum Asari).—It is yellow, glutinous, lighter than water, and has an acrid burning taste, and a penetrating valerian-like odour. It is slightly soluble in water, more so in alcohol, ether, and the oils (volatile and fixed). Its constituents are C^8H^4O.

β. Asarite of Gräger.—In small needles of a silky lustre. It is odourless and tasteless. It is fusible and volatilisable by heat; its vapour being white and very irritating. It is soluble in alcohol, ether, and the volatile oils, but not in water. Both nitric and

[1] *Eng. Flora.*
[2] *Ibid.*
[3] Pfaff, *Mat. Med.* Bd. iii. S. 229.
[4] *Journ. de Pharm.* t. vi. p. 561.
[5] *Ibid.* t. xiv. p. 200.
[6] Goebel and Kunze, *Pharm. Waarenk.*

sulphuric acids dissolve the crystals without the evolution of gas : if water be added to the sulphuric solution, the asarite is thrown down unchanged.

γ. *Asarum-camphor.*—Is distinguished from asarite by the following characters :—Water throws it down from its alcoholic solution in cubes or six-sided prisms, whereas asarite is precipitated in delicate flexible needles. It dissolves in nitric acid without effervescence. Water added to its sulphuric solution throws down a brown resin. After fusion it has the form of a crystalline, striated mass. Its composition is $C^8H^5O^2$. Blanchet and Sell regard it as the hydrate of the liquid volatile oil.

2. BITTER PRINCIPLE OF ASARABACCA (*Asarin* of Gräger and of some other pharmacologists).—Brownish, very bitter, soluble in alcohol.

PHYSIOLOGICAL EFFECTS.—Every part of the plant possesses acrid properties. Applied to the mucous membrane of the nose, it excites sneezing, increased secretion of mucus, and even a discharge of blood. Swallowed, it causes vomiting, purging, and griping pains. It is also said to possess diuretic and diaphoretic properties. Dr. Cullen has enumerated it in his list of diuretics, but expresses his doubts whether it possesses any specific power of stimulating the renal vessels.

USES.—Asarabacca has been employed in medicine to excite vomiting, and as an errhine. As an emetic, it is now superseded by ipecacuanha and tartarised antimony. As an errhine, to excite irritation and a discharge of mucus from the nasal membrane, it has been used in certain affections of the brain, eyes, face, mouth, and throat, on the principle of counter-irritation : thus in paralytic affections of the mouth and tongue, in toothache, and in ophthalmia.

ADMINISTRATION.—We may administer either the root or leaves, recollecting that the latter are somewhat milder than the former. As an *emetic,* the dose is half a drachm to a drachm. As an *errhine,* one or two grains of the root, or three or four grains of the dried leaves, are snuffed up the nostrils every night.—The powder of this plant is supposed to form the basis of *cephalic snuff.*

COMPOUND POWDER OF ASARABACCA. (Asarabacca Leaves, dried, ℥j. ; Lavender Flowers, dried, ℨj. Reduce them together to powder.)—Used as an errhine in headache and ophthalmia. Dose, from grs. v. to grs. viij. [This was formerly a preparation of the Dublin Pharmacopœia.—ED.]

145. Aristolochia rotunda, *Linn.;* **et A. longa,** *Linn.*—**Round and Long Birthwort.**

Sex. Syst. Gynandria, Hexandria.

(Radix.)

Both of these plants are natives of the South of Europe. Their roots are still kept in the shops. *The long aristolochia root* is several inches in length, one or two inches broad, and has a more or less cylindrical form. *The round aristolochia root* has a more rounded and knobby form. Both kinds are bitter and acrid, and have, especially when powdered, a disagreeable odour. They contain extractive matter and starch. Lassaigne found ulmin in the long species. Their effects are stimulant and tonic. Their stimulant effects are supposed by some to be principally directed to the abdominal and pelvic viscera. They have been employed in amenorrhœa as an emmenagogue. Their dose is from Əj. to ℨj. Round aristolochia root is a constituent of the *Duke of Portland's powder for the gout,* which consisted of equal quantities of the roots of *Gentian* and Birthwort

(*Aristolochia rotunda*), the tops and leaves of Germander (*Chamædrys*), Ground Pine (*Chamæpitys*), and lesser Centaury (*Chironia Centaurium*), powdered and mixed together.[r]

ORDER XXXV. LAURACEÆ, *Lindley.*—LAURELS.

LAURI, *Jussieu.*—LAURINEÆ, *Vent.* and *Rob. Brown.*

CHARACTERS.—*Calyx* 4- to 6-cleft, with imbricated æstivation, the limb sometimes obsolete. *Petals* 0. *Stamens* definite, perigynous opposite the segments of the calyx, and usually twice as numerous; the 3 innermost, which are opposite the 3 inner segments of the calyx, sterile or deficient; the 6 outermost scarcely ever abortive; *anthers* adnate, 2- to 4-celled; the cells bursting by a longitudinal persistent valve from the base to the apex; the outer anthers valved inwards, the inner valved outwards [or both valved inwards, *Lindley*]. *Glands* usually present at the base of the inner filaments. *Ovary* single, superior, 1-celled [formed of 3 valvate carpellary leaves, and as many rib-like placentæ stationed at the sutures, all generally imperfect except one, *Endl.*], with 1 or 2 single pendulous ovules; *style* simple; *stigma* obtuse, 2- or 3-lobed. *Fruit* baccate or drupaceous, naked or covered. *Seed* without albumen; *embryo* inverted; *cotyledons* large, plano-convex, peltate near the base! *radicle* very short, included, superior; *plumule* conspicuous, 2-leaved.—*Trees*, often of great size. *Leaves* without stipules, alternate, seldom opposite, entire, or very nearly lobed. *Inflorescence* panicled or umbelled (*Rob. Brown*).

PROPERTIES.—The plants of this Order owe their most important qualities to the presence of volatile oil, which is found, more or less abundantly, in all parts of the vegetable. This oil is sometimes liquid and highly aromatic, as oil of cinnamon; at others it is solid at ordinary temperatures, and is endowed with narcotic properties, as camphor. The acrid principle of some species is probably a volatile oil. In the bark and leaves the volatile oil is usually associated with tannic acid, which gives them astringency, as in cinnamon. In the fruit and seeds, on the other hand, it is usually combined or mixed with fixed oil, as in bay-berries. Besides the officinal lauraceous barks, presently to be described, there are several others which have obtained considerable celebrity, in the countries producing them, on account of their aromatic qualities.

Two of these bear the name of *clove bark*, on account of their odour. The *Indian clove bark* or *cortex culilawan* is a large flat bark, and is obtained from *Cinnamomum Culilawan*, Blume, a native of the Indian islands. Its properties are analogous to those of Cassia-lignea.[2] It is rarely met with in London. I have received from Dr. Martiny, of Hesse Darmstadt, a bark marked *Culilawan papuanus*. It is, 1 presume, the produce of *Cinnamomum xarthoneuron* of Blume.

The *Brazilian clove bark* or *clove cassia bark*, *cortex cassiæ caryophyllatæ*, is the produce of *Dicypellium caryophyllatum*, and grows in Para and Rio Negro. Its bark occurs in tubular quills.

Massoy bark (in commerce *Misoi*) is the *cortex oninus* of Rumphius. It is used in the cosmetics of the natives of India.[3] I have never found it in the London shops.

Sintoc bark is the produce of *Cinnamomum Şintoc*, Blume. Its properties are analogous to those of Culilawan.

The *folia malabathri* of India are obtained from *Cinnamomum nitidum*, Hooker and Blume; and from *C. Tamala*. They are aromatic tonics, but are not found in the London market.

---

[1] See Dr. Clephane's *Inquiry into the Origin of the Gout Powder*, in the *Med. Observ. and Inq.*, vol. i. Lond. Dr. Clephane concludes that "Cælius Aurelianus's *diacentaureon* and Aëtius's *antidotus ex duobus centaureæ generibus* were the same medicine, and are the old names for the Duke of Portland's Powder."

[2] See Pereira, in Lindley's *Flora Medica*, p. 331.

[3] Crawford, *Hist. of the Ind. Archip.* vol. i. p. 510.

146. CINNAMOMUM ZEYLANICUM, *Nees*—THE CEYLON CINNAMON.

Laurus Cinnamomum, *Linn.*

Sex. Syst. Enneandria, Monogynia.

(Cortex ; et Oleum e cortice destillatum, *L.*—Bark ; and volatile oil of the bark, *E.*—The bark, *D.*)

HISTORY.—Cinnamon (*Kinman,* Hebr.) is mentioned in the Old Testament,[1] about 1490 years before Christ. In all probability the Hebrews received it from the Arabians, who must, therefore, have had commercial dealings with India at this early period.[2] The first notice of cinnamon (κιννάμωμον) by the Greek writers occurs in Herodotus,[3] who died 413 years before Christ. Probably both the Hebrew and Greek names for this bark are derived from the Cingalese *cacyn-nama* (*dulce lignum*), or the Malayan *kaimanis.*[4] Hippocrates[5] employed cinnamon externally. Dioscorides[6] decribes several kinds of cinnamon.

BOTANY. **Gen. Char.**—*Flowers* hermaphrodite or polygamous. *Calyx* 6-cleft, with the limb deciduous. *Stamina* 12, in 4 rows; the 9 external ones fertile, the 3 inner ones capitate, abortive; the three most internal of the fertile stamina having 2 sessile glands at the base : *anthers* 4-celled, the 3 inner turned outwards. *Ovary* 1-celled, with 1 ovule. *Fruit* (a berry) seated in a cup-like calyx. *Leaves* ribbed. *Leaf-buds* naked. *Flowers* panicled, rarely fascicled. (Condensed from Endlicher.[7])

Sp. Char.—*Branches* somewhat 4-cornered, smooth. *Leaves* ovate or ovate-oblong, tapering into an obtuse point, triple-nerved, or 3-nerved, reticulated on the under side, smooth, the uppermost the smallest. *Panicles* terminal and axillary, stalked. *Flowers* hoary and silky; segments oblong, deciduous in the middle (Nees[8]).

FIG. 173.

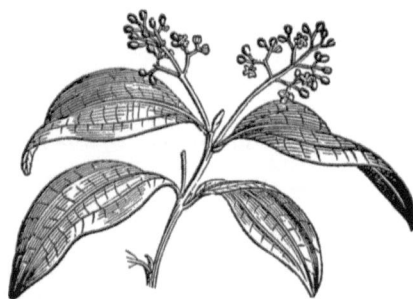

Cinnamomum zeylanicum.

Botanists admit several varieties of this species : the most important are—

α. *Broad-leaved,* Moon;[9] *Mŭ-pat* (Cingalese). — The plant above described.

β. *Narrow-leaved,* Moon; *Cinnamomum zeylanicum* var. γ; *Cassia,* Nees; *Heen-pat* (Cingalese). — This variety, which I have received from Ceylon under the name of *Bastard Cinnamon,* has oblong or elliptical leaves, much tapering to the point, and acute at the base.

Percival[10] mentions four varieties which are barked : 1st, *Rasse curundu,* or *honey cinnamon,* with broad leaves, yields the best bark ; 2dly, *Nai curundu,* or *snake cinnamon,* also with large leaves, not greatly inferior to the former; 3dly, *Capura curundu,* or *camphor cinnamon,* an inferior kind; 4thly, *cabatte curundu,* or *astringent cinnamon,* with smaller leaves ; its bark has a harsh taste.

Hab.—Cultivated in Ceylon and Java.

---

[1] *Exod.* xxx. 23.
[2] *Pictorial Bible,* vol. i. p. 222.
[3] *Thalia,* cvii. and cxi.   [and 141.
[4] Royle, *Essay on Hindoo Medicine,* pp. 84
[5] Pp. 265, 575, and 609, ed. Fœs.

[6] *Lib.* i. cap. 13.
[7] *Gen. Plant.*
[8] *Systema Laurinarum.*
[9] *Cat. of Ceylon Plants.*
[10] *Account of the Island of Ceylon.*

PRODUCTION.—The cinnamon bark of Ceylon is obtained by the cultivation of the plant. The principal *cinnamon gardens* lie in the neighbourhood of Columbo.[1] The bark-peelers, or *choliahs*, having selected a tree of the best quality, lop off such branches as are three years old, and which appear proper for the purpose. Shoots or branches, much less than half an inch, or more than two or three inches in diameter, are not peeled. The peeling is effected by making two opposite, or when the branch is thick three or four, longitudinal incisions, and then elevating the bark by introducing the peeling-knife beneath it. When the bark adheres firmly, its separation is promoted by friction with the handle of the knife. In twenty-four hours the epidermis and greenish pulpy matter (rete mucosum) are carefully scraped off. In a few hours the smaller quills are introduced into the larger ones, and in this way a congeries of quills formed, often measuring forty inches long. The bark is then dried in the sun, and afterwards made into bundles with pieces of split bamboo twigs.[2]

Cinnamon walking-sticks.—The hazel-like walking-sticks so much esteemed by visitors to Ceylon, are obtained from the shoots which spring almost perpendicularly from the roots after the parent bush or tree has been cut down.[3]

COMMERCE.—Cinnamon is imported in bales, boxes, and chests, from Ceylon principally; but in part also from Madras, Tellicherry, and rarely from Java and other places. In order to preserve and improve the quality of the bark, black pepper is sprinkled among the bales of cinnamon in stowing them at Ceylon (Percival). Mr. Bennett states that ships are sometimes detained for several weeks, through the want of pepper to fill the interstices between the bales in the holds. When cinnamon arrives in London, it is unpacked and examined; all the mouldy and broken pieces are removed from it. It is then re-made into bales. These are cylindrical, 3 feet 6 inches long, but of variable diameter, perhaps 16 inches on the average. These bales are enveloped by a coarse cloth, called *gunny*. The cinnamon in boxes and chests is usually the small, inferior, and mouldy pieces. [The quantity of cinnamon imported in the seven years from 1844 to 1850 was as follows :—

	lbs.		*lbs.*
1844	951,220	1848	347,368
1845	636,759	1849	759,088
1846	408,603	1850	700,001—ED.]
1847	383,642		

DESCRIPTION.—Four kinds of cinnamon[4] are distinguished in the London market; namely, *Ceylon, Tellicherry, Malabar,* and *Java* cinnamon. The latter, however, is rarely met with. A fifth kind, called *Cayenne*, occurs in French commerce.

The *Chinese cinnamon* of Continental writers is *Cassia lignea* of English commerce.

1. **Ceylon Cinnamon** (*Cinnamomum zeylanicum* seu *Cinnamomum acutum*). — This is the most esteemed kind. The fasciculi or compound quills, of which the bales are made up, are about 3 feet 6 inches long, slen-

---

[1] See Percival's *Account of Ceylon*, 2d ed. 1805.

[2] Percival, *op. cit.;* and Marshall, in *Thomson's Ann. of Philosophy*, vol. x.
Bennett, *Ceylon and its Capabilities*, 1843.

[4] In the years 1839 and 1840 I examined above 1000 bales of cinnamon in the Dock warehouses. In 1840 I was kindly assisted in my examination by Mr. Carroll, of Mincing Lane, one of the most experienced London dealers, who attended with me, and from whom I derived much practical information.

der, and shivery, and are composed of several smaller quills inclosed one within the other. The bark is thin (the finest being scarcely thicker than drawing paper), smooth, of a light yellow-brown or brownish-yellow, moderately pliable, with a splintery fracture, especially in the longitudinal direction. The inner side or *liber* is darker and browner, and contains, according to Nees, small medullary rays filled with a red juice, and which he regards as the peculiar bearers of the aroma. The odour of the bark is highly fragrant. The flavour is warm, sweetish, and agreeable. Inspection and tasting are the methods resorted to for ascertaining the qualities of cinnamon.[1]

Ceylon cinnamon is characterised by being cut obliquely at the bottom of the quill, whereas the other kinds are cut transversely. In the London market three qualities of Ceylon cinnamon are distinguished; viz. *first, seconds,* and *thirds.* Inferior kinds are thicker, darker, browner, and have a pungent, succeeded by a bitter taste.

Thin, very much convoluted, the smaller quills being enclosed in larger ones.—*Ph. Lond.*

2. Tellicherry or Bombay Cinnamon is grown on one estate only, at Tellicherry, by Mr. Brown, and is wholly consigned to Messrs. Forbes and Co. Only 120 or 130 bales were annually imported [but the quantity has increased of late years.—Ed.] In appearance it is equal to the Ceylon kind; but the internal surface of the bark is more fibrous, and the flavour is inferior. It is superior to the Malabar variety.

3. Madras or Malabar Cinnamon is of inferior quality. It is grown, I am informed, on the Coromandel coast. It is coarser and inferior in flavour to the other kinds. In thickness it approximates to Cassia lignea. Its quality has annually deteriorated since its introduction into the market. It does not meet with a ready sale, and it is expected that its importation will cease.

4. Java Cinnamon.—This is, according to some authorities, equal in quality to the Ceylon sort[2] [but we are informed by those who are experienced in the trade, that this is not correct. It has much less flavour, and fetches invariably a lower price: hence its quality is inferior. It ranks between Ceylon and Tellicherry in flavour, but it is generally of a brownish colour, while the Tellicherry has a pale yellow colour.—Ed.]

[Java cinnamon being the produce of a Dutch colony, is imported almost exclusively into Holland, and is thence distributed throughout Europe; while the other descriptions are confined to the London market, the Ceylon sort forming the bulk.—Ed.]

5. Cayenne Cinnamon.—This is unknown in the London market. Its volatile oil is more acrid and peppery than the oil from Ceylon cinnamon.[3]

Substitution.—In commerce, Cassia lignea (called on the continent Chinese cinnamon) is frequently substituted for cinnamon. It is distinguished by its greater thickness, its short resinous fracture, its less delicacy but greater strength of flavour, its shorter quills, and its being packed in small bundles. Moreover, it may be distinguished chemically by the action of iodine on its infusion (see *infra*). The difference of flavour is best distinguished when the barks are ground to powder. The great consumers

---

[1] See Percival, *op. supra cit.*; also Marshall, *op. supra cit.*
[2] *Proceedings of the Committee of Commerce and Agriculture of the Asiatic Society,* p. 147.
[3] Vauquelin, *Journ. de Pharm.* t. iii. p. 434.

of cinnamon are the chocolate-makers of Spain, Italy, France, and Mexico, and by them the difference of flavour between cinnamon and cassia is readily detected.   An extensive dealer in cinnamon informs me that the Germans, Turks, and Russians prefer cassia, and will not purchase cinnamon, the delicate flavour of which is not strong enough for them.   In illustration of this, I was told that some cinnamon (valued at 3s. 6d. per lb.) having been by mistake sent to Constantinople, was unsaleable there at any price; while cassia lignea (worth about 6d. per lb.) was in great request.

COMPOSITION.—In 1817 Vauquelin[1] made a comparative analysis of the cinnamons of Ceylon and Cayenne.   The constituents of both were found to be *volatile oil, tannin, mucilage, colouring matter* (partially soluble in water and in alcohol, but insoluble in ether), *resin, an acid*, and *ligneous fibre*.   *Starch* is a constituent of cinnamon, though not mentioned in this analysis.

CHEMICAL CHARACTERISTICS.—Sesquichloride of iron causes a greenish flocculent precipitate (*tannate of iron*) in infusion of cinnamon.   Solution of gelatine also occasions a precipitate (*tannate of gelatine*) in the infusion. A decoction of cinnamon may be distinguished from a decoction of cassia lignea by tincture of iodine; which gives a blue colour (*iodide of starch*) with the latter, but not with the former.   Both barks contain starch, but cinnamon appears to contain a larger proportion of some principle (tannic acid?) which destroys the blue colour of iodide of starch; for if the decoction of cassia-lignea rendered blue by iodine be added to the decoction of cinnamon, the blue colour disappears.

PHYSIOLOGICAL EFFECTS.—Cinnamon produces the effects of the spices, already described.   *In moderate doses* it stimulates the stomach, produces a sensation of warmth in the epigastric region, and promotes the assimilative functions.   The repeated use of it disposes to costiveness.   *In full doses* it acts as a general stimulant to the vascular and nervous systems.   Some writers regard it as acting specifically on the uterus.[2]

USES.—The uses of cinnamon are those of the species generally, and which have been before noticed.   It is employed by the cook as an agreeable condiment.   In medicine, it is frequently added to other substances,—as to the bitter infusions, to improve their flavour; and to purgatives, to check their griping qualities.   As a cordial, stimulant, and tonic, it is indicated in all cases characterised by feebleness and atony.   As an astringent, it is employed in diarrhœa, usually in combination with chalk, the vegetable infusions, or opium.   As a cordial and stimulant, it is exhibited in the latter stages of low fever.   In flatulent and spasmodic affections of the alimentary canal, it often proves a very efficient carminative and antispasmodic.   It checks nausea and vomiting.   It has also been used in uterine hemorrhage.

ADMINISTRATION.—The dose of it in substance is from ten grains to half a drachm.

1. OLEUM CINNAMOMI, L. E. D.; *Oleum Cinnamomi veri* offic.; *Oil of Cinnamon.*   (Obtained in Ceylon by macerating the inferior pieces of the

---

[1] *Journ. de Pharmacie*, t. iii. p. 433.
[2] Sundelin, *Heilmittel.* Bd. ii. S. 199, 3tte Aufl.; and Wibmer, *Wirk. d. Arzn. u. Gifte*, Bd. ii. S. 137.

bark, reduced to a gross powder, in sea-water for two days, when both are submitted to distillation.)—As imported, the oil varies somewhat in its colour from yellow to cherry-red: the paler varieties are most esteemed; hence London druggists frequently submit the red oil of cinnamon to distillation, by which they procure two pale yellow oils; one lighter (amounting to about a quarter of the whole), the other heavier than water. The loss on this process is considerable, being near 10 per cent. Percival says that the oil obtained from the finer sorts of cinnamon is of a beautiful gold colour, while that from the coarser bark is darker and brownish. Its odour is pleasant, and purely cinnamomic. Its taste is at first sweetish, afterwards cinnamomic, burning, and acrid.

Cinnamon oil of commerce is a complex substance, consisting of a mixture or compound of two or more bodies. The principal constituent, and which is considered to be cinnamon oil properly so called, is the *hydruret of cinnamyle*, whose formula, according to Mulder,[1] is $C^{20}H^{11}O^2$; but, according to Dumas and Peligot,[2] is $C^{18}H^8O^2$. Mulder[3] supposes that the differences in these formulæ depend on the oil analysed by Dumas and Peligot not having been quite fresh.

By exposure to the air, oil of cinnamon absorbs oxygen, and produces cinnamic acid, two resins, and water.

$$3(C^{20}H^{11}O^2) \quad + \quad 8O \quad = \quad C^{18}H^7O^3 \quad + \quad C^{12}H^5O \quad + \quad C^{39}H^{15}O^4 \quad + \quad 6HO$$

Oil of cinnamon.	Oxygen.	Cinnamic acid.	α resin.	β resin.	Water.

With nitric acid oil of cinnamon combines to form a white crystalline nitrate $(C^{18}H^8()^2,NO^5)$ and a red oil. With ammonia the oil unites to form a crystalline solid amide called *cinnhydramide*, whose formula is $C^{54}H^{24}N^2$. [4]

On account of their great difference in commercial value, and resemblance in physical and chemical properties, oil of cassia is sometimes substituted for, or admixed with, genuine oil of cinnamon. The finer and more delicate odour of the latter is the chief distinction between them. The Edinburgh College gives the following characters of oil of cinnamon:—

"Cherry-red when old, wine-yellow when recent; odour purely cinnamomic; nitric acid converts it nearly into a uniform crystalline mass."

These characters, however, are not peculiar to this oil, as they are also possessed by oil of cassia. Zetter[5] says that oil of cinnamon is a thinner and specifically lighter oil, which does not become turbid at a lower temperature than the oil of cassia. Most, if not all, the other characteristic differences which he has given, probably relate rather to particular samples of the oils than to their peculiar natures.

Oil of cinnamon root.—In 1848 some of this oil was imported. Its colour was pale yellow, and its odour that of cinnamon; but not so delicate as the oil of the bark.

Oil of cinnamon is sometimes employed as a powerful stimulant in paralysis

---

[1] *Berlinisches Jahrbuch für d. Pharmacie*, Bd. xxxviii. p. 176, 1837.

[2] *Ann. de Chim. et de Phys.*

[3] *Pharmaceutisches Central-Blatt für* 1839, p. 879.

[4] [Strecker has found that *styron*, obtained by treating styracin with potash, when mixed with platinum black, and exposed to the air for a few days, is converted by oxidation to oil of cinnamon.—ED.]

[5] *Jahrbuch für praktische Pharmacie*, Bd. xix. S. 3, and General-Tabelle, 1849.

of the tongue, in syncope, or in cramp of the stomach. But its principal use is as an adjuvant to other medicines. The dose of it is from one to three minims.

2. **OLEUM CINNAMOMI FOLIORUM**; *Oil of Cinnamon Leaf.*—It is exported from Ceylon, and is sometimes called, on account of its odour, *clove oil.* I was informed by a gentleman on whose estate in Ceylon it is obtained, that it is procured by macerating the leaves in sea-water, and afterwards submitting both to distillation. It is a yellow liquid, heavier than water, and has an odour and taste analogous to those of oil of cloves. Bennett[1] considers it to be equal in aromatic pungency to the oil made from the clove at the Molucca Islands. Oil of cinnamon leaf is, however, specifically lighter than genuine oil of cloves; but, like the latter, yields a dark blue colour with the tincture of the sesquichloride of iron. Its effects and uses are similar to those of oil of cloves.

[This oil has been recently examined by Mr. Stenhouse. The sample was two or three years old. It had a brownish colour, and a sp. gr. of 1·053, an aromatic and penetrating odour, and an exceedingly pungent taste. It had an acid reaction, and formed a butyraceous crystalline magma when treated with solutions of potash or ammonia. Like the oils of cloves and pimento, it is essentially a mixture of eugenic acid and a neutral hydrocarbon having the formula $C^{20}H^{16}$. Cinnamon-leaf oil, however, is remarkable for containing a small quantity of benzoic acid. By the action of potash, a colourless highly refractive liquid was obtained, the greater portion of which was distilled over between 320° and 329°. Its specific gravity was 0·862, and its smell closely resembled that of *cymene.* The results of its analysis agree exactly with the formula $C^{20}H^{16}$. The portion of the oil which was dissolved by potash (eugenate of potash) was heated for a considerable time with agitation, in order to drive off the last portions of hydrocarbon which might be adhering to it. It was next saturated with sulphuric acid, and the liberated eugenic acid still further purified. It agreed perfectly in its characters with those ascribed to eugenic acid by Bonastre, Ettling, and Boeckmann. Its specific gravity was 1·076, and its boiling point 467°.[2] Its formula is $C^{24}H^{16}O^{5}$.—Ed.]

3. **AQUA CINNAMOMI,** L. E. D.; *Cinnamon Water.* (Cinnamon, bruised, lb. iss.; Water, Cong. ij. Let a gallon distil. [Or, Oil of Cinnamon, ʒij.; Powdered Flint, ʒij.; Distilled Water, Cong. j. Diligently rub the oil first with the flint, afterwards with the water, and strain the liquor, *L.* Cinnamon Bark, bruised, ℥xviij.; Water, Cong. ij.; Rectified Spirit, ℥iij. Mix them together, and distil off one gallon, *E.* Essence of Cinnamon, fʒj.; Distilled Water, Cong. ss. Mix with agitation, and filter through paper, *D.* Take Oil of Cinnamon, fʒss.; Carbonate of Magnesia, ʒj. Distilled Water, Oij. Rub the oil of cinnamon first with the carbonate of magnesia, then with the water gradually added, and filter through paper, *U.S.*]) — This water is usually prepared in the shops by diffusing the oil through water by the aid of sugar or carbonate of magnesia. Cinnamon water is principally employed as a vehicle for other medicines. It is aromatic and carminative. Goeppert says it is poisonous to plants. By dissolving iodine and iodide of potassium in cinnamon water, a crystalline compound is produced, consisting of iodide of potassium 12·55, iodine 28·14, oil of cinnamon 59·31.[3]

4. **SPIRITUS CINNAMOMI,** L. E.; *Spirit of Cinnamon.* (Oil of Cin-

---

[1] *Ceylon and its Capabilities,* p. 70, 1843.
[2] [*Pharmaceutical Journal,* January 1855, p. 320.]
[3] Apjohn, *Athenæum,* No. 517, for 1837; and No. 559, 1838.

namon, ʒij.; Proof Spirit, Cong. j. Dissolve, *L.* Cinnamon, in coarse powder, lb. j.; Proof Spirit, Ovij. Macerate for two days in a covered vessel;
add a pint and a half of water; and distil off seven pints, *E.*)—Stimulant.
Dose, fʒj. to fʒiv.

5. ESSENTIA CINNAMOMI, D.; *Essence of Cinnamon.* (Oil of Cinnamon,

fʒj.; Rectified Spirit, fʒix. Mix with agitation.)—Used in the preparation
of *Aqua Cinnamomi.*

6. TINCTURA CINNAMOMI, L. E.; *Tincture of Cinnamon.* (Cinnamon,

bruised, ʒiiiss. [in moderately fine powder, *E.*]; Proof Spirit, Oij. Macerate
for fourteen days, and strain. [Proceed by percolation or digestion, as directed
for tincture of cassia, *E.*])—Commonly used as an adjuvant to cretaceous,
astringent, tonic, or purgative mixtures. It has also been employed in uterine
hemorrhage.[1] Dose, fʒj. to fʒiv.

7. TINCTURA CINNAMOMI COMPOSITA, L. E. D.; *Compound Tincture of*

Cinnamon. (Cinnamon, bruised [in fine powder, if percolation be followed,
E.], ʒj.; Cardamom, bruised, ʒss. [ʒj. *E.*]; Long Pepper, powdered [ground
finely, *E.*], ʒiiss. [ʒiij. *E.*]; Ginger, ʒiiss. [not used by the *Edinburgh
College*]; Proof Spirit, Oij. Macerate for fourteen days, and strain, *L.*
" This tincture is best prepared by the method of percolation, as directed for
the compound tincture of cardamom. But it may also be made in the
ordinary way by digestion for seven days, straining and expressing the liquor,
and then filtering it," *E.* Cinnamon, bruised, ʒij.; Cardamom Seeds, bruised,
ʒj.; Ginger, ʒss.; Proof Spirit, Oij. Macerate for fourteen days, and strain,
D.)—Cordial and aromatic. Used in the same cases as the last. Dose, fʒj.
to fʒij.

8. PULVIS CINNAMOMI COMPOSITUS, L.; *Pulvis Aromaticus,* E. D.;

Compound Powder of Cinnamon; Aromatic Powder. (Cinnamon, ʒij.;
Cardamom, ʒiss.; Ginger, ʒj.; Long Pepper, ʒss. Rub them together, so
that a very fine powder may be made, *L.* Cinnamon, Ginger, of each
ʒij.; Cardamom Seeds freed from their capsules, Nutmeg, of each ʒj. Rub
each separately to powder, and, having mixed them by trituration, pass through
a fine sieve. When prepared, the powder should be kept in well-stopped
bottles, *D.*) The *Edinburgh College* employs cinnamon, cardamom seeds,
and ginger, of each equal parts.)—Aromatic and carminative. Dose, grs. x.
to grs. xxx. Principally employed as a corrigent of other preparations.

9. CONFECTIO AROMATICA, L. D.; *Electuarium Aromaticum,* E.;

Aromatic Confection. (Cinnamon, Nutmegs, each ʒij.; Cloves, ʒj.; Cardamom Seeds, ʒss.; Saffron, ʒij.; Prepared Chalk, ʒxvj.; Sugar, lb. ij.
Rub the dry ingredients together to a very fine powder, and keep them in a
closed vessel. Whenever the confection is to be used, add to each ounce of
the powder two fluidrachms of water, and mix all well together, *L.* The
Dublin College orders Aromatic Powder, ʒv.; Dried Saffron, in fine powder,
ʒss.; Oil of Cloves, fʒss.; Simple Syrup, fʒv.; Clarified Honey, *by weight,*
ʒij. Rub the aromatic powder with the saffron, add the syrup and honey,
and beat them together till thoroughly mixed; lastly, add the oil of cloves, *D.*

---

[1] Voigtels, *Arzneim.* Bd. ii. S. 465.

The *Edinburgh College* orders of Aromatic Powder, *one part;* Syrup of Orange-peel, *two parts.* Mix and triturate them into a uniform pulp.)—The preparation of the London Pharmacopœia differs essentially from the aromatic confection of the Edinburgh and Dublin Pharmacopœias, in containing chalk. The London College directs the water to be added when the preparation is wanted, with the view of preventing fermentation, to which the preparation is subject. Some druggists substitute a strong infusion of saffron for the solid saffron; the volatile oils of the spices for the spices themselves; and precipitated carbonate of lime for chalk.

Aromatic confection, Ph. L. and D., is antacid, stimulant, and carminative. It is usually added to the ordinary chalk mixture in diarrhœa, and is employed on various other occasions where spices are indicated. Dose, grs. x. to ʒj.

147. CINNAMOMUM CASSIA, *Blume, E.*—THE CINNAMON CASSIA.

Cinnamomum aromaticum, *Nees.*

Sex. Syst. Enneandria, Monogynia.

(Cassia-bark. Oil of Cassia, *E.*—Cassia-lignea, and Cassia buds, *offic.*)

HISTORY.—It is highly probable that the bark, now called *cassia-lignea,* was known to the ancient Greeks and Romans; but we cannot positively prove this. The barks termed by the ancients cinnamomum (κιννάμωμον) and cassia[1] (κάσσια), as well as the trees yielding these substances, are too imperfectly described to enable us to determine with precision the substances referred to. The Cassia tree is called in Chinese *Kwei (Qui).* Cassia-lignea is called *Kwei Pe,* or Cassia skin; while Cassia buds are termed *Kwei Tsze,* or Cassia seeds. Cinnamon is called *Yuh Kwei* (vulgarly Yoke Qui), or Precious Cassia. It is not a product of China.

BOTANY. **Gen Char.**—Vide *Cinnamomum zeylanicum.*

Sp. Char.—*Leaves* opposite, sometimes alternate, oblong-lanceolate, triple-nerved; the nerves vanishing at the point of the leaf. *Petioles* and younger branches silky-tomentose. *Stem* arborescent (Blume).[2]

Hab.—China; cultivated in Java.

The tree known in Ceylon as the *Dawul Kurunda* was erroneously supposed by Linnæus to be the source of cassia bark, and hence he termed it *Laurus Cassia.* The Dublin College has been led into the same error. Many years since, Mr. Marshall[3] stated that the bark of Dawul Kurunda was not aromatic, like cinnamon, but had the bitter taste and the odour of myrrh. This tree is the *Litsæa Ceylanica* of recent botanists.[4] Mr. Marshall declares[5] that in Ceylon it is never decorticated, and that the coarse cinnamon (*i. e.* cinnamon procured from thick shoots or large branches of Cinnamomum zeylanicum) "has been imported into England, and sold under the denomination of cassia." It has been erroneously inferred from this statement that the cassia-lignea of European commerce was merely coarse cinnamon; but if this were the case, it would be somewhat remarkable that cassia-lignea is not imported from Ceylon. It is not at all improbable that coarse Ceylon cinnamon may have been sold in the London market as cassia-lignea; [but those who are accustomed to the drug trade can easily distinguish them. There is now no duty levied on cinnamon exported from Ceylon.—ED.]

---

[1] *Psalm* xlv. 9.

[2] *Bijdrag.*

[3] *Ann. of Phil.* vol. x. 1817.

[4] C. G. Nees ab Esenbeck, *Syst. Laurinarum,* Berol. 1836 ; also Dr. Wright, in Jameson's *Journal,* vol. xxviii. Edinb. 1840.

Op. cit.

In the *Pun tsaou* (a Chinese herbal) is a drawing of the Cassia tree. It is represented growing on a hill, and as having a very crooked and knotted stem.

DESCRIPTION.—Two substances are believed to be obtained from this species; namely, the bark called *cassia-lignea*, and the flower buds termed *cassia buds*.

1. Cassia-lignea *(cortex cassiæ)* is regarded on the continent of Europe, and in America,[1] as a sort of cinnamon. In English commerce it is always distinguished. It is imported in chests. It resembles cinnamon in many of its qualities. It is made up in bundles, which are tied with slips of bamboo. It has the same general appearance, smell, and taste, as cinnamon; but its substance is thicker, its appearance coarser, its colour darker, browner, and duller; its flavour, though cinnamomic, is much less sweet and fine than that of Ceylon cinnamon, but is more pungent, and is followed by a bitter taste; it is less closely quilled, and breaks shorter, than genuine cinnamon (see *ante*, p. 439). It is imported from Singapore, Calcutta, Bombay, and Manilla. [It comes originally from China, and the largest quantity is now imported directly from Canton.—ED.]

1. *China cassia-lignea* (sometimes called *China cinnamon*) is the best kind. Mr. Reeves[2] says vast quantities of both cassia buds and cassia-lignea are annually brought to Canton from the province of Kwangse, whose principal city (*Kwei Lin Too*), literally the city of the Forest (or Grove) of Cassia trees, derives its name from the forests of cassia around it. The Chinese themselves use a much thicker bark (which they call *Gan Kwei Pe*), unfit for the European market. Mr. Reeves informs me that they esteem it so highly as to pay nearly 10 dollars per lb. for it. A very fine quality is occasionally met with, and commands the enormous price of 100 dollars per catty (1⅓ lb.) A specimen of it, with which he has kindly furnished me, is straight, semi-cylindrical, 11 inches long, rather more than an inch wide, and about one-sixth or one-eighth of an inch thick. Externally it is warted, and covered with crustaceous lichens. Internally it is deep brown. Its odour and flavour are those of cassia. Mr. Reeves also informs me that the best cassia-lignea is cut in the 3rd or 4th moon, the second sort in the 6th or 7th moon.

2. *Malabar cassia-lignea.*—This is brought from Bombay. It is thicker and coarser than that of China, and is more subject to foul packing; hence each bundle requires separate inspection.[3] It may perhaps be coarse cinnamon; for Dr. White states that the bark of the older branches of the genuine cinnamon plant is exported from the Malabar coast as cassia. [We are informed that there is a coarse kind which is called indifferently Malabar cassia or cinnamon. It has little flavour, but a slightly sweetish taste, and is, therefore, more like coarse cinnamon.—ED.]

3. *Manilla cassia-lignea.*—This, I am informed, is usually sold in bond for Continental consumption. I have received a specimen of bark ticketed "Cassia vera from Manilla," the epidermis of which was imperfectly removed. [Manilla cassia-lignea in bundles comes originally from China. There is a very fine sort of cassia vera also imported, which is probably grown in the Manillas. This is nearly equal in quality to cassia-lignea. The cassia vera, as it is known to merchants, is an aromatic bark, and appears to be a very

---

[1] In the American Pharmacopœia both cinnamon and cassia-lignea are included under the name of cinnamon.

[2] *Trans. Med.-Bot. Society* for 1828, p. 26.

[3] Milburn's *Orient. Comm.*

coarse sort of cinnamon. The best comes from Batavia. It also comes in large quantities from Calcutta, and occasionally from Madras.—Ed.]

4. *Mauritius cassia-lignea.*—This is occasionally met with. [It is nothing more than the China cassia-lignea.—Ed.]

[Commerce.—The quantity of cassia-lignea imported in the seven years from 1844 to 1850 was as follows:—

	lbs.			lbs.
1844	1,278,413		1848	510,247
1845	1,422,236		1849	472,693
1846	995,490		1850	988,017—Ed.]
1847	342,693			

2. Cassia buds (*flores cassiæ immaturæ; clavelli cinnamomi*) are not contained in any of the British Pharmacopœias. They are the produce of China, and are probably procured from the same plant which yields cassia-lignea. Mr. Reeves states that he has always understood and has no doubt that both cassia buds and cassia-lignea are obtained from the same trees. The buds are gathered, in the 8th or 9th moon. Dr. T. W. C. Martius[1] says " that according to the latest observations which the elder Nees has made known, cassia buds are the calyces (*Fruchtkelche*) of *Cinnamomum aromaticum*, about one-fourth of their normal size. It is also said that they are collected from *Cinnamomum dulce* (Nees), which is found in China." Cassia buds bear some resemblance to cloves, but are smaller,—or to nails with round heads; they have the odour and flavour of cassia-lignea or cinnamon. The exports from Canton in 1831 were 177,866 lbs., and the imports into Great Britain in 1832 were 75,173 lbs.[2] In 1840, 6,406 lbs. paid duty. Cassia buds have not yet been analysed; their constituents are similar to those of cassia-lignea; they yield a volatile oil by distillation, and contain tannic acid.

Composition.—*Cassia-lignea* was analysed by Bucholz,[3] who obtained the following results:—*Volatile oil* 0·8, *resin* 4·0, *gummy (astringent) extractive* 14·6, *woody fibre with bassorin* 64·3, *water* and loss 16·3 = 100·0.

Chemical Characteristics.—Sesquichloride of iron renders decoction of cassia-lignea dark green, and causes a precipitate (*tannate of iron*). Gelatine also produces a precipitate (*tannate of gelatine*). If tincture of iodine be added to it, a blue colour (*iodide of starch*) is produced. By this cassia-lignea may be distinguished from genuine cinnamon (see *ante*, p. 441).

Physiological Effects.—Similar to those of cinnamon. Sundelin[4] regards it as being more astringent.

Uses.—Are the same as those of cinnamon.

Administration.—Dose, gr. x. to ʒss.

1. OLEUM CASSIÆ, E.; *Oil of Cassia; Oil of Chinese Cinnamon.* (Obtained from cassia-lignea by distillation with water.)—Its properties and composition are similar to those of oil of cinnamon already described. Its odour and flavour, however, are inferior to those of the latter. Its colour is usually pale yellow. Nitric acid converts it into a crystalline mass. Its effects and uses are similar to those of oil of cinnamon. It is employed in the preparation of *Aqua* and *Spiritus Cassiæ.*—Dose, gtt. j. to gtt. iv.

---

[1] *Pharmacognosie*, S. 213.
[2] M'Culloch's *Dict. of Comm.*
[3] *Parliam. Returns*, No. 50, Sess. 1829; No. 367, Sess. 1832; No. 550, Sess. 1833.
[4] *Heilmittell.* Bd. ii. S. 119, 3tte Aufl.

[*Adulterations.*—This oil is frequently adulterated with oil of cloves. For the detection of this, M. Ulex advises that a drop of the oil should be heated on a watch-glass. Genuine cassia oil evolves a fragrant vapour possessing but little acridity: when, however, clove oil is present, the vapour is very acrid, and excites coughing. With fuming nitric acid cassia oil merely crystallises. If clove oil be present, it swells up, evolves a large quantity of red vapour, and yields a thick reddish-brown oil. Cassia oil, when pure, solidifies with concentrated potash, but not when mixed with clove oil.[1] A mixture of these oils is used for precipitating silver upon glass under the new silvering process.—Ed.]

2. AQUA CASSIÆ, E.; *Cassia Water.* (Cassia Bark, bruised, ℥xviij.; Water, Cong. ij.; Rectified Spirit, f℥iij. Mix them together, and distil off one gallon.)—Used as an aromatic vehicle for other medicines. It is usually prepared from the oil in the same way that cinnamon water is commonly made.

3. SPIRITUS CASSIÆ, E.; *Spirit of Cassia.* (Cassia, in coarse powder, lb. j.; Proof Spirit, Ovij. Macerate for two days in a covered vessel, add a pint and a half of water, and distil off seven pints.)—Dose f℥j. to f℥iv. It is usually prepared by adding oil of cassia to proof spirit.

4. TINCTURA CASSIÆ, E.; *Tincture of Cassia.* (Cassia, in moderately fine powder, ℥iiiss.; Proof Spirit, Oij. Digest for seven days, strain, express the residuum strongly, and filter. This tincture is more conveniently made by the process of percolation, the cassia being allowed to macerate in a little of the spirit for twelve hours before being put into the percolator.)—Dose, f℥j. to f℥ij. Used as an adjuvant to tonic infusions.

148. CAMPHORA OFFICINARUM, *Nees.*—THE CAMPHOR LAUREL.

Laurus Camphora, *Linn.*

Sex. Syst. Enneandria, Monogynia.

(Concretum e ligno sublimatione comparatum, *L.*—Camphor. *E, D.*)

History.—The ancient Greeks and Romans do not appear to have been acquainted with camphor. C. Bauhin and several subsequent writers state that Aëtius speaks of it; but I have been unable to find any notice of it in his writings; and others[2] have been equally unsuccessful in their search for it. Avicenna[3] and Serapion[4] call it *cáfúr*: the latter erroneously cites Dioscorides. Symeon Seth,[5] who lived in the 11th century, describes it, and calls it καφουρά (the name by which it is designated in the *Pharmacopœa Grœca*, 1837); and his description is considered, both by Voigtels[6] and Sprengel,[7] to be the earliest on record.

Botany. **Gen. Char.**—*Flowers* hermaphrodite, panicled, naked. *Calyx* 6-cleft, papery, with a deciduous limb. *Fertile stamens* 9, in 3 rows; the inner with 2, stalked, compressed glands at the base; *anthers* 4-celled, the outer turned inwards, the inner outwards. 3 *sterile stamens*, shaped like the last, placed in a whorl alternating with the stamens of the second row;

---

[1] [*Pharmaceutical Journal*, June 1853, p. 602.]
[2] Alston, *Lect. on the Mat. Med.* vol. ii. p. 406.
[3] Lib. ii. tract. ii. cap. 134.
[4] *De temp. simpl.* cccxxxiv.
[5] *De aliment. facult.*
[6] *Arzneim.* Bd. i. S. 83.
[7] *Hist. de la Méd.* t. ii. p. 228.

3 others stalked, with an ovate, glandular head. *Fruit* placed on the ob-conical base of the calyx. *Leaves* triple-nerved, glandular in the axils of the principal veins. *Leaf-buds* scaly (*Lindley*).

Sp. Char.—*Leaves* triple-nerved, shining above, glandular in the axils of the veins. *Panicles* axillary and terminal, corymbose, naked.

Flowers smooth on the outside (*Nees*).

Young *branches* yellow and smooth. *Leaves* evergreen, oval, acuminate, attenuate at the base, bright green and shining above, paler beneath. *Petioles* from 1 to 1½ inch long. *Panicles* axillary and terminal, corymbose. *Flowers* small, yellowish-white. *Berry* round, blackish-red, size of a black currant. *Seed* solitary.

Every part of the tree, but especially the flower, evinces by its smell and taste that it is strongly impregnated with camphor.

Hab.—China, Japan, and Cochin China. Introduced into Java from Japan.

EXTRACTION AND DESCRIPTION.—Two kinds of *unrefined* or *crude camphor* (*camphora cruda* vel *rudis*) are known in commerce; one is the produce of Japan, the other of China.

1. Japan Camphor.—This is always brought to Europe by the Dutch, and is, therefore, called *Dutch camphor.* Kæmpfer[1] and Thunberg[2] have described the method of extracting this kind of camphor in the provinces of Satzuma, and the islands of Gotho in Japan. The roots and wood of the tree, chopped up, are boiled with water in an iron vessel, to which an earthen head, containing straw, is adapted. The camphor sublimes and condenses on the straw.

Japan or Dutch camphor is brought to Europe by way of Batavia. It is imported in tubs (hence it is called *tub camphor*) covered by matting, and each surrounded by a second tub, secured on the outside by hoops of twisted cane. Each tub contains from 1 cwt. to 1¼ cwt. or more. It consists of pinkish grains, which, by their mutual adhesion, form various-sized masses. It differs from the ordinary crude camphor in having larger grains, in being cleaner, and in subliming (usually) at a lower temperature. In consequence of these properties it generally fetches 10s. per cwt. more. There is not much brought to England, and of that which does come the greater part is re-shipped for the Continent.

[Dutch camphor now fetches only from 2s. 6d. to 5s. per cwt. more than China, the present value of it being only one-half of what it used to be; the refiners evidently expecting from two to five per cent. more yield than from the Chinese. It is found by experience that newly-imported camphor generally loses in the first year of warehousing about four to five per cent. in weight; in the second year, about two per cent.; and after that, one per cent. each succeeding year.—Ed.]

2. China Camphor; *Formosa Camphor.*—This is the *ordinary crude camphor.* The method of obtaining crude camphor in China has been described by the Abbé Grosier,[3] Dentrecolles,[4] and Davies.[5] The chopped branches are steeped in water, and afterwards boiled, until the camphor begins to adhere to the stick used in stirring. The liquid is then strained,

---

[1] *Amœn. Exot.* p. 772.
[2] *Fl. Japonica.*
[3] *Hist. Gén. de la Chine*, t. xiii. p. 335.
[4] Quoted by Davies.
[5] *The Chinese*, vol. ii. p. 355, 1835.

and, by standing, the camphor concretes. Alternate layers of a dry earth, finely powdered, and of this camphor, are then placed in a copper basin to which another inverted one is luted, and sublimation effected. This kind of crude camphor is imported from Singapore and Bombay, in square chests lined with lead-foil, and containing from $1\frac{1}{4}$ to $1\frac{1}{2}$ cwt. It is chiefly produced in the island of Formosa, and is brought by the Chin-Chew junks in very large quantities to Canton, whence foreign markets are supplied.[1] It consists of dirty-greyish grains, which are smaller than those of Dutch camphor. Its quality varies: sometimes it is wet and impure, but occasionally it is as fine as the Dutch kind.[2] [The importation of camphor in the ten years from 1835 to 1844 amounted to 19004 chests, and the consumption to 5928 chests, making the average importation annually 1900 chests, and the annual consumption 592 chests, of about one hundredweight each.—Ed.]

REFINEMENT.—Crude camphor is refined by sublimation. Formerly this process was carried on only at Venice. Afterwards it was successfully practised in Holland.[3] The method at present adopted in this metropolis is, as I am informed, as follows :[4]—The vessels in which this sublimation is effected are called *bomboloes* (bombola, *Ital.*, βομβυλιὸς). They

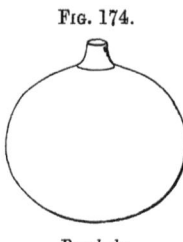

FIG. 174.

Bombolo.

are made of very thin flint glass, and weigh about 1 lb. each. Their shape is that of an oblate spheroid, whose shorter or vertical axis is about ten inches, and the longer or horizontal axis about twelve inches. They are furnished with a short neck.[5] When filled with crude camphor, they are imbedded in the sand-bath, and heated. To the melted camphor lime is added, and heat raised so as to make the liquid boil. The vapour condenses on the upper part of the vessel. As the sublimation proceeds, the height of the sand around the vessel is diminished. In about forty-eight hours the process is usually completed. The vessels are then removed, and their mouths clothed with tow; water is sprinkled over them by watering-pots, by which they are cracked. When quite cold, the cake of camphor (which weighs about eleven pounds) is removed, and trimmed by paring and scraping. In this process the lime retains the impurities and a portion of the camphor; hence, to extract the latter the lime is submitted to a strong heat in an iron pot with a head to it, and the sublimed product refined by a second sublimation. [We have witnessed this process at a large chemical factory in the neighbourhood of London. The bombolo was not there used in the mode described by the author, but the short neck was fitted to the mouth of the subliming-pot, which was imbedded in sand. The thin glass globe receives the pure

---

[1] Reeves, *Trans. Med.-Bot. Soc.* for 1828, p. 26 ; Gutzlaff and Reed, *China Opened*, vol. ii. p. 84, 1888.

[2] [The reader will find a complete history of the camphor tree of Borneo and Sumatra (Dryobalanops), by Dr. De Vriese, of Leyden, in the *Pharmaceutical Journal* for July 1852, p. 22.—Ed.]

[3] Ferber (*Journ. de Pharm.* t. i. p. 136, 1815) has described the refining process as practised by the Dutch.

[4] Dossie, in his *Elaboratory laid Open*, 1758, has described the mode of refining camphor.

[5] Clemandot (*Journ. de Pharm.* t. iii. p. 321, 1817) has described and figured another sort of subliming apparatus. $2\frac{1}{4}$ lbs. of crude camphor, mixed with 6 drachms of powdered quicklime, are placed in a flat-bottomed squat bottle with a short neck on a sand-bath : the neck of the bottle fits into a conical tin-plate head, into which the camphor is sublimed.

sublimed camphor in a thick crust. The glass vessel is then broken, and a hollow globe of camphor is removed from it.—ED.]

PROPERTIES.—*Refined camphor* (*camphora raffinata* vel *elaborata; camphora* officin.) is met with in the form of large hemispherical or convex-concave cakes, perforated in the middle. It is translucent, has a crystalline granular texture;[1] a strong, peculiar, not disagreeable, aromatic odour, and an aromatic, bitter, afterwards cooling taste. It is solid at ordinary temperatures, soft, and somewhat tough, but may be readily powdered by the addition of a few drops of rectified spirit. It evaporates in the air at ordinary temperatures; but in closed vessels, exposed to light, sublimes and crystallises on the sides of the bottle. It burns in the air like the volatile oils generally. It fuses at 347° F., and forms a transparent liquid, which boils at 400° F., and in close vessels condenses unchanged. It is lighter than water, its sp. gr. being 0·9867; or, according to some, 0·996.[2] Small pieces,. when thrown on this liquid, are violently agitated, and present a gyratory motion, which ceases directly a drop of oil is let fall on the water. If a cylinder of camphor, of the ¼th or ⅓th of an inch in diameter, be placed vertically in water, it communicates a to-and-fro movement to this liquid, and in a few days becomes deeply notched at the surface of the water. These phenomena are due to the simultaneous evaporation of the camphor and water, and which is most active where the two bodies are in contact.

Camphor is but very slightly soluble in water; 1000 parts of the latter dissolving only one part of camphor at the ordinary pressure of the atmosphere. But under augmented pressure it becomes more soluble.

Alcohol readily dissolves camphor; but if water be added to the solution, the camphor is precipitated. Ether, bisulphuret of carbon, chloroform, the oils (both fixed and volatile), and the acids, also dissolve it. The liquid obtained by dissolving camphor in nitric acid is sometimes termed *camphor oil:* it is a *nitrate of camphor,* and is decomposed by water, the camphor being precipitated. Camphor absorbs sulphurous and hydrochloric acid gases, with which it unites and forms respectively a *sulphite* and a *hydrochlorate of camphor.* Camphor is insoluble in alkaline solutions. The vapour of camphor passed over red-hot lime is converted into a naphthaline and an oily liquid called *camphrone.*

COMPOSITION.—Camphor is represented by the formula $C^{20}H^{16}O^2$, and has the following composition:—

	Atoms.	Eq. Wt.	Per Cent.	Dumas.	Blanchet and Sell.
Carbon	20	120	78·94	78·02	77·96
Hydrogen	16	16	10·53	10·39	10·61
Oxygen	2	16	10·53	11·59	11·43
Camphor	1	152	100·00	100·00	100·00

Dumas has suggested that camphor may be regarded as an oxide of a base (as yet hypothetical) which he calls *camphogen,* and whose composition is $C^{10}H^8$.

---

[1] A crystal of native camphor in the wood (probably not *laurel camphor,* but *Borneo or dryobalanops camphor*) in the collection of Materia Medica at the College of Physicians, appears as a flat octohedron, but its primary form is a right rhombic prism (W. Phillips, in Paris's *Pharmacologia*).

[2] The density of camphor varies considerably, according to the temperature. At 32° it is said to be denser than water (*Pharmaceutical Journal,* vol. v. p. 473, 1846). [When saturated with water, it sinks in this liquid at a temperature below 40°. By raising the temperature of the water, the camphor again rises to the surface.—ED.]

CHEMICAL CHARACTERISTICS.—In its combustibility, volatility, powerful odour, solubility in alcohol and ether, and almost insolubility in water, camphor agrees with the volatile oils. Being concrete or solid at ordinary temperatures, it obviously belongs to the class of *stearoptenes*, or *solid volatile oils*. It is further distinguished by the remarkable character of its odour, by its not blackening in burning, and by its not being converted into resin by the oxygen of the air or by nitric acid. By repeatedly distilling nitric acid from camphor, the latter is converted into *camphoric acid* ($C^{20}H^{14}O^6$, 2HO). Before the whole of the camphor has been converted into camphoric acid, there are produced intermediate compounds of camphor and this acid, which we may regard as camphorates of camphor. The camphor here described may be designated *common* or *laurel camphor*, in order to distinguish it from *Borneo camphor*, or *camphor of the Dryobalanops*, as well as from *artificial camphor*.

Common or laurel camphor absorbs hydrochloric acid gas, and forms a transparent colourless liquid; Borneo camphor, on the contrary, is scarcely acted on by this acid gas. If Borneo camphor be boiled in nitric acid, it is converted into common camphor.

Artificial camphor (see OIL OF TURPENTINE) usually evolves some hydrochloric acid when volatilised, and burns in the air with a greenish sooty flame : if the flame be blown out, the evolved vapour has a terebinthinate odour. By these characters artificial camphor may be distinguished from laurel camphor. [Mr. Bailey has applied polarised light to the distinction of artificial from natural camphor. The artificial camphor is a hydrochlorate of camphene. If small fragments of each be placed separately on glass slides, and a drop of alcohol added to them, they are dissolved, and by the evaporation of the alcohol speedily crystallise. If the crystallisation of natural camphor is watched by means of the microscope and polarised light, a most beautiful display of coloured crystals is seen, while with the artificial product nothing of the kind is witnessed.[1]—ED.]

OIL OF LAUREL CAMPHOR.—Pelouze and Fremy state that when the branches of Camphora officinarum are distilled with water, a mixture of camphor and a liquid essential oil is obtained, which is called *oil of camphor*.—This oil has a density of 0·910 : its composition is $C^{20}H^{16}O$. By exposure to oxygen gas or to the action of nitric acid, it absorbs oxygen, and becomes solid camphor, $C^{20}H^{16}O^2$. It is probable, therefore, that its formation precedes that of solid camphor in the camphor tree. I have met with this oil in commerce under the name of *oil of camphor*. By keeping, it deposits crystals of camphor, and by this circumstance it may be distinguished from the *oil of Borneo camphor* (see Dryobalanops). By the action of hydrochloric acid I find that these crystals liquify, like common or laurel camphor. A considerable quantity of the oil was purchased some years ago by a London manufacturer of scented soap, who submitted it to distillation, and obtained from 60 lbs. of it 40 lbs. of colourless liquid oil, and 20 lbs. of crystalline camphor. The oil has been described and analysed by Dr. Th. Martius.[2]

PHYSIOLOGICAL EFFECTS. *α. On Vegetables.*—Goeppert[3] has satisfactorily shown—first, that solutions of camphor act in the same deleterious manner on plants as the volatile oils; secondly, that they destroy the mobility of contractile parts without previously exciting them; thirdly, that they have no influence either on the germination of phanerogamia, or the vegetation of the

[1] [*Silliman's Journal*, May 1851 ; and *Pharmaceutical Journal*, September 1851, p. 122.]
[2] *Berlinisches Jahrbuch für d. Pharmacie*, Bd. xl. S. 455, 1838.
[3] Poggendorff, *Ann. d. Phys. u. Chem.* 1828.

cellular cryptogamia; and fourthly, that the vapour only is sufficient to destroy fleshy plants and ferns. Miquet[1] has confirmed these results.[2]

β. *On Animals generally.*—The action of camphor on animals has been the subject of numerous experiments made by Hillefield,[3] Monro,[4] Menghini and Carminati,[5] Viborg, Hertwich,[6] Orfila,[7] and Scudery.[8]

Air impregnated with the vapour of camphor proves injurious to *insects* (the Tineæ, which destroy wool, excepted). Sooner or later it causes frequent agitation, followed by languor, insensibility, convulsions, and death (Menghini). To *amphibials* (frogs) the vapour also proves noxious. It produces preter-natural movements, difficult respiration, trembling, and stupor (Carminati). Given to *birds* and *mammals*, in sufficient doses, camphor proves poisonous; but the symptoms which it gives rise to, do not appear to be uniform. Indeed, there are few remedies whose action on the animal economy is so variable as that of camphor. Three drachms dissolved in oil and given to a dog, the œsophagus being tied, caused violent convulsions, somewhat analogous to those of epilepsy, followed by insensibility and death (Orfila). When admi-nistered in substance, it inflamed the digestive tube, caused ulceration, and after its absorption gave rise to convulsions (Idem). Given to horses, in doses of two drachms, it excited spasmodic movements, and quickened the pulse, but did not determine any serious result.[9] Tiedemann and Gmelin[10] detected the odour of camphor in the blood of the vena portæ and of the mesenteric vein of a horse to which they had given camphor; but they could recognise it neither in the chyle nor in the urine. It is evolved from the system principally by the bronchial surfaces; for the breath of animals to which this substance has been administered has a strong odour of camphor. Moiroud[11] observed that the skin of a horse into whose jugular vein camphor had been injected, smelt of this substance.

"The general sedative effects of camphor on animals are rarely well-marked; however, when administered in a proper dose, and in cases really requiring its use, it sometimes causes a diminution in the force and frequency of the pulse, and seems to allay pain" (Moiroud). Scudery[12] observed that the convul-sions caused in animals by camphor were accompanied with a peculiar kind of delirium, which caused them to run up and down without apparent cause. He also found the urinary organs generally affected, and for the most part with strangury.

γ. *On Man.*—No article of the materia medica has had more contradictory statements made respecting its effects and mode of action, than camphor. These, however, have principally referred to its influence over the functions

---

[1] Meyen's *Report on the Progress of Vegetable Physiology during the year* 1837, p. 139, trans-lated by W. Francis.

[2] [Camphor appears to prevent the growth of various kinds of mould. It may be thus usefully employed for preventing ink from becoming mouldy.—ED.]

[3] Quoted by Wibmer, *Wirk. d. Arzneim. u. Gifte*, Bd. iii. S. 215.

[4] *Essays and Observ., Phys. and Lit.* vol. iii. p. 351.

[5] Wibmer, *loco cit.*

[6] *Ibid.*

[7] *Toxicol. Gén.*

[8] Wibmer, *op. cit.*

[9] Moiroud, *Pharm. Vétér.*

[10] *Versuche üb. d. Wege auf welchen Subst. aus d. Mag. u. Darmk. ins Blut gelang.* S. 24 and 25.

[11] *Op. cit.*

[12] Quoted by Dr. Christison.

of circulation and calorification; for, with regard to the modifications which it induces in the other functions, scarcely any difference of opinion prevails.

Its local action on the mucous surfaces, the denuded dermis, and ulcers, is that of an *acrid.* A piece of camphor held in the mouth for half an hour caused the mucous lining of this cavity to become red, hot, swollen, and painful; and it is highly probable that, had the experiment been persevered in, ulceration would have followed.[1] The pain and uneasiness which camphor, when swallowed in substance, sometimes produces in the stomach, is likewise imputed to its local action as an acrid. Rubbed on the skin covered with cuticle, Dr. Cullen says that it causes neither redness nor other mark of inflammation;[2] but Dr. Clutterbuck[3] declares this to be " undoubtedly a mistake." When applied to the denuded dermis, or to ulcers, it produces pain, and appears to act as an irritant. These observations respecting the local action of camphor on man are confirmed by the ascertained effects of this substance on other animals. Camphor has been charged with producing brittleness of the teeth when it has been used for a considerable time as a dentifrice,[4] but I believe without any valid foundation.

Camphor becomes absorbed, and is thrown out of the system by the bronchial membrane principally, but also by the skin. Trousseau and Pidoux[5] recognised its odour in every case in the pulmonary exhalation, but failed to detect it in the cutaneous perspiration. Cullen, however, says[6] that " Mr. Lasonne, the father, has observed, as I have done frequently, that camphor, though given very largely, never discovers its smell in the urine, whilst it frequently does in the perspiration and sweat." The non-detection of it in the urine agrees with the observation of Tiedemann and Gmelin with regard to horses, already noticed.

Camphor specifically affects the nervous system.—Regarding the symptoms of this effect, but little difference of opinion prevails. In moderate doses it exhilarates, and acts as an anodyne.[7] Its exhilarating effects are well seen in nervous and hypochondriacal cases. In large doses it causes disorder of the mental faculties, the external senses, and volition; the symptoms being lassitude, giddiness, confusion of ideas and disordered vision, noise in the ears, drowsiness, delirium or stupor, and convulsions. These phenomena, which have been observed in several cases, agree with those noticed in experiments on brutes. In its power of causing stupor, camphor agrees with opium; but it differs from the latter in its more frequently causing delirium and convulsions. Epilepsy has been ascribed to the use of camphor.

The quality of the influence which camphor exercises over the vascular system has been a subject of much controversy. From my own limited observations of its use *in small* or *medium doses* (from five to ten grains), I am disposed to regard its leading effect as that of a vascular excitant, though I am not prepared to deny that slight depression may not have preceded this effect. Combined with diaphoretic regimen (warm clothing and tepid diluents),

---

[1] Trousseau and Pidoux, *Traité de Thérap.* t. i. p. 43.
[2] *Mat. Med.* vol. ii. p. 298.
[3] *Inquiry into the Seat and Nature of Fever*, 2d edit. p. 424.
[4] See *Lond. Med. Gaz.* N.S. vols. iii. and iv. 1846–7 ; and *Pharm. Journ.* vol. vi. p. 234, 1846.
[5] *Op. supra cit.* p. 49.
[6] *Op. cit.* p. 305.
[7] Harrup, *On the Anodyne Effects of Camphor*, in *The London Medical Review*, vol. iv. p. 200. Lond. 1800.

I have seen camphor increase the fulness of the pulse, raise the temperature of the surface, and operate as a sudorific. If opium be conjoined, these effects are more manifest.[1]

In *excessive doses* it acts as a powerful poison. One of the earliest cases reported is that of Mr. Alexander,[2] who swallowed two scruples of camphor in syrup of roses. In about twenty minutes he experienced lassitude and depression of spirits, with frequent yawnings : at the end of three-quarters of an hour his pulse had fallen from 77 to 67. Soon after he felt giddy, confused, and almost incapable of walking across the room. He became gradually insensible, and in this condition was attacked with violent convulsions and maniacal delirium. From this state he awoke as from a profound sleep; his pulse was 100, and he was able to reply to interrogatories, though he had not completely recovered his recollection. Warm water being administered, he vomited the greater part of the camphor, which had been swallowed three hours previously; and from this time he gradually recovered. In another case,[3] a man swallowed four ounces of camphorated spirits containing 160 grains of camphor. The symptoms were burning heat of skin, frequent, full, and hard pulse, brilliancy of the eyes, redness of the face, heaviness of the head, anxiety, agitation, violent sense of heat in the stomach; then intense headache, giddiness, indistinctness of sight, and ocular hallucinations. The patient complained of heat only, which he said was intolerable. In the night copious sweating came on, followed by sleep. The pulse continued full and frequent, and the voiding of urine difficult.

[The following case is reported by Mr. Hallett, of Axminster :—A woman swallowed in the morning about a scruple of camphor dissolved in rectified spirits of wine, and mixed with tincture of myrrh. In half an hour she was suddenly seized with languor, giddiness, occasional loss of sight, delirium, numbness, tingling and coldness of the arms and legs, as well as loss of muscular power, so that she could hardly walk. The pulse was quick, and respiration difficult, but she suffered no pain in any part. On the administration of an emetic, she vomited a yellowish liquid smelling strongly of camphor. In the evening the symptoms were much diminished, but she had slight convulsive fits during the night. The next day she was convalescent : the difficulty of breathing, however, continued more or less for several weeks. The dose did not probably exceed *twenty grains :* this is the smallest dose of camphor which appears to have been attended with serious symptoms. In a case which occurred to Wendt, of Breslau, eight scruples were swallowed by a drunkard, dissolved in spirit. The symptoms were giddiness, dimness of sight, delirium, and burning pain in the stomach. There was *no vomiting :* the man recovered. In another, reported by Mr. Stookes, a woman swallowed *half an ounce* of camphor dissolved in oil. In two hours she was delirious; her face pale ; pupils dilated ; hands and feet cold; pulse 120. There was neither pain, vomiting (except as the result of emetics), nor purging. She recovered in a few hours.[4] These and other cases show that camphor cannot

---

[1] See Vol. I. for some remarks on the comparative operation of ammonia and camphor.
[2] *Experimental Essays*, p. 128, 1768.
[3] *Lond. Med. Gaz.* vol. v. p. 635, from Rust's *Magazin.*
[4] [*Med. Times*, June 10, 1848, p. 88.]

be regarded as a very active poison.[1] In Orfila's experiments on animals, the mucous membrane of the stomach was found inflamed.[2]

In three cases reported by Dr. Schaaf, the symptoms caused by camphor were those of a narcotico-irritant poison. A woman gave about thirty grains (half a tea-spoonful) of powdered camphor to each of her three children as a vermifuge. Two of the children were respectively of the ages of three and five years, the third was an infant aged eighteen months. The first symptoms were paleness of the face, with a fixed and stupid look. Delirium followed, with a sense of burning in the throat, and great thirst. Vomiting, purging, and convulsions supervened; and in one child the convulsions were most violent. The two elder children, after suffering thus for three hours, fell into a comatose sleep, and on awaking the symptoms passed off. The infant died in seven hours, not having manifested any return of consciousness from the first occurrence of convulsions.[3]—ED.]

In some other well-reported cases, camphor, in large doses, caused depression of the vascular system. In the instances related by Fred. Hoffmann,[4] Pouteau,[5] Griffin,[6] Cullen,[7] Callisen,[8] Edwards,[9] and Trousseau and Pidoux,[10] sedation of the vascular system was observed. It was manifested by a languid, small, and slower pulse, coldness of the surface, and pallid countenance; in some cases with cold sweat. In some of these instances symptoms of vascular excitement followed those of depression. The pulse became more frequent and fuller than natural, and the heat of the surface augmented. Trousseau and Pidoux[11] ascribe the symptoms of sedation to the depressing influence which camphor exerts over the system by sympathy; while the sanguineous excitation they refer to the passage of camphor into the blood, and the efforts of the organism to eliminate this unassimilable principle. But in some of the cases in which excessive doses of camphor have been taken, no symptoms of depression were manifested; as in the instance mentioned by Dr. Eickhorn (in which great heat, rapid but small pulse, copious sweating, and agreeable exhilaration, were produced by 120 grains[12]), by Dr. Wendt,[13] by Scudery,[14] and by Bergondi.[15]

Camphor has long been celebrated as an anaphrodisiac; the smell of it even is said to be attended with this effect; hence the verse of the School of Salernum—" *Camphora per nares castrat odore mares.*" Trousseau and Pidoux[16] experienced the anaphrodisiac property of 36 grains of camphor

---

[1] [Wibmer, *Arzneim. u. Gifte,* iii. 212.]
[2] [*Toxicologie,* ii. 493.]
[3] [*Med. Gazette,* xlvii. p. 219.]
[4] *Op. omnia,* t. iv. p. 26, Geneva, 1748.
[5] Murray, *App. Med.* vol. iv.
[6] Quoted by Alexander.
[7] *Mat. Med.* vol. ii. p. 295.
[8] Murray, *App. Med.*
[9] Orfila, *Tox. Gén.*
[10] *Traité de Thérap.* t. i. p. 48.
[11] *Op. cit.* p. 51.
[12] *Lond. Med. Gaz.* vol. xi. p. 772.
[13] Quoted in Dr. Christison's *Treatise on Poisons,* p. 810.
[14] Wibmer, *op. supra cit.*
[15] *Ibid.*
[16] *Op. cit.* p. 48.

taken into the stomach. Strangury has also been ascribed to this substance by Heberden,[1] by Scudery,[2] and others.

USES.—The discrepancy among authors as to the physiological effects of camphor has had the effect of greatly circumscribing the use of this substance. Indeed, until its operation on the system be more satisfactorily ascertained, it is almost impossible to lay down general rules which should govern its exhibition. The following are the principal maladies in which it has been found useful :—

1. *Fever.*—Camphor has been employed in those forms of fever which are of a typhoid type. It is chiefly valuable by causing determination to the surface, and giving rise to diaphoresis. Hence those remedies should be conjoined with it which promote these effects : such as ipecacuanha, emetic tartar, and the vegetable alkaline salts. Opium greatly contributes to the sudorific effects of camphor; and, when it is admissible, benefit is sometimes obtained by the administration of one grain of opium with five or eight of camphor. But in a great number of cases of fever the cerebral disorder forbids the use of opium. From its specific influence over the cerebral functions, camphor has been frequently used in fever to allay the nervous symptoms,—such as the delirium, the watchings, and the subsultus tendinum; but it frequently fails to give relief. Dr. Home[3] did not find any advantage from its use in low nervous fever; and Dr. Heberden[4] has seen one scruple of camphor given every six hours, without any perceptible effect in abating the convulsive catchings, or composing the patient to rest.

2. *In inflammatory diseases.*—In the latter stages of inflammation of internal important parts (as the serous and mucous membranes, the stomach, intestines, and uterus), after proper evacuations have been made in the earlier periods of the disease, when great exhaustion is manifested by a small feeble pulse and a cold flaccid skin, small but repeated doses of camphor have been employed to determine to the skin, and to promote diaphoresis. It is particularly serviceable in rheumatic inflammation, especially when produced by metastasis.[5]

3. *In the exanthemata.*—Camphor has been employed in small-pox, as also in measles, scarlatina, and miliary fever; but it is admissible only when the circulation flags, and the temperature of the surface falls below the natural standard. In such cases it is sometimes employed, with a diaphoretic regimen, to determine to the skin. It is to be carefully avoided when inflammation of the brain or its membranes is feared. It has been asserted that if a camphorated ointment be applied to the face, no small-pox pustules will make their appearance there; but the statement is not correct.

4. *In mania, melancholia, and other forms of mental disorder.*—Camphor is occasionally taken to cause exhilaration. I was acquainted with two persons (females), both of nervous temperament, who used it for this purpose. To relieve despondency I have often found it serviceable. In mania and melancholia it has now and then proved useful by its narcotic effects : it induces mental quiet and causes sleep. It was used in these affections by

---

[1] *Comment.* art. *Stranguria.*
[2] *Supra cit.*
[3] *Clin. Hist.* p. 36.
[4] *Comment.* art. *Febris.*
[5] Sundelin, *Handb. d. spec. Heilmittell.* Bd. ii. S. 145.

Paracelsus and several succeeding writers,[1] especially, in more modern times, by Dr. Kinneir,[2] and by Avenbrugger.[3] The latter regards it as a specific in the mania of men, when accompanied with a small contracted penis, corrugated empty scrotum, or when both testicles are so retracted that they appear to be introduced into the abdominal cavity !

5. *In spasmodic affections.*—The narcotic influence of camphor has occasionally proved serviceable in some spasmodic or convulsive affections; viz. spasmodic cough, epilepsy, puerperal convulsions, hysteria, and even tetanus : its use, however, requires caution.

6. *In irritation of the urinary or sexual organs.*—A power of diminishing irritation of the urinary organs has long been assigned to camphor. In strangury and dysury, especially when produced by cantharides, it is said to have been used with benefit,—a statement apparently inconsistent with that more recently made, of its producing irritation of the urinary organs. In satyriasis, nymphomania, and onanism, it is said to have proved advantageous by its anaphrodisiac properties. In dysmenorrhœa it sometimes proves serviceable as an anodyne.

7. *In poisoning.*—Small doses of camphor (administered by the mouth or by the rectum) have been exhibited with apparent benefit in cases of poisoning by opium.[4] It has also been employed to mitigate the effects of cantharides, squills, and mezereon;[5] but toxicologists, for the most part, do not admit its efficacy : at any rate, further evidence is required to establish it. Nor does there appear any valid testimony for believing that camphor possesses the power of checking mercurial salivation, as some have supposed.

8. *In chronic rheumatism and gout.*—A mixture of camphor and opium, in the proportions before mentioned, is useful in chronic rheumatism, by its sudorific and anodyne properties. Warm clothing and diluents should be conjoined. In chronic gout, also, camphor is said to have proved beneficial.

9. *In cholera.*—The combination of camphor and opium above referred to, I have seen used with benefit in cholera.

10. *Externally,* camphor is employed in the form of vapour, in solution, or, more rarely, in the solid state. The *vapour* is occasionally inhaled in spasmodic cough, and is applied to the skin to alleviate pain and promote sweat, constituting the *camphor fumigations* (*fumigationes camphoræ*). Dupasquier[6] recommended these fumigations in chronic rheumatism. The patient may be in bed, or seated in a chair; and, in either case, is to be enveloped in a blanket tied round the neck. About half an ounce of camphor is then to be placed on a metallic plate, and introduced within the blanket (under the chair, if the patient be seated). In *solution,* camphor is used either as an anodyne or a local stimulant. The nitric solution of camphor is used to relieve toothache. A solution of camphor in oil has been used as an injection into the urethra, to relieve ardor urinæ in gonorrhœa, and into the rectum to mitigate tenesmus arising from ascarides or dysentery. The acetic and alcoholic solutions of camphor are mostly employed as stimulants. In

---

[1] Murray, *App. Med.* vol. iv. p. 499.
[2] *Phil. Trans.* vol. xxxv.
[3] *Experim. de remed. specif. in mania virorum,* Vind. 1776.
[4] Orfila, *Toxicol. Gén.*
[5] Hahnemann, and Van Bavegem, in Marx's *Die Lehre v. d. Giften,* Bd. ii. S. 202 and 358. *Revue Méd.* t. ii. p. 218, 1826.

substance, camphor is not frequently used. A scruple or half a drachm "added to a poultice, and applied to the perineum, allays the chordee, which is a painful attendant upon gonorrhœa."[1] Powdered camphor is a constituent of some tooth-powders, to which it communicates its peculiar odour.

[It has been employed successfully, for the prevention of pitting from small-pox, by Mr. Henry George, of Kensington. On the second day of a confluent case of small-pox, he covered one half of the face with wadding well sprinkled with powdered camphor, over which he placed oil-silk. The remainder of the face and the whole of the body were covered with powdered calamine. The side of the face which had been covered with camphor was free from pitting, while on the opposite side, a month afterwards, the areolæ and indentations of the pustules still remained.[2]—ED.]

The foregoing are some only of the maladies in which camphor has been extensively used and lauded. I must refer to the work of Murray[3] for various other uses which have been made of this substance.—It is scarcely necessary to add that camphor-bags possess no prophylactic properties against contagion.

ADMINISTRATION.—The medium dose of it is from five to ten grains; but it is frequently exhibited in much smaller doses (as one grain); and occasionally a scruple has been employed. It is given in the form of a pill or emulsion. That of *pill* is said to be objectionable, " as in this state the camphor is with difficulty dissolved in the gastric liquors, and, floating on the top, is apt to excite nausea, or pain or uneasiness at the upper orifice of the stomach."[4] It has even been charged with causing ulceration of the stomach when given in the solid form. The *emulsion* is made by rubbing up the camphor with loaf-sugar, gum-arabic, and water; and the suspension will be rendered more complete by the addition of a little myrrh.[5]

ANTIDOTE.—In a case of poisoning by camphor, first evacuate the contents of the stomach. Hufeland[6] recommends the use of opium to relieve the effects of camphor. Phœbus[7] directs chlorine water to be administered as the antidote, and afterwards purgatives and clysters. Vinegar and coffee, he states, promote the poisonous operation. Wine assists the patient's recovery.

1. MISTURA CAMPHORÆ, L. E. D.; *Aqua Camphoræ; Camphor Mixture.* (Camphor, ℨss.; Rectified Spirit, ♏x.; Water, Oj. First rub the camphor with the spirit, then with the water gradually poured in, and strain through linen, L. The *Dublin College* employs Tincture of Camphor, fℨj.; Water, Oiij. Shake the tincture and water together in a bottle, and, after the mixture has stood for twenty-four hours, filter through paper, D. The *Edinburgh College* employs Camphor, ℈j.; Sweet Almonds, and Pure Sugar, of each ℨss.; Water, Oj. Steep the almonds in hot water, and peel them; rub the camphor and sugar well together in a mortar; add the almonds; beat the whole into a smooth pulp; add the water gradually, with constant stirring, and then strain, E.)—The *camphor mixture* kept in the shops is often prepared by suspending camphor in water without the intervention of any third body. The

[1] *United States Dispensatory.*
[2] [*Med. Times and Gazette*, Aug. 14, 1852.]
[3] *App. Med.* vol. iv.
[4] *United States Dispensatory.*
[5] *Ibid.*
[6] Marx, *Die Lehre von d. Gift.* Bd. ii. S. 202.
[7] *Handb. d. Arzneiverord.* 2te Ausg.

quantity of this substance dissolved is exceedingly small. The rectified spirit employed by the London and Dublin Colleges serves to promote the pulverisation, and, very slightly perhaps, the solution of the camphor. Sugar also assists its diffusion through water. The preparation of the Edinburgh Pharmacopœia is, in fact, an emulsion. None of these artificial mixtures, however, are very permanent, and the quantity of camphor which remains in solution is so small, that the liquid can scarcely be said to possess more than the flavour and odour of camphor. Hence its principal value is as a vehicle for the exhibition of other medicines. Its usual dose is from f℥j. to f℥ij.

2. MISTURA CAMPHORÆ CUM MAGNESIA, E.; *Camphor Mixture with Magnesia*.

(Camphor, gr. x.; Carbonate of Magnesia, gr. xxv.; Water, f℥vj. Triturate the camphor and carbonate of magnesia together, adding the water gradually.)—The carbonate of magnesia promotes the solution of the camphor in water. This mixture, therefore, holds a larger quantity of camphor in solution than the previous one. A minute portion of magnesia is also dissolved. As the magnesian carbonate is not separated by filtration, it gives to the mixture antacid properties, in addition to those qualities which this preparation derives from the camphor. "In addition to the uses of the simple camphor mixture, this preparation has been found very beneficial in the uric acid diathesis, and also in irritations of the neck of the urinary bladder,—particularly when given in combination with hyoscyamus."[1] The dose is from f℥ss. to f℥j.

Murray's Fluid Camphor.—This is a solution of camphor in fluid magnesia. Each ounce contains three grains of camphor and six grains of bicarbonate of magnesia. Its sp. gr. is 1·0026.[2]

3. SPIRITUS CAMPHORÆ, L. E.; *Tinctura Camphoræ*, sive *Spiritus Camphoratus*, D.; *Spiritus Camphoræ; Spirit of Camphor; Camphorated Spirits of Wine*, offic.

(Camphor, ℥v. [in small fragments, ℥j. D.; ℥iiss. E.]; Rectified Spirit, Oij. [f℥viij. D.] Mix, that the camphor may be dissolved.)—The principal use of this preparation is as a stimulant and anodyne liniment in sprains and bruises, chilblains, chronic rheumatism, and paralysis. Water immediately decomposes it, separating the greater part of the camphor, but holding in solution a minute portion; thereby forming an extemporaneous camphor mixture. By the aid of sugar or mucilage, the greater part of the camphor may be suspended in water. Employed in this form, we may give tincture of camphor internally in doses of from ♏x. to f℥j.

"Spiritus camphoræ is miscible with liquor plumbi diacetatis in the proportion of two parts of the former to one of the latter, and in this form it is a convenient preparation, sometimes ordered as a concentrated lotion, to which water is to be added by the patient. But if a larger proportion of liquor plumbi be added, the camphor is partially precipitated."[3]

4. TINCTURA CAMPHORÆ COMPOSITA, L.; *Compound Tincture of Opium; Tinctura Opii camphorata*, E. D.; *Elixir Paregoricum; Paregoric Elixir*, offic.

(Camphor, ℈iiss.; Opium, powdered [sliced, E.], gr.

[1] Dr. Montgomery, *Observ. on the Dubl. Pharm.*
[2] *Lancet*, 1847, vol. ii. p. 553; *Pharmaceutical Journal*, vol. vii. p. 367, 1848.
[3] Mr. Jacob Bell, *Pharmaceutical Journal*, vol. iv. p. 313, 1844.

lxxij. [Ʒiv. *E.*] ; Benzoic Acid, gr. lxxij. [Ʒiv. *E.*] ; Oil of Anise, fʒj. ; Proof Spirit, Oij. Macerate for fourteen [seven, *E.*] days, and filter, *L.* Opium, in coarse powder; Benzoic Acid, of each ʒiss. ; Camphor, ʒj. ; Oil of Anise, fʒj. ; Proof Spirit, Oij. Macerate for fourteen days, strain, express, and filter, *D.*)—This is a very valuable preparation, and is extensively employed both by the public and the profession. Its active ingredient is opium. The principal use of it is to allay troublesome cough unconnected with any active inflammatory symptoms. It diminishes the sensibility of the bronchial membrane to the influence of cold air, checks profuse secretion, and allays spasmodic cough. Dose, fʒj. to fʒiij. A fluidounce contains nearly two grains of opium. The name given to this preparation by the London College, though less correct than that of the Edinburgh and Dublin Colleges, is, I conceive, much more convenient, since it enables us to prescribe opium without the knowledge of the patient,—no mean advantage in cases where a strong prejudice exists in the mind of the patient or his friends to the use of this important narcotic. Furthermore, it is less likely to give rise to serious and fatal errors in dispensing. In a case mentioned by Dr. M. Good,[1] laudanum was served by an ignorant dispenser for *tinct. opii camph.* The error proved fatal to the patient.

5. **LINIMENTUM CAMPHORÆ,** L. E. D.; *Camphor Liniment,* offic. (Camphor, ʒj. ; Olive Oil, fʒiv. Dissolve, *L.* Dissolve the camphor in the oil with a gentle heat, *D.* Rub them together in a mortar, *E.*)—A stimulant and anodyne embrocation in sprains, bruises, and rheumatic and other local pains. In glandular enlargements it is used as a resolvent.

6. **LINIMENTUM CAMPHORÆ COMPOSITUM,** L. D. (Camphor, ʒiiss. ; Oil of Lavender, fʒj. ; Rectified Spirit, ʒxvij. ; Stronger Solution of Ammonia, ʒiij. Dissolve the camphor and the oil in the spirit, then add the ammonia, and shake them together until they are mixed, *L.* Camphor, ʒv. ; Oil of Lavender, fʒij. ; Rectified Spirit, Oiss. ; Stronger Solution of Ammonia, Oss. Dissolve the camphor and oil of lavender in the spirit, then add the solution of ammonia, and mix with agitation, *D.*)—A powerful stimulant and rubefacient, producing, when freely used, considerable irritation and inflammation. It is applicable in the same cases as the simple *camphor liniment* and the *liniment of ammonia.* From both of these compounds it differs in not being greasy. "I have used," says Dr. Montgomery,[2] "a liniment composed of two parts of this and one of turpentine, with children, as a substitute for a blister, and with good effect ; or, with equal parts of the *anodyne liniment* I have found it highly beneficial in the removal of those distressing pains in the back which so frequently annoy women about the close of their pregnancy."

---

[1] *Hist. of Med.* 1795, App. p. 14.
[2] *Op. supra cit.*

149. SASSAFRAS OFFICINALE, *Nees.*—THE SASSAFRAS TREE.

Laurus Sassafras, *Linn.*
Sex. Syst. Enneandria, Mouogynia.
(Radix, *L.*—The Root, *D. E.*)

History.—Sassafras wood is mentioned by Monardes,[1] who states that it had been recently introduced into Spain from Florida. It was, however, first brought to Europe by the French.[2]

Botany. **Gen. Char.**—Diœcious. *Calyx* 6-parted, membranous; segments equal, permanent at the base. Males : *Fertile stamens* 9, in 3 rows, the 3 inner with double-stalked distinct glands at the base. *Anthers* linear, 4-celled, all looking inwards. Females with as many sterile stamens as the male, or fewer; the inner often confluent. *Fruit* succulent, placed on the thick fleshy apex of the peduncle, and seated in the torn unchanged calyx. *Flowers* yellow, before the leaves. *Leaves* deciduous (*Lindley*).

Sp. Char.—Leaves thin, oblong, entire, 2—3-lobed.

A small tree or bush. Leaves smooth above, finely downy beneath. Racemes with subulate downy bracts.

Hab.—Woods of North America, from Canada to Florida.

Description.—The root (*radix sassafras*) is used in medicine. Its bark (*cortex radicis sassafras* vel *cortex sassafras*) occurs in rather small pieces, which are light, odorous, not fibrous, but spongy or corky. The epidermis is brownish-grey : the cortical layers and inner surface reddish cinnamon-brown, or almost rust-red, becoming darker by age. Sometimes small, white, micaceous crystals (like those found on *sassafras nuts*) are observed on the inner surface of the bark. *Sassafras wood* (*lignum radicis sassafras* vel *lignum sassafras*) occurs in the form of large stems or branches, frequently more or less covered with the bark. The wood is soft or spongy, light, of a greyish-reddish tint, and has a fragrant aromatic odour. It is usually sold cut up into chips (*sassafras chips*).

Brazilian Sassafras; *Páo Sassafras.*—This is the produce of *Nectandra cymbarum* of Nees, the *Ocotea amara* of Martius. It grows in Rio Negro. Its bark is bitter and aromatic, and is used as a tonic and carminative.

Sassafras Nuts; *Pichurim Beans; Fabæ Pichurim.*—These seeds (or rather cotyledons) are the produce of *Nectandra Puchury major* of Nees, and *Nect. Puchury minor* of Nees,—trees growing in the province of Rio Negro. "They were imported from Brazil into Stockholm in the middle of the last century, and were found a valuable tonic and astringent medicine : during the continental war they were used as a bad substitute for nutmegs."[3] They are still to be found in some of the old drug-houses of London. By keeping in a bottle, small micaceous crystals form on their surface. These seeds have been analysed by Bonastre.[4] Their aromatic qualities depend on a volatile oil.

---

[1] *Hist. Simpl. Med.* 1569–74.

[2] Alston's *Lect. on the Mat. Med.* vol. ii. p. 51.

[3] [The statement here made by the author led to a claim on the part of the Custom House for the same duty on a few casks of sassafras nuts (lately imported from Holland) as that which was levied on nutmegs. The Custom House authorities must, however, have had a weak case, if they could assign no better reason than this for levying a heavier duty. The author describes them, not as nutmegs, but as a bad substitute. Quassia is a bad substitute for hops, but this would not be a satisfactory reason for charging quassia with the same duty as hops. There is no similarity of flavour in the two nuts, and it is probable that the substitution only occurred when, during the war with the Dutch, nutmegs could not be obtained in this country at any price.—Ed.]

[4] *Journ. de Pharm.* vol. xi. p. 1, 1825.

COMPOSITION.—Neither the bark nor the wood have been analysed. They contain *volatile oil, resin,* and *extractive matter.*

PHYSIOLOGICAL EFFECTS.—The wood and the bark are stimulant and sudorific. Taken in the form of infusion, and assisted by warm clothing and tepid drinks, they excite the vascular system, and prove sudorific. They owe their activity to the volatile oil, which possesses acrid properties.

USES.—Sassafras is employed as a sudorific and alterative in cutaneous, rheumatic, and venereal diseases. On account of its stimulant properties it is inadmissible in febrile or inflammatory conditions of the system. It is rarely or never used alone, but generally in combination with sarsaparilla and guaiacum.

ADMINISTRATION.—Sassafras is administered in the form of *oil* or *infusion.* The dose of the oil is from two to ten drops. *Sassafras tea,* flavoured with milk and sugar, is sold at day-break in the streets of London, under the name of *saloop.* Sassafras is a constituent of the *Decoctum Sarzæ compositum;* but the volatile oil is dissipated by boiling.

OLEUM SASSAFRAS, U. S.; *Volatile Oil of Sassafras officinale,* E. ; *Oil of Sassafras.* (Obtained by submitting the wood to distillation with water.) —It is colourless, but by keeping becomes yellow or red. Its smell is that of sassafras ; its taste hot. Sp. gr. 1·094. Water separates it into two oils ; one lighter, the other heavier than water. By keeping, it deposits large crystals (stéaroptène; *sassafrol,* $C^{10}H^5O^2$), which are readily soluble. Oil of sassafras is rendered orange-red by nitric acid. It is said to be adulterated with oil of lavender or oil of turpentine ;[1] but the statement, I suspect, does not apply to the oil found in English commerce. Oil of sassafras is stimulant and diaphoretic. It may be employed in chronic rheumatism, cutaneous diseases, and venereal maladies. It is a constituent of the *Compound Extract of Sarsaparilla.*

150. LAURUS NOBILIS, *Linn.*—THE SWEET BAY.

Sex. Syst. Enneandria, Monogynia.

(Fructus, *L.*)

HISTORY.—The " green bay-tree" is mentioned, though erroneously, in our translation of the Bible ;[2] the Hebrew word translated *bay,* meaning *native.*[3] Hippocrates[4] used both the leaves and berries of the bay-tree (δάφνη) in medicine. Bay-leaf is analogous to the *malabathrum* of the ancients.[5]

BOTANY. **Gen. Char.**—*Flowers* diœcious or hermaphrodite, involucrated. *Calyx* 4-parted ; segments equal, deciduous. *Fertile stamens* 12, in 3 rows ; the outer alternate with the segments of the calyx ; all with 2 glands in the middle or above it. *Anthers* oblong, 2-celled, all looking inwards. *Female flowers,* with 2 to 4 castrated males, surrounding the ovary. *Stigma* capitate. *Fruit* succulent, seated in the irregular base of the calyx. *Umbels*

[1] Bonastre, *Journ. de Pharm.* vol. xiv. p. 645, 1828.
[2] *Psalms,* xxxvii. 35, 36.
[3] Carpenter's *Script. Nat. Hist.*
[4] *Opera,* p. 267, 623, 621, &c., ed. Fœs.
[5] Royle, *Hindoo Med.* pp. 32 and 85.

axillary stalked. *Leaf-buds* with valvate papery scales. *Leaves* ever-green (*Lindley*).

Sp. Char.—The only species.

A *bush* or *small tree. Bark* aromatic, rather bitter. *Leaves* alternate, lanceolate, acute, or acuminate, wavy at the edge, somewhat coriaceous. *Flowers* yellowish. *Fruit* (called by Nees a 1-seeded flesh berry; by De Candolle, a drupe) bluish-black, oval, size of a small cherry. *Seed* pendulous; *funiculus* compressed, ascending from the base of the fruit, and attached at the top of the testa; *testa* papery; *tunica interna* very thin; *embryo* exalbuminous, composed of two large oleaginous *cotyledons* inclosing superiorly the *radicle.*

Hab.—South of Europe. Cultivated in gardens.

Description.—Bay leaves (*folia lauri*) have a bitter aromatic taste, and a somewhat aromatic odour. Their infusion reddens litmus. Dried bay berries (*baccæ lauri* offic.) are covered externally by a dark-brown brittle coat, which is produced by the epidermis and succulent covering of the fruit.

Composition.—In 1824 bay berries were analysed by Bonastre,[1] who found the constituents to be—*Volatile oil* 0·8, *laurin* 1·0, *fixed oil* 12·8, *wax* (stearin) 7·1, *resin* 1·6, *uncrystallisable sugar* 0·4, *gummy extractive* 17·2, *bassorin* 6·4, *starch* 25·9, *woody fibre* 18·8, *soluble albumen* traces, *an acid* 0·1, *water* 6·4, *salts* 1·5.—The ashes (amounting to 1·2) consisted of carbonate of potash and the carbonate and phosphate of lime.

1. Volatile Oil of Laurel Berries ; *Oil of Sweet Bay.*—Obtained from the berries by distillation with water. The crude oil is pale yellow, transparent, readily soluble in alcohol and ether. By redistillation it yields two isomeric oils ($C^{20}H^{16}O$) ; one having a sp. gr. of 0·857, the other 0·855, while a brown balsamic matter remains in the retort.[2]

2. Laurin ; *Camphor of the Bay Berry.*—A crystalline solid, fusible and volatile. Has an acrid bitter taste, and an odour analogous to that of the volatile oil. It is soluble in ether and in boiling alcohol. Sulphuric acid renders it yellow; nitric acid liquifies it. Alkalies are without action on it. It is extracted from bay berries by rectified alcohol.

3. Fixed Oil of Bays (see *post*).

Physiological Effects.—The berries, leaves, and oil, are said to possess aromatic, stimulant, and narcotic properties. The leaves, in large doses, prove emetic.[3]

Uses.—Bay berries or leaves are rarely, if ever, used in medicine in this country. They might, therefore, with great propriety be expunged from the Pharmacopœia. The leaves are employed by the cook on account of their flavour. Both leaves and berries have been used to strengthen the stomach, to expel flatus, and to promote the catamenial discharge.

Administration.—Both berries and leaves are used in the form of infusion.

OLEUM LAURI ; *Oleum Lauri expressum ; Oleum Laurinum ; Laurel Fat ; Oil of Bays.*—This may be obtained from either the fresh or dried berries. Duhamel[4] states that it is obtained from the fresh and ripe berries by bruising them in a mortar, boiling them for three hours in water, and then pressing them in a sack. The expressed oil is mixed with the decoction,

---

[1] *Journ. de Pharm.* x. 30.
[2] Brandes, *Pharmaceutisches Central-Blatt für* 1840, S. 344.
[3] Mérat and De Lens, *Dict. Univ. de Mat. Méd.* t. iv. p. 62.
[4] *Traité des Arbres et Arbustes qui se cultivent en France en pleine Terre,* t. i. p. 351.

on which, when cold, the butyraceous oil is found floating. From the dried berries it is procured by exposing them to the vapour of water until they are thoroughly soaked, and then rapidly subjecting them to the press between heated metallic plates. By the latter method they yield one-fifth of their weight of oil.[1] Oil of bays is imported in barrels from Trieste. In 1839, duty was paid on 1737 lbs. of it. It has a butyraceous consistence and a granular appearance. Its colour is greenish ; its odour is that of the berries. It is partially soluble in alcohol, completely so in ether. With alkalies it forms soaps. It is occasionally employed externally as a stimulating liniment in sprains and bruises, as well as in paralysis. It has also been used to relieve colic, and against deafness.[2] Its principal use, however, is in veterinary medicine.

OLEUM LAURI ÆTHEREUM NATIVUM ; *Native Oil of Laurel*, Hancock, Trans. of the Medico-Bot. Society of Lond. p. 18, 1826 ; *Laurel Turpentine*, Stenhouse, Mem. of the Chemical Society, vol. i. p. 45, 1843.—Imported from Demerara : obtained by incision in the bark of a large tree, called by the Spaniards "*Azeyte de Sassafras*," growing in the vast forests between the Orinoco and the Parime. By Dr. Hancock this tree was thought to belong to the nat. ord. Lauraceæ ; but Mr. Stenhouse thinks that it is a species of Pine. The oil is transparent, slightly yellow, and smells like turpentine, but more agreeable, and approaching to the oil of lemons. Its sp. gr. at 56° F. is 0·8645. The commercial oil consists of two or more oils isomeric with each other and with oil of turpentine, $C^{20}H^{16}$. Its yellow colour is due to a little resin. A volatile acid (formic acid ?) is also present in very small quantity. In its medicinal qualities it resembles turpentine ; being stimulant, diuretic, and diaphoretic. It has been used externally as a discutient in rheumatism, swellings of the joints, cold tumours, and paralytic disorders. It is an excellent solvent for caoutchouc.

151. NECTANDRA RODIÆI, *Schomburgk.*—THE BIBIRU OR GREENHEART TREE.

Sex. Syst. Dodecandria, Monogynia.

(Cortex.)

HISTORY.—In 1769, Bancroft[3] noticed the valuable quality of the wood of this tree, which he called the *Greenheart* or *Sipeira*. In 1834, Dr. Roder[4] discovered that the bark was a good substitute for cinchona, and that both it and the fruit contained an alkaloid, which he used with great success in intermittents : he terms the tree the *Bebeeru*, and the alkaloid *Bebeerine*. In 1843,[5] Dr. Douglas Maclagan published an account of the chemical and therapeutical properties of the bark, and confirmed the discoveries of Dr. Roder. The following year a full botanical description of the tree, which he terms *Bibiru* or *Sipiri*, was drawn up by Sir Robert Schomburgk, aided by Mr. Bentham.[6]

BOTANY.   Gen. Char.—*Flowers* hermaphrodite. *Calyx* 6-parted, rotate ; segments deciduous, the 3 outer rather the broadest. *Stamens* 12, in 4

---

[1] Soubeiran, *Nouveau Traité de Pharmacie*, t. ii. p. 32, 2de éd.
[2] Murray, *Apparatus Medicam.* vol. iv. p. 533.
[3] *Natural History of Guiana*, 1769.
[4] See the circular issued by Dr. Roder, and dated November 22, 1834 ; also, Sir Andrew Halliday's notice of Dr. Roder's discoveries, in the *Edinb. Med. and Surg. Journal*, vol. xliv. Oct. 1835.
[5] *Transactions of the Royal Society of Edinburgh*, vol. xv. p. 423, 1843.
[6] Hooker's *London Journal of Botany*, December 1844, p. 624.

series; the 9 outer fertile, the 3 inner sterile; glands in pairs, globose, sessile, at the base of the 3 inner fertile stamens; the anthers in the first and second series turned inwards, those of the third series turned outwards, all ovate, nearly sessile, with 4 cells arranged in a curve, and distinct from the tip of the anther, with as many ascending dehiscing valves; sterile stamens either tooth-shaped and biglandular at the base, or glandless, and then with a small ovule head. *Ovary* 1-celled, with 1 ovule in each cell. *Style* very short; *stigma* short and truncated. *Berry* 1-seeded, more or less immersed in the tube of the calyx changed into a truncated cup.—*Trees* of tropical America, with alternate, feather-veined *leaves,* and panicled or corymbose, axillary, lax, ample *flowers* (*Endlicher*).

Sp. Char.—[*Leaves* opposite, oblong, acute, entire, shining, undulated, about 5 inches long, with reverted margins, on short petioles. Inflorescence a cyma, generally axillary, appears at the equinoxes, each flower about 2 lines in diameter, on short peduncles, internally snow-white, and thickly studded with minute glands; has a strong jessamine odour. Specific character and synonymes not ascertained.—ED.] *Panicles* few-flowered, axillary, much shorter than the leaves, finely downy; *anthers* all thick oblong, without glands (*Bentham*).

A large forest *tree,* of 60 or more feet high, with a trunk frequently above 50 feet high, undivided by branches till near the top, and covered by an ash-grey smooth bark. *Leaves* 5 or 6 inches long, and 2 or 3 inches broad. *Flowers* yellowish-white. *Berry* somewhat obovate, globular, slightly compressed, the longer extension 7½ inches in circumference, the less about 6¼ inches: the pericarp greyish-brown, speckled with whitish dots, hard, very brittle, and about a line in thickness. *Seed* 1 in each fruit, about the size and shape of a walnut, and containing 2 large plano-convex cotyledons.

Hab.—British Guiana: on rocky hill-sides on the borders of rivers (the Essequibo, Cuyuni, Demerara, Pomeroon, and Berbice). [This tree is found in the greatest perfection immediately behind the alluvial soil of the coast and rivers, on clay hills but little elevated above the level of the ocean, and degenerates as it extends into the interior, till on the more elevated region of the Cinchonas it disappears. It seems almost peculiar to British Guiana.

The tree generally stands single, and rises on an erect cylindrical, gently tapering stem, to a height of 80 or 90 feet, to 40 or 50 without a branch, by a circumference of 9 or even 12 feet. It is recognised at a distance by its dense glossy foliage, and comparatively white trunk. On striking it with the edge of the cutlass, the bark flies like sandstone, and is very bitter.—ED.] The timber is used for ship-building, under the name of *Greenheart.*

[The wood is extremely strong, hard, and heavy, sinking in water, and taking a high polish. Neither the white ants on land, nor the Teredo in the water, affect it much; it has stood on wharves totally unprotected for sometimes thirty years in the tides-way. Its various shades of colour, from black to yellow, cannot be ascertained until the sapwood be cut through, which is invariably of a pale yellow colour. No difference in their botanical character or medicinal virtue has been observed. It appears to be of slow growth, for from the detritus accumulated around the old trees, and from the young trees in the formerly exhausted ground, having in seventy years scarcely attained the size of a spar (8 inches diameter), it is supposed that several hundred years would be required for its growth.—ED.]

DESCRIPTION.—*Bibiru* or *beeberu bark* (*cortex bibiru*) is derived from the trunk. It consists of large, flat, heavy pieces, from 1 to 2 feet long, from 2 to 6 inches broad, and about 3 or 4 lines thick. It is covered externally with a brittle greyish-brown epidermis. Internally its colour is dark cinnamon-brown. The fracture is rough and somewhat fibrous. The taste is strong, persistent, bitter, with considerable astringency, but with aroma, pungency, or acridity. [The bark is hard, heavy, and brittle, fracture short like sandstone, covered externally with a white exfoliating epidermis, and is of a bright cinnamon colour within; it adheres firmly to the tree, even when full of sap, requiring to be gently beaten so as to crush the liber or inner rind, when it can be parted in flat pieces of 6 to 12 inches square, and from ⅛ to ¼ of an inch thick. It has a very bitter taste.

On subjecting it to the process by which quinine is usually made, two alkaloids are obtained; and the term *bibirine* has been applied to them collectively. One of these only, when combined with slight excess of sulphuric acid, and the solution reduced to the consistence of syrup, *appeared* to form small acicular crystals, which could not be separated from the mass.

Its infusion, like that of the cinchonas, reddens litmus-paper, is clearer though darker-coloured than the latter, and deposits much less sediment on standing. Its productiveness, compared to that of yellow cinchonas, appears to be nearly as 3½ to 5. When long subjected to a boiling temperature (212°), or long contact with alkaline or caustic earthy substances, its bitterness is destroyed.—ED.]

The *fruit* (*fructus bibiru*), commonly called a nut, has been described above. The *seeds* (*semina bibiru*) yield starch, which is used as food by the Indians.[1] A section of the cotyledons, when moist and fresh, was of a pale yellow colour, and became brown by exposure to the air. The juice had an acid reaction, and was intensely bitter.

COMPOSITION.—The bark and seeds have been analysed by Dr. Maclagan, and his results are as follows :—

	Bark.	Seeds (much dried by keeping).
Alkalies [bibirina and sipirina] (not quite pure)	2·56	2·20
Tannic acid and resinous matter	2·53	4·04
Soluble matter (gum, sugar, and salts)	4·34	9·40
Starch	—	53·51
Fibre and vegetable albumen	62·92	11·24
Ashes (chiefly calcareous)	7·13	0·31
Water	14·07	18·13
Loss	6·45	1·17
Total	100·00	100·00

1. BIBIRINA; *Beebeerina; Biberine; Bebeerine*, $C^{35}H^{20}NO^6$.—Obtained by decomposing commercial sulphate of bibirina by ammonia: the precipitate is washed with cold water, triturated, while still moist, with moist hydrated oxide of lead, and the magma dried on a water-bath, and exhausted by rectified spirit. In this way is obtained an alcoholic solution of

---

[1] [The Indians, when their provisions fail, have from time immemorial used this nut as food (bread). They first break and part the shell from the kernel, which they then scrape and grate as they do cassava, throw the pulp into an open basket placed over a pail, and pour water over it so as to wash away the bitter; and this is repeated five times or oftener.

It is then *invariably* mixed with about one-third part its bulk of decayed wallaba (a wood containing tannic acid), powdered, and sifted; or a like quantity of cassada pulp put into the matappe or press, and the farinaceous substance thus expressed baked into bread.—ED.]

bibirina and sipirina, while the oxide of lead, tannic acid, and other impurities, are left behind. The alcohol is to be distilled off, and the resinous-looking residue treated with pure ether, which dissolves the bibirina, but leaves the sipirina.

Bibirina is uncrystallisable. When obtained by evaporation from its ethereal solution, it is a yellow, amorphous, resinous-looking substance; but in the form of powder it is white. It is very soluble in alcohol, less so in ether, and very sparingly in water. Its alcoholic solution reacts as an alkali on reddened litmus-paper. It dissolves in acids, and neutralises them, forming amorphous yellow salts. Colourless or crystallised salts have not yet been procured. According to Maclagan and Tilley,[1] its composition is identical with morphia. Winckler[2] says that bibirina resembles in many respects paracine, but it differs from the latter in the circumstance of its hydrate being gelatinous. [M. Planta has described a process for obtaining pure bibirine from the commercial sulphate. He describes it as a colourless inodorous powder, unalterable in the air, highly electric, and when ignited on platinum foil burning without leaving any carbonaceous residue. It melts at 355° F., and on cooling becomes a vitreous mass. Above this temperature it is decomposed, without being volatilised. It has a strong alkaline reaction, and completely neutralises the acids, forming uncrystallisable salts. It is very slightly soluble in water, but dissolves more readily in ether, and is soluble in alcohol in all proportions. The formula for bibirine, according to Planta, is $C^{38}H^{21}NO^6$. It is not, therefore, according to him, isomeric with morphia.[3]—ED.]

2. SIPIRINA; *Sipeerina; Sipirine; Sipeerine.*—This substance, which Dr. Maclagan at first thought to be a second alkaloid, he now regards as a product of the oxidation of bibirine.

3. BIBIRIC ACID; *Bebeeric Acid.* — A white, crystalline, deliquescent, volatile acid obtained from the seeds.

4. STARCH.—I am indebted to Dr. Maclagan for some of the starch obtained from the seeds of this plant. It is greyish-white, and almost tasteless. When examined by the microscope, it was found to consist of particles which were somewhat smaller than those of cassava starch, but in their external form quite agreed with the latter. Schomburgk states that the Indians are obliged to live for months on it. It is prepared by grating the seeds and immersing them in water. Repeated washing, he found, did not deprive the starch of its bitterness. The starch mixed with decayed wood, chiefly of the Wallaba tree (*Eperna falcata*), is baked into cakes. Winckler has discovered starch in the bark as well as in the seeds.

5. TANNIC ACID.—This agrees very much with that found in the cinchona bark; and, like the latter, it yields a green colour with the salts of iron.

PHYSIOLOGICAL EFFECTS.—Bibiru bark appears to possess the tonic, anti-periodic, febrifuge, and astringent properties of cinchona barks. Like the latter, its bitter, tonic, and antiperiodic powers reside in a vegetable alkaloid; and its astringent property in that kind of tannic acid which strikes a green colour with the salts of iron.

Sufficient experience has not yet been obtained with bibiru bark, and its alkaloid (*bibirine*), to enable us to form an accurate opinion of their thera-peutical power in comparison with cinchona bark and quinia. In some cases bibirina has appeared to produce its peptic and tonic effects with less tendency to cause headache, giddiness, ringing in the ears, and feverishness, than quinia; and it can in consequence be administered to some patients with whom quinia disagrees. On the other hand, it appears inferior to the latter in febrifuge and antiperiodic power. [Bebeerine, when properly administered, according to Mr. Rodie, generally cures intermittents when quinine has failed, seems not to affect the head, nor to produce its effects by counter-morbid action, as the alkaloids of the cinchonas are supposed to do.—ED.]

USES.—Bibiru bark and bibirina (in the form of sulphate) have been used

---

[1] *Pharmaceutical Journal,* vol. v. p. 228, 1845.

[2] *Ibid.* vol. vi. p. 493, 1847 ; also, Buchner's *Repert.* 2ter Reihe, Bd. xlvi. p. 231, 1846.

[3] *Ibid.* September 1851, p. 36.

as a peptic in anorexia and dyspepsia; as a general tonic in debility, protracted phthisis, and strumous affections; as a febrifuge in intermittent and remittent diseases; and as an antiperiodic in periodical headache and intermittent neuralgias.[1]

BIBIRINÆ SUBSULPHAS; *Bebeerinæ Sulphas; Sub-sulphate of Bibirine; Sulphate of Bebeerine.*—The process for obtaining this is essentially the same as that of the Edinburgh Pharmacopœia for sulphate of quinia. The bark is first boiled with a solution of carbonate of soda, to remove the tannic acid and colouring matter; it is boiled with water acidulated with sulphuric acid, by which sulphate of bibirine is obtained in solution. To the strained liquor carbonate of soda is added, and the impure bases thus thrown down washed, dissolved and neutralised with sulphuric acid, and the solution decolorised by animal charcoal, concentrated, filtered, and finally evaporated in flat open vessels; excess of acid being avoided in order to prevent charring on evaporation.

There are two compounds of sulphuric acid and bibirina,—the sulphate ($BiSO^3$) and sub-sulphate (Bi^2SO^3): the latter is the commercial salt which has been prepared for medicinal use by Mr. Macfarlane, of Edinburgh:—

	Maclagan (Trans. Royal Soc. Edinb.)		*Macfarlane's* *basic commercial sulphate.*
Bibirina	86·39		90·83
Sulphuric acid	13·61		9·17
Neutral sulphate of bibirina ...	100·00	Sub-sulphate of bibirina	100·00

The sub-sulphate of bibirina (Macfarlane's basic commercial sulphate of beeberine) is not absolutely pure. It contains sub-sulphate of sipirina, sulphate of lime, and colouring matter. It occurs in brownish-yellow, thin, glittering scales, which form a yellow powder, and by incineration leave a mere trace of ash only. It has a very persistent bitter taste. It is soluble in alcohol. It is slightly soluble in cold water, with which it yields a turbid solution, partly from the excess of base, partly from the decomposing tendency of the sipirina. Its solution in water is rendered more complete by a few drops of sulphuric acid. Its effects and uses have already been alluded to.

It may be administered in doses of from one to three grains as a tonic, and from five to twenty grains as a febrifuge. In substance it is given in the form of pill, made with conserve of roses; and in solution with dilute sulphuric acid. The following is given as a convenient form for its exhibition as a tonic:—Sub-sulphate of Bibirine, ʒss.; Diluted Sulphuric Acid, ℥xxv.; Syrup, ʒj.; Tincture of Orange-peel, ʒj.; Water, ℥iv. Dose, one tablespoonful three times a day.

It has been recommended as an economical substitute for quina; its price being about 6s. per ounce, while disulphate of quina has been lately more than double that price.

---

[1] For further information respecting the therapeutical value of bibiru bark and bibirina, the reader is referred to Dr. Maclagan's papers on this subject in the *Trans. of the Royal Society of Edinburgh*, vol. xv. 1843; Cormack's *Lond. and Edinb. Monthly Journal of Medical Science* for August 1843; and the *Edinb. Med. and Surg. Journal*, No. 163. In these papers will be found the observations not only of Dr. Maclagan, but also of Drs. Rodie and Watt of Demerara, Drs. Bennett and Simpson of Edinburgh, and of several army medical officers serving in the East Indies.

Order XXXVI. MYRISTICACEÆ, *Lindley.*—NUTMEGS.

Myristiceæ, *R. Brown.*

CHARACTERS.—*Flowers* completely unisexual. *Calyx* trifid, rarely quadrifid; with valvular æstivation. *Males:—Filaments* either separate, or completely united in a cylinder. *Anthers* 3 to 12, 2-celled, turned outwards, and bursting longitudinally; either connate or distinct. *Females:—Calyx* deciduous. *Ovary* superior, sessile, with a single erect ovule; *style* very short; *stigma* somewhat lobed. *Fruit* baccate, dehiscent, 2-valved. *Seed* nut-like; *albumen* ruminate, between fatty and fleshy; *embryo* small; *cotyledons* foliaceous; *radicle* inferior; *plumule* conspicuous.—*Tropical trees*, often yielding a red juice. *Leaves* alternate, without stipules, not dotted, quite entire, stalked, coriaceous; usually, when full-grown, covered beneath with a close down. *Inflorescence* axillary or terminal, in racemes, glomerules, or panicles; the *flowers* often each with one short cucullate bract. *Calyx* coriaceous, mostly downy outside, with the hairs sometimes stellate, smooth in the inside (*Lindley*, from R. Brown chiefly).

PROPERTIES.—The bark and pericarp contain an acrid juice. The seed (?) and arilloid abound in an aromatic volatile oil, which is mixed with a fixed oil.

152. MYRISTICA FRAGRANS, *Houtt.*—THE TRUE NUTMEG TREE.

Sex. Syst. Diœcia, Monadelphia.

(Semen putamine nudatum. Oleum e semine expressum concretum, *L.*—Kernel of the fruit; volatile oil from the kernel; concrete expressed oil from the kernel, *E.*—The kernel of the fruit, *D.*)

SYNONYMES.—*Myristica fragrans*, Houttuyn, Nat. Hist. (1774), vol. ii. part iii. p. 333; Blume, Rumphia, i. 180, 1835; *M. officinalis*, L., Linn. (1781); Hooker, Bot. Mag. vol. i. N. S. tab. 2756 and 2757; *M. moschata*, D., Thunberg (1782); *M. aromatica*, Lamarck (1788).

HISTORY.—Both nutmegs and mace[1] were unknown to the ancient Greeks and Romans,—unless, indeed, the nutmeg be the aromatic Arabian fruit used in unguents, and which Theophrastus[2] calls κώμακον. Pliny[3] says that the *cinnamum quod comacum appellant* is the expressed juice of a nut produced in Syria. Does he refer to the expressed oil of nutmeg, as some have suggested? Both mace and nutmegs are referred to by Avicenna.[4]

The modern Greek names for the nutmeg and mace are respectively μοσχοκάρυα and μοσχομάκερ.

BOTANY. **Gen. Char.**—*Anthers* united throughout their whole length into a cylindrical column. *Stigma* emarginate, somewhat 2-lobed. *Cotyledons* folded (*Blume*).

Sp. Char.—Leaves oblong, subacute at the base, smooth. Peduncles axillary, few-flowered. Calyx urceolate. Fruit nodding, obovoid, globose, smooth (*Blume*).

A *tree* from 20 to 25 feet high, similar in appearance to a pear tree. *Bark* dark greyish-green, smooth, with a yellowish juice. *Leaves* aromatic.

---

[1] The μάκερ of Dioscorides (lib. i. cap. 110), the *macir* of Pliny (lib. xii. cap. 16), was an astringent bark, and not, as some have supposed, our mace.

[2] *Hist. Plant.* lib. ix. cap. 7. Fraas (*Syn. Plant. Fl. classicæ*, p. 135, 1835) considers κώμακον to be our nutmeg.

[3] *Hist. Nat.* lib. xii. cap. 63, ed. Valp.

[4] Lib. ii. tract. ii. cap. 436 and 503.

Racemes axillary. *Peduncles* and *pedicels* glabrous, the latter with a quickly deciduous ovate *bract* at its summit, often pressed close to the flower. *Flowers* usually diœcious, sometimes monœcious. *Males:*—3 to 5 on a peduncle ; *calyx* fleshy, pale yellow, with a reddish pubescence. *Females:*—scarcely different from the males, except that the pedicel is frequently solitary. *Fruit* pyriform, smooth externally, about the size of a peach, marked by a longitudinal groove. *Pericarp* fleshy, dehiscing by two nearly equal longitudinal valves. *Arillode*[1] (false aril), commonly called *mace*, large, fleshy, branching, scarlet ; when dry, yellow, brittle, and somewhat horny. *Seed* (*nutmeg in the shell*, offic.) within the arilloid, oval or ovate : its outer coat (*testa, tunica externa*, or *shell*) is dark brown, hard, glossy ; its inner coat (*endopleura* seu *tunica interna*) closely invests the seed, and dips down into the substance of the albumen, giving it a marbled or *ruminated* appearance. The *nucleus* or *nut* (the *round* or *true nutmeg* of the shops) consists chiefly of the oleaginous *albumen ;* the so-called veins of which are processes of the endopleura, which have a reddish-brown colour, and abound in oil ; the *embryo* is at the base of the seed ; *radicle* inferior, hemispherical ; *cotyledons* 2, large, flat, foliaceous, fan-shaped ; *plumule* 2-lobed.

Hab.—Molucca islands, especially the group called the Banda or Nutmeg isles.[2] Cultivated in Java, Sumatra, Penang (Prince of Wales Island), Singapore, Bengal, Bourbon islands, Madagascar, and some parts of the West Indies.[3]

MYRISTICA FATUA, Houtt., Blume ; *M. tomentosa*, Thunberg ; *M. dactyloides*, Gærtn. (the synonymes excluded) ; *Nux moschata fructu oblongo*, C. Bauh. ; *Nux myristica mas*, Clusius.—A native of the Banda isles.—Fruit elongated, ellipsoidal, rusty, tomentose. Seed elongated, ellipsoidal, covered by a membranaceo-fleshy, orange-coloured, insipid arilloid (mace) ; outer coat (*testa*) dark brown, hard ; nucleus acerb, slightly aromatic, greyish ash-coloured, cylindrical, ellipsoidal, rugous, marked by a furrow. Yields the *long nutmeg* of the shops.

Closely allied to this is the M. MALABARICA, Lam., or *Malabar Nutmeg ;* it is the *Panam-pálca* of Rheede (Hist. Malab. part iv. tab. 5). The latter authority says that the nucleus resembles the *date* in size and figure. Unlike the male or long nutmeg, it has scarcely any flavour or odour. Rheede adds that "the Turkish and Jewish merchants mix these nutmegs with the true long ones, and the mace with good mace, selling them together. They also extract from these inferior articles an oil, with which they adulterate that of a more genuine quality." The Malabar nutmeg, according to Rheede, differs from the long nutmegs in size, hardness, and especially in flavour.

---

[1] The laciniate envelope of the nutmeg, usually called the aril, and which constitutes the substance called *mace*, is said by M. Plauchon to be nothing but an expansion of the exostome, and, therefore, an *arillode* or *false aril.*

[2] The Dutch endeavoured to confine the growth of the nutmeg to three of the Banda isles ; viz. Lantoir or Banda proper, Banda-Neira, and Way (Pulo Ay) ; but their attempts were partly frustrated by a pigeon, called the *nutmeg bird* or *nut-eater* (a species of *Carpophaga*), which, extracting the nutmeg from its pulpy pericarp, digests the mace, but voids the nutmeg in its shell, which, falling in a suitable situation, readily germinates. Young plants thus obtained are used for transplanting into the *nutmeg parks.* During the time that the English had possession of the Molucca islands (namely, from 1796 to 1802 ; and again from 1810 to 1814), they exported plants to Bencoolen in Sumatra, to Penang, India, and other places. In 1819, the nutmeg tree was sent from Bencoolen to Sumatra, where it is now largely cultivated. (For a sketch of the culture and trade in nutmegs, and of the monopolising policy of the Dutch, the reader is referred to Crawford's *History of the Indian Archipelago*, vol. i. p. 505 ; vol. ii. p. 437 ; vol. iii. p. 406). To keep up the price of this spice, the Dutch used to burn nutmegs when the crops were superabundant ! (See Hooker's *Bot. Mag.* vol. i. N. S. 1827, t. 2756-7 ; also Stephenson and Churchill's *Med. Bot.* vol. iii. pl. 104.)

[3] [The reader will find an interesting account of the cultivation of nutmegs at Bencoolen and Singapore, in the *Pharmaceutical Journal* for May 1852, p. 516-20.—ED.]

CURING.—In the Banda isles there are three harvests annually; namely, the principal one in July or August, the second in November, and the third in March or April. The ripe fruit is gathered by means of a barb attached to a long stick; the mace separated from the nut, and both separately cured.

Mace is prepared for the market by drying it for some days in the sun. Some flatten it by the hands in single layers; others cut off the heels, and dry the mace in double blades.[1] In rainy weather artificial heat is employed for drying it. At first the mace is crimson or blood-red, but after a few months acquires the golden colour preferred by the dealers.[2] The Dutch sprinkle the mace with salt water prior to packing it in the sacks called *sokkol*.[3]

Nutmegs require more care in curing, on account of their liability to the attacks of an insect (the *nutmeg insect*). It is necessary to have them well and carefully dried in their shells, as in this state they are secure from the attack of this insect.[4] In order to effect this, they are placed on hurdles or gratings, and smoke-dried for about two months by a slow wood-fire, at a heat not exceeding 140° F. (In the Banda isles they are first sun-dried for a few days.) When thoroughly dried, the nuts rattle in the shells, which are then cracked with wooden mallets, and the worm-eaten and shrivelled nuts thrown out.

To prevent the attacks of the insect, the nuts are frequently limed. For the English market, however, the brown or unlimed nutmegs are preferred. The Dutch lime them by dipping them into a thick mixture of lime and water; but this process is considered to injure their flavour. Others lime them by rubbing them with recently-prepared well-sifted lime. This process is sometimes practised in London.

After being garbled, the nutmegs are packed for transportation in tight casks, the insides of which have been smoked and covered with a coating of fresh water and lime. Newbold says the unlimed nutmegs are mixed with cloves.

The dried produce of a nutmeg tree consists of nutmeg, mace, and shell, in the following proportions:—In 15 parts of the whole produce there are 2 parts of mace, 5 of shell, and 8 of nutmegs. Hence, although nutmegs in the shell may keep better than the clean or shelled nutmegs, yet the heavy allowance required for the shell (viz. about one-third) is a serious objection to their preservation in this form.

DESCRIPTION. 1. **Of Nutmegs** (*Nuces moschatæ*). — In commerce two kinds of nutmegs are met with; one called the *true* or *round*, the other the *long* or *wild*.

a. True or Round Nutmeg; the *female nutmeg; nux myristica fæmina,* Clusius; *nux moschata fructu rotundo,* C. Bauh.—This sort is the produce of Myristica fragrans. It is about an inch in length. Its shape is roundish or elliptical, like that of the French olive. Externally it is marked with reticular furrows. The colour of the *unlimed* or *brown* nut-

---

[1] Newbold, *Polit. and Statist. Account of the British Settlements in the Straits of Malacca,* vol. i. 1839.

[2] Oxley, *Some Account of the Nutmeg and its Cultivation,* in the *Journal of the Indian Archipelago and Eastern Asia,* October 1848, p. 641, Singapore.

[3] C. B. Valentini, *Indiæ Literatæ,* Epist. xxv., contained in M. B. Valentini's *Historia Simplicium reform.* 1716.

[4] Crawford, *Hist. of the Ind. Archip.*

megs is ashy-brown; that of *limed* nutmegs is brown on the projecting parts, and white (from the presence of lime) in the depressions. Internally, nutmegs are pale reddish-grey, with red veins. The odour is strong, but pleasant, peculiar, and aromatic. The taste is agreeable and aromatic.

FIG. 175.

Occasionally the round nutmeg is imported *in the shell.* This is dark and shiny.

A very small nutmeg, not larger than a pea, has been described under the name of the *royal nutmeg* (*nux moschata regia*).

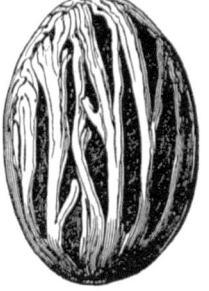

In the London market the following are the sorts of round nutmegs distinguished by the dealers :—

1. *Penang nutmegs.*—These are unlimed or brown nutmegs, and fetch the highest price. They are sometimes limed here for exportation, as on the Continent the limed sort is preferred. According to Newbold, the average amount annually raised at Penang is 400 piculs (of 133½ lbs. each) : [but it is considered to be much greater at the present time,—probably five times the quantity here stated.—ED.]

True or Round Nutmeg in the shell, surrounded by its mace (from a specimen preserved wet).

2. *Dutch or Batavian nutmegs.*—These are limed nutmegs. In London they scarcely fetch so high a price as the Penang sort.

3. *Singapore nutmegs.*—These are a rougher, unlimed, narrow sort, of somewhat less value than the Dutch kind. According to Mr. Oxley, 4,085,361 nutmegs were produced at Singapore in 1848, or about 252 piculs (of 133½ lbs. each); but the greater number of the trees had not come into full bearing, and it was estimated that the amount would, in 1849, be 500 piculs.

β. *Long or Wild Nutmegs ;*[1] the *male nutmeg ; nux myristica mas,* Clusius ; *nux moschata fructu oblongo,* C. Bauhin.—This is the produce of Myristica fatua. It is met with in commerce in three forms :— in the shelled or clean state (*long* or *wild nutmegs*), contained within the shell (*long* or *wild nutmegs in the shell*), and with the mace dried around them (*long* or *wild nutmegs covered with mace*).

FIG. 176.

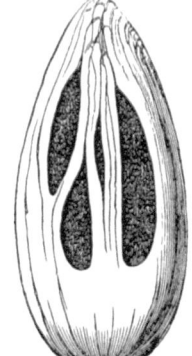

The long or wild nutmeg in the shell in shape is oblong, like that of the date; its length about an inch and a half. The shell is bony, somewhat brittle, externally shiny and brown, internally dull greyish-white. The contained seed is paler-coloured and less aromatic than in the preceding sort. Some specimens are almost insipid. Are these the *Malabar wild nutmegs* before referred to (see *ante,* p. 471)? The mace which is sometimes found in the long nutmeg is insipid.

Long or Wild Nutmeg in the shell, surrounded by its mace (from a dry commercial specimen).

2. **Of Mace** (*Macis*).—Two kinds of mace are found in commerce; one called *true* or *genuine,* the other *wild* or *false.*

α. *True* or *genuine mace.*—This is the produce of the round or true nutmeg. It occurs in single or double blades, flat, irregularly slit, smooth,

---

[1] Sir J. E. Smith (Rees's *Cyclopædia*) says that in 1797 they were received from Banda under the name of *New Guinea nutmegs.* A specimen of the fruit and leaves, preserved in spirit in the Banksian Collection, is marked the *long nutmeg from Sumatra.*

slightly flexible or brittle membrane, of a pale cinnamon-yellow or golden-yellow colour, and an odour and taste analogous to those of nutmegs. Although the natural colour of mace is red, yet red-coloured mace is looked on suspiciously.

The London dealers distinguish three sorts of genuine mace :—

1. *Penang mace.*—This fetches the highest price. It is flaky and spread. The annual quantity produced in Penang is about 130 piculs (of 133⅓ lbs. each).

2. *Dutch or Batavian mace.*—This is a fleshy sort. It scarcely fetches so high a price as the Penang sort.

3. *Singapore mace.*—This is a somewhat inferior kind.

β. *Wild or false mace.*—This is a dark red mace, the produce of the long or wild nutmeg, and is also devoid of aromatic flavour.   [It has a very strong coarse flavour, although not like that of mace.—Ed.]

[Commerce.—The quantity of mace and nutmegs annually imported during a period of seven years was as follows :—

	Mace.	*Nutmegs.*
1844	33,898 lbs.	152,110 lbs.
1845	35,551 „	444,706 „
1846	33,104 „	405,679 „
1847	60,265 „	367,936 „
1848	47,572 „	336,420 „
1849	45,978 „	224,021 „
1850	76,365 „	312,418 „ —Ed.]

Composition.—Nutmegs were analysed in 1823 by Bonastre.[1]   In 1824 an analysis of mace was made by N. E. Henry.[2]

NUTMEG.		MACE.
Bonastre's Analysis.		*N. E. Henry's Analysis.*
Volatile oil	6·0	Volatile oil.
Liquid fat	7·6	Red fat oil soluble in alcohol.
Solid fat	24·0	Yellow fat oil insoluble in alcohol.
Acid (?)	0·8	Alcoholic extractive.
Starch	2·4	Amidin.
Gum	1 2	Ligneous fibre with lime.
Ligneous fibre	54·0	
Loss	4·0	
Nutmeg	100·0	Mace.

The *volatile oils* and the *fats* will be noticed hereafter, as they are employed in medicine. The *starch* occurs in small compound grains.

Chemical Characteristics.—The presence of starch in both nutmegs and mace may be detected by a solution of iodine, which gives them a blue tint (*iodide of starch*). Both of these substances yield, by distillation with water, *a volatile oil*, characterised by its peculiar odour ; and both yield by expression a *fixed butyraceous oil*.

Physiological Effects.—The activity of both nutmegs and mace depends on the volatile oil which they contain. Swallowed *in moderate quantities*, they produce the before-described effects of the spices (see Vol. 1). *In large doses* they prove narcotic, and cause giddiness, delirium, præcordial anxiety, sleepiness, or actual stupor. Instances of this kind are mentioned

---

[1] *Journ. de Pharm.* t. ix. p. 281, 1823.
[2] *Ibid.* t. x. p. 281, 1824.

by Bontius,[1] Rumphius,[2] Lobel,[3] Schmid,[4] and Cullen.[5] In the case related by the last-mentioned authority, two drachms of powdered nutmegs produced drowsiness, which gradually increased to complete stupor and insensibility. The patient continued for several hours alternately delirious and sleeping, but ultimately recovered. Purkinje[6] has confirmed these statements by experiments made on himself. I am acquainted with a case in which the narcotic effects of a whole nutmeg have been several times experienced.

Uses.—The principal consumption of nutmegs and mace is for dietetical purposes. They serve to flavour, and, by their stimulant properties, to assist the digestive process. Food highly seasoned with these substances may prove injurious in cerebral affections (apoplexy, for example), on account of their narcotic properties.

Medicinally they are used, like other spices, as stimulants, carminatives, and flavouring ingredients. Nutmeg is an important constituent in the *confectio aromatica* so frequently employed as a cordial and antacid in bowel complaints. In mild cases of diarrhœa I have frequently employed nutmeg as a substitute for opium. It may be taken in warm brandy and water, unless the use of spirit be contraindicated.

Administration.—Either nutmeg or mace may be taken to the extent of a scruple or half a drachm, in powder obtained by grating; or the volatile oil of these substances may be used in doses of ℥j. to ℥v.

1. **OLEUM MYRISTICÆ**, L. E.; *Oleum Nucis Moschatæ; Oleum Nucistæ æthereum; Essential Oil of Nutmeg.* (Procured by submitting Nutmegs and Water to distillation.)—The usual produce of volatile oil in the distillations at Apothecaries' Hall, London, is 4·5 per cent.; but the oil is generally imported. It is colourless or pale yellow, has the odour and taste of nutmegs, and a viscid consistence. By agitation with water it separates into two oils,— one lighter, the other heavier than water. By keeping, it deposits crystals of stéaroptène (*myristicine*), which are fusible at 212° F., volatile, soluble in alcohol, in ether, and in boiling water: from the latter liquid myristicine is separated in a crystalline form as the liquid cools. According to Mulder, the stéaroptène consists of $C^{16}H^{16}O^5$. Volatile oil of nutmegs is seldom employed medicinally. Its dose is ℥j. to ℥v., taken on sugar or dissolved in spirit. [According to Mitscherlich, the volatile oil of nutmegs is a strong poison, affecting the heart and lungs, and producing death without convulsions.[7]—Ed.]

2. **OLEUM MACIDIS**; *Essential Oil of Mace.*—This is colourless or of a pale yellow colour, lighter than water, and has the flavour and odour of mace. Its composition, effects, and uses are similar to those of nutmegs.

3. **MYRISTICÆ ADEPS**, E.; *Myristicæ Oleum expressum*, L.;[8] *Oleum*

---

[1] *De Med. Indor.*
[2] *Herb. Amboyn.* vol. ii. p. 21.
[3] Quoted by Murray, *App. Med.* vol. vi. p. 145.
[4] *Ibid.*
[5] *Mat. Med.* vol. ii. p. 204.
[6] Quoted by Wibmer, *Die Wirk. d. Arzneim. u. Gifte*, Bd. iii. S. 308.
[7] [*Pharmaceutical Journal*, January 1851, p. 350.]
[8] This oil is used in the preparation of *Emplastrum Picis*. The Edinburgh College has committed an error respecting it; for while in the list of Materia Medica it is called *Myristicæ Adeps*, in the formula for the preparation of Emplastrum Picis it is termed *Oil of Mace*.

vel *Balsamum Nucistæ; Butter of Nutmegs; Expressed* or *Concrete Oil of Nutmegs.*—In the shops it is usually denominated *expressed oil of mace.* It is prepared by beating the nutmegs to a paste (which is to be inclosed in a bag, and then exposed to the vapour of water), and afterwards expressing by heated plates. It is imported in oblong cakes (covered by some monocotyledonous leaves, commonly called *flag leaves*), which have the shape of common bricks, but whose size is somewhat smaller. Its colour is orange, its consistence firm, its odour fragrant, like that of the seeds from which it is obtained. In 1804 it was examined by Schrader,[1] who found that 16 parts of concrete oil, expressed by himself, consisted of 1 part of volatile oil, 6 parts of brownish-yellow fat, and 9 parts of white fat. In 16 parts of the commercial concrete oil he found $\frac{2}{3}$ volatile oil, $8\frac{1}{3}$ yellow fat, and 7 parts of white fat. The volatile oil and yellow fat are soluble in both cold alcoho and cold ether. The white fat (known by the name of *corpus pro balsamis,* or *mater balsamorum*) is soluble in boiling alcohol and boiling ether, but is insoluble in cold alcohol and ether. It has been more recently examined by Dr. L. Playfair,[2] who calls it *myristine* (formerly *sericine*). By saponification it yields glycerine and myristic acid ($C^{28}H^{27}O^3,HO$). Playfair mentions a false butter of nutmegs, composed of animal fat, boiled with powdered nutmegs, and flavoured with sassafras. The specimen may be relied on as pure, if it dissolve in four times its weight of strong boiling alcohol, or half that quantity of ether.

Expressed oil of nutmegs is occasionally employed externally in chronic rheumatism and palsy. It is a constituent of *Emplastrum Picis.*

4. SPIRITUS MYRISTICÆ, L. E.; *Spirit of Nutmeg.* (Nutmegs, bruised, ʒiiss.; Proof Spirit, Cong. j.; Water, Oj. Mix them, then [with a slow fire, *L.*] let a gallon distil.)—It is frequently prepared by mixing volatile oil of nutmegs with proof spirit. It is cordial and carminative, and is employed, in doses of fʒj. to fʒiv., as a pleasant addition to stimulant, narcotic, or purgative draughts.

5. ESSENTIA MYRISTICÆ MOSCHATÆ, D. (Oil of Nutmeg, fʒj.; Stronger Spirit, fʒix. Mix with agitation.)

ORDER XXXVII. THYMELACEÆ, *Lindl.*—DAPHNADS.

THYMELEÆ, *Jussieu.*—DAPHNOIDEÆ, *Endl.*

CHARACTERS.—*Calyx* inferior, tubular, coloured; the limb 4-cleft, seldom 5-cleft, with an imbricated æstivation. *Corolla* 0, or sometimes scale-like petals in the orifice of the calyx. *Stamens* definite, inserted in the tube or its orifice, often 8, sometimes 4, less frequently 2; when equal in number to the segments of the calyx, or fewer, opposite to them; *anthers* 2-celled, dehiscing lengthwise in the middle. Ovary composed of a single carpel, with 1 solitary pendulous anatropal ovule; *style* 1; *stigma* undivided. *Fruit* hard, dry, and nut-like, or drupaceous. *Albumen* 0, or thin and fleshy; *embryo* straight; *cotyledons* plano-convex, sometimes lobed and crumpled; *radicle* short, superior; *plumule* inconspicuous.—*Stem* shrubby, very seldom herbaceous; with tenacious bark. *Leaves*

[1] *Berlinisches Jahrbuch für d. Pharmacie,* 1804, p. 83.
[2] *Lond. Ed. Dub. Phil. Mag.* vol. xviii. p. 102, 1841; and *Ann. de Chim. et de Phys.* 3me sér. t. iii. p. 228, 1841.

without stipules, alternate or opposite, entire. *Flowers* capitate or spiked, terminal or axillary, occasionally solitary, sometimes unisexual by abortion, often inclosed in an involucre (*R. Brown*, with some additions).

PROPERTIES.—The prevailing property of the plants of this Order is acridity. This depends on a principle contained in the bark and pericarp. The liber of many species is remarkably tough, and is applied to various useful purposes; as for making ropes, whips, and a kind of cloth.—The LAGETTA LINTEARIA, or the *Lace Bark Tree*, which possesses the medicinal properties of mezereon, and has been used in the same cases,[1] is provided with a bark which may be separated into 20, 30, or more laminæ, which are fine and white, like gauze; and of these, caps, ruffles, and even whole suits of ladies' clothes, have been made.[2] Some few years since, a quantity of the stiffened lagetta cloth was imported into Liverpool under the name of *guana*.

153. DAPHNE MEZEREUM, *Linn.*—COMMON MEZEREON OR SPURGE-OLIVE.

Sex. Syst. Octandria, Monogynia.

(Radicis cortex, *L.*—Root-bark, *E. D.*)

HISTORY.—Tragus[3] is the earliest author who mentions this plant.[4]   He calls it *Thymelæa*. The *Mezereon* of Avicenna,[5] and of other Arabian authors, is declared by C. Bauhin to be *Chamelæa tricocca* (now called *Cneorum tricoccon*), a plant of the order Euphorbiaceæ; but it is probably identical with the χαμελαία of Dioscorides, which is stated by Sibthorp[6] and Fraas[7] to be *Daphne oleoides*.

BOTANY. **Gen. Char.**—*Flowers* hermaphrodite. *Calyx* funnel-shaped; limb in 4 segments; throat without scales. *Stamina* 8, inclosed within the tube, inserted in 2 rows near the throat. Hypogynous *scales* 0. *Ovary* 1-celled. *Style* terminal, very short; *stigma* capitate. *Drupe* baccate, 1-seeded, naked, with a crustaceous putamen or stone. *Seed* inverted.; *albumen* 0 ; *embryo* orthotropal ; *cotyledons* plano-convex (*Endlicher*).

Sp. Char.—*Flowers* naked on the stem, sessile, about 3 together. *Leaves* lanceolate, deciduous (*Smith*).

Stem bushy, 4 or 5 feet high, with upright, alternate, smooth, tough, and pliant branches ; leafy while young. *Leaves* scattered, stalked, lanceolate, smooth, 2 inches long, appearing after the flowers, and soon accompanied by flower-buds for the next season. *Flowers* highly, and to many persons too powerfully, fragrant, seated in little tufts on the naked branches, with several brown, smooth, ovate bracteas underneath. *Calyx* like a corolla in texture, crimson all over; the tube externally hairy. *Berries* scarlet.

Hab.—Indigenous. Plentiful near Andover. Flowers in March.   Collected for medicinal purposes in Kent and Hampshire.

Var. *flore albo* has white flowers and yellow fruit.
Var. *autumnale* has larger leaves, and flowers in the autumn.

DESCRIPTION OF THE BARK.—The *root-bark* (*cortex radicis mezerei*) is alone employed in this country.   It is tough, pliable, and when dry

---

[1] Wright's *Med. Plants of Jamaica.*
[2] Sloane's *Nat. Hist. of Jamaica*, vol. ii. p. 22.
[3] *Hist. Stirpium*, 1532.
[4] Sprengel, *Hist. Rei Herb.* Præf. xi.
[5] Lib. 2ndus, tract. 2ndus, cap. 464.
[6] *Prod. Fl. Græcæ.*
[7] *Synops. Plant. Fl. Classicæ*, 1845.

fibrous; externally brown and corrugated; internally white, tough, and cottony. It occurs in strips of several inches long. When chewed, the taste is at first sweetish; afterwards an acrid burning sensation is felt in the mouth and fauces, and extends to the gullet and stomach if the bark and saliva be swallowed. This sensation continues for several hours. The odour of the fresh root is faint, but marked.

The *stem-bark* (*cortex caudicis* vel *caulis mezerei*) is usually considered to be somewhat less active than the root-bark; but in the Dublin, United States, and most of the continental Pharmacopœias, the bark of both root and stem is included under the general name of *mezereon bark* (*cortex mezerei*). The stem-bark, in the fresh state, is externally somewhat darker and rougher than the root-bark; but it is most readily recognised, in the fresh state, by the green colour of the cellular integument beneath the epidermis.

In Germany the bark of the stem and larger branches is removed in spring, folded in small bundles, and dried for medicinal use. It is imported from Hamburgh. I have been informed that the root-bark commands nearly three times the price of the stem-bark. The bark is stripped from the crushed roots while fresh and soft. Sometimes the entire root (bark and wood) of mezereum is used instead of the root-bark: but this proceeding is highly objectionable, as the wood possesses only a feeble acridity.

The bark of other species of *Daphne* (as of *D. Gnidium* and *D. Laureola*) is said to be sometimes substituted for that of the mezereon.

Mr. Squire[1] states that

13¾ lbs. of fresh mezereon ⎱ 3¼ lbs. of wood.
    root produced by drying ⎰ 3½ lbs. of bark, dry; equivalent to 8½ lbs. of fresh bark.
3 lbs. of stems produced ¾ lb. of dried bark.

COMPOSITION.—The bark of the stem was analysed by C. G. Gmelin and Bär,[2] and found to consist of *wax, an acrid resin, daphnin*, a trace of *volatile oil, yellow colouring principle, uncrystallisable but fermentable sugar, nitrogenous gummy matter, reddish-brown extractive, woody fibre, free malic acid*, with the *malates of potash, lime*, and *magnesia*.

1. ACRID RESIN.—Obtained by boiling the bark in alcohol: when the solution cools, some wax is deposited. The supernatant liquid is to be evaporated, and the residual extract washed with water. The resin then left behind is dark green, and soluble in both alcohol and ether. To this substance mezereon owes its acridity. There is, however, some reason to suspect that this resin is itself a compound of two principles, viz. an acrid, vesicating, fixed oil, and another substance. The resin is rendered soluble in water by means of the other constituents of the bark. Mr. Squire could not obtain any blistering effect from the resin extracted by alcohol.

2. DAPHNIN.—A peculiar crystalline principle, having a bitter, slightly astringent taste. It is soluble in alcohol and ether, but possesses neither basic nor acid properties. Gmelin and Bär consider it to be analogous to asparagin. It is not the active principle of mezereon.

3. ACRID VOLATILE OIL?—According to Mr. Squire, mezereon contains a volatile acrid substance which is carried off by the vapour of water, but not by the vapour of alcohol. He says that "the pungent odour given off by boiling mezereon root in water over a lamp is so powerful, that, after holding my head over it for a short time, great irritation was produced, and it was difficult to carry on respiration."

PHYSIOLOGICAL EFFECTS.—All parts of the plant, but more especially the

---

[1] *Pharmaceutical Journal*, vol. i. p. 395, 1842.
[2] L. Gmelin, *Handb. d. Chem.* Bd. ii. S. 1317.

bark and the fruit, are endowed with excessive acridity ; in virtue of which they cause irritation and inflammation in tissues to which they are applied. When swallowed, therefore, in large quantities, they prove poisonous. The topical action of mezereon bark is that of an irritant, and, when the bark has been applied to the skin, vesicant.

A decoction of mezereon bark, taken in moderate quantities, sometimes appears to promote the action of the secreting and exhaling organs (especially the kidneys and the skin). But Dr. Alex. Russell[1] could not observe, upon the strictest inquiry, " that it sensibly increased any of the secretions, more than the same quantity of any small liquor would do." In some cases it proves laxative, where the patients are easily moved, and large doses disturb and irritate the stomach. Richter[2] says that under the long-continued use of mezereon the saliva acquires a peculiar odour. In larger doses it causes dryness and heat in the throat, increased saliva, pain in the stomach and bowels, and sometimes vomiting and purging,—the stools being occasionally bloody. The urinary organs are sometimes specifically affected by it ; irritation, analogous to that produced by cantharides, being set up by it. An affection of the cerebro-spinal system (marked by great feebleness, giddiness, incapability of keeping the erect posture, and slight convulsive movements) is occasionally brought on.[3] I am unacquainted with any cases which have proved fatal from the use of mezereon bark. Vicat[4] mentions the case of a dropsical patient in whom the wood caused diarrhœa, pain, and vomiting, which continued for six weeks.

Uses.—In this country mezereon is scarcely ever employed alone. It is usually administered in conjunction with sarsaparilla, and is employed as a sudorific and alterative in venereal, rheumatic, scrofulous, and chronic cutaneous diseases. Decoction of the root-bark of mezereon was recommended to the notice of the profession, by Dr. Alexander Russell,[5] as a very efficacious remedy in cases of venereal nodes and nocturnal pains. Dr. Home[6] also speaks of it as " a powerful deobstruent in all venereal tumours, of the scirrhous kind, where mercury has failed." But Mr. Pearson,[7] after many years' observation of it, says, " I feel myself authorised to assert unequivocally, that the mezereum has not the power of curing the venereal disease in any one stage, or in any one form." Dr. Cullen[8] employed it with success in some cutaneous diseases.

As a topical remedy, it is sometimes applied to relieve toothache. It is occasionally used as a *masticatory*. Dr. Withering[9] cured a case of difficulty of swallowing (arising from a paralytic affection) by mezereon, which he directed to be chewed frequently. In France the bark of both *Daphne Mezereum* and *D. Gnidium* is used as a vesicatory.[10] The mode of applying

---

[1] *Med. Observ. and Inq.* vol. iii. p. 194.
[2] *Ausführ. Arzneimittell.* Bd. ii. S. 193.
[3] Vogt, *Pharmakodynamik*, Bd. ii. S. 305, 2te Aufl.
[4] Orfila, *Toxicol. Gén.*
[5] *Op. supra cit.* vol. iii. p. 189.
[6] *Clin. Exper. and Hist.*
[7] *Observ. on the Effects of various Articles of the Mat. Med.* 1800.
[8] *Mat. Med.*
[9] *Arrangement of Brit. Plants*, vol. ii. pp. 490, 7th edit.
[10] J. A. Leroy, *Essai sur l'Usage de l'Ecorce du Garou, ou Traité des Effets des Exutoires employés contre les Maladies rebelles*, Paris, 1774.

it is this :—First soften the bark by soaking it in hot vinegar and water, and then apply it to the part by a compress and bandage. The application is to be renewed night and morning until vesication is produced.

Administration.—Mezereon is usually administered internally in the form of *decoction*. It is a constituent of the *decoctum sarzæ compositum*.

As a *masticatory*, a few grains of the bark may be chewed.

For external use, an *ointment* prepared with the *extract* is sometimes employed.

Antidote.—In a case of poisoning by mezereon, evacuate the contents of the stomach as speedily as possible, and give emollient drinks, opiates, and the vegetable acids. To counteract inflammatory symptoms, the usual anti-phlogistic treatment should be adopted.

1. DECOCTUM MEZEREI, E.; *Decoction of Mezereon*. (Mezereon Bark, in chips, ʒij.; Liquorice Root, bruised, ʒss.; Water, Oij. Mix them, and boil down with a gentle heat to a pint and a half, and strain.)—Stimulant and sudorific. Used in chronic rheumatism and secondary syphilis. Dose, fʒiv. to fʒviij. three or four times a day. From Mr. Squire's observations, already referred to, it appears that ebullition is injurious to the action of mezereon, by dissipating a volatile active principle.

2. EXTRACTUM MEZEREI ALCOHOLICUM; *Alcoholic* or *Spirituous Extract of Mezereon*.—A tincture of mezereon is first made with rectified spirit, and the spirit then drawn off by distillation. In the Prussian Pharmacopœia, the alcoholic extract is directed to be digested in ether, and from the ethereal tincture is obtained by distillation the *extractum mezerei æthereum*.

Extract of mezereon is greenish or brownish-green-coloured, and is insoluble in water. Mr. Squire obtained a drachm of dry resin (alcoholic extract) by digesting half an ounce of the bruised bark in ten ounces of alcohol, and then distilling off the alcohol. During the distillation none of the pungency of the root came over. Extract of mezereon is used for the preparation of a blistering ointment or tissue.

3. UNGUENTUM MEZEREI, U.S.; *Mezereon Ointment*. (The Prussian Pharmacopœia directs this to be prepared by mixing ʒj. of the ethereal extract of mezereon with ʒj. of wax ointment. In the Hamburgh Codex, it is prepared by dissolving ʒij. of the spirituous extract in a small quantity of spirit, and then mixing ʒviij. of purified lard and ʒj. of white wax; [and the directions of the United States Pharmacopœia are as follows :—Take of Mezereon, sliced transversely, ʒiv.; Lard, ʒxiv.; White Wax, ʒij. Moisten the mezereon with a little alcohol, and beat it in an iron mortar until reduced to a fibrous mass: then digest it, by means of a salt-water-bath, with the lard and the wax, previously melted together, for twelve hours. Strain with strong expression, and allow the strained liquid to cool slowly, so that any undissolved matters may subside. From these separate the medicated ointment.—Ed.]) —The ointment is used as an irritant. Applied to ulcers or wounds, it serves to excite suppuration. Mr. Squire states that an ointment made by boiling the root in lard soon spoils by keeping.

154. Daphne Laureola, *Linn.*—Spurge-laurel.

(Cortex.)

Laureola, Gerard ; Parkinson, 205.—This is another indigenous species of Daphne. It has drooping axillary racemes of green flowers, evergreen lanceolate leaves, and black berries.   Mr. Squire says that 7 lbs. of the root yielded 4 lbs. 5 oz. of fresh bark, or 1 lb. 1¼ oz. of dry bark; and 11 lbs. of the stems yielded 1¾ lb. of fresh bark, which, when dried, weighed ¾ lb. The liber is remarkably tough.   In odour and irritating effect on the throat, the bark of the spurge-laurel appeared to him to be weaker than that of mezereon.   Half an ounce of the bruised bark yielded him 45 grs. of alcoholic extract.   In its effects spurge-laurel resembles mezereon.   Parkinson mentions its emmenagogue properties.—Some years ago a farrier gave a girl, æt. 17, three pills to procure abortion.   They caused violent vomiting, convulsions (during which she aborted), coma, and paralysis, from which she slowly recovered.   A microscopic examination of the fragments of leaves in the pills led the late Mr. Edwin Quekett to believe that the poison was this plant.

155. Daphne Gnidium, *Linn.*—The Flax-leaved Daphne.

(Cortex.)

Θυμελαία, Dioscorides, lib. iv. cap. 173.   The berries were the κόκκοι γνιδίοι, *grana gnidia*, or *gnidian berries*, used by Hippocrates.[1] The properties of this species of Daphne resemble those of Mezereon.   In France the bark (called *garou*) is used in the way before described (see *Daphne Mezereum*) as a vesicatory.

ORDER XXXVIII. POLYGONACEÆ, *Lind.*—BUCK-WHEATS.

POLYGONEÆ, *Jussieu.*

CHARACTERS.—*Calyx* free, often coloured, imbricated in æstivation. *Stamens* very rarely perigynous, usually definite and inserted in the bottom of the calyx ; *anthers* dehiscing lengthwise. *Ovary* free, usually formed by the adhesion of 3 carpels, 1-celled, with a single erect ovule, whose foramen points upwards : *styles* and *stigmas* as many as the carpels. *Ovules* orthotropal. *Nut* usually triangular, naked, or protected by the calyx. *Seed* with farinaceous albumen, rarely with scarcely any : *embryo* inverted, generally on one side, sometimes in the axis ; *radicle* superior, long.—*Herbaceous* plants, rarely *shrubs*. *Leaves* alternate, their stipules cohering round the stem in the form of an ochrea (or boot); when young, rolled backwards, occasionally wanting. *Flowers* occasionally unisexual, often in racemes (*Lindley*).

PROPERTIES.—The herbaceous plants are distinguished by their acidulous character. They owe this to the presence of vegetable acids, chiefly oxalic acid.   This is found in the form of a superoxalate of potash (or soda), which communicates to the leaves and petioles refreshing and refrigerant qualities.   The roots contain colouring and astringent matter, and often oxalate of lime.   Some of them are purgative.   The seeds of some species serve as a kind of corn for cattle, and, in times of scarcity, for man.

156. RHEUM.—RHUBARB.

Sex. Syst. Enneandria, Monogynia.

(Rheum Sinense ; Rhei species incerta ; Radix, *L.*—The root, *E. D.*)

HISTORY.—Dioscorides[2] speaks of a root which he calls *rha* or *rheon* ('ρᾶ 'ρῆον), and which has been regarded by some as identical with our

---

[1] See also Paulus Ægineta, Syd. Soc. edit. by Dr. Adams, vol. iii. p. 179.
[2] Lib. iii. cap. 11.

rhubarb. *Rha*, by some called *rheon*, grows," says Dioscorides, " in those countries which are beyond the Bosphorus, and from which it is brought. It is a root which is black externally, like to great centaury, but smaller and redder, odourless, loose or spongy, and somewhat smooth internally." Pliny[1] gives a similar account of it, under the name of *rhacoma*: it comes, he says, from the countries beyond Pontus, resembles the black costus, is odourless, and has a hot, astringent taste. Prosper Alpinus[2] was of opinion that the *rha* of Dioscorides was the root of Rheum rhaponticum, which Alpinus obtained from Thracia in 1608 A.D., and cultivated at Pavia. The later Greek writers are supposed to have been acquainted with our rhubarb. Alexander of Tralles[3] is the first who speaks of it. He used it in weakness of the liver and dysentery. Paulus Ægineta says that in the crudities and vomiting of pregnant women we may give "the knot-grass, boiled in water, for drink; and likewise dill, and the *pontic root, called* rha *in the dialect of its native country;*"[4] and, in noticing the practice of the ancients, he says, "alvine discharges they promoted by giving turpentine to the extent of an olive, when going to rest; or, when they wished to *purge* more effectually, by adding a little *rhubarb*" [rheon].[5] This is the first notice of the purgative properties of rhubarb.

In one of the Arabian authors (Mesue the younger) we find three kinds of rhubarb mentioned :—The *Indian*, said to be the best; the *Barbarian;* and the *Turkish*, which is the worst of all.

BOTANY. **Gen. Char.**—*Calyx* petaloid, 6-parted, withering. *Stamina* about 9, inserted into the base of the calyx. *Styles* 3, reflexed. *Stigmas* peltate, entire. *Achenium* 3-cornered, winged, with the withered calyx at the base. *Embryo* in the centre of the albumen (*Lindley*).

It is not yet ascertained what species of *Rheum* yields the officinal rhubarb. Several species now cultivated in this country have been at different times declared to be partially or wholly the source of it. Formerly *Rheum Rhaponticum* was supposed to yield it.[6]

In 1732 *R. undulatum* was sent from Russia to the Messrs. Jussieu, at Paris, and to Rand, of Chelsea, as the true rhubarb. This is the species which Linnæus described as *R. Rhabarbarum.*[7] About 1750, at the desire of Kauw Boerhaave, first physician to the Emperor of Russia, the senate commissioned a Tartarian merchant, a dealer in rhubarb, to procure them some seeds of the genuine plant. This he did, or pretended to do; and, on sowing them, two species of *Rheum* were obtained; namely, the *undulatum* and the *palmatum.*[8] In 1762, seeds of the latter species were received by Dr. Hope, of Edinburgh, from Dr. Mounsey, at Petersburg : they were sown, and the plants cultivated with success.[9] The root of this species being found to agree, in many of its characters, with that of genuine rhubarb, led to the belief that the *palmatum* was the true species. The inquiries of Pallas, however, raised some doubts about the correctness of this opinion; for the Bucharians declared themselves unacquainted with the leaves of the palmatum, and described the true plant as having round leaves, with a few incisions only at the margin. This description agreed best with *Rheum compactum*, the roots of which

---

1 *Hist. Nat.* lib. xxvi. cap. 105, ed. Valp.
2 *De Rhapontico*, 1612.
3 Lib. viii. cap. 3.
4 Paulus Ægineta, Syd. Soc. edit. by Dr. Adams, vol. i. book i. sect. 1, p. 1.
5 *Ibid.* book i. sect. 43, p. 54. See also vol. iii. pp. 317 and 478.
6 Alston, *Mat. Med.* vol. i. p. 502.
7 *Ibid.*
8 Murray, *App. Med.* vol. iv. p. 363.
9 Hope, *Phil. Trans.* vol. lv. for the year 1765, p. 290.

were declared by Millar, who cultivated the plant, to be as good as foreign rhubarb.[1] Georgi says that a Cossack pointed out to him the leaves of the R. undulatum as the true species.[2] These accounts were not satisfactory to the Russians ; and, in consequence, in 1790 Sievers, an apothecary, went to Siberia, under the auspices of Catherine II., with a view of settling the question ; but after four years of persevering attempts to reach the country where the true rhubarb grew, or even to obtain the seeds, he was obliged to be satisfied with negative results only. "My travels," says he, "as well as acquaintance with the Bucharians, have satisfied me that as yet nobody—that is, no scientific person—has seen the true rhubarb plant. All that is said of it by the Jesuits is miserably confused stuff ; all the seeds procured under the name of true rhubarb are false ; all the plantations, from those of the Knight Murray down to the flower-pot of a private individual, will never yield true rhubarb. Until further determination, I hereby declare all the descriptions in all the Materia Medicas to be incorrect."[3] Calau,[4] apothecary in the rhubarb factory at Kiachta, and who, from his appointment, might be expected to know the origin of the rhubarb he receives from the Bucharians, says, "All that we know of the rhubarb plant or its origin is defective and wrong ; every sacrifice to obtain a true plant or the seed has been in vain ; nor has the author been enabled to obtain it. A severe prohibition from the Chinese government prevents all possibility of eliciting the truth."

Himalayan rhubarb is obtained from several species of Rheum : viz. *R. Emodi*, Wallich ;[5] *R. Webbianum*, Royle ;[6] *R. spiciforme*, Royle ; and *R. Moorcroftianum*, Royle ; but there are no reasons for supposing that they yield any of the rhubarb of European commerce. It is not improbable that the species yielding the officinal rhubarb is yet undescribed. Dr. Royle,[7] after referring to the accounts of different authors as to the precise locality of the country yielding Russian rhubarb, concludes that it is within 95° of E. long. in 35° of N. latitude,—that is, in the heart of Thibet. And he adds, "as no naturalist has visited this part, and neither seeds nor plants have been obtained thence, it is as yet unknown what species yields this rhubarb." The late Mr. Anderson, of the Apothecaries' Botanic Garden, Chelsea, furnished me with the fresh roots of thirteen species of *Rheum ;* viz. *R. palmatum, undulatum, compactum, Rhaponticum, Emodi, crassinervium, caspicum, tataricum, hybridum, confluens, Fischeri, bardanifolium,* and *bullatum.* Having carefully dried these by artificial heat, I found that one species only, viz. *R. palmatum,* closely resembled Asiatic rhubarb in the combined qualities of odour, colour, and marbling : *R. undulatum* agreed tolerably well in colour and marbling, but not in odour. It deserves, however, to be noticed, that the specimens examined were of unequal ages, some forming the root-stock, others root-branches of the respective plants,—a circumstance which considerably diminishes the value of a comparative examination of them. Furthermore, all the samples were probably injured by the wet season. The root-branches of *R. crassinervium* (from a strong plant of six or seven years old, but which had not flowered) did not resemble Asiatic rhubarb either in colour or odour.[8]

Species.—1. *With compound racemes.*

1. RHEUM PALMATUM, Linn., L. D. ; *Palmated Rhubarb ;* commonly known to gardeners as the *True Turkey Rhubarb.*—"*Leaves* roundish-cordate, half-palmate ; the lobes pinnatifid, acuminate, deep dull green, not wavy, but uneven, and very much wrinkled on the upper side, hardly scabrous at the edge, minutely downy on the under side ; sinus completely closed ; the lobes of the leaf standing forwards beyond it. *Petiole* pale green, marked with short purple lines, terete, obscurely channelled quite at the upper end. *Flowering stems* taller than those of any other species" (*Lindley*).—Perennial.

---

[1] Murray, p. 365-6.
[2] *Ibid.* p. 360.
[3] Duncan, *Suppl. to the Edinb. New Disp.* p. 89.
[4] *Pharm. Journ.* vol. ii. p. 658, 1843.
[5] *Bot. Mag.* t. 3508.
[6] *Illust. of the Bot. of the Himal. Mount.*
[7] *Op. cit.*
[8] In 1834, Geiger (*Pharm. Central-Blatt für* 1834, S. 209) made a comparative examination of the roots of *R. Emodi, compactum, undulatum,* and *Rhaponticum.*

Grows spontaneously in the Mongolian empire, on the confines of China.[1] Its leaf-stalks make excellent tarts and puddings.

Prof. Guibourt[2] observes that out of the roots of *R. palmatum, undulatum, compactum,* and *Rhaponticum,* those of the first species possess only the exact odour and taste (grittiness excepted) of the China rhubarb.

2. RHEUM UNDULATUM, Linn., D.; *Wave-leaved Rhubarb.*—" *Leaves* oval, obtuse, extremely wavy, deep green, with veins purple at the base, often shorter than the petiole, distinctly and copiously downy on each side, looking as if frosted when young, scabrous at the edge; sinus open, wedgeshaped, with the lower lobes of the leaves turned upwards. *Petiole* downy, bloody, semicylindrical, with elevated edges to the upper side, which is narrower at the upper than the lower end" (*Lindley*).—Perennial. Grows in Siberia (*Georgi* and *Pallas,* cited by Murray[3]) and China (*Ammann,* quoted by Lindley). Cultivated in France, and yields part of the *French rhubarb.*[4] It was formerly cultivated in Siberia as the real officinal plant; but, as genuine rhubarb could not be procured from it, its cultivation has been given up.[5]

FIG. 177.   FIG. 178.

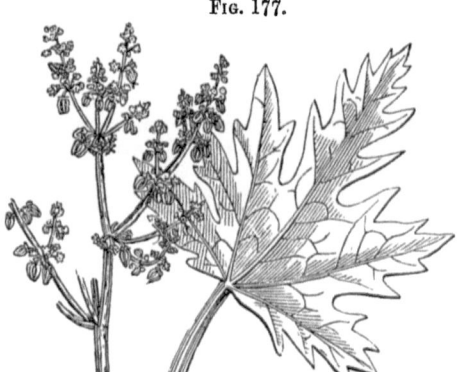

Rheum palmatum.

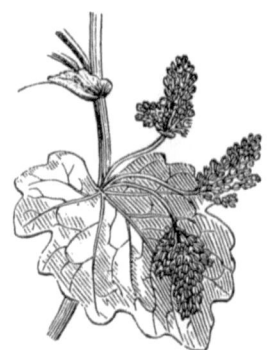

Rheum compactum.

3. RHEUM COMPACTUM, Linn.; *Thick-leaved Rhubarb.*—" *Leaves* heartshaped, obtuse, very wavy, deep green, of a thick texture, scabrous at the margin, quite smooth on both sides, glossy and even on the upper side; sinus nearly closed by the parenchyma. *Petiole* green, hardly tinged with red, except at the base, semicylindrical, a little compressed at the sides, with the upper side broad, flat, bordered by elevated edges, and of equal breadth at each end" (*Lindley*).—Perennial. Grows in Tartary and China. Cultivated in France, and yields part of the *French rhubarb.*[6] This rhubarb is a very fair imitation of that from China; but it is distinguished by its reddish tint, its different odour (common to it, to *R. undulatum,* and *R. Rhaponticum*), its close and radiated marbling, its not tinging the saliva, and its not grating under the teeth.

---

[1] Murray, *App. Med.* vol. iv. p. 363.
[2] *Hist. des Drogues.*
[3] *App. Med.*
[4] Guibourt, *Hist. des Drogues.*
[5] *Ibid.*
[6] Guibourt, *supra cit.*

4. RHEUM EMODI, Wallich; *R. australe*, Don.—"*Leaves* cordate, acute, dull green, but little wavy, flattish, very much wrinkled, distinctly rough, with coarse short hairs on each side; sinus of the base distinctly open, not wedge-shaped, but diverging at an obtuse angle, with the lobes nearly turned upwards. *Petioles* very rough, rounded angular, furrowed; with the upper side depressed, bordered by an elevated edge, and very much narrower at the upper than the lower end" (*Lindley*). Perennial. Grows on the Himalayas. It yields part of the *Himalayan rhubarb*. Its stalks make excellent tarts and puddings.

FIG. 179.

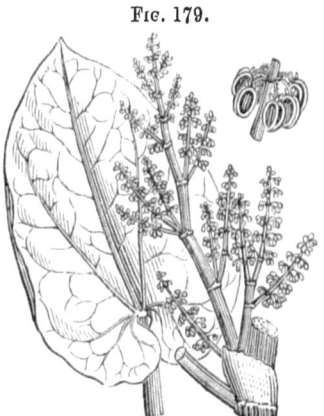

Rheum Emodi.

5. RHEUM WEBBIANUM, Royle.—Choor Mountain, Niti Pass. Yields part of the *Himalayan rhubarb*.

6. RHEUM RHAPONTICUM, Linn.; *Common or Rhapontic Rhubarb.*—Grows in Thrace; borders of the Euxine sea; north of the Caspian and Siberia. Cultivated in this country for the leaf-stalks, which are used for tarts and puddings; whence it is frequently termed *culinary* or *tart rhubarb*. Grown largely at Banbury, in Oxfordshire, on account of its roots, which, when dried, constitute *English* or *Banbury rhubarb*.[1] Cultivated also in France, and yields part of the *French rhubarb*.

7. R. CRASSINERVIUM, Fischer.—Habitation unknown. Sent from St. Petersburgh to the Apothecaries' Garden, Chelsea. Its roots possess, according to the late Mr. Anderson, the colour and odour of Turkey rhubarb.[2]

8. R. LEUCORRHIZUM, Pallas; *R. nanum*, Sievers, Ledebour, Fl. Pl. Ross. t. 492.—Deserts of the Kirghis, and south of Siberia and Altai mountains. Said to yield *white* or *imperial rhubarb*.

9. R. HYBRIDUM, Murray, Comm. Gott. t. i.—Cultivated as a culinary rhubarb.

II. *With spiciform racemes.*

10. RHEUM SPICIFORME, Royle.—Kherang Pass, and other places in Kunawar. Also Thibet.

11. RHEUM MOORCROFTIANUM, Royle; *Small-stalked Rhubarb.*—Niti Pass, in the Himalayas. This and the preceding species have denser and more yellow roots than the two other Himalayan species of Rheum above noticed (viz. *R. Emodi* and *R. Webbianum*).

PREPARATION.—The method of curing or preparing Asiatic rhubarb for the market varies somewhat in different localities. In China it is as follows:—The roots are dug up, cleansed, cut in pieces, and dried on stone tables, heated beneath by a fire. During the process the roots are frequently turned. They are afterwards pierced, strung upon cords, and further dried in the sun.[3]

---

[1] See a note by the author in the *Pharmaceutical Journal*, vol. vi. p. 76, 1846; also a paper by Mr. W. Bigg, in the same volume, p. 74.
[2] Lindley, *Fl. Med.*
[3] Du Halde, *Descript. Géograph. et Hist. de la Chine*, t. iii. p. 492.

In Tartary the Moguls cut the roots in small pieces, in order that they may dry the more readily, and make a hole in the middle of every piece, through which a cord is drawn, in order to suspend them in any convenient place. They hang them, for the most part, about their tents, and sometimes on the horns of their sheep.[1] Sievers, however, states that the roots are cut in pieces, strung upon threads, and dried under sheds, so as to exclude the solar rays; and the same author tells us that sometimes a year elapses from the time of their collection until they are ready for exportation.[2]

VARIETIES AND DESCRIPTION.—The various sorts of rhubarb (*radix rhei*) of commerce may be conveniently arranged in four divisions, respectively distinguished as *Muscovitic* or *Russian, Canton, Himalayan,* and *European.*

1. Muscovitic or Russian Rhubarb (*Radix Rhei Muscovitici, Ruthenici* vel *Rossici*).—Under this head are included those sorts of Asiatic rhubarb which are brought into Europe by way of Russia. The principal and chief sort is the *crown rhubarb.* Two other inferior sorts, called respectively *Bucharian* and *Siberian Rhapontic rhubarb,* are occasionally imported, but are not found in the shops. *Taschkent* and *white rhubarb* are other Russian sorts which I have not met with.

1. *Russia Crown Rhubarb.*—This is Chinese rhubarb which is taken in exchange, on behalf of the Russian crown, at Kiachta. In Russia it is known as *Chinese rhubarb:* and on the Continent it is called *Russian rhubarb.* It might with propriety be termed *Chinese-Russian rhubarb.* In English commerce it is commonly called *Turkey rhubarb* (*radix rhei turcici*), because formerly this description of rhubarb came into Europe by way of Natolia.[3]

The barter of rhubarb is carried on by the Russian government under a contract made with Bucharians at Kiachta for ten years, and confirmed by the Chinese government. According to this contract, the Bucharians undertake to furnish a certain quantity of rhubarb annually to the Russian crown, for a certain quantity of goods of a certain quality, and to deliver up all rhubarb not approved of, without remuneration, and permit it to be burnt by the Russian government.

The rhubarb grows wild in Chinese Tartary, especially in the province Kansu. It is collected on that long chain of mountains of Tartary, destitute for the most part of woods, and which arises not far from the town of Selin, and extends to the south as far as the lake Kokonor, near Thibet.[4] It is generally gathered in summer, from plants of six years of age. When the root is dug up, it is washed, to free it from earthy particles, peeled, bored through the centre, strung on a thread, and dried in the sun. In autumn, all the dried rhubarb collected in the province is brought in horse-hair sacks, containing about 200 lbs., to Sinin (the residence of the dealers), loaded on camels, and sent over Mongolia to Kiachta, Canton, Macao, and partly to Pekin. All the rhubarb brought to Kiachta undergoes an examination, prescribed by the Imperial Russian Medical Council, according to directions of the Russian government. The selection of the rhubarb bartered for by Russian merchants takes place in the custom-house at Kiachta; and of that for the crown, in a house for that purpose on the Chinese borders.

In this selection the following rules are chiefly to be observed :[5]—

a. To reject pieces obtained from dead plants, which are porous, of a grey colour, and, besides fibre and oxalate of lime, contain little of the other constituents of rhubarb.

---

[1] Bell, *Travels from St. Petersburgh to divers parts of Asia,* vol. i. p. 311.
[2] Duncan, *Suppl. to the Edinb. New Disp.* p. 88.
[3] Murray, *App. Med.* vol. iv. p. 379.
[4] Pallas, *Voyages en différ. Prov. de l'Empire de Russie,* t. iv. p. 216, et seq.
[5] Calau, *Pharm. Journ.* vol. ii. p. 658, 1843.

b. To reject pieces that are small, derived from young plants, and which are of a pale colour, and without much virtue.

c. To reject roots of other plants which are casually or purposely mixed with the rhubarb.

d. To pare the rhubarb. This is done, first, to remove remaining portions of the bark and the upper part of the root ; and secondly, to cleanse those parts that may be stained with the sweat of the camels.

e. To perforate all pieces, and examine their interior.

f. To re-dry those roots which may be moist.

As the rhubarb taken in exchange by the crown is not permitted to be imported into the European part of Russia, except in quantities of 1,000 poods, or 40,000 pounds, the roots approved of, after the examination, are packed in bags, and placed where there is a free current of air, until the necessary quantity has accumulated, which is then packed in cases capable of containing 4—5 poods. These chests are covered with linen, and pitched, then sewed into skins, and marked with the year of the importation of the root, and sent to Moscow.

Crown rhubarb is imported in chests holding from 156 to 160 lbs. each. Each chest is pitched on the outside, and covered with a hempen cloth and a hide. On the outside of the chest is a printed paper, stating the year in which the rhubarb was imported into Russia, and the weight of the chest. The following is a literal copy (reduced in size) of one of these papers :[1]—

The best prices are obtained for those chests whose rhubarb is in small pieces (for retailing), has a bright colour, and is sound and hard. The shapes of the pieces are various, being angular, rounded, or irregular. The flat surfaces and angles which the pieces present, show that the cortical portion of the root has been removed by slicing (and not by scraping, as in the Canton

---

[1] The following is a translation of the above label :—

rhubarb). Holes are observed, in some of the pieces, extending completely through : they have been made for the purpose of hanging the pieces to dry; but all traces of the cord have been carefully removed, and the holes scraped or filed to get rid of all decayed portions. The holes which extend only partially through the pieces are borings which have been made to examine the condition of the interior of the pieces. Externally the pieces are covered with a bright-yellow-coloured powder, usually said to be produced by the mutual friction of the pieces in the chests during their passage to this country; though many druggists believe it is derived from the process of *rouncing* (that is, shaking in a bag with powdered rhubarb), before its exportation. The odour is strong and peculiar, but somewhat aromatic. It is considered by druggists to be so delicate, that in all wholesale drug-houses a pair of gloves is kept in the Russian rhubarb drawer, with which only are the assistants permitted to handle the pieces. When chewed, it feels gritty under the teeth, from the presence of numerous crystals of oxalate of lime: it communicates a bright yellow colour to the saliva, and has a bitter, slightly astringent taste.

Beneath the dust with which the pieces are covered, the surface has a reddish-white tint, owing to the intermixture of white and red parts. The yellowish-white parts have the form of lines or veins, which, by their union with each other, assume a reticular form. Irregularly scattered over the surface we observe small star-like spots and depressions of a darker colour. The transverse fracture is uneven, and presents numerous brownish-red or dark carmine-coloured undulating veins. The longitudinal fracture is still more uneven, and shows the longitudinal direction of the veins, which are often interrupted with white. The surface obtained by cutting is more or less yellow, and frequently exposes the veins, disposed in groups.

By boiling very thin slices of the root in water, and then submitting them to the microscope, we observe cellular tissue, annular ducts, and numerous *conglomerate raphides* (clumps of crystals of oxalate of lime). From 100 grs. of Russian rhubarb, the late Mr. Edwin Quekett procured between 35 and 40 grs. of these raphides.[1] Turpin considered the presence of these crystals sufficient to distinguish Russian and Chinese rhubarb from that grown in Europe; but in some specimens of English rhubarb I have met with them in as great abundance as in foreign rhubarb. According to Raspail,[2] they are situated in the interstices of the elongated tissue; but this statement is erroneous, the situation of the crystals being in the interior of the cells.

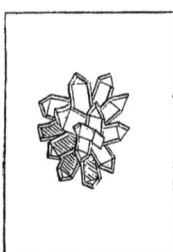

Fig. 180.

Crystals of Oxalate Lime in Russian Rhubarb.

The small pieces of crown rhubarb are usually picked out and sold as *radix rhei turcici electa;* the larger pieces and dust being employed for powdering.

The powder of Russian rhubarb is of a bright yellow colour, with a reddish tint; but, as met with in the shops, it is almost invariably mixed with the powder of English rhubarb.

2. *White or Imperial Rhubarb.*—When Pallas was at Kiachta, the Bucharian mer-

---

[1] Lindley's *Introduction to Botany*, 3d ed. p. 553.
[2] *Chim. Organ.*

chants who supplied the crown with rhubarb bought some pieces of rhubarb as white as milk, with a sweet taste, and the same properties as rhubarb of the best quality.[1] It is not met with in English commerce as a distinct kind; and it is almost unknown in Russia.[2] But in the chests of Russian rhubarb there are occasionally found pieces having an unusually white appearance : these I presume to be the kind alluded to.[3]

3. *Taschkent Rhubarb.*—This is the refuse of the true Russian rhubarb, which comes by way of Taschkent. It differs but little from the crown rhubarb. On account of its cheapness, it, like the Bucharian sort, is employed for purposes for which the crown rhubarb of Russia is too expensive. I have not met with it in English commerce.

4. *Bucharian Rhubarb* (*Rheum bucharicum*).—[It is called Bucharian, not because it is the growth of Bucharia, but from the circumstance of a few Bucharian families having been the purveyors of it to the Russian crown for a century.—ED.] Grassmann, an apothecary at St. Petersburg, who has described this sort,[4] considers it to be the rhubarb which, according to Pallas, is obtained from *Rheum undulatum*. As it is not under the control of the crown in Russia, it undergoes no examination, and inferior and rotten pieces, therefore, are often met with. On account of its cheapness it is used, in Russia, in veterinary medicine. [Bucharian rhubarb is described by Guibourt under the name of *Rhubarbe de Perse.* It is the only description of rhubarb that comes by Persia or Turkey into Europe.—ED.]

In 1840, some of it was received here by Mr. Faber, from Russia, to whom I am indebted for samples of it. It is described as being carried into the latter country by way of Nischny, where it is trimmed for the Moscow market.

This kind of rhubarb is intermediate between the Chinese and Russian or Muscovite rhubarb, but is of inferior quality. The pieces are more or less rounded or flattened, and weigh from one to two ounces each. Some of them appear to have been deprived of their cortical portion by scraping, as in the Chinese rhubarb; but in others the cortex has been removed by slicing. Most of them are perforated by a hole, apparently for the purpose of drying them : but in none of the holes are there any remains of the cord used in suspending the roots. The holes, moreover, appear to have been cleaned out, as in the Russian rhubarb, for no portion of decayed rhubarb is seen in them. Some of the pieces are dense, but most of them are lighter than good Russian rhubarb. Internally, they are often decayed and dark-coloured. Their texture is similar to that of genuine rhubarb. The odour is also like that of rhubarb, but much feebler; the taste is bitter and astringent. When chewed, this rhubarb feels gritty under the teeth. Its colour is darker than that of good Russian rhubarb.

5. *Siberian Rhubarb ; Rheum sibiricum.*[5]—This is the sort which Grassmann has described as *Siberian rhapontic rhubarb.* In 1845, three chests of it came to England from St. Petersburg, and were sold by public sale at 6d. per lb. In its general appearance it agreed with rhubarb grown in this country, and known as English stick rhubarb. It had been decorticated, though imperfectly so, as portions of the dark brown cortex were here and there left adherent. The pieces were all more or less cylindrical, seldom exceeding four inches in length and an inch in diameter, and on the average weighed about 100 grains each : the longest piece was six inches in length, and an inch and a half in diameter. The broadest piece was somewhat flattened, and about three inches in its broadest diameter. Its colour was in general darker than that of the ordinary rhubarb, but was of the same kind of tint. Its odour was remarkably sweet, similar to what I have perceived when drying the roots of different species of Rheum cultivated in England. When chewed, it was not gritty. Its taste was mucilaginous, bitterish, but not astringent. The fracture of the smaller and sound pieces was similar to that of English stick rhubarb : the larger pieces were decayed, dark brown, and tasteless in the centre. [Twelve chests of this rhubarb were imported from St. Petersburg, and offered

---

[1] *Voyages*, t. iv. p. 218.

[2] Grassmann, Buchner's *Repert.* Bd. xxxviii. S. 179, 1831. [It has been now clearly ascertained that white rhubarb has no existence as a separate kind. The idea that it was a different kind appears to have originated with Pallas, who acknowledged that a few such pieces were picked out of a large quantity. Most parcels of Russian and Chinese rhubarb yield such pieces.—ED.]

[3] Consult Goebel and Kunze, *Pharm. Waarenkunde.*

[4] Buchner's *Repertorium*, Bd. xxxviii. S. 179, 1831.

[5] For a notice of this and two preceding varieties, see a paper by the author in the *Pharmaceutical Journal*, vol. iv. pp. 445 and 500, 1845.

for sale in London, in December 1853. This rhubarb was said to be of the crop of 1793, and the produce of plants raised in Siberia from seeds obtained in the country of the China rhubarb by order of the Empress Catherine II. of Russia. A few packages had remained in the Russian government warehouses until this year, when it was determined to dispose of them. The rhubarb was, generally speaking, in small pieces, the larger flat or somewhat cylindrical or semi-cylindrical, from two and a half to three and a half inches long, and from one inch to one and a half inch broad. The smaller pieces were evidently from the younger roots. The larger pieces were perforated. The colour was good, and the fracture showed the hue and markings of the best rhubarb. The odour had nothing peculiar; the taste was nauseous and bitter, in some pieces sweetish. In many pieces the grittiness of oxalate of lime was perceptible.[1]—Ed.]

2. Canton Rhubarb.—This, like the Russian crown rhubarb, is the produce of China, but is exported from Canton. It is usually known in English commerce as *Chinese* or *East Indian rhubarb* (*radix rhei chinensis* seu *indici*). It is imported either directly from Canton, or indirectly by Singapore and other parts of the East Indies, and is probably the produce of the province of Se-tchuen (Du Halde), of Hoo-nan and Hoo-pih, as well as of other provinces (Gutzlaff and Reed).

Three kinds of Canton rhubarb are known in commerce : these arc,—The *untrimmed,* or *half-trimmed*; the *trimmed,* sometimes called the *Dutch-trimmed*; and what I have called *stick rhubarb.*

6. *Half-trimmed* or *untrimmed Canton Rhubarb.* — This is usually *Chinese* or *East Indian rhubarb* of the shops. It is called " untrimmed," or " half-trimmed," because the cortical portion of the root has been incompletely scraped (not sliced) off; and consequently the pieces have a rounded character, and are devoid of the flat surfaces and angles produced by slicing (as in the Russian and Dutch-trimmed rhubarbs). The inferior pieces present the remains of the greenish-brown or blackish cortex. The pieces are frequently cylindrical or roundish, but sometimes flattened; in trade they are distinguished as *rounds* and *flats.* They are generally perforated with holes, in many of which we find portions of the cords by which they were suspended. These holes are smaller than those observed in Russian rhubarb, and that portion of the root forming their sides is usually dark-coloured, decayed, and of inferior quality. The best pieces are heavier and more compact than that of the Russian kind; and are covered with an easily separable dust. When this is removed we observe that the surface is not so regularly reticulated, is of a more yellowish-brown than reddish-white colour, and has coarser fibres than Russian rhubarb. On the finer pieces we notice numerous star-like spots or depressions. The fracture is uneven; the veins, especially towards the middle, have a less determinate direction, and are of a duller or reddish-brown colour, and, in very bad pieces, of an amber-brown colour, with a grey substance between the veins. The odour of this species is much less powerful than that of Russian rhubarb, and is somewhat less aromatic. The taste, grittiness when chewed, and microscopic appearances, are similar to those of Russian rhubarb. The colour of the powder is of a more dull yellow or brownish cast.

This sort of rhubarb is imported in chests and half-chests : the former contain one picul (133½ lbs.), the latter half a picul. The chests are oblong, have been coarsely put together, and, except in shape, resemble tea-chests ; and, like the latter, are lined with sheet lead. The cover is a double one.

---

[1] [*Pharmaceutical Journal*, January 1854, p. 329.]

When this sort arrives in London, it is hand-picked, tared, and sorted into three qualities,—bright and sound, dark and horny, and worm-eaten. This is not done with Russian rhubarb.

7. *Dutch-trimmed* or *Batavian Rhubarb*, offic.—This kind of rhubarb is closely allied to, if it be not identical with, the preceding in its texture. In commerce, however, it is always regarded as distinct. It is imported from Canton and Singapore in chests, each containing one picul (133½ lbs.) It has been dressed or trimmed to resemble the Russian crown rhubarb, which it does in shape, size, and general appearance; for the cortical portion of the root seems to have been separated by slicing, and hence the pieces have the same angular appearance on the surface that the Russian rhubarb has. The pieces are frequently perforated, and in the holes are found the remains of the cord by which the root has been suspended; in this it differs from the Russian crown rhubarb. In the drug trade this kind of rhubarb is said to be trimmed, and, according to the shape of the pieces, they are called *flats* or *rounds*. The colour and weight of the pieces are variable.

8. *Canton Stick Rhubarb.*[1]—In 1844 five cases of this rhubarb were imported from Canton, and were sold by public sale at 8d. per lb.
All the pieces but one of my sample were cylindrical, about two inches long, from half to three-quarters of an inch in diameter, and weighed each, on the average, about 100 grains. The piece to which I have referred as forming the exception was shaped like a flattened cylinder, cut obliquely at one end; its greatest length was about two and a half inches, its greatest breadth two inches and a quarter; while its depth was about one inch, and its weight about two ounces. Mr. Faber, from whom I received it, informed me that on the examination of a quantity of Canton stick rhubarb he found several such pieces.
Most of the pieces are decorticated. These resemble English stick rhubarb in their texture and colour, except that they are, perhaps, somewhat paler. The taste is bitter, and somewhat astringent, but considerably less so than that of good half-trimmed Canton rhubarb. In chewing it, little or no grittiness is perceptible.
This kind of rhubarb is probably obtained from the root-branches of the plant which yields the usual Canton rhubarb.

3. Himalayan Rhubarb (*Radix Rhei Himalayanensis; Radix Rhei Indici*).—Rhubarb, the produce of the Himalayas, which makes its way through the plains of India, through Khalsee, Almora, and Butan, is probably, from its usual dark colour and spongy texture, the produce of either or both *R. Emodi* and *R. Webbianum;* the roots of *R. spiciforme* and *R. Moorcroftianum* being lighter-coloured, and more compact in structure.
I have met with two sorts of Himalayan rhubarb :—

9. *Large Himalayan Rhubarb; Rhubarb* from *Rheum Emodi?*—I am indebted to Dr. Wallich for some specimens of this sort of rhubarb. He obtained them from the inhabitants of the Himalayas, who had strung the pieces around the necks of their mules. It has scarcely any resemblance to the officinal rhubarb. The pieces are cylindrical, and are cut obliquely at the extremities; the cortex of the root is not removed; the colour is dark brown, with a slight tint of yellow; they are without odour, and have a coarse fibrous texture. In November 1840, when China rhubarb was very scarce and dear, nineteen chests of Himalayan rhubarb were imported from Calcutta into this country. The chests were of the usual Calcutta kind, made of the hard, heavy, brittle Bengal wood. The weight per chest was gross 1 cwt. 2 qrs. 26 lbs.

---

[1] See a paper by the author in the *Pharmaceutical Journal*, vol. iv. p. 446, 1845.

The pieces varied considerably in size and shape; some were twisted, cylindrical and furrowed, cut obliquely at the extremities, about four inches long, and an inch and a half in diameter. Others were circular discs, about three inches in diameter, two inches thick, and weighed about four ounces each. Besides these, semicylindrical, angular, and other-shaped pieces were met with, and were obviously obtained by slicing the root. Some of the pieces were decorticated, others were coated. The general colour was dark brown; the prominent decorticated and paler parts having an ochre-brown tint. It had a feeble rhubarb odour, and a bitter astringent taste. When broken, it did not present the marbled texture characteristic of ordinary rhubarb. In chewing it, little or no grittiness was perceived. It was exceedingly light, and worm-eaten.

This was the first shipment of Himalayan rhubarb ever made to this country. Two chests sold at 4d. per lb.; the remainder at 1d. per lb.[1]

10. *Small Himalayan Rhubarb; Rhubarb from Rheum Webbianum.* —I am indebted to Dr. Royle for this sort. It is the same as that referred to in the experiments of Mr. Twining.[2] The pieces are short transverse segments of the root-branches, of a dark-brownish colour, odourless, or nearly so, with a very bitter astringent taste, and in quality they do not essentially differ from the roots given me by Dr. Wallich.

4. European Rhubarb (*Radix Rhei Europæi*).—This is rhubarb cultivated in Europe. The only two sorts with which I am acquainted are the English and French.

11. *English Rhubarb* (*Radix Rhei Anglici*).—This is the produce of Rheum Rhaponticum, cultivated in the neighbourhood of Banbury, in Oxfordshire.

The history of this rhubarb is not a little curious. It appears that Mr. Wm. Hayward, an apothecary at Banbury, was the original cultivator of rhubarb in that locality. From his own statement[3] it appears that he began to cultivate it about the year 1777.[4] In 1789 he obtained a silver medal, and in 1794 a gold medal, from the Society of Arts, for the cultivation of what he terms "the true Turkey rhubarb;"[5] the plant for which the Society offered the premium being the "R. palmatum, or true rhubarb."[6] Mr. Hayward died in 1811, and his plants were purchased by the father of one of the present cultivators.

There were lately three cultivators of Banbury rhubarb; viz. Mr. R. Usher of Overthorpe and Bodicott, Mr. T. Tustian of Milcombe, and Mr. E. Hughes of Neithorp. These parties grew altogether about 12 acres of rhubarb. Only one species was in cultivation, namely the R. Rhaponticum. I examined specimens of it sent to me by Mr. Rye, surgeon of Banbury, and to the Pharmaceutical Society by Mr. W. Bigg. Mr. Usher states that no other species was ever cultivated at Banbury, and that he cannot produce English rhubarb from the "Giant rhubarb," or any other sort.[7]

At Banbury, the rhubarb is obtained from roots of three or four years old. They are dug up in October or November, freed from dirt, deprived of their outer coat by a sharp knife, exposed to the sun and air for a few days,

---

[1] Dr. Royle (*Illust. of the Botany of the Himalayan Mountains*, p. 316) says that the Himalayan rhubarb sells for only one-tenth of the price of the best rhubarb, resembling in quality the Russian, which is found in India.

[2] *Trans. Med. and Phys. Soc. of Calcutta*, vol. iii. p. 441.

[3] *Trans. Society of Arts*, vol. viii. pp. 75 and 76, 1790.

[4] The cultivation of rhubarb in Britain was long since recommended by Sir William Fordyce, in a work entitled *The Great Importance and proper Method of Cultivating and Curing Rhubarb in Britain, for Medical Purposes*, Lond. 1784.

[5] *Trans. Society of Arts*, vol. xii. p. 225-9, 1794.

[6] *Ibid.* vols. vii. p. 281, and xi. p. 285.

[7] For further details, see Mr. Bigg's *Answers to Queries* (drawn up by the author), and the author's *Note on Banbury Rhubarb*, in the *Pharmaceutical Journal*, vol. vi. pp. 73, 74, and 76.

and dried on basket-work in drying-houses heated by stove-pipes or brick flues. Mr. Hayward accelerated the curing process by scooping a hole in the largest pieces, and dried both these and the smaller pieces strung on packthread, and hung in a warm room.

The root-stock yields the *trimmed English rhubarb :* the root-branches yield the *cuttings,* or *stick English rhubarb.* The produce of the process of trimming is called *raspings,* and serves for powdering.

Trimmed or *dressed English rhubarb* is the kind frequently observed in the show-bottles of druggists' windows, and was formerly sold in Cheapside and the Poultry for " *Turkey rhubarb,*" by persons dressed up as Turks. It occurs in various-sized and shaped pieces, which are trimmed and frequently perforated, so as to represent foreign rhubarb :[1] some of the pieces are cylindrical in their form, and are evidently segments of cylinders; others are flat. This kind of rhubarb is very light, spongy (especially in the middle of the large flat pieces), attractive of moisture, pasty under the pestle, and has a reddish or pinkish hue not observed in the Asiatic kinds. Internally it has usually a marbled appearance ; the streaks are pinkish, parallel, and have a radiated disposition ; and in the centre of some of the larger pieces the texture is soft and woolly, and may be easily indented by the nail. Its taste is astringent and very mucilaginous ; it is not at all, or only very slightly, gritty under the teeth : its odour is feeble, and more unpleasant than either the Russian or East Indian kinds. The microscope discovers in it, for the most part, very few crystals of oxalate of lime.

The *common stick English rhubarb* (called at Banbury the *cuttings*) occurs in angular or roundish pieces, of about five or six inches long, and an inch thick. When fractured, it presents the radiated appearance and the red-coloured streaks of the kind last mentioned. Its taste is astringent, but very mucilaginous ; it is not gritty under the teeth ; it breaks very short.

English rhubarb is extensively employed by druggists to adulterate the powder of Asiatic rhubarb.

12. *French Rhubarb* (*Radix Rhei Gallici*).—This kind of rhubarb is procured from *Rheum Rhaponticum, undulatum,* and especially *compactum.*[2] These are cultivated at Rheumpole, a place not far from Lorient, in the department of Morbihan. *Rheum palmatum* is no longer cultivated there. I received from Professor Guibourt two kinds of French rhubarb. One of these he called *flat,* and is probably the produce of *R. Rhaponticum ;* the other he termed *round,* and is the produce of *R. compactum.*

[COMMERCE.—The quantity of rhubarb imported annually into this country during a period of seven years, was as follows :—

	lbs.
1843	268,766
1844	206,015
1845	323,416
1846	427,694
1847	305,736
1848	116,005
1849	94,914.—ED.]

---

[1] Specimens in the Russian or Dutch style of trimming, in the Chinese or East India style of trimming, and of small trimmed (pieces like truncated cones) and fine trimmed Banbury rhubarb, are contained in the museum of the Pharmaceutical Society.

[2] Guibourt, *op. supra cit.*

COMPOSITION.—Few, if any, articles of the materia medica have been so frequently the subject of chemical investigation, as rhubarb. Many chemists have submitted it to examination for the purpose of discovering all its proximate principles. Among these may be mentioned Schrader[1] in 1807, N. E. Henry[2] in 1814, Brande[3] in 1821, Hornemann[4] in 1822, Peretti[5] in 1826, Buchner and Herberger[6] in 1831, Lucae[7] in 1833, O. Henry[8] in 1836, Brandes[9] in 1836, and Schlossberger and Doepping in 1844.[10]

But several of the more important chemical examinations of rhubarb have been made with the view chiefly of discovering the one or more active principles of rhubarb. Among these I include the investigations of Trommsdorff,[11] Pfaff,[12] Nani,[13] Caventou,[14] Carpenter,[15] Dulk,[16] and especially of Schlössberger and Doepping, before quoted.

One hundred grains of the finest Russian rhubarb, according to Mr. Brande, lost 44·2 grs. by being repeatedly digested in alcohol (sp. gr. 0·815). By evaporation the alcoholic solution yielded a residue of 36 grains (the loss 8·2 grs. may be ascribed to water), of which 10 grains (resin ?) were insoluble in water.

The rhubarb left after the action of alcohol weighed, when dried at 212° F., 55·8 grs. It yielded to water 31 grs. (gum ?). The insoluble residue, weighing 24·8 grs., must have consisted of woody fibre, oxalate of lime, &c.

Brandes's Analysis. (Chinese Rhubarb.)		*Schlössberger and Doepping's Analysis.* (Moscow and Chinese Rhubarb.)
Pure rhabarberic acid	2·0	1. Chrysophanic acid.
Impure rhabarberic acid	7·5	2. Three resins (*aporetine, phæoretine*, and *erythroretine*).
Gallic acid, with some rhabarberic acid ...	2·5	
Tannic acid	9·0	3. Extractive matter.
Colouring extractive	3·5	4. Tannic acid.
Uncrystallisable sugar, with tannic acid ...	11·0	5. Gallic acid.
Starch and pectic acid	4·0	6. Sugar.
Gummy extractive taken up by caustic potash	14·4	7. Pectine.
Pectic acid	4·0	8. Oxalate of lime.
Malate and gallate of lime	1·1	9. Ashes (containing potash, soda, silica and sand, traces of sesquioxide of iron, phosphate of lime and magnesia, sulphuric, muriatic (chlorine), phosphoric and carbonic acids.
Oxalate of lime	11·0	
Sulphate of potash, and chloride of potassium	1·5	
Phosphate of lime with oxide of iron	0·5	
Silica	1·0	
Woody fibre	25·0	
Water	2·0	
Rhubarb	100·0	Rhubarb.

[1] *Berlinisches Jahrbuch f. d. Pharmacie* auf das J. 1807, p. 123.
[2] *Bull. de Pharm.* vi. 87, 1814.
[3] *Quarterly Journ. of Science*, vol. x. p. 288, 1821.
[4] *Berl. Jahrb.* Bd. xxiii. p. 252, 1822.
[5] *Journ. de Pharm.* xiv. 536, 1828.
[6] Buchner's *Repertor.* Bd. xxxviii. p. 337, 1831.
[7] *Ibid. für* 1834, p. 78.
[8] *Journ. de Pharm.* xxii. 393, 1836.
[9] *Pharm. Central-Blatt für* 1836, p. 482.
[10] *Ann. der Chem. u. Pharm.* Bd. l. p. 196, 1844; and *Pharm. Journal*, vol. iv. p. 136, 1844.
[11] *Journ. de Pharm.* iii. 1, p. 106.
[12] *Syst. d. Mat. Med.* Bd. iii. p. 23, 1814; and Bd. vi. p. 308, 1821.
[13] *Biblioth. Univ.* xxxiii. 232.
[14] *Journ. de Pharm.* t. xii. p. 22, 1826.
[15] *Philadelphia Journal of Pharmacy*, vol. i. p. 139.
[16] *Arch. d. Pharm.* Bd. xvii. p. 26; also, *Pharm. Central-Blatt für* 1839, p. 102.

	Hornemann's Analyses.			Lucae's Analysis.
	Russian.	English [Chinese ?]	Sicilian [English ?]	Rheum Emodi.
Bitter principle of Pfaff	16·042	14·375	10·156	4·220
Yellow colouring matter of Henry	9·583	9·166	2·187	7·500
Astringent extractive	14·687	16·458	10·417	6·458
Oxidised tannic acid	1·458	1·249	0·833	0·469
Mucilage	10·000	8·333	3·542	6·250
Substance extracted by potash ley	28·333	30·416	41·042	55·833
Oxalic acid	1·042	0·833	...	1·302
Woody fibre	14·583	15·416	8·542	16·364
Moisture	3·333	3·125	6·042	...
Rhaponticin	...	...	1·042	...
Starch	...	...	14·583	...
Loss [water and odorous matter ?]	0·939	0·629	1·614	1·604
Rhubarb	100·000	100·000	100·000	100·000
The woody fibre being incinerated, yielded—				
Potash	trace	trace	The quantities of potash, lime, alumina, and magnesia, were too small to be accurately determined.	...
Charcoal	0·208	0·208		0·208
Silica	2·416	0·416		0·155
Carbonate of magnesia	0·208	0·208		0·208
Alumina with oxide of iron	0·208	0·208		0·572
Carbonate of lime	5·883	7·083		3·854
Ashes	8·873	8·123	...	4·997

Schlössberger and Doepping conclude that the flavour, relation to chemical reagents, and therapeutical properties of rhubarb, depend on the conjoint operation of the resin, the colouring matter, and the extractive,—modified perhaps, in some degree, by the other ingredients.

1. ODOROUS MATTER OF RHUBARB (*Volatile Oil ?*).—In none of the analyses of rhubarb is any mention made of a distinct odorous principle; yet it appears to me that such must exist. As the colour and odour bear no proportion to each other in different kinds of rhubarb, it is tolerably clear that they cannot depend on one and the same principle. The odorous principle is probably a volatile oil, but it has not hitherto been isolated. A few years since, Dr. Bressy announced to the *Académie de Médecine* that he had separated it, but the committee appointed to repeat his experiments was unable to procure it by his process.[1] Zenneck[2] says that the rhubarb odour is imitated by a mixture of nitric acid, aloes, and chloride of iron.

2. YELLOW CRYSTALLINE GRANULAR MATTER OF RHUBARB; *Chrysophanic Acid* (so called from χρυσός, *gold;* and φαίνω, *I shine*); *Rheic Acid;* $C^{10}H^8O^3$.—Found in Russian and Canton rhubarb, in the roots of Rheum Rhaponticum and Rumex obtusifolius, and in Parmelia parietina. In the pure or more or less impure state, it has been long known under the names of *rhabarbaric acid, rheumin, rhabarberin,* and *rhein.* It may be procured from rhubarb by means of ether in Robiquet's displacement apparatus.

Pure chrysophanic acid is a beautiful, clear, yellow, odourless and tasteless substance, which is separated in granular masses, and shows little disposition to crystallise. It is tolerably soluble in hot rectified spirit of wine; not very soluble in ether, even when boiling; and almost insoluble in cold water, but more soluble in boiling water. Heated, it evaporates, emits yellow fumes, which condense and form yellow flocculi, and at the same time a part becomes carbonised. It dissolves in alkalies, producing a beautiful red colour: if the potash solution be evaporated to dryness, the red colour changes to violet, and then to a beautiful blue. It dissolves in oil of vitriol, forming a beautiful red solution, from which water precipitates yellow flocculi.

---

[1] *Dict. des Drog.* t. iv. p. 425.
[2] *Pharm. Central-Blatt für* 1832, S. 237.

3. Resins.—According to Schlössberger and Doepping, rhubarb contains three resins, soluble in alcohol, but insoluble in water.

α. *Aporetine* (from ἀπο, *from ;* and ῥητίνη, *resin*).—Is a product or deposit of the resin of rhubarb. It is black and shining when dry; slightly soluble in hot spirit, ether, cold and hot water ; very soluble in ammonia and potash.

β. *Phæoretine* (from φαιός, *red brown ;* and ῥητίνη); *Brown resin* of rhubarb; $C^{16}H^8O^7$.— It is yellowish-brown, very slightly soluble in water and ether ; very soluble in spirit and its alkalies, and may be thrown down from the latter solution by the mineral acids.

γ. *Erythroretine* (from ἐρυθρός, *red ;* and ῥητίνη) ; *Red resin* of rhubarb; $C^{19}H^9O^7$ —It is yellow, soluble in ether, very soluble in alcohol; forms rich purple combinations with potash and ammonia, which are very soluble in water. To this resin, as well as to chrysophanic acid, rhubarb chiefly owes its colour.

4. Bitter Principle ; *Extractive ?*—Rhubarb contains a bitter principle; but most of the substances which have been announced as the bitter principle of rhubarb, under the name of *caphopicrite* (? from καφέω, *I exhale ;* and πικρός, *bitter*), or *rhabarberin*, are themselves compounded of two or more principles. Schlössberger and Doepping describe the extractive matter of rhubarb as having a bitter taste, but not the flavour of rhubarb.

5. Astringent Matter (*Tannic and Gallic acids*).—The red veins are the seat of the astringent matter. This is proved by brushing the cut surface of rhubarb with a weak solution of a ferruginous salt ; the red veins, only, undergo a change of colour.

6. Indifferent Substances.—Rhubarb contains a considerable quantity of *starch* and *pectine* or vegetable jelly. The starch consists of small grains, with a very distinct nucleus or hilum, and arranged in groups, each of 2, 3, or more grains. *Sugar* also may be detected by Trommer's test and the process of fermentation. *Cellulose* and *mucilage* also are present.

7. Oxalate of Lime.—The conglomerate raphides before noticed (see *ante*, p. 488) are crystals of oxalate of lime. They may be separated in great abundance by boiling Russian or China rhubarb in water until the cohesion of the tissue is completely destroyed. When the decomposed tissue is well shaken with water, the crystals fall to the bottom of the vessel. Heated to redness, they are changed into carbonate of lime. A solution of them in diluted nitric acid, or a solution obtained by boiling the crystals with a solution of carbonate of soda, forms with nitrate of silver a white precipitate (*oxalate of silver*), which detonates when heated. It has been already stated that the late Mr. Edwin Quekett obtained from 35 to 40 per cent. of oxalate of lime from Russian rhubarb.

8. Rhaponticin.—A yellow, crystallisable, odourless, tasteless substance, obtained from the root of European [English ?] rhubarb. It is insoluble in cold water, ether, and the volatile oils, but soluble in twenty-four times its weight of boiling water, and twice its weight of absolute alcohol.[1]

Chemical Characteristics.—If the powder of rhubarb be heated in a glass capsule over a lamp, an odorous yellow vapour (*oil ?* or *resin with chrysophanic acid*) is obtained, which communicates a red colour to a solution of caustic potash. The aqueous infusion of rhubarb is rendered green by the sesquichloride of iron (*tanno-gallate of iron*) ; with a solution of gelatin it yields a copious yellow precipitate (*tannate of gelatin*), which is dissolved on the application of heat, or by the addition of an excess of gelatin ; with a solution of disulphate of quina, a yellowish precipitate (*tannate of quina*); with the alkalies (potash, soda, and ammonia), a red-coloured solution (*soluble alkaline chysophanates*) ; with lime-water, a reddish precipitate (*chrysophanate of lime*) ; with the acids (the acetic excepted), precipitates ; and with various metallic solutions (as of acetate of lead, protochloride of tin, protonitrate of mercury, and the nitrate of silver), precipitates (principally *metallic chrysophanates* and *tannates*).

[Adulterations.—Dr. R. D. Thompson stated in his evidence before the

---

[1] Berzelius, *Traité de Chim.* vi. 205.

Committee on the Adulteration of Drugs, in July 1855, that the adulteration of rhubarb was carried to such an extent that samples frequently contained as much as fourteen pounds of flour and eight ounces of turmeric in a hundred-weight.—ED.]

Distinguishing characteristics of rhubarb and turmeric. — Paper stained by a strong decoction of tincture of rhubarb is not affected by boracic acid, or by the borates rendered acid, whereas turmeric paper is reddened by these agents.[1] Hence the presence of turmeric in powdered rhubarb may be detected by this means.

Differential characteristics of the commercial sorts of rhubarb.—All the different commercial sorts of rhubarb contain the same constituents,· but in different proportions : hence the differential characteristics are founded on relative or comparative, and not on absolute differences. English rhubarb usually contains a smaller quantity of crystals of oxalate of lime, and a larger quantity of starch. It, therefore, is less gritty between the teeth. In general, a decoction of Russian, Dutch-trimmed, or of China rhubarb, becomes, with a solution of iodine, greenish-blue (*iodide of starch*) : after a few minutes the colour disappears, and no iodine can be detected in the liquor by starch, unless nitric acid be previously added. A decoction of English rhubarb, however, is rendered, by a solution of iodine, intensely blue (*iodide of starch*), the colour not completely disappearing by standing. These peculiarities, however, are not constant. Some specimens of Russian rhubarb contain so much starch that they react on iodine, like those of English rhubarb.

PHYSIOLOGICAL EFFECTS. *α. On Animals.*—On the *solipedes* rhubarb acts as a tonic, confining its action principally to the stomach, whose digestive power it augments. On the *carnivora* it operates, in doses of half a drachm, in the same way ; but in doses of several drachms, as a purgative. On the larger *herbivora* it may be given to the extent of several ounces without causing purgation.[2] Tiedemann and Gmelin[3] detected it by its yellow colour in the serum of the blood of the mesenteric, splenic, and portal veins, and in the urine of dogs to which rhubarb had been administered by the mouth. They failed to recognise it in the chyle.

β. On Man.—*In small doses* (as from four to eight grains) it acts as an astringent tonic, its operation being principally or wholly confined to the digestive organs. In relaxed conditions of these parts it promotes the appetite, assists the digestive process, improves the quality of the alvine secretions, and often restrains diarrhœa. *In large doses* (as from a scruple to a drachm) it operates, slowly and mildly, as a purgative, sometimes causing slight griping. It never inflames the mucous membrane of the alimentary canal, as jalap, scammony, colocynth, and some other drastic purgatives, are capable of doing. The constipation which follows its cathartic effect has been ascribed to the operation of its astringent matter. In febrile complaints and inflammatory diseases it sometimes accelerates the pulse and raises the temperature of the body ; whence the impropriety of its use in these cases.

Under the use of rhubarb, the secretions, especially the urine, become coloured by it. According to Heller, the colour which the urine acquires

---

[1] Faraday, *Quart. Journ. of Science*, vol. vi. p. 152.
[2] Moiroud, *Pharm. Vétér.* p. 260.
[3] *Versuche üb. d. Wege auf welch. Subst. aus d. Magen u. Darmk. gelang.* S. 10–12.

under the employment of this medicine depends on the acid or alkaline condition of this secretion : if acid, it is yellow ; if alkaline, it becomes reddish-yellow or blood-red. From Schlössberger's experiments[1] it appears that the colour is communicated to the urine by the phæoretine and erythro-retine, and not by the chrysophanic acid, which, when pure, neither operates on the bowels nor colours the urine. Urine coloured by rhubarb stains the linen, and is reddened by caustic potash. The cutaneous secretion (especially of the arm-pits) also becomes coloured under the use of rhubarb. The milk of nurses who have taken it is said to acquire a purgative property.

Rhubarb has for a long period been considered to possess a specific influence over the liver, to promote the secretion of bile, and to be used in jaundice. These opinions, which, as Dr. Cullen[2] correctly observed, have no foundation either in theory or practice, arose from the absurd doctrine of signatures. Considered in relation to other medicinal agents, rhubarb holds an interme-diate rank between the bitter tonics on the one hand, and the drastics on the other. From the first it is distinguished by its purgative qualities ; from the latter, by its tonic operation and the mildness of its evacuant effects. As a purgative, it is perhaps more closely allied to aloes than to any other ca-thartic in ordinary use ; but is distinguished by its much milder operation, and its want of any specific action on the large intestines.

The comparative power of the several kinds of rhubarb has scarcely been ascertained with precision. The remarks above made apply to the Russian and Chinese varieties, whose power is about equal. From experiments made by Dr. Parry at the Bath Hospital, it appears that the purgative qualities of the English rhubarb are scarcely so strong as those of the Russian and Chi-nese varieties ; but the difference is not great.[3] For several years past English rhubarb has been exclusively employed at the London Hospital ; and no com-plaints have been made respecting its operation. Himalayan rhubarb is, according to Dr. Twining,[4] almost equal to Russian rhubarb in its purgative effects ; but is less aromatic, though more astringent.

USES.—The remedial value of rhubarb depends on the mildness and safety of its operation, and on its tonic and astringent influence over the alimentary canal.

1. *As a purgative.*—There are many cases in which the above-mentioned qualities render rhubarb peculiarly valuable as a purgative. In mild cases of *diarrhœa* it sometimes proves peculiarly efficacious, by first evacuating any irritating matter contained in the bowels, and afterwards acting as an astrin-gent. Given at the commencement of the disease, it is a very popular remedy ; and though doubtless it is often employed unnecessarily (since, as Dr. Cullen has justly observed, in many cases no further evacuation is neces-sary or proper than what is occasioned by the disease), yet it rarely, if ever, does harm. Sulphate of potash is a very useful adjunct to it, and promotes its purgative operation. Antacids (as chalk or magnesia) are frequently conjoined with it. It is not fitted for inflammatory or febrile cases. As *an infant's purgative* it is deservedly celebrated. It is well adapted for a variety of children's complaints ; but is peculiarly adapted to scrofulous sub-

---

[1] *Pharmaceutical Journal*, vol. viii. p. 190, 1848.
[2] *Mat. Med.*
[3] Stephenson and Churchill, *Med. Bot.*
[4] *Trans. Med. and Phys. Soc. of Calcutta*, vol. iii. p. 441.

jects, and those afflicted with enlargement of the mesenteric glands, accompanied with tumid belly and atrophy. Magnesia, sulphate of potash, or calomel, may be associated with it, according to circumstances. *For an ordinary purgative in habitual costiveness* it is scarcely adapted, on account of the constipation which follows its purgative effect.

2. *As a stomachic and tonic.*—In *dyspepsia*, accompanied with a debilitated condition of the digestive organs, small doses of rhubarb sometimes prove beneficial, by promoting the appetite and assisting the digestive process. In *scrofulous* enlargement of the lymphatic glands in children, rhubarb, in small doses, is often combined with mercurial alteratives (as the *hydrargyrum cum cretâ*), or with antacids (as magnesia or chalk), and frequently with apparent advantage.

3. *As an external application.*—Sir Everard Home[1] used it as a topical application to promote the healing of indolent non-painful ulcers. The powder is to be lightly strewed over the ulcer, and a compress applied. In irritable ulcers an eighth part of opium is to be added. When applied to large ulcers it has produced pretty active purging.[2] The powder of rhubarb, incorporated with saliva and rubbed on the abdomen, proves purgative.[3]

ADMINISTRATION.—The powder of Russian or China rhubarb may be exhibited, as a stomachic and tonic, in doses of from five to ten grains; as a purgative, from a scruple to a drachm. The dose of indigenous rhubarb should be about twice as much as the above.

" By roasting it with a gentle heat till it becomes friable [*rheum torrefactum*], its cathartic power is diminished, and its astringency supposed to be increased" (Lewis).

1. INFUSUM RHEI, L. E. D.; *Infusion of Rhubarb.* (Rhubarb, sliced [in coarse powder, *E.*], ʒiij. [ʒj. *E.*] ; Boiling [distilled, *L.*] Water, Oj. [f℥xviij. *E.*] ; Spirit of Cinnamon, fʒij. *E.* Macerate for two hours [twelve hours, *E.*] in a lightly-covered vessel, and strain [through linen or calico, *E.*] [The *Dublin College* orders of Rhubarb Root, in thin slices, ʒij. ; Boiling Water, f℥ix. Infuse for one hour in a covered vessel, and strain. The product should measure about eight ounces.—ED.])—Boiling water extracts from rhubarb, chrysophanic acid, resin, tannic and gallic acids, sugar, extractive, and starch. As the liquor cools it becomes turbid. Infusion of rhubarb is stomachic and gently purgative. It is usually employed as an adjunct to, or vehicle for, other mild purgatives or tonics. The alkalies or magnesia are sometimes conjoined. The stronger acids, and most metallic solutions, are incompatible with it. Dose, fʒj. to f℥ij.

2. TINCTURA RHEI, E. ; *Tincture of Rhubarb.* (Rhubarb, in moderately fine powder, ℥iiiss.; Cardamom Seeds, bruised, ʒss.; Proof Spirit, Oij. Mix the rhubarb and cardamom seeds, and proceed by the process of percolation, as directed for tincture of cinchona. This tincture may also be prepared by digestion.)—The alcoholic tincture of rhubarb contains chrysophanic acid, tannic acid, resin, and uncrystallisable sugar. Cordial, stomachic, and mildly purgative. Dose, as a stomachic, fʒj. to f℥iij. ; as a purgative, f℥ss. to f℥j.

---

[1] *Pract. Observ. on the Treatment of Ulcers*, p. 96, 1801.
[2] Arnemann, *Chirurg. Arzneim.* 6ste Aufl. S. 224.
[3] Alibert, *Nouv. Elém. de Thérap.* t. ii. p. 275, et. seq. 5me éd.

3. TINCTURA RHEI COMPOSITA, L. D. ; *Compound Tincture of Rhubarb.* (Rhubarb, sliced, ʒiiss. [ʒiij. *D.*] ; Liquorice, bruised, ʒvj. [ʒss. *D.*] ; Saffron, ʒiij. [ʒij. *D.*] ; Ginger, bruised, ʒiij. [Cardamom Seeds, ʒj. *D.*] ; Proof Spirit, Oij. Macerate for fourteen days, and strain [filter, *D.*]—Cordial, stimulant, stomachic, and mildly purgative. A popular remedy in various disordered conditions of the alimentary canal, especially at the commencement of diarrhœa, also in flatulent colic. It is a very useful adjunct to purgative mixtures, in cases in which the use of a cordial and stomachic cathartic is required. Dose, as a stomachic, fʒj. to fʒiij. ; as a purgative, fʒss. to fʒiss.

4. TINCTURA RHEI ET ALOES, E. ; *Tincture of Rhubarb and Aloes.* (Rhubarb, in moderately fine powder, ʒiss. ; Socotrine or East Indian Aloes, in moderately fine powder, ʒvj. ; Cardamom Seeds, bruised, ʒv. ; Proof Spirit, Oij. Mix the powders, and proceed as for the tincture of cinchona.)—A cordial and stomachic purgative in doses of from fʒss. to fʒj.

5. TINCTURA RHEI ET GENTIANÆ, E. ; *Tincture of Rhubarb and Gentian.* (Rhubarb, in moderately fine powder, ʒij. ; Gentian, finely cut or in coarse powder, ʒss. ; Proof Spirit, Oij. Mix the powders, and proceed as directed for tincture of c nchona.)—Stomachic, tonic, and feebly purgative. Dose, as a tonic, fʒj. to fʒiij. ; as a very mild purgative, fʒss. to fʒj.

6. VINUM RHEI, E. D. ; *Wine of Rhubarb.* (Rhubarb, in coarse powder, ʒv. [ʒiij. *D.*] ; Canella, in coarse powder, ʒij. ; Proof Spirit, fʒv. ; Sherry, Oj. and fʒxv. [Sherry Wine, Oij. *D.*] Digest for seven days [fourteen, *D.*], strain, express strongly the residuum, and filter the liquors.)—Cordial, stomachic, and mildly purgative. Used in the same cases as the *compound tincture of rhubarb.* Dose, as a stomachic, fʒj. to fʒiij. ; as a purgative, fʒss. to fʒj.

7. EXTRACTUM RHEI, L. E. D. ; *Extract of Rhubarb.* (Rhubarb, powdered, ʒxv. [lb. j. *E. D.*] ; Proof Spirit, Oj. ; Distilled Water, Ovij. [Water, Ov. *E. D.*] Macerate for four days [twenty-four hours, *E. D.*] with a gentle heat, afterwards strain, and set by, that the dregs may subside. Pour off the liquor, and evaporate it, when strained, to a proper consistence, *L. D.*—The process of the *Edinburgh College* is as follows :—Take of Rhubarb, lb. j. ; Water, Ov. Cut the rhubarb into small fragments ; macerate it for twenty-four hours in three pints of the water, filter the liquor through a cloth, and express it with the hands or otherwise moderately ; macerate the residuum with the rest of the water for twelve hours at least ; filter the liquor with the same cloth as before, and express the residuum strongly. The liquors, filtered again if necessary, are then to be evaporated together to a proper consistence in a vapour-bath. The extract, however, is obtained of finer quality by evaporation in a vacuum with a gentle heat.) [The process of the *Dublin College* is similar to this.— Ed.]

The Edinburgh and Dublin Colleges, it will be observed, employ no spirit in the above process. Great care is required in the preparation of this extract, as both the purgative and tonic properties of rhubarb are very apt to become deteriorated by the process. Some extract prepared *in vacuo* more than twenty years retained the proper odour and flavour of rhubarb. The dose of extract of rhubarb, as a purgative, is from grs. x. to ʒss.

[8. EXTRACTUM RHEI FLUIDUM, U.S. ; *Fluid Extract of Rhubarb.*

(Take of Rhubarb, in coarse powder, ʒviij.; Sugar, ʒv.; Tincture of Ginger, ʒss.; Oil of Fennel, Oil of Anise, each ♏iv.; Diluted Alcohol, a sufficient quantity. To the rhubarb, previously mixed with an equal bulk of coarse sand, add twelve fluidounces of diluted alcohol, and allow the mixture to stand for twenty-four hours. Transfer the mass to a percolator, and gradually pour upon it diluted alcohol, until the liquid which passes has little of the odour or taste of the rhubarb. Evaporate the tincture thus obtained, by means of a water-bath, to five fluidounces; then add the sugar, and after it is dissolved mix thoroughly with the resulting fluid extract, the tincture of ginger holding the oils in solution.)—This is an excellent and efficient preparation in doses of ʒj. to ʒij. It may be given to children in small doses. By addition to magnesia, it constitutes an effective combination.—ED.]

9. PILULÆ RHEI, E.; *Rhubarb Pills.* (Rhubarb, in fine powder, *nine parts;* Acetate of Potash, *one part;* Conserve of Red Roses, *five parts.* Beat them into a proper mass, and divide it into five-grain pills.)—Stomachic and purgative. The acetate of potash is employed, I presume, to prevent the pills becoming hard by keeping. Each pill contains nearly three and a half grains of rhubarb.

10. PILULA RHEI COMPOSITA, L. E.; *Pilulæ Rhei compositæ,* D.; *Compound Pills of Rhubarb.* (Rhubarb, powdered, ʒj. [*twelve parts,* E.]; Socotrine Aloes, powdered, ʒvj. [*nine parts,* E.]; Myrrh, powdered, ʒij. [*six parts,* E.]; Soft Soap, ʒss. [*six parts,* E.]; [Oil of Caraway, ♏xv. *L.*; Oil of Peppermint, *one part,* E.]; Treacle, q. s. [Conserve of Red Roses, *five parts,* E.] Mix them, and beat them into a proper mass [and divide this into five-grain pills. This pill may be also made without oil of peppermint, when so preferred, *E.* [The *Dublin College* orders Rhubarb, in fine powder, ʒiss.; Hepatic Aloes, in fine powder, ʒix.; Myrrh in fine powder, Castile Soap, of each ʒvj.; Oil of Peppermint, fʒj.; Treacle, by weight, ʒij. Reduce the soap to fine powder, and triturate it with the rhubarb, aloes, and myrrh: then add the treacle and oil of peppermint, and beat the whole into a uniform mass, *D.*—ED.]—Tonic and mildly purgative. Dose, Əj., or to four pills. [This is used as a dinner pill.—ED.]

11. PILULÆ RHEI ET FERRI, E.; *Pills of Rhubarb and Iron.* (Dried Sulphate of Iron, *four parts;* Extract of Rhubarb, *ten parts;* Conserve of Red Roses, about *five parts.* Beat them into a proper pill-mass, and divide into five-grain pills.)—Tonic. Dose, two to four pills.

12. PULVIS RHEI COMPOSITUS, E. D.; *Compound Powder of Rhubarb.* (Magnesia, lb. j. [ʒvj. *D.*]; Ginger, in fine powder, ʒij. [ʒj. *D.*]; Rhubarb, in fine powder, ʒiv. [ʒij. *D.*] Mix them thoroughly, and preserve the powder in well-closed bottles.)—A very useful antacid and mild stomachic purgative, especially adapted for children. Dose, for adults, Əj. to ʒss.; for children, grs. v. to grs. x.

[**13. SYRUPUS RHEI, U.S.;** *Syrup of Rhubarb.* (Take of Rhubarb, bruised, ʒij.; Boiling Water, Oj.; Sugar, lb. ij. Macerate the rhubarb in the water for twenty-four hours, and strain; then add the sugar, and proceed in the manner directed for syrup.)—This is a mild astringent and laxative, and may be used in bowel affections. The dose is from ʒj. to ʒj.—ED.]

[**14. SYRUPUS RHEI AROMATICUS, U.S.;** *Aromatic* or *Spiced Syrup of Rhubarb.* (Take of Rhubarb, bruised, ʒiiss.; Cloves, bruised, Cinnamon, bruised, each 3ss.; Nutmeg, bruised, 3ij.; Diluted Alcohol, Oij.; Syrup, Ovj. Macerate the rhubarb and aromatics in the diluted alcohol for fourteen days, and strain; then, by means of a water-bath, evaporate the liquor to a pint, and while it is still hot mix it with the syrup previously heated: or it may be made by displacement.)—This syrup is cordial, carminative, and slightly laxative. It is well adapted to weak and relaxed conditions of the bowels; as in chronic diarrhœa, dysentery, and infantile bowel complaints with feeble action. The dose is 3j. to 3ss.—ED.]

157. RUMEX ACETOSA, *Linn.*—COMMON SORREL.

Sex. Syst. Hexandria, Trigynia.

HISTORY.—Dioscorides[1] mentions this as the fourth sort (τέταρτον εἶδος) of λάπαϑον, which some call ὀξαλίς.

BOTANY. **Gen. Char.**—*Sepals* 6, the 3 inner (petals) larger, subsequently becoming enlarged (enlarged or permanent petals), converging, and finally concealing the nut. *Stamens* 6. *Stigmas* in many fine tufted segments. *Embryo* lateral.

Sp. Char.—*Leaves* oblong, sagittate or hastate, veiny. *Flowers* diœcious. *Inner sepals* (petals) roundish, cordate, with a very minute tubercle at the base.

Hab.—Indigenous. Woods, and pastures common. Perennial. Flowers in June.

DESCRIPTION.—Sorrel leaves have an agreeably acid and slightly astringent taste.

COMPOSITION.—I am unacquainted with any analysis of this plant. The leaves are composed of *superoxalate of potash, tartaric acid, mucilage, fecula, chlorophylle, tannic acid,* and *woody fibre.*

PHYSIOLOGICAL EFFECTS.—Slightly nutritive. Refrigerant and diuretic. Esteemed antiscorbutic.

USES.—Employed as a pot-herb and salad: from the latter use of it, it has been termed *green sauce.*[2] Rarely applied medicinally. A decoction of the leaves may be administered in whey, as a cooling and pleasant drink, in febrile and inflammatory diseases. In some parts of Scandinavia bread is made of it in times of scarcity.[3] But the use of aliments containing oxalic acid may, as suggested by Laugier, under some circumstances, dispose to the formation of mulberry calculi.

158. RUMEX HYDROLAPATHUM, *Hudson.*—GREAT WATER DOCK.

Sex. Syst. Hexandria, Trigynia.

HISTORY.—This is not the *R. aquaticus* of Linnæus.

BOTANY. **Gen. Char.**—See *Rumex acetosa.*

Sp. Char.—*Inner sepals* (petals) ovate-triangular, entire or slightly toothed, all tubercled. *Racemes* panicled, leafless. *Leaves* lanceolate, narrowed at the base; petiole flat on the upper side.—Stem 3-5 feet high. Leaves often more than a foot long.

Hab.—Indigenous. Ditches and river-sides. Perennial. Flowers in July and August.

---

[1] Lib. ii. cap. 140.
[2] Withering, *Bot.* vol. ii.
[3] Clarke, *Travels in Scandinavia*, Part 3, S. ii. p. 90, 1823.

DESCRIPTION.—The herb and root were formerly used under the name of *herba et radix britannicæ.* The root is inodorous, but has an acrid bitter taste. The flowers are called by Pliny[1] *vibones.*

COMPOSITION.—I am unacquainted with any analysis of the plant. The root contains *tannic acid.*

PHYSIOLOGICAL EFFECTS.—The root is astringent, and is reputed anti-scorbutic.

USES.—Scarcely employed. Has been exhibited internally in scurvy, skin diseases, and rheumatism. The powdered root has been used as a dentifrice; the decoction of the root as an astringent gargle for ulcerated or spongy gums. The Druids entertained a superstitious veneration for this plant.

159. POLYGONUM BISTORTA, *Linn.*—GREAT BISTORT OR SNAKE-WEED.

Sex. Syst. Octandria, Trigynia.

(Radix, *D.*)

HISTORY.—It is doubtful by whom this plant is first mentioned. It was certainly noticed by the herbalists of the 16th century.

BOTANY. **Gen. Char.**—*Calyx* 4-5-cleft, more or less coloured. *Stamens* 5-8, in 2 rows, generally with glands at the base. *Styles* 2-3, more or less united at the base. *Nut* 1-seeded, lenticular or 3-cornered, inclosed by the calyx. *Embryo* lateral, incurved; cotyledons not contorted.

Sp. Char.—*Stem* simple. *Leaves* oblong-ovate, somewhat cordate and wavy; petioles winged. *Spike* dense, terminal.—*Flowers* flesh-coloured. *Stem* 1-1½ foot high.

Hab.—Indigenous. Meadows. Perennial. Flowers in June.

DESCRIPTION.—Bistort root (*radix bistortæ*) is twice bent on itself: hence its name,—from *bis,* twice; and *torta,* twisted or bent. It is rugous and brown externally, reddish internally; almost inodorous; it has an austere, strongly astringent taste.

COMPOSITION.—This root has not been analysed. The principal constituents are *tannic acid, starch, oxalate of lime, colouring matter,* and *woody fibre.*

PHYSIOLOGICAL EFFECTS.—The local effect is that of a powerful astringent, depending on the tannic acid which it contains; its remote effects are those of a tonic. The presence of starch renders the root nutritive: hence in Siberia it is roasted and eaten.

USES.—It is but little employed. A decoction of the root is sometimes employed as an astringent injection in leucorrhœa and gleet; as a gargle in spongy gums and relaxed sore-throat; and as a lotion to ulcers attended with a profuse discharge.

Internally it has been employed, in combination with gentian, in intermittents. It has also been used as an astringent in passive hemorrhages and chronic alvine fluxes.

ADMINISTRATION.—The dose of the powder is from ℈j. to ʒss. The *decoction* (prepared by boiling ʒij. of the root in Oiss. of boiling water) may be administered in doses of from fʒj. to fʒij.

---

[1] *Hist. Nat.* lib. xxv. cap. vi. ed. Valp.

ORDER XXXIX. SALSOLACEÆ, *Moquin.*—SALTWORTS.

ATRIPLICES, *Jussieu.*—CHENOPODEÆ, *R. Brown.*—CHENOPODIACEÆ, *Lindl.*

CHARACTERS. — *Calyx* deeply divided, persistent, with an imbricated æstivation. *Corolla* 0. *Stamens* usually inserted into the receptacle or base of the calyx, opposite the segments of the latter, and equal to them in number, or fewer. *Staminodia* (squamulæ hypogynæ) in a few genera, very minute, alternate between the filaments and with the segments of the calyx. *Ovary* single, superior, or occasionally adhering to the tube of the calyx, with a single amphitropal ovule attached to the base of the cavity; *style* in 2 or 4 divisions, rarely simple; *stigmas* undivided. *Fruit* membranous, utriculate, sometimes a caryopsis, rarely a berry. *Seed* with or without farinaceous albumen; *embryo* curved or annular (*cyclolobeæ*), or in a flat spiral (*spirolobeæ*).—*Herbs* or *under-shrubs* sometimes jointed. *Leaves* usually alternate, without stipules. *Flowers* very small, regular, hermaphrodite, or sometimes by abortion unisexual (from *Lindley* chiefly).

PROPERTIES.—The plants of this family are characterised by the large quantity of alkali which they contain, and which is combined with an organic acid. Those which inhabit salt marshes are called *halophytes* (from ἅλς, *salt ;* and φυτόν, *a plant*), and by combustion yield *barilla* (see Vol. i. *Soda*). Those in most common use for this purpose belong to the genera *Salsola, Salicornia,* and *Chenopodium.*

Many of the plants are esculent, and some of them are used as pot-herbs or salads ; as spinach (*Spinacea oleracea*) and beet (*Beta vulgaris*). The latter is extensively cultivated and employed as a source of sugar ; and a variety of it, called Mangold-Wurzel, is used for feeding cattle. The seeds of *Chenopodium Quinoa* are employed in Peru as food, under the name of *petty rice :* their starch-grains are the smallest known.

Volatile oil is found in several, which owe their aromatic, carminative, stimulant, and anthelmintic properties to it.

160. Chenopodium Vulvaria, *Linn.*—Stinking Orache.

Sex. Syst. Pentandria, Digynia.

(Herba.)

Chenopodium olidum, Smith, Eng. Flora ; *Atriplex fœtida,* Cullen, Mat. Med. vol. ii. p. 365 ; *Stinking Goosefoot.*—Indigenous. Cultivated at Mitcham. Sold in the herb-shops as a popular emmenagogue and "strengthener of the womb." In the fresh state it has a nauseous state, and a strong offensive odour like that of putrid fish. By drying, it loses its smell, and probably its medicinal qualities also : Dr. Houlton and Mr. Churchill[1] declare that the popular notion of its emmenagogue powers is well founded. Dr. Cullen regarded it as a powerful antispasmodic in hysteria. The recent plant has been used in the form of infusion or tea, and conserve. Mr. Churchill gave the inspissated juice or extract in doses of from five to fifteen grains.

CHENOPODIUM AMBROSIOIDES, *Linn.,* is said to be used indiscriminately with the preceding. Its odour is weaker and less offensive.

CHENOPODIUM BOTRYS, *Linn.* This is considered to have anthelmintic properties.

[161. Chenopodium anthelminticum, *Linn.*—Wormseed.

Sex. Syst. Pentandria, Digynia.

(Fructus.)

Gen. Char.—*Calyx* 5-parted, with 5 angles. *Corolla* 0. *Style* bifid, rarely trifid. *Seed* 1, lenticular, horizontal, covered by the closing calyx (*Nuttall*).

Sp. Char.—*Leaves* oblong, lanceolate, sinuate, and dentate, rugose. *Racemes* naked. *Style* 1, 3-cleft (*Elliot*).

---

[1] Stephenson and Churchill's *Medical Botany,* vol. iv. pl. clxxvi. 1831.

The common names by which this plant is known in the United States are Jerusalem Oak, Goosefoot, and Stinkweed.

DESCRIPTION.—The root of the plant is perennial and branched. Stem upright, herbaceous, much branched, deeply grooved, from 2 to 4 feet high. Branches fastigiate, giving to the plant a shrubby appearance. Leaves sessile, scattered, and alternate, attenuate at each end, with strongly marked nervures, oval or oblong, deeply sinuate, studded beneath with small globular, oleaginous dots. Flowers small, numerous, of a yellowish-green colour, and collected in long, axillary, dense, leafless spikes.

Hab.—This species of Chenopodium is found in most parts of the United States. It flowers in old fields, along roadsides, in moist and sandy situations. It flowers in June and July; and from August until cold weather the seeds may be collected.

The seeds are small, not larger than the head of a common-sized pin, irregularly spherical, very light, of a dull greenish-yellow colour, approaching to brown, and having a bitterish, somewhat aromatic, pungent taste. The odour and taste are due to the volatile oil that they contain; this is found in other parts; in fact, the whole plant contains it, and hence the uniform flavour possessed by them.

The properties of the seeds are vermifuge, which appears to have been known soon after the establishment of the British Colonies in America, especially in Virginia, where they were first used for this purpose. The herb is spoken of by Schoepf and Kalm, with others, in terms of commendation. The vermifuge power, by long trial, has been decidedly proved. As an antispasmodic it has also been used. Plenck employed it with success in five or six cases of chorea,[1] and this success has been confirmed by other writers.

The Chenopodium anthelminticum has sometimes been confounded with the C. ambrosioides, which is a smaller plant, and distinguished by the leafy spikes of flowers. The sensible properties are similar.

The seeds are given in the form of an electuary, pulverised and mixed with molasses or syrup; but the quantity required to be taken is liable to produce nausea and sickness. Dose, Əj. to Əij. given twice or thrice daily.

The expressed juice is sometimes administered; the dose is ℥ss. : or a decoction of the leaves may be employed; this is best prepared with milk, in the proportion of ℥j. leaves to Oj. of milk or water. It may be flavoured with aromatics.

OLEUM CHENOPODII, U.S.; *Oil of Wormseed.*—This oil is of a light yellow colour when distilled, but its colour deepens by age and exposure. It has in a high degree the flavour of the plant. Its sp. gr. is 0·908. It is obtained by distilling the seeds; but the whole plant may be used for this purpose, as the oil is abundant in the glands. Sometimes it is adulterated with spirit of turpentine, or other inferior volatile oils; this must be determined by the odour. From the readiness with which it may be given, it is the best for exhibition, as it possesses the vermifuge properties in the smallest possible compass. The dose is from 10 to 20 drops on a lump of sugar, or in emulsion. After several doses have been given, a purgative, as castor oil, may be interposed.[2]—ED.]

SUB-DIVISION II. COROLLIFLORÆ, *De Cand.*

MONOPETALÆ COROLLA HYPOGYNA, *Juss.,* ET COROLLA PERIGYNA (partim).
GAMOPETALÆ, *Endl.* (partim).

Calyx gamosepalous, i. e. sepals more or less united at the base. Petals mostly united, distinct at the base from the calyx. Stamens usually adnate to the corolla. Ovary mostly free, rarely adnate to the calyx.

ORDER XL. LABIATÆ, *Jussieu.*—LABIATES.

LAMIACEÆ, *Lindley.*

CHARACTERS.—*Calyx* tubular, inferior, persistent, the odd tooth being next the axis; regular 5- or 10-toothed, or irregular bilabiate or 3- to 10-toothed. *Corolla* monopeta-

---

[1] Griffith, *On Chem. Anthel.* in *Am. Journ. of Pharm.* vol. v. p. 180.
[From the American Edition, by Dr. Carson.]

FIG. 181.

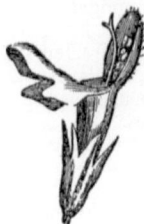

Bilabiate Flower.

lous, hypogynous, bilabiate; the upper lip undivided or bifid, overlapping the lower, which is larger and 3-lobed. *Stamens* 4, didynamous, inserted upon the corolla, alternately with the lobes of the lower lip, the 2 upper sometimes wanting; anthers 2-celled; sometimes apparently unilocular, in consequence of the confluence of the cells at the apex: sometimes 1 cell altogether obsolete, or the 2 cells separated by a bifurcation of the connective. *Ovary* deeply 4-lobed, seated in a fleshy hypogynous disc; the lobes each containing 1 erect ovule; *style* 1, proceeding from the base of the lobes of the ovary; *stigma* bifid, usually acute. *Fruit* 1 to 4 small nuts, inclosed within the persistent calyx. *Seeds* erect, with little or no albumen; *embryo* erect; *cotyledons* flat.—*Herbaceous* plants or *undershrubs*. Stem 4-cornered, with opposite ramifications. *Leaves* opposite, divided or undivided, without stipules, replete with receptacles of aromatic oil. *Flowers* in opposite, nearly sessile, axillary cymes, resembling whorls; sometimes solitary, or as if capitate (*Lindley*).

PROPERTIES.—The medicinal activity of the plants of this family depends on volatile oil, bitter extractive, and astringent matter.

The *volatile oil* resides in small receptacles (by some called *globular glands*) contained in the leaves. " These glands are placed quite superficially, or rather in depressed points, and are commonly of a shining yellow colour. We may regard them as oleo-resinous matter separated from glands lying on the under surface. When macerated in strong spirit of wine, they remain unchanged, and appear under the microscope as transparent, probably cellular, vesicles, filled with a yellow granular matter."[1]

The *bitter extractive* is found, in greater or less quantity, in all the Labiatæ. It is this principle which communicates the bitterness to the watery infusion of these plants.

The presence of *astringent matter* is shown by the green colour produced when a ferruginous salt is added to the infusion of some of the Labiatæ.

The volatile oil gives to these plants aromatic, carminative, and slightly stimulant properties. The bitter extractive renders them tonic and stomachic. The astringent matter is usually in too small a quantity to communicate much medicinal activity, though it must contribute to the tonic operation.

The perfumer uses some labiate plants on account of their fragrant odour; the cook employs others for their flavour and condimental properties; the medical practitioner administers them to relieve nausea and colicky pains, to expel wind, to cover the taste of nauseous medicines, and to prevent or relieve griping pains.

The following species, enumerated by Loudon,[2] are cultivated in this country as *sweet herbs:*—Common or Garden Thyme (*Thymus vulgaris*, Linn.), Lemon Thyme (*T. citriodorus*, Schreb.), Sage (*Salvia officinalis*, Linn.), Clary (*S. Sclarea*, Linn.), Peppermint (*Mentha piperita*, Linn.), Spearmint (*M. viridis*, Linn.), Pennyroyal (*M. Pulegium*), Common Marjoram (*Origanum vulgare*, Linn.), Winter Sweet Marjoram (*O. heracleoticum*, Linn.), Sweet Marjoram (*Majorana hortensis*, Mœnch.), Pot Marjoram (*M. Onites*, Benth.), Winter Savory (*Satureja montana*, Linn.), Summer Savory (*S. hortensis*, Linn.), Sweet or Larger Basil (*Ocimum Basilicum*, Linn.) Bush or Least Basil (*O. minimum*, Linn.), Rosemary (*Rosmarinus officinalis*, Linn.), and Garden Lavender (*Lavandula vera*, De Cand.) Some of these species have been, or are, used in medicine, and several of them are officinal.

Besides the labiate plants contained in the British pharmacopœias, and to be noticed, a considerable number of other species have been at different times introduced into medicinal use. Some of these are deficient in volatile oil, but abound in a bitter principle, on which account they have been employed as stomachics and tonics: such are Water Germander (*Teucrium Scordium*, Linn.), Wall Germander (*T. Chamædrys*, Linn.), and Ground Pine (*Ajuga Chamæpitys*, Smith); the two last of which have been used, as I have elsewhere mentioned, as anti-arthritic remedies. Others abound in essential oil, and are consequently more aromatic, stimulant, and carminative: such are Cat-Thyme (*Teucrium Marum*, Linn.), Common Hyssop (*Hyssopus officinalis*, Linn.), and Dittany of Crete (*Amaracus Dictamnus*, Benth.). *Teucrium Polium* has been used in diarrhœa, dysentery, and cholera.

---

[1] Nees and Ebermaier, *Handb. d. med.-pharm. Bot.* Th. i. S. 524.
[2] *Encycl. of Gardening.*

Tribe I. Ocimoideæ, *Benth.*

Stamens bent downwards.

162. LAVANDULA VERA, *De Cand.*—COMMON OR GARDEN LAVENDER.

Lavandula angustifolia, *Ehrenberg.*

Sex. Syst. Didynamia, Gymnospermia.

(Oleum e flore destillatum, *L.*—The flowers, *D.*—The flowering heads ; and volatile oil of ditto, *E.*)

History.—No plant is mentioned, under the name of Lavender, by Hippocrates, Theophrastus, Dioscorides, or Pliny. It is not improbable, however, that lavender may be alluded to, under some other name, by one or more of these authors; but it is impossible now to identify it with any certainty. Sprengel[1] declares, on the authority of Heyschius, that the ἴφνον of Theophrastus[2] is *Lavandula Spica.* The στιχάς or στοιχάς of Dioscorides,[3] the *stœchas* of Pliny,[4] is the *L. Stœchas*, Linn.

Botany. **Gen. Char.**—*Calyx* ovate-tubular, nearly equal, 13- or rarely 15-ribbed, shortly 5-toothed, with the 4 lower teeth nearly equal, or the 2 lower narrower; the upper either but little broader than the lateral ones, or expanded into a dilated appendage. *Corolla* with the tube exserted, the throat somewhat dilated, the limb oblique and bilabiate; upper lip 2-lobed; lower 3-lobed; all the divisions nearly equal. *Stamens* 4, inclosed in the tube of the corolla, bent downwards. *Filaments* smooth, distinct, not toothed. *Style* shortly bifid at the apex ; the lobes complanate, subconnate. *Disc* concave, with 4 fleshy scales at the margin. *Nuts* smooth, adnate to the scales of the disc (*Bentham*).

Sp. Char.—*Leaves* oblong-linear or lanceolate, quite entire, when young hoary and revolute at the edges. *Spikes* interrupted. *Whorls* of 6 to 10 flowers. *Floral leaves* rhomboid-ovate, acuminate, membranous, all fertile, the uppermost shorter than the calyx. *Bracts* scarcely any (*Bentham*).—An *undershrub* 1 to 2 feet high. *Flowers* purplish-grey.

Hab.—South of Europe. Extensively cultivated at Mitcham, in Surrey, from which place the London market is chiefly supplied.

Lavandula Spica, De Cand. (*L. latifolia*, Villars), or *French Lavender*, formerly considered as a variety only of the preceding species, is not used in medicine. It is distinguished by its lower habit, whiter colour, the leaves more congested at the base of the branches, the spike denser and shorter, the floral leaves lanceolate or linear, and the presence of bracts (Bentham). It yields by distillation *oil of spike* (*oleum spicæ*), sometimes called *foreign oil of lavender*,—or, in order to distinguish it from the oil of *Lavandula Stœchas*, the *true oil of spike* (*oleum spicæ verum*). This oil is distinguished from the genuine oil of *Lavandula vera* by its darker green colour, and its less grateful odour. It is used by painters on porcelain, and by artists in the preparation of varnishes.

Properties.—*Lavender flowers* (*flores lavandulæ*) have a bluish-grey colour, a pleasant odour, and a pungent bitter taste. The flowering stems

---

[1] *Hist. Rei Herb.* t. i. p. 96.
[2] *Hist. Plant.* lib. vi. cap. 6.
[3] Lib. iii. cap. 31.
[4] *Hist. Nat.* lib. xxvii. cap. 107.

are collected in June or July, dried in the shade, and made up into bundles for sale. A cold infusion of the flowers is deepened in colour (*tannate of iron*) by sesquichloride of iron.

Composition.—The principal constituents of the flowers are *volatile oil, resin* (?), *tannic acid,* a *bitter principle,* and *woody fibre.*

Physiological Effects.—The flowers are carminative, mildly stimulant, and somewhat tonic. Kraus[1] says that when taken internally they cause griping.

Uses.—Lavender flowers are sometimes employed as errhines.

1. OLEUM LAVANDULÆ, E.D.; *Oleum Lavandulæ veræ; Oleum Lavandulæ (Anglicum),* L.; *English Oil of Lavender,* offic. (Prepared by submitting lavender flowers to distillation with water.)—It has a pale yellow colour, a hot taste, and a very fragrant odour. Its sp. gr. varies from 0·877 to 0·905; the lightest oil being the purest. It boils at 397° F., and is composed, according to Dr. Kane, of $C^{15}H^{14}O^2$. 1 lb. of oil is obtained from 50 to 70 lbs. of the flowers. 1973 lbs. of the flowers, carefully separated from the stalks, yielded Mr. Jacob Bell,[2] at thirteen distillations, 28½ lbs. of oil,—or 1 lb. of oil from 69¼ lbs. of flowers. When the stalks and leaves are distilled with the flowers, the odour of the oil is considerably deteriorated.[3] It is a stimulant and stomachic, and is sometimes given in hysteria and headache, but is more commonly employed as a perfume for scenting evaporating lotions, ointments, or liniments. [It is thus used in the preparation of the *Linimentum Camphoræ compositum,* L. D.—Ed.]—Dose, gtt. ij. to gtt. v.

2. SPIRITUS LAVANDULÆ, E.; *Spirit of Lavender.* (Fresh Lavender, lb. iiss.; Rectified Spirit, Cong. j. Mix them, and with the heat of a vapourbath let seven pints distil.)—The dried may be substituted for the fresh flowers. Druggists frequently prepare this compound by dissolving a few drops of oil of lavender in a fluidounce of rectified spirit. Employed in the preparation of the *Tinctura Lavandulæ composita.*

Lavender Water.—The fragrant perfume sold in the shops under the name of *lavender water (aqua lavandulæ)* is a solution of the oil of lavender and of other odoriferous substances in spirit. It is in fact, therefore, a *compound spirit of lavender;* but this name is already appropriated to another preparation. There are various formulæ for its preparation, scarcely two manufacturers adopting precisely the same one. The following yields a most excellent product :—Oil of Lavender, Oil of Bergamot, aa. f3iij.; Otto of Roses, Oil of Cloves, aa. gtt. vj.; Musk, gr. ij.; Oil of Rosemary, f3j.; Honey, 3j.; Benzoic Acid, 9ij.; Rectified Spirit, Oj.; Distilled Water, 3iij. Mix, and after standing a sufficient time (the longer the better), filter. This agreeable perfume may be employed for scenting spirit washes, but it is principally consumed for the toilette.

3. TINCTURA LAVANDULÆ COMPOSITA, L. D.; *Compound Tincture of Lavender; Spiritus Lavandulæ compositus,* E.; *Lavender Drops,* or *Red Lavender Drops,* offic. (Oil of Lavender, 3iss.; Oil of Rosemary, mx.; Cinnamon, bruised, and Nutmeg, bruised, of each 3iiss.; Red Saunders Wood, sliced, 3v.; Rectified Spirit, Oij. Macerate the cinnamon, nutmeg, and red Saunders wood in the spirit for seven days, then press out and strain, and dissolve the oils in the strained tincture, *L.* Take of Spirit of Lavender, Oij.;

---

[1] *Heilmittell.* p. 473.
[2] *Pharm. Journal,* vol. viii. p. 276, 1848.
[3] Brande, *Dict. of Mat. Med.* pp. 387-8; J. Bell, *op. cit.*

Spirit of Rosemary, ʒxij.; Nutmeg, bruised, ʒss.; Cinnamon, in coarse powder, ʒj. Let the whole macerate for seven days : then strain the liquor through coarse calico, *E.* Oil of Lavender, fʒiij.; Oil of Rosemary, fʒj.; Cinnamon, bruised, ʒj.; Nutmeg, bruised, ʒss.; Cloves, bruised, Cochineal, in powder, of each ʒij.; Rectified Spirit, Oij. Macerate for fourteen days, strain, express, and filter, *D.* [The United States Pharmacopœia directs Spirit of Lavender, Oiij.; Spirit of Rosemary, Oj.; Cinnamon, bruised, ʒj.; Cloves, bruised, ʒij.; Nutmeg, bruised, ʒss.; Red Saunders, rasped, ʒiij. Macerate for fourteen days, and filter through paper, *U.S.*—Ed.])—Stimulant, cordial, and stomachic. Employed to relieve gastric uneasiness, flatulence, low spirits, languor, and faintness. A favourite remedy with hysterical and hypochondriacal persons. —Dose, from fʒss. to fʒij. administered in water or on sugar. The red Saunders wood is merely a colouring ingredient.

Tribe II. Satureieæ, *Benth.*

Stamens distant, straight, straggling, or converging under the upper lip, 4 or 2 (in that case the anthers 2-celled, and the connective not filiform). Lobes of the *corolla* flat.

163. Pogostemon Patchouli, *Pellet.*—Pucha Pat, or Patchouli.

Sex. Syst. Didynamia, Gymnospermia.

(Herba.)

Patchouly, Virey, Journ. de Pharm. t. xii. p. 61, 1826 ; *Puchá Pát*, Wallich, Trans. Med. and Phys. Soc. of Calcutta, 1835 ; *Pogostemon intermedius*, Bentham, in Wall. Cat. n. 2327 ; *Patchouli* or *Puchá Pát*, Pereira, Pharm. Journ. vol. iv. p. 80, 1844 ; *Pogostemon Patchouly*, Pelletier-Sautelet, in Mém. de la Soc. Roy. des Sc. d'Orl. tom. v. p. 274, 1845, cum Ic.; also Pharm. Journ. vol. viii. p. 574 ; Benth. in De Cand. Prodr. t. xii. p. 153 ; *Pogostemon suavis*, Tenore ; *Pogostemon Patchouli*, Hooker, Journ. of Bot. and Kew Gard. Miscell. vol. i. p. 329, c. Ic.

A pubescent undershrub. Branches vague, decumbent or ascending. Leaves with stalks, opposite, rhomboid-ovate, somewhat obtuse; the lobes crenato-dentate. Spikes terminal and axillary, dense, pedunculated, interrupted at the base. Bracts ovate. Calyx hirsute, twice as long as the bracts, with lanceolate teeth. Corolla bilabiate, smooth and whitish. Stamens 4, didynamous, nearly equal in length ; the filaments bearded with violet or bluish-purple hairs; the anthers pale yellow, after flowering whitish. Style pale purplish, whitish at the lower part, at the apex deeply cleft. Ovaries 4, distinct.—A native of Silhet, Penang, and the Malayan peninsula.

The wild plant is collected at Penang and the Malayan peninsula, and dried in the sun. If too much dried, it becomes crisp and brittle, and is liable to crumble to dust in packing.

The dried tops (*summitates patchouli*) are imported into England in boxes of 110 lbs. each, and in half-boxes. They are a foot or more in length. The large stems are round and woody, and, when cut transversely, show the pith surrounded with a thick layer of wood, which is remarkable for its distinct medullary rays ; the smaller branches are obscurely 4-angled. The leaves are covered, especially on their inferior surface, with a soft pallid pubescence, which gives the plant a greyish appearance. The odour is strong, persistent, peculiar, and somewhat analogous to that of *Chenopodium anthelminticum*. It is said to smell more strongly in dry than in damp places. One writer describes the smell of it as being dry, mouldy, or earthy ; and states that the Chinese or Indian ink owes its characteristic odour to it. The taste of the dried plant is very slight.

The plant, which has not been analysed, contains *volatile oil, green resin, extractive matter,* and *tannic acid.* By distillation it yields about 2 per cent. of volatile oil (*essential oil of patchouli*), which possesses the odour of the herb.

Patchouli is almost exclusively used as a perfume. To its excessive employment ill effects have been ascribed. "Very recently," says a French writer,[1] "a young lady was seized with a passion for patchouli. Her linen, her dresses, and her furniture, were saturated with it. In a short time she lost her appetite and sleep; her complexion got pale, and she became subject to nervous attacks."[2] In India, patchouli is used as an ingredient in tobacco, for smoking. The *sachets de patchouli* of the perfumers consist of a few grains of the coarsely-powdered herb mixed with cotton wool and folded in paper. Placed in drawers, they are said to drive away insects from linen, shawls, and other articles of dress. *Oil of patchouli* is in common use in India for imparting the peculiar fragrance of the leaf to clothes among the superior classes of natives. *Essence de patchouli* is used by perfumers principally for mixing with other scents in the preparation of compounded perfumes, for which purpose it is considered very useful.

164. MENTHA VIRIDIS, *Linn.*—SPEARMINT.

Sex. Syst. Didynamia, Gymnospermia.

(Herba florens recens et exsiccata, *L.*—The herb, *E. D.*)

HISTORY.—See *Mentha piperita.*

BOTANY. **Gen. Char.**—*Calyx* campanulate or tubular, 5-toothed, equal or somewhat 2-lipped, with the throat naked inside, or villous. *Corolla* with the tube enclosed, the limb campanulate, nearly equal, 4-cleft; the upper segment broader, nearly entire or emarginate. *Stamens* 4, equal, erect, distinct; *filaments* smooth, naked; *anthers* with 2 parallel cells. *Style* shortly bifid, with the lobes bearing stigmas at the points. *Nucules* dry, smooth (*Bentham*).

Sp. Char.—*Stem* erect, smooth. *Leaves* subsessile, ovate-lanceolate, unequally serrated, smooth; those under the flowers all bract-like, rather longer than the whorls; those last and the calyxes hairy or smooth. *Spikes* cylindrical, loose. *Whorls* approximated, or the lowest or all of them distant. Teeth of the *calyx* linear subulate (*Bentham*).—Creeping-rooted.

Var. β *angustifolia*, Bentham.—Leaves of the branches with short petioles. Distinguished from *M. piperita* by the slender elongated spikes.

Var. γ *crispa*, Bentham; *Curled Mint.*—Cultivated in gardens.

Hab.—Marshy places. Indigenous. A native of the milder parts of Europe; also of Africa and America. Perennial. Flowers in August. Selected for medicinal use when about to flower.

PROPERTIES.—The whole herb, called *green mint* or *spearmint* (*herba menthæ viridis*), is employed in medicine. It has a strong but peculiar odour, and an aromatic, bitter taste, followed by a sense of coldness when air is drawn into the mouth. Sesquichloride of iron communicates a green colour (*tannate of iron*) to the cold watery infusion.

COMPOSITION.—Its odour and aromatic qualities depend on *volatile oil.* It also contains *tannic acid*, *resin* (?), a *bitter principle*, and *woody fibre.*

PHYSIOLOGICAL EFFECTS.—Aromatic, carminative, mildly stimulant and tonic. Feebler than peppermint. Said, though without sufficient foundation, to check the secretion of milk, and to act as an emmenagogue.[3]

USES.—Employed as a salad and sweet herb. In medicine it is principally

---

[1] *Annuaire de Thérapeutique* pour 1847, p. 75.

[2] For some remarks on the sensitiveness of some female constitutions to odorous emanations, see Vol. i.

[3] Linnæus, in Murray's *App. Med.* vol. ii. pp. 180–1.

used as a flavouring ingredient, and to alleviate or prevent colicky pains. The following are its officinal preparations, with their uses :—

1. INFUSUM MENTHÆ VIRIDIS, D. ; *Infusion of Spearmint; Spearmint Tea.* (Spearmint, dried, and cut small, ʒiij. ; Boiling Water, Oss. Infuse for fifteen minutes in a covered vessel, and strain. The product should measure about eight ounces.)—Stomachic and carminative. Used in irritable conditions of the stomach, but is ordinarily a vehicle for other remedies. Dose, fʒj. to fʒij., or *ad libitum.*

2. OLEUM MENTHÆ VIRIDIS, L. E. D. ; *Oil of Spearmint; Oleum ex herbâ florente destillatum,* L. (Obtained by submitting the fresh herb to distillation with water.)—It is of a pale yellowish colour, but becomes reddish by age. It has the odour and taste of the plant, and is lighter than water; sp. gr. 0·914. It boils at 320° F. ; and is composed, according to Dr. Kane, of $C^{35}H^{28}O$. The average produce of the essential oil is not more than 1-500th of the fresh herb.[1] It is carminative and stimulant.[2] Dose, gr. ij. to gtt. v. rubbed with sugar and a little water.

3. SPIRITUS MENTHÆ VIRIDIS, L. ; *Spirit of Spearmint.* (Oil of Spearmint, ʒiij. ; Proof Spirit, Cong. j. ; Water, Oj. Dissolve. Dose, fʒss. to fʒij.)—This preparation is similar to the *essence of spearmint* of the shops.

4. ESSENTIA MENTHÆ VIRIDIS, D. ; *Essence of Spearmint.* (Oil of Spearmint, fʒj. ; Stronger Spirit, fʒix. Mix with agitation, *D.*—In the same way are made, with the respective oils, ESSENTIA MENTHÆ PIPERITÆ, *D.* ; ESSENTIA MENTHÆ PULEGII, *D.* ; and ESSENTIA ROSMARINI, *D.*)

It may be coloured green by spearmint or spinach leaves. Dose, gtt. x. to gtt. xx. taken on sugar or in water.

5. AQUA MENTHÆ VIRIDIS, L. E. D. ; *Spearmint Water.* (Spearmint Leaves, if dried, lb. ij. ; if fresh, lb. iv. ; Rectified Spirit, fʒiij. *E.* ; Water, Cong. ij. Mix. Let a gallon distil. Prepared in the same manner as *Aqua Menthæ piperitæ,* L. The *Dublin College* employs Essence of Spearmint, fʒj. ; Distilled Water, Cong. ss. Mix with agitation, and filter through paper, *D.*—In the same way are made, with the respective essences, AQUA MENTHÆ PIPERITÆ, *D.* ; and AQUA PULEGII, *D.*)—Spearmint water is usually made extemporaneously by suspending or dissolving a drachm of the oil in four pints of distilled water, by means of a drachm of rectified spirit and a lump of sugar. Spearmint water is carminative and stomachic. It is commonly used as a vehicle for other medicines. Its dose is fʒj. to fʒiij.

165. MENTHA PIPERITA, *Linn.*—PEPPERMINT.

Sex. Syst. Didynamia, Gymnospermia.

(Herba florens recens et exsiccata, *L.*—The herb, *D.*—Herb ; Volatile oil, *E.*)

HISTORY.—The ancient Greeks[3] employed in medicine a plant which they called Μίνθος, or Μίνθη, and which, on account of its very agreeable odour,

---

[1] Brande, *Dict. Mat. Med.* p. 328.
[2] [Spearmint oil is obtained in England. It is also imported from America, but the American oil is less pure.—ED.]
[3] Hippocrates, *De victûs rat.* lib. ii. p. 359, ed. Fœs. ; Dioscorides, lib. iii. cap. 36.

was also termed 'Ηδύοσμον, or the *sweet-smelling herb*. It was probably a species of *Mentha*, and, according to Fraas,[1] was the *M. piperita*, Linn., the 'Ηδύοσμον πεπερῶδες of the modern Greek Pharmacopœia.

Peppermint came into use in England in the last century: at least Hill,[2] in 1751, says that it "has lately got into great esteem;" and Geiger[3] says it was introduced into Germany as a medicine, through the recommendations of the English, in the latter half of the last century.

BOTANY. **Gen. Char.**—See *Mentha viridis.*

Sp. Char.—*Stem* smooth. *Leaves* petiolated, ovate-oblong, acute, serrate, rounded-crenate at the base, smooth. *Spikes* lax, obtuse, short, interrupted at the base. *Pedicels* and *calyxes* at the base smooth; teeth hispid (*Bentham*).—Creeping-rooted.

Var. β *sub-hirsuta*, Bentham; *M. hirsuta* δ, Smith.—The nerves of the under surface of the leaves, as well as the petioles, hairy.

Hab.—Watery places. Indigenous. Extensively cultivated at Mitcham,[4] in Surrey, from whence the London market is principally supplied. Found in various parts of Europe; also in Asia, Africa, and America.

PROPERTIES.—The whole herb (*herba menthæ piperitæ*) is officinal. It has a peculiar aromatic odour, and a warm, burning, bitter taste, followed by a sensation of coolness when air is drawn into the mouth. Sesquichloride of iron communicates a green colour (*tannate of iron*) to the cold infusion of peppermint.

COMPOSITION.—The principal constituents are *volatile oil, resin ?, a bitter principle, tannic acid*, and *woody fibre.*

PHYSIOLOGICAL EFFECTS.—Peppermint is an aromatic or carminative, stimulant, and stomachic. It is the most agreeable and powerful of all the mints.

USES.—It is employed in medicine for several purposes, but principally to expel flatus, to cover the unpleasant taste of other medicines, to relieve nausea, griping pain, and the flatulent colic of children. The following are the officinal preparations, with their uses:—

1. OLEUM MENTHÆ PIPERITÆ, L. E. D.; *Oleum ex herbâ florente destillatum*, L.; *Oil of Peppermint*. (Obtained by submitting the fresh herb to distillation with water.)—It is colourless, or nearly so, sometimes having a pale yellow or greenish tint, and becoming reddish by age. It has a penetrating odour, like that of the plant, and a burning aromatic taste, followed by a sensation of cold. The vapour of it, applied to the eye, causes a feeling of coldness.

Oil of peppermint consists of two isomeric oils,—one liquid, the other solid: the latter is called *peppermint camphor*, or the stearoptene of oil of peppermint. Its composition is $C^{20}H^{20}O^2$. It is in colourless prisms, which have the odour and taste of peppermint, are almost insoluble in water, but readily soluble in alcohol and ether, and are fusible at 92° F. Under the

---

[1] *Synop. Plant. Fl. Classicæ*, 1845.
[2] *Hist. of the Mat. Med.* p. 358.
[3] *Handb. d. Pharm.* Bd. iii. S. 1230.
[4] [For an account of the cultivation of this plant at Mitcham, see *Pharmaceutical Journal*, January 1851, p. 340. About fifty acres of mint, and fifty of lavender, are grown at Carshalton, in Surrey.—ED.]

influence of phosphoric acid, peppermint camphor loses $2HO$, and becomes a colourless liquid oil, called *menthene, $C^{20}H^{18}$.*

I have met with three varieties of oil of peppermint :—

α. English Oil of Peppermint.—This is the finest sort. Its sp. gr. is 0·902. It is obtained at Mitcham. In a warm, dry, and favourable season, the produce of oil, from a given quantity of the fresh herb, is double that which it yields in a wet and cold season. The largest produce is three drachms and a half of oil from two pounds of fresh peppermint ; and the smallest, about a drachm and a half from the same quantity.[1] I was informed by a distiller at Mitcham, that twenty mats of the herb (each mat containing about 1 cwt.) yield about seven lbs. of oil. [English oil of peppermint is obtained, not only from Mitcham (the purest quality), but also from the neighbourhood of Cambridge.—ED.]

β. American Oil of Peppermint.—In odour and flavour it is inferior to the preceding sort. It is said to be prepared from the dried plant gathered when in flower (Brande). It yields a considerable quantity of camphor. [The American oil is often adulterated with oil of turpentine, which is perceptible to the smell. The adulterated oil gives a black smoky flame in burning.—ED.]

γ. China Oil of Peppermint ; Po-ho-yo.—For a sample of this I am indebted to Dr. Christison. It comes from Canton. It consists chiefly of peppermint camphor, and forms a white crystalline solid even in summer.

Oil of peppermint is said to be adulterated with oil of rosemary :[2] the odour would probably serve to distinguish the fraud.

Oil of peppermint is carminative and stimulant, and is used occasionally as an antispasmodic. It is taken on sugar in doses of from gtt. ij. to gtt. v.

2. SPIRITUS MENTHÆ PIPERITÆ, L. ; *Spiritus Menthæ,* E. ; *Spirit of Peppermint.* (Prepared with the Oil of Peppermint, in the same way as the *Spiritus Menthæ viridis,* L., before described. The *Edinburgh College* prepares it thus :—Peppermint, fresh, lb. iss. ; Proof Spirit, Ovij. Macerate for two days in a covered vessel ; add a pint and a half of water ; and distil off seven pints.)—A solution of the oil of peppermint has with great propriety been substituted for the former preparation of the Pharmacopœias. The spirit of peppermint is given in doses of from f𝔷ss. to f𝔷ij.

3. ESSENTIA MENTHÆ PIPERITÆ, D. ; *Essence of Peppermint.* (Oil of Peppermint, 𝔷j. ; Stronger Spirit, f℥ix. Mix with agitation.)—Some persons add peppermint or spinach leaves, to communicate a green colour. The dose of this essence is from gtt. xx. to gtt. xxx. on sugar.

4. AQUA MENTHÆ PIPERITÆ, L. E. D. (Take of Peppermint, dried, lb. ij. ; Water, Cong. ij. Let a gallon distil. If the fresh herb be employed, twice the weight is to be used, *L.* Take of Essence of Peppermint, 𝔷j. ; Distilled Water, Cong. ss. Mix with agitation, and filter through paper, *D.* To be prepared like *Aqua Menthæ viridis, E.*)—Carminative and stimulant. Used to relieve flatulency, and as a vehicle for other medicines. Dose f𝔷j. to f℥ij.

Besides the above, there are several popular preparations of peppermint extensively used.

α. Infusum Menthæ piperitæ (Peppermint Tea) is prepared in the same way as spearmint tea.

β. Elæosaccharum Menthæ piperitæ, Ph. Bor., is prepared by mixing 𝔷j. of the whitest sugar, in powder, with gtt. xxiv. of the oil of peppermint.

γ. Rotulæ Menthæ piperitæ (in plano-convex masses, called *peppermint drops ;* in flat-

---

[1] Brande, *Dict. of Mat. Med.* p. 356.
[2] *Pharmaceutical Journal,* vol. i. p. 263, 1841.

2 L

tened circular discs, termed *peppermint lozenges*) should consist of sugar and oil of peppermint only, though flour or plaster of Paris is sometimes introduced.

The *liqueur* sold at the spirit-shops as *mint* or *peppermint* is used as a cordial.

166. MENTHA PULEGIUM, *Linn.*—PENNYROYAL.

Sex. Syst. Didynamia, Gymnospermia.

(Herba florens recens et exsiccata, *L.*—The herb, *E. D.*)

History.—This plant was employed in medicine by the ancient Greeks and Romans. It is the Γλήχων of Hippocrates[1] and Dioscorides,[2] and the *Pulegium* of Pliny.[3]

Botany. **Gen. Char.**—See *Mentha viridis.*

Sp. Char.—*Stem* very much branched, prostrate. *Leaves* petiolated, ovate. *Whorls* all remote, globose, many-flowered. *Calyxes* hispid, bilabiate, villous in the inside of the throat (*Bentham*).—Creeping-rooted.

Hab.—Wet commons and margins of brooks. Indigenous. A native of most parts of Europe, of the Caucasus, Chili, and Teneriffe.

Properties.—The herb with the flowers (*herba* seu *summitates pulegii*) is employed in medicine. It has a strong but peculiar odour; a hot, aromatic, bitter taste, followed by a feeling of coolness in the mouth. Sesquichloride of iron causes a green colour (*tannate of iron*) with the cold infusion of pennyroyal.

Composition.—Its principal constituents are *volatile oil, a bitter matter, resin ?, tannic acid,* and *woody fibre.*

Physiological Effects.—Its effects are analogous to the other mints. Emmenagogue and antispasmodic properties are ascribed to it by the public, and formerly by medical practitioners.

Uses.—A popular remedy for obstructed menstruation, hysterical complaints, and hooping-cough. Rarely employed by the professional man. The following are its officinal preparations, with their uses :—

1. OLEUM PULEGII ; *Oleum Menthæ Pulegii,* E. D. ; *Oleum Pulegii* offic.; *Oleum ex herbâ florente destillatum,* L.; *Oil of Pennyroyal.* (Obtained by submitting the herb to distillation with water.)—It has a pale colour, a warm taste, and the peculiar odour of the herb. It boils at 395° F. Its sp. gr. is 0·925 ; and it is composed, according to Dr. Kane, of $C^{10}H^8O$. The fresh herb yields from 1-120th to 1-100th of its weight of oil.[4] It is stimulant and carminative, and is used, as an antispasmodic and emmenagogue, in doses of from gtt. ij. to gtt. v. taken on sugar.

2. SPIRITUS PULEGII, L.; *Spiritus Pulegii; Spirit of Pennyroyal.* (Prepared with Oil of Pennyroyal, as the *Spiritus Menthæ viridis.*—Oil of Pulegium, fℨiij. ; Proof Spirit, Cong. j. Dissolve.)—Stimulant and carminative. Employed as an antispasmodic and carminative. Dose, fℨss. to fℨij.

---

[1] P. 359, &c. ed. Fœs.
[2] Lib. iii. cap. 36.
[3] *Hist. Nat.* lib. xx. cap. 54, ed. Valp.
[4] Brande, *Dict. Mat. Med.* p. 357.

3. ESSENTIA MENTHÆ PULEGII, D. ; *Essence of Pennyroyal.* (Take of Oil of Pennyroyal, f3j.; Rectified Spirit, f3ix. Mix with agitation.)—This essence may be given in doses of from gtt. x. to gtt. xx.

4. AQUA PULEGII, L. ; *Aqua Menthæ Pulegii,* E. D., offic. ; *Pennyroyal Water.* (Prepared with the herb or oil, like *Aqua Menthæ viridis.*)— Carminative and stomachic.   Dose, f3j. to f3iij.

The liquid sold in the shops as Pennyroyal and Hysteric Water is prepared by adding f3ss. of the *compound spirit of bryony* to Oss. of pennyroyal water.

167. ORIGANUM VULGARE, *Linn.*—COMMON OR WILD MARJORAM.

Sex. Syst. Didynamia, Gymnospermia.

(Herb, *E.*)

History.—Fraas[1] is of opinion that this plant is the ὀρίγανον μέλαν of Theophrastus,[2] the ἀγριορίγανος of Dioscorides.[3]

Botany.   **Gen. Char.** — *Calyx* ovate-campanulate, nearly 13-nerved, 5-toothed or 2-lipped, the upper lip entire or 3-toothed, the inferior lip 2-toothed, truncated, or altogether deficient, the calyx being then obcompressed-flat.   Tube of the *corolla* enclosed or exserted, the upper lip emarginate or slightly 2-cleft, the lower lip longer, spreading, 3-cleft.   *Stamens* 4, ascending or straggling at the apex, or distant at the base ; anthers with 6 distinct diverging or straggling cells.   Lobes of the *style* acute, the posterior one usually shorter.   Floral *leaves* bract-like.   *Flowers* in spikes (*Bentham*).

Sp. Char.—Erect, villous.   *Leaves* petiolate, broad-ovate, obtuse, subserrate, broad-rounded at the base, green on both sides.   *Spikes* oblong or cylindrical, clustered in corymbose panicles.   *Bracts* (floral leaves) ovate, obtuse, coloured (commonly glandless), half as long again as the calyx (*Bentham*).—Creeping-rooted.   *Flowers* light purple.

Hab.—In bushy places, on a limestone and gravelly soil.   Indigenous. A native of several parts of Europe ; also of Asia.   Flowers in July and August.

Properties.—The whole herb (*herba origani*) is officinal.   It has a peculiar aromatic odour, and a warm, pungent taste.   Sesquichloride of iron produces a green colour (*tannate of iron*) with the cold infusion of origanum.

Composition.—*Volatile oil, resin ?, tannic acid, a bitter principle,* and *woody fibre,* are the principal constituents of this plant.

Physiological Effects.—Stimulant and carminative, like the other labiate plants.

Uses.—Principally employed to yield the volatile oil.   The dried leaves have been used as a substitute for China tea.[4]   The infusion of origanum has been used in chronic cough, asthma, and amenorrhœa.

---

[1] *Synops. Plant. Fl. Classicæ,* 1845.
[2] *Hist. Plant.* lib. vi. cap. 2.
[3] Lib. iii. cap. 34.
[4] Murray, *App. Med.* vol. ii. p. 173.

OLEUM ORIGANI, E.; *Oil of Common Marjoram.* (Obtained by submitting the herb to distillation with common water.)—The average produce of essential oil from the herb is one pound from two hundredweight; but it varies exceedingly with the season and culture of the plant.[1] According to Dr. Kane, its sp. gr. is 0·867, its boiling point 354° F., and its composition $C^{50}H^{40}O$.

This oil is a powerful acrid and stimulant, and is applied to carious teeth, by means of lint or cotton, to relieve toothache. Mixed with olive oil, it is frequently employed as a stimulating liniment against alopecia or baldness, rheumatic or paralytic affections, sprains and bruises.

The red volatile oil usually sold in the shops as *oleum origani,* or *oil of thyme,* is obtained from *Thymus vulgaris,* and is imported from the south of France (see *Thymus vulgaris*).

[According to Mr. D. Hanbury,[2] oil of origanum is distinguished from oil of thyme by the following characters:—1. Odour, which is somewhat analogous to that of oil of peppermint, and entirely dissimilar from that of oil of thyme; 2. Colour, which in oil of origanum is bright yellow, while the ordinary kind of oil of thyme is more or less deep reddish-brown. The sp. gr. of the two oils is so nearly alike as to furnish no distinctive criterion: that of oil of origanum is ·8854, of oil of thyme (average of three samples) 8934 at 62° F.—ED.]

168. ORIGANUM MAJORANA, *Linn.*—SWEET OR KNOTTED MARJORAM.

Marjorana hortensis, *Mœnch.*
Sex. Syst. Didynamia, Gymnospermia.

HISTORY.—Fraas[3] is of opinion that the ἀμάρακον of Theophrastus,[4] the σάμψυχος of Dioscorides,[5] and the *Amaracam* or *Sampsuchum* of Pliny,[6] are identical with our sweet marjoram.

BOTANY. **Gen. Char.**—See *ante,* p. 515.

Sp. Char.—*Branches* smoothish, racemose-paniculate. *Leaves* petiolate, oblong-ovate, obtuse, quite entire, on both sides hoary-tomentose. *Spikelets* oblong, on sessile crowded branchlets. *Calyx* nearly toothless, cleft anteriorly (*Bentham*).—*Flowers* purple or white.

Hab.—Africa and Asia. Cultivated in kitchen-gardens.

PROPERTIES.—The whole plant (*herba majoranæ*) has a warm aromatic flavour, and a peculiar savoury smell. Its watery infusion is deepened in colour (*tannate of iron*) by sesquichloride of iron.

COMPOSITION.—By distillation the plant yields *volatile oil.* The other constituents are *tannic acid, resin?, bitter matter,* and *woody fibre.*

OIL OF SWEET MARJORAM (*Oleum Majoranæ*) is pale yellow or brownish, with the strong odour and taste of marjoram.

PHYSIOLOGICAL EFFECTS.—Tonic and mild stimulant.

---

[1] Brande, *Dict. Mat. Med.* p. 401.
[2] [*Pharmaceutical Journal,* January 1851, p. 324.]
[3] *Hist. Plant. Fl. Class.* p. 183, 1845.
[4] *Hist. Plant.* lib. vii. cap. 7.
[5] Lib. iii. cap. 47.
[6] *Hist. Nat.* lib. xxi. cap. 35, ed. Valp.

Uses.—Principally employed as a sweet herb by the cook. Its powder is sometimes used, either alone or mixed with some other powder, as an errhine. *Marjoram tea* is occasionally employed as a popular remedy for nervous complaints.

169. THYMUS VULGARIS, *Linn.*—COMMON OR GARDEN THYME.

Sex. Syst. Didynamia, Gymnospermia.

(Herba.)

History.—The true thyme, Θύμος of the ancients, is the *Thymus capitatus,* Hoffm. et Link (*Satureia capitata,* Linn.)

Botany. **Gen. Char.**—*Calyx* ovate, 10—13-nerved, 2-lipped; upper lip 3-toothed, spreading; lower lip 2-cleft, with ciliate, subulate segments; throat villous inside. *Corolla* having the tube enclosed by the calyx or imbricated bracts, naked inside; limb sub-bilabiate; upper lip straight, emarginate, flattish; lower lip spreading, 3-cleft, with equal lobes, or the middle one largest. *Stamens* exserted, or rarely enclosed, straight, distant, nearly equal or didynamous, the lower 2 being the longest. *Anthers* with 2 parallel or at length diverging cells. *Style* about equally bifid at the apex, with subulate lobes (*Bentham*).

Sp. Char.—Erect or procumbent at the base. *Leaves* sessile, linear, or ovate-lanceolate, acute, with revolute edges, fascicled in the axils. *Bracts* (floral leaves) lanceolate, obtuse. *Whorls* loose, rather distant. Teeth of the upper lip of the *calyx* lanceolate; the segments of the lower lip subulate ciliated (*Bentham*).—Shrub much branched, ½ to 1 foot high, rather hoary with a short down. Flowers purplish.

Var. *a latifolius;* Broad-leaved Garden Thyme.—Cultivated in gardens for culinary purposes.

Var. *β angustifolius;* Narrow-leaved Garden Thyme.

A variegated variety is cultivated for ornament. Lemon Thyme, which is cultivated for culinary purposes, is *T. Serpyllum* var. *vulgaris,* Bentham.

Hab.—South-west of Europe, in dry, arid, uncultivated places. Cultivated as a sweet herb in England.

Description.—The flowering tops of garden thyme (*herba et summitates thymi*) are dried, and sold in the shops as one of the herbs used for culinary purposes. The odour is fragrant, and to most persons agreeable.

Composition.—Similar to that of Origanum vulgare. The odour and condimentary properties depend on volatile oil (*oleum thymi*).

Effects and Uses.—Similar to the other sweet herbs. Chiefly used by the cook for soups, stuffings, and sauces. In the south of France the herb is used for distillation, to yield the oil of thyme.

OLEUM THYMI ; *Oil of Thyme.*—At Milhaud, Aujargues, Souvignargues, and near the village of Fontanes, as well as at several other places in the neighbourhood of Nismes, in the department of Gard, in the south of France, this oil is largely distilled, and is imported into England and sold as *oleum origani.* Mr. Daniel Hanbury, who visited this district in the summer of 1849, found that the plant grew spontaneously in abundance on the arid, rocky, waste hills of that neighbourhood.[1] The entire plants, whether in flower or not, are collected, and, either in the fresh or dried state, submitted to distillation with water. The oil, which is of a reddish-brown colour, is called *red oil of thyme* (*huile rouge de thym*), becomes much paler by redistillation, and is then called *white oil of thyme* (*huile blanche de thym*). The specimen of red oil of thyme obtained by Mr. D. Hanbury is identical with the oil sold as *oleum origani* in the London shops, all of which is imported.[2] Specimens of the plant which yields the oil have been examined by Mr. Bentham, Dr. Lindley, and others; and by all have been pronounced undoubtedly *Thymus vulgaris*.

[M. Lallemand finds that this oil contains a large quantity of a stearoptene, which he calls *Thymol*. It is a crystalline substance, melting at 108°, and remaining liquid for a considerable time at the ordinary temperature. It has no rotatory action on polarised light: in the crystalline state it behaves like the other birefractive media. Its composition is expressed by the formula $C^{20}H^{14}O^2$, differing from the camphor of the Lauraceæ by two atoms of hydrogen.

Thymene, the other constituent of oil of thyme, is isomeric with turpentine, $C^{20}H^{16}$. It does not exert any rotatory action on a ray of polarised light.[3]—ED.]

The medicinal properties and uses of oil of thyme are the same as those of the *oleum origani*, for which it is usually employed.

170. MELISSA OFFICINALIS, *Linn.*—COMMON BALM.

Sex. Syst. Didynamia, Gymnospermia.

(Herba, *E.*)

HISTORY.—Both Smith[4] and Sprengel[5] consider this plant to be the μελισσόφυλλον or μελίτταινα of Dioscorides;[6] but Fraas[7] is of opinion that the *Melissa altissima* is the species referred to by Dioscorides.

BOTANY. **Gen. Char.**—*Calyx* tubular-campanulate, 13-ribbed, 2-lipped, the upper lip nearly flat, 3-toothed, the inferior lip bifid, the throat naked within. Tube of the *corolla* recurved-ascending, enlarged from above, naked within, limb 2-lipped, upper lip emarginate erect, lower ones spreading, 3-cleft, the lobes flat, the middle one entire or emarginate. *Stamens* 4, arched-converging; cells of the anthers at length straggling. Lobes of the *style* nearly equal, subulate. *Nucules* dry, smooth (*Bentham*).

Sp. Char.—Erect, branching. *Leaves* broad-ovate, crenate, truncate or cordate at the base; the floral ones nearly similar to the cauline ones. *Whorls* axillary, loose, 1-sided. *Bracts* (floral leaves) few, ovate. *Corolla* longer by half than the calyx (*Bentham*).

Hab.—South of France.

---

[1] [We have seen it covering the whole of the rocky soil around Marseilles.—ED.]
[2] The price at which the oil is sold by M. Sagnier, and other exporters at Nismes, is so low as to preclude its distillation in England.
[3] [*Pharm. Journal*, January 1854, p. 342.]
[4] *Floræ Græcæ Prodromus*, vol. i. p. 423, 1806.
[5] *Hist. Rei Herb.* t. i. p. 100.
[6] Lib. iii. cap. 118.
[7] *Synopsis Plantarum Fl. Classicæ*, p. 182, 1845.

PROPERTIES.—The fresh herb (*herba melissæ*) has a strong, peculiar odour, which is somewhat similar to that of lemons. By drying, this is, for the most part, lost. The taste is aromatic, bitter, and somewhat austere. Sesquichloride of iron gives a greenish colour (*tannate of iron*) to the cold infusion.

COMPOSITION.—The principal constituents of balm are *volatile oil, resin, bitter matter, gum, tannic acid*, and *woody fibre*.[1]

OIL OF BALM (*Oleum Melissæ*) is pale yellow, and has the peculiar odour of balm. Its sp. gr. is 0·975. Oil of lemon is said to be frequently substituted for it.

PHYSIOLOGICAL EFFECTS.—The effects of balm are similar to, though milder than, those of the labiate plants already described. The mildness of its operation arises from the small quantity of volatile oil which the plant contains.

USES.—*Balm tea* is sometimes employed as a diaphoretic in fevers, as an exhilarating drink in hypochondriasis, and as an emmenagogue in amenorrhœa and chlorosis.

TRIBE III. MONARDEÆ, *Benth.*

Stamens 2, straight or ascending; cells of the anthers oblong-linear, or solitary, or separated by the filiform connective (very rarely approximate in Perowskia).

171. ROSMARINUS OFFICINALIS, *Linn.*— COMMON ROSEMARY.

Sex. Syst. Diandria, Monogynia.

(Oleum e cacumine florente destillatum, *L.*—The tops, *E. D.*)

HISTORY.—The Λιβανωτὶς στεφανωματικὴ, or *Libanotis coronaria* of Dioscorides,[2] is supposed to be our officinal rosemary, which received its name, Λιβανωτὶς (from Λίβανος, *Thus*), on account of its odour, and στεφανωματικὴ (στεφανωματικός, *coronarius*) from its use in making garlands.[3] Pliny[4] calls it *Rosmarinum.* The flowers are termed *anthos* (from ἄνθος, *a flower*), signifying they are *the flowers* par excellence,—just as we call cinchona *the bark*, and the inspissated juice of the poppy, *opium* (i. e. *the juice*).

BOTANY. **Gen. Char.**— *Calyx* ovate-campanulate, 2-lipped; the upper lip entire, the lower bifid, the throat naked within. *Corolla* with a protruding tube, smooth and not ringed on the inside, somewhat inflated in the throat; limb 2-lipped; lips nearly equal, the upper one erect and emarginate, the lower spreading, trifid, with the lateral lobes oblong, erect, somewhat twisted; the middle lobe very large, concave, and hanging down. No rudiments of the superior *stamina:* fertile (inferior) ones 2, ascending, protruding: *filaments* inserted in the throat of the corolla, shortly-toothed near the base: *anthers* linear, subbilocular; the cells straggling, confluent,

---

[1] Pfaff, *Mat. Med.* Bd. iv. S. 270.
[2] Lib. iii. cap. 89.
[3] The Arabian name signifies "royal crown."
[4] *Hist. Nat.* lib. xix. cap. 62, cd. Valp.

connate at the margin.   Upper lobe of the *style* very short.   *Nucules* dry, smooth (*Bentham*).

Sp. Char.—The only species.—*Leaves* sessile, linear, revolute at the edge, hoary beneath.   *Calyx* purplish.   *Corolla* white or pale purplish-blue.

Hab.—South of Europe; also Asia Minor.

PROPERTIES.—The flowering tops (*cacumina rosmarini*) are the officinal parts.   They have a strong and remarkable odour, and a warm bitter taste.

COMPOSITION.—The peculiar odour and flavour of this plant depend on *volatile oil*.   Besides this, the tops contain *tannic acid, a bitter matter, resin ?*, and *woody fibre*.

PHYSIOLOGICAL EFFECTS.—Carminative and mildly stimulant, analogous to the other labiate plants.

USES.—Rarely employed medicinally.   *Infusion of rosemary* (*rosemary tea*) is sometimes used as a substitute for ordinary tea by hypochondriacal persons.   The admired flavour of Narbonne honey depends on the bees collecting this substance from rosemary plants, which abound in the neighbourhood of Narbonne: hence sprigs of rosemary are sometimes added to the honey of other places, in order to imitate the flavour of Narbonne honey.

1. OLEUM ROSMARINI (Anglicum, L.), L. E. ;   *Oleum Anthos* offic. ; *English Oil of Rosemary*.   (Prepared by submitting the rosemary tops to distillation with water.)—This oil was first procured by Raymond Lully.[1] It is transparent and colourless, with the odour of rosemary, and a hot, aromatic taste.   Its sp. gr. is 0·897, and it boils at 365° F.   It consists, according to Dr. Kane, of $C^{45}H^{38}O^2$.   One pound of the fresh herb yields about one drachm of oil.[2]   It is rarely taken internally, but is not unfrequently used externally, in conjunction with other substances, as a stimulating liniment; for example, in alopecia or baldness, and also as a perfume.   Dose, gtt. ij. to gtt. v.

2. SPIRITUS ROSMARINI, L. E. ;   *Spirit of Rosemary*.   (Oil of Rosemary, ʒij. ;   Rectified Spirit, Cong. j.   Dissolve, *L.*   The *Edinburgh College* submits the tops (lb. iiss.) to distillation with a gallon of Rectified Spirit, so as to obtain seven pints of the distilled spirit.)—It is usually prepared merely by dissolving the oil in spirit, distillation being superfluous.   Seldom employed internally.   Its principal use is as an odoriferous adjunct to lotions and liniments.   It is a constituent of the *Linimentum Saponis* and *Tinctura Lavandulæ composita*.

[**3. ESSENTIA ROSMARINI**, D. ;   *Essence of Rosemary*.   (Oil of Rosemary, fʒj. ;   Rectified Spirit, fʒix.   Mix with agitation.)—Its uses are the same as those of the spirit.—ED.]

AQUA HUNGARICA ;   *Aqua Rosmarini* seu *Anthos composita ; Hungary Water*.—Various formulæ for the preparation of this perfume have been given.   The following is from the *Pharm. Wurtem.* and *Bavar.:*—Take of fresh Rosemary, in blossom, lb. iv. ; fresh Sage, in blossom, ʒvj. ; Zingiber, ʒij.   Cut into pieces, and add Rectified Spirit, lb. xij. ; Common Water, Oij.   Let eleven pints distil by a gentle heat.   A hermit is said to have given the formula for the preparation of this perfume to a Queen of Hungary ; whence this water has been called the *Queen of Hungary's Water* (*Aqua Reginæ Hungariæ*).[3]

---

[1] Thomson's *Hist. of Chem.* vol. i. p. 41.
[2] Brande, *Dict. of Mat. Med.* p. 466.
[3] For the history of Hungary water see Beckmann's *History of Inventions*, translated by Wm. Johnston, vol. ii. p. 107, 1791.

Hungary water is frequently imitated by mixing Spirit of Lavender, f℥vij., with Spirit of Rosemary, f℥iv.—This liquid is employed principally as a perfume for the toilette; also as an excitant and restorative in fainting. Externally it is used as a stimulating liniment.

TRIBE IV. STACHYDEÆ, *Benth.*

Stamens 4, ascending under the helmet (which is usually concave).

172. MARRUBIUM VULGARE, *Linn.*—WHITE HOREHOUND.

Sex. Syst. Didynamia, Gymnospermia.

(Herba.)

HISTORY.—This is the plant which is called Πράσιον by Hippocrates, Theophrastus, and Dioscorides;[1] and *Marrubium* by Pliny.[2]

BOTANY. **Gen. Char.**—*Calyx* tubular, 5—10-nerved, equal; teeth 5—10, acute, somewhat spinous, nearly equal, erect, or often spreading at maturity. *Corolla* with an enclosed tube, which is naked inside, or somewhat annulated, and a 2-lipped limb; the upper lip erect, flattish or concave, entire or shortly bifid; the lower lip trifid, spreading, the middle lobe the broadest, often emarginate. *Stamens* enclosed within the tube of the corolla; anthers with 2 straggling, somewhat confluent cells, all nearly alike. *Style* bifid at the apex, with short obtuse lobes. *Nucules* obtuse, not truncate at the apex (*Bentham*).

Sp. Char.—*Branches* white-woolly. *Leaves* ovate or rounded, softly villous, greenish or white-woolly beneath, crenate. *Whorls* many-flowered. *Calyx* villose, woolly, with 10 subulate, recurved-spreading or woolly teeth. *Corolla* with an oblong helmet, bifid at the point (*Bentham*).—*Flowers* white.

Hab.—Dry waste grounds. Indigenous. Grows in most parts of Europe; also in Asia and America. Flowers in July.

PROPERTIES.—The whole herb (*herba marrubii*) is used in medicine. It has an aromatic odour and a bitter taste. Sesquichloride of iron communicates an olive-green tint (*tannate of iron*) to the cold watery infusion.

COMPOSITION.—Its bitterness depends on *extractive;* its aromatic properties, on *volatile oil.* Besides these principles it contains *resin, tannic acid, bitter matter,* and *woody fibre.*

PHYSIOLOGICAL EFFECTS.—Horehound is tonic, mildly stimulant, and, in large doses, laxative. Taken in the form of infusion, it promotes the secretions of the skin and kidneys. It was formerly supposed to possess emmenagogue properties.

USES.—It is rarely employed by medical practitioners. As a domestic remedy it is used in chronic pulmonary complaints, especially catarrh. It was formerly given in uterine and hepatic affections.

ADMINISTRATION.—*Horehound tea* (prepared by infusing an ounce of the

---

[1] Lib. iii. cap. 119.
[2] *Hist. Nat.* lib. xx. cap. 89, ed. Valp.

herb in a pint of boiling water) is taken in the dose of a wine-glassful. *Syrup of horehound* (prepared with the infusion and sugar) is a popular remedy, and is kept in the shops. *Candied horehound* ought to be made of the same ingredients.

BALLOTA NIGRA, Linn., or *Stinking Black Horehound*, possesses similar properties to the *Marrubium vulgare*.

ORDER XLI. SCROPHULARIACEÆ, *Lindley.*
FIGWORTS.

PEDICULARES ET SCROPHULARIÆ, *Juss.*—SCROPHULARINEÆ, *R. Brown.*

CHARACTERS. — *Flowers* hermaphrodite, usually irregular. *Calyx* free, persistent, 5—4-merous. *Corolla* gamopetalous (monopetalous), hypogynous, pentamerous or (the upper petals being united) tetramerous, very rarely 6—7-merous, or 2-lobed, the lobes being united; bilabiatedly or irregularly imbricated, very rarely (in a few didynamous or diandrous genera) plaited in æstivation. *Stamens* inserted on the corolla, alternate with its lobes; the upper stamen usually, and the 2 anterior or posterior ones sometimes, sterile or deficient : *anthers* 2-celled, or by growing together, or by half disappearing, 1-celled ; the cells dehiscing by a longitudinal slit. *Ovary* free, 2-celled ; ovules in each cell many (very rarely 2 together), inserted on the dissepiment near the axis, anatropal or amphitropal. *Style* simple, or very shortly bifid, at the apex ; the stigmatic part either very thin, or incrassate, entire, or 2-lobed. *Fruit* capsular, dehiscing, variously or rarely baccate. *Placentæ* 4, separate by dehiscence, or united variously with each other, with the edges of the valves, or with the central column. *Seeds* albuminous, indefinite with the radicle towards the basilar hilum, or few and definite, with a more or less lateral hilum, and the radicle towards the apex of the fruit ; embryo straight, or rarely curved.—*Herbs, under-shrubs,* or rarely *shrubs. Leaves* opposite, whorled, or alternate. *Stipules* commonly absent. *Inflorescence* centrifugal or centripetal. *Bracts* 2, opposite, or solitary ; *bractlets* none, or 1 or 2, alternate, or nearly opposite (*Bentham*).

PROPERTIES.—Juice watery, frequently bitter, astringent or narcotic.

173. VERBASCUM THAPSUS, *Linn.*—GREAT MULLEIN OR HIGH TAPER.

Sex. Syst. Pentandria, Monogynia.
(Folia.)

HISTORY.—This plant is, according to both Smith[1] and Fraas,[2] the φλόμος λευκή ἤ ἄρρην of Dioscorides.[3]

BOTANY. **Gen. Char.**—*Calyx* deeply 5-cleft or 5-partite, rarely 5-toothed. *Corolla* flat, expanded, or rotate, rarely concave ; the segments scarcely unequal. *Stamens* 5 ; the filaments either the 3 posterior ones, or all woolly or bearded, rarely (abnormally?) naked. *Style* compressed-dilated at the apex, rather thick. *Capsule* globose, ovoid or oblong, dehiscing (*Bentham*).

Sp. Char—Nearly simple, densely yellowish or whitish, tomentose. Radical *leaves* oblong, crenulate ; those of the stem decurrent, winged, acuminate. *Raceme* dense, or interrupted at the base. Throat of the *corolla* concave.

---

[1] *Fl. Græcæ Prodr.* vol. i. p. 149.
[2] *Synopsis Plant. Fl. Class.* p. 191, 1845.
[3] Lib. iv. cap. 104.

Anthers inferior, shortly decurrent *(Bentham).—Corolla* golden-yellow; *stamens* red; *stigma* green.

Hab.—Indigenous : on banks and waste ground. Biennial. Flowers in July and August.

DESCRIPTION.—The leaves (*folia verbasci*) have a mucilaginous, bitterish taste, and a very slight odour. They communicate their virtues to water.

COMPOSITION.—Morin[1] analysed the flowers of Verbascum Thapsus, and obtained *a yellow volatile oil, a fatty acid, free malic and phosphoric acids, malate and phosphate of lime, acetate of potash, uncrystallisable sugar, gum, chlorophylle,* and *yellow resinous colouring matter.*

PHYSIOLOGICAL EFFECTS.—Emollient, demulcent, and supposed to be feebly narcotic. Fishes are stupified by the seeds of Verbascum.[2]

USES.—In the form of decoction (prepared of ℥ij. of the leaves and Oij. of water) mullein has been used in catarrhs and diarrhœas : the dose is f℥iv. Dr. Home[3] found it serviceable in the latter complaint only. Fomentations and cataplasms made of great mullein have been used as applications to hemorrhoidal tumours and indurated glands.

174. SCROPHULARIA NODOSA, *Linn.*—KNOTTY-ROOTED FIGWORT.

Sex. Syst. Didynamia, Angiospermia.

(Folia.)

HISTORY.—The earliest notice of this plant occurs in the work of Brunfels.[4]

BOTANY. Gen. Char.—*Calyx* deeply 5-cleft or 5-partite. Tube of the *corolla* ventricose, globular, or oblong; segments of the limb short, the 4 upper ones erect the lower one spreading, 2 upper ones usually longest. *Stamens* didynamous, declinate, cells of the anthers united transversely into one : the rudiment of a fifth sterile stamen at the apex of the squamiform tube often present. *Capsule* usually acute, the valves entire or bifid at the apex. *Seeds* ovoid, rugose (*Bentham*).

Sp. Char.—Smooth. *Stem* angular. *Leaves* ovate, ovate-oblong, or the upper ones lanceolate, acute, serrate or somewhat incised, broadly cordate or rounded at the base. *Thyrsus* oblong, beardless, or scarcely clothed with leaves at the base. *Cymes* pedunculate, loosely many-flowered. Segments of the *calyx* broadly ovate, obtuse, with the margin very narrow. The sterile *anther* broadly orbiculate (*Bentham*).—*Corolla* dull green, with a livid purple lip.

Hab.—Indigenous : hedges, woods, and thickets. Perennial. Flowers in July.

DESCRIPTION.—The fresh leaves (*folia scrophulariæ nodosæ*) have, when bruised, a fetid odour: their taste is bitter, and somewhat acrid. Water extracts the virtues of the plant : the infusion is darkened by the sesquichloride of iron, but is unchanged by tincture of nutgalls.

---

[1] *Journ. de Chim. Méd.* t. ii. p. 223.
Bergius, *Mat. Med.*
[3] *Clin. Exp. and Hist.*
[4] Sprengel, *Hist. Rei Herb.* Præf. xi.

COMPOSITION.—The whole plant (root and herb) was analysed in 1830 by Grandoni.[1] He obtained *brown bitter resin* 0·31, *extractive with gum* 4·84, *extractive having the odour of benzoic acid* 0·88, *chlorophylle* 1·58, *starch* 0·23, *greenish fecula* 0·18, *mucilage* 0·27, *inulin* 0·16, *malic acid* 0·15, *pectic acid* 0·15, *acetic acid* 0·13, *woody fibre* 19·80, *water* 70·31, *sulphate* and *carbonate of potash* 0·59, *alumina* 0·20, *oxalate* and *carbonate of lime* 0·46, *magnesia* 0·26, *silica* 0·07, *odorous matter* and *loss* 0·31.

PHYSIOLOGICAL EFFECTS.—But little known. Judging from their taste, the leaves possess acrid properties. When swallowed, they occasion vomiting and purging. They are said to be diuretic and narcotic.

USES.—Rarely employed. In the form of a fomentation, the leaves are sometimes applied to piles and other painful tumours. The ointment is used in skin diseases. The tuberous root was formerly esteemed in scrofula.[2]

UNGUENTUM SCROPHULARIÆ; *Ointment of Scrophularia.* (Fresh Leaves of Scrophularia nodosa, Prepared Hogs' Lard, of each lb. ij.; Prepared Mutton Suet, lb. j. Boil the leaves in the fat until they become crisp, then strain by expression.)—Recommended by Dr. W. Stokes[3] for the cure of a disease of children commonly termed *burnt-holes,* and which he calls *Pemphigus gangrenosus* [*Rupia escharotica ?*]. It has also been used in tinea capitis, impetigo, and other cutaneous affections.[4] [It was formerly an article of the Dublin Pharmacopœia, but is now excluded.—ED.]

175. Gratiola officinalis, *Linn.*—Officinal Hedge Hyssop.

Sex. Syst. Diandria, Monogynia.

(Herba.)

A perennial plant, native of the south of Europe. Cultivated in England, and formerly contained in the British Pharmacopœias. The herb (*herba gratiolæ*) is cathartic, diuretic, and emetic, acting in large doses as an acrid poison. It has been used in visceral obstructions, liver affections, dropsies, scrofula, and venereal diseases.—Dose of the *powder*, gr. xv. to ʒss.; of the *infusion* (prepared with ʒij. of the dried herb and Oss. of boiling water), f℥ss. to f℥j. three times a day.[5]

176. DIGITALIS PURPUREA, *Linn.*—PURPLE FOXGLOVE.

Sex. Syst. Didynamia, Angiospermia.

(Herba agrestis.—Folium caulinum recens et exsiccatum, *L.*—Leaves, *E. D.*)

HISTORY.—It appears very improbable that the ancients should have overlooked so common and elegant a plant as foxglove; yet in none of their writings can we find any plant whose description precisely answers to the one now under examination. Fabricius Columna[6] thought that it was the Ἐφήμερον of

---

[1] *Pharm. Central-Blatt für* 1831, S. 446.
[2] Murray, *App. Med.* vol. ii. p. 224.
[3] *Dubl. Med. Essays,* p. 146.
[4] Dr. Montgomery, *Observ. on the Dubl. Pharm.*
[5] Thomson, *Lond. Dispensat.*
[6] Quoted by Mentzelius, *Index Nom. Plant.* p. 104.

Dioscorides,[1] but the description of the latter does not at all agree with foxglove. The Βάκκαρις[2] of the same writer has also been referred to, but with little more probability of correctness. The term Foxer-glope occurs in a MS., *Glossarium Ælfrici*, probably written before the Norman Conquest (A.D. 1066), and in a MS. Saxon translation of L. Apulius; both of which are among the Cottonian manuscripts in the British Museum.[3] Fuchsius[4] is usually regarded as the earliest botanist who mentions this plant, which he named Digitalis (from *Fingerhut*, a finger-stall; on account of the blossoms resembling the finger of a glove). Fuchsius states that until he gave it this appellation the plant had no Greek or Latin name.

BOTANY. **Gen. Char.**—*Calyx* 5-partite, imbricate. *Corolla* declinate; tube ventricose or campanulate, frequently constricted above the base; upper segment of the limb short, broad, emarginate or bifid, spreading, the external lateral ones narrower, the lowermost one longer than the others, extended. *Stamens* 4, didynamous, ascending, shorter than the corolla, and frequently enclosed within the tube; *anthers* approximated in pairs, their cells diverging and confluent. *Style* briefly bilobed at the apex; the lobes stigmatic within. *Capsule* ovate, 2-valved, with septicidal dehiscence; the valves entire, curved inwards at the margins, half exposing the placentiferous column. *Seeds* numerous, minute, oblong, somewhat angular (*Bentham*).

Sp. Char.—*Leaves* ovate-lanceolate or oblong, crenate, rugose; the under surface, or both surfaces, as well as the stem, tomentose or woolly. *Raceme* long, lax. Segments of the *calyx* ovate or oblong. *Corolla* enlarged above, campanulate; its segments obtuse, shorter than broad, the lower one longer than the lateral ones.

Herbaceous. *Root* of numerous long and slender fibres; biennial. *Stem* erect, 3 or 4 feet high, commonly simple, roundish, with several slight angles, downy. *Leaves* alternate, downy, veiny, of a dull green; tapering at the base into winged foot-stalks; lower ones largest. *Raceme* terminal, erect, one-sided, simple, of numerous, large, pendulous, odourless flowers. *Corolla* crimson, elegantly marked with eye-like spots, as well as hairy, within.

Var. *albiflora.*—A variety with white flowers, spotted with shades of cream-colour or pearl, is met with in gardens : it remains tolerably constant from seed.

Hab.—Indigenous : in pastures and about hedges or banks, on a gravelly or sandy soil.

DESCRIPTION.—The officinal parts are the leaves and seeds : the latter, however, are rarely employed. As some doubts have been expressed as to the equal activity of cultivated specimens, wild or native plants are to be preferred.

1. *Foxglove leaves (folia digitalis).*—The leaves should be gathered when the plant is in the greatest perfection,—that is, just before or during the period of inflorescence; and those are to be preferred which are full-grown and fresh. As the petioles possess less activity than the laminæ or expanded portions of the leaves, they ought to be rejected. Dr. Withering[5] directs the leaves to be dried either in the sunshine, or in a tin pan or pewter dish before the fire; but the more usual, and, I believe, better mode of pro-

---

[1] Lib. iv. cap. 85.
[2] Lib. iii. cap. 51.
[3] Lye, *Dict. Saxon.*
[4] *Hist. Stirp.* 1542.
[5] *Account of the Foxglove*, p. 181, 1785.

ceeding, is to dry them in baskets in a dark place, in a drying-stove. Both dried leaves and powder should be preserved in well-stoppered bottles, covered externally by dark-coloured paper, and kept in a dark cupboard. As both undergo changes by keeping, whereby their medicinal activity is considerably diminished, they ought to be renewed annually. Dried foxglove leaves have a dull green colour, a faint odour, and a bitter, nauseous taste.

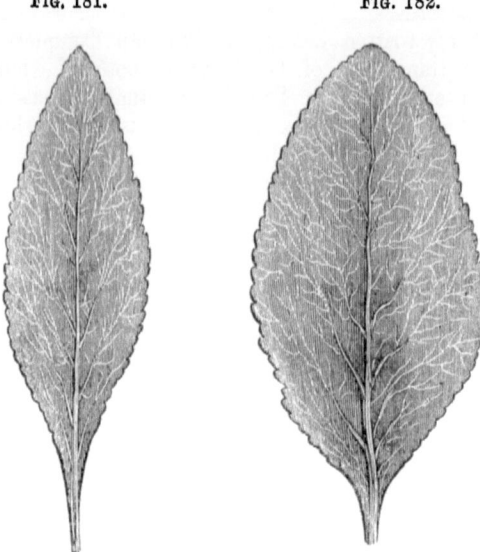

Fig. 181.   Fig. 182.

First year's leaf.   Second year's leaf.

Foxglove Leaves.

Although the leaves should be collected just before or at the period of inflorescence,—that is, in the second year of the plant's growth,—yet not unfrequently first year's leaves, which are considered to be of inferior activity, are sometimes substituted for them.

The first year's leaves are frequently more tapering than those of the second year's growth; but this character is not much to be relied on; and, therefore, to avoid the substitution, the best and safest plan is to purchase the fresh leaves at the proper season,—namely, just before or at the period of inflorescence (which is from the middle of June to the end of July). [The efficacy of the leaves of digitalis appears to depend on the season at which they are gathered. Nineteen ounces of leaves gathered in the month of May yielded three ounces of dry leaves, = 15·8 per cent. One hundred and fourteen and a half ounces gathered in July yielded twenty ounces of dry leaves, = 17·4 per cent.[1]—Ed.]

"Subsessile or shortly petiolated, ovate-lanceolate or oblong; narrowed at the base; crenated; wrinkled and veined. The under or both sides woolly. Let it be gathered before the terminal flowers are unfolded. The petiole and midrib being removed, dry the lamina."—*Ph. Lond.*

The leaves of *Inula Conyza*, De Cand., or *Ploughman's Spikenard,* closely resemble those of foxglove; but, when rubbed, are readily distinguished by their odour, which by some is called aromatic, by others fetid. Moreover, they are rougher to the touch, and are less divided on the edge.

2. *Foxglove seeds (semina digitalis).*—The seeds of the foxglove are small, roundish, and of a greyish-brown colour.

[Dr. Buchner[2] has published the results of his examination of the seeds of

---

[1] [Experiments of Von Hees, *Pharmaceutical Journal*, May 1852, p. 528.]
[2] [*Pharmaceutical Journal*, March 1852, p. 419.]

digitalis. The seed was found to lose by drying at 162° F., 9·26 per cent. of water. In his opinion, the seeds are preferable to the leaves for medicinal use, as they not only contain a larger amount of digitaline, but are more easily dried and preserved without experiencing any alteration. The oily compound, containing the digitaline, may be separated from the seed by ether. This oily compound amounts to about forty per cent. of the weight of the seed. It belongs to the siccative oils.—Ed.]

Composition.—Purple foxglove has been the subject of repeated chemical examination, but, until very recently, with no satisfactory results. Memoirs on its composition, or on its active principle, have been published by Destouches,[1] Bidault de Villiers,[2] Rein and Haase,[3] Le Royer,[4] Dulong d'Astafort,[5] Meylink,[6] Welding,[7] Radig,[8] Brault and Poggiale,[9] Lancelot,[10] Trommsdorff,[11] Homolle,[12] Nativelle,[13] and by Morin.[14] Homolle's memoir gained the prize offered by the Société de Pharmacie of Paris for the isolation of the active principle.

Radig's Analysis.		Brault and Poggiale's Analysis.	Nativelle's Analysis.
Picrin (digitaline of Le Royer) ...	0·4	Resin.	Digitaline combined with tannic
Digitaline (of Lancelot)	8·2	Fatty matter.	acid.
Scaptin (acrid extractive)........	14·7	Chlorophylle.	Crystallisable substance.
Chlorophylle.......................	6·0	Starch.	Aromatic principle.
Oxide of iron	3·7	Gum.	Crystallisable resinous matter.
Potash	3·2	Lignin.	Fixed oil.
Acetic acid	11·0	Tannic acid.	Sugar.
Vegetable albumen	9·3	Salts of lime and potash.	Red colouring matter soluble in
Woody fibre	43·6	Volatile oil.	water.
		Fixed oil.	Chlorophylle.
		Oxalate of potash.	Extractive.
			Albumen.
			Salts containing vegetable acids.
			Salts containing inorganic acids.
Foxglove leaves................100·1		Foxglove leaves.	Foxglove leaves.

Morin found a peculiar volatile acid (*antirrhinic acid*), and a peculiar non-volatile acid (*digitalic acid*).

1. Digitaline; *Bitter Principle of Foxglove; Picrin.*—Homolle's process for obtaining digitaline, as simplified by M. Ossian Henry,[15] is as follows :—Digest 2½ lbs. of carefully dried and powdered foxglove leaves with rectified spirit, and express the tincture strongly in a press. Draw off the spirit in a still, and treat the residual extract with half a pint of water acidulated with about two drachms of acetic acid. Digest with a gentle heat, add some animal charcoal, and filter. Dilute the filtered liquor with water, partly neutralise with ammonia, and add a fresh-made strong infusion of nutgalls : by this

[1] *Bull. de Pharm.* t. i. p. 123.
[2] *Essai sur les Propr. méd. de la Digit. pourp.* 3e édit. 1812.
[3] *Diss. de Digit. purp.* 1812 ; quoted in Schwartze's *Pharm. Tabell.*
[4] *Bibl. Univers. des Sciences,* t. xxvii. p. 102, 1824, Genève.
[5] *Journ. de Pharm.* t. xiii. p. 379, 1827.
[6] *Buchner's Repert. für d. Pharm.* Bd. xxviii. p. 237, 1828.
[7] *Journ. of the Philadelphia Coll. of Pharm.* July 1833.
[8] *Pharm. Central-Blatt für* 1835, S. 209.
[9] *Journ. de Pharm.* t. xxi. p. 130, 1835.
[10] *Pharm. Central-Blatt für* 1833, p. 620.
[11] *Ibid.* 1837, p. 663.
[12] *Journ. de Pharm. et de Chim.* 3e sér. t. vii. p. 57.
[13] *Journ. de Chim. Méd.* 2e sér. t. xi. p. 62, 1845.
[14] *Journ. de Pharm. et de Chim.* 3e sér. t. vii. p. 295, 1845.
[15] *Ibid.* 3e sér. t. vii. p. 460, 1845.

means tannate of digitaline is precipitated. Wash the precipitate with water, mix it with a little alcohol, and carefully rub it with finely-powdered litharge. Expose the mixture to a gentle heat, digest with alcohol, decolourise the tincture by animal charcoal, and draw off the alcohol by a gentle heat. The residual extract is then to be treated with sulphuric ether, which takes up some foreign matters and leaves the digitaline. From 1 kilogramme (about 2½ lbs. 8 oz. troy) of the leaves, O. Henry obtained from 140 to 150 grs. of digitaline.

Digitaline is white, inodorous, difficultly crystallisable, and usually occurs in porous mammillated masses, or in small scales. It is intensely bitter when in solution, and excites violent sneezing when it is pulverised. It is soluble in about 2000 parts of water, is very soluble in alcohol, but almost insoluble in ether. It does not contain nitrogen ; nor does it neutralise acids. Concentrated sulphuric acid blackens it, and then dissolves it, forming a blackish-brown solution, which, in a few days, becomes successively reddish-brown, smoky amethyst, pure amethyst, and ultimately a beautiful crimson. If during this time a small quantity of water be added, a limpid, beautiful, green solution is obtained. In concentrated and colourless hydrochloric acid digitaline dissolves, forming a solution, which passes from yellow to a fine green. This reaction Homolle considers to be sufficiently delicate for medico-legal researches.

The effects of digitaline on both animals and the human subject have been examined by Homolle, and by Bourchardat and Sandras.[1] From their experiments it appears that its effects are similar to those of the plant; but that it is at least 100 times as powerful as the powder of the dried plant. In the human subject, doses of from 2 to 6 milligrammes (from about 1-32nd to 1-11th of an English grain) diminished the frequency of the pulse, and caused nausea, vomiting, griping, purging, and increased secretion of urine.

Digitaline has been employed in medicine, as a substitute for the plant, in doses of from 1-60th to 1-30th of a grain. It may be administered in substance in the form of pills, or dissolved in alcohol and given in the form of mixture or syrup. But the difficulty of adjusting these small doses, as well as the uncertainty of the purity and activity of the remedy, are great drawbacks to its use.

2. Scaptin.—Radig has applied the term scaptin to a brown, almost tasteless extractive, which leaves an acrid sensation in the throat.

3. Empyreumatic Oil of Foxglove (Pyrodigitaline).—By the destructive distillation of the dried leaves of foxglove, Dr. Morries[2] obtained a coloured, disagreeable, empyreumatic oil, which was semi-solid at 60° F., and soluble in boiling alcohol and ether : the solution, on cooling, let fall a flocculent precipitate composed of two substances,—one crystalline, the other globular. Given to a rabbit, it caused paralysis of the hind legs, convulsions, laborious and rapid breathing, and accelerated action of the heart. It does not contain the sedative principle of foxglove.

Chemical Characteristics.—Sesquichloride of iron causes a dark precipitate (tanno-gallate of iron) with decoction of foxglove leaves, as well as with the tincture diluted with water. A solution of gelatine, added to the decoction, causes, after some time, a scanty precipitate (tannate of gelatine). Tincture of nutgalls has scarcely any effect (perhaps a slight turbidness) when added to the decoction or to the tincture diluted with water.

(By the action of sulphuric or hydrochloric acid on the tincture or decoction of foxglove, I have not been able to detect the presence of digitaline.)

Physiological Effects. α. On Vegetables. — Marcet[3] found that a solution of the watery extract of foxglove killed a haricot plant (Phaseolus vulgaris) in twenty-four hours.

β. On Animals generally.—The effects of foxglove have been tried on dogs,[4] horses, rabbits,[5] turkeys,[6] the domestic fowl, and frogs ; and on all it

[1] Annuaire de Thérapeutique pour 1845, p. 60.
[2] Ed. Med. and Surg. Journ. vol. xxxix. p. 377.
[3] Ann. de Chim. et de Phys. vol. xxix. p. 200.
[4] Orfila, Toxicol. Gén.
[5] Le Roger, Bibl. Univ. June 1824.
[6] Salerne, Hist. de l'Acad. des Scien. 1748, p. 84.

has been found to act as a poison. One drachm of the powder may be given to horses as a sedative in inflammation.[1] Two ounces have produced death in twelve hours.[2] According to the experience of Orfila, the first symptoms of poisoning observed in [carnivorous] animals is vomiting. The influence of the poison over the heart does not appear to be uniform ; for in some cases he found the pulsations of this viscus unaltered, in others accelerated, while occasionally they were retarded. In a horse killed by two ounces of foxglove, the pulse was 130 per minute a short time before death (Moiroud) ; the standard pulse of the horse being 40 or 42 per minute. The cerebro-spinal symptoms observed in animals are diminished muscular power, con-vulsive movements, tremors, and insensibility. The powder acts as a local irritant, giving rise to inflammation of parts to which it is applied (Orfila).

γ. *On Man.*—We may, for convenience, establish three degrees of the operation of foxglove.

In the first degree, or that produced by *small and repeated doses,* fox-glove sometimes affects what are termed the organic functions, without disor-dering the animal or cerebro-spinal functions. Thus we sometimes have the stomach disordered, the pulse altered in frequency, and sometimes also in fulness and regularity ; and the secretion of urine increased, without any other marked symptoms. The order in which the symptoms just mentioned occur is not uniform : sometimes the diuresis, at others nausea, and occasionally the affection of the circulation, being the first obvious effect.

The influence of foxglove over the circulation is not at all constant. In some cases the frequency of the pulse is augmented, in others decreased, while in some it is unaffected. Lastly, in a considerable number of instances the pulse becomes irregular or intermittent under the use of foxglove.[3] A few drops of the tincture will, in some cases, reduce the frequency of the pulse, and render it irregular and intermittent, while in other instances much larger doses may be taken without any obvious effect on it. Dr. Withering[4] mentions one case in which the pulse fell to 40 ; and I have several times seen it reduced to 50. In some cases the slowness of the pulse is preceded by an increased activity of the vascular system. From Sandras's reports[5] this would appear to occur more frequently after small than large doses of fox-glove. Dr. Sanders,[6] indeed, asserts that foxglove invariably excites the pulse, and refers to an experience of 2000 cases in proof. He says that he has seen the pulse rise from 70 to 120 under the use of foxglove, and at the end of twenty-four hours, or sooner, fall with greater or less rapidity to 40, or even below this. But an experience of the use of foxglove in only twenty cases will, I believe, convince most persons that Dr. Sanders has fallen into an error in the sweeping assertion which he has made. A great deal, how-ever, depends on the position of the patient. If it be desired to reduce the frequency of the pulse, the patient should be kept in a recumbent posture. The important influence of posture was first pointed out, I believe, by Dr. Baildon.[7] His own pulse, which had been reduced by this plant from 110

---

[1] Youatt, *The Horse,* in *Libr. of Usef. Knowledge.*
[2] Moiroud, *Pharm. Vétér.* p. 354.
[3] See the statistical *resumé* of Sandras, *Bull. de Thérap.* t. vi.
[4] *Account of the Foxglove,* p. 73, 1785.
[5] *Op. cit.*
[6] *Treat. on Pulm. Consumption,* ed. 1808.
[7] *Ed. Med. and Surg. Journ.* vol. iii. p. 270.

to 40 beats per minute while he was in the recumbent position, rose to 70 when he sat up, and to 100 when he stood. We have a ready explanation of this fact. In a state of health the pulsations of the heart are more frequent (usually to the extent of five or six in the minute) in the erect than in the horizontal position; and it is very obvious that greater force is required to carry on the circulation in the former than in the latter, since in the erect position the heart and arteries have to send blood to the head against gravity. Now the power of the heart being enfeebled by foxglove, when a demand is made on this viscus for an increase in the force of contractions by the change from the recumbent to the standing attitude, it endeavours to make up for its diminished force by an increase in the frequency of its contractions. I need scarcely add, that the sudden change of position in those who are much under the influence of this medicine is attended with great danger, and in several instances has proved fatal; for, in consequence of the heart not having sufficient power to propel the blood to the head against gravity, fatal syncope has been the result.[1] The influence of digitalis over the pulse is more marked in some individuals or cases than in others; thus the reduction of the frequency of the pulse is in general more readily induced in weak and debilitated constitutions than in robust and plethoric ones. Occasionally no obvious effect on the number, force, or regularity of the pulse is produced, though the foxglove may be given to an extent sufficient to excite vomiting and cerebral disorder. Shroek[2] experienced, from two grains of foxglove, nausea, headache; small, soft, and quick pulse; dryness of the gums and throat, giddiness, weakness of limbs, and increased secretion of saliva. Some hours after, he observed sparks before the eyes, his vision became dim, and he experienced a sensation of pressure on the eye-balls.

A most important fact connected with the repeated uses of small doses of it, is the *cumulative effect* sometimes observed. It has not unfrequently happened that, in consequence of the continued use of small doses of this medicine, very dangerous symptoms, in some cases terminating in death, have occurred. The most prominent of these were great depression of the vascular system, giddiness, want of sleep, convulsions, and sometimes nausea and vomiting.[3] A knowledge of its occasional occurrence impresses us with the necessity of exercising great caution in the use of this remedy, particularly with respect to the continuance of its administration and increase of dose; and it shows that after the constitutional effect has become obvious, it is prudent to suspend from time to time the exhibition of the remedy, in order to guard against the effects of this alarming accumulation. I may add, however, that I have used it, and seen others employ it, most extensively, and in full doses, and have rarely seen any dangerous consequences; and I believe, therefore, the effects of accumulation to be much less frequent than the statements of authors of repute would lead us to expect. The experience of Dr. Holland[4] is to the same effect. "Though employing the medicine somewhat largely in practice," he observes, "I do not recollect a case in which I have seen any injurious consequences from this cause."

---

[1] For some interesting remarks on the *Effects produced by Posture on the Pulse*, by Dr. Graves, consult *Dubl. Hosp. Rep.* vol. x. p. 561.

[2] Quoted by Wibmer, *Wirk. d. Arzneim. u. Gifte*, Bd. ii. S. 311.

[3] See the cases published by Dr. Withering, *op. cit.*; also a fatal case recorded by Dr. Blackall, *On Dropsy*, p. 175, 4th ed.

[4] *Med. Notes and Reflections*, p. 544.

The diuretic operation for which we employ foxglove is very inconstant. Dr. Withering stated that this medicine more frequently succeeds as a diuretic than any other, and that if it fail, there is but little chance of any other remedy succeeding. My experience, however, is not in accordance with Dr. Withering's. I have frequently seen foxglove fail in exciting diuresis, and have often found the infusion of common broom (*Cytisus scoparius*) subsequently succeed. It has been asserted by some that the diuretic effect of foxglove was only observed in dropsical cases, and that it, therefore, depended on the stimulus given to the absorbent vessels, and not to any direct influence exerted over the kidneys; but the statement is not true, since foxglove is sometimes found acting as a diuretic even in health. In some cases the bladder has appeared more irritable than usual, the patient having a frequent desire to pass his urine.

An increased flow of saliva is an occasional consequence of the continued use of moderate doses of foxglove. Dr. Withering[1] first noticed this effect. Dr. Barton[2] has also seen it produced from ordinary doses.

2. The *second degree of operation* of digitalis, or that ordinarily resulting from the use of too large or too long-continued doses, is manifested by the disordered condition of the alimentary canal, of the circulating organs, and of the cerebro-spinal system. The more ordinary symptoms are nausea or actual vomiting, slow and often irregular pulse, coldness of the extremities, syncope, or tendency to it, giddiness, and confusion of vision. Sometimes the sickness is attended with purging, or even with diuresis; at other times the patient is neither vomited nor purged, and the principal disorder of system is observed in the altered condition of the nervous and vascular organs. External objects appear of a green or yellow colour; the patient fancies there is a mist, or sparks, before his eyes; a sensation of weight, pain, or throbbing of the head, especially in the frontal region, is experienced; giddiness, weakness of the limbs, loss of sleep, occasionally stupor or delirium, and even convulsions, may also be present. The pulse becomes feeble, sometimes frequent, sometimes slow; there may be actual syncope, or only a tendency to it, and profuse cold sweats. Salivation is sometimes produced by poisonous doses of foxglove. It was observed in a case narrated by Dr. Henry,[3] and has been known to last three weeks.[4]

The quantity of digitalis that may be given to a patient without destroying life, is much greater than is ordinarily imagined. In one instance I saw twenty drops of the tincture given to an infant labouring under hydrocephalus, three times daily for a fortnight, at the end of which time the little patient had completely recovered, without one untoward symptom. I have frequently given a drachm of the tincture (of the best quality) three times daily to an adult, for a fortnight, without observing any marked effect. I know that some practitioners employ it in much larger doses (as an ounce or half an ounce of the tincture) with much less effect than might be imagined. The following communication on this subject, from my friend Dr. Clutterbuck, illustrates this point:—" My first information on this subject was derived from an intelligent pupil, who had been an assistant to Mr. King,

---

[1] *Op. cit.* p. 184.
[2] Beck's *Med. Jurisprudence.*
[3] *Ed. Med. and Surg. Journ.* vol. vii. p. 148.
[4] *Rust's Magazin*, xxv. 578.

a highly respectable practitioner at Saxmundham, in Suffolk, who, on a subsequent occasion, personally confirmed the statement. This gentleman assured me that he had been for many years in the habit of administering the tincture of digitalis to the extent of from half an ounce to an ounce at a time, not only with safety, but with the most decided advantage, as a remedy for acute inflammation,—not, however, to the exclusion of blood-letting, which, on the contrary, he previously uses with considerable freedom. To adults he often gives an ounce of the tincture (seldom less than half an ounce), and awaits the result of twenty-four hours, when, if he does not find the pulse subdued, or rendered irregular by it, he repeats the dose; and this, he says, seldom fails to lower the pulse in the degree wished for; and when this is the case, the disease rarely fails to give way, provided it has not gone the length of producing disorganisation of the part. He has given as much as two drachms to a child of nine months. Sometimes vomiting quickly follows these large doses of the digitalis, but never any dangerous symptom, so far as his observation has gone, which has been very extensive. In less acute cases he sometimes gives smaller doses, as thirty drops, several times in a day.

"Such is the account I received from Mr. King himself, and which was confirmed by his assistant, who prepared his medicines. I do not see any ground for questioning the faithfulness of the report. I have myself exhibited the tincture to the extent of half an ounce (never more), in not more than two or three instances (cases of fever and pneumonia). To my surprise, there was no striking effect produced by it; but I did not venture to repeat the dose. In numerous instances I have given two drachms; still more frequently one drachm; but not oftener than once in twenty-four hours, and not beyond a second or third time. Two or three exhibitions of this kind I have generally observed to be followed by slowness and irregularity of pulse, when I have immediately desisted." Dr. T. Williams[1] states that a man in a state of intoxication took two ounces of tincture of foxglove in two doses, in quick succession, without the slightest inconvenience.

3. The *third degree* of the operation of foxglove, or that resulting from the use of *fatal doses*, is characterised usually by vomiting, purging, and griping pain in the bowels; slow, feeble, and irregular pulse, great faintness, and cold sweats; disordered vision; at first giddiness, extreme debility; afterwards insensibility and convulsions, with dilated insensible pupils.

If we compare the effects of foxglove with those of other medicinal agents, we find they approximate more closely to those of tobacco than of any other cerebro-spinant. These two agents especially agree in their power of enfeebling the action of the heart and arteries. Green tea agrees with foxglove in its property of preventing sleep. Considered as a diuretic, foxglove is, in some respects, comparable with squills. I have already pointed out the peculiarities attending the operation of each of these.

[In his lectures on Materia Medica, delivered in 1855 at the Royal College of Physicians, Dr. Bence Jones gives the following summary of the properties of digitaline, and its effects, as contrasted with those of digitalis itself:[2]—

" *Digitaline*, the most active ingredient of the digitalis, is prepared pure by extracting the neutral principles with ether and alcohol of specific gravity

---

[1] *Lond. Med. Gaz.* vol. i. p. 744.
[2] [*Med. Times and Gazette*, April 21, 1855.]

780.   This dissolves the digitaline and the digitalose; the ethereal solution is then evaporated, the residue treated with alcohol, again evaporated and treated with weak alcohol : the digitaline remains dissolved.   On gentle evaporation, it does not crystallise, but forms a resinous-looking mass of a pale yellow colour, unchangeable in the air, and very bitter; slightly soluble in water, very soluble in alcohol.   It is a neutral substance.   It becomes emerald-green with strong hydrochloric acid.   The best test of its quality is its bitterness.   This is best determined by taking one centigramme of the powder of digitaline, and dissolving it in two grammes of alcohol, and continuing to dilute this solution with water until the bitterness is found to disappear.   From the quantity of water required, the goodness of the digitaline may be estimated : if the digitaline be good, more than three pints of water will be required to be added before the bitterness becomes imperceptible.

" The best form for keeping and giving the digitaline as medicine is in granules, and not in tincture.   Thus it keeps best, and is more certain in composition.   It is thus most easily given, as its bitter taste is concealed.   Each granule is made to contain one milligramme.   This is equal to ·015 grain of digitaline.

" MM. Homolle and Quevenne state that one of them took four of these granules daily for eight days.   The average healthy pulse of the person experimented on was 67·5 ; after taking the granules the pulse fell to 50.   The difference is 17·5 beats, which are equal to one quarter the beats of the heart.   Two dogs were given from 2 to 11 granules daily.   In the first dog the pulse fell from 60 to 51 ; in the second, from 87 to 70.

" The comparison between the digitaline and digitalis is remarkable.   The differences are given in this table :—

Digitaline.	*Digitalis.*
1st. Type unalterable; to this all digitaline may be reduced.	1st. No standard of comparison.
2nd. Constant action.	2nd. Uncertain action ; depends on the quality of the plant.
3rd. Possibility of determining comparative excellence by the bitterness.	3rd. No mode of determining the quality of different specimens.
4th. Agreeable form.	4th. Disagreeable smell and odour.

" M. Bouillaud states that during four or five years not a day has passed without his employing digitaline on many patients affected with diseases of the heart or vessels.   He has given it to from 150 to 200 patients of all ages.   In all, excepting three, the pulse was reduced.   Two of these had endocarditis and pericarditis.   If the pulse was irregular previous to the taking of the digitaline, it became regular as the medicine took effect.   In fifteen cases taken at hazard, in La Charité, the maximum pulse before the action of the digitaline was 96 ; after the medicine, 41 pulsations less.   In three cases the pulse was reduced 80, 102, and 106 beats.   The minimum reduction in three other cases was 12, 14, 16.   The number of granules taken daily was from 2 to 7 ; the number of days on which the granules were taken usually, 13 to 14.   One patient took 70 granules in 18 days; another, 82 in 14 days; a third, 98 granules in 20 days ; a fourth, 164 granules in 40 days, without harm.   As soon as pain in the head, vertigo, or nausea came on, the medicine was stopped."—Ed.]

Uses.—We employ foxglove for various purposes, as,—1st, to reduce the frequency and force of the heart's action; 2dly, to promote the action of the absorbents; 3dly, as a diuretic; and 4thly, sometimes on account of its specific influence over the cerebro-spinal system. In the following remarks on the uses of foxglove in particular diseases, I refer to the administration of this remedy in the doses in which it is ordinarily employed. I have no experience of its therapeutical effects when given in the enormous quantities mentioned by Dr. Clutterbuck.

1. *In fever.*—Digitalis is occasionally useful in fever to reduce the frequency of the pulse when the excitement of the vascular system is out of proportion to the other symptoms of fever, such as the increased temperature and the cerebral or gastric disorder. It cannot, however, be regarded, in the most remote way, as a curative means; on the other hand, it is sometimes hurtful. Thus, not unfrequently it fails to reduce the circulation; nay, occasionally it has the reverse effect,—accelerates the pulse, while it increases the cerebral disorder, and perhaps irritates the stomach. In estimating its value as a remedial agent for fever, we must not regard it as a sedative means (I refer now to the vascular system) merely,—it is an agent which exercises a specific influence over the brain; and, therefore, to be able to lay down correct indications or contra-indications for its use in disordered conditions of this viscus, we ought to be acquainted, on the one hand, with the precise nature of the influence of the remedy, and, on the other, with the actual condition of the brain in the disease which we wish to relieve. Now, as we possess neither of these data in reference to fever, our use of foxglove is, with the exception of the sedative influence over the circulation, empirical; and experience has fully shown us it is not generally beneficial. But, I repeat, where the frequency of pulse bears no relation to the local or constitutional symptoms of fever, foxglove may be serviceable.

2. *Inflammation.*—Foxglove has been employed in inflammatory diseases, —principally on account of its power of reducing the frequency of the pulse, though some have referred part of its beneficial operation to its influence over the absorbent system. Inflammation, of a chronic kind, may be going on in one part of the body to an extent sufficient to produce complete disorganisation, and ultimately to cause the death of the patient, without the action of the larger arterial trunks (*i. e.* of the system generally) being remarkably increased. In such cases digitalis is, for the most part, of little use. Again, in violent and acute inflammation, accompanied with great excitement of the general circulation, especially in plethoric subjects, foxglove is, in some cases, hurtful; in others it is a trivial and unimportant remedy; and we therefore rely, in our treatment, on blood-letting and other powerful antiphlogistic measures; and foxglove, if serviceable at all, can only be used after the other means. As a remedy for inflammation, foxglove is principally useful in less violent cases, particularly when accompanied with increased frequency of pulse, and occurring in subjects not able to support copious evacuations of blood. Moreover, it has more influence over inflammation of some parts of the body (as the arachnoid membrane, the pleura, the pericardium, and the lungs) than of others. In gastric and enteritic inflammation it would appear to be objectionable, on account of its irritant properties; while its specific influence over the brain would make it a doubtful remedy in phrenitis. In arachnitis of children it is certainly a most valuable agent.

In conclusion, then, it appears that digitalis, as a remedy for inflammation, is principally valuable where the disease has a tendency to terminate in serous effusion. But in no case can it be regarded as a substitute for blood-letting. Its powers as an antiphlogistic remedy have, I suspect, been greatly over-rated.

3. *Dropsy.*—Of all remedies for dropsy, none have gained more, and few so much, celebrity as foxglove. It has been supposed to owe its beneficial operation to its repressing arterial excitement, to its promoting the functions of the absorbent vessels, and particularly to its diuretic effects. Whatever may be its *modus operandi*, its powerful and salutary influence in many dropsies cannot be a matter of doubt. Dr. Withering has observed that " it seldom succeeds in men of great natural strength, of tense fibre, of warm skin, of florid complexion, or in those with a tight and cordy pulse." " On the contrary, if the pulse be feeble or intermitting, the countenance pale, the lips livid, the skin cold, the swollen belly soft and fluctuating, or the anasarcous limbs readily pitting under the pressure of the finger, we may expect the diuretic effects to follow in a kindly manner." In those with a florid complexion blood-letting and purgatives will often be found useful preparatives for foxglove. In some forms of dropsy foxglove is more serviceable than in others. Thus anasarca, ascites, hydrothorax, and phlegmasia dolens, are sometimes benefited by it; whereas ovarian dropsy and hydrocephalus are not relieved by it. Its diuretic effect is greatly promoted by combining other diuretics with it, especially squills (as in the *Pilulæ Digitalis et Scillæ*, Ph. Ed.), calomel, or the saline diuretics (as the acetate of potash). A combination of vegetable bitters (as infusion of gentian or calumba) with foxglove forms, I think, a valuable form of exhibition in many old dropsical cases. Infusion of common broom (*Cytisus scoparius*) might probably be advantageously conjoined with foxglove where a powerful diuretic is required. In old cases of general dropsy, in œdematous swellings from debility, and in anasarca following scarlet fever, where, together with weakness, there is still left an excited and irritable state of the arterial system, chalybeates (as the *tinctura ferri sesquichloridi*) may be conjoined with foxglove with the happiest effects.[1]

4. *In hemorrhages.*—In active hemorrhages from internal organs, accompanied with a quick, hard, and throbbing pulse, foxglove as a sedative is oftentimes serviceable. Epistaxis, hæmoptysis, and menorrhagia, are the forms of hemorrhage more frequently benefited by the use of foxglove.

5. *Diseases of the heart and great vessels.*—An important indication in the treatment of many diseases of the heart and great vessels, is to reduce the force and velocity of the circulation. The most effectual means of fulfilling this indication are,—the adoption of a low diet, repeated blood-letting, and the employment of foxglove. There are, perhaps, no diseases in which the beneficial effects of foxglove are more marked than in those of the heart and great vessels. In *aneurism of the aorta* our only hope of cure is by the coagulation of the blood in the aneurismal sac, and the consequent removal of the distensive pressure of the circulation. To promote this, we endeavour to retard the movement of the blood within the sac by diminishing the quantity of blood in the system generally, and by reducing the force and velocity with which it circulates. Blood-letting and digitalis are, in these

---

[1] Holland, *Med. Notes and Reflect.* p. 546.

cases, very important agents; and under their use cases now and then recover. Again, in *simple dilatation* of the cavities of the heart our objects are to remove, if possible, the cause (usually obstruction in the pulmonic or aortic system), to strengthen the muscular fibres of the heart, and to repress any preternatural excitement of the vascular system. Digitalis is useful to us in attaining the latter object. In *simple hypertrophy*, or *hypertrophy with dilatation*, we have to reduce the preternatural thickness of the heart's parietes; and this we do by removing, when it can be done, any obstruction to the circulation, by using a low diet, by repeated blood-letting, and by the employment of foxglove. No means, says the late Dr. Davies,[1] excepting the abstraction of blood, diminishes the impulsion of the heart so completely and so certainly as digitalis. "I have been," adds he, "in the habit of using it for several years for these affections, and have rarely seen it fail in producing at least temporary relief." "The enlarged and flaccid heart," observes Dr. Holland,[2] "though, on first view, it might seem the least favourable for the use of the medicine, is, perhaps, not so. At least, we have reason to believe that in dropsical affections, so often connected with this organic change, the action of digitalis as a diuretic is peculiarly of avail." *In some disordered conditions of innervation of the heart and great vessels*—as in angina pectoris, nervous palpitation of the heart, and augmented arterial impulsion—foxglove is also at times beneficial. In patients affected with an intermittent or otherwise irregular pulse, I have several times observed this medicine produce regularity of pulsation,—a circumstance also noticed by Dr. Holland. Besides the preceding, there are *various other affections of the heart* in which foxglove may be found serviceable, either by its sedative influence over the circulation, or by its power of relieving dropsical effusion through its diuretic property.

6. *In phthisis.*—Digitalis has been declared capable of curing pulmonary consumption, and numerous cases of supposed cures have been published. Bayle[3] has collected from the writings of Sanders,[4] Kinglake, Fowler, Beddoes,[5] Drake, Mossman,[6] Maclean, Ferriar,[7] Magennis, Moreton, and others, reports of 151 cases treated by foxglove. Of these, 83 are said to have been cured, and 35 relieved. But a more accurate and extended experience has fully proved that this medicine possesses no curative, and very slightly palliative, powers in genuine phthisis: it is totally incapable of preventing or of causing the removal of tubercular deposits, and has little, if any influence, in retarding the progress of consumption. Its power of diminishing the rapidity of the circulation cannot be doubted; but this effect is, as Dr. Holland[8] justly remarks, " of less real moment than is generally supposed."

7. *In insanity and epilepsy.*—In these maladies foxglove may prove occasionally serviceable, by repressing excessive vascular excitement, which sometimes accompanies them. Furthermore, the specific influence of this remedy over the cerebro-spinal system may now and then contribute to the

---

[1] *Lond. Med. Gaz.* vol. xv. p. 790.
[2] *Med. Notes and Reflect.* p. 574.
[3] *Bibl. Thérap.* t. iii. p. 362.
[4] *Op. ante cit.*
[5] *Observations on the Management of the Consumptive*, 1801.
[6] *Essay to elucidate the Nat. Orig. and Connex. of Scrof. and Gland. Consumption.*
[7] *On Digitalis.*
[8] *Op. cit.* p. 551.

beneficial operation of foxglove. But the precise nature of this influence not having as yet been accurately ascertained, while the pathology of the above-mentioned diseases is involved in considerable obscurity, it follows that the therapeutic value of this influence can only be ascertained empirically. In insanity, Dr. Hallaran[1] recommends foxglove to reduce vascular action after the employment of depletion and purgation. It has been used in this disease, with success, by Dr. Currie,[2] and by Fanzago.[3] In epilepsy it is, I conceive, less likely to be serviceable, because this disease is less frequently accompanied with the vascular excitement against which foxglove is most successful. Accordingly, while in some cases it has appeared to act beneficially,[4] in others it has either been unsuccessful,[5] or has only given temporary relief.[6]

8. *In various other diseases.*—Besides the preceding, there are several other maladies against which foxglove has been employed with occasional benefit, as *scrofula*[7] and *asthma*.[8] For other diseases relieved by foxglove, I must refer the reader to the works of Murray[9] and Bayle.[10]

ADMINISTRATION.—The ordinary dose of foxglove, *in powder*, is from gr. ss. to gr. iss. repeated every six hours.

ANTIDOTES.—In a case of poisoning by foxglove, or its preparations, expel the poison from the stomach by the stomach-pump, or by emetics if vomiting should not have already commenced; assist the vomiting, when it is established, by the use of diluents; and counteract the depressing influence of the poison on the circulation, by the use of ammonia and brandy; and keep the patient in a recumbent posture, to guard against syncope. I am unacquainted with any chemical antidote for foxglove; perhaps infusion of nutgalls might prove serviceable, by the tannic acid which it contains.

1. **INFUSUM DIGITALIS**, L. E. D.; *Infusion of Foxglove.* (Foxglove Leaves, dried, ʒj. [ʒij. *E.*]; Spirit of Cinnamon, fʒj. [fʒij. *E.*]; Boiling [distilled, *L.*] Water, Oj. [fʒxviij. *E.*] Macerate the foxglove leaves in the water for four hours, in a vessel lightly covered, and strain [through linen or calico, *E.*]; then add the spirit of cinnamon, *L.* Foxglove Leaves, dried, ʒj.; Boiling Water, ʒix. Infuse for one hour in a covered vessel, and strain. This product should measure about eight ounces, *D.*)—I believe this, when properly made, to be the most effectual of the preparations of foxglove. The dose of the London infusion is from fʒss. to fʒj. repeated every six hours; [of the Dublin and Edinburgh infusions, ʒij. to ʒss.—ED.] I have known it given to the extent of fʒij.

2. **TINCTURA DIGITALIS**, L. E. D.; *Tincture of Foxglove.* (Foxglove Leaves, dried [in moderately fine powder, *E.*], ʒiv.; Proof Spirit, Oij. Mace-

---

[1] *Inquiry, &c., with Observ. on the Cure of Insanity,* 1810.
[2] *Mem. of the Med. Soc. of London,* vol. iv.
[3] Quoted by Bayle, *Bibl. Thérap.* t. iii. p. 320.
[4] Scott, *Ed. Med. and Surg. Journ.* Jan. 1827; Dr. E. Sharkey, *On the Efficacy of Digitalis in the Treatment of Idiopathic Epilepsy,* 1841.
[5] Percival, *ibid.* vol. ix. p. 274.
[6] Currie, *op. supra cit.*
[7] Haller, Merz, Schiemann, and Hufeland; quoted by Bayle, *Bibl. Thér.* t. iii. p. 369.
[8] Ferriar, *On Digitalis,* 1799; Fogo [asthma cured by an overdose of foxglove], *Ed. Med. and Surg. Journ.* vol. xviii. p. 345.
[9] *App. Med.* vol. i.
[10] *Op. supra cit.*

rate for seven [fourteen, *E.*] days, and strain, *L.* Foxglove Leaves, dried, and in coarse powder, ʒv.; Proof Spirit, Oij. Macerate for fourteen days, strain, express, and filter, *D.* "This tincture is best prepared by the process of percolation, as directed for the tincture of capsicum. If forty fluidounces of the spirit be passed through, the density is 944 [0·944], and the solid contents of a fluidounce amount to twenty-four grains. It may also be made by digestion," *E.*)—The usual dose of this preparation, for an adult, is ♏x. cautiously increased to ♏xl., repeated every six hours. I usually begin with ♏xx. The largest dose I have employed is fʒj.; but, as I have already stated, it has been given to the extent of one ounce! The colour of this preparation is somewhat affected by exposure to strong solar light.

Succus Digitalis.—*The preserved juice of foxglove* may be employed as a substitute for the tincture. From 1 cwt. 2 qrs. 26 lbs. of digitalis gathered in May, 49 pints of juice have been obtained.

3. EXTRACTUM DIGITALIS, E.; *Extract of Foxglove.* ("This extract is best prepared from the fresh leaves of digitalis, by any of the processes indicated for extract of conium," *E.*)—The preparation of this extract requires very great care and attention, or the virtues of the plant may be destroyed during the process. Dose, gr. j. cautiously increased.

4. PILULÆ DIGITALIS ET SCILLÆ, E.; *Pills of Foxglove and Squill.* (Digitalis, Squill, of each *one part;* Aromatic Electuary, *two parts.* Beat them into a proper mass with conserve of red roses, and divide the mass into four-grain pills.)—A valuable diuretic compound. Used in dropsies. Dose, one or two pills.

Order XLII. SOLANACEÆ, *Lindley.*—NIGHTSHADES.

Solaneæ, *Jussieu.*

Characters.—*Calyx* 5-parted, seldom 4-parted, persistent, inferior. *Corolla* monopetalous, hypogynous; the limb 5-cleft, seldom 4-cleft, regular, or somewhat unequal, deciduous; the æstivation plaited or imbricated. *Stamens* inserted upon the corolla, as many as the segments of the limb, with which they are alternate : *anthers* bursting longitudinally, rarely by pores at the apex. *Ovary* 2-celled, composed of a pair of carpels right and left of the axis, rarely 4—5- or many-celled, with polyspermous placentæ; *style* continuous; *stigma* simple; *ovules* numerous, amphitropal. *Pericarp* with 2 or 4 or many cells, either a capsule with a double dissepiment parallel with the valves, or a berry with the placentæ adhering to the dissepiment. *Seeds* numerous, sessile; *embryo* straight or curved, often out of the centre, lying in a fleshy *albumen;* *radicle* next the hilum.— *Herbaceous* plants or *shrubs.* *Leaves* alternate, undivided, or lobed, sometimes collateral; the floral ones sometimes double, and placed near each other. *Inflorescence* variable, often out of the axil; the *pedicels* without bracts (*Lindley*).

Properties.—The narcotic properties which many members of this Order possess depend on the presence of vegetable alkaloids; but the narcotism which they induce is very different to that caused by opium :[1] hyoscyamus, belladonna, and stramonium, give rise to phantasms and dilatation of the pupil (see the *Solanacea mydriatica*) : nicotiana is a nauseating cardiaco-vascular sedative. An acrid resin is found in many species; on this the hot, pungent, burning qualities of capsicum depend. A bitter principle confers on some species (as *S. pseudoquina* and *crispum*) tonic properties. Starch abounds in potatoes, which owe their nutritive qualities chiefly to it.

---

[1] The generalisations of some late French writers (Trousseau and Pidoux, *Traité de Thérap.* t. i. p. 206) with respect to the identity of the operation of the narcotic Solaneæ, do not appear to me to be founded in fact.

177. HYOSCYAMUS NIGER, *Linn.*—COMMON HENBANE.

Sex. Syst. Pentandria, Monogynia.

(Herbæ biennis folium caulinum recens et exsiccatum, *L.*—Leaves, *E. D.*)

History.—This plant is the Ὑοσκύαμος μέλας of Dioscorides,[1] the *hyoscyamus niger* of Pliny.[2]

Botany. **Gen. Char.**—*Calyx* urceolate, 5-toothed. *Corolla* funnel-shaped; the limb plaited, 5-lobed; the lobes obtuse, unequal. *Stamens 5,* inserted in the lower part of the tube of the corolla, enclosed or exserted, declinate; *anthers* dehiscing longitudinally. *Ovary* 2-celled; placentæ fixed to the dorsal dissepiment; ovules numerous; *style* simple; *stigma* capitate. *Capsule* enclosed by the persistent often enlarged calyx, narrowed from the ventricose base, membranous, 2-celled, circumscissile at the apex, with a 2-celled lid. *Seeds* many, kidney-shaped; *embryo* in fleshy albumen, almost peripherical, curved (*Endlicher*).

Sp. Char.—*Leaves* oblong, pinnatifid, or sinuate sessile, and subamplexicaul; lower leaves stalked. *Flowers* nearly sessile, axillary, unilateral (*Babington*).

Root spindle-shaped. *Stem* bushy. *Leaves* soft and pliant, sharply lobed. Whole herbage glandular, downy, and viscid, exhaling a powerful fetid and oppressive odour.

[" Sessile, oblong, acutely sinuous, subpubescent, with viscid fœtid hairs. To be gathered and dried as directed for Foxglove. The plant which grows spontaneously in old rubbish and in highways is to be preferred to that which is cultivated in gardens."—*Ph. Lond.*]

Flowers numerous from the bosoms of the crowded upper leaves, drooping, almost entirely sessile, of an elegant straw colour, usually pencilled with dark purple veins.

Hab.—Indigenous: waste ground, banks, and commons. Flowers in July. There are two varieties of this species,—one biennial, the other annual. Both are cultivated at Mitcham.

Var. *a biennis; Biennial Black Henbane.*—This is larger, stronger, more branched, more clammy, than the annual variety. Its root is biennial. Cultivated at Mitcham.—During the first year of its growth the plant has no aerial stem, all the leaves being radical and stalked. It is less odorous and clammy than the mature plant; and Dr. Houlton[3] states that it yields less extract. In the autumn the leaves die, but the root survives during the winter, and in the following spring sends up an aerial stem, which grows to the height of from two to four feet. The leaves of the second year are large, deeply sinuate, or pinnatifid. It flowers towards the end of May, or in June. As this variety is more highly developed than the annual sort, it probably possesses more medicinal activity, and, therefore, should be preferred. I am, however, unacquainted with any experiments demonstrative of its superiority. This variety flowers earlier than the annual sort. The surest plan of obtaining it, therefore, is to purchase it fresh while in flower.

Var. *β annua*, Sims, Bot. Mag. 2394; *H. agrestis*, Kitaibel, ex Schult. Fl. Austr. ed. 2, p. 383; *H. niger* var. *β minor*, Brandt u. Ratzeburg, Deutschl. phan. Giftgewächse; *H. niger*, var. *β agrestis*, Nees, in Linn. Trans. xvii. 77; *Annual* or *Field Henbane.*—Root annual; stem simple, downy; leaves smoothish, sinuately toothed; flowers sessile; corolla reticulated.—Indigenous: South of Europe; North of India.—Cultivated at Mitcham for medicinal use.—Flowers in July and August.

---

[1] Lib. iv. cap. 69.
[2] *Hist. Nat.* lib. xxv. cap. 17, ed. Valp.
[3] *Pharmaceutical Journal*, vol. iii. p. 578, 1844.

The plant is smaller, the leaves less deeply sinuated (not pinnatifid), less hairy, clammy, and fetid, than var. *a biennis*.

   * *Corolla non violaceo-reticulata ; H. pallidus*, Koch, Babing. Man. of Br. Botany. This is a sub-variety of *β annua*, with yellow corolla, without any purple veins.— It is said to grow wild at Esher, in Surrey.

Hyoscyamus albus, Linn.; 'Υοσκύαμος λευκός, Diosc. lib. iv. cap. 69.—Leaves petiolate ; lower ones orbicular, entire ; the rest from cordate to ovate at the base, sinuated ; flowers sessile.—South of Europe. Annual. Its medicinal properties resemble those of H. niger, for which it has sometimes been employed in medicine.[1]

Description.—The herb (*herba hyoscyami*), when fresh, has a strong, unpleasant, narcotic odour, a mucilaginous, slightly acrid taste, and a clammy feel. It should be gathered when in full flower. By drying, it almost wholly loses these properties. One hundred pounds of the fresh herb yield about fourteen pounds when dried.[2] The *leaves* (*folia hyoscyami*), when fresh, are pale dull green. The seeds (*semina hyoscyami*) are small, compressed, uniform, roundish, finely dotted, of a yellowish-grey colour, and have the odour of the plant, and an oleaginous, bitter taste.

Composition.—The seeds of Hyoscyamus niger were analysed in 1816 by Kirchof,[3] and in 1820 by Brandes.[4] The extract of the herb was analysed by Lindbergson.[5]

Brandes's Analysis.		Lindbergson's Analysis.
Fatty oil	24·2	Narcotic extractive soluble in water and alcohol.
Waxy fat	1·4	
Resin insoluble in ether	3·0	Bitter extractive.
Malate of hyoscyamia with malates of lime and magnesia, and a salt of potash and ammonia ...	6·3	Gummy extractive.
Uncrystallisable sugar	a trace	Malates, phosphates, sulphates, and muriates of magnesia.
Gum 1·2, bassorin 2·4, and starch 1·5	5·1	
Albumen	4·5	Extract of the herb.
Vegeto-animal matter	3·4	
Malate, phosphate, sulphate, and muriate of potash	0·4	
Malates of lime and magnesia	0·6	
Phosphates of lime and magnesia	2·4	
Woody fibre	26·0	
Water	24·1	
Seeds of hyoscyamus	101·4	

The ashes contained carbonate, phosphate, sulphate, and muriate of potash, carbonate and much phosphate of lime, much silica, manganese, iron, and minute traces of copper.

1. Hyoscyamia or Hyoscyamina.—This term has been applied to a vegetable alkali procured from the seeds and herbs of Hyoscyamus niger by Brandes,[6] whose statements have been confirmed by Geiger and Hesse, as well as by Mein.[7] However, Chevallier, as well as Brault and Poggiale,[8] have failed to procure it. The properties assigned to it are almost identical with those of atropia, from which it differs in being more soluble in water. It is crystallisable, has an acrid taste, and, when volatilised, yields ammonia. Reisinger[9] says that a drop of a solution of one grain of this substance in ten grains of

[1] Fouquier, *Archiv. Gén. de Méd.* Mars 1823 ; Chevallier, *Journ. de Chim. Méd.* t. ii. p. 36.
[2] Martius, *Pharmakogn.*
[3] *Berl. Jahrb.* Bd. xvii. S. 144.
[4] *Ibid.* Bd. xxi. S. 280.
[5] Gmelin, *Handb. d. Chem.* ii. 1303.
[6] *Pharm. Central-Blatt für* 1822, S. 479.
[7] *Journ. de Pharm.* t. xx. p. 87 ; and *Pharm. Central-Blatt für* 1835, S. 83.
[8] *Ibid.* t. xxi. p. 134.
[9] *Arch. Gén. de Méd.* t. xviii. p. 301.

water caused dilatation of the pupil, but did not give rise to irritation of the eye. A solution of double this strength acted as an irritant.

1. EMPYREUMATIC OIL OF HENBANE (*Pyro-Hyoscyamia ?*).—This was obtained by Dr. Morries[1] by the destructive distillation of henbane. Its chemical properties are identical with those of the empyreumatic oil of foxglove. It proved a powerful narcotic poison.

PHYSIOLOGICAL EFFECTS. *α. On Vegetables.*—Water holding in solution extract of henbane proved poisonous to Hyoscyamus niger.[2]

β. On Animals.—Its effects on herbivorous animals are slight. Given to horses in large quantities, it causes dilatation of the pupils, spasmodic movements of the lips, and frequency of pulse.[3] On dogs its effects appear to be analogous to those on man.[4] It does not cause any local irritation. Its constitutional effects are dilatation of pupil, weakness of the posterior extremities, staggering, and insensibility.

γ. On Man.—*In small and repeated doses* henbane has a calming, soothing, and tranquillising effect. This is especially observed in persons suffering from great nervous irritability, and from a too active condition of the sensorial functions. In such it frequently causes quietude, with a tendency to sleep. It frequently allays irritation and preternatural sensibility existing in any organ. It does not quicken the pulse, check secretion, or cause constipation. *Large doses* sometimes induce sleep. Fouquier,[5] however, denies this. He says henbane causes headache, giddiness, dimness of sight, dilatation of pupil, a greater or less tendency to sleep, and painful delirium. In some cases these symptoms are followed by thirst, nausea, griping, and either purging or constipation; and in a few instances febrile heat and irritation of skin are induced. But I have frequently seen sleep follow its use, although its hypnotic properties are neither constant nor powerful. It more frequently fails to occasion sleep in those accustomed to the use of opium. Very large doses are apt to be followed by delirium rather than by sleep. Its power of alleviating pain and allaying spasm is greatly inferior to that of opium. *In poisonous doses* it causes loss of speech, dilatation of pupil, disturbance of vision (presbyopia), distortion of face, coma, and delirium, generally of the unmanageable, sometimes of the furious kind, and phantasms; and paralysis, occasionally with convulsive movements. Irritation of the stomach and bowels (manifested by nausea, vomiting, pain, and purging) is occasionally induced.[6] One author[7] says hyoscyamus renders the hair grey, while another[8] states that it darkens it.

In its operation on the body henbane presents several peculiarities. From opium it is distinguished by the sedative rather than stimulant effects of small doses; by its not confining the bowels; by the obscurity of vision (presbyopia); and, when swallowed in large doses, by its producing dilatation of the pupil, and by its being more apt to occasion delirium with phantasms. Furthermore, in some individuals opium causes headache and other distressing symptoms

[1] *Ed. Med. and Surg. Journ.* vol. xxxix. p. 379.
[2] Macaire, quoted by De Candolle, *Phys. Vég.* p. 1354; also Miguel, quoted in Meyen's *Report on the Progress of Vegetable Physiology during the year* 1837, translated by W. Francis, p. 139.
[3] Moiroud, *Pharm. Vét.* p. 349; see also Viborg, in Wibmer's *Wirk. d. Arzn. u. Gift.* Bd. iii. S. 156.
[4] Orfila, *Tox. Gén.*
[5] *Arch. Gén. de Méd.* t. i. p. 297.
[6] For abstracts of cases illustrative of these effects, consult Orfila, *Toxicol. Gén.*; and Wibmer, *Wirk. d. Arzneim. u. Gift.*
[7] Hühnerwolf, quoted by Wibmer, *op. cit.* S. 148.
[8] Most, *Encykl. der gesamm. med. u. chir. Praxis*, art. Cosmetica, Bd. i. S. 498, Leipzig, 1836.

which henbane is not so apt to produce. From belladonna and stramonium, to which it is in several respects closely allied, it is distinguished by the very rare occurrence of any symptoms of gastro-intestinal irritation after the ingestion of large doses of it. Sundelin[1] says "that it wants the resolvent operation, and the stimulant influence over the vascular system, which belladonna possesses." Vogt[2] ranks hyoscyamus between belladonna and hydrocyanic acid. But, with every respect for the opinions of so profound a writer, I cannot concur in the propriety of this arrangement. I have never seen, from the use of hydrocyanic acid, the same tranquillising and soothing influence over the mind and external senses which I have repeatedly witnessed from the use of small doses of hyoscyamus; and the effects of poisonous doses of these two agents more strikingly display the difference of their operation; for while hydrocyanic acid causes insensibility and convulsions, henbane produces delirium and paralysis.

Uses.—Hyoscyamus is said to alleviate pain and irritation in various organs, to promote sleep, to procure quietude, and to obviate spasm. For any of these objects it is greatly inferior to, and less confidently to be relied on, than opium. Yet it is, on various occasions, preferred to the latter; as where opium causes headache or other distressing cerebral symptoms, or where it occasions constipation. Again, the stimulant influence of small doses of opium over the vascular system, and the tendency of this narcotic to lock up the secretions and excretions, form objections to its use in the maladies of children: in such, therefore, hyoscyamus is frequently preferred. Fouquier, to whose observations with respect to the effects of henbane I have already had occasion to refer, can find in this narcotic no useful property, and he thinks it ought to be banished from the Materia Medica.[3]

The following are the principal purposes for which it is ordinarily employed in this country :—

1. *As an anodyne* where opium disagrees, or is from any circumstance objectionable. It may be used in neuralgia, rheumatism, gout, periostitis, the milk abscess, painful affections of the urino-genital organs, scirrhus, and carcinoma.

2. *As a calmer* and *soporific* it is available in sleeplessness accompanied with great restlessness and mental irritability, and where opium, from its stimulant or other properties, proves injurious. Sometimes, where it fails to cause actual sleep, it proves highly serviceable by producing a calm and tranquil state conducive to the well-doing and comfort of the patient.

3. *As an antispasmodic* it occasionally proves serviceable in spasmodic affections of the organs of respiration (*e. g.* spasmodic asthma) and of the urino-genital apparatus (*e. g.* spasmodic stricture and spasm of the sphincter vesicæ). Notwithstanding the favourable reports of Storck to the contrary, it is rarely calculated to be of any service in epilepsy.

4. *As a sedative,* to allay irritation and preternatural sensibility. In troublesome cough it sometimes proves useful, by dulling the sensibility of the bronchial membrane to the influence of the cold air. In nephritic and vesical irritation, and in gonorrhœa, it is sometimes a useful substitute for opium. In the irritation of teething it is valuable, from its power of

---

[1] *Handb. d. sp. Heilm.* Bd. i. S. 463, 3te Aufl.
[2] *Lehrb. d. Pharmakod.* Bd. i. S. 170, 2te Aufl.
[3] *Op. cit.* p. 312.

relieving pain and convulsion. Its advantages over opium, in the disorders of children, have been already pointed out.

5. *To dilate the pupil* the extract may be used as a substitute for extract of belladonna, than which it is less powerful.

6. *As a topical sedative and anodyne,* fomentations of the herb or the extract are sometimes applied to painful glandular swellings, irritable ulcers, hemorrhoids, and parts affected with neuralgia. In irritation of the rectum or bladder it is sometimes used per anum.

ADMINISTRATION.—The *powder* of the leaves is rarely employed: the dose is from three to ten grains. The *extract* and *tincture* are the preparations commonly used.

ANTIDOTES.—The treatment of a case of poisoning by henbane is the same as that by opium.

1. TINCTURA HYOSCYAMI, L. E. D.; *Tincture of Henbane.* (Henbane Leaves, dried [in moderately fine powder, *E.*], ℥v.; Proof Spirit, Oij. Macerate for seven [fourteen, *D.*] days, strain, express, and filter. "This tincture is best prepared by the process of percolation, as directed for tincture of capsicum; but it may also be obtained, though with greater loss, by the process of digestion," *E.*)—Dose, f℥ss. to f℥ij.

SUCCUS HYOSCYAMI.—*The preserved juice of henbane* may be substituted for the tincture. The following are the quantities of juice obtained from henbane leaves:—

	Imperial Quarts of Juice.
July 24th. 3 *cwt.* of leaves	42
July 28th. 2 *cwt.* of leaves	22
Aug. 3rd. 2 *cwt.* of leaves	25

2. EXTRACTUM HYOSCYAMI, L. E. D.; *Extract of Henbane.* ("Prepare this extract by the process ordered for extract of aconite," *L.* "This extract is to be prepared from the fresh leaves of hyoscyamus by any of the processes directed for extract of conium," *E.* The *Dublin College* orders it to be prepared from the fresh hyoscyamus leaves collected when the plant begins to flower. The method of preparation is the same as for extract of belladonna, *D.*)—The average produce of extract is stated by Mr. Brande[1] to be from 4 to 5 lbs. from 112 lbs. of the fresh herb. Mr. Squire[2] states the following as the products (obtained by a common screw-press and water-bath) from 112 lbs. of matured hyoscyamus, gathered dry and in good order; the season, however, being rather more rainy than the average:—

	Weight. lbs.	Yielded of Juice. lbs.		Yielded of Extract. lbs. oz.
The leaves, the very fine summits of the stalks, the flowers and seed-vessels already formed, weighed	70	42	=	4 10
The stalks weighed	35	17½	=	0 15
Waste leaves and dirt	3½	—		—
Lost by evaporation during the two hours occupied by picking	3½	—		—
	112	59¼		5 9

The quality of the extract met with in the shops is extremely variable. This arises principally from the unequal care with which it has been prepared.[3]

---

[1] *Dict. Mat. Med.* p. 312.

[2] *Pharmaceutical Transactions,* p. 97.

[3] [For some remarks on the preparation of this extract, by Mr. Cracknell, see *Pharmaceutical Journal,* March 1851, p. 439.—ED.]

The dose is from gr. v. to Əj. Occasionally very much larger doses have been taken without any injurious effects. It is a valuable addition to the compound extract of colocynth, whose operation it renders milder, though not less efficacious. It is sometimes used as a topical application to inflamed or tender parts : thus, alone, or in the form of ointment, it is applied to painful hemorrhoids; spread on linen, it forms a plaster which has been used in neuralgia, rheumatic pains, and painful glandular swellings.

My friend Dr. William Lobb, and nearly a dozen other persons, in 1841 experienced symptoms like those of poisoning by belladonna, from the employment of several grains of an extract sold by a most respectable country chemist as that of hyoscyamus. The greater part of the extract sold by this chemist had been most carefully prepared by himself; but not having made sufficient for the year's consumption, he purchased some in London, and the extract used on these occasions *might have been* that which was bought. The extract employed had an unusually greenish colour, and the hyoscyamus odour. The effects produced were difficulty of swallowing, a sensation as if the parts about the throat had been powdered with tow-dust, impaired vision (presbyopia), eyes bloodshot, pupils dilated, feeling of suffocation, strangury, cessation of cough and expectoration, which had been previously troublesome. The vision was greatly improved by the use of a magnifier. The third day the symptoms had disappeared, but great prostration of strength supervened. In some of the patients an eruption like that of scarlatina appeared, with intense redness of the palms of the hands.

[3. **EXTRACTUM HYOSCYAMI ALCOHOLICUM,** U.S. (Take of Henbane Leaves, in coarse powder, lb. j. Diluted Alcohol, Oiv. Moisten with half a pint of alcohol, and having allowed the mixture to stand twenty-four hours, transfer to an apparatus for displacement, and gradually add the remainder of the diluted alcohol. When the last portion shall have penetrated the leaves, pour in sufficient water from time to time to keep the powder covered. Cease to filter when the liquid which passes begins to produce a precipitate as it falls. Distil off the alcohol from the filtered liquor, and evaporate the residue to a proper consistence.)—This preparation is intended as a substitute for the preceding, as the fresh herb cannot be obtained in sufficient quantity in the United States. It is a fine, clear, dark, shining extract, is possessed of the active properties of the drug, and may be employed in place of the common extract. The dose is gr. j. to grs. v., or in larger quantities if required.—Ed.]

178. ATROPA BELLADONNA, *Linn.*—COMMON DWALE; DEADLY NIGHTSHADE.

Sex. Syst. Pentandria, Monogynia.

(Folium recens et exsiccatum, *L.*—Leaves, *E.*—The leaves and root, *D.*)

History.—Belladonna, being a native of both Greece and Italy, was doubtless known to, and described by, the ancient Greek and Roman writers. Modern botanists, however, have been unable to identify it with certainty. Fraas[1] is of opinion that it is the Μανδραγόρας of Theophrastus,[2] the Στρύχνος μανικός ("ἄνθος μέλαν") of Dioscorides,[3] the third sort of *Strychnos* (*Solanum*) of Pliny.[4] But this notion is not without its difficulties. The

[1] *Synops. Plant. Fl. Class.* p. 166, 1845.
[2] *Hist. Plant.* lib. vi. cap. 2.
[3] Lib. iv. cap. 74.
[4] Lib. xxi. cap. 105 ; and lib. xxviii. cap. 108, ed. Valp.

plant which Theophrastus mentions under the above name had a stem like the νάρθηζ (*ferula*), and a black racemose fruit with a vinous taste. Now the stem of belladonna certainly does not resemble that of an umbelliferous plant, nor is the fruit racemose. Sibthorp and Smith[1] have, in my opinion, only exercised a proper precaution in not assigning any ancient synonyme to belladonna. The earliest undoubted notice of belladonna occurs in the work of Tragus (A.D. 1532), who calls it *Solanum hortense nigrum*.[2] It has been supposed that it was this plant which produced such remarkable and fatal effects on the Roman soldiers during their retreat from the Parthians.[3] Buchanan[4] relates that the Scots mixed the juice of this plant with the bread and drink, which, by their truce, they were to supply the Danes, which so intoxicated them, that the Scots killed the greatest part of Sweno's army while asleep. Shakspeare[5] is supposed to allude to it under the name of the *insane root*.

BOTANY. **Gen. Char.**—*Calyx* 5-parted. *Corolla* hypogynous, funnel-shaped, campanulate ; the limb plaited, 5-10-cleft. *Stamens* 5, inserted into the lower part of the corolla, exserted, or nearly so ; filaments filiform ; anthers dehiscing longitudinally. *Ovary* 2-celled ; placentæ inserted in a line on the dorsal dissepiment ; ovules numerous ; *style* simple ; *stigma* peltato-depressed. *Berry* supported by the spreading calyx, 2-celled. *Seeds* many, subreniform ; *embryo* in fleshy albumen, subperipherical, arched or annular (*Endlicher*).

Sp. Char.—*Stem* herbaceous. *Leaves* broadly-ovate, entire. *Flowers* solitary, axillary on short stalks (*C. C. Babington*).

Root fleshy, creeping. Whole plant fetid when bruised, of a dark and lurid aspect, indicative of its deadly narcotic quality. *Stems* herbaceous, 3 feet high, round, branched, leafy, slightly downy. *Leaves* lateral, mostly 2 together of unequal size, ovate, acute, entire, smooth. *Flowers* imperfectly axillary, solitary, stalked, drooping, dark full purple in the border, paler down-wards, about an inch long. *Berry* of a shining violet black, the size of a small cherry, sweetish, and not nauseous (*Smith*).

" Leaves oval, acute, entire, smooth, fœtid when bruised. The herb which grows spontaneously in hedges and uncultivated places is to be preferred to that cultivated in gardens."—*Ph. Lond.*

Hab.—Indigenous : hedges and waste ground, on a calcareous soil. Flowers in June.

DESCRIPTION.—The root (*radix belladonnæ*), when fresh, is one or more inches thick, and sometimes a foot or more long : it is branching, fleshy, internally white, externally greyish or brownish-white. Its taste is slight, sweetish : its odour feeble. It may be collected in the autumn or early in the spring. The flowering stems (*herba belladonnæ*) are collected in June or July ; they are then deprived of leaves (*folia belladonnæ*), which are to be carefully dried. The leaves, when fresh, have a feeble, bitterish, sub-acid taste.

[1] *Prod. Fl. Græcæ.*
[2] Bauhin, *Pinax.*
[3] See Plutarch's *Life of Antony.*
[4] *Rerum Scot..Hist.* lib. vii.
[5] *Macbeth*, Act i. Scene 3d.

COMPOSITION.—The *leaves* of belladonna were analysed, in 1808, by Melandri;[1] the *expressed juice*, in 1809, by Vauquelin;[2] and the *dried herb*, in 1819, by Brandes.[3] Besides these, there have been several less complete examinations of this plant by other chemists, which have yielded more or less interesting results.

Brandes's Analysis.

Supermalate of atropia	1·51
Pseudo-toxin with malate of atropia and potash salts	16·05
Wax	0·70
Chlorophylle	5·84
Phytocolla (a nitrogenous substance insoluble in alcohol)	6·90
Gum	8·33
Starch	1·25
Albumen	10·70
Lignin	13·70
Salts	7·47
Water	25·50
Loss	2·05
Dried herb of Belladonna	100·00

1. ATROPIA.—(See p. 556.)

2. PSEUDOTOXIN.—A substance obtained by Brandes from the watery extract of belladonna. It is brownish-yellow, soluble in water, insoluble in absolute alcohol and ether, is coloured green by the salts of iron, and is totally precipitated from its watery solution by the salts of lead and by tincture of galls.[4]

3. BELLADONNIN.—Under this name, Luebekind[5] has described a volatile vegetable alkali, which, he says, is distinct from atropia. It is crystallisable, and has an ammoniacal odour. It consists of *carbon* 28·5, *hydrogen* 22·4, *nitrogen* 32·1, *oxygen* 17·0. The crystals contain three equivalents of water. Two grains caused extreme heat in the throat, and constriction of the larynx.

4. ATROPIC ACID.—This name has been given by Richter[6] to a volatile, crystallisable acid, distinguished from benzoic acid by its not precipitating the salts of iron.

PHYSIOLOGICAL EFFECTS. *α. On Vegetables.*—An aqueous solution of extract of belladonna is poisonous to plants.[7]

β. On Animals generally.—Belladonna proves poisonous to mammalia and birds; but much less so to herbivorous than to carnivorous animals. Eight pounds (Troy) of the leaves have been eaten by a horse without any ill effects.[8] The late Mr. Anderson told me that blackbirds ate the seeds at the Chelsea Garden with impunity. A pound of ripe berries has been given to an ass with very little effect.[9] Given to dogs belladonna causes dilatation of pupil, plaintive cries, efforts to vomit, weakness of the posterior extremities, staggering, frequent pulse, a state like intoxication, and death.[10] Forty or fifty grains of the watery extract, injected into the jugular vein of a dog, have

---

[1] *Ann. de Chim.* lxv. 222.

[2] *Ibid.* lxxii. 53.

[3] Gmelin's *Hand. d. Chem.* ii. 1305.

[4] *Ibid.* ii. 1032.

[5] *Pharm. Central-Blatt für* 1839, S. 448.

[6] *Ibid. für* 1837, S. 614.

[7] Marcet, *Ann. Chim. et Phys.* vol. xxix. p. 200 ; and Schübler and Zeller, *Schweigger's Journ. f. d. Chem.* 1827, Bd. 50, S. 54–66.

[8] Moiroud, *Pharm. Vét.* p. 344.

[9] Viborg, in Wibmer, *Wirk. d. Arz. u. Gifte,* Bd. i. S. 366.

[10] Orfila, *Toxicol. Gen.*

proved fatal.[1] Flourens[2] thinks that the *tubercula quadrigemina* are the parts of the nervous centres on which this poison specifically acts. His inferences were drawn from experiments made on birds. The topical action of belladonna is that of an acrid, although not a very violent one.[3]

γ. *On Man.*—*In the first degree* of its operation, belladonna diminishes sensibility and irritability. This effect (called by some, *sedative*) is scarcely obvious in the healthy organism, but is well seen in morbid states, when these properties are preternaturally increased. A very frequent, and sometimes the earliest, obvious effect of belladonna is dryness of the mouth and throat, frequently attended with thirst. The other secretions and the circulation are oftentimes not affected, though occasionally they are augmented. Mr. Bailey[4] " asserts that belladonna affects neither the stomach nor bowels, nor any of the secretions nor excretions, those of the salivary glands excepted." The asserted influence of belladonna over the organic functions is said to be shown by its power of inducing, in some cases, resolutions of swellings and tumours of various kinds, as will be presently noticed.

In the second degree of its operation, belladonna manifests, both in healthy and morbid conditions, its remarkable influence over the cerebrospinal system. It causes dilatation of the pupils (mydriasis), presbyopia or long-sightedness, with obscurity of vision, or absolute blindness (amaurosis), visual illusions (phantasms), suffused eyes, occasionally disturbance of hearing (as singing in the ears), numbness of the face, confusion of head, giddiness, and delirium, which at times resembles intoxication, and may be either combined with or followed by sopor. These symptoms are usually preceded by a febrile condition, attended with a remarkable affection of the mouth, throat, and adjacent parts. Besides dryness of these parts, it causes difficulty of deglutition and of articulation, a feeling of constriction about the throat, nausea, and sometimes actual vomiting, with, now and then, swelling and redness of the face. The pulse is usually hurried and small. The cutaneous, renal, and mucous secretions are frequently augmented. An exanthematous eruption, like that of scarlet fever, has been noticed; and irritation of the urinary organs has in some instances occurred.[5]

In some cases very severe effects have been induced by the application of the extract to abraded surfaces.[6] The continued application of it to the sound skin has also been attended with similar effects.[7]

In the third degree of its operation, belladonna produces effects similar to the preceding, but in a more violent form. The following are the symptoms experienced by above 150 soldiers, who were poisoned by the berries of belladonna, which were gathered at Pirna, near Dresden :—" Dilatation and immobility of the pupil; almost complete insensibility of the eye to the presence of external objects, or at least confused vision; injection of the conjunctiva with a bluish blood; protrusion of the eye, which in some appeared as if it were dull, and in others ardent and furious; dryness of the lips, tongue, palate,

---

[1] Orfila, *Toxicol. Gen.*
[2] *Rech. Exper.* 1824.
[3] Orfila, *supra cit.*
[4] *Observations relative to the Use of Belladonna*, p. 9, 1818.
[5] Jolly, *Nouv. Méd.* iii. 1828 ; and *Lancet*, vol. i. p. 45, 1828-9.
[6] Wade, *Med. and Phys. Journ.* vol. lvii. p. 289, 1827 ; Davies, *Lectures on Diseases of the Lungs and Heart*, p. 496.
[7] Bacot, *Lond. Med. and Phys. Journ.* vol. xxiv. p. 383, 1810.

and throat; deglutition difficult or even impossible; nausea not followed by vomiting; feeling of weakness, lipothymia, syncope; difficulty or impossibility of standing, frequent bending forward of the trunk; continual motion of the hands and fingers; gay delirium, with a vacant smile; aphonia or confused sounds, uttered with pain; probably ineffectual desires of going to stool; gradual restoration to health and reason, without any recollection of the preceding state."[1]

Seven cases (two of which proved fatal) of poisoning by belladonna berries have occurred under my notice in the London Hospital: of these a report has been published by Dr. Letheby.[2] The phenomena were tolerably uniform. The following symptoms especially attracted my attention:—

1. *Dryness of the fauces.*—The excessive dryness of all the parts about the throat contributed greatly to the difficulty of swallowing and alteration of voice.

2. *Scarlet eruption.*—In several cases a scarlet eruption appeared on the arms and legs.

3. *Mydriasis and presbyopia.*—Mydriasis or dilatation of the pupil was present in every case: and was accompanied, in all the cases in which the patient was in a fit state for observation, with presbyopia or long-sightedness. These two symptoms depend, as I have elsewhere stated, on the paralysing influence of the belladonna on the muscular fibres of the iris, by which mydriasis is produced, and on the ciliary muscle, by which the adjusting power of the eye is impaired. I strongly suspect that the impaired vision which has been ascribed to the use of belladonna is chiefly or entirely presbyopia. In one of the patients (a woman) above alluded to, the vision was so much impaired that she could not see to read; and when I placed the prayer card in her hand, she held it upside down, and declared her inability to distinguish the letters or words on it. But after trying several pairs of spectacles, borrowed of patients and others in the ward, she found one (magnifiers) which enabled her to read with ease. This agrees with the results of experiments of Müller[3] on himself. This physiologist found that by the local action of belladonna on one eye, he caused presbyopia of that eye, and thus gave rise to an unequal refractive power of the two eyes. Moreover, it accords with the effects experienced on his own person by Dr. Lobb (see *ante*, p. 544), who informs me that he could see objects at a distance (as on the opposite side of the street), but could not distinguish a letter or a word in a book; but by the aid of a magnifying-glass or powerful spectacles he could read distinctly the smallest print.

Delirium; Phantasms.—The delirium was of the cheerful or wild sort, amounting in some cases to actual frenzy. In some of the patients it subsided into a kind of sleep attended with pleasant dreams, which provoked laughter. The delirium was attended with phantasms; and in this respect resembled that caused by alcohol (*delirium é potu*); but the mind did not run on cats, rats, and mice, as in the case of drunkards. Sometimes the phantasms appeared to be in the air, and various attempts were made to catch or chase them with the hands: at other times they were supposed to be on the bed. One patient (a woman) fancied the sheets were covered with cucumbers. The production of phantasms by belladonna was known to Linnæus,[4] who calls this agent "*a phantastic.*"

5 *Convulsions; Paralysis; Sopor* or *Coma.*—In most of the cases the power of the will over the muscles was so far disordered, that the muscular movements were somewhat irregular, causing a kind of staggering or jerking; but actual convulsions were not general. There was sopor, which terminated in coma, with a weakened or paralytic condition of the muscles.

The active principle of belladonna becomes absorbed and is thrown out of the urine, in which secretion both Runge and Dr. Letheby have detected it.

In comparing the operation of belladonna with that of other cerebro-spinals, the most remarkable symptoms which attract our attention are the

---

[1] Gaultier de Claubry, in Orfila's *Toxicol. Gén.*
[2] *Pharmaceutical Times*, vol. i. p. 25, 1846.
[3] *Elements of Physiology*, translated by Dr. Baly, vol. ii. pp. 1144 and 1153, 1842.
[4] *Materia Medica.*

dilatation of the pupils, with insensibility of the irides to light, disturbance of vision (presbyopia), giddiness, staggering, the delirium (extravagant, pleasing, or furious), with phantasms, followed by sopor, and the remarkable affection of the mouth and throat (dryness of the throat, difficulty of deglutition and of articulation).   Convulsions are rare, and, when they occur, are slight.   Lethargy or sopor occurs subsequently to the delirium.   Local irritation is not well marked.

These characters distinguish the effects of belladonna from those of any other substance, except henbane, stramonium, and perhaps from some other solanaceous species.

When applied to the eyebrow, belladonna causes dilatation of the pupil, without necessarily affecting the other eye, or disturbing vision.   Segalas[1] thought that absorption or imbibition was essential to this effect; but the action on the iris depends, according to Müller,[2] not on the operation of the belladonna on the central organs of the nervous system, but on its topical, paralysing influence on the ciliary nerves.   When, however, belladonna is swallowed, it is obvious that the irides can become affected through the general system only; and in this case the dilatation of the pupil is accompanied with disturbance of vision.[3]   The pneumogastric nerve is obviously concerned in producing the affection of the mouth, and the difficulty of deglutition and articulation.

The disorder of the intellect and of the external senses caused by belladonna proves that the influence of this agent is not limited to the excito-motory system, but is extended to those portions of the nervous centres which are the seat of the intellect and of sensibility.   I have, therefore, classed it among the phrenics and anæsthetics.

USES.—Belladonna has been employed to allay pain and nervous irritation (erethismus nervosus, of some authors); to diminish the sensibility of the retina to the impression of light; to produce dilatation of the pupil; to counteract that condition of brain which is accompanied with contraction of the pupil; and to lessen rigidity and spasmodic contraction of muscular fibres.   These uses obviously arise out of the ascertained physiological effects of the remedy.   There are others, however, which may be regarded as altogether empirical: such as its employment to resolve or discuss scirrhous tumours.

The indications and contra-indications for its use are not sufficiently established to induce us to place much confidence in them.   My own experience leads me to believe that it is not a remedy fitted for plethoric constitutions, or for febrile or acute inflammatory cases; and I am not disposed to admit the observations of Dr. Graves, hereafter to be mentioned, as offering any valid objections to these statements.

1. To allay pain and nervous irritation.—As an anodyne in most internal pains, no remedy hitherto proposed is equal to opium; but this agent totally fails us in many of those external pains known as neuralgia, proso-

---

[1] Lancet, 1826-7, vol. xii. p. 170.
[2] Physiology, vol. i. p. 630.
[3] For some interesting observations on the associated functions of the retina and iris, consult Grainger's Observations on the Structure and Functions of the Spinal Cord, p. 72, et seq.—The power which belladonna possesses of dilating the pupil was discovered by J. A. H. Reimarus, and was made known by Daries in 1776 (Marx, Lond. Med. Gaz. N. S. vol. i. p. 185, 1844-5).

palgia, or *tic douloureux.* In such, belladonna occasionally succeeds in abating, sometimes in completely removing, pain; while it totally fails to give relief in the internal pains for which experience has found opium so efficacious. It is remarkable, therefore, that while both these cerebro-spinals (narcotics, *auctor.*) agree in lessening pain, they totally disagree as to the cases in which they succeed, and for which they are individually applicable. In the treatment of neuralgia, belladonna is employed both internally and externally. I believe that, to be successful, it requires, in many cases, to be persevered in until dryness of the throat, dilatation of pupil, and some disorder of vision, are produced. Just as in many diseases for which mercury has been found a most efficient remedy, it is necessary to continue the use of this mineral until the mouth be affected, and often even to use it for some time afterwards. Of the success of belladonna in the treatment of neuralgia, we have abundant evidence in the published cases of Mr. Bailey,[1] and of several other practitioners.[2] My own experience of the use of this remedy leads me to regard it as very much inferior to aconite as a local remedy for this disease.

Besides neuralgia, there are many other painful affections against which belladonna is used as a local anodyne. Such are, arthritic pains, painful ulcers, and glandular enlargements which are tender to the touch. Dr. Osborne[3] says that, given internally, it causes an immediate cessation of the migratory or flying pains of rheumatism, without producing any effect on the fixed pains.

[M. Grandi has lately published the following summary of his observations on the physiological effects of atropia. He has administered atropia with some success to patients suffering from epilepsy. The dose was gradually increased from 1-16th grain to 1 grain. Then it might be reduced to 1-8th grain. The following are the phenomena which M. Grandi observed, in their order of appearance :—

Dryness of the mouth and fauces.—This phenomenon appears to be at first purely nervous; but subsequently the parts become really dry, and then there is diminution of the salivary secretion.

Dysphagia.—Difficulty of deglutition immediately follows dryness of the mouth. The patient cannot swallow, except after long efforts of the muscles of the neck and the pharynx.

Embarrasssd utterance from quasi-paralysis of the tongue.—After many days' action of the atropia, there manifested itself a slowness and embarrassment of articulation of words, as MM. Bouchardat and Stuart have noted among the principal effects of the solaneæ.

Mydriasis, or dilatation and subsequent immobility of the pupil.—Dilatation of the pupil is one of the most constant and early effects of atropia. It is also the last to disappear, being usually more or less evident for eight days after the suspension of the remedy.

Obscurity of vision.—Objects appear at first enveloped in a white vapour; the contours are no longer distinct. The patient is unable to read, to sew. If the dose is increased, almost complete blindness may ensue.

---

[1] *Observ. relat. to the Use of Belladon. in painful Disord. of the Head and Face*, 1818.
[2] Bayle, *Bibl. Thérap.* t. ii.
[3] *Lond. Med. Gaz.* Feb. 21, 1840.

Torpor and paralytic tremblings.—In proportion as the doses of atropia augment, the limbs, and especially the lower, although still under the control of the will, become heavy and inactive. If the dose be increased, sensation is lost, and the movements of the muscles are automatic and convulsive.

Intellectual confusion.—At first a slowness of intelligence; ideas and replies are imperfect and indifferent. Then comes vertigo and confusion, as of drunkenness.

Hallucination of hearing and sight.—Perceptions of noise, tinkling sounds, as of bells, &c.; distorted countenances of persons standing around; extraordinary and gigantic phantoms; the buzzing of insects of black colour, &c.

Delirium or stupor.—Upon every occasion, when a larger dose than proper of atropia is taken, there ensues delirium, followed by stupor. The delirium may be of a lively or of a loquacious character, with forgetfulness of all surrounding objects, with transport and imagination of distant objects, with incoherent actions, movements, and discourse.[1]—ED.]

2. *As an antispasmodic.*—To relieve rigidity and spasmodic contraction of muscular fibres, belladonna sometimes proves serviceable as a topical remedy. *In rigidity of the os uteri*, during lingering labours or puerperal convulsions, the extract or an ointment of belladonna (see *unguentum belladonnæ*) has been applied to the part by way of friction. Though the practice has been lauded by Chaussier,[2] and adopted by Velpeau,[3] Conquest,[4] and others, yet it has not found much favour with British practitioners. It cannot be regarded as a substitute for, but only an adjuvant to, depletion; and its use is not devoid of danger : for, not to insist on the possibility of absorption, and the consequent injurious effects therefrom, it is obvious that the long-continued friction of the tender womb, and the removal of the lubricating mucus, may dispose to inflammation. *In spasmodic stricture of the urethra, and of the sphincters of the bladder and rectum, as well as in spasmodic contraction of the uterus*, the topical use of the extract (smeared on a bougie, applied to the perineum or other parts, or employed by way of a clyster) has in some cases appeared to give relief.[5] *In strangulated hernia* it has been employed to produce relaxation of the abdominal muscles.[6]

In a case of angina pectoris, unconnected with organic disease, the application of a belladonna plaster to the chest (before the ulcerations caused by tartar emetic ointment had healed) produced alarming signs of poisoning ; but when these had subsided, all symptoms of the angina had totally disappeared.[7]

Considerable relief has been gained in several cases of *hooping-cough* by the use of belladonna.[8] Its occasional efficacy depends in part, probably, on

---

[1] *Bulletino delle Scienze Mediche, di Bologna*, 1854.; also *Med. Times and Gaz.* Jan. 6, 1855.
[2] *Consid. sur. les Convuls. qui attaq. les Femmes enceint.*, 2d ed. 1824.
[3] *Traité compl. des Accouchem.*
[4] *Outlines of Midwifery.*
[5] *Brit. and For. Med. Rev.* vol. ii. p. 261.
[6] Van Looth, Köhler, and Pages, quoted by Bayle, *Bibl. Thérap.* t. ii., and *Brit. and For. Med. Rev.* vol. ii. p. 262-3.
[7] Davies, *Lect. on Diseases of the Lungs and Heart*, p. 496.
[8] See the observations of Schaeffer and Wetzler, of Meglin, and of Raisin, quoted by Bayle, *Bibl. Thér.* t. ii.

its lessening the necessity of respiration,[1] as well also on its power of obviating spasm of the bronchial tubes, and of decreasing the susceptibility of
the bronchial membrane to the influence of the exciting causes of the paroxysms. But, like all other vaunted specifics for this peculiar disease, it
frequently fails to give the least relief.

3. *In maladies of the eyes.*—Belladonna is applied to the eye for two
purposes : the first, and the most common, is to dilate the pupil ; the other
is to diminish the preternatural sensibility of the retina to the impression of
light. *Dilatation of the pupil* is sometimes produced, in certain diseases
of the eye, in order to enable us to examine the condition of the refractive
humours, and thereby to ascertain the nature and extent of the malady ; as
in cases of incipient cataract, which might otherwise be occasionally confounded
with glaucoma or amaurosis. In the operation of cataract by solution or
absorption (*keratonyxis*), the full dilatation of the pupil belladonna is
essential.[2] In *iritis*, dilatation of the pupil is important, in order to prevent,
or in recent cases to rupture, adhesions of the uvea to the capsule of the
crystalline lens. Some surgeons consider it an objectionable remedy during
the early stage of the disease. In *prolapsus iridis*, benefit is, under some
circumstances, gained by the use of belladonna ; as, where there is opacity of
the cornea covering the pupil, the dilatation of the aperture, so as to get its
circumference beyond the opaque spot, is attended with an improvement of
vision. These are some of the cases in which dilatation of the pupil by belladonna is advisable. It is usually effected by applying the extract (see
extractum belladonnæ) to the parts around the eye, or to the conjunctiva.
The dilatation usually takes place within a few minutes, and sometimes
continues for twenty-four hours.

Belladonna is sometimes employed in inflammatory and other affections of
the eye, to diminish the morbid sensibility of this organ to the influence of
light.[3]

4. *As a resolvent or discutient.*—In enlargement and induration of the
lymphatic glands, in scirrhus and cancer (or diseases which have been supposed to be such), belladonna has gained no slight repute from its supposed
resolvent or discutient properties. That it may give relief by its anodyne
powers we can easily understand, but that it has any real resolvent or discutient properties in the diseases just enumerated, may be reasonably doubted,
notwithstanding the favourable reports of Gataker,[4] Cullen,[5] Blackett,[6] and
others.[7] Bromfield[8] and others have reported unfavourably of it, and no one,
I think, now places any reliance on it.

5. *As a prophylactic against scarlatina.*—The introduction of belladonna into practice as a preventive of scarlet fever, is owing to the absurd
homœopathic axiom of "*similia similibus curantur;*" for as this plant
gives rise to an affection of the throat, and sometimes to a scarlet rash on the

---

[1] Laennec, *Treat. on Dis. of the Chest,* by Forbes, pp. 77 and 99.
[2] Lawrence, *Lect.* in *Lancet,* for Sept. 9, 1826.
[3] Lisfranc, *Rev. Med.* t. i. p. 17, 1826; and t. ii. p. 384.
[4] *Observations on the Internal Use of Solanum,* 1757.
[5] *Mat. Med.*
[6] *Essay on the Use of Atropa Belladonna,* 1826.
[7] See Bayle, *Bibl. Thér.* t. ii.
[8] *Account of the English Nightshades,* 1757.

skin, its power of guarding the system against the reception of scarlet fever
has been assumed; and the assumption has been endeavoured to be established
by an appeal to experience. Bayle[1] has collected from various publications
2,027 cases of persons who took this medicine, and were exposed to the
contagion; of these, 1,948 escaped. Oppenheim[2] gave it to 1,200 soldiers,
and only twelve became affected. To the authorities here referred to may be
added Hufeland[3] and Koreff,[4] who admit, from their own personal observations, the efficacy of the remedy, though they have not specified the number
of cases in which they have tried it. But bearing in mind the well-known
capriciousness evinced by scarlet fever (as indeed by other contagious disorders)
in regard to the subjects of its attacks, and the large number of those who,
though exposed to its influence, escape, the best evidence hitherto adduced
in favour of the notion must be admitted to be inconclusive. While,
therefore, the facts brought forward in favour of the existence of this prophylactic power are only negative, those which can be adduced against it are
positive; for I conceive twenty cases of failure are more conclusive against
the opinion here referred to, than one thousand of non-occurrence are in
favour of it. Now Lehman,[5] Barth,[6] Wendt,[7] Muhrbeck,[8] Hoffmann,[9]
Bock,[10] and many others that I could refer to, declare it has failed in their
hands to evince its prophylactic powers. In this country we have no extended
series of observations to quote; but the cases with which I am acquainted
are decidedly against the efficacy of the remedy. A remarkable failure is
mentioned by Dr. Sigmond[11] of a family of eleven persons who took the
supposed specific, yet every individual contracted the disease.

6. *In fever, with contraction of the pupil.*—Dr. Graves[12] has recently
proposed the use of belladonna in those cases of fever with cerebral disease
which are attended with contraction of the pupil. It is not unreasonable,
he observes, "to suppose that the state of the brain which accompanies
dilatation of the pupil is different from that which accompanies contraction;
and if belladonna has an effect in producing that cerebral state which is
attended with dilatation, it is not going too far to infer, that its administration
may do much towards counteracting the opposite condition; neither is it
unphysiological to conclude, that if a remedy be capable of counteracting,
or preventing, one very remarkable effect of a certain morbid state of the
brain, it may also counteract other symptoms connected with the same condition." This line of argument, it must be admitted, is ingenious and
plausible, and is supported by reference to several apparently successful cases
treated on the principles here laid down. But I would observe, if the above
reasoning were valid, opium should be serviceable in cerebral diseases attended

---

[1] *Bibl. Thérap.* t. ii. p. 504.
[2] *Lond. Med. Gaz.* vol. xiii. p. 814.
[3] *Lancet*, May 2, 1829.
[4] *Lond. Med. Gaz.* vol. iv. p. 297.
[5] Bayle, *Bibl. Thérap.* t. ii. p. 417.
[6] *Ibid.*
[7] Rust and Casper's *Krit. Repert.* Bd. xxii. S. 27.
[8] Rust's *Magaz.* Bd. xxiv. S. 495.
[9] *Ibid.* Bd. xxv. S. 115.
[10] *Ibid.* S. 80.
[11] *Lancet*, vol ii. p 78, 1836-7.
[12] *Dubl. Journ. of Med. Science*, July 1, 1838.

with dilatation of pupil, since it causes contraction of this aperture. Now this is in direct opposition to our every-day experience of the uses of this important narcotic.

7. *In other diseases.*—Cruveilhier[1] found that belladonna-smoking relieved some cases of *phthisis.* The fresh leaves were infused in a strong solution of opium, and then dried like tobacco : the patients began by smoking two pipes a day, and the quantity was gradually increased to six pipes. Perhaps this practice would be beneficial in spasmodic asthma and old catarrhs.—In *hydrophobia,* notwithstanding the asserted prophylactic powers of this medicine,[2] there is no valid ground for believing in its efficacy. I tried it in one case without success. In *epilepsy, mania, hysteria, chorea,* and some other maladies of the cerebro-spinal system, occasional benefit has resulted by the use of belladonna. In *ileus*[3] it has been most successfully used in the form of clyster, as a substitute for tobacco, which is objectionable on account of the horrible sickness and great depression which it causes. [In *profuse saliva-tion* it is stated to have been found highly beneficial. A woman who had been treated profusely with mercury for the cure of enteritis, had violent salivation from the use of the drug. Extract of belladonna was ordered by Espenbeck, in doses of $2\frac{1}{2}$ grains in an emulsion ; and the following day the salivation was found to be completely arrested, and the mouth dry. When the administration of the belladonna was suspended, the ptyalism returned, and again it disappeared when the use of the drug was resumed. Espenbeck has also employed it successfully as a prophylactic against salivation.[4]—ED.]

ADMINISTRATION.—The dose of the *powder* for an adult is one grain, which should be gradually increased until dryness of the throat, dilatation of pupil, or some head symptoms, are produced. For children, the dose at the commencement should be one-eighth of a grain. For internal as well as external use the *extract* or *tincture* is, however, commonly employed. For external use an *infusion* of the leaves is sometimes used as a fomentation, or is made into a poultice with bread or linseed meal.

ANTIDOTES.—Similar to those for opium. After the use of evacuants the vegetable acids have appeared to give great relief. Decoction of nutgalls or green tea might probably prove serviceable.

1. EXTRACTUM BELLADONNÆ, L. E. D. ; *Extract of Belladonna.* (Prepare this in the same manner as directed for Extract of Aconite, *L.*—The *Edinburgh College* directs the expressed juice to be filtered, and then to be evaporated, in the vapour-bath, to the consistence of firm extract, stirring constantly towards the close.—The *Dublin College* gives the following process :—Fresh Belladonna Leaves, collected when the plant begins to flower, any convenient quantity. Crush them in a mortar, express the juice, and allow it to stand for twenty-four hours. Pour off the clear liquor, and set it aside for subsequent use ; and having placed the sediment on a calico filter, wash it with an equal bulk of distilled water, and mix the washings with the decanted liquor. When, by the application of a water-heat, coagulation has occurred, skim off the coagulated matter, filter the hot liquid through flannel,

---

[1] *Lancet,* vol. i. p. 520, 1828–.9
[2] See the authorities quoted by Bayle, *Bibl. Thér.* t. ii., and Richter, *Ausf. Arzneim.* Bd. ii.
[3] *Brit. and For. Med. Rev.* vol. iv. p. 223.
[4] [Hannover, *Corresp. Blatt,* June 1853 ; also *Edinb. Monthly Journal,* Oct. 1854.]

mix in now the washed sediment, and evaporate to the consistence of a firm extract by a steam or water bath, constantly stirring, particularly towards the close of the evaporation. *D.*)—[Mr. Squire, in commenting on the lengthened directions of the Dublin College, observes that they ought to have some advantages over the processes of the other Colleges. The first step, however, in the process, during hot weather, would allow of incipient fermentation, and perhaps ruin the product. The washing of the fecula is another great objection, and tends to no purpose, since it is afterwards added to the extract. It may be said that this is to remove entirely the albumen; but, according to this gentleman, except in very wet seasons this principle need never be removed at all.[1]—Ed.] 1 cwt. of fresh belladonna yields from 4 to 6 lbs. of extract.[2] Dose, gr. j. to gr. v. cautiously increased. As the strength of the extract is extremely variable, some writers recommend only one-quarter or one-half of a grain to be given at the commencement of its use, to be repeated three times a day; and the dose to be increased until the well-known effects of the remedy are produced.[3] Mr. Bailey observes that he at first began with one grain, and repeated it every four hours until relief followed; but further experience induced him to commence with three times that quantity, and, if a repetition were necessary, to give it in diminished doses afterwards. Spread upon leather, the extract is frequently used as a plaster to relieve neuralgic and other pains (see *Emplastrum Belladonnæ*). Diluted with water to the consistence of cream, it is applied to the eyebrow to produce dilatation of the pupil; or an aqueous solution of the extract is dropped between the lids. Mixed with lard or spermaceti ointment, it is used as a topical anodyne and antispasmodic in various diseases (see *Unguentum Belladonnæ*). A bougie smeared over with the extract and oil is sometimes used with benefit in stricture.[4] A drachm or two of the extract, either alone or in the form of ointment, may be applied to the os uteri to diminish rigidity. In irritation of the bladder, urinary organs, or rectum, clysters holding in solution the extract are sometimes used. Rubbed into the perineum or over the track of the urethra, the extract or ointment is useful in preventing chordee, and alleviating spasm of the neck of the bladder.

2. [**EXTRACTUM BELLADONNÆ ALCOHOLICUM**, U.S.—As the fresh leaves of belladonna are with difficulty procured in the United States, the States' Pharmacopœia directs an extract to be made from the dried leaves by means of diluted alcohol. The formula is, Belladonna in coarse powder, lb. j.; Diluted Alcohol, Oiv. Moisten first with half a pint of the alcohol, and allow the liquid to stand twenty-four hours; then transfer to a percolator and displace, driving over the last quantity of fluid with water. Evaporate the solution to a proper consistence.—Ed.]

3. **EMPLASTRUM BELLADONNÆ**, L. E. D.; *Plaster of Belladonna.* (Extract of Belladonna, ʒiij. [ʒiss. *E.*] [ʒj. *D.*]; Plaster of Soap, ʒiij. [Plaster of Resin, ʒiij. *E.*] [ʒij. *D.*] Add the extract to the plaster, melted

---

[1] [*New London Pharmacopœia*, 1851.]
[2] Brande, *Man. of Pharm.* 3d edit. p. 401.
[3] [For warding off scarlatina, according to Dr. Christison, a solution of five grains in an ounce of cinnamon water is given in the dose of fifteen drops twice or thrice a-day to children about ten years old.—Ed.]
[4] *Lond. Med. Gaz.* vol. v. p. 735.

by the heat of a water-bath, and mix.)—Anodyne and antispasmodic. Applied for the relief of neuralgic, rheumatic, and other pains. It is said to relieve the pain of dysmenorrhœa when applied to the sacrum. In spreading it, care must be taken not to employ a very hot spatula, or the properties of the extract will be injured.

4. UNGUENTUM BELLADONNÆ, L.; *Ointment of Belladonna*. (Lard, ʒj.; Extract of Belladonna, ʒj. Rub together.)—Though not contained in two of the British pharmacopœias, it is a very useful preparation; and may be used as an anodyne and antispasmodic in some of the before-mentioned cases.

5. TINCTURA BELLADONNÆ, L.; *Tinctura foliorum Belladonnæ*, D.; *Tincture of Belladonna*. (Belladonna leaves, dried, ʒiv.; Proof Spirit, Oij. Macerate for seven days, express, and strain.)—Is contained in two of the British pharmacopœias.—Dose ♏iij. to ♏xx. The *Dublin College* employs ʒv. of the leaves to Oij. of the proof spirit, and directs that the maceration continue for fourteen days, *D*. Mr. Blacket[1] prepared a *saturated tincture of belladonna* by macerating, for fourteen days, ʒx. of extract of belladonna in lb. j. of proof spirit; then straining. The dose of this is ♏ij. or ♏iij. gradually increased: in the form of lotion, a drachm of it was added to eight ounces of liquid.

Succus Belladonnæ.—*The Preserved Juice of Belladonna* may be substituted for the tincture. From 2 cwt. of belladonna leaves gathered towards the end of June, 36 imperial quarts of juice have been procured.

6. ATROPIA, L.;+*Alkali e radice comparatum; Atropina; Atropine*. Symbol At. Formula $C^{34}H^{23}NO^6$. Eq. Wt. 289. — Found in all parts of the plant. Discovered in 1819 by M. Brandes. The most improved processes for the preparation of this alkaloid are those of Mein[2] and Richter.[3] The following is a sketch of Mein's process as modified by Liebig :—

Fresh dried and powdered belladonna root is to be exhausted by alcohol, sp. gr. 0·822. To the tincture add slacked lime (in the proportion of one part of lime to 24 parts of dried root). Digest for 24 hours, frequently shaking. Add, drop by drop, sulphuric acid to the filtered liquor till there is a slight excess; then filter again, and distil off rather more than half of the spirit. To the residue add some water, and evaporate the remainder of the alcohol as rapidly as possible, but *by a very gentle heat;* filter again, and continue the evaporation until the liquid is reduced to the 1-12th part of the weight of the root employed. To the cold liquid, add, drop by drop, a concentrated solution of carbonate of potash, to throw down a dark greyish-brown precipitate, taking care not to render the liquid alkaline. In a few hours filter again; add carbonate of potash as long as a precipitate (atropia) is produced; and in from 12 to 24 hours collect the crystallised atropia on a filter, press it between folds of blotting-paper, and dry it. To purify the dry but impure atropia, make it into a paste with water, and again squeeze between folds of blotting-paper : dry it, and dissolve in five times its weight of alcohol. The filtered liquor is to be decolourised by shaking it with purified animal

---

[1] *Lond. Med. Rep.* vol. xix. p. 458.
[2] *Journ. de Pharm.* t. xx. p 87, 1834; also *Thomson's Chemistry of Organic Bodies*, p. 273, 1838.
[3] *Pharm. Central-Blatt für* 1837, p. 613.

charcoal, then deprived of the greater part of its alcohol by distillation, and afterwards evaporated by a gentle heat, so as to allow the atropia to crystallise : or draw off half of the spirit, add, gradually, water (3 or 4 parts), which renders the liquid milky, heat to boiling, and allow it to cool slowly ; or add to the spirituous solution 6 or 8 times its volume of cold water, which renders the liquid milky, and, in from 12 to 24 hours, the atropia crystallises and is to be dried on blotting-paper.

In this process the alcohol extracts from the belladonna root a salt of atropia : this is decomposed by the lime, which removes the organic acid and colouring extractive matter. Sulphuric acid is then added, to unite with the disengaged atropia ; for this alkaloid, when free, and especially when in contact with alkalies, readily undergoes decomposition by heat. The solution of sulphate of atropia must be evaporated by a very gentle heat, because the atropia salts, especially in the impure state, easily undergo decomposition. A small quantity of carbonate of potash is necessary, to separate a resinous substance which impedes the crystallisation of the atropia. An excess of a concentrated solution of carbonate of potash is required to precipitate, as speedily as possible, the atropia, as by long contact with watery fluids this alkaloid disappears.

Messrs. Bourchardat and Cooper[1] recommend the following mode of preparing atropia :—The atropia is to be precipitated by a watery solution of iodine in iodide of potassium, and the ioduretted hydriodate of atropia decomposed by zinc and water. The metallic oxide is separated by means of carbonate of potash, and the alkaloid dissolved in alcohol.

[Mr. Luxton has recently suggested the following process for the preparation of atropia. A pound of the dry leaves of the belladonna are to be boiled in distilled water sufficient to cover them, for two hours, and the decoction strained off through a coarse cloth into a large precipitating jar. The leaves are again boiled in a second water and the decoctions mixed, to which two drachms of strong sulphuric acid are now added : the vegetable albumen is precipitated, and the clear liquor is now drawn off with a syphon to a filter. A clear, sherry-coloured solution comes through, which is to be decomposed either by passing gaseous ammonia through it, or by suspending in it a lump of sesquicarbonate of ammonia. In either case, the colour becomes changed to black ; and crystals of atropia are slowly formed and deposited. At the expiration of a day or two, the supernatant liquor may be drawn off with a syphon, and the crystals thrown on a filter to dry. By this process, Mr. Luxton has obtained forty grains of atropia from a pound (avoirdupois) of leaves, which gives 5⅘ grs. to 1000 of plant, instead of 3 to 1000.[2] The fixed alkalies, potash and soda, convert atropia to ammonia : hence ammonia is preferable as the precipitating agent.—Ed.]

Atropia crystallises from its concentrated hot, watery, or spirituous solution in white, transparent, silky prisms : from its solution in dilute spirit, in needles like those of sulphate of quinia. It is odourless, and has a very bitter, acrid, somewhat metallic taste. Impure atropia is not crystalline, is more or less coloured, and has an unpleasant odour. One part of atropia requires 200 parts of cold water, or 54 parts of hot water, to dissolve it. It is soluble in

---

[1] *Annuaire de Thérapeutique pour* 1849.
[2] [*Pharmaceutical Journal,* January 1855, p. 299.]

1½ times its weight of cold alcohol, but requires, at ordinary temperatures, 25 parts of ether to dissolve it, or 6 parts of boiling ether.

It reacts on vegetable colours as an alkali, fuses by heat, and at a higher temperature is partly volatilised and partly decomposed. Nitric acid dissolves it, forming a yellow solution. Cold oil of vitriol dissolves it without colour; but if heat be applied, the mixture acquires a red colour. When heated with a solution of potash or soda, atropia undergoes decomposition, and gives out ammonia.

"White in the form of prisms, soluble in water and rectified spirit. There are no certain tests for the purity of this substance."—*Ph. Lond.*

Atropia possesses the property of left-handed circular polarisation; but its rotating power is feeble, though it is unaffected by the presence of acids.

A watery solution of a salt of atropia is reddened by tincture of iodine; yields a citron-yellow precipitate with a chloride of gold; a whitish, flocculent precipitate with tincture of nutgalls; and a yellowish-white with chloride of platinum. The *sulphate, hydrochlorate,* and *acetate of atropia,* are crystalline salts.

Atropia is a most energetic poison. Its effects are similar to, but more powerful than, those of belladonna. Dogs are readily poisoned by it; but rabbits are less under its influence. A very minute (imponderable) quantity applied to the eye is sufficient to dilate the pupil. Given to dogs it excites vomiting, dilatation of the pupil, and stupor. On man the effect is much stronger. One centigramme (about 1-6th of a grain) produces the following symptoms :—At first, acceleration of the pulse by eight to twenty strokes; after from fifteen to thirty minutes, an affection of the brain is produced. The first and most constant symptom is dry throat, with difficulty of swallowing. The second is dilatation of pupils, with dimness of sight, also giddiness, noise in the ears, hallucination, delirium, and occasionally strangury : numbness of the limbs, a sensation of formication in the arms, rigidity of the thighs, depression of the pulse. The voice is sometimes weakened; or there may be complete aphonia. The unfavourable symptoms disappear after from twelve to twenty hours.

Atropia has recently been employed medicinally (chiefly as an external agent) as a substitute for belladonna; to which it is considered superior, on account chiefly of the uncertainty of the latter. It is of course much more energetic, and, for external use especially, is much cleaner than the extract. As a topical agent it has been employed as a mydriatic or dilator of the pupil, by Reisinger, Mr. W. W. Cooper,[1] and Dr. Brookes,[2] in cataract, &c. The last-mentioned writer states, that in a case of glaucoma he succeeded in causing dilatation of the pupil with an ointment of atropia when belladonna had failed. As an anæsthetic or anodyne he used the same preparation with success in a painful affection of the face (neuralgia ?).—The local pain which atropia produces when used endermically is of very short duration, and is unattended with any ill consequences. Internally atropia has been employed in hooping-cough, chorea, and some other nervous diseases.

The dose of atropia for internal use is from about 1-30th to 1-6th of a grain.

---

[1] *Lancet,* June 8th, 1844.
[2] *Ibid.* January, 30th 1847.

Its employment requires great caution. The safest mode of administration is in solution, on account of the facility with which the dose may be adjusted : but it has also been given, mixed with sugar, in the form of powder ; and, mixed with the powder of marshmallow root and honey, in the form of pills. It may be employed endermically in doses of about the $\frac{1}{30}$th of a grain gradually increased to $\frac{1}{10}$th of a grain. For a collyrium, to dilate the pupil, one grain may be dissolved in 400 grs. of water ; and a few drops of the solution applied to the eye.

1. *Tinctura Atropiæ ;* Tincture of Atropine.—Dissolve one grain of atropia in one fluidrachm of rectified spirit, and then add seven fluidrachms of distilled water. Dose, from fifteen minims gradually and cautiously increased to eighty minims. One drop of this solution applied to the eye, night and morning, was used by Mr. W. W. Cooper to keep up dilatation of the pupil.

2. *Solutio Atropiæ Hydrochloratis ;* Solution of Muriate of Atropine. —Dissolve one grain of atropia in a fluidrachm of water acidulated with one minim of hydrochloric acid ; then add seven fluidrachms of water. Dose from fifteen to eighty minims.

[3. *Solutio Atropiæ Nitratis.*—This may be prepared by adding two grains of atropia to one minim of strong nitric acid (sp. gr. 1·5), and to this add one drachm of water. It is an uncrystallisable compound. This has been found by Mr. Luxton to be a most useful preparation for the relief of the severe paroxysms of facial neuralgia. The affected portion of the face is to be painted with the above solution, and the pain is frequently subdued in from three to five minutes. Sometimes a second, third, or fourth application may be required. Its chief efficacy is witnessed in those cases in which the neuralgia has arisen from exposure to vicissitudes of temperature or other external causes.[1]—Ed.]

4. *Unguentum Atropiæ ;* Ointment of Atropine.—Atropia, five grains ; lard, three drachms ; attar of roses, one drop : mix.—The size of a pea to be applied three times a day. Used by Dr. Brookes, with great success, in a painful affection of the face, and to dilate the pupil.

[7. ATROPIÆ SULPHAS, L. ; *Sulphate of Atropia.* This salt is introduced into the last edition of the London Pharmacopœia, and the following formula is given for its preparation :—Dilute Sulphuric Acid, fℨij. ; Atropia, ℈viiss. or q. s. ; Distilled Water, ℥ss. To the acid and water mixed, add by degrees the Atropia until the acid is saturated. Let the solution be strained and evaporated at a gentle heat in order that crystals may be formed.

This salt is intended for external use only. It is employed in the form of solution, by dissolving one or two grains in a fluid ounce of distilled water, and dropping it into the eye to produce dilatation of the pupil. For an ointment five grains or more may be rubbed up with half an ounce of lard.

The sulphate of atropia may be regarded as one of the best preparations of belladonna. In a weak solution it has no irritant effect, and is free from that mechanical action which may be objected to in the extract of belladonna, while, owing to its uniform composition, it can be applied in a precisely regulated strength. We find the following practical remarks by Dr. Donders, on its local action in dilating the pupil, in the Edinburgh Monthly Journal for December, 1854.

---

[1] [*Pharmaceutical Journal,* January 1855, p. 300.]

The English were the first to introduce this preparation into practice. In London it is generally used in the proportion of 4 grs. of sulphas atropiæ to an ounce of distilled water. A single drop of this, retained in contact with the cornea and conjunctiva for only a few instants, produces, in twenty to twenty-five minutes, a *complete dilatation, with immoveabilitg of the pupil.*

Such a dilatation is desirable and even necessary to obviate synechia, synizesis, prolapsus iridis, &c., and as preparatory to the operation for cataract, in which the pupil has so great a tendency to contract. It would also be highly advantageous, when it is wished to dilate the pupil, in order to examine the deeper seated parts, the lens, the vitreous humour, the retina, and the choroide, with the aid of the ophthalmoscope; but there is here an important counter-indication, in the marked disturbance of vision which is temporarily induced by it. Besides the intolerance of light, which annoys some, the seeing of small objects, as in reading, is rendered almost impossible for from four to eight days, in cases where this could be accomplished readily in ordinary states of the pupil; so that most persons complain of it bitterly. In cases of amplyopia also the patient becomes usually less able to distinguish objects during several days; and shows unnecessary alarm lest the instillation should have injured the sight permanently, notwithstanding the forewarning, which I have never neglected, that the effect was merely of a temporary nature.

The objection, thus occasioned, led me to the inquiry, whether it was not possible to fulfil our purpose without exposing the patient to the inconvenience of which he thus justly complains. One obvious course was, to employ weaker solutions; and yet I continued for a long time, like others, to pursue the old routine, and to use in all cases the solution of gr. iv. to the ounce of water. Dr. De Ruiter[1] had already stated, that a drop of a solution, in which was contained not more than $\frac{1}{129600}$ of sulphate of atropia, when kept some time in contact with the eye of a dog, sufficed to produce a dilatation lasting for twenty hours. Farther experiments on dogs have shown him, that a solution with a proportion of $\frac{1}{3600}$ of sulphate of atropia, induces powerful dilatation in from ten to fifteen minutes, which disappears only at the end of four days; that a solution with $\frac{1}{21600}$, five to ten minutes in contact with the eye, causes also strong dilatation and even sometimes immoveability; that a solution with $\frac{1}{129600}$, kept five minutes in contact, gave a good dilatation at the end of an hour, which lasted eighteen hours; that with a threefold dilution, and the same time of application, a perceptible dilatation still followed, and that it was only upon a sixfold dilution, and therefore with $\frac{1}{772800}$, that the effect became doubtful. The sensitiveness of the eye to atropia, indeed, excites astonishment, when we consider that of the single drop of the attenuated solution, which suffices to produce dilatation, probably not a fiftieth part is absorbed.

At my request, Dr. De Ruiter has also investigated the sensibility of the human eye to atropia. It seems to be somewhat smaller than in the dog; yet is so strong that, where it is desired to examine the internal parts of the eye, a much weaker solution than that ordinarily employed is sufficient to produce a good result. I consider it superfluous to communicate the various trials made upon man. It is enough that they have led me to adopt the following solutions.

---

[1] *Nederlandsch Lancet*, 1854, p. 464.

1st. Of gr. iv. of sulph. atropia to an ounce of distilled water, as preparatory to operations, to prevent threatening synechia, synizesis, or prolapsus iridis, and to increase the capacity of sight in central cataract, or in central opacity of the cornea, &c.

2d. One part of this solution, diluted with fifteen parts of water, in order to induce full dilatation, with transient immoveability of the pupil, with a view to a full examination of the internal parts, in all directions. The dilatation ensues after thirty to forty-five minutes ; and ordinarily, in twenty-four hours, it ceases to disturb the vision.

3d. The same solution, diluted with eighty parts of water,—that is, one part of sulph. atropia with 9600 parts of water ; of this I make use in the largest proportion of cases. One or two drops of this solution, held for a few seconds between the eyelids, causes in thirty to sixty minutes a dilatation sufficient for the examination of the greater number of eyes. The dilatation, however, is not so strong as perceptibly to injure vision, and in eight to thirty-six hours it has wholly passed away. I esteem it a great advantage, in common cases, to make use of this dilute solution.[1]—ED.]

179. DATURA STRAMONIUM.—COMMON THORN-APPLE.

Sex. Syst. Pentandria, Monogynia.

(Folium et semen, *L.*—Herb, *E.*—The seeds, *D.*)

HISTORY.—This plant, being a native of Greece, must have been known to the ancient Greek botanists ; though it is impossible now to identify it, with certainty, with any of the plants described by them. It appears, however, to agree tolerably well with the στρύχνος μανίκός of Theophrastus.[2] Datura Stramonium is mentioned by Fuchsius in 1542.

BOTANY. **Gen. Char.**—*Calyx* tubular, frequently angular, 5-cleft at the apex, or longitudinally slit, falling off by a circular horizontal incision above the peltate base. *Corolla* hypogynous, funnel-shaped, with a large, spreading, plaited 5—10-toothed limb. *Stamens* 5, inserted into the tube of the corolla, inclosed or somewhat exserted ; anthers dehiscing longitudinally. *Ovary* incompletely 4-celled, the alternate dissepiment being lost above the middle, the other one complete ; the middle on both sides placentiferous. *Style* simple ; *stigma* bilamellate. *Capsule* ovate or sub-globose, muricate or aculeate, rarely smooth, half 4-celled, incompletely 4-valved at the septa. *Seeds* numerous, reniform. *Embryo* within fleshy albumen, subperipherical, arched (*Endlicher*).

Sp. Char.—Annual. Leaves ovate, angulate-dentate, wedge-shaped at the base, rather smooth. Fruit ovate, erect, densely spinous. Calyx equal to the diameter of the limb of the corolla (*Nees*).

A bushy, smooth, fetid *herb*. *Stem* much branched, forked, spreading,

---

[1] [From Dr. F. C. Donders, in *Nederlandsch Lancet*, Maart, 1854, p. 533 ; quoted from the *Edin. Monthly Journal*, December 1854.]

[2] *Hist. Plant.* lib. ix. cap. 12.

leafy. *Leaves* from the forks of the stem, large, unequal at the base, variously and acutely sinuated and smooth, simple-ribbed, veiny, of a dull green. *Flowers* axillary, erect, white, sweet-scented, especially at night, about 3 inches long. *Fruit* as big as a walnut, in its outer coat very prickly. *Seeds* black (*Smith*).

Hab.—Indigenous: in waste ground and on dunghills. Annual. Flowers in July.

Several other species of Datura are used in the East.

DATURA FEROX, Linn.—Annual. Leaves ovate, angulate-dentate, cuneiform at the base, glaucous. Fruit ovate, erect, pyramidate-spinous. Calyx longer than the diameter of the limb of the corolla (*Nees*).—Nepal. In 1802 General Gent introduced this species into this country as a remedy for asthma. It was employed by smoking it.[1] Waitz[2] says that half an upright capsule acted violently on a girl.

DATURA FASTUOSA, Mill.—Annual. Leaves ovate, acuminate, repandly-toothed, unequal at the base, and are, as well as the stem, somewhat downy. Fruit nodding, tuberculated (*Nees*).—East Indies. In 1811 Dr. Christie[3] directed attention to this species. Mr. Skipton[4] administered the decoction of the root of this plant; and Dr. Adams[5] used a tincture (prepared as tincture of digitalis, *Ph. L.*)

DATURA TATULA, Linn.—Annual. Leaves cordate-ovate, angulate-dentate, unequal at the base, smooth. Fruit ovate, erect, spinous (*Nees*).—Schubarth[6] gave half a pound of the bruised leaves of this species to a horse without effect; twenty-one ounces of the half-ripe fruit caused dejection, increased secretion, and loss of appetite. Cigars for the use of asthmatics are made of this species.

DATURA ALBA, Rumph.; *D. Metel*, Roxb. — Annual. Leaves ovate, acuminate, repandly-dentate, unequal at the base, rather smooth. Fruit nodding, spinous.—East Indies. Both this and the preceding species have been employed, especially in the East, to cause intoxication for criminal and licentious purposes.[7]

[DATURA SANGUINEA, Ruiz et Pav.—The Indians of Darien, as well as those of Chocò in Central America, prepare from the seeds of this plant a decoction which is given to their children to produce a state of excitement in which they are supposed to possess the power of discovering gold. According to Hooker, in any place where the unhappy patients happen to fall down, digging is commenced; and as the soil nearly every where contains gold-dust, an amount of more or less value is obtained. In order to counteract the effects of the poison a beer of made Indian corn is administered.[8]—Ed.]

DESCRIPTION.—The herb (*herba stramonii*) should be collected when the plant is in flower. The leaves (*folia stramonii*) are then to be carefully dried. In the fresh state, their odour, when bruised, is unpleasant and narcotic; their taste nauseous and bitter. By drying, the odour is lost, but the bitter taste remains. The seeds (*semina stramonii*) are small, compressed, kidney-shaped, roughish, dark-brown or blackish, dull, and odourless: they have a bitter, nauseous, somewhat acrid taste.

COMPOSITION.—The herb was analysed in 1815, by Promnitz;[9] the seeds in 1820, by Brandes.[10]

---

[1] *Ed. Med. and Surg. Journ.* vol. viii. p. 365.
[2] Wibmer, *Wirk. d. Arzn. u. Gifte*, Bd. ii. S. 286.
[3] *Ed. Med. and Surg. Journ.*, vol. vii. p. 158.
[4] *Trans. Med. and Phys. Soc. Calcutta*, vol. i. p. 121.
[5] *Ibid.* p. 370.
[6] Wibmer, *op. cit.* p. 300.
[7] *Lond. Med. and Phys. Journ.* vol. xxv. p. 383–4; and vol. xxvi. p. 22.
[8] [*Pharmaceutical Journal*, October 1851, p. 170.]
[9] Gmelin's *Handb. d. Chem.* Bd. ii. S. 1305.
[10] *Ibid.*

Promnitz's Analysis.	
Resin	0·12
Extractive [containing the daturia]	0·60
Gummy extractive	0·58
Green fecula	0·64
Albumen	0·15
Phosphatic and vegetable salts of lime and magnesia	0·23
Water	91·25
Woody fibre	5·15
Loss	1·28
Fresh herb of stramonium	100·00

Brandes's Analysis.	
Malate of daturia with some uncrystallisable sugar	1·80
Fixed oil with some chlorophylle	16·05
Wax	1·40
Resin insoluble in ether	9·90
Extractive	0·60
Gummy extractive	6·00
Gum and bassorin with some salts	11·30
Albumen and phytocolla	6·45
Glutenoin	5·50
Malates of daturia, potash, and lime, and acetate of potash	0·60
Woody fibre	23·35
Water	15·10
Loss	1·95
Seeds of stramonium	100·00

1. DATURIA (*Datura* or *Daturine*).—A vegetable alkali found in stramonium. The properties assigned to it by Geiger and Hesse[1] are the following : It crystallises in colourless, odourless, brilliant prisms, which have at first a bitterish, then a tobacco-like flavour. It requires 288 parts of cold, or 72 parts of boiling, water to dissolve it : it is very soluble in alcohol, less so in ether. In most of its properties it agrees with hyosciamia (atropia ?). It strongly dilates the pupil, and has a poisonous action on animals.

[It appears that, like the active principles of other poisonous plants, daturine is absorbed and carried into the blood. It is eliminated in the urine. In 1847, Mr. Allan detected daturia in the urine taken from the bladder of a man who had been poisoned by stramonium. He has subsequently detected it in two other cases of poisoning ; that of a man aged forty years, and that of his son aged twelve years. In both cases the daturin was detected by Henry's method.[2] Daturia has been minutely examined by Dr. Planta, and he finds that it not only possesses the properties of atropia, but that it is isomeric with that alkaloid, its formula, according to him, being $C^{34}H^{23}NO^6$, which precisely corresponds to the formula for atropia, based on Liebig's analysis (see *ante*, p. 556). Dr. Planta finds that atropia and daturia both crystallise in colourless needles, are permanent in the air, inodorous, heavier than water, and not very soluble in that liquid. They are very soluble in alcohol, but less soluble in ether. Both alkaloids melt at about 190°, without losing in weight or undergoing decomposition. At a higher temperature they are decomposed. The aqueous solution of each has a strong alkaline reaction. Both alkaloids form neutral uncrystalline salts with sulphuric and hydrochloric acids, very soluble in water and alcohol, but not easily dissolved by ether. Chemical reagents produce similar results with the solutions. The two alkaloids resemble each other physiologically in their power of causing dilatation of the pupil.[3]—ED.]

2. EMPYREUMATIC OIL OF STRAMONIUM (*Pyrodaturia ?*).—Resembles tar and the aqueous fluid which distils along with its acid. This arises from the woody part of the plant having been employed. The oil itself does not differ, in its physical and chemical properties, from the empyreumatic oil of foxglove already described.[4]

PHYSIOLOGICAL EFFECTS. *α. On Vegetables.*—A branch of stramonium was killed by immersing it in a watery solution of the extract of its own species.[5] *β. On Animals generally.*—Its influence on herbivorous animals is much less than that on man. Five ounces of the expressed juice given to a horse cause merely slight drowsiness and gaping.[6] Two pounds and a half

---

[1] *Pharm. Central-Blatt für* 1835, p. 85.
[2] [See *Pharmaceutical Journal*, Feb. 1, 1851, p. 516 ; also Taylor *On Poisons*, p. 786.]
[3] [*Ibid.* May 1851, p. 561.]
[4] Morries, *Ed. Med. and Surg. Journ.* vol. xxxix. p. 379.
[5] Macaire, quoted by De Candolle, *Phys. Vég.* p. 1354.
[6] Moiroud, *Pharm. Vét.* p. 350.

of the seeds killed a horse in fifty-two hours.[1] From Orfila's experiments on dogs,[2] it does not appear to act powerfully as a local irritant. Its effects were very similar to those caused by belladonna.

γ. On Man.—The symptoms produced on man closely resemble those caused by belladonna. *In small but gradually increased doses* it diminishes sensibility, and thereby frequently alleviates pain. It does not usually affect the pulse; it slightly and temporarily affects the pupil, and has no tendency to cause constipation, but rather relaxation. Though it allays pain it does not usually produce sleep. *In larger doses* it causes thirst, dryness of the throat, nausea, giddiness, nervous agitation, dilatation of the pupil, obscurity of vision, headache, disturbance of the cerebral functions, perspiration, occasionally relaxation of bowels, and in some cases diuresis. It has no direct tendency to induce sleep, and hence it cannot be called *soporific.* But indirectly, by alleviating pain, and thereby producing serenity and ease, it often disposes to sleep. *In fatal doses* the leading symptoms are flushed countenance, delirium (usually maniacal), dilatation of the pupil, dryness of the throat, loss of voice, difficulty of deglutition, convulsions, and, in some cases, palsy. A very interesting fatal case of poisoning by 100 seeds is related by Mr. Duffin.[3] The patient (his own child) was two years and a quarter old. In addition to the preceding symptoms, there were a hot, perspiring skin, flushed, slightly swollen face, pulse almost imperceptible, but, as far as could be felt, it was natural in regard to frequency; and coldness of the inferior extremities. The anterior fontanelle was neither tense, hot, nor in the slightest degree raised by the cerebral pulsations; so that there did not seem to be any active determination of blood to the brain. During the continuance of the coma the pulse became extremely rapid. Death occurred twenty-four hours after swallowing the seeds.

Vogt[4] says stramonium is probably distinguished from belladonna by the following peculiarities :—

1. Its effects are more similar to those of acid vegetables, especially of *Helleborus.*
2. It operates more strongly, but more in the manner of the acrid substances, on the nervous system, especially on the central organs, viz. the ganglia, spinal cord, and brain.
3. Its secondary effects on the irritable system are not so marked; for most observers have failed to detect any alteration of pulse, and a slow pulse is more frequently mentioned than a quick one.
4. It operates on the organic life more strongly. It more strongly and directly promotes all the secretions, especially the secretion of the skin.
5. Marcet[5] and Begbie[6] have inferred, from numerous observations, that it possesses an anodyne property, which it frequently evinces where opium and belladonna fail.

Uses.—A more extended experience of this plant is requisite to enable us to speak with much confidence of its employment. The similarity of its effects with those of belladonna would lead us to expect a similarity of uses. Like the last-mentioned plant, it has been successfully employed to diminish sensibility, and thereby to relieve external pain. Some of the other uses

---

[1] Viborg, in Wibmer's *Wirk. d. Arzneim. u. Gifte*, Bd. ii. S. 292.
[2] *Toxicol. Gén.*
[3] *Lond. Med. Gaz.* vol. xv. p. 194.
[4] *Pharmakodyn.* Bd. i. S. 164.
[5] *Med.-Chir. Trans.* vols. vii. and viii.
[6] *Trans. of the Med. Soc. Edinb.* vol. i.

made of it require a more impartial examination ere we can form any just estimate of their value. The indications and contra-indications for its employment are probably similar to those of belladonna. In persons disposed to apoplexy it is a very dangerous remedy.

In *neuralgia* (*tic douloureux, sciatica,* &c.) it has been employed with considerable success by Lentin,[1] Marcet,[2] and Begbie.[3] It was given internally in the form of extract. Its external application has scarcely been tried. In *rheumatism* it has frequently proved serviceable from its anodyne qualities.[4] In *enterodynia* (that is, spasmodic pain of the bowels unconnected with inflammatory action or the presence of irritating substances), Dr. Elliotson[5] found it most successful. In some cases of *spasmodic asthma,* smoking the herb has given at least temporary relief :[6] but the practice requires very great caution, as it has proved highly injurious, and in some instances fatal. Dr. Bree[7] tried it in 82 asthmatic cases ; in 58 of these it had no permanent effect, and in the remaining 24 it acted injuriously. General Gent, who was instrumental in introducing the practice, fell a victim to it.[8] Aggravation of the dyspnœa, paralytic tremblings, epilepsy, headache, and apoplexy, are some of the evils said to have been induced in the cases above referred to. In persons disposed to head affections, and in aged persons, it is, therefore, a highly dangerous practice.

The diseases in which stramonium has been principally used are *mania* and *epilepsy.* Bayle[9] has collected from the works of Storck, Schemalz, Razoux, Reef, Meyer, Odhelius, Durande, Maret, Bergius, Greding, Schneider, Bernard, and Amelung, fifty-five cases of the first, and forty-five of the latter malady, treated by stramonium : in both diseases a considerable majority of cases are said to have been either cured or relieved by it. Without denying the occasional benefit of stramonium in these diseases, I believe the cases in which it is serviceable to be very rare, while those in which it is calculated to be injurious are very common. Dr. Cullen[10] observes, that he has no doubt that narcotics may be a remedy for certain cases of mania and epilepsy ; but he very justly adds, "I have not, and I doubt if any other person has, learned to distinguish the cases to which such remedies are properly adapted."

Stramonium has been used to *dilate the pupil* and *to diminish the sensibility of the retina to the influence of light ;* but for both of these purposes belladonna is preferred by British oculists. Wendt[11] used it *to lessen venereal excitement,* as in nymphomania. An ointment (made with ʒj. of the powdered leaves, and ʒiv. of lard) has been used as an anodyne application to *irritable ulcers* and to *painful hemorrhoids.* The application of the leaves to *burns* has been attended with dangerous results.[12]

---

[1] Bayle, *Bibl. Thér.* t. ii.
[2] *Med.-Chir. Trans.* vols. vii. and viii.
[3] *Trans. Med.-Chir. Soc. of Edinb.* vol. i.
[4] See the reports of Kirckhoff, Engelhart, Van Nuffal, and Amelung, in Bayle, *op. cit.* ; also Eberle, *Mat. Med.*
[5] *Lancet,* 1826-7, vol. xii.; and 1827-8, vol. ii.
[6] English, in *Edinb. Med. and Surg. Journ.* vol. vii. ; and Dr. Sims, *ibid.* vol. viii.
[7] *Lond. Med. and Phys. Journ.* vol. xxvi. p. 51.
[8] *Ibid.* vol. xxvi. p. 49.
[9] *Bibl. Thérap.* t. ii.
[10] *Mat. Med.*
[11] Rust's *Magaz.* Bd. xxiv. S. 302.
[12] *Journ. de Chim. Méd.*

ADMINISTRATION.—The dose of the powdered *leaves* is one grain; of the *seeds* half a grain. These doses are to be repeated twice or thrice a day, and to be gradually increased until some obvious effect is produced.

ANTIDOTES.—The same as for belladonna.

1. EXTRACTUM STRAMONII, L. E.; *Extract of Thornapple.* (Thornapple Seeds, ℥xv.; Boiling Distilled Water, Cong. j. Macerate for four hours in a vessel slightly covered, near the fire; afterwards take out the seeds, and bruise them in a stone mortar: return them, when bruised, to the liquor. Then boil down to four pints, and strain the liquor while hot. Lastly, evaporate to a proper consistence, *L.* The directions of the *Edinburgh College* are as follows:—Take of the seeds of stramonium, any convenient quantity; grind them well in a coffee-mill. Rub the powder into a thick mass with proof spirit; put the pulp into a percolator, and transmit proof spirit till it passes colourless; distil off the spirit, and evaporate what remains in the vapour-bath to a proper consistence.)—Of the above modes of preparation, that of the Edinburgh College is doubtless the best, as yielding a more efficient extract. The product, according to the London process, is about 12 per cent.[2] Recluz[3] states, that 16 oz. of the seeds yield 2 oz. 2 dr. by maceration in dilute alcohol: this is about 14 per cent. The dose of extract of stramonium, at the commencement, is about a quarter of a grain, which should be gradually increased until some obvious effect is produced.

[**2. EXTRACTUM STRAMONII FOLIORUM, U.S.**; *Extract of Stramonium Leaves.* (Take of Stramonium Leaves, lb. j. Bruise them in a stone mortar, sprinkling on them a little water; then express the juice, and having heated it to the boiling point, strain and evaporate to the proper consistence.)—This affords a fine green extract endowed with the odour and properties of the plant. The dose is from one to five grains.—ED.]

3. TINCTURA STRAMONII, D. U.S.; *Tincture of Thornapple.* (Stramonium Seeds, bruised, ℥v.; Proof Spirit, Oij. Macerate for fourteen days, strain, express, and filter, *D.* Stramonium Seeds, bruised, ℥ij.; Proof Spirit, Oij. Macerate for fourteen days, and filter through paper. U.S. Dose, ♏x. to ♏xx. twice or thrice a day, gradually increased until it occasions some obvious effect on the system).—This preparation is applicable to all the cases for which stramonium is used.

4. [UNGUENTUM STRAMONII, U.S.; *Ointment of Stramonium.* (Take of fresh Stramonium Leaves, cut into pieces, lb. j.; Lard, lb. iij.; Yellow Wax, lb. ss. Boil the stramonium leaves in the lard until they become friable, then strain through linen: lastly, add the wax previously melted, and stir them until they are cold.)—This ointment is used for the same purposes as the belladonna ointment.—ED.]

---

[1] Barker, *Observ. on the Dublin Pharm.*
[2] *United States Dispensatory.*

180. NICOTIANA TABACUM.—VIRGINIAN TOBACCO.

Sex. Syst. Pentandria, Monogynia.

(Folium.—The leaves, *E. D.*)

HISTORY.—The inhalation of the fumes of burning vegetable substances, both for causing inebriation and for medicinal purposes, seems to have been very anciently practised. Herodotus[1] tells us that the Babylonians and Scythians intoxicated themselves by this means ; and both Dioscorides[2] and Pliny[3] speak of the efficacy of smoking Tussilago in obstinate cough.

Humboldt[4] says that the tobacco plant has been cultivated, from time immemorial, by the natives of Oronoko. It does not appear, however, to have been known to Europeans prior to the discovery of America ; although it is not improbable that the Asiatics were acquainted with it long before that time, as Pallas, Rumphius, and Loureiro have supposed. It is not, however, probable that the Europeans learned the use of it from the Asiatics, as Ulloa has endeavoured to show. When Columbus and his followers arrived at Cuba, in 1492, they, for the first time, beheld the custom of smoking cigars.[5] Hernandez de Toledo introduced the plant into Spain and Portugal ; and from the latter place Joan Nicot sent the seeds or the plant to France, about 1559-60.[6] In 1586, on the return of Sir Francis Drake, with the colonists, from Virginia, the practice of smoking was introduced into England ; and, being adopted by Sir Walter Raleigh and other courtiers, soon became common.[7]

Various attempts, by writings, imposts, or bodily punishments, have been made in Europe to restrict or put down its use.[8] It is said that upwards of a hundred volumes[9] were written to condemn its employment ; and not the least curious of these is the celebrated *" Counterblaste to Tobacco"* of James I.[10] Despite, and partly, perhaps, as a consequence of the attempts, the use of tobacco rapidly spread, and is now universal throughout the world.[11]

The generic appellation, Nicotiana, is obviously derived from Nicot, the name of an individual above referred to. The origin of the specific name, Tabacum, is less satisfactorily ascertained. It is probable, however, that the word is derived from *tabac,* an instrument used by the natives of America in smoking this herb ; though some derive it from *Tobago,* others from *Tabasco,* a town in New Spain.

BOTANY. **Gen. Char.**—*Calyx* tubular-campanulate, half 5-cleft. *Corolla* hypogynous, funnel-shaped or hypocrateriform ; limb plaited, 5-lobed. *Stamens* 5, inserted on the tube of the corolla, inclosed, of equal length ;

[1] Lib. i. *Clio,* ccii. ; lib. iv. *Melpomene,* lxxiv. and lxxv.
[2] Lib. ii. cap. 126.
[3] *Hist. Nat.* lib. xxvi. cap. 16, ed. Valp.
[4] *Personal Narrative,* vol. v. p. 666.
[5] W. Irving, *Hist. of the Life and Voyages of Columbus,* vol. i. p. 287 ; also the Narrative of Don Fernando Colon, son-in-law of Columbus, *Hist. del Amir.* cap. 27, in Barcia, *Hist. prim. de las Indias occid.* vol. i. p. 24.
[6] Bauhin's *Pinax.*
[7] *Biograph. Brit.* vol. v. p. 3471 ; and Clusius, *Exotic.* p. 310.
[8] Don's *Gardener's Dictionary,* vol. iv. p. 462.
Adam Clarke, *Dissert. on the Use and Abuse of Tobacco,* 1797 ; *Med. and Phys. Journ.* vol. xxiv. p. 451 ; and C. C. Antz, *Tabaci Hist. Dissert. Inaug.* Berol. 1836.
[10] *Works,* p. 214, fol. 1616.
[11] *Asiat. Journ.* vol. xxii.

anthers dehiscing longitudinally. *Ovary* bilocular ; placentæ adnate to the dorsal dissepiment ; ovules numerous ; *style* simple ; *stigma* capitate. *Capsule* covered by the persistent calyx, bilocular, septicidal-bivalved at the apex ; the valves ultimately bifid, retaining the separated placentæ. *Seeds* many, small ; the embryo slightly arched, in the axis of fleshy albumen (*Endlicher*).

Sp. Char.—*Stem* herbaceous. *Leaves* sessile (the lower ones decurrent), oblong-lanceolate, acuminate. Throat of the *corolla* inflated-ventricose ; the segments of the limb acuminate (*Nees*).

A viscid *herb*. *Root* branching, fibrous. *Stem* 3 to 6 feet high, erect, round, hairy, branching at the top. *Leaves* very large, pale green, with glandular short hairs. *Bracts* linear, acute. *Flowers* panicled on the end of the stem and branches. *Calyx* hairy. *Corolla* rose-coloured. *Ovarium* ovate ; *style* long and slender ; *stigma* capitate, cloven. *Capsule* 2-celled, opening cross-wise at the top, loculicidal. *Seeds* numerous, small, somewhat reniform, brown.

Hab.—America. Extensively cultivated in most parts of the world, especially the United States of America. Virginia is the most celebrated for its culture. North of Maryland the plant is rarely seen.[1] In England the cultivation is restricted, not more than half a pole being allowed " in a physic or university garden, or in any private garden for physic or chirurgery."[2]

This is the only species employed in medicine ; but the tobacco used for smoking, chewing, and snuff, is derived from several species, the most important of which are the following :—

1. N. Tabacum, Linn. ; *Common* or *Virginian Tobacco.*—Of this species several varieties are cultivated.[3] The Virginian and most other sorts of tobacco imported from the United States of America, as also Columbian tobacco, are obtained from it.

2. N. latissima, Miller ; *N. macrophylla*, Sprengel ; *Large-leaved* or *Oronoko Tobacco.*—This species is very closely allied to, if indeed it be not a variety of, the preceding species.[4] Nees[5] describes the leaves as being more erect or horizontal than those of N. Tabacum, which droop somewhat, and are thicker and more strongly ribbed. Moreover, the lateral nerves of the midrib of N. latissima, proceed, he says, at right angles ; whereas those of N. tabacum are given off at an acute angle.[6] Furthermore, the flowers of N. latissima form a dense contracted panicle ; whereas those of N. Tabacum form a loose spreading one.

This species, like the preceding, has varieties, with broader or smaller, shorter or longer, sessile or stalked leaves. To the latter variety probably belong *N. fruticosa*, Linn., and *N. chinensis*, Fischer.

According to Mr. G. Don,[7] this species probably yields the large Havannah cigars.

---

[1] *United States Dispensatory.*

[2] Loudon's *Encyclopædia of Agriculture.*

[3] Schrank (*Botan. Zeitung*, 1807) makes eight varieties, which he respectively calls *attenuatum, macrophyllum, pallescens, alipes, serotinum, gracilipes, Verdon*, and *Lingua ;* but it is doubtful whether or not some of these are identical with plants which by others have been described as distinct species.

The cultivated varieties differ in the degree of the thickness of the ribs, of the size and smoothness of the leaf, and in the absence or presence of a petiole (*N. Tabacum* var. *petiolata* is figured in Zeuker's *Naturgesch. d. vorzugl. Handelspflanzen*, Bd. ii. Taf. xxxix. 1832).

N. Loxensis, HBK., is probably a variety of N. Tabacum.

[4] Sprengel, who, in 1807, regarded it as a distinct species, has subsequently (in 1825) declared it to be merely a variety (*Syst. Veget.* vol. i. p. 616).

[5] Geiger's *Handb. d. Pharm.* 2te Aufl. 1839.

[6] Nees says that by this character several of the commercial sorts of tobacco may be recognised. By himself and other German writers this species is called " Maryland tobacco ;" but I find that, though the lateral nerves of the Maryland tobacco of British commerce are given off at a less acute angle than those of the Virginian tobacco, I cannot find any that proceed at a right angle.

[7] *Gardeners' Dictionary*, vol. iv.

3. N. RUSTICA, Linn.; *Common Green Tobacco.*—Stem, herbaceous, terete. Leaves petiolate, ovate, quite entire. Tube of the corolla cylindrical, longer than the calyx; segments of the limb roundish obtuse.—Corolla greenish-yellow.—Indigenous in America; grows wild in Europe, Asia, and Africa. It grows quicker, ripens earlier, and is more hardy than N. Tabacum; and hence it is frequently cultivated in gardens in England, and in several other parts of the world. It is used by peasants as a substitute for the Virginian sort, and by gardeners for the destruction of insects. Nees says that, in smoking, it may be readily distinguished by a peculiar violet odour. Parkinson[1] says that, though it is a milder tobacco,[2] yet he has known Sir W. Raleigh, when prisoner in the Tower, prefer it to make good tobacco.—It yields the tobacco of Salonica (the ancient Thessalonica), and probably also that of Latakkia (Laodicea), which is so much esteemed. The tobacco called Turkish, grown on the coasts of the Mediterranean, and highly valued in India, is the produce of this species.

4. N. PERSICA, Lindl., Bot. Reg. 1592.—Native of Persia. Yields the celebrated Shiraz or Persian tobacco.[3]

5. N. REPANDA, Willd.—Native of Cuba, near Havannah. The small Havannah cigars, or Queen's, are said to be made of this species.

6. N. QUADRIVALVIS, Parsh.—Cultivated and spontaneous on the Missouri; principally among the Mandan and Ricara nations.—The tobacco prepared from it is excellent. The most delicate is prepared by the Indians from the dried flowers.

7. N. NANA, Lindl., Bot. Reg. t. 833.—Rocky mountains of North America. The Indians are said to prepare the finest of their tobacco from the leaves of this species.

8. N. MULTIVALVIS, Lindl., Bot. Reg. t. 1057.—Cultivated by the Indians who inhabit the banks of the Columbia for tobacco, for which purpose the calyx, which is very fetid, is selected in preference to any other part.

CULTURE.—In Virginia and Maryland the seeds are thickly sown in beds of finely-prepared earth. When the young plants have five or six leaves, exclusive of the seminal leaves, they are transplanted into fields during the month of May, and set three or four feet apart, in rows. During the whole period of growth the crop requires constant attention; and, to promote the development of leaves, the tops are pinched off, by which the formation of flowers and seeds is prevented. The harvest is in August. The ripe plants are cut off above their roots, dried under cover, stripped of their leaves, tied in bundles, and packed in hogsheads.[4]

DESCRIPTION.—In commerce two states of tobacco are distinguished: in the one it is called *unmanufactured* or *leaf tobacco*, in the other it is termed *manufactured tobacco*.

1. UNMANUFACTURED or LEAF TOBACCO (*Folia Nicotianæ*).—Tobacco in this state consists of dried leaves, which have a brownish colour, a strong narcotic but peculiar odour, and a bitter nauseous taste. The darker-coloured sorts are the strongest. For medicinal purposes, Virginian tobacco in leaf (*folia tabaci*) should be employed.

In trade various sorts of unmanufactured or leaf tobacco are met with, and are distinguished by the name of the country from which they are imported, into the United Kingdom. The differences between them depend on the species or variety of plant cultivated, on the soil and climate, and on the mode of curing.

1. UNITED STATES LEAF TOBACCO.—This constitutes by far the greater proportion of unmanufactured tobacco imported into the United Kingdom. In 1843 no less than 41,038,597 lbs. were imported.

---

[1] *Theatrum Botanicum,* p. 712, 1640.

[2] Endlicher (*Medicinal-Pflanzen,* p. 338, 1842) declares that it is more stupifying than other species of Nicotiana.

[3] For a notice of the cultivation of Shiraz tobacco, see a paper by Dr. Riach, in the *Trans. of the Horticultural Society,* 2d series, vol. i. p. 205, 1885.

[4] Loudon's *Encyl. of Agricult.;* Carver, *Treatise on the Cult. of the Tobacco Plant,* 1779.

Several kinds, named from the States where respectively grown, are distinguished in trade: they are as follows:—

The *Virginian* is one of the strongest kinds, and is, therefore, not for cigars, but is adapted for pipes and snuff, and for medicinal use. It is imported in leaves or heads contained in hogsheads. Its colour is deep mottled brown; the leaves feel unctuous. The *Maryland* is paler, yellower, weaker, and adapted for smoking: the *pale cinnamon* is the best, the *scrubs* the commonest. The *Kentucky* is intermediate between the two preceding: it is paler and weaker than the Virginian. The *Carolina* is less frequently met with, and is of inferior quality. The *Missouri* and the *Ohio* are other sorts imported from the United States.

2. CUBA LEAF TOBACCO.—In 1843, 494,954 lbs. of leaf tobacco were imported from the island of Cuba. The *Havannah* sort is most esteemed for smoking: its colour is yellowish-brown; its odour is musky or spicy. It is imported in heads. The *Cuba* is an excellent kind; it is darker than the Havannah. Both these kinds, as well as the Columbian, are remarkable for the light yellow spots on the leaves.

3. ST. DOMINGO LEAF TOBACCO.—In 1843, 93,114 lbs. of leaf tobacco were imported from St. Domingo (Hayti). It comes over in leaves, and is deficient in flavour.

4. PORTO-RICO LEAF TOBACCO.—Small quantities of tobacco in rolls are sometimes imported from this island. In quality this sort is allied to the Varinas.

5. COLUMBIAN LEAF TOBACCO.—In 1843, 1,556,206 lbs. of unmanufactured tobacco were imported from Columbia. Three commercial sorts are brought from that country. Like the Cuba sorts, the leaves are marked with light yellow spots. The *Columbian* is imported in heads and leaves, and is much esteemed for cigars, for which it is more used than any other kind. It is dark brown, but not mottled like the Virginian. The *Varinas*[1] is brought over in rolls and in hands. It is a mild tobacco, suitable for smoking only. The third sort imported from Columbia is that called *Cumana*. *Orinoco* comes over in leaves.

6. BRAZILIAN LEAF TOBACCO.—In 1843, 128,329 lbs. of unmanufactured tobacco were imported from the Brazils.

7. DUTCH OR AMERSFOORT LEAF TOBACCO.—In 1843, 55,686 lbs. of unmanufactured tobacco were imported from Holland. Dutch tobacco is very mild, and deficient in flavour. The darker kind is the strongest, and is much esteemed for snuff; while the lighter and weaker kind is employed in the manufacture of the commonest cigars.

8. LEVANT LEAF TOBACCO.—*Turkey* tobacco is pale and yellowish. It occurs in small, short, broad leaves, and is the produce of N. rustica. It is a weak tobacco, and is cut for smoking. *Latakkia* (Laodicea) is an esteemed Syrian tobacco, the produce of the same species. *Salonica* is also yielded by N. rustica. *Persian* or *Shiraz* tobacco is delicate and fragrant. It is the produce of N. persica.

9. EAST INDIAN LEAF TOBACCO.—*East Indian tobacco* has never obtained a high repute, doubtless from inattention to its culture and curing.[2] In 1843, 59,158 lbs. were imported.

10. MANILLA LEAF TOBACCO.—In 1843, 2038 lbs. of unmanufactured tobacco were imported from the Philippine Islands. *Manilla* tobacco is dark coloured, and is much esteemed for cheroots.

2. MANUFACTURED TOBACCO.—Under this head are included the different forms of tobacco prepared for chewing and smoking, and for taking as snuff.

1. **Chewing and Smoking Tobaccos.**—Manufacturers distinguish chewing tobaccos and those used in pipes into two kinds, called respectively cut and roll tobacco. For smoking in the pipe, cut tobacco is principally used in England; the roll in Scotland and Ireland. Cigars and cheroots form a third kind.

1. CUT TOBACCOS.—These sorts are manufactured by moistening and compressing the leaves of tobacco, and cutting the compressed mass, with knife-edged chopping stamps, into small pieces or shreds varying from 16 to 100 cuts in the inch. By the addition of

---

[1] Sir H. Sloane (*Jamaica*, vol. i. p. lxiii.) says that the tobacco "from Nuevo Reyno de Grenada (corruptly called *Verinas* or *Tabac de Verine*) is reckoned the best."
[2] Royle, *Essay on the Productive Resources of India*, 1840.

water (or the *liquor*[1]), cut tobacco increases in weight from 8 to 16 per cent., according to circumstances. *Shag* tobacco is chiefly prepared from the Virginian and Kentucky sorts deprived of their stalks or midribs. *Returns*[2] is a lighter coloured and milder smoking tobacco. It derives its name from its being formerly prepared by returning shag for re-cutting. *Bird's-eye* is prepared like shag, with the exception that it contains the midribs of the leaves, the slices of which have been compared to the eyes of birds. *Maryland* is another kind of cut tobacco. *Canaster* or *Kanaster* is a favourite kind. It received its name from *canastra* (a Spanish word, signifying *a basket*), because it was imported in baskets. It is prepared from Varinas tobacco. *Orinoco, Turkey, Persian,* and *Varinas,* are also cut tobaccos.

2. SPUN, ROLL, OR TWIST TOBACCOS.—These are prepared by twisting tobacco into a kind of rope, which is moistened with liquor,[3] and is usually made up into cylindrical or barrel-shaped rolls or sticks, which are subjected to pressure before they are considered fit for sale. *Pig-tail, Negro-head, Bogie, Alloa, Cavendish,* and *Irish twist,* are roll tobaccos for chewing and smoking. During its manufacture roll tobacco increases in weight from 15 to 25 per cent.

3. CIGARS AND CHEROOTS.—These are small rolls of tobacco permeable to air and adapted for smoking. *Cigars* were originally derived from the New World. They are distinguished from cheroots by their pointed extremity, called the *curl* or *twist.* The *Havannah cigars* are in great request by smokers. Cigars, however, are extensively made in London. *Cheroots* were originally derived from the East. They are characterised by their truncated extremities. *Manilla cheroots* are much valued by smokers. Cheroots, however, like cigars, are extensively manufactured in London.

2. **Snuffs.**—In the manufacture of snuff, tobacco, cut in small pieces, is first fermented by placing it in heaps and sprinkling it with water or a solution of salt : the latter prevents the tobacco becoming mouldy. The heaps soon become hot and evolve ammonia. The extent to which this process is allowed to proceed varies with different kinds of snuff. The usual time is two or three months, seldom less than one month. The fermented tobacco is then ground in mills, or powdered with a kind of pestle and mortar. The Scotch and Irish are prepared for the most part from the midribs ; the Strasburgh, French, and Russian snuffs from the soft part of the leaves. The siftings, sometimes termed *thirds,* are usually reground. Sal ammoniac is occasionally added to snuffs.

The theory of the *tobacco fermentation* is imperfectly known. Decomposition probably first commences in the albuminous constituent, which yields carbonate of ammonia. The organic salts (malates) next suffer change, and are converted into carbonates. The lignin is the last to decompose : it becomes friable, yields ulmic acid, which colours the tobacco, and a little acetic acid. A portion (perhaps two-thirds) of the nicotina disappears during the process, being either decomposed or volatilised by the aid of the carbonate of ammonia. Moreover, while in the fresh plant the nicotina is found in the state of a salt (malate ?) insoluble in ether, in the fermented plant it is found chiefly in the state of acetate or sub-acetate soluble in ether. The immense varieties of snuffs found in the shops are reducible to two kinds,—dry and moist snuffs.

a. Dry Snuffs.—These derive their characteristic property from being dried at a high temperature previous to being ground. *Scotch, Irish,* and *Welsh,* are well-known high-dried snuffs. The latter frequently contains lime, the particles of which may be usually

---

[1] It is said that tobacconists employ, in the preparation of tobacco, a solution of sea-salt (sp. gr. 1·107), which is termed the *sauce* or *liquor ;* but I am assured that this is not generally the case. This liquor, it is further stated, is sometimes coloured by treacle or liquorice.

[2] " Returns of tobacco are the small pieces of broken leaf, and the dust and siftings, produced in the various processes of manufacture" (*Tobacco Report*).

[3] Water and oil are alone allowed by law to be used in the manufacture of roll tobacco ; but sugar, molasses, and liquorice, are frequently employed.

distinguished by the naked eye: hence its desiccating effect on the pituitary membrane.[1] *Spanish* snuff is also a dry snuff. *Brown Scotch* is Scotch snuff moistened after being ground.

β. *Moist Snuffs; Rappees.*—These are snuffs which have been prepared by grinding the tobacco to powder in a moist state. It is sometimes said that pearlash is added to these snuffs to keep them moist, but several respectable manufacturers assure me this is not usual. The rappees of the shops may be divided into three classes:—*Simple Rappees,* —as *Brown, Black, Cuba, Carotte,* and *Bolangero: Mixed Rappees,*—as *Hardham's Genuine* No. 37; and *Scented Rappees*—as *Prince's Mixture* and *Princeza,* &c.

COMPOSITION.—The juice of the fresh leaves of tobacco was analysed in 1809 by Vauquelin.[2] Subsequently this chemist analysed manufactured tobacco.[3] In 1821 Hermbstädt[4] discovered *nicotianin.* In 1827 the leaves were analysed by Posselt and Reinmann,[5] and in 1831 by Dr. Conwell.[6] In 1845 Messrs. Brande and Cooper[7] made a series of experiments to ascertain the proportion of soluble and insoluble matters in eight samples of tobacco.

Vauquelin's Analysis.

An acrid volatile principle (*nicotina*).
Albumen.
Red matter, soluble in alcohol and water.
Acetic acid.
Supermalate of lime.
Chlorophylle.
Nitrate of potash and chloride of potassium.
Sal ammoniac.
Water.

Expressed juice of the leaves.

The *leaves* contained, in addition to the above, *woody fibre, oxalate* and *phosphate of lime, oxide of iron,* and *silica.* The two latter substances were obtained from the ashes. *Manufactured tobacco* contained the same principles, and, in addition, *carbonate of ammonia* and *chloride of calcium,* perhaps produced by the reaction of sal ammoniac and lime, which are added to tobacco to give it pungency.

Posselt and Reinmann's Analysis.

Nicotina	0·06
Concrete volatile oil (*nicotianin*)	0·01
Bitter extractive	2·87
Gum with malate of lime	1·74
Chlorophylle	9·267
Albumen and gluten	1·308
Malic acid	0·51
Lignin and a trace of Starch	4·969
Salts (sulphate, nitrate, and malate of potash, chloride of potassium, phosphate and malate of lime, and malate of ammonia)	0·734
Silica	0·088
Water	88·280
Fresh leaves of tobacco	100·836

Conwell's Analysis.

Gum.
Mucilage soluble in both water and alcohol.
Tannic acid.
Gallic acid.
Chlorophylle.
Green pulverulent matter, soluble in boiling water.

Yellow oil, having the odour, taste, and poisonous properties of tobacco.
Pale yellow resin (large quantity).
Nicotina.
A substance analogous to morphia.
An orange-red colouring matter.
Nicotianin.

1. NICOTINA (*Nicotine*). Symbol $\overset{+}{Ni}$. Formula $C^{20}H^{14}N^2$. Eq. Wt. 162—Exists not only in the leaves (both fresh and fermented), but also in the root[8] and in the seeds,[9] as well as in the smoke of tobacco.—It is obtained by digesting an aqueous extract of the leaves in rectified spirit, which takes up the nicotina salts. The decanted tincture is to

[1] The Act of Parliament allows lime-water to be used in the manufacture of Irish and Welsh snuffs; but Mr. Foot (*Tobacco Report*) states that the Lundyfoot or "high-toast snuff" is made of the stalks and leaves of tobacco and water (which latter is afterwards got rid of by drying) without lime.

[2] *Ann. de Chim.* lxxi. 139.

[3] *Annal. du Mus. d'Hist. Nat.* t. xiv.

[4] Schwcigger's *Journ. für Chem.* xxxi. 441.

[5] Gmelin, *Handb. d. Chem.* ii. 1303.

[6] Silliman's *Journ.* xvii. 369.

[7] Brande's *Manual of Chemistry,* p. 1623, 1848.

[8] E. Davy, *Lond. and Ed. Phil. Mag.* vol. vii. p. 393.

[9] Buchner, *Report.* Bd. xxxii.

be concentrated, mixed with a solution of potash, and briskly shaken with ether, which dissolves the nicotina set free by the potash.—To purify the alkaloid, add gradually to its solution oxalic acid in powder : oxalate of nicotina, insoluble in ether, forms, at the bottom of the vessel, a syrupy layer, which is to be repeatedly shaken with pure ether. The nicotina may be separated by potash and ether, as before. The ethereal solution is to be distilled in a salt-water bath, then transferred to a retort, through which a current of dry hydrogen circulates; exposed to a temperature of 284° F. in an oil bath, in order to entirely get rid of the water, ether, and ammonia : lastly, the temperature is to be raised to 356°, when the nicotin distils over drop by drop. From 28 lbs. of Virginia tobacco, at least 4 per cent. of nicotina can be procured by this process. [Nicotine may also be obtained by passing the vapour of tobacco into water acidulated with sulphuric acid. Sulphate of nicotine is thus produced, and this may be decomposed by potash or soda, and the nicotine separated by distillation. In cases of poisoning the following process for procuring nicotine has been recommended by Orfila. The contents of the stomach and intestines, or the viscera themselves, finely cut up, are to be digested in water acidulated with sulphuric acid in the proportion of about five drops to a concentrated acid to seven ounces of distilled water. After twelve hours' digestion the acid liquid may be filtered : it may contain some sulphate of nicotine as well as organic matter. It may then be concentrated almost to dryness in a close vessel over a water-bath. Add distilled water to dissolve the sulphate of nicotine, then hydrate of potash or soda, and distil to separate the nicotine. Orfila states that he has thus detected nicotine in the livers of animals poisoned by twelve or fifteen drops of the alkaloid.[1]—ED.]

Nicotina is a colourless liquid alkaloid, with an acrid odour and an acrid burning taste. [The vapours of this alkaloid have the irritating and peculiar odour of tobacco in a most powerful degree.—ED.] Its density is 1·024 (1·048 Orfila). It restores the blue colour of reddened litmus, and renders turmeric brown. It does not solidify at 14° F. : it boils at 482° F., and at the same time undergoes decomposition. By exposure to the air it becomes brown and thick. It is readily combustible with the aid of a wick. It is soluble in water, ether, alcohol, and the oils (fixed and volatile). [Ether readily separates it from its aqueous solution.—ED.] It combines with acids, and forms very deliquescent salts : the *sulphate, phosphate, oxalate,* and *tartrate,* are crystallisable ; the *acetate* is not. A dilute aqueous solution of nicotina yields a white flocculent precipitate (double chloride) with a solution of bichloride of mercury, and a yellow granular precipitate with chloride of platinum.

[In addition to the above properties it may be observed that this is one of the three natural volatile vegetable alkaloids, the other two being *conicine* and *theobromine*. Nicotine, like hydrocyanic acid, is a compound of nitrogen, carbon, and hydrogen. The fact that this alkaloid is soluble in water and ether is a peculiarity, since an alkaloid which is easily dissolved by one of these liquids is not readily dissolved by the other. Concentrated sulphuric acid strikes a wine red colour with nicotine in the cold. If heated, it darkens, becomes black, and sulphurous acid is evolved. It gives white fumes with hydrochloric acid, precisely like ammonia. Heated with the acid it acquires a deep violet colour. Nitric acid colours it orange yellow, and vapours of deutoxide of nitrogen are given off when the mixture is heated. It forms a soluble soap with stearic acid. The simple salts of nicotine are deliquescent, and are difficultly crystallisable. The compound salts with metallic oxides are more readily crystallised. In many of its reactions nicotine resembles ammonia. Among other differences it may be mentioned that iodine water which is decolorised by ammonia produces a yellow precipitate with a solution of nicotine ; and pure tannic acid, which gives a reddish colour with ammonia, throws down a copious white precipitate in a solution of nicotine.—ED.]

Nicotina is an energetic poison, almost equalling in activity hydrocyanic acid. [The following experiment, performed by Orfila, will show the effects produced by this poison. A middling sized dog was made to swallow twelve drops of nicotine. In a few seconds there was giddiness, and the animal fell upon its right side. Convulsions followed, at first slight, but passing rapidly to a tetanic state, with opisthotonos. The animal fell into a state of stupor, and uttered no cry. There was neither vomiting nor purging. The pupils were dilated. The animal died in *ten minutes*. On inspection, the abdomen and chest when cut into, were found to evolve powerfully the odour of tobacco. The heart contained much blood, dark coloured, and coagulated. The right cavities contained

---

[1] [For further details, see Orfila's *Mémoire sur la Nicotine* : Baillière, 1851.]

more than the left. The stomach contained a quantity of a yellow thick frothy liquid, and some points of the mucous membrane were inflamed. The œsophagus, intestines, liver, spleen, and kidneys, were in a natural state. The epithelium of the tongue was readily detached, and its base scarred and slightly excoriated. The brain was more injected than the membrane, and the pons varolii was also injected. This poison has been used for the purpose of murder. The Count de Bocarmé was tried, convicted, and executed at Mons in 1851 for poisoning his brother-in-law with nicotine. He procured the poison by distillation.[1]—Ed.]

The amount of nicotina in leaf or manufactured tobacco may be estimated by Schloesing's process :[2] exhaust two drachms of tobacco by ammoniacal ether in a continuous distillatory apparatus, expel the ammoniacal gas from the nicotina solution by boiling, then decant, and, after the evaporation of the ether, estimate the amount of nicotina in the residue by the quantity of diluted sulphuric acid of known strength required to saturate it.

The following are the amounts found in various French and American tobaccos :—

100 *Parts of Tobacco dried at* 212°.	*Nicotina.*
Virginia	6·87
Kentucky	6·09
Maryland	2·29
Havannah (cigares primera), less than	2·00
Lot	7·96
Lot-et-Garonne	7·34
Nord	6·58
Ile-et-Vilaine	6·29
Pas-de-Calais	4·94
Alsace	3·21
Tobacco in powder	2·04

2. Acids of Tobacco.—Tobacco is very rich in malic acid : it also contains citric and phosphoric acids, and, according to M. Barral, a peculiar acid which he terms *nicotianic acid.*

3. Concrete Volatile Oil of Tobacco (*Nicotianin,* Hermbstädt ; *Tobacco-camphor,* Gmelin).—Obtained by submitting tobacco leaves, with water, to distillation. Six pounds of the leaves yielded eleven grains of oil, which swims on the surface of the liquor. This oil is solid, has the odour of tobacco, and a bitter taste. It is volatile, insoluble in water and the dilute acids, but soluble in ether and caustic potash. According to Landerer,[3] fresh tobacco leaves yield no nicotianin, which, therefore, would appear to be developed by the drying of the leaves under the influence of air and water. Nicotianin excites, in the tongue and throat, a sensation similar to that caused by tobacco smoke. Hermbstädt swallowed a grain of it, and experienced, soon after, giddiness, nausea, and inclination to vomit. Applied to the nose, it causes sneezing.

4. Ashes of Tobacco.—Tobacco yields a very large amount of ashes, the quantity and quality of which vary considerably. The ashes obtained from the leaves (including the ribs) vary from 17 to 27 per cent.[4]

5. Tobacco Smoke.—The constituents of tobacco smoke, according to Raab,[5] are much *carbonate of ammonia, acetate of ammonia* (nicotine) *nicotianin, empyreumatic oil, carbonaceous matter* (soot), *moisture,* and several *gases.* Unverdorben obtained,[6] by the dry distillation of tobacco, water, oil, and resin. These products consisted of *a volatile oil, an oleaginous acid, an empyreumatic acid* (Brandsäure), *resin,* traces of *a powder insoluble in potash and acids,* a small quantity of *odorin,* a *base soluble in water* (nicotin ?), *fuscin, red matter* soluble in acids, and *two extractive matters,* one forming a soluble, the other an insoluble compound with lime. Zeise,[7] more recently, has submitted tobacco smoke to a careful analysis, and gives the following as its constituents :—A *peculiar empyreumatic oil, butyric acid, carbonic acid, ammonia, paraffine, empyreumatic resin,* water, probably some *acetic acid,* more or less *carbonic oxide,* and *carburetted hydrogen.* To the absence of

---

[1] [See Orfila's *Mémoire,* above quoted.—Ed.]
[2] *Chemical Gazette,* vol. v. p. 41, 1847.
[3] *Pharm. Central-Blatt für* 1835, S. 890.
[4] Johnston's *Lectures on Agricultural Chemistry,* p. 391, 1847.
[5] Zenker and Schenk, *Naturgesch. d. vorzug. Handelspfl.* Bd. ii. S. 75.
[6] Poggendorff's *Annalen,* viii. 399.
[7] *Annal. d. Chemie u. Pharm.* vol. xlvii. p. 212, 1843.

creasote is, perhaps, to be ascribed the less acrid quality of tobacco smoke than of wood smoke. Melsens[1] has subsequently detected *nicotina* in tobacco smoke.

The purified *empyreumatic oil of tobacco* passes over colourless, but soon becomes yellowish, and ultimately brownish. Its sp. gr. is 0·870. It is soluble in alcohol and in ether, but not in water. Its composition is $C^{11}H^{11}O^2$.—In the impure state, Dr. Morries[2] describes the oil as being rather less solid than the empyreumatic oil of foxglove ; but it is undistinguishable from the latter by either taste or smell. In this state it probably contained some nicotina. It has been suggested that this oil is *"the juice of cursed hebenon,"* alluded to by Shakspeare,[3] who also calls it a *"distilment."*

CHARACTERISTICS.—The characteristics of tobacco leaves are partly botanical, partly chemical. The *botanical* characters which apply to large and perfect leaves have been before stated (see *ante,* p. 568) : those used to detect small fragments will be noticed under the head of adulterations (see *infra*).

The following are the *chemical* characters, as given by Dr. Ure,[4] of a filtered cold infusion of tobacco, prepared by macerating 100 grs. of dried Virginia tobacco in 1000 grains of distilled water :—" Infusion pale-brown; acid reaction with litmus paper ; nitrate of barytes, 0 ; nitrate of silver, a faint opalescence, but no curdy precipitate ; oxalate of ammonia, a faint cloud of calcareous matter ; water of ammonia, 0 ; chloride of tin, a faint white precipitate—hence no sulphuretted hydrogen present ; chloride of platinum, a copious white precipitate, from the ammoniacal salt present ; acetate of lead, an abundant whitish precipitate, soluble in nitric acid ; chloride of iron caused a green tint, and sulphate of copper an olive brown, both resulting from the yellow of the iron, and blue of the copper solutions, with the brown of the tobacco."

The mode of determining the per centage quantity of nicotina in tobacco has been already mentioned (see *ante,* p. 574).

The peculiar odour of tobacco smoke, as well as the remarkable sensation of acridity which both it and tobacco leaf excite in the throat, may sometimes aid in the detection of tobacco. (See, on this subject, *Lobelia inflata.*)

ADULTERATION.—From the evidence laid before a Committee of the House of Commons in 1844, it appears that the adulteration of tobacco has been (and probably still is) very general, and has varied from 5 to 40 per cent. ; in some cases being carried as far as 100 per cent. of the tobacco.

The substances used for adulterating it are numerous and various. *Water* being necessary in the manufacture of tobacco, and being allowed by law, can scarcely be called an adulterating ingredient, although it serves to increase the weight of the tobacco. In the preparation of Shag tobacco, about 12 per cent. of water is used in this country.[5] *Saccharine matter* (sugar, molasses, or honey), which is the principal adulterating ingredient, is said to be used both for sophistication and for rendering the tobacco more agreeable. *Vegetable leaves* (as of rhubarb and beech), *mosses, bran, malt-combs,* sprout of the malt), *beetroot dregs, liquorice, terra japonica, rosin, salts* (nitre, common salt, and sal-ammoniac), *yellow ochre, fuller's earth,* and

---

[1] *Ann. de Chim. et de Physiq.* 3me sér. t. ix. p. 465.

[2] *Edinb. Med. and Surg. Journ.* vol. xxxix. p. 379.

[3] *Hamlet,* Act i. Scene 5.

[4] *Supplement to his Dictionary,* p. 251.

[5] On the continent tobacco is more coarsely cut, and, therefore, less water is required in its manufacture.

sand, are stated (see the *Tobacco Report*) to have been employed as adulterating ingredients.[1]

The detection of adulteration is in some cases easy, in others difficult, if not
impossible.[2]   Two methods of analysis have been resorted to ; one mechanical,
the other chemical.[3]   The presence of foreign bodies may sometimes be
detected by the naked eye, at other times the use of a magnifying glass or
microscope is necessary to detect them.   Tobacco leaves present several
remarkable (though not peculiar) characters which lend important aid
in detecting adulterations : these are—1st, the horse-shoe or crescentic
mark seen on a transverse section of the leaf-stalk ;[4] 2dly, the glandular
character of the hairs ;[5] 3dly, the size and shape of the meshes or reticulations
of the epidermis ;[6] 4thly, the size, shape, and number, in a given space, of
stomata.

The chemical characters or tests on which reliance has been placed in
detecting adulterations are chiefly the following : 1st, the relative proportions
of matters soluble and insoluble in water.   The substances insoluble in water
are called by the excise officers "ligneous matters," and for Virginia, Missouri,
and Kentucky tobacco amount to from 45 to 55 per cent.   Porto Rico
tobacco, however, yields 70 per cent. of ligneous matters.   The matters
soluble in water are termed " extractive," and, of course, make up the difference.
It is obvious, however, that no reliance can be placed on this test (on account
of the great variations in the proportions of the two constituents) unless a
portion of the pure leaf, from which the suspected manufactured tobacco was
made, can be obtained for comparison.[7] 2dly, genuine tobacco mixed with
yeast and water, and submitted to a proper temperature, does not undergo the
vinous fermentation ; but tobacco which has been adulterated with saccharine
matter undergoes this kind of fermentation, and yields alcohol.[8]   Trommer's

---

[1] [A return moved for in the Session of 1855, and printed by order of the House of Commons,
in the Session of 1855, gives a list of the seizures made and of prosecutions for breach of the
tobacco laws in the years 1852, 1853, and 1854, with a list of the offenders.   It appears that about
69 persons or firms were so prosecuted in England and 31 in Ireland during the said period.   The
offences included the hawking of tobacco and cigars, and having adulterated or smuggled tobacco in
possession, and having spurious tobacco.   The cases of adulterated tobacco are very numerous, and
the materials for adulterating it consisted of sugar, alum, lime, flour of meal, rhubarb leaves,
saltpetre, fullers' earth, starch, malt combings, chromate of lead, peat-moss, treacle, common
burdock leaves, common salt, endive leaves, lampblack, gum and red dye, and black dye, composed
of vegetable red, iron, and liquorice.—Ed.]

[2] Dr. Ure in his evidence (Quest. 8849), states that he is quite sure that he " could so adulterate
tobacco as to elude every chemical and microscopical examination."

[3] Mr. Richard Phillips, Professor Graham, and Mr. George Phillips, employed mechanical means
chiefly in the analysis of various samples (some adulterated, others unadulterated) of tobacco submitted to their examination by the Parliamentary Committee (Quest. 7511–12).

[4] The horse-shoe or crescentic mark seen in the centre of the leaf-stalk of tobacco is the mass of
woody fibres and vessels which eventually make the veins of the leaf.   This character, though much
relied on by the excise officers, is not peculiar to tobacco,—being found in stramonium, belladonna,
and some other leaves.   It is, however, absent in rhubarb leaves.

[5] The hairs of tobacco leaves are tipped by a small spherical or ellipsoidal gland.   In rhubarb
and potato leaves, the hairs are lymphatic, not glandular.

[6] In tobacco, the meshes seen on the epidermis are bound by sinuous lines.

[7] Dr. Ure (Quest. 8770) declares that the amount of residuum or ligneous matter is as variable
from the genuine tobacco as from adulterated specimens furnished him by the Parliamentary Com-
mitte ; and he, therefore, declares this test as good for nothing.

[8] Dr. Ure objects to the fermentation test that it might be rendered nugatory by adding to the
tobacco substances which are known to prevent fermentation in sugar.   Thus it has been long

test is employed to distinguish grape sugar and molasses from cane sugar (see SUGAR). 3dly, treating the samples with alcohol, and examining the alcoholic solution and the parts insoluble in alcohol. 4thly, incinerating the suspected sample, and determining the amount and nature of the ashes. According to Mr. Johnston,[1] the per-centage of ash left by dry tobacco leaf varies from 19 to 27 per cent. of its whole weight ; Pelouze and Frémy,[2] on the other hand, state that for leaves and ribs dried at 212° it varies from 17 to 24 per cent., and for stalks from 6 to 16 per cent. The nature and solubility of the ashes, and the proportion of silica in them, are subject to great variation.[3] 5thly, the determination of the amount of nitrogen ; but Dr. Ure,[4] who suggested this line of research, has satisfied himself that this method can serve no good purpose. 6thly, special tests are required for the detection of particular substances suspected to be present. Thus for terra japonica the tests employed are the salts of iron and gelatine, by which the presence of astringent matter is indicated.

PHYSIOLOGICAL EFFECTS. *α. On Animals generally.*—In the *carnivora* tobacco causes nausea, vomiting, sometimes purging, universal trembling, staggering, convulsive movements, and stupor. Five drachms and a half of rappee introduced into the stomach of a dog, and secured by a ligature on the œsophagus, caused death in nine hours. In another experiment, two drachms applied to a wound killed the animal in an hour.[6] Sir B. Brodie[6] found that the infusion of tobacco, thrown into the rectum, paralysed the heart, and caused death in a few minutes. But if the head of the animal be previously removed, and artificial respiration kept up, the heart remains unaffected ; proving that tobacco disorders this organ through the medium of the nervous system only. In the *herbivora* the effects of tobacco, as of other vegetable poisons, are much less marked : vomiting does not occur. Schubarth[7] gave four ounces of the leaves to a horse, at three times, within two hours. The pulse became irregular, then slower, afterwards quicker : respiration and the pupils were scarcely affected. For two days the stools and urine were more frequent. Moiroud[8] observed no remarkable effect from the exhibition of a decoction of four ounces of tobacco to a horse.

It is remarkable that the *empyreumatic oil of tobacco* does not possess the same power of paralysing the heart. Applied to the tongue of a cat, one drop caused convulsions, and in two minutes death : on opening the body, the heart was beating regularly and with force.[9] Its operation, therefore, is

---

known in Burgundy that a little red precipitate of mercury, when added to must (juice of the grape), prevents fermentation. He also observes (*Supplement to his Dictionary*, p. 253), that it would seem from experiments made by Professor Graham and Messrs. Phillips, that infusions of tobacco without sugar, when mixed with brisk yeast, and placed for forty hours in a temperature of about 80° F., undergoes a certain degree of decomposition, attended with diminution of their specific gravity ; or, in the language of the Excise, they suffer attenuation.

[1] *Lectures on Agricultural Chemistry*, p. 391, 1847.
[2] *Cours de Chimie Générale*, t. iii. p. 232, 1850.
[3] Will and Fresenius, *Mem. of the Chemical Society*, vol. ii. p. 191 ; and Beauchef, in Pelouze and Frémy, *op. supra cit.* pp. 233 and 234.
[4] *Tobacco Report*, p. 460 ; and *Supplement to his Dictionary*, p. 250, 1844.
[5] Orfila, *Tox. Gén.*
[6] *Phil. Trans.* for 1811, p. 178.
[7] Wibmer, *Wirk. d. Arzneim. u. Gift.* Bd. iii. S. 336.
[8] *Pharm. Vét.* p. 364.
[9] Brodie, *op. cit.*

analogous to that of hydrocyanic acid. Dr. Morries[1] says it has less tendency to induce convulsions than the empyreumatic oils of foxglove, henbane, or the thornapple.

β. *On Man.*—*In small doses* tobacco causes a sensation of heat in the throat, and sometimes a feeling of warmth at the stomach : these effects, however, are less obvious when the remedy is taken in a liquid form, and largely diluted. By repetition it usually operates as a diuretic, and less frequently as a laxative. Accompanying these effects are oftentimes nausea and a peculiar feeling usually described as giddiness, but which scarcely accords with the ordinary acceptation of this term. As dropsical swellings sometimes disappear under the use of these doses, it has been inferred that the remedy promotes the operation of the absorbents. *In larger doses* it provokes nausea, vomiting, and purging. Though it seldom gives rise to abdominal pain, it produces a most distressing sensation of sinking at the pit of the stomach. It occasionally acts as an anodyne, or more rarely promotes sleep. But its most remarkable effects are languor, feebleness, relaxation of muscles, trembling of the limbs, great anxiety, and tendency to faint. Vision is frequently enfeebled, the ideas confused, the pulse small and weak, the respiration somewhat laborious, the surface cold and clammy, or bathed in a cold sweat, and, in extreme cases, convulsive movements are observed. *In excessive doses* the effects are of the same kind, but more violent in degree. The more prominent symptoms are nausea, vomiting, and in some cases purging, extreme weakness and relaxation of the muscles, depression of the vascular system (manifested by feeble pulse, pale face, cold sweats, and tendency to faint), convulsive movements, followed by paralysis and a kind of torpor, terminating in death.

Taken in the form of *snuff*, its principal effect is topical. It causes increased secretion of nasal mucus, and, in those unaccustomed to its use, sneezing. Getting into the throat it produces a feeling of acridity, and sometimes nausea. From some kinds of rappee I have experienced giddiness and great prostration of strength. Lanzoni[2] states that an individual fell into a state of somnolency, and died lethargic on the twelfth day, in consequence of taking too much snuff. Reasonable doubt, however, may be entertained, I think, whether these accidents really arose from snuff. The habitual use of this substance blunts the sense of smell and alters the tone of voice ; but I am unacquainted with any other well-ascertained effects, though Cullen[3] ascribes loss of appetite and dyspepsia to it, and Dr. Prout[4] observes, that "the severe and peculiar dyspeptic symptoms sometimes produced by inveterate snuff-taking are well known ; and I have more than once seen such cases terminate fatally with malignant diseases of the stomach and liver." I have known several inveterate snuff-takers who, after many years' use of this substance, have discontinued it with impunity ; but Dr. Cullen thinks that when the discharge of mucus is considerable, the ceasing or suppression of it, by abstaining from snuff, is ready to occasion the very disorders of headache, toothache, and ophthalmia, which it had formerly relieved. There do not appear to be any

---

[1] *Ed. Med. and Surg. Journ.* vol. xxxix. p. 383.
[2] Christison, *On Poisons.*
[3] *Mat. Med.* ii. 274.
[4] *On the Nature and Treatment of Stomach and Urinary Diseases*, p. 25, Lond. 1840.

good grounds for the supposed baneful effects of the manufacture of snuff on the workmen.[1]   Sir W. Temple[2] recommends the introduction of a tobacco leaf into the nostrils for the relief of affections of the eyes and head.

The *smoking* of tobacco by those unaccustomed to it gives rise to all the before-described effects of large and excessive doses.   A very interesting case, which had almost terminated fatally, is related by Dr. Marshall Hall.[3]   It was that of a young man, who, for his first essay, smoked two pipes.   Gmelin[4] mentions two cases of death from smoking, in the one of seventeen, in the other of eighteen pipes at a sitting.

In habitual smokers, the practice, when employed moderately, provokes thirst, increases the secretion of saliva and buccal mucus, and produces a remarkable soothing and tranquillising effect on the mind, which has made it so much admired and adopted by all classes of society, and by all nations, civilised and barbarous.   I am not acquainted with any well-ascertained ill effects resulting from the habitual practice of smoking.   A similar observation is made by Dr. Christison.[5]   Yet Dr. Prout says it "disorders the assimilating functions in general, but particularly, as I believe, the assimilation of the saccharine principle.   I have never, indeed, been able to trace the development of oxalic acid to the use of tobacco; but that some analogous and equally poisonous principle (probably of an acid nature) is generated in certain individuals by its abuse, is evident from their cachectic looks, and from the dark and often greenish-yellow tint of their blood."[6]   There do not appear to be any good grounds for supposing that smoking is a prophylactic against contagious and epidemic diseases,—an opinion at one time entertained.

The practice of *chewing* tobacco is principally confined to sailors, and is less frequently submitted to our observation; so that we are not so competent to speak of its effects, which, probably, are similar to those caused by smoking.

The application of tobacco to abraded surfaces is a very dangerous practice, and has in some instances been attended with violent or even fatal results.   Mr. Weston[7] has related a case in which the expressed juice of tobacco was applied to the head of a boy, aged eight years, for the cure of tinea capitis.   Death took place three hours and a half after the application. In the form of *clyster* tobacco has frequently proved fatal, sometimes from the use of inordinate doses by ignorant persons,[8] and occasionally in the hands of the well-informed practitioner.   Dessault[9] has witnessed the smoke prove fatal.   Sir A. Cooper[10] has seen two drachms, and even one drachm, destroy life.   In a case related by Sir Charles Bell[11] death probably occurred from the same cause.   Dr. Copland[12] saw half a drachm in infusion prove fatal.

---

[1] Christison, *op. cit.*
[2] *Letters*, p. 286, folio, 1720.
[3] *Edinb. Med. and Surg. Journ.* vol. xii. p. 11.
[4] Quoted by Christison.
[5] *Op. cit.* p. 774.
[6] *Op. supra cit.* p. 25.
[7] *Med. and Phys. Journ.* vol. xiv. p. 305.
[8] Christison, *op. cit.*
[9] *Œuvres Chir.* t. ii. p. 344.
[10] *Anatomy and Treatment of Hernia*, p. 24.
[11] *Surgical Observations*, part ii. p. 189.
[12] *Dict. of Pract. Med.* art. *Colic*, vol. i. p. 371.

The operation of tobacco resembles that of *Lobelia inflata* (see LOBE-LIACEÆ). With foxglove tobacco agrees in several circumstances, especially in that of enfeebling the action of the vascular system, although its power in this respect is inferior to that of foxglove. In its capability of causing relaxation and depression of the muscular system, and trembling, tobacco surpasses foxglove; as it does, also, in its power of promoting the secretions. From belladonna, stramonium, and hyoscyamus, it is distinguished by causing contraction of the pupil, both when applied to the eye and when taken internally in poisonous doses; and also by the absence of delirium and of any affection of the parts about the throat. Vogt[1] and Sundelin[2] have considered the effects of tobacco as closely allied to those of aconite; but to me the resemblance is less obvious (see RANUNCULACEÆ). The power possessed by the last-mentioned substance of paralysing the sentient nerves sufficiently distinguishes it from tobacco.

USES.—The principal remedial value of tobacco consists in its power of relaxing muscular fibres, whereby it becomes a valuable antispasmodic. As a purgative, but especially as an antispasmodic and purgative conjoined, it is exceedingly serviceable in alvine obstructions. As a sedative to the vascular system it has not been much used. I tried it somewhat extensively a few years since, as a substitute for blood-letting in inflammatory affections; but, while it produced such distressing nausea and depression that it was with difficulty I could induce patients to persevere in its use, I did not find its antiphlogistic powers at all proportionate, and eventually I discontinued its employment. As an anodyne, diuretic, or emetic, it is much inferior to many other articles of the Materia Medica.

1. *In colic, ileus (volvulus), strangulated hernia, and constipation.*— The efficacy of tobacco in these diseases depends principally on its power of relaxing muscular fibres and on its purgative properties. These effects are usually accompanied by nausea and giddiness. The remedy is applied in the form of clyster, consisting either of the infusion or of the smoke. The latter was at one time supposed to be more efficacious. Heberden[3] says it causes less giddiness than the infusion. It probably extends farther up the intestines than the liquid enema, and, therefore, acts on a larger surface; but the difficulties and inconvenience of applying it, and the uncertainty of its effects, have led, for the most part, to the discontinuance of its use. In *ileus* the tobacco clyster has been recommended by Sydenham,[4] by Heberden,[5] by Abercrombie,[6] and by several other distinguished authorities. The earlier it is resorted to, the more successful is it likely to prove. Indeed, when employed in the last stage of the disease, it sometimes hastens the fatal termination by exhausting the already depressed vital powers. As it is occasionally necessary to repeat the injection, it is of importance to begin cautiously. Dr. Abercrombie uses only fifteen grains of tobacco infused in six ounces of boiling water for ten minutes, and he repeats this in an hour if no effect have been produced. I have generally employed a scruple, and have not

---

[1] *Pharmakodyn.*.
[2] *Handb. d. spec. Heilmittell.*
[3] *Comment. on the Hist. and Cure of Diseases*, 3d edit. p. 270, 1806.
[4] *Whole Works*, 4th edit. by Peachey, p. 428.
[5] *Op. cit.*
[6] *On Diseases of the Abdominal Viscera.*

experieneed any dangerous effects from its application; and it is possible that, in persons long accustomed to the use of tobacco, a somewhat larger dose might be required: but I have never met with any cases in which a scruple did not produce the full effect on the system that was desired.   In *strangulated hernia* the tobacco clyster has frequently effected the return of the protruded parts when the operation appeared almost inevitable; and every surgical writer speaks in the highest terms of its use.   A tense hernial tumour sometimes becomes soft and relaxed by the diminished force of circulation produced by tobacco.   Notwithstanding these facts, this remedy is much less resorted to than formerly.   Three circumstances have, I suspect, led to the infrequency of its use:—first, the dangerous, if not fatal, consequences which have sometimes resulted from its employment; secondly, the frequency of its failure and the consequent loss of time, by which the chance of recovery is diminished; thirdly, the operation for hernia being much less dreaded now than formerly, for experience has fully proved that death rarely (Mr. Pott says only once in fifty times) results from it.   In *colic* from lead, and in *obstinate constipation* from spasmodic constriction, the tobacco clyster has sometimes proved most beneficial.   Of the application, in lead colic, of compresses soaked in a strong decoction of tobacco, to the abdomen, as recommended by Dr. Graves,[1] I have had no experience.   The practice is, of course, calculated to be beneficial, but is less certain and speedy in its effect than tobacco clysters.

2. *In ischuria and dysury.* — When retention of urine arises from spasm of the neck of the bladder or from spasmodic stricture, tobacco, by its powerfully relaxing properties, is an agent well calculated to give relief. Mr. Earle[2] has published several cases illustrative of its efficacy.   In dysury, also, tobacco proves serviceable; it abates pain, relaxes the urinary passages, promotes the secretion of urine, and, by diminishing the sensibility of the parts, facilitates the expulsion of calcareous matter.[3]

3. *Tetanus.*—The relaxing influence over the muscular system possessed by tobacco, suggested the employment of this remedy in tetanus.   Its effects have been, like those of most other medicines in this disease, unequal.   Sir J. Macgrigor[4] says that in the advanced stage of the malady the tobacco clyster had no effect.   Mr. Earle,[5] however, thought it afforded temporary alleviation in a case in which he tried it.   Since then, several cases have been successfully treated by tobacco.   Dr. O'Beirne[6] obtained most marked relief by its use.   He employed it in the form of clyster (containing a scruple of tobacco), which was repeated once or thrice or oftener daily during eighteen days: and it was observed that if by design or accident the remedy was discontinued, the spasms recurred with force.   Mr. Anderson[7] employed a decoction of the fresh leaves in the form of enema, and both with good effect. Mr. Curling[8] has collected accounts of nineteen cases (including those of Earle, O'Beirne, and Anderson, above referred to) treated by tobacco: of these, nine recovered; and in seven of the fatal cases the remedy had not a fair

---

[1] *Dublin Hospital Reports*, vol. iv.
[2] *Med.-Chir. Trans.* vol. vi. p. 82.
[3] Fowler, *Med. Rep. of the Effects of Tobacco*, 1785.
[4] *Med.-Chir. Trans.* vol. vi. p. 456.
[5] *Ibid.* p. 92.
[6] *Dublin Hospital Reports*, vol. iii.
[7] *Edinb. Med.-Chir. Trans.* vols. i. and ii.
[8] *Treatise on Tetanus*, p. 168, 1836.

trial; while in the eighth, organic disease of the brain was found. Mr. Curling observes, that "more has now been advanced in proof of the efficacy of tobacco than can be adduced in favour of any other remedy yet resorted to. I have not," he adds, "succeeded in finding a single case in which, being fully and fairly tried before the constitution had given way, it has been known to fail."[1]

4. *Other spasmodic diseases.*—The success attending the use of tobacco in tetanus has led to its employment in *hydrophobia,* but hitherto without avail. In a case of periodical *epilepsy,* Dr. Currie[2] prevented the return of the disease by the application of a tobacco cataplasm to the scrobiculus cordis half an hour before the expected paroxysm. In a very bad case of *spasm of the rima glottidis,* which resisted powerful depletion by the lancet, Dr. Wood[3] applied with success a tobacco cataplasm to the throat. In *spasmodic asthma,* tobacco, either smoked or taken internally, in nauseating doses, has been found occasionally to give relief. My own observation is unfavourable to the use of tobacco smoke, which I have repeatedly found to bring on convulsive cough and spasmodic difficulty of breathing in persons afflicted with chronic catarrh. Dr. Sigmond[4] says the tincture of tobacco has been sold and used to a great extent under the name of tincture of lobelia, and that it had proved successful in spasmodic asthma. In *rigidity of the os uteri,* a tobacco clyster failed to produce relaxation, while it caused alarming constitutional symptoms.[5]

5. *In dropsy.*—Tobacco was recommended as a diuretic in dropsy by Dr. Fowler,[6] who published a number of cases of anasarca and ascites which had been relieved by it.[7]   Whatever benefit may have been obtained, in these cases, by the use of tobacco, should be ascribed, I suspect, rather to the sedative powers of this agent than to its influence over the kidneys. In small doses it is an uncertain diuretic, and in large doses it causes such distressing nausea and depression, that practitioners have long since ceased to use it in dropsical cases. The ashes of the tobacco plant have also been used in dropsy.[8]

6. *As a topical remedy.*—Dr. Vetch[9] recommends the infusion as an anodyne and sedative topical application, in gouty and rheumatic inflammation of the joints, testicle, and sclerotic coat of the eye, and in erysipelatous inflammation. Bergius[10] recommends a fomentation of tobacco leaves in phymosis and paraphymosis. An infusion or ointment of tobacco has been used in porrigo and other skin diseases, as well as in some obstinate ulcers. The smoke, applied to the hair, is a popular means of destroying pediculi, and has been used, in the form of clyster, to destroy ascarides. Dr. Sigmond[11] says tobacco promotes the growth of the hair. Toothache has been relieved by tobacco smoke.

---

[1] *Op. cit.* p. 117.
[2] *Med. Rep.* vol. i. p. 163.
[3] *United States Dispensatory.*
[4] *Lancet* for 1836-7, vol. ii. p. 253–4.
[5] Dr. Dewees, *Comp. Syst. of Midwif.* p. 378, 1825.
[6] *Op. supra cit.*
[7] See also Garnett, in Duncan's *Med. Comment.* for 1797, Dec. 11, vol. vi.
[8] Garden, in Duncan's *Med. Comment.* Dec. 1, vol. iii.
[9] *Med.-Chir. Trans.* vol. xvi. p. 356.
[10] *Mat. Med.* i. 222.
[11] *Lancet,* vol. ii. p. 249, 1836–7.

In addition to the preceding, there are various other diseases against which tobacco has been employed. Thus in *soporose affections* and *asphyxia* tobacco clysters have been employed; but they are more likely to do harm than good. Tobacco has also been used as an *anthelmintic.*

ADMINISTRATION.—Tobacco is rarely administered *in substance.* Five or six grains of snuff have been taken as an emetic, and are said to have operated as effectually as two grains of emetic tartar. For internal administration the *wine of tobacco* is generally employed. Dr. Fowler used an *infusion* (prepared with an ounce of Virginian tobacco to a pound of boiling water), which he gave in doses of from sixty to a hundred drops. The best time for administering it he found to be two hours before dinner, and at bed-time. The usual *tobacco enema* is the infusion prepared according to the Pharmacopœia. The *tobacco-smoke clyster* (*clyster e fumo tabaci*) is applied by means of a proper apparatus, formerly kept by the instrument-makers. Various extemporaneous methods of employing it have been devised.[1] For external use tobacco is used in the form of *cataplasm* (made of the leaves and water and vinegar), *infusion* (the *tobacco water* of the shops), *smoke,* and *ointment :* all these, however, require great caution in their use, especially when applied to abraded surfaces.

ANTIDOTES.—If the poison have been swallowed, let the contents of the stomach be withdrawn as speedily as possible, No chemical antidote has as yet been demonstrated; but the vegetable astringents (infusion of nutgalls, or green tea), deserve examination. As anti-narcotics, the vegetable acids and coffee may be administered. The other parts of the treatment must be adapted to circumstances. When the depression of the vascular system is extreme, ammonia and brandy may be administered with good effect, and frictions employed : even acupuncture of the heart (!) has been suggested.[2] Artificial respiration should not be omitted when other means have failed. If apoplectic symptoms present themselves, blood-letting may, perhaps, be requisite, as in the case related by Dr. M. Hall.

1. ENEMA TABACI, L. E. D. ; *Tobacco Clyster.* (Tobacco, Əj. *L. D* [grs. xv. to ʒss. *E.*] ; Boiling Water, Oss. [f℥viij. *E. D.*] Macerate for an hour [half an hour, *E.*], and strain.)—The want of uniformity in the formulæ of the British Colleges is greatly to be regretted ; and I cannot but think that the latitude permitted by the Edinburgh College, in the quantity of tobacco employed, is highly objectionable, and calculated to lead to serious errors in dispensing. The tobacco clyster is used, as I have already stated, in ileus (volvulus), strangulated hernia, obstinate constipation, and retention of urine. It is not to be forgotten that two drachms, one drachm, and even half a drachm of tobacco infused in water, have proved fatal, as I have before mentioned. The cautious practitioner, therefore, will not use more than 15 or 20 grains. [The United States Pharmacopœia has the old formula of the London College ; namely, ʒj. of tobacco to Oj. of boiling water.—ED.]

2. VINUM TABACI, E. U.S.; *Wine of Tobacco.* (Tobacco, ℥iiiss.; Sherry,

---

[1] Murray, *App. Med.* t. i.
[2] Stephenson and Churchill, *Med. Bot.*

Oij. Digest for seven days, strain, express strongly the residuum, and filter the liquors. [The United States Pharmacopœia directs Tobacco, ℥j.; Wine, Oj. Digest for fourteen days, and filter.—ED.])—Sedative and diuretic. Employed in dropsy and dysury. Rarely used. Dose, from ♏x. to ♏l.

3. UNGUENTUM TABACI, Ph. United States; *Ointment of Tobacco.* (Fresh Tobacco, cut in pieces, ℥j.; Lard, lb. j. Boil the tobacco in the lard, over a gentle fire, until it becomes friable; then strain through linen.)—Employed as an application to irritable ulcers and skin diseases, especially tinea capitis; but its use requires great caution.

An *ointment,* prepared with twenty drops of the empyreumatic oil of tobacco and an ounce of simple ointment, has been applied with advantage, by American practitioners, to indolent tumours and ulcers; but, like all other preparations of tobacco, when employed externally it must be used with great caution."[1]

181. SOLANUM TUBEROSUM, *Linn.*—COMMON POTATO.

Sex. Syst. Pentandria, Monogynia.

(Herba; Tuber.)

HISTORY.—Pedro de Cieça, in his *Chronica del Peru,* published at Seville in 1553, is the first writer who mentions potatoes. They probably first came into Europe from the neighbourhood of Quito to Spain. In 1586 they were brought to England from Virginia by the colonists sent out by Sir Walter Raleigh in 1584.

BOTANY. **Gen. Char.**—*Calyx* 5-10 cleft. *Corolla* hypogynous, rotate or rarely campanulate; tube short; limb plaited, 5-10-, rarely 4-6-cleft. *Stamens* 5, rarely 4 or 6, inserted in the throat of the corolla, exserted; filaments very short; anthers equal or sometimes unequal, converging, dehiscing by two pores at the apex. *Ovary* 2-, rarely 3-4-celled; the placentæ attached to the dissepiments, adnate, with numerous ovules. *Style* simple; *stigma* obtuse. *Berry* 2-, rarely 3-4-celled. *Seeds* numerous, subreniform. *Embryo* peripherical, spiral, inclosing fleshy albumen (*Endlicher*).

Sp. Char.—Tuberous. Stem herbaceous. Leaves interruptedly pinnate, downy; leaflets entire. Pedicels articulated. Flowers white.

Hab.—West coast of South America. Cultivated everywhere.

The cultivated varieties of the potato are very numerous. They are distinguished according to their precocity, lateness, form, size, colour, and quality.

DESCRIPTION.—1. The part of the plant which is used as food is the *tuber* (*tuber solani tuberosi*) attached to the subterranean stem, of which, in fact, it may be regarded as a part in a state of excessive development. It is provided with a number of buds, commonly called *eyes,* which, with contiguous portions of the potatoes, are used, under the name of *sets,* for multiplying the species.

---

[1] *United States Dispensatory.*

The tubers vary in shape; being round, oblong, or kidney-shaped. When boiled, they vary in quality; being watery, waxy, or mealy. When examined by the microscope, the tissue of the potato is found to consist of a mass of cells, between and within which is an albuminous juice. Each cell also contains about ten or twelve starch grains[1] (fig. 309, *a*). By boiling,the cells are separated, the starch grains absorb the albuminous liquid, swell up, and completely fill the cells; while the albumen coagulates and forms irregular fibres, which are placed between the starch grains (fig. 309, *b*). Potatoes in which these changes are complete are called *mealy*, while those in which the liquid is only partially absorbed, and the coagulation imperfectly effected, are denominated *doughy* or *watery*.[2] By boiling in water, potatoes do not form a jelly or mucilage like mere starch, because the starch grains in the tubers are protected partly by the coats of the cells in which they are contained, and partly by a layer of coagulated albumen.

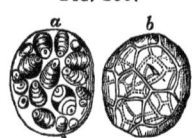

FIG. 183.

Cells of the Potatoes.

a. Cell before boiling, containing the starch particles.
b. Cell of a mealy potato after boiling.

2. For medicinal purposes the *herb* (*herba solani tuberosi*), including both stems and leaves, has been employed.

COMPOSITION. — Potatoes have been repeatedly subjected to chemical examination. The following are the results of analyses made by Michaelis[3] and by Johnston.[4]

(*Michaelis.*)	Natural.	MEAN OF NUMEROUS ANALYSES MADE IN 1846.		
		(*Johnston.*)		
			Natural.	Dry.
Water	66·875	Water	75·52 ...	—
Starch and amylaceous fibre..............	30·469	Starch	15·72 ...	64·20
Albumen	0·503	Dextrin (gum)	0.55 ...	2·25
Gluten	0·055	Sugar	3·30 ...	13·47
Fat	0·056	Albumen, casein, gluten ...	1·41 ...	5·77
Gum...	0·020	Fat	0·24 ...	1·00
Asparagin..................................	0·063	Fibre...........................	3·26 ...	13·31
Extractive	0·921			
Chloride of potassium	0·176			
Silicate, phosphate, and citrate of iron, manganese, alumina, soda, potash, and lime (of these potash and citric acid are the prevailing ingredients)	0·815			
Free citric acid.................	0·047			
Red variety of potato ....100·000		100·00 ... 100·00		

As a portion of both albumen and gluten adheres to the fibre, and of both, with some of the casein, to the starch, the true per-centage of protein matters is somewhat understated in the above table; and Johnston, therefore, gives the following as the representation, in round numbers, of the composition of the dry potato : *starch* 64, *sugar and gum* 15, *protein compounds* 9, *fat* 1, and *fibre* 11. The proportion of water, starch, and protein matters in

---

[1] See Turpin's *Mémoire sur l'Organisation intérieure et extérieure des tubercles du Solanum tuberosum*, in the *Mémoires du Muséum d'Hist. Naturelle*, t. xix. Paris, 1830.

[2] Fritzsche, in Poggendorff's *Ann. d. Phys. u. Chem.* Bd. xxxii. S. 159; and *Pharm. Central-Blatt für* 1834, pp. 927 and 943.

[3] *Archiv d. Pharm.* xiii. 233 ; and *Pharm. Central-Blatt für* 1838.

[4] *Lectures on Agricultural Chemistry*, 2d edit. p. 906, 1847.

the potato, according to the investigations of Horsford and Krocker,[1] have been already given.

The ultimate composition of the potato, according to Boussingault,[2] is as follows :—

	Natural.		Dry.
Water	75·9	Carbon	44·0
Solid matter, viz. :—		Hydrogen	5·8
Carbon	10·6040 ⎫	Oxygen	44·7
Hydrogen	1·3978 ⎪	Nitrogen	1·5
Oxygen	10·7727 ⎬ 2·41	Ashes	4·0
Nitrogen	0·3615 ⎪		
Ashes	0·9640 ⎭		
	100·0		100·0

Baup,[3] Spatzier,[4] and Otto,[5] have found solanina in potatoes.

1. SOLANINA; *Solanine; Potato-Solanin.*—Found chiefly in the buds and shoots (sprouts) of the potato; also in the leaves, stalks, and fruits. Even sound ripe potatoes (the tubers) contain traces of it; but diseased potatoes, according to Liebig,[6] do not yield it. (For the properties of *Solanina,* see *Solanum Dulcamara.*)

2. STARCH (see p. 588).

3. PROTEINE COMPOUNDS; *Albumen, Gluten,* and *Casein.*—The juice of the potato coagulates when heated, owing to the albumen which it contains. If the washings of a grated potato be heated to coagulate the albumen, and a little acetic acid be added to the strained liquor when cold, a white substance, called casein, is precipitated. If dry potato in powder be boiled in alcohol, the solution evaporated, and water added to it, a substance resembling the gluten of wheat is obtained. In potatoes which have been kept for some time the proportion of proteine matters is diminished.—In diseased potatoes the proteine compounds appear to be the constituents chiefly affected: the albumen is diminished in quantity and altered in quality, becoming dark, especially on coagulating; while, according to Liebig, the casein is augmented in quantity.

4. FAT.—Ether extracts from dried sliced potatoes a minute portion of fatty matter.

5. GUM (*Dextrine*) and SUGAR.—Healthy potatoes contain small portions of that variety of gum called dextrine, and also of sugar. When the quantity of these ingredients is unusually large, as in diseased potatoes, the quantity of starch is proportionately small.

6. CELLULOSE; *Fibre; Lignin.*—The proportion of this constituent of the potato is subject to great variation. As usually obtained, it contains some adherent starch and proteine matters: hence the nutritive qualities of the pulp of potato mills, which is used for feeding cattle.

7. ACIDS and SALTS.—The vegetable acid which exists in potatoes, and which several chemists[7] have declared to be citric acid, is, according to Ilisch, *malic acid.*[8] He also detected *phosphoric* and *hydrochloric acids.* By the microscope crystals of *oxalate of lime* can be detected.[9]

The quantity of ash obtained by drying and burning the potato varies from 0·76 to 1·58 of the weight of the potato in the natural state. It consists, in large proportion, of *potash* salts, with some *soda* and *lime* salts. These bases are combined with carbonic acid (produced by the decomposition of the malic and oxalic acids), phosphoric acid, sulphuric acid (formed by the oxidation of the sulphur of the proteine matters), and hydrochloric acid.

---

[1] *Ann. der Chemie u. Pharm.* Bd. xlviii. 1846.

[2] *Ann. de Chimie et Physique.*

[3] *Ann. de Chimie,* 1826.

[4] Buchner's *Repert.* Bd. xxxix. p. 480, 1831.

[5] *Journ. für prakt. Chemie,* Bd. i. p. 58; and Buchner's *Repert.* Bd. xlviii. p. 336, 1834.

[6] *Pharmaceutical Journal,* vol. v. p. 263, 1845.

[7] Baup (Buchner's *Repert.* 2te Reihe, Bd. iii. p. 390, 1835) says that the potato yields sufficient citric acid to admit of its being employed for the preparation of this acid for commercial purposes. He also states that he found succinic acid and a new acid, which he calls *solano-tuberic acid,* in potatoes.

[8] *Annal. der Chem. u. Pharm.* Bd. li. p. 246, 1844.

[9] Johnston's *Lectures on Agricultural Chemistry,* 2d edit. p. 905, 1847.

DISEASES OF THE POTATO.—The potato is subject to various diseases, the chief of which are the *curl*, the *scab*, and two sorts of *rot*—one called the *dry rot*, the other the *wet rot*.   Martius[1] mentions two other maladies also ; namely, the *rust* and the *blue pock ;* but they are imperfectly known.   The disease, called the *potato murrain* or *potato blight*, which recently raged epidemically among the potatoes of Europe and America,[2] was a kind of rot, usually of the humid or wet kind.   The cause of this, as of the other maladies of the potato, is very obscure.[3]

The *scab* (*porrigo tuberum solani*) is characterised by the surfaces of the tubers be-coming " covered with pustules, which at length become cup-shaped, and are powdered within with an olive-yellow meal, consisting of the spores of a fungus," which Martius calls *Protomyces Tuberum Solani*, but which Mr. Berkeley terms *Tuburcinia Scabies* (Sub-order Hyphomycetes,—see *ante*, p. 38).

In the *dry rot* (*gangræna sicca tuberum solani*) "the tubers, when stored for winter use, or when planted, become impregnated with a kind of mould, and are at length so hard that they can scarcely be broken, and, instead of producing shoots, merely throw out a few small misshapen tubers." In 1830 this disease was first noticed in Germany. Martius ascribes it to the growth of a peculiar fungus, the *Fusisporium Solani* (Sub-order Hyphomycetes,—see *ante*, p. 38).

The *wet rot* (*gangræna humida tuberum solani*) differs from the preceding in the circum-stance that the tubers become soft instead of hard ; and parasitic fungi, referred by Fries to his genus *Periola* (Sub-order Gasteromycetes,—see *ante*, p. 49), appear, for the most part, under the form of hemispherical masses bursting through the cuticle.

The *potato murrain*, or *potato blight*, commonly called the *potato disease*, is closely allied to, if it be not identical with, the rot,—usually the wet rot.   But according to Mr. Berkeley it is characterised by the presence of *Botrytis infestans* (Sub-order Hyphomy-cetes,—see *ante*, p. 38.)   The malady commences in the leaves, and extends from thence by the stems to the tubers.   Both on the inferior surface of the leaves and in the tubers a peculiar fungus has been discovered, called by Dr. Montagne the *Botrytis infestans*, which has been very fully described and figured by Mr. Berkeley.—The malady seems to affect chiefly the proteine constituents of the potato.   Liebig[4] states that a part of the vegetable albumen which usually prevails in the potato has become converted into casein. The starch appears to be unaltered in quality.

PHYSIOLOGICAL EFFECTS.   1. *Of the herb.*—An extract obtained from the stalks and leaves of the potatoes was declared by Dr. J. Latham[5] to possess narcotic properties in doses of two or three grains ; but the cases adduced are not satisfactory.   Furthermore, his experiments were repeated by Dr. Worsham[6] with very different results, for 100 grains produced no sensible effects.   The observations of Nauche,[7] however, tend to confirm Latham's statements.

2. *Of the tubers.*—Potatoes, when in good condition, and cooked by

---

[1] *Die Kartoffel-Epidemie der letzten Jahre oder die Stockfäule und Räude der Kartoffeln, geschildert und in ihren ursachlichen Verhältnissen erörtert,* von Dr. C. Fr. Ph. v. Martius, München, 1842.

[2] The first notice of the disease in England was by Dr. Bell Salter, in the *Gardener's Chronicle*, Aug. 16, 1845.

[3] The fungal hypothesis of the potato blight has been ably advocated by Mr. Berkeley in a paper entitled *Observations, Botanical and Physiological, on the Potato Murrain,* published in the *Journal of the Horticultural Society*, vol. i. p. 9, 1846.   Most authors ascribe the disease to peculiar atmospherical or meteorological conditions.   Mr. Smee (*The Potato Plant, its Uses and Properties, together with the Cause of the Present Malady,* 1846) attributes it to an animal parasite, the *Aphis vastator,*—a species of hemipterous insect, which punctures the leaf, sucks the sap, and thus, by exhausting the plant, causes the death of the leaf or of some other part.

[4] *Pharmaceutical Journal,* vol. v. p. 263, 1845.

[5] *Med. Trans.* vol. i. p. 92.

[6] *United States Dispensatory.*

[7] Nauche, *Journ. de Chim. Méd.* t. vii. p. 373.

boiling, form a nutritious and easily digestible article of food. The starch, sugar, gum (dextrine), and fat, serve for the production of fatty matters, sugar, lactic acid, and, by combustion, of heat and carbonic acid. The proteine matters (albumen, gluten, and casein) are plastic elements of nutrition, and serve for the production of fibrinous, albuminous, and gelatigenous tissues. According to Gunsford, the non-digestible constituents of the potato, which he found in the excrements, are the cellular, fibrous, and vascular tissues, with which some undigested starch grains were intermixed. Potatoes are valuable antiscorbutics. Sir G. Blane, Julia Fontanelle, Nauche, Dr. Baly, and others, have testified to their valuable preservative qualities against scurvy.[1] These have been ascribed to the vegetable acids contained in the tubers; but Dr. Garrod attributes them to the presence of a large quantity of potash.

From an experiment made at the Glasgow Bridewell, it would appear that baked potatoes are less nourishing than boiled ones.

The process of cooking potatoes is useful in two ways; by effecting changes in the nutritive principles (e. g. rendering the starch digestible), and by extracting some noxious matter (solanina). The water in which potatoes are boiled possesses some noxious properties: Nauche found that it augmented the renal and biliary secretions, and slightly affected the nervous system.

Uses. 1. Of the herb.—The extract has been used as a narcotic and antispasmodic to allay cough, spasm, rheumatic pains, &c. The dose is from one-eighth to half a grain.

2. Of the tubers.—Scraped potato is a popular application to burns and scalds. Boiled potatoes have been used for the formation of emollient poultices. They have been recommended as an antidote for poisoning by iodine: but on what principle it is difficult to understand. For dietetical purposes potatoes are valuable anti-scorbutics. In diabetes, however, they are objectionable on account of the large quantity of starch which they contain. But bread made of potato and cellulose (rasped potatoes deprived, by washing, of starch) has been employed as a *bread for diabetic patients*.[2]

Potatoes are used by bakers in the preparation of the ordinary loaf bread of London. [The dried pulp has been largely employed as an article for exportation. When mixed with from two to three parts of water it is softened: it swells into a pulp, and forms a palatable article of food.—Ed.]

1. AMYLUM SOLANI TUBEROSI; *Potato Starch.*—Obtained by washing potatoes, then rasping or grinding them to a pulp, and repeatedly washing the latter with water. The washings are strained through a sieve to separate the fibre or cellular tissue, and then allowed to stand at rest, by which the starch is deposited, and is afterwards washed and dried. The quantity of starch yielded by potatoes varies with the variety or sort, the soil, the climate, and the season. Payen found the same variety of potato to yield, in October, 17·2 per cent. of starch; in November, 16·8; in December, 15·6; in January,

---

[1] See my *Treatise on Food and Diet*, 1843.
[2] Percy, *Chemical Gazette*, vol. vii. p. 119, 1849.—The following is Mr. Palmer's receipt for making this bread: "Take the ligneous matter of 16 lbs. of potatoes washed free from starch, ¾ lb. of mutton suet, ½ lb. of butter, 12 eggs, ½ oz. of carbonate of soda, and 2 oz. of dilute hydrochloric acid. This quantity to be divided into eight cakes, and in a quick oven baked until nicely browned." Care must be taken to procure pure hydrochloric acid, as some commercial sorts contain arsenic.— This bread may be regarded as a substitute for the *bran bread* already described.

15·5 ; in February, 15·2 ; in March, 15·0 ; and in April, 14·5. In general the centre of the potato yields the smallest portion, the heel end which is attached to the rootlet the most, and the rose or upper end an intermediate portion of starch.

Potato starch is white and pulverulent, and, on account of the large size of its particles,[1] has a satiny or glistening character. The smaller grains are circular or globular; the larger ones elliptical, oblong, ovate, or obtusely triangular. Frequently their shape is irregular, and approximates to that of an oyster-shell, or a mussel-shell. Their nucleus, central cavity, or hilum, is very distinct; and their laminated structure is indicated by a system of concentric or excentric rings or zones surrounding the nucleus. It is most allied in appearance to the starches of Marantaceæ. The characters by which they are distinguished from West Indian arrow-root and from tous-les-mois have been already pointed out. The mode of distinguishing potato starch from wheat starch has likewise been stated (see WHEAT STARCH).

In its general chemical properties potato starch agrees with other starchy bodies. In cold water it is insoluble. If 1 part of potato starch be mixed with 15 parts of water, and heated, the liquid begins to be thick and mucilaginous at about 140° F. ; and as the heat augments, especially from 162° F. to 212° F., it acquires a pasty or gelatinous consistence. Starch-paste or starch mucilage is not, however, a true solution of starch in water : the starch grains are burst and exfoliated, the coats or laminæ being hydrated and enormously swollen. In cold water to which a small quantity of caustic potash or soda has been added, they become enormously swollen. Starch-mucilage in the cold becomes intensely blue on the addition of iodine : the colour is destroyed by heat, caustic alkalies, corrosive sublimate, sulphurous acid, and other reagents.

The greater facility with which potato starch gelatinises when rubbed in a mortar with a mixture of equal parts of commercial hydrochloric acid and water ;[2] the strong smell of formic acid emitted when it is rubbed with hydrochloric acid ; the dove-grey colour which it assumes when exposed to the vapour of iodine ;[3] and the transparency of the mucilage which it forms with boiling water (whence it has been termed *soluble starch*,),—are characters by which it has been attempted to distinguish potato starch from other sorts of starch, but with no great success, as they are not to be relied on.

Potato starch, in the pure or anhydrous state, consists of $C^{12}H^9O^9$: but, as found in commerce, it contains water.

COMPOSITION OF POTATO STARCH.

Anhydrous starch (as combined with oxide of lead)	$= C^{12}H^9O^9$
Starch dried in a vacuum at from 212° to 248° F.	$= C^{12}H^9O^9,HO$
Starch dried in a vacuum at 68° F.	$= C^{12}H^9O^9,3HO$
Starch air-dried at 68° F. (hygr. 0·5)	$= C^{12}H^9O^9,5HO$
Starch dried in air saturated with humidity	$= C^{12}H^9O^9,11HO$
Starch drained as much as possible	$= C^{12}H^9O^9,16HO$

---

[1] The following measurements, in parts of an English inch, of ten particles of potato starch, were made for me by Mr. George Jackson :—

Length.	Breadth.		Length.	Breadth.		Length.	Breadth.
1. ...... 0·0023	× 0·0016	4. ...... 0·0011	× 0·0009	7. ...... 0·0005	× 0·0005
2. ...... 0·0021	× 0·0014	5. ...... 0·0009	× 0·0007	8. ...... 0·0004	× 0·0004
3. ...... 0·0018	× 0·0013	6. ...... 0·0007	× 0·0006	9. ...... 0·0003	× 0·0003
					10. ...... 0·0002	× 0·0002

[2] Scharling, *Pharm. Journ.* vol. ii. p. 417, 1842.

[3] Gobley, *Journ. d. Pharm.* sér. 3me, t. v. p. 299, 1844.

Potato starch is sometimes adulterated. M. Dietrich[1] mentions having received some which was adulterated to the extent of 50 per cent. with comminuted fibre, and which prevented the employment of the starch in the fabrication of yeast for a distillery.

Potato starch possesses the alimentary properties of other starchy substances. It does not, however, yield so firm a jelly as some other starches, and has been said to be apt to occasion acidity, especially in infants. It is sold under the various names of *potato flour, English arrow-root, Bright's nutritious farina,* &c.; and is used as a farinaceous food for infants and invalids, as well as for the preparation of puddings and soufflés, and, as a thickening ingredient, in gravies and sauces.

Potato starch is used in the production of a factitious sago (see SAGO, p. 148), in the preparation of dextrine, and in the manufacture of *potato sugar* (see *ante*, p. 129).

2. DEXTRINA ; *Dextrine ; Dextrinum ; Starch-gum.* Formula $C^{12}H^9O^9,HO.$—This substance is called " dextrine" from its property of rotating to the right a ray of plane polarised light. There are three modes of procuring it from starch ; viz. by torrefaction, by the action of dilute acids (usually nitric acid), and by the action of diastase. The impure dextrine obtained by torrefying or roasting starch is termed *roasted starch,* or *leicomme* (from λεῖος, *smooth ;* and *gomme,* the French name for gum !). This sort of dextrine resembles British gum, is pulverulent, and has the aspect of starch, but it usually possesses a yellowish tint in consequence of being over-roasted. A second method consists in moistening 1000 parts of potato starch with 300 parts of water to which 2 parts of nitric acid have been added. The mixture is to be allowed to dry spontaneously, and is afterwards heated, for one or two hours, in a stove at 212° F. or 230° F : the transformation is then complete.

Dextrine is soluble in water and in dilute spirit, but is insoluble in alcohol. Its solution is perfectly limpid ; and, by concentration and solidification, it is obtained in an amorphous form like gum arabic. It is sometimes made up in tear-like masses in imitation of gum arabic, and in this state is called *artificial gum.* This, when fresh, has an odour like that of a cucumber ; but, by keeping, I find that it loses this smell. The solution of dextrine yields with acetate of lead a precipitate (*dextrinate of lead*). As usually found in the shops, the solution strikes a violet or reddish tint with iodine ; but in this case the starch has been incompletely converted into dextrine, which, when pure, is not coloured by iodine.[2]

Dextrine in many of its characters resembles ordinary gum ; from which, however, it is distinguished by its right-handed rotation of a ray of plane polarised light, and by its yielding oxalic acid, but not mucic acid, when heated with nitric acid. Saccharine matter, when mixed with dextrine, may be separated by strong spirit, which more readily dissolves sugar than dextrine. The freedom of dextrine from starch is readily shown by the iodine test.[3]

Dextrine is used in the arts as a substitute for gum, size, and paste. The

---

[1] *Chemical Gazette,* vol. ii. p. 20, 1844.

[2] [All the samples of dextrine which we have examined have assumed a wine red colour on the addition of iodine water to their solutions.— ED.]

[3] [Starch strikes a rich blue colour, dextrine a wine red, while gum and sugar are unchanged by iodine.—ED.]

saccharine solution of dextrine obtained by the action of diastase (contained in the infusion of malt) on potato starch is used in Paris in the manufacture of *pains de luxe*, and for the fabrication of beer and other alcoholic liquors. In medicine, dextrine is employed as a nutritient, as an emollient, and as an agglutinant.   In the French hospitals it is used in *tisanes* as a substitute for gum.   Devergie has employed it with benefit in the treatment of eczema. Velpeau has employed dextrine, as a substitute for gum arabic or starch, in the preparation of bandages for maintaining the reduction of fractures by what is called "the immoveable apparatus." For this purpose 100 parts of dextrine are moistened first with a small quantity of spirit of camphor, and then mixed with 40 parts of water. The bandages are soaked in the thick mucilage thus obtained.[1]

182. SOLANUM DULCAMARA, *Linn.*—WOODY NIGHT-SHADE ; BITTERSWEET.

Sex. Syst. Pentandria, Monogynia.

(Ramus novellus, *L.*—The twigs, *E. D.*)

HISTORY.—Fraas[2] declares this plant to be the στρύχνος ὑπνωτικός of Dioscorides (lib. iv. cap. 73).   Sprengel[3] considers it to be the *Citocatia* of the Abbess Hildegard, of Bingen, who died A. D. 1180.   But the derivation of the word Citocatia (*cito* and *cacare*) negatives, in my opinion, this suppo- sition.   The first undoubted notice of Dulcamara occurs in the work of Tragus.[4]

BOTANY.   **Gen. Char.**—See *ante*, p. 584.

Sp. Char.—Stem shrubby, zigzag.   Leaves cordate-ovate ; upper ones auriculate-hastate.   Flowers drooping (*Babington*).

Root woody.   *Stem* twining, branched, rising (when supported) to the height of many feet.   *Leaves* acute, generally smooth ; the lower ones ovate or heart-shaped ; upper, more or less perfectly halbert-shaped ; all entire at the margin.   *Clusters* either opposite to the leaves or terminal, drooping, spreading, smooth, alternately subdivided.   *Bracts* minute.   *Flowers* elegant, purple, with two round green spots at the base of each segment.   *Berries* oval, scarlet, juicy.

Hab.—Indigenous.   In hedges and thickets, especially in watery situations. Flowers in June and July.

Var. *β tomentosum*, Koch.—Stem round, almost glabrous throughout.—Woods and hedges ; common.

Var. *γ marinum*, Babington ; *S. lignosum* seu *Dulcamara marina*, Ray.—Branches of the present year, and leaves fleshy and usually clothed with hairs incurved upwards.   Stem angular, prostrate, diffuse, much branched.   Leaves all (?) cordate, not hastate.—Pebbly sea beach.   Renville, Cunnamara, Galway ; Lizard Point, Cornwall ; Shoreham, Sussex (glabrous).

DESCRIPTION.—The annual stems (*caules* seu *stipites dulcamaræ*) are

---

[1] Mr. Smee (*London Medical Gazette*, N.S. vol. i. Feb. 23, 1839), in his paper " *On the Forma- tion of Moulding Tablets for Fractures*," says that " a mixture of carbonate of lime with the solu- tion of dextrine made a composition which answered very well," but it was not equal to a composition of gum and whiting.   [Whiting is nothing more than carbonate of lime.—ED.]

[2] *Synopsis Plant. Fl. Classicæ*, p. 168, 1845.

[3] *Hist. Rei Herb.* vol. i. p. 227.

[4] Sprengel, *op. cit.* p. 319.

collected in the autumn, after the leaves have fallen.   When fresh, they have an unpleasant odour, which they lose by drying.   Their taste is at first bitter, afterwards slightly acrid and sweet.   The epidermis is greenish-gray, the wood light, and the pith very light and spongy.

COMPOSITION.—The stems have been analysed by Pfaff.[1]   100 parts of the air-dried stems lost 17·4 parts of water when completely dried.   From 100 parts of perfectly dried stems Pfaff obtained *bittersweet extractive (picroglycion)* 21·817, *vegeto-animal matter* 3·125, *gummy extractive* 12·029, *gluten with green wax* 1·4, *resin containing benzoic acid* 2·74, *gummy extractive, starch, sulphate* and *vegetable salts of lime,* 2·0, *oxalate* and *phosphate of lime with extractive* 4·0, and *woody fibre* 62·0 (excess 9·111). Desfosses[2] discovered *solanina* in the stems.

1. DULCAMARIN; *Picroglycion,* Pfaff; *Dulcarin,* Defosses.—Crystalline; has both a bitter and a sweet taste, is fusible, soluble in water, alcohol, and acetic ether, and is not precipitated from its solution by either infusion of nutgalls or metallic salts.[3]   Pelletier[4] thinks that it is sugar combined with solanina   +

2. SOLANINA; *Solania; Solanine.*   Symbol So.   Formula $C^{84}H^{68}NO^{28}$.   Eq. Weight. 810 ?—This alkaloid has been discovered in several species of Solanum; viz. S. Dulcamara, S. tuberosum, S. nigrum, and S. verbascifolium.   It resembles sulphate of quina, but its needle-like crystals are finer and shorter.   It restores the blue colour of litmus paper reddened by an acid.   It dissolves in acids, and is precipitated from its solution by the caustic alkalies.   Some of the salts (as the acetate and hydrochlorate) have a gummy appearance when evaporated to dryness; others (as the phosphate and sulphate) are crystallisable.   Iodine strikes a characteristic turbid brown colour with a solution of solanina or of its salts, owing to the formation of the insoluble brown iodide of solanina.[5] If Blanchet's analysis be correct, solanina differs from the other vegetable alkalies in the small quantity of nitrogen which it contains. and in its very high atomic weight.   A grain of solanina dissolved in dilute sulphuric acid killed a rabbit in six hours: four grains of the sulphate caused, in an hour, paralysis of the hind legs; and in eight hours, death.[6] Soubeiran says it does not dilate the pupils like the other alkalies of Solanaceæ.

CHEMICAL PROPERTIES.—A strong   decoction of dulcamara is slightly darkened by tincture of iodine.   Iodic acid had no effect on it.   Iodide of potassium rendered it feebly yellow.   Tincture of galls had no effect.

PHYSIOLOGICAL EFFECTS.—Not very obvious.   Its decoction operates as a diaphoretic and diuretic.   It is said also to promote secretion from the mucous surfaces, and to diminish sensibility.   In excessive doses, dulcamara is stated to have acted as an acro-narcotic.[7]   Chevallier[8] says a young man experienced narcotism from carrying a bundle of the plant on his head.   But the accuracy of all these observations has been called in question by Jos. Frank,[9] by Dunal, and by Fages.[10]   The first gave the decoction, the latter the extract and fruit, in very large doses, without any obvious effects.

USES.—Dulcamara has been thought serviceable in chronic pulmonary catarrhs, in rheumatic and gouty complaints, in chronic skin diseases, and in various cachectic conditions of the system, in which sarsaparilla has been

---

[1] *Syst. d. Mat. Med.* Bd. vi. S. 506.
[2] *Journ. de Pharm.* t. vii. p. 414.
[3] Soubeiran, *Traité de Pharm.* t. ii. p. 52.
[4] *Journ. de Pharm.* vii. 416.
[5] Baumann, *Pharmaceutical Journal,* vol. iii. p. 354, 1844.
[6] Otto, *Pharm. Central-Blatt für* 1834, p. 455.
[7] Murray, *App. Med.* t. i. p. 60; and Schlegel, Hufeland's *Journal,* Bd. liv. St. 2, S. 27.
[8] *Dict. des Drog.* t. ii. p. 228.
[9] *Handb. d. Toxicol.* S. 61, 1803.
[10] Orfila, *Toxicol. Gén.*

found beneficial. As a remedy for lepra, it was introduced to the notice of British practitioners by Dr. Crichton. For this disease it has been declared a most effectual remedy by Bateman ;[1] while Rayer[2] speaks of its good effects in eczema and psoriasis. In the few cases in which I have tried it, it proved useless.

DECOCTUM DULCAMARÆ, L. E. D.; *Decoction of Bittersweet.* (Stems of Woody Nightshade [Dulcamara, chopped down, *E.*], ʒx. [ʒj. *E.*] ; [Twigs of Woody Nightshade, ʒss. *D.*] ; Water [distilled, *L.*], Oiss. [fʒxxiv. *E.* ; Oss. *D*]. Boil down to a pint, and strain. Mix them, boil and concentrate by evaporation to fʒxvj. *E.* Boil for ten minutes in a covered vessel, and strain. The product should measure about ʒviij. *D.*)—Diaphoretic and diuretic. The usual dose stated in books is fʒss. to fʒj. But I have given fʒiv. for a dose. Rayer has given four ounces of the root in twenty-four hours.

183. Solanum nigrum, *Linn.*—Black Nightshade.

Sex. Syst. Pentandria, Monogynia.

(Herba.)

Στρύχνος κηπαῖος, Dioscorides (lib. iv. cap. 71) ; *Common* or *Garden Nightshade.*—Stem herbaceous, with tubercled angles ; a foot or more high. Leaves ovate, obtusely dentate or wavy, attenuated below. Flowers lateral, drooping, sometimes with a musky scent ; corolla white. Berries globular, black or rarely green when ripe.—Indigenous : waste grounds.—No complete analysis of it has been made. Desfosses[3] has found malate of solanina in the fruit. Black nightshade possesses narcotic properties, but its powers appear to be neither great nor uniform. Its emanations are said to be soporific; and in Bohemia a handful of the fresh plant is sometimes placed in the cradles of infants to promote sleep.[4] In England this plant has been employed as a resolvent.[5] Smith[6] says a grain or two of the dried leaf has sometimes been given to promote various secretions, possibly, he adds, by exciting a great and rather dangerous agitation in the viscera.

184. CAPSICUM ANNUUM, *Linn.* (FASTIGIATUM, *Ph. L.*) COMMON CAPSICUM OR CHILLY PEPPER.

Sex. Syst. Pentandria, Monogynia.

(Fructus, *L.*—Fruit of Capsicum annuum and other species ; Capsicum or Chillies, *E.*—The fruit, D.)

HISTORY.—The *piperitis* or *siliquastrum* of Pliny[7] is declared by Sprengel[8] to be undoubtedly Capsicum annuum. But confidence in this opinion is greatly diminished by the doubt entertained as to this plant being a native of Asia.[9] Of course, if it be exclusively a native of America, there is no reason

---

[1] *Synopsis of Cutaneous Diseases.*
[2] *Treatise on Diseases of the Skin,* by Dr. Willis, p. 91.
[3] *Journ. de Pharm.* t. vii. p. 414, 1821.
[4] Weitenweber, quoted by Dierbach, *Die neuesten Entdeck. in d. Mat. Med.* Bd. ii. p. 907, 1843.
[5] Gataker, *Obs. on the Use of Solanum,* 1757 ; Bromfield, *Account of the Engl. Nightshades,* 1757.
[6] *English Flora,* vol. i. p. 318, 1824.
[7] *Hist. Nat.* lib. xix. cap. 62 ; and lib. xx. cap. 66, ed. Valp.
[8] *Hist. Rei Herb.* vol. i. p. 201.
[9] Roxburgh, *Fl. Ind.* vol. i. p. 573 ; Royle, *Illustr.* p. 27.

for supposing that Pliny could have been acquainted with it. Fraas[1] considers it to have been Capsicum longum DC., which Theophrastus[2] terms πέπερι ἀπόμηκες. The term capsicum (κάψικον) occurs first in Johannes Actuarius.

Botany. Gen. Char.—*Calyx* 5-6-cleft. *Corolla* hypogynous, rotate; tube very short; limb plaited, 5-6-cleft. *Stamens* 5-6, inserted in the throat of the corolla, exserted; filaments very short; anthers connivent, dehiscing longitudinally. *Ovary* 2-, 3-, 4-celled; the placentæ adnate to the base of the dissepiment or central angle. *Style* simple, subclavate; *stigma* obtuse, obsoletely 2-3-lobed. *Berry* juiceless, polymorphous, incompletely 2-3-celled, placentæ and septa deliquescent superiorly. *Seeds* many, reniform; embryo within fleshy albumen, peripherical, hemicyclical (*Endlicher*).

Sp. Char.—Fruit oblong, pendulous, and erect. Petioles glabrous. Stem herbaceous. Calyx obsoletely 5-toothed.

Herbaceous annual, 1 to 2 feet high. *Leaves* ovate or oblong, acuminate, long-stalked, almost entire, sometimes hairy on the veins underneath. *Flowers* white. *Berry* scarlet, yellow, variegated with red and yellow, or dark green; variable in shape, being oblong, round, or cordate.

Hab.—America. A doubtful native of the East Indies. Cultivated in England.

Description.—The dried fruit, sold by druggists as *chillies* (*fructus* vel *baccæ capsici annui*), is flat, more or less shrivelled, oblong, blunt or pointed at one end, while the calyx or stalk is usually attached at the other end. The length of the berry (independent of the stalk) is two or three inches, the breadth one-half to three-quarters of an inch, the colour yellowish or reddish-brown, the taste hot and pungent, the odour none. The epidermis is tough and leathery; the seeds are flattened and whitish. The recent fruit, called *capsicum* or *chillies*, grown in this country, and sold for pickling, is, when ripe, yellow or red, but it is frequently gathered green: its size and shape are variable, and it is distinguished as long-podded, short-podded, and heart-shaped.

Besides Capsicum annuum, several other species of Capsicum are employed dietetically and medicinally.

Capsicum frutescens, Linn., yields the capsules sold by druggists as *Guinea pepper* or *bird pepper* (*baccæ capsici*), as I have satisfied myself by comparing the commercial article with the East Indian Solanaceæ belonging to the Linnean Society. These capsules do not exceed an inch in length, and are about two or three lines broad: their colour is orange-red, their odour aromatic and pungent. Their properties are similar to those of chillies, than which they are much hotter and more fiery. Their powder is *Cayenne pepper*, so extensively employed as a condiment. *Cayenne lozenges* and *essence of cayenne* (an alcoholic tincture) are kept in the shops.

Capsicum cerasiforme, Willd.—The fruit of this species is called *cherry chilly* or *cherry pepper*. It is small, round, and cherry-shaped.

Capsicum grossum, Linn.; *Bell Pepper.*—Fruit large, oblong or ovate, red or yellow.

Composition.—The fruit was analysed, in 1816, by Maurach;[3] in the same year by Bucholz;[4] and in the following year by Braconnot.[5]

---

[1] *Synops. Plant. Fl. Cl.* p. 169, 1845.
[2] *Hist. Plant.* lib. ix. cap. 22.
[3] *Berl. Jahrb.* Bd. xvii. S. 63.
[4] Gmelin, *Handb. d. Chem.* ii. 1310.
[5] *Ann. de Chim. Phys.* vi. 122.

Bucholz's Analysis.		*Braconnot's Analysis.*	
Acrid soft resin (*capsicin*)	4.0	Acrid oil...........................	1·9
Wax	7·6	Wax with red colouring matter...........	0·9
Bitter aromatic extractive	8·6	Brownish starchy matter	9·0
Extractive with some gum.................	21·0	Peculiar gum	6·0
Gum	9·2	Animalised matter........................	5·0
Albuminous matter	3·2	Woody fibre	67·8
Woody fibre	28·0	Salts (citrate of potash 6·0, phosphate of	
Water	12·0	potash and chloride of potassium 3·4) .	9·4
Loss	6.4		
Fruit of Capsicum annuum without seeds 100·0		Fruit of Capsicum annuum .... 100·0	

CAPSICIN, Bucholz; *Acrid Soft Resin ; Acrid Oil*, Braconnot.—Obtained by digesting the alcoholic extract in ether, and evaporating the etherial solution. It is a thick liquid, of a yellowish-red or reddish-brown colour, which becomes very fluid when heated, and, at a higher temperature, is dissipated in fumes. Half a grain of it, volatilised in a large room, causes all who respire the air of the room to cough and sneeze. By exposure to air and light it solidifies. It is decolorised by chlorine. It is slightly soluble in water and in vinegar; but very much so in alcohol, ether, oil of turpentine, and the caustic alkalies. With baryta it forms a solid acrid combination.

PHYSIOLOGICAL EFFECTS.—Capsicum belongs to the spices, and is more closely allied, by its effects, to the peppers than to any other article of the Materia Medica. Sundelin,[1] however, considers it to be more related to pyrethrum. Its active principle is more fixed, and its operation is more permanent and violent, than mustard or horse-radish. Its hot and fiery taste is familiar to every one. Applied to the skin, capsicum acts as a rubefacient and vesicant. Swallowed *in small doses*, it creates a sensation of warmth in the stomach; and in torpid and languid habits proves a valuable stimulant, and a promoter of the digestive functions. Taken *in somewhat larger quantities*, it produces a glow over the body, excites thirst, and quickens the pulse : the latter effect, however, is not in proportion to its local effect. Like the peppers, it is said to exercise a stimulant influence over the urino-genital organs. *In excessive doses*, we can easily believe that vomiting, purging, abdominal pain, and gastric inflammation, ascribed to it by Vogt,[2] may be induced by it, though I am not acquainted with any cases in which these effects have occurred. Richter[3] mentions, in addition to the symptoms just mentioned, a paralysed and altered condition of the nervous influence, an affection of the head, drunkenness, and giddiness, as being produced by large doses.

USES.—Capsicum is more employed as a *condiment* than as a medicine. It is added to various articles of food, either to improve their flavour, or, if difficult of digestion, to promote their assimilation, and to prevent flatulence. The inhabitants of tropical climates employ it to stimulate the digestive organs, and thereby to counteract the relaxing and enervating influence of external heat.

As a *medicine*, it is principally valuable as a local stimulant to the mouth, throat, and stomach. Its constitutional not being in proportion to its topical effects, it is of little value as a general or diffusible stimulant. Administered internally, capsicum has long been esteemed in cases of *cynanche maligna.*

---

[1] *Handb. d. sp. Heilm.* Bd. ii. S. 44, 3tte Aufl.
[2] *Pharmakodyn.* Bd. ii. S. 581, 2te Aufl.
[3] *Ausf. Arzneim.* Bd. ii. S. 179.

It was used, in 1786, with great success by Mr. Stephens[1] and by Mr. Collins.[2] It promoted the separation of the sloughs, and soon improved the constitutional symptoms. Mr. Headby[3] also employed it both internally and by way of gargle. Its use has been extended to *scarlatina anginosa*.[4] As a gargle, in relaxed conditions of the throat, its efficacy is undoubted. The powder or tincture may be applied, by means of a camel's-hair pencil, to a relaxed uvula. It is a very useful gastric stimulant in enfeebled, languid, and torpid conditions of the stomach. Thus in the dyspepsia of drunkards, as well as of gouty subjects, it has been found useful.[5] In various diseases attended with diminished susceptibility of stomach, capsicum is an exceedingly useful adjunct to other powerful remedies, the operation of which it promotes by raising the dormant susceptibility of this viscus ; as in cholera, intermittents, low forms of fever, and dropsies. Dr. Wright[6] speaks in high terms of it as a remedy for obviating the black vomit—a symptom of the fever of tropical climates, at one time considered fatal. A capsicum cataplasm may be used with advantage to occasion rubefaction in any cases in which a rubefacient counter-irritant is indicated ; as in the coma and delirium of fever, and in chronic rheumatism : unless kept on for a long period, it does not vesicate.

ADMINISTRATION.—The *powder* of capsicum is usually given in doses of from gr. v. to gr. x., made into pills with crumbs of bread. The dose of the *tincture* will be mentioned presently. The *infusion* (prepared by digesting ʒij. of capsicum in f℥x. of boiling water for two hours) may be administered in doses of f℥ss. But, in malignant sore-throat and scarlatina, capsicum has been employed in much larger doses. *Stephen's pepper medicine* consisted of two table-spoonfuls of small red pepper [*Capsicum frutescens*], or three of the common Cayenne pepper, and two tea-spoonfuls of fine salt digested in half a pint of boiling water. To the liquor, strained when cold, half a pint of very sharp vinegar is added. A table-spoonful of this mixture to be given to an adult every half hour. The *capsicum gargle* is prepared by infusing ʒss. of capsicum in a pint of boiling water; or by adding f℥vj. of the tincture to f℥viij. of the infusion of roses ; or, in some cases, Stephen's pepper medicine may be used as a gargle.

TINCTURA CAPSICI, L. E. D.; *Tincture of Capsicum.* (Capsicum, bruised [or, if percolation be followed, in moderately fine powder, *E.*], ʒx. [Cayenne Pods, f℥iss., *D.*] ; Proof Spirit, Oij. [Oj., *D.*] Digest for seven [fourteen, *D.*] days, and strain [strain, squeeze the residuum, and filter the liquors. This tincture is best prepared by percolation; which may be commenced so soon as the capsicum is made into a pulp with a little of the spirit, *E.*] [The United States Pharmacopœia directs Capsicum, in powder, ℥j.; Diluted Alcohol, Oij.—ED.]). Dose, ℞x. to f℥j. Employed in the low stage of typhus and scarlet fevers, and in gangrenous sore-throat, and to prevent the nausea which oil of turpentine is apt to occasion. Properly diluted, it may be used as a gargle, as above mentioned. Externally, it is sometimes used as a local stimulant.

---

[1] Duncan's *Med. Comment.* vol. ii. Dec. 2d. 1788.
[2] *Med. Communications*, vol. ii. p. 372, 1790.
[3] *Lond. Med. and Phys. Journ.* vol. v. p. 425, 1801.
[4] Kreysig, *U. d. Scharlachfieber*, 1803, in Voigtel's *Arzneim.*
[5] Chapman's *Elem. of Therap.* vol. ii.
[6] *Med. Facts and Observ.* vol. vii.

185. Mandragora officinarum, *Linn.*—Common Mandrake.

Sex. Syst. Pentandria, Monogynia.

(Radix.)

Μανδραγόρας μέλας, ἀντίμηλον, κιρκαία, &c., Dioscorides, lib. iv. cap. 76; *Mandragora*, Pliny, Hist. Nat. lib. xxv. cap. 94, ed. Valp.; *Atropa Mandragora*, Linn.—South of Europe. Mandrake is an acro-narcotic poison: when swallowed, it purges violently.[1] The roots, from their fancied resemblance to the human form, were called *anthropomorphon*, and were supposed to prevent barrenness.[2] The root of *Bryonia dioica* is sold at the herb-shops as a substitute for mandrake. Dr. Sylvester[3] has recently drawn attention to the ancient uses of this plant as an anæsthetic.

ORDER XLIII. BORAGINACEÆ, *Lindl.*—BORAGEWORTS.

BORRAGEÆ, *DC.*—BORAGINEÆ, *Endl.*

CHARACTERS.—*Calyx* persistent, with 4 or 5 divisions. *Corolla* hypogynous, monopetalous, generally regular, 5-cleft, sometimes 4-cleft, with an imbricated æstivation. *Stamens* inserted upon the corolla, equal to the number of its lobes, and alternate with them. *Ovary* 4-parted, 4-seeded, or 2-parted, 4-celled; ovules attached to the lowest point of the cavity, amphitropal. *Style* simple, arising from the base of the lobes of the ovary; *stigma* simple or bifid. *Nuts* 2 or 4, distinct. *Seed* separable from the pericarp, destitute of albumen; embryo with a superior radicle; cotyledons parallel with the axis, plano-convex, sometimes 4 (!) in Amsinckia.—*Herbaceous* plants or *shrubs*. *Stems* round. *Leaves* alternate, often covered with asperities consisting of hairs proceeding from an indurated enlarged base. *Flowers* in 1-sided gyrate spikes or racemes, or panicles, some solitary and axillary (*Lindley*).

PROPERTIES.—The plants of this order are characterised by their mucilaginous quality: they are, therefore, mostly harmless and inert.

Formerly several borageworts were used in medicine; for example, *Symphytum officinalis* Linn., *Borrago officinalis* Linn., *Cynoglossum officinale* Linn., *Pulmonaria officinalis* Linn., *Lithospermum officinale* Linn., and *Echium vulgare* Linn. They possess little medicinal value (though formerly many virtues were ascribed to them), and are now obsolete. The only boragewort still found in pharmaceutists' shops is *Alkanna tinctoria* Linn.

186. Alkanna tinctoria, *Tausch.*—Dyer's Alkanet.

Sex. Syst. Pentandria, Monogynia.

(Radix.)

Ἄγχουσα, Dioscorides, lib. iv. cap, 23; *Lithospermum tinctorium*, Linn., Herb. Sp. ed. i. non ed. ii.; *Anchusa tinctoria*,[5] Desf., Atl. i. p. 156; Hayne, Arzneigew., 10, t. ii.; *Alcanna tinctoria*, Nees, Offic. Pflanz., Suppl. ii. t. 6; Handb. ii. 591; *Alkanna tinctoria*, Tausch, in Florâ, 1824.—A deciduous herbaceous plant with a perennial, dark blood-red root. This, when dried, constitutes the *alkanet root* (*radix alkannæ tinctoriæ*) of the shops, and which is sometimes called *spurious alkanet root* (*radix alkannæ spuriæ*) to distinguish it from the *henna* or *al-henna* of the Arabs (*Lawsonia alba*, Lam.), whose root is called the *true alkanet* (*radix alkannæ veræ*). The plant grows on the shores of the Mediterranean, in Asia Minor and Greece. [Alkanet root is imported from the Mediter-

---

[1] Brandt and Ratzeburg, *Deutsch. phan. Giftgewächse*, S. 79.
[2] Matthiolus, *Comm. Dioscor.*
[3] *Pharmaceutical Journal*, vol. vii. p. 519, 1848.
[4] Smith (*Prodr. Fl. Græcæ*, i. 116) and Gussone (*Syn.* p. 218) declare the *Anchusa tinctoria* Linn., Herb. Sp. ed. ii. p. 192 (*Alkanna controversa* DC., Prodr. x. 103), to be entirely different from the *Alkanna tinctoria* Tausch.

ranean : it is not the produce of Italy, but of Hungary, whence it is taken to Trieste for shipment.—ED.]

Alkanet root was analysed by John,[1] who found the constituents to be *a peculiar colouring matter* (pseudo-alkannin) 5·50, *extractive* 1·00, *gum* 6·25, *matters extracted by caustic potash* 65·00, *woody fibre* 18·00=95·75 [loss 4·25]. The colouring matter resides in the cortical part of the root, and was regarded by Pelletier[2] as a kind of fatty acid (*anchusic acid*); but it is now usually considered to be a resinoid (*anchusine*), whose composition is $C^{35}H^{20}O^8$. It is of a dark red colour, fusible at 140° F., insoluble in water, but very soluble in alcohol and in acetic acid. The alkalies colour it blue. Acetate and subacetate of lead, protochloride of tin, the salts of iron and alumina, precipitate it : chlorine and strong acids destroy it.—Alkanet root communicates its colouring matter to oily and fatty substances ; and hence is used by the pharmaceutist to colour *lip salve* (*unguentum labiale*), *hair oil*, and various cosmetics.

ORDER XLIV. CONVOLVULACEÆ, *R. Brown.*—BINDWEEDS.

CONVOLVULI, *Jussieu.*

CHARACTERS.—*Calyx* persistent, in 5 divisions, remarkably imbricated, as if in more whorls than 1, often very unequal. *Corolla* monopetalous, hypogynous, regular, deciduous ; the limb 5-lobed, plaited ; the tube without scales. *Stamens* 5, inserted into the base of the corolla, and alternate with its segments. *Ovary* simple, with 2 or 4 cells, seldom with 1 ; sometimes in 2 or 4 distinct divisions ; few-seeded ; the ovules definite and erect, when more than 1 collateral ; *style* 1, usually divided at the top, or as many as the divisions of the ovary, and arising from their base ; *stigmas* obtuse or acute. *Disc* annular, hypogynous. *Capsule* with from 1 to 4 cells, succulent or capsular ; the valves fitting, at their edges, to the angles of a loose dissepiment, bearing the seeds at its base. *Seeds* with a small quantity of mucilaginous albumen ; *embryo* curved ; *cotyledons* leafy, shrivelled ; *radicle* inferior next the hilum.—*Herbaceous plants* or *shrubs*, usually twining and milky, smooth, or with a simple pubescence ; sometimes erect bushes. *Leaves* alternate, undivided or lobed, seldom pinnatifid, with no stipules. *Inflorescence* axillary or terminal ; peduncles 1- or many-flowered, the partial ones generally with 2 bracts, which sometimes enlarge greatly after flowering (*Lindley*).

PROPERTIES.—The roots and seeds only have been used in medicine.

The tuberous roots of some species (as of jalap and scammony) contain an acrid, milky, purgative juice, which owes its medicinal qualities to the contained resin. *Mechoacan* and *Turpeth* (*Ipomæa Turpethum*) roots, formerly used as purgatives, are now obsolete. In other tuberous roots (as of *Batatas edulis*) the resin is deficient or absent, and starchy matter predominates ; in consequence of which they become edible, and are cultivated for the table.

The seeds of some species (as of *Pharbitis cærulea*) are cathartic.

187. CONVOLVULUS SCAMMONIA, *Linn.* — THE SCAMMONY.

Sex. Syst. Pentandria, Monogynia.

(Gummi-resina e resectâ radice emissa, *L.*—Gum-resinous exudation from incisions into the root, *E. D.*)

HISTORY.—A purgative substance called scammony (Σκαμμώνιον) was known to the Greeks long before the time of Hippocrates.[3] The Father of Medicine, who frequently employed it, says that it evacuates both upwards

---

[1] *Chemische Schriften*, iv. 85 ; Kunze, *Waarenkunde*, ii. 37.
[2] *Bull. de Pharm.* vi. 445, 1814 ; *Journ. de Pharm.* xix. 105, 1833.
[3] Voigtels, *Arzneimittell.* Bd. i. S. 17 ; Bischoff, *Handb. d. Arzneimittell.* Bd. i. S. 40.

and downwards, bile and mucus, and expels flatus.[1] Dioscorides[2] notices the plant which yields scammony, and terms it Σκαμμώνια.[3] Pliny,[4] also, speaks of scammony, which he calls *scammonium*. Dr. Sibthorp[5] refers the scammony of Dioscorides to *C. farinosus*, a Madeira species!—on what ground does not appear, as this supposed species is not in his herbarium.[6] If the ordinary reading of the text of Dioscorides be correct, this author represents the scammony as having hairy branches and leaves; which applies better to *C. sagittifolius* (*C. Sibthorpii*, Roemer and Schultes), found by Sibthorp in Samos[7] and other islands of the Grecian Archipelago. This species is with great probability adopted by Dierbach[8] as the source of the ancient scammony.[9]

BOTANY. **Gen. Char.**—*Sepals* 5. *Corolla* campanulate. *Style* 1. *Stigmas* 2, linear-cylindrical, often revolute. *Ovary* 2-celled, with 4 ovules. *Capsule* 2-celled (*Choisy*).

Sp. Char. — Stem smooth. Leaves sagittate, posteriorly truncate, with entire or elongated slashed auricles. Peduncles very long, many-flowered. Sepals coloured, ovate, obtusely truncated, mucronulate, the external ones a little smaller, 2-3 lines long. Corolla campanulate, an inch long (*Choisy*).

Root perennial, tapering, 3 or 4 feet long, with an acrid, milky juice. *Stem* numerous, twining, herbaceous, smooth. *Leaves* on long petioles, acuminate, with pointed lobes at the base. *Peduncles* solitary, scarcely twice so long as the leaves. *Bracts* awl-shaped. *Sepals* obovate, truncated, with a reflex point, coloured at the edge. *Corolla* pale yellow, with purple stripes [or white, with red external stripes.—ED.] *Stamina* shorter than the corolla; *anthers* erect, sagittate. *Style* as long as the stamens; *stigmas* white.

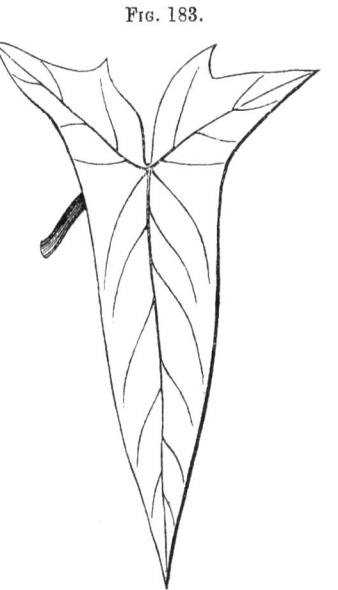

FIG. 183.

Leaf of Convolvulus Scammonia.

[1] *De Morb. Mul.* p. 597, ed. Fœs.
[2] Lib. iv. cap. 171.
[3] [The scammony plant is called by the Turks, as well as by the Greeks of Anatolia, *Mamoutià.*—ED.]
[4] *Hist. Nat.* lib. xxvi. cap. 38, ed. Valp.
[5] *Prod. Fl. Græcæ.*
[6] Lindley, *Fl. Medica.*
[7] [According to Maltass, scammony is not produced in Samos, nor do the peasants of that island know of any plants existing there, although it is not improbable that a few may be found. Some of the Samians, he informs us, still collect the drug, but they cross over to the mainland and work in the neighbourhood of Sochia, on the Mæander, Scala nova, and Ephesus. They usually carry it for sale to Smyrna, but occasionally sell it in Samos.—ED.]
[8] *Arzneimittell. d. Hippokrates*, S. 138.
[9] Tournefort (*Voyage into the Levant*, vol. ii. p. 96, 1741) says that the scammony of Samos is collected from a bindweed (*convolvulus*) whose leaves are larger, hairy, and slashed at their basis not so prettily as those of the Syrian scammony (*C. Scammonia*). This doubtless is *C. sagittifolius*, which Sibthorp found in Samos.

[We are indebted to Mr. Maltass[1] for a more detailed history of the growth and diffusion of the scammony plant, than that given by the author. This gentleman resided at Smyrna for a period of eighteen years, and made himself practically conversant with all that relates to this drug. The scammony plant grows wild in all parts of Anatolia, as well as in Syria and in some of the Greek and Turkish islands of the Archipelago. It is found in mountainous districts, in the plains, and in the open ground, flourishing most luxuriantly among the Juniper, Arbutus, and wild Valonea bushes. These afford shelter and support to its branches, and their decayed leaves produce a soil favourable to its growth. The *root* is succulent, and shaped like a carrot: when about four years old, it is generally one or two inches in diameter at the crown, whence it tapers gradually to the extremity, with occasional fibres, its length varying from ten inches to two or three feet, according to the depth of the soil. In some instances it is found to have four or even five inches diameter at the crown. The root is the same, whether the flower be yellow or white; and there is no apparent difference in the leaf. The yellow-flowered plant is more abundant, but the scammony is indifferently collected from the roots, without regard to the colour of the flower. The only perceptible difference in quality is to be ascribed to the soil. The scammony which has the strongest odour is that produced in mountainous districts, and on a poor soil: rich soils and marshy ground produce a scammony-juice containing a larger proportion of water, which, when dry, forms a scammony of a greyish-black colour, and of less specific gravity.—Ed.]

Hab.—Hedges and bushy places in Greece and the Levant. [The scammony district extends from Adalia on the south, to Broussa or Mount Olympus on the north, and even as far as Angora. Sochia, or the district of the river Mæander, produces a large quantity; but Kirkagatch and Demirgik, in the plain of Mysia, furnish the largest quantity of all. But little comes from Konieh or Kutaya. A pure scammony, but of inferior quality, is also produced at Melissa or Melas.—Ed.]

Preparation.—The method of procuring scammony is, according to Dr. Russel,[2] as follows:—Having cleared away the earth from the upper part of the root, the peasants cut off the top in an oblique direction, about two inches below where the stalks spring from it. Under the most depending part of the slope they affix a shell, or some other convenient receptacle, into which the milky juice flows. It is then left about twelve hours, which time is sufficient for the drawing-off the whole juice : this, however, is in small quantity, each root affording but a few drachms. This milky juice from the several roots is put together, often into the leg of an old boot, for want of some more proper vessel, when in a little time it grows hard, and is the genuine scammony. Of this entirely pure scammony, says Dr. Russel, but very little is brought to market, the greater part of what is to be met with being adulterated, if not by those who gather it, by those who buy it of them abroad; for the chief part of what is brought hither passes through the hands of a few people, chiefly Jews, who make it their business to go to the villages of any note near which the scammony is collected (as Antioch, Shogre, Elib, and Maraash), and then, buying it while it is yet soft, they have an op-

---

[1] [*Pharmaceutical Journal*, 1853, p. 264.]
[2] *Med. Obs. and Inq.* vol. i. p. 13, 1776.

portunity of mixing it with such other things as suit their purpose best,—as wheat-flour, ashes, or fine sand, all of which he found mixed with it : but there seems, he adds, some other ingredient (possibly the expressed juice), which makes it so very hard and indissoluble that he was not able to discover it to his satisfaction.

Dioscorides thus describes the mode of procuring it :—The head being separated, the root is to be excavated in the form of a dome (or vault) by a knife, so that the juice may flow into the cavity, from which it is to be taken out in shells. Others excavate the earth, and having incised the root, let the juice run into the cavity, which has been previously lined with walnut leaves : when the scammony is dry, it is removed.

I have been informed by a Turkey merchant, who formerly resided at Smyrna, that scammony is brought into Smyrna, in the soft state, on camels. Here it is mixed with various impurities by persons (Jews) who are denominated scammony makers, and who adulterate it, and thereby lower its value to suit the market. [The account given by Dr. Russel in 1776, and quoted by the author, is not so complete as that with which Mr. Maltass has more recently furnished us. Scammony is collected solely from the *Convolvulus Scammonia*. During the summer months, when the plant is in flower, the Greek and Turkish peasants, having cleared away the bushes which shelter it, remove the earth from the root to the depth of three or four inches. The root is then cut through, in a slanting direction, with a sickle-shaped knife, at the distance of about one inch to one inch and a half below the crown : a mussel-shell is immediately stuck into the root under the lower part, and the sap or milk runs into it. A stone is then placed to windward of the root, to protect the shell from the loose earth and dust which might be otherwise blown into it by the high winds prevalent during summer. The sap flows freely early in the morning and late in the evening, but ceases during the hottest part of the day. One plant will not generally fill a shell; but it sometimes happens that a good root will fill two or three shells : in this case the peasant removes the first as soon as it is full, and places another, and so on until he perceives that the root is nearly drained. The quantity afforded by one root varies according to soil, position, and age. In some districts, one hundred roots produce but ten drachms of scammony : in others the average of each root is one drachm : and in a good soil a four-year plant will produce two drachms. A root four inches in diameter has been known to produce as much as twelve drachms ; but those cut by Mr. Maltass himself did not produce above one drachm, and some afforded none at all. The shells are usually left till the evening, when they are collected, and the cut part of the root is scraped with a knife to remove the dry, or partially dry, drops of scammony which exude after the first part has run off. These drops are called by the peasants *Kaimak*, or cream, while the sap which flows into the shell is called γάλα, or milk. The peasants then empty the shells (from which they carefully blow the dust) into copper vessels, and work up the drops scraped from the roots together with the contents of the shells. This is done with a knife, and continued until the whole is so well mixed that it forms a string when run off the knife. If it be too dry, then water is added; but in that case it must be done during the hottest part of the day, when Fahrenheit's thermometer stands at 86° to 90° in the shade; otherwise it will not amalgamate properly. This is the *pure Lachryma scammony*. That which the Greeks collect is far better than that which is collected by the Turks : the latter, with their usual apathy, do not trouble themselves to screen the shells from the dust, nor do they blow off any of that which may have accumulated on the hardened surface of the scammony in the shell. They show equal carelessness by scraping the roots too roughly in order to remove the drops, and small pieces of the root thus frequently fall into the receiving vessels. The scammony brought to market by the Greek peasants is almost the only pure sort that can be obtained. It does not exceed three hundred *okes* yearly, or about seven hundredweight, and is sold at a high price to a few dealers who know its superiority. When purchased, it is placed in a room having the windows open, to allow the wind to blow over it; care being taken to prevent the rays of the sun from striking upon it. Here it is spread upon sheep-skins, flattened if moist, and turned occasionally, to prevent it becoming mouldy underneath. When nearly dry, it is broken into irregular pieces, and allowed to remain a few days longer, until quite dry: it is then shipped in small cases containing about thirty pounds each.[1]—Ed.]

DESCRIPTION.—Scammony (*scammonium; gummi-resina scammonii*) is usually imported from Smyrna. Occasionally it comes by way of Trieste. Still more rarely it is brought from Alexandretta (also called Scanderoon or Iskenderún), the port of, and road to Aleppo. It comes over in boxes and drums, which are frequently lined with tin.

[The quantity of scammony annually sold in Smyrna amounts to about 3000 Turkish okes, or 7500 lbs. weight. Out of this quantity about seven hundredweight of pure can be obtained, the remainder being of different qualities, the quantity of resin that they contain varying from one ounce to fifteen ounces in every pound. If the whole crop were brought to market *unadulterated*, it is doubtful whether the annual quantity would exceed 3000 lbs. weight.[2]—Ed.]

The different sorts of scammony of commerce may be arranged under three heads: 1st, pure scammony; 2dly, adulterated scammony; 3dly, factitious scammony.[3]

1. PURE SCAMMONY (*Scammonium purum*).—In English commerce one sort only is known under this name—namely, the virgin scammony. Scammony in shells is probably a pure scammony, but is unknown in trade. Trebizond or Samos scammony, though perhaps a pure scammony, differs so much in its external appearance from the ordinary commercial sorts, that it is unsaleable here.

---

[1] ⌜See the paper above quoted, in the *Pharmaceutical Journal*, 1853.⌝

[2] ⌞Maltass, in *Pharmaceutical Journal*.⌟

[3] Marquart (*Pharm. Central-Blatt für* 1837, p. 671), who has published an elaborate paper on scammony. He arranges the various sorts as follows:—

    1. *Scammony from the Convolvulaceæ.*—Under this head he includes
        α. Aleppo scammony. Of this he makes five sorts.
        β. Antioch scammony. Of this he makes three sorts.
        γ. Samos scammony.
    2. *Scammony from the Asclepiadeæ.*
        δ. French or Montpellier scammony.
    3. *Scammony from the Apocyneæ.*
        ε. Smyrna scammony of commerce. Of this he makes four sorts.

But the foundation of this arrangement is erroneous. Smyrna scammony is not the produce of Apocyneæ, but of a smooth-leaved Convolvulus, as Sherard (Geoffroy, *Tract. de Mat. Med.* ii. 667) has shown. Under the head of Smyrna scammony, Marquart includes adulterated and factitious commercial sorts. In English commerce no distinction of Aleppo, Antioch, and Smyrna scammony is made.

a. Virgin Scammony (Lachryma¹ Scammony ; Superior Aleppo Blackish Scammony, Guib.)—It usually occurs in amorphous pieces ; but a careful examination of some large lumps has led me to believe that they formed portions of a mass, which, when in the soft state, had a rounded form. The whitish-gray powder, which covers some of the pieces, effervesces with hydrochloric acid ; and I have no doubt, therefore, that the masses have been rolled in chalk. Virgin scammony is friable; easily reduced to small fragments between the fingers, or by the pressure of the nail, and has, according to my experiments, a sp. gr. of 1·210. Its fractured surface is resinous, shining, greenish-black (see p. 609, *post*); presents small air-cavities, and numerous gray semi-transparent splints, or fragments, when examined by a magnifying glass ; and does not effervesce on the addition of hydrochloric acid. When rubbed with the finger moistened with ether, water, or saliva, it readily forms a milky liquid. If we examine thin fragments, or splinters, by transmitted light, we observe them to be semi-transparent at the edges, and of a grey-brown colour. In the same pieces we sometimes find some portions shining, and blackish, as above described ; while others are dull-greyish. This difference depends probably, as Dr. Russel has suggested, on different methods of drying. Virgin scammony readily takes fire, and burns with a yellowish flame. Its odour is peculiar, somewhat analogous to old cheese ; its taste is slight at first, afterwards acrid. The decoction of its powder, when filtered and cold, is not rendered blue by tincture of iodine. When incinerated in a crucible, it leaves a minute portion only of ash. This sort of scammony is usually imported from Smyrna.

β. *Scammony in shells* or *calebashes (Scammonium in testis ; Sc. in calebassis).*—Unknown in English commerce. It is described by continental writers as a very pure sort. [Maltass states that scammony is never sold in shells. When dry, it would be difficult to empty them. The peasants who collect the juice, however, frequently keep a few for their own use, as this drug is much employed by them for the purpose of staunching blood and healing wounds. They also use it as a purgative. The contents of a shell amount, on the average, to one drachm.—ED.]

γ. *Trebizond Scammony.*—In 1832 a substance was imported into London, from Trebizond, under the name of scammony, which was unsaleable here. The sample which I received is a portion of cake apparently round, flat below, and convex above. Its colour is light-grayish or reddish-brown ; when moistened, the surface becomes glutinous and odorous; its taste is sweet, nauseous, and somewhat bitter. In its external appearance it has more resemblance to benzoin than scammony.

This probably is the *Scammony of Samos* mentioned by Tournefort;[2] the *Scammony from Mysia* of Dioscorides. It would appear to be obtained from a species of Convolvulus (*C. sagittifolius*) different from that which yields the Aleppo and Smyrna scammony ; for both Dioscorides and Tournefort state that the leaves are hairy.

2. ADULTERATED SCAMMONY (*Scammonium adulteratum*).—Under this head are included the various sorts of scammony commonly found in the shops, and which English dealers distinguish as *seconds, thirds,* &c. To

---

[1] The term "lachryma scammony" I have heard applied to this sort of scammony by a Turkey merchant. It is remarkable that a somewhat similar term was used by the ancients. Cælius Aurelianus (*Acut. Morb.* lib. ii. cap. xxix.) speaks of " succum scamoniæ quam diagridium appellamus." Now *diagridium* is a corruption from δακρύδιον, *lachrymula*, a little tear. The word diagridium was also applied to a preparation of scammony. [The lachryma scammony sold as such in London is of mixed quality. It is in irregular pieces, and not in cakes, like pure Greek scammony. It is collected by the Jews. Some good pieces, it is said, may be picked out, but it is greatly inferior to Greek scammony. Some of the best pieces contain seventy-six per cent. of resin.—ED.]

[2] *A Voyage into the Levant*, vol. ii. p. 96, 1741.

this division belongs the so-called *Antioch scammony* (*scammonium Antiochum*) of continental writers. What is sometimes called on the continent *Smyrna scammony* (*scammonium Smyrnense*), is either adulterated or factitious scammony. The term *Aleppo scammony* (*scammonium Halepense* seu *Aleppicum*) is applied by the same writers to virgin scammony, and to the better sorts of adulterated scammony.[1] The different sorts of adulterated scammony more frequently occur in round flattened or plano-convex cakes of variable size, usually an inch or two in thickness, and about five inches in diameter. Some are met with in amorphous, irregular lumps; others in large cylindrical or drum-shaped masses. The different sorts of adulterated scammony vary considerably in appearance, but pass so insensibly the one into the other, that it is impossible to classify them according to their physical characters. I shall, therefore, arrange them according to their chemical characters.

A. *Adulterated scammony which effervesces on the addition of hydrochloric acid.*—This is sophisticated with carbonate of lime, and sometimes with starch or dextrine.

α. *Calcareous, chalky, or cretaceous scammony.*—Occurs in round flat cakes, or in irregular lumps. It is more ponderous than the virgin sort, and usually breaks with a dull, earthy fracture. Its colour is ash-grey, like common secondary limestone. A specimen in irregular lumps I found to have the sp. gr. of 1·463. Its chemical characters are as follows: hydrochloric acid applied to a fractured surface causes effervescence; iodine produces no change of colour when added to the filtered decoction after it has become cold. Lumps of crystallised carbonate of lime are sometimes found in this sort of scammony. [Mr. Maltass states that most of the peasants adulterate scammony before it is brought to the market. One process is as follows:—The scammony is brought to a liquid state by admixture with water, and a quantity of white chalky earth (probably carbonate of lime) is added. The earth is previously sifted through a silk handkerchief, so as to prevent detection by the touch. The quantity used varies from 10 to 150 per cent.! The colour of soft moist scammony is not affected by the addition, unless the proportion exceeds 20 per cent.: when dry, it is then apparent to anyone acquainted with the drug. This adulterated kind of Smyrna scammony is sold in London as Lachryma scammony,—a name which is much misapplied (see footnote, *ante*, p. 603).—ED.]

β. *Calcareo-amylaceous scammony.*—This, like the preceding, occurs in round flat cakes or in irregular lumps, which contain carbonate of lime and either wheat or barley starch or meal.[2] I have also met with it in cylindrical or drum-shaped masses.

αα. *In irregular lumps.*—It sometimes resembles pure scammony in its glossiness and dark resinous appearance; but usually it has a waxy lustre and greyish colour.

---

[1] A specimen of scammony was sent to a friend of mine for sale from Aleppo, which was so adulterated that no offer could be obtained for it. It was in thin flat cakes, having a sweet smell, and containing the starch of either wheat or barley,—probably the former.

[2] Dioscorides states that the Syrian scammony is adulterated with τιθύμαλος (*euphorbia* or *spurge*) and ὀρόβινον ἄλευρον (*meal of the ervil* or *bastard lentil*, the *Ervum Ervilia* of Linn.) A careful microscopic examination of amylaceous and calcareo-amylaceous scammony has satisfied me that the starch or flour used for adulterating these sorts of scammony, at the present day, is that of either wheat or barley,—probably wheat.

ββ. In cylindrical or drum-shaped masses.—This kind is imported either in boxes or drums, into which it seems to have been introduced when soft, and to have hardened subsequently: hence its form is that of the package in which it was imported. A sample of a circular cake (about 12 inches in diameter, and several inches thick) presents a dull-greyish fracture. Its sp. gr., according to my experiments, is 1·359.

γγ. In circular flat cakes.—I have received this sort of scammony in the form of circular flat cakes, about five inches in diameter, and one inch thick. They are heavy, dense, and much more difficult to fracture than the preceding kinds. The fractured surface, in some samples, is resinous and shining, in others dull; it has air-cavities, and numerous small white specks (chalk); its colour is greyish to greyish-black. The sp. gr. varies, in different samples, from 1·276 to 1·543. I have received portions of five cakes of this variety of scammony, on which were marked the actual quantity of chalk which had been intermixed in each sample. In 100 parts of the cakes the proportions of chalk were respectively as follows:—13·07, 23·1, 25·0, 31·05, and 37·54. These numbers were furnished by the Levant importer to one of our most respectable wholesale druggists, from whom I received them.

The chemical characters of calcareo-amylaceous scammony are as follows :—Hydrochloric acid applied to a fractured surface causes effervescence; iodine produces a blue colour when added to the filtered decoction after it has become cold.

γ. Calcareo-dextrinous scammony.—This sort differs from the preceding in the circumstance that iodine produces a reddish-purple tint when added to the filtered decoction after it has become cold. It appears to contain carbonate of lime and dextrine.

B. *Adulterated scammony which does not effervesce on the addition of hydrochloric acid.*—This sort of scammony is usually sophisticated with wheat-meal.

δ. *Amylaceous scammony.*—This sort of scammony is adulterated with the starch or flour of either wheat or barley—probably the former: it is of less frequent occurrence than the calcareo-amylaceous kind. It occurs in irregular lumps and round flat cakes, which sometimes have a resinous fracture and a dark colour like pure scammony, but which more commonly have a waxy lustre and a greyish colour. It contains starch and ligneous matter, but not chalk. It does not, therefore, effervesce with hydrochloric acid. Its decoction, when filtered and cooled, strikes a blue colour on the addition of iodine. [The scammony collected near Smyrna is rarely adulterated with starch by the peasants. In other instances, however, starch is used mixed more or less with other substances. The usual mixture, we are told, is wheat-starch, wood-ashes, earth (not always calcareous), and gum arabic, or gum tragacanth; occasionally, wax, yolk of egg, pounded scammony, roots and leaves, flour or resin, are added. These mixtures vary so much that it is almost impossible to find two parcels exactly alike. This adulterated scammony is put into drums, and scammony nearly pure, and about as liquid as honey, is poured on the top to give it a good appearance, and to prevent detection, which, without this precaution, would not be difficult, the surface of the adulterated drug being always dry. A variety of adulterated scammony called *skilip* is prepared at Angora, and sent to Constantinople for sale. It is composed of from 30 to 40 per cent. of scammony, and from 60 to 70 per cent. of starch. This quality is, we are informed by Maltass, much used in Austria, where cheap drugs are required without much reference to their medicinal efficacy !—Ed.]

ε. *Selenitic* or *Gypseous Scammony.*—This kind has been described by Marquart. Its sp. gr. 1·731, and it contained no less than 52 per cent. of gypsum (sulphate of lime).

ζ. *Bassorin Scammony.*—Marquart met with a scammony which had a horny consistence and a sp. gr. of 1·167. After it had been deprived of its resin and extractive, it swelled up in boiling water. The constituent which thus swelled up was soluble in caustic potash : Murquart regarded it as bassorin.

In the Museum of the Pharmaceutical Society is a specimen of scammony which is supposed to be adulterated with tragacanth and some resin.

η. *Indian Scammony.*—From my friend Dr. Royle I have received a sample of scammony met with in the Indian bazaars. It is light, porous, of a greenish-gray colour; gritty under the teeth, as if containing a considerable quantity of sand, and having a balsamic olibanum-like odour.

3. Factitious Scammony (*Scammonium factitium*).—To this division belongs part of the so-called *Smyrna scammony* of continental commerce, as well as *French* or *Montpellier scammony*. I have met with three samples of factitious scammony.

α. Under the name of *Smyrna scammony*, I purchased of a London dealer a sort of scammony in the form of circular flat cakes, about half an inch thick. It is blackish, and has, externally, a slaty appearance ; it breaks with difficulty ; its fracture is dull and black. Its sp. gr. is 1·412. Moistened and rubbed it evolves the smell of guaiacum. Boiled with water, it yields a turbid liquor (which is not rendered blue by iodine), and deposits a blackish powder : the latter, boiled with alcohol, yields a solution which becomes greenish-blue on the addition of nitric acid, showing the presence of guaiacum.

It is probably the *common Smyrna scammony* (Scammonium smyrnense factitium) of Gray,[1] who directs it to be made with Aleppo Scammony, 1 lb. ; extract of jalap, 5 lbs. ; guaiacum resin, 10 lbs. ; and ivory black, 4 lbs.

β. Under the name of *Scammonium Smyrnense medicinale venale*, M. Batka has presented to the Pharmaceutical Society a spurious scammony said to be made up of gum, bread, scammony, guaiacum, benzoin, wax, sand, and wood.[2]

γ. *French* or *Montpellier Scammony* (*Scammonium Gallicum* seu *Monspeliacum*) —This substance is made, in the southern part of France, with the expressed juice of *Cynanchum monspeliacum*, mixed with different resins and other purgative substances. It occurs in semi-circular, blackish, hard, compact cakes, which frequently have the smell of balsam of Peru.

[Having thus described the three commercial varieties of pure, adulterated, and factitious scammony, it may be interesting to inquire what are the qualities of the drug as it is usually employed in medical practice in Great Britain. It is stated by Mr. Maltass that the two kinds largely used in England and Scotland are called *first* and *second quality prepared.* The better kind, termed *first quality prepared,* is made up into thick smooth cakes or loaves, and shipped in cases or drums. When packed, the cakes are sometimes broken up. This kind is *prepared* (!) principally by the Jews, and in Smyrna only. The following is the process :—A quantity of scammony of *inferior* kind, containing earth, woody substances, and occasionally gum, as brought from the interior, is mixed with about 40 per cent. of *skilip*, or inferior

---

[1] *Supplement to the Pharmacopœia*, 3d edit. 1824.

[2] [Another mixture is made from refuse scammony, after the extraction of the resin, with the addition of gum arabic and *rosin*. Such a vile compound, it is said, will fetch in the London market ten shillings per pound.—Ed.]

Angora scammony, already containing, as it has been above stated, from 60 to 70 per cent. of starch. This mixture having been made by pounding, warm water is added, and the mixture is then placed in a shallow iron dish, beneath which another of the same shape, but of larger proportions, and half filled with water, is set over a charcoal fire, to act as a water-bath. When the scammony has melted, and the two adulterated kinds have become thoroughly incorporated—an operation which usually requires about half an hour— the contents of the dish are removed on a sheepskin, and rolled with the hands until cold. It is then made into flat or oval cakes or loaves, with rounded tops, which are next *washed over with a solution of pure scammony, to give them a gloss;* and lastly, placed in a room with open windows to dry. This scammony usually contains about 50 per cent. of pure resin : in other words, it is about one-half scammony and one-half a compound of starch, woody fibre, gum, and earthy matters, including chalk !

The other kind, called *second quality prepared,* is made in a similar manner. It is composed of about 60 per cent. of Angora scammony, 30 per cent. of a better kind from the neighbourhood of Smyrna, to which are added about 10 per cent. of gum arabic and black lead. This scammony is said to contain 30 per cent. of resin, 50 per cent. of starch and white earth; the remainder being made up of gum, woody substances, &c. Other proportions are occasionally used. It contains less than one-third scammony, and more than two-thirds impurity !

The quantity of scammony resin extracted from *dry* commercial scammony by ether or alcohol will afford a test of the purity of this drug; but it is adulterated to such a large extent by the peasants who extract it, and the Jew dealers who export it, that it is hopeless to seek for a pure specimen except in pharmaceutical museums.—ED.]

COMPOSITION. *a.* **Of the Root.**—The dried root of Convolvulus Scammonia was analysed, in 1837, by Marquart,[1] who obtained from it the following substances :—*resin* 4·12, *sugar, convolvulin,* and *extractive* 13·68, *resin and wax* 0·55, *gum* 5·8, *extractive* 2·4, *starch* 7·0, *extractive* soluble in hot, but not in cold, water 1·4 [*salts* and *woody fibre* 65·05]. The resin, the wax, and a portion of the gum, are contained in the milky juice of the latex vessels (*vasa laticis*); while the sugar, gum, extractive, and salts dissolved in water, constitute the juice of the cells; and in this juice the starchglobules float.

1. RESIN.—This is analogous to that of the scammony of commerce.

2. CONVOLVULIN.—A substance supposed by Marquart to be a vegetable alkali. It reacts feebly as a vegetable alkali, and is precipitated from its watery solution by tincture of nutgalls. Marquart thinks it probably exists in jalap.

β. **Of Scammony.**—Bouillon-Lagrange and Vogel[2] analysed two kinds; one called Aleppo, the other Smyrna scammony. Marquart[3] analysed twelve kinds : of these, eight sorts (five called *Aleppo,* and three *Antioch scammony*) he considers to be the produce of *Convolvulus Scammonia;* while the remaining four, which, he says, are called in commerce *Smyrna scammony,* he erroneously ascribes to *Periploca Secamone,* Linn. Three of these, however, appear to be adulterated sorts, and one (the 12th) is obviously factitious.

[1] *Pharm. Central-Blatt für* 1837, S. 687.
[2] *Bulletin de Pharmacie,* t. i. p. 421, 1809.
[3] *Pharm. Central-Blatt für* 1837, p. 687.

ALEPPO SCAMMONY, Marq.

	No. 1. In shells. Sp. gr. 1.2.	No. 2. Irregular pieces. Sp. gr. 1.239.	No. 3. Broken cakes. Sp. gr. 1.403.	No. 4. Flat pieces. Sp. gr. 1.421.	No. 5. Irregular pieces. Sp. gr. 1.731.
Resin	81·25	78·5	77·0	50·0	32·5
Wax	0·75	1·5	0·5	—	—
Extractive	4·50	3·5	3·0	5·0	3·0
Extractive with salts	...	2·0	1·0	3·0	4·0
Gum with salts	3·00	2·0	1·0	1·0	6·75
Starch	...	1·5	—	5·0	52·00
Starchy envelopes, bassorin, and gluten	1·75	1·25	—	5·0	2·0
Albumen and woody fibre	1·50	3·5	3·5	4·5	
Ferruginous alumina, chalk, and carbonate of magnesia	3·75	2·75	12·5	22·5	1·5
Sulphate of lime	...	—	—	—	
Sand	3·50	3·5	2·0	4·0	—
	100·00	100·00	100·5	100·0	101·75

ANTIOCH SCAMMONY, Marq. / SMYRNA SCAMMONY, Marq.

	No. 6. Round cakes. Sp. gr. 1.174.	No. 7. Angular pieces. Sp. gr. 1.120.	No. 8. Flat cakes. Sp. gr. 1.167.	No. 9. Round cakes. Sp. gr. 1.428.	No. 10. Round cakes. Sp. gr. 1.503.	No. 11. Broken pieces. Sp. gr. 1.863.	No. 12. Round cakes. Sp. gr. 1.376. (Fictitious.)
Alpha resin, with traces of wax	18·5	16·0	8·5	4·50	5	5·00	25·00
Beta resin	—	0·5	—	1·50	1	2·00	12·00
Extractive taken up by alcohol	7·0	10·0	8·0	3·00	11	15·00	4·00
Extractive taken up by water	6·0	5·0	12·0	10·00	18	8·00	13·00
Gum, with sulphate of lime	2·5	3·0	8·0	21·00	20	7·00	5·00
Mucilage	15·5	36·0	17·0	19·50	5	9·00	13·00
Starch	7·0	12·5	24·0		23	15·00	5·00
Colouring matter	6·5	12·5	16·5	—	2	—	—
Woody fibre, oxides, extractive, &c.	12·5	1·5	1·0	33·00	11	35·00	18·00
Inorganic salts, silica, &c.	22·5	3·0	4·0	7·50	4	4·00	5·00
Sand	2·0						
	100·5	100·0	99·0	100·00	100	100·00	100·00

Dr. Christison[1] has analysed both pure and adulterated scammony. His results are as follows :—

	PURE SCAMMONY.			ADULTERATED SCAMMONY.					
	Old.	Old.	Moist.	Calcareous.			Amylaceous.		Calcareo-Amylaceous.
Resin	81·8	83·0	77·0	64·6	56·6	43·3	37·0	62·0	42·4
Gum	6·0	8·0	6·0	6·8	5·0	8·2	9·0	7·2	7·8
Starch (fecula) ...	1·0	—	—	—	1·4	4·0	20·0	10·4	13·2
Lignin and sand...	3·5	3·2	5·0	5·2	7·1	7·8	22·2	13·4	9·4
Chalk..............	—	—	—	17·6	25·0	31·6	—	—	18·6
Water	7·7	7·2	12·6	6·4	5·2	6·4	12·2	7·5	10·4
	100·0	101·4	100·6	100·6	100·3	101·3	100·2	100·5	101·8

ADULTERATION.—The characters of good scammony are as follows :—It readily fractures between the fingers, or by the pressure of the nail ; its sp. gr. is about 1·2 ; its fracture is dark, glistening, and resinous ; its fractured surface should not effervesce on the addition of hydrochloric acid ; the decoction of the powder, filtered and cooled, is not rendered blue or purplish by tincture of iodine ; paper moistened with an alcoholic or ethereal tincture of scammony should undergo no change of colour when exposed to brown nitrous fumes (produced by pouring a drachm of strong nitric acid over some filings of zinc, iron, or copper, contained in a tumbler or wine-glass) ; 100 grains, incinerated with nitrate of ammonia, yield about three grains of ashes (according to my experiments) ; sulphuric ether separates at least 78 per cent. of resin (principally), dried at 280° F.

" Fracture glistening, almost resinous, if the specimens be old and dry : muriatic acid does not cause effervescence on its surface : the decoction of its powder, filtered and cooled, is not rendered blue by tincture of iodine. Sulphuric ether separates at least 80 per cent. of resin dried at 280°."—*Ph. Ed.*

[Pure scammony, according to Maltass, is easily recognised, when dry, by the following characters :—It is light, and breaks easily with a glossy fracture. If no water have been added by the peasants, the colour of the fracture is reddish-black. If water have been added, or the scammony has been collected in shady places, the fracture is black, and very glossy. If it have been put in tins or skins, the fracture is black, and not so glossy. If the dry drops, or Kaimak, scraped from the roots, be not worked up with the γὰλα or milk, pieces will be found of a light red colour resembling rosin. An emulsion is immediately produced by application of the tongue, excepting when water has been added without the assistance of the sun's rays, in which case the emulsive property becomes impaired. One of the best characters of genuine scammony is its golden-reddish colour when reduced to small fragments. *Black* scammony is indeed to be met with, but it is uncommon (unless it be adulterated) ; and it is not to be considered perfectly pure. The scammony collected by the Turkish peasants is black, heavy, and does not so readily break as that above described. It is procured by making a decoction of the cut and drained roots :

---

[1] *Dispensatory.*

the larger pieces of the root are thrown away, while the decoction, with the smaller portions of root, are thrown upon the scammony and worked up with it. This accounts for the quantity of vegetable fibre found in some samples.[1] Mr. D. Hanbury, in some useful practical remarks on scammony, describes the characters of pure natural scammony—*i. e.* the unmixed inspissated juice of the root—as follows :—It should have a pale yellowish-brown colour ; it should be transparent, very brittle, readily afford a white emulsion when rubbed with water, and leave but a small quantity of white residue when treated with ether.[2]—Ed.]

Hydrochloric acid detects the presence of carbonates : iodine added to the cooled decoction of scammony detects starch and dextrine ; by nitrous fumes the presence of guaiacum resin may be detected, for they give a blue colour to paper which has been moistened with tincture of guaiacum ; incineration detects an abnormal amount of inorganic matter, as chalk, gypsum, or sand; ether determines the amount of resinous matter present.[3] The microscope serves to detect the presence and sort of starch or meal used for adulterating. Hitherto, the only starch I have detected in adulterated scammony is that of a cereal, either wheat or barley,—probably the former.

[According to M. Thorel, resin of jalap, owing to its comparative cheapness, has been used for adulterating resin of scammony. This fraud may be detected by digesting the suspected substance in rectified ether. Jalap resin is quite insoluble in this menstruum, while the resin of scammony is soluble in it in all proportions. Resin of scammony is sometimes adulterated with resin of guaiacum ; this may be detected by nitrous gas. If the adulteration be caused by colophony this may be dissolved out and separated from scammony resin by oil of turpentine. Sulphuric acid gives with colophony immediately on contact an intense red colour; with scammony resin only a wine red slowly produced.[4]—Ed.]

PHYSIOLOGICAL EFFECTS.   *α. On Animals generally*.—The experiments of Orfila[5] lead us to infer that scammony is not poisonous. " We have," says he, " frequently administered four drachms of it to dogs who had the œsophagus afterwards tied, and have only observed alvine evacuations." On horses and other herbivorous animals its operation is very uncertain. Gilbert[6] states that six drachms killed a sheep in twenty days, without having caused purging. Viborg[7] says half an ounce given to a dog caused several loose stools : the same dose had no effect on a badger. It is probable, however, that in all the experiments now referred to, adulterated scammony was employed.

β. On Man.—The effects of pure scammony are those of a powerful and drastic purgative. As the greater part of the commercial drug is largely adulterated, practitioners are, I suspect, scarcely acquainted with the operation of the genuine article, which appears to me to possess nearly double the activity of that usually found in commerce. As the evacuant properties of scammony depend on its local irritation, it operates more energetically when there is a

---

[1] [*Pharmaceutical Journal*, loc. cit.]
[2] [*Ibid.* 1853, p. 270.]
[3] For further details, see a paper *On the Adulteration of Scammony*, by the author, in the *Pharmaceutical Journal*, vol. iv. p. 267, 1845.
[4] [*Pharmaceutical Journal*, December 1851, p. 278. For some valuable notes, by Mr. D. Hanbury, on the adulterations of this drug, we refer the reader to the same *Journal* for December 1853, p. 268.—Ed.]
[5] *Toxicol. Gén.*
[6] Moiroud, *Pharm. Vét.* p. 271.
[7] Wibmer, *Wirk. d. Arzn. u. Gifte*, Bd. ii. S. 181.

deficiency of intestinal mucus, and is then very apt to gripe; and, *vice versá*, when the intestines are well lined with secretion, it passes through with much less effect. In its operation scammony is closely allied to jalap, than which it is more active, while its odour and taste are less nauseous. It is less irritant than gamboge.

USES.—Scammony is, of course, inadmissible in inflammatory conditions of the alimentary canal, on account of its irritant qualities. It is well adapted for torpid and inactive conditions of the abdominal organs, accompanied with much slimy mucus in the intestines. It is principally valuable as a smart purgative for children, on account of the smallness of the dose necessary to produce the effect, the slight taste, and the energy, yet safety, of its operation. When used for them, it is generally associated with calomel. Where a milder purgative is required, it may be conjoined with rhubarb, sulphate of potash, and an aromatic. It may be employed to open the bowels in constipation; to expel worms, especially of children; to act as a hydragogue purgative, on the principle of counter-irritation, as in affections of the head and dropsies; and for any other purpose for which an active cathartic may be required.

ADMINISTRATION.—For an adult, the usual dose of commercial scammony is ten grains to a scruple; but, of virgin scammony, from ten to fifteen grains. In order to diminish its irritant and griping qualities, it should be finely divided. For this purpose it may be intimately mixed with some bland powder (as gum, starch, or sugar), or made into an emulsion with milk.[1]

1. PULVIS SCAMMONII COMPOSITUS, L. E. D.; *Compound Powder of Scammony.* (The *London College* directs it to be prepared with Scammony, Hard Extract of Jalap, of each ℥ij.; Ginger, ℨss. Rub them separately to very fine powder; then mix them. The *Edinburgh College* directs it to be made of equal parts of Scammony and Bitartrate of Potash, triturated together to a very fine powder.—The *Dublin College* directs Scammony, in fine powder, ℥j.; Compound Powder of Jalap, ℥iij. Mix thoroughly by trituration, and pass the powder through a fine sieve.)—The effects of scammony and of extract of jalap being very similar, little or no advantage can be obtained by the intermixture of these substances. The ginger is intended to correct the griping of the other ingredients. The bitartrate of potash, used by the Edinburgh College, can do little more than serve to divide the scammony. Compound powder of scammony is cathartic, and is used as a smart purge for children, especially where much mucous slime is contained in the bowels, and in worm cases.—The dose of the London preparation, for an adult, is from grs. x. to ℈j.; for children under a twelvemonth old, from grs. iij. to grs. v. The dose of the Edinburgh and Dublin preparations, for an adult, is is from grs. xv. to ℨss. The Dublin preparation is the weakest of the three.

2. PULVIS SCAMMONII CUM CALOMELANE; *Powder of Scammony with Calomel.* (Scammony, ℥j.; Calomel, Sugar, of each ℨss. Mix.)—Though

---

[1] [The usual dose of scammony as a purgative, among the Greek and Turkish peasants who collect it, is, according to Maltass, a shell, or one drachm. It is stated that a Greek peasant, while collecting scammony in 1852, near Macri, opposite the island of Rhodes, had an application made to him by a Turk for a dose of scammony. He gave him a shell-full. The Turk thinking that if the contents of *one* shell would prove salutary, that of a *greater number* would be proportionally of greater benefit, stole three or four more from the Greek, took the whole, and died the same day from the effects.— ED.]

this preparation is not contained in any of the British Pharmacopœias, yet the frequency of its employment in the diseases of children is a sufficient apology for its introduction here.   Dose, for an adult, grs. x. to grs. xx.; for children, from grs. iv. to grs. x., according to the age of the patient.

This preparation may be employed as a substitute for the old *Pulvis Basilicus* or *Royal Powder,* which consisted of equal parts of scammony, calomel, cream of tartar, and antimonic acid.

3. CONFECTIO SCAMMONII, L. D.; *Confection of Scammony.* (Scammony, powdered, ℥jss.; Cloves, bruised, Ginger, powdered, each ʒvj.; Oil of Caraway, fʒss.; Syrup of Roses, as much as may be sufficient.   Rub the dry ingredients together to very fine powder, and preserve them in a covered vessel; then, whenever the confection is to be used, the syrup being poured in, rub again; lastly, the oil being added, mix them all together, *L.*   The *Dublin College* directs Scammony, in fine powder, ℥iij.; Ginger, in fine powder, ℥iss.; Oil of Caraway, fʒj.; Oil of Cloves, fʒss.; Simple Syrup, f℥iij.; Clarified Honey, by weight, ℥iss.   Beat the powders with the syrup and honey into a uniform mass, then add the oils, and mix all well together.)— A warm or aromatic cathartic.   Dose, for an adult, ℈j. to ʒj.; for children, grs. iij. to grs. x.   It is seldom employed.

4. EXTRACTUM *sive* **RESINA SCAMMONII,** E.; *Extract* or *Resin of Scammony.* (Take any convenient quantity of scammony in fine powder; boil it in successive portions of proof spirit till the spirit ceases to dissolve any thing; filter; distil the liquid till but little water passes over.   Then pour away the watery solution from the resin at the bottom; agitate the resin with the successive portions of boiling water till it is well washed; and, lastly, dry it at a temperature not exceeding 204°.)—To obtain pure resin of scammony, alcohol or ether should be used instead of proof spirit.   It is brownish, and in thin layers transparent; when heated, it evolves a peculiar, not disagreeable odour; it is fusible and combustible.   It is soluble in alcohol, ether, and oil of turpentine.

Resin of jalap is insoluble in oil of turpentine, and nearly so in ether; whereas scammony resin is readily soluble in these liquids. By these peculiarities the two resins may be distinguished from each other (see *ante,* p. 610).

The alcoholic solution of scammony resin is feebly acid; the addition of water causes a white precipitate (*hydrate of resin*).   Precipitates (*metallic scammoniates ?*) are also produced by alcoholic solutions of the acetate of lead and the acetate of copper.   Caustic potash deepens the colour of the solution.[1]   Scammony resin may be decolorised by animal charcoal without having its purgative qualities affected.[2]   Its composition, according to Mr. Johnston,[3] is $C^{40}H^{33}O^{20}$.   It is "remarkable for containing the largest quantity of oxygen of any resin hitherto analysed" (Johnston).   When pure or virgin scammony can be obtained, the extract or resin is an unnecessary preparation.   Scammony resin is a drastic cathartic.   Dose, grs. viij. to grs. xij. When administered, it should be intimately divided, either by some bland powder, or still better by an emulsion.

---

[1] Marquart, *op. cit.*
[2] *Journ. de Pharm.* t. xiii. p. 589.
[3] *Phil. Trans.* for 1840, p. 341.

5 TINCTURA SCAMMONII ; *Tincture of Scammony; Tincture de Scammonée,* Codex Pharm. Française, 1837. (Aleppo Scammony, 1 part; Rectified Spirit, 4 parts by weight : macerate for fifteen days and filter.)— Dose, fʒss. to fʒj., diffused throughout a mucilaginous mixture or milk.

6. MISTURA SCAMMONII, E.; *Mixture of Scammony.* (Resin of Scammony, gr. vij.; Unskimmed Milk, fʒiij. Triturate the resin with a little of the milk, and gradually with the rest of it till a uniform emulsion is formed.)—This is an imitation of *Planche's purgative potion,* except that two drachms of sugar and three or four drops of cherry-laurel water are omitted. It is one of the most agreeable draughts that can be taken.

188. EXOGONIUM PURGA, *Bentham.*—TRUE JALAP.

Sex. Syst. Pentandria, Monogynia.

(Tuber, *L.*—Root, *E. D.*)

HISTORY.—De Paiva[1] thinks that jalap was known to Dodoens in 1552, to Monardes in 1568, and to Clusius in 1574.[2] But Bauhin[3] (who calls it *Bryonia Mechoacana nigricans*) says it was brought from India, under the name of *Chelapa,* or *Celapa,* about eleven years before the time he wrote (the date of the preface to his work is 1620) : that is, about 1609 or 1610. Its name seems to be derived from Xalapa, a town of Mexico.

The jalap plant has been successively declared to be a *Mirabilis,* a *Convolvulus,* an *Ipomæa,* and an *Exogonium.*

The *Convolvulus Jalapa* described and figured by Woodville[4] and Desfontaines,[5] is now well known to yield none of this drug. The real jalap plant was first described by Mr. Nuttall;[6] but the name (*Ipomæa Jalapa*) which he gave to it had been already applied by Pursh to another plant. In the same year Dr. Schiede[7] and Dr. Wenderoth[8] noticed it : the latter called it first *Convolvulus Purga,* and afterwards *Ipomæa Purga.* In 1832 it was described and figured by Zuccarini,[9] under the name of *Ipomæa Schiedeana.* Choisy, in De Candolle's *Prodromus* (vol. ix. p. 374), has adopted Wenderoth's name of *Ipomæa purga ;* but as the jalap plant has a salver-shaped (hypocrateriform) corolla and exserted stamens, it certainly cannot be an Ipomæa, a part of whose character is a campanulate corolla and enclosed stamens.

BOTANY. **Gen. Char.**—*Sepals* 5. *Corolla* tubular. *Stamens* exserted. *Style* 1. *Stigma* capitate, 2-lobed. *Ovary* 2-celled; the cells 2-seeded (*Choisy*).

---

1 Voigtels' *Arzneimittell.* Bd. i. S. 117.
2 See some remarks on this subject in *Pharm. Central-Blatt für* 1834, S. 955-6.
3 *Prodromus,* p. 135.
4 *Med. Bot.* p. 59.
5 *Ann. Mus. d'Hist. Nat.* t. ii.
6 *American Journal of Medical Sciences for February* 1830.
7 *Linnæa,* v. 3, July 1830, p. 473 ; and *Pharm. Central-Blatt für* 1830, p. 408.
8 *Pharm. Central-Blatt für* 1830, p. 456 ; and *Linnæa,* viii. 515.
9 *Acta Acad. Reg. Monacensis,* vol. x.

Sp. Char.—*Root* tuberose; incrassated, perennial. *Stems* annual, twining, branched, smooth. *Leaves* ovate, acuminate, cordate at the base, quite entire, and smooth on both sides. *Peduncles* 1- to 3-flowered. *Sepals* unequal, obtuse, smooth. *Corolla* salver-shaped, with a subclavate, cylindrical tube, and a subpentagonal, horizontally-expanded limb.

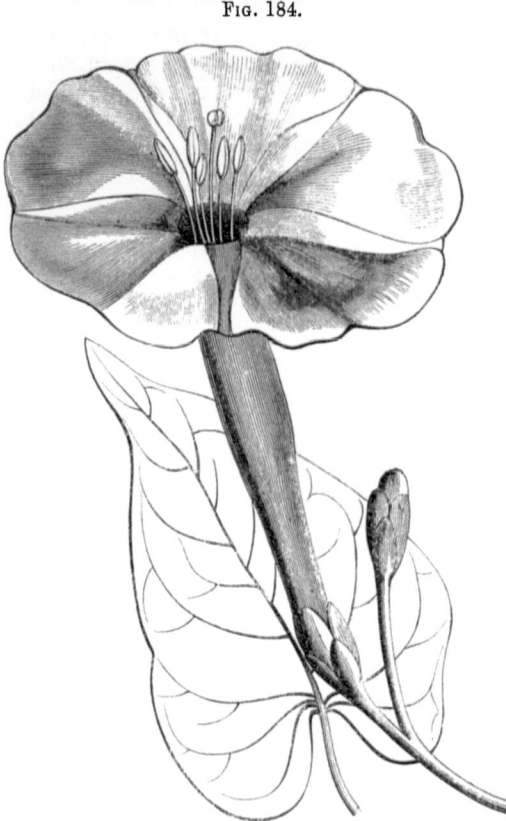

Fig. 184.

Root perennial, irregularly ovate-conical, terminating inferiorly in some subcylindrical fibrous branches; covered by a very thin, dirty, blackish epidermis; internally white and fleshy. *Stem* herbaceous. *Leaves* alternate, petioled. Tube of the *corolla* purplish-violet (red lake).

Hab.—In the woods of the Mexican empire, near Chicanquiaco, at an elevation of nearly 6,000 feet above the level of the sea. Jalapa is the only market for the root, from whence it is exported to Europe by way of Vera Cruz.

Flower and Leaf of Exogonium Purga.

IPOMÆA ORIZABENSIS, Ledanois; *Convolvulus orizabensis;* Pelletan, Journ. de Chim. Méd. t. x. p. 10, 1834; *Ipomæa batatoides,* Bentham, Botan. Regist. Jan. 1841; *Ipomæa? Mestitlanica,* Choisy, De Cand. Prodr. ix. 389.—This plant grows in the environs of Orizaba and near Mestitlan in Mexico. It yields an inferior sort of jalap, called *light, fusiform,* or *male jalap.*

DESCRIPTION.—1. The dried tubers of true jalap (*radix jalapæ; rad· jalapæ tuberosæ* vel *ponderosæ*) found in commerce rarely exceed a pound each in weight. They vary in size from that of the fist to that of a nut. When entire, they are usually more or less oval, and pointed at the two opposite extremities. The larger tubers are frequently incised,—apparently to facilitate desiccation. They are covered with a thin, brown, wrinkled cuticle. They should be heavy, hard, and difficult to powder. When broken, good tubers should present a deep yellowish-grey colour, interspersed with deep brown concentric circles. The slices vary in their shape, colour, and other properties. Those of inferior quality are light, *whitish,* friable; they usually appear to be quarter segments of transverse slices, and are sometimes called *spurious jalap*, or, from their shape, *cocked-hat jalap*.   Jalap is very apt to become worm-eaten; but the insects which attack it devour the amylaceous matter and ligneous matter, and leave the resin.   Hence *worm-eaten jalap* is well adapted for the preparation of extract.

2. A *spurious jalap*, called in Mexico *male jalap*, is sometimes found intermixed with the genuine sort.   It was first described by Mr. D. B. Smith,[1] and has been termed by Guibourt *light* or *fusiform jalap*.   It is the kind sometimes called in English commerce *woody jalap* or *jalap wood*, and which in Germany has been termed *jalap stalks* (*stipites jalapæ*).   It is the produce of *Ipomæa orizabensis*, Ledanois.   As met with in commerce, it is in slices or segments which are more fibrous or woody than genuine jalap. The cut surface is often darker from exposure to the air, and uneven from the unequal shrinking in the drying process.   Internally the colour is whitish. The odour and taste are similar to, but feebler than, the true jalap.

[MICROSCOPICAL CHARACTERS.—This spurious article differs essentially from the true jalap, inasmuch as it is a true root, and not a tuber : it consists of slices or segments of the root, some extremely fibrous, and others heavy, solid, and resinous.   According to Mr. Evans, when microscopically examined, it presents large quantities of oval or rounded cells with thin walls, filled with minute starch grains.   Empty or collapsed cells are nearly absent : numerous cells filled with sugar, and a great number containing a greenish-yellow resin soluble in ether, are abundant.   These cells are more of an elongated or cubical form than those containing starch or sugar.   There are also cells filled with a resin insoluble in ether, but much less numerous.   The epidermis consists of a continuous membrane composed of large irregularly angular cells, with thick walls slightly pitted : no oval epidermal cells are found, as in the true jalap.[2]—ED.]

3. Guibourt[3] has described a *false rose-scented jalap*.   It is in tubercles which are not so dark-coloured as the genuine drug.   They are deeply furrowed ; the prominent parts of the furrows being white, from the friction of the pieces against each other ; the depressions being dark-coloured.   The pieces are but slightly resinous, are amylaceous and saccharine, and have rather an agreeable sweetish odour, which Guibourt compares to that of oil of rhodium or of the rose.   It possesses scarcely any purgative action.   It is probably the kind known in the American market as *overgrown jalap*.

[There are four descriptions of jalap in English commerce, of which the first two are genuine, and the remaining two false : viz. 1, the dark and heavy description ; 2, less heavy, and of a lighter colour, evidently less resinous, and worth 20 per cent. less than the best ; 3, white or false jalap, of which a few pieces may at times be found mixed with the true sort, but which, latterly, has arrived in separate bales without finding buyers ; 4, jalap stalk or jalap wood, cut into pieces of the size of the root, but which cannot be mistaken for it, the shape being less rounded off, and the weight and colour being much lighter than the true root.—ED.]

SELECTION.—Jalap is more active as a cathartic in proportion to the

[1] *American Journal of Pharmacy*, vol. ii. p. 22.
[2] [*Pharmaceutical Journal*, March 1854, p. 410.]
[3] *Ibid.* vol. ii. p. 331, 1842.

quantity of resin which it contains : plump, firm, heavy, resinous pieces, there-fore, are preferable.   Light, whitish, amylaceous, shrivelled, or woody pieces, are objectionable.

[Commerce. — The importation of jalap amounted, in the ten years 1835—1844, to 2,303 bales, and the consumption to 448,326 pounds, making the annual importation, on an average, 230 bales of two to two and a half hundredweight each, and the annual consumption 44,832 pounds. We subjoin the annual importation in pounds during a period of seven years :—

	Pounds imported.
1843	67,587
1844	47,548
1845	38,113
1846	73,199
1847	53,178
1848	68,829
1849	82,519.—Ed.]

Composition.—Jalap was analysed, in 1817, by Cadet de Gassicourt,[1] and more recently by Gerber.[2]   Other less complete analyses have been made by Henry,[3] by Ledanois,[4] by Nees v. Esenbeck, and Marquart.[5]   In 1835 Cannobio analysed a variety of jalap called *gialappone*,[6] similar in appearance to galanga.

Gerber's Analysis.

Hard resin	7·8
Soft resin	3·2
Slightly acrid extractive	17·9
Gummy extractive	14·4
Colouring matter	8·2
Uncrystallisable sugar .	1·9
Gum, with some salts .	15·6
Bassorin	3·2
Vegetable albumen	3·9
Starch	6·0
Water	4·8
Malic acid, and malates of potash and lime	2·4
Chlorides of calcium and potassium	1·4
Phosphates of magnesia and lime	1·7
Carbonate (?) of lime .	3·0
Loss	4·6
Jalap	100·0

Henry's Analyses.

	Light.	Sound.	Worm-eaten.
Resin	12	9·6	14·4
Extractive	15	28·0	25·0
Starch	19	20·4	20·6
Woody fibre	54	42·0	40·0
Jalap	100	100·0	100·0

Nees v. Esenbeck and Marquart's Analyses.

	Root of *Exogonium Purga.*	Commercial Jalap.	False Jalap.
Extractive	20·416	27·50	6·66
Resin	12·083	13·33	18·33
Matters insoluble in alcohol	67·500	59·16	75·00
	100·000	100·00	100·00

The following are analyses by Ledanois and Guibourt :—

[1] *Journ. de Pharm.* t. iii. p. 495.
[2] Gmelin, *Handb. d. Chemie*, Bd. ii. S. 1299.
[3] *Bull. de Pharm.* t. ii. p. 87.
[4] *Journ. de Chim. Méd.* t. v. p. 508.
[5] *Pharm. Central-Blatt für* 1834, S. 695.
[6] *Ibid. für* 1835, S. 304.

Ledanois's Analysis.		Guibourt's Analyses.		
Male, light, or fusiform Jalap.			**Officinal Jalap.**	**False rose-scented Jalap.**
Resin	8·0	Resin	17·65	.... 3·23
Gummy extract.	25·6	Liquid sugar by alcohol	19·00	.... 16·47
Starch	3·2	Brown saccharine extract obtained by water..	9·05	.... 5·92
Albumen	2·4	Gum	10·12	.... 3·88
Woody fibre	58·0	Starch	18·78	.... 22·69
Water and loss..	2·8	Woody fibre....................................	21·60	.... 46·00
		Loss...	3·80	.... 1·81
Jalap ......100·0		Jalap......................	100·00	.... 100·00

1. JALAP RESINS.—The resinous portion of jalap is the most important, because it is the active ingredient of this root. The substance generally known as *jalap resin* is obtained by mixing the alcoholic tincture of jalap (prepared by percolation or digestion) with water. The precipitated resin is to be washed with warm water, and then dissolved in alcohol. By evaporation the tincture yields the resin. Planche[1] has proposed another process. By digestion with animal charcoal the alcoholic solution of the resin is rendered nearly colourless, and by evaporation yields an almost colourless resin (*resina jalapæ alba* of Martius).[2] Jalap resin is soluble in alcohol, but insoluble in water. Triturated with milk, it does not form an emulsion, but its particles unite into a solid mass. By this it may be distinguished from scammony resin.[3] It is insoluble in the fixed and volatile oils. Its insolubility in oil of turpentine is a means of detecting the intermixture of some other resins, as of scammony and turpentine.[4] Jalap resin is sometimes adulterated with guaiacum.[5] This, unlike jalap resin (rhodeoretin), is soluble in ether: and paper moistened with its alcoholic solution is rendered blue by nitrous gas. Decolorised jalap is composed, according to Goebel,[6] of *carbon* 36·62, *hydrogen* 9·47, and *oxygen* 53·91; but Johnston[7] declares this analysis to be incorrect, and gives the following as the formula for the resin:—$C^{40}H^{34}O^{18}$. According to Buchner and Herberger,[8] as also Kayser,[9] the so-called jalap resin consists of two distinct resins,—one soluble in ether, the other insoluble in this liquid.

a. Jalapin; Rhodeoretin (from ῥόδεος, rose-red; ῥητίνη, resin); $C^{42}H^{35}O^{20}$.—Is this the jalapin of Mr. Hume?[10] This resin is insoluble in ether. Kayser obtained it by boiling purified jalap resin in ether, which took up the jalapic acid and left the jalapin. According to Buchner and Herberger, it constitutes not quite nine-tenths of jalap resin. It is a transparent, colourless, odourless, and tasteless resin; very soluble in alcohol, but insoluble in water and in ether. It does not possess basic properties, as Buchner and Herberger supposed; but, on the contrary, possesses acid properties, reddens litmus, and is soluble in ammonia and acetic acid. If the salt which it forms with oxide of lead be decomposed by sulphuretted hydrogen, the resin is then found to have combined with the elements of water, and to have become converted into *hydrorhodeoretin*, $C^{42}H^{36}O^{21}$. [Mayer has recently examined this substance, which he calls rhodeoretine. He states that it is without smell, taste, or colour; softening at 266°, and melting at 302°. Its formula, according to him, is $C^{72}H^{60}O^{37}$: and it is identical with the jalapine of Buchner and Herberger, above described, and the β resin of Sandrock. It appears to be the active principle of jalap: three or four grains caused repeated and violent purging. Chemically, it has not the characters of an acid, although by the action of bases it is converted into rhodeoretinic acid, the formula of which is, according to Mayer, $C^{72}H^{64}O^{40}$. Sulphuric acid, hydrochloric acid, and emulsine, convert rhodeoretine into an oily substance—rhodeoretinic acid and sugar. When acted upon by nitric acid, rhodeoretinic acid yields oxalic

[1] Soubeiran, *Traité de Pharm.* t. ii. p. 28.
[2] *Pharm. Central-Blatt für* 1835, S. 557.
[3] Planche, *Journ. de Pharm.* t. xviii. p. 181–5.
[4] *Pharm. Central-Blatt für* 1832, 837; and *für* 1838, S. 904.
[5] *Pharmaceutical Journal*, vol. iii. p. 132, 1843.
[6] *Pharm. Waarenk.* Bd. ii. S. 59.
[7] *Phil. Trans.* for 1840, p. 343.
[8] *Pharm. Central-Blatt für* 1831, S. 284.
[9] *Ann. der Chem. u. Pharm.* Bd. li. p. 81, 1844; and *Pharm. Journal*, vol. iv. p. 327, 1845.
[10] *Med. and Phys. Journ.* for April 1824, p. 346.

acid, and a white crystalline non-nitrogenous acid—ipomic acid—perhaps identical with the sebacic. Its formula is $C^{10}H^8O^4$. Mayer is of opinion that rhodeoretinic acid is a conjugate compound—rhodeoretinolic acid and sugar.[1]—Ed.]

β. Jalapic Acid; Odorous Principle of Jalap?.—Constitutes thirteen per cent. of jalap resin. It is a brown, soft, and greasy substance, which reacts as an acid, has the odour of jalap, and an acrid taste. By long contact with water it crystallises. It is soluble in ether, in alcohol, and in alkaline solutions; but is insoluble in hydrochloric acid. It is either a crystallisable soft resin or a fatty acid.

Pararhodeoretin; $C^{42}H^{34}O^{18}$.—This is a simple resin, and is obtained from the male or fusiform jalap (Ipomæa orizabensis). It is soluble in both alcohol and ether. If jalap resin (rhodeoretin or pararhodeoretin) be digested in a watch-glass with oil of vitriol, a crimson-coloured solution is obtained, from which in a few hours a brown viscid resin will separate. By this test jalap resin is distinguished from other resins.

2. Starch.—The starch-grains vary in size. Their shapes are spheres, semi-spheres, or that of mullers. The hilum is very distinct.

[Adulterations.—The chief source of adulteration in jalap is the substitution of the Mexican male jalap (*Ipomæa orizabensis*) for the tuber of the *Exogonium Purga*. The microscopical characters of the root of Ipomæa, as observed by Mr. Evans, have been elsewhere described (*ante*, p. 615). The principal grounds of distinction are the general coarseness of the male jalap, the large thick-walled cells of its epidermis, its abundant woody tissue, small muller-shaped starch-grains, with abundance of resins soluble in ether. Linseed meal, wheat flour, and guaiacum dust, are also used for adulterating the true jalap powder. These admixtures may be distinguished by the microscope.

In the jalap of commerce, tubers of very different qualities are met with; some having been gathered before, and others after the flowering of the plant: the former may be considered as immature, the latter as mature jalap.

Microscopical Characteristics.—In the *mature* jalap there are many large rounded cells with thin walls filled with starch-grains, tightly packed with others of the same character, but empty and collapsed. These form the substance of the tuber, but interspersed among them there are many large elongated or angular cells with thin walls filled with resinous matter insoluble in ether. This is the resin peculiar to jalap, and to which it owes its purgative properties. It is secreted from the elaborated juice of the plant. The epidermis consists of a layer of elongated angular cells, with thick pitted walls firmly adherent to one another. Starch-grains are numerous, of small size, contained for the most part within cells, but frequently loosely distributed in the tissue. Associated with these are numerous stellated groups of raphides. In the *immature* tubers the epidermis consists of much larger and very irregularly shaped angular cells with thick walls. The cells of the cellular tissue are generally empty and collapsed, with but little starch and much sugar, a paucity of resin, and that which is found differing from the true resin of jalap in being partially soluble in ether.[2]—Ed.]

Physiological Effects. *a. On Animals generally.* — Jalap root in powder, as well as the resin obtained from it, is a local irritant. Its operation on the bowels is well seen in the *carnivora*. Cadet de Gassicourt[3] found that the resin applied to the pleura, peritoneum, or intestinal canal of dogs, caused fatal inflammation. Two drachms introduced into the stomach, the œsophagus being afterwards tied, killed a dog in a few hours. It is remarkable, however, that the same experimenter observed no particular effect from the application of a drachm of the finely-powdered resin to the cellular tissue of the back. Moreover, 24 grains, with the yelk of an egg, injected into the jugular vein, had, he says, a very slight effect; indeed, at first none was observed, but the two following days the animal had soft, pale evacuations, and lost his appetite, though he soon recovered from this state. In the *her-*

---

[1] [*Pharmaceutical Journal*, April 1853, p. 502.]
[2] [See a paper by Mr. Evans in the *Pharmaceutical Journal*, March 1854, p. 409.]
[3] Wibmer, *Wirk. d. Arzn. u. Gifte*, Bd. iii. S. 181.

bivora it proves a very uncertain purgative. Gilbert[1] gave two ounces to a sheep without observing any effect. Donné[2] administered two or three ounces to horses without observing any remarkable effect except increased secretion of urine.

β. *On Man.*—In the human subject jalap acts as a powerful and drastic purgative, producing copious liquid stools; and, when judiciously exhibited, is both safe and efficacious. Its objectionable effects are, that while in the stomach it causes frequently nausea, and sometimes vomiting; while, after it has passed into the intestines it oftentimes gripes. It is tolerably certain in its operation,—more so, indeed, than many other purgatives. In the proper dose it may be given without the least hesitation to children, in any case requiring an active purge. It has an advantage over some other evacuants, that it does not stimulate or heat the system, its effect being confined principally to the alimentary canal—the peristaltic motion, secretions, and exhalations of which, it promotes; and it is said that constipation less frequently succeeds its use than of some other purgatives.

My own experience of jalap would lead me to regard it as a perfectly safe, though active cathartic; but Dr. Christison[3] says that "severe and even dangerous effects have followed its incautious use in the hands of the practical joker." I am not acquainted with any cases, in the human subject, in which its employment has been attended by serious consequences. It is a more drastic purgative than senna. To scammony it is closely allied, not only by its effects, but also by botanical affinities and chemical properties. It is much less irritant to the intestinal mucous membrane than gamboge; and, therefore, is a much safer purgative. Vogt[4] regards it as exceeding the last-mentioned substance, but as being inferior to aloes, in its stimulant influence over the abdominal and pelvic blood-vessels; and Sundelin[5] observes that while it is more irritant it is less heating than aloes or senna.

USES.—Daily experience proves the value of jalap, as an active purgative, in various diseases both of children and adults. Of course its irritant properties unfit it for exhibition in inflammatory affections of the alimentary canal, as well as after surgical operations about the abdomen and pelvis. Moreover, it is not an appropriate purgative in irritation of, or hemorrhage from, the uterus; or in piles, stricture, and prolapsus of the rectum. On the other hand, its use is indicated in torpid and overloaded conditions of the intestinal canal, as well as in constipation attended with retention of the catamenia. When the object is to relieve cerebral congestion and dropsical affections, by a counter-irritant influence on the mucous membrane, jalap is well adapted to fulfil it, both by the energy and safety of its operation. The following are some of the cases in which it is employed :—

1. *In constipation.*—When this condition is not dependent on, or connected with, irritation or inflammation of the alimentary canal or pelvic organs, jalap is admissible. Its efficiency is much increased by association with calomel. It may be employed in febrile and inflammatory diseases (those above mentioned excepted), as well as in chronic maladies.

---

[1] Moiroud, *Pharm. Vét.* p. 269.
[2] *Ibid.*
[3] *On Poisons,* p. 554.
[4] *Pharmakodyn.* Bd. ii. S. 230, 2te Aufl.
[5] *Handb. d. spec. Heilmittell.* Bd. ii. S. 26, 3te Aufl.

2. *As a vermifuge.*—The compound of jalap and calomel is a most efficacious anthelmintic, and may be used with the most happy effects in children,
especially where there is an excessive secretion of mucus.   " Jalap," says
Bremser,[1] " is, without contradiction, in verminous diseases, one of the best
purgatives, and which, perhaps, possesses, at the same time, greater anthelmintic virtues than any other."

3. *In cerebral affections.*—Jalap, in combination with calomel, is used
with the best effect, on the principle of counter-irritation, to relieve cerebral
congestion.   In inflammatory affections of the brain or its membranes, or in
hydrocephalus, it is a valuable purgative.

4. *In dropsies.*—In dropsical affections it is frequently desirable to promote
watery stools.   Jalap, especially in combination with cream of tartar, may be
used for this purpose with the best effects.   Marggrave[2] calls it a *panacea
hydropicorum.*

5. *In retention of the catamenia, or of the hemorrhoidal flux,* jalap is
one of the purgatives adapted, from their stimulant influence over the pelvic
vessels, to promote these discharges.

ADMINISTRATION.—The dose of jalap, *in powder,* is, for an adult, from ten
to thirty grains : a scruple usually acts smartly and safely : for children under
twelve months old the dose is from two to five grains.   Fifteen grains of jalap,
and two or three grains of calomel, form an efficient, yet safe, purgative for
an adult; but this combination very readily produces salivation by repetition.
From two to five grains of ipecacuanha are sometimes substituted for the calomel.
To children jalap is sometimes exhibited in gingerbread cakes.   *Purgative
cakes* of this kind are kept in the shops.   The *Biscuits purgatifs* (*Panes
saccharati purgantes*) are composed of Jalap, ʒxx. ; Flour, ʒij. ; 24 Eggs ;
and Sugar, lb. j.   This quantity is sufficient for 60 biscuits.[3]

1. PULVIS JALAPÆ COMPOSITUS, L. E. D. ; *Compound Powder of Jalap.*
(Jalap, ʒiij. ; Bitartrate of Potash, ʒvj. ; Ginger, ʒij.   Rub them separately
to powder; then mix them, *L.*   The *Edinburgh College* uses the same proportions of jalap and bitartrate of potash, but the ginger is omitted.   The
Dublin College orders Jalap, in fine powder, ʒij. ; Bitartrate of Potash, ʒiiiss. ;
Ginger, in fine powder, ʒss.   Mix thoroughly by trituration, and pass the
powder through a fine sieve.)—Hydragogue purgative.   Used in habitual
costiveness, verminal diseases, and dropsies.   Dose for an adult, ϶j. to ʒj.

2. TINCTURA JALAPÆ, L. E. D. ; *Tincture of Jalap.* (Jalap, coarsely powdered, ʒv. [in moderately fine powder, ʒvij. *E.*] ; Proof Spirit, Oij.   Macerate
for seven days, then press out and strain, *L.*   " This tincture may be prepared
either by digestion or percolation, as directed for tincture of cinchona," *E.*   The
Dublin College orders Jalap Root, in coarse powder, ʒv. ; Proof Spirit, Oiss.
Macerate for fourteen days, strain, express, and filter.)—An active cathartic.
Rarely used alone : generally employed as an adjunct to purgative draughts;
the activity of which it promotes.—Dose, fʒj. to fʒiv.   As an adjuvant to a
cathartic draught, the dose rarely exceeds fʒij.

---

[1] *Traité sur les Vers Intest.* p. 440.
[2] *Mat. Med. contr.* p. 46, ed. 2nda.
[3] Jourdan, *Pharmacopée Universelle.*

3. EXTRACTUM JALAPÆ, L.; *Extractum* sive *Resina Jalapæ*, E.; *Extract of Jalap.* (Jalap Root, powdered, lb. iiss.; Rectified Spirit, Cong. j.; Distilled Water, Cong. ij. Macerate the jalap root in the spirit for four days, and pour off the tincture. Boil down the residue in the water to half a gallon; afterwards strain the tincture and the decoction separately, and let the latter be evaporated, and the former distil, until each thickens. Lastly, mix the extract with the resin, and evaporate to a proper consistence, *L.* This extract should be kept *soft*, which may be fit to form pills; and *hard*, which may be rubbed to powder, *L.* The directions of the *Edinburgh College* are the following:—"Take any convenient quantity of jalap, in moderately fine powder; mix it thoroughly with enough of the rectified spirit to moisten it well; put it in twelve hours into a percolator, and exhaust the powder with rectified spirit; distil off the greater part of the spirit, and concentrate the residuum over the vapour-bath to a due consistence." In this process the alcohol extracts the resin, and the water subsequently used by the London College takes up the gummy extractive : the alcoholic tincture is distilled to save the spirit, while the aqueous decoction is evaporated.)—The preparation of the *Edinburgh College* is the impure resin of jalap; whereas that of the *London College* is a mixture of resin with the gummy extractive. It was formerly, and indeed is now by many persons, supposed that the combination of these ingredients was necessary for the full cathartic effect of jalap. It is, however, well known that the watery extract is inert as a purgative, though it is said to be diuretic : the only advantage, therefore, that can attend the mixture of the two extracts (the watery and the alcoholic) is, that the resin is intimately divided, and thereby prevented from causing violent irritation and griping in any one part of the intestinal tube. But it is obvious that the same advantage can be obtained by mixing the resin with some mild agent (as almonds, sugar, or saline matter, as sulphate of potash). Mr. Brande[1] says that jalap yields about 66 per cent. of extract; that is, 16 of alcoholic, and 50 of watery extract. According to this statement, therefore, the extract of the Edinburgh College possesses four times the activity of that of the London College.—The dose of the *resin* (Ph. Ed.) is from grs. iij. to grs. vj., in a minute state of division, as above directed; of the extract (Ph. L.), from grs. x. to Əj.

189. Pharbitis Nil, *Choisy.*

Sex. Syst. Pentandria, Monogynia.

(Semina.)

Convolvulus Nil, Linn.—A tropical plant, with purgative seeds.—The *Pharbitis cærulea*, Wallich (*Ipomæa cærulea*, Kœnig, in Roxb. Fl. Ind. vol. i. p. 501) is probably only a variety of it. Its seeds are sold in India under the name of *kala dana, hub ul nil*, and *mirchai*. They are black, angular, and weigh, on an average, half a grain each. Their taste is sweetish, and subsequently acrid. They consist of resin, gum, starch, bland fixed oil, vegetable fibre, and colouring matter. They yield from 15 to 20 per cent. of alcoholic brown extract containing resin and oil. In doses of from 30 to 40 grains the seeds act as a quick and safe cathartic; in some few cases they occasion vomiting and griping. The alcoholic extract may be given in doses of ten grains. The effects of the seeds and

---

[1] *Dict. Mat. Med.* p. 331.

extract resemble those of jalap, for which they may be substituted.[1] Roxburgh directs the seeds to be gently roasted, like coffee, then powdered, and given in any convenient vehicle.

ORDER XLV. GENTIANACEÆ, *Lindley.*—GENTIANWORTS.

GENTIANEÆ, *Jussieu.*

CHARACTERS.—*Calyx* divided, inferior, persistent. *Corolla* monopetalous, hypogynous, usually regular and persistent; the limb regular, sometimes furnished with delicate fringes, its lobes of the same number as those of the calyx, generally 5, sometimes 4, 6, 8, or 10; occasionally extended at the base into a bag or spur, with a plaited, or folded, or imbricated twisted æstivation. *Stamens* inserted upon the corolla; all in the same line, equal in number to the segments, and alternate with them; some of them occasionally abortive. *Ovary* composed of 2 carpels, 1- or partly 2-celled, many-seeded. *Style* 1, continuous with the ovary; *stigmas* 2, right and left of the axis; *ovules* indefinite, anatropal, parietal. *Capsule* or *berry* many-seeded; when 2-valved, the margins of the valves turned inwards, and bearing the seeds; in the 2-celled genera, inserted into a central placenta. *Seeds* small; *testa* single; *embryo* minute in the axis of soft fleshy *albumen; radicle* next the hilum.—*Herbaceous* plants, seldom *shrubs,* generally smooth, sometimes twining. *Leaves* opposite, entire, without stipules, sessile, or having their petioles confluent in a little sheath, in most cases 3-5-ribbed; very rarely brown and scale-like; sometimes alternate. *Flowers* terminal or axillary, regular, or very seldom irregular (*Lindley*).

PROPERTIES.—This Order contains a bitter principle, which is especially abundant in the roots.   On this substance depend the stomachic, tonic, and febrifuge properties of the different species.

190. GENTIANA LUTEA, *Linn.* — COMMON OR YELLOW GENTIAN.

Sex. Syst. Pentandria, Digynia.

(Radix, *L.*—Root, *E. D.*)

HISTORY.—Gentian is said to owe its name, and introduction into medical use, to Gentius, king of Illyria, who was vanquished by the Romans about 160 or 169 years before Christ.   It is, therefore, not noticed by either Hippocrates or Theophrastus, but is mentioned by Dioscorides,[2] who calls it γεντιανὴ; and by Pliny.[3]

BOTANY.   Gen. Char.—*Calyx* 5-4-parted or split, sometimes dimidiate-spathaceous, valvate. *Corolla* withering, rarely glandular, without epipetalous hollows; the limb 5-4-parted, or spuriously 10-parted. *Stamens* 5-4, inserted in the tube of the corolla; filaments equal at the base. *Ovary* 1-celled; the ovules in rows next the suture.   *Stigmas* 2, terminal, revolute, or, if contiguous, funnel-shaped; *style* 0, or persistent with the stigmas. *Capsule* 2-valved, septicidal, 1-celled; the placentæ membranous. *Seeds* immersed in the placentæ (condensed from *Grisebach*).

Sp. Char.—Stem tall, straight.   Leaves oval and ovate, smooth at the

---

[1] O'Shaughnessy, *Bengal Dispensatory.*
[2] Lib. iii. cap. 3.
[3] *Hist. Nat.* lib. xxv. cap. 34, ed. Valp.

margin. Cymes umbelliform, dense-flowered, axillary or terminal, pedunculate. Corollas yellow; the segments oblong-linear, acuminate (*Grisebach*).

Root perennial, cylindrical or spindle-shaped, simple or somewhat branched, ringed, wrinkled, externally brown, internally yellow and fleshy. *Stem* simple, erect, 2-3 feet high, roundish, hollow, smooth. *Leaves* pale green, opposite, ovate or oval, pointed, entire, smooth, 5-7-ribbed, plaited; lower ones on short, sheathing petioles; upper ones amplexicaul; those next the flowers becoming concave yellowish-green *bracts*. *Flowers* on smooth peduncles of 4-6 lines long. *Calyx* yellow. *Corolla* yellow; segments 5-7, lanceolate. *Stamens* as long as the corolla. *Ovary* conical, with 5 greenish glands at the base. *Capsule* conical, 2-valved. *Seeds* numerous, roundish, albuminous, with membranous margins.

Hab.—Subalpine and mountainous meadows, 6500-8000 feet above the level of the sea, of Central and Southern Europe.

Collection.—The roots are collected and dried by the peasants of Switzerland, the Tyrol, Burgogne, and Auvergne. They are imported into this country in bales from Havre, Marseilles, and other ports.

Description.—Gentian root (*radix gentianæ*) is imported in cylindrical, usually more or less branched pieces, varying in length from a few inches to a foot or more, and in thickness from half an inch to one or two inches. These pieces are marked by transverse annular wrinkles and longitudinal furrows. Externally the root is yellowish-brown, internally it is brownish-yellow; its texture is spongy; its odour, in the fresh state, peculiar and disagreeable; its taste is intensely bitter. The roots of other species of Gentiana are said to be frequently mixed with those of the officinal species : their effects, however, are analogous.

Martius[1] says that the roots of *G. purpurea* have strong longitudinal furrows, and are of a darker brown colour internally, but want the transverse wrinkles. The roots of *G. pannonica* are similar to those of *purpurea*. Both kinds are met with in Bavaria, and serve in Switzerland for the preparation of a spirit. *Gentiana punctata* has roots which are just as bitter, but of a more yellow colour : they are dug up in great abundance in Moravia. The roots of both the last-mentioned species are dug up at, and exported from, Salzburg : in the fresh state they are white when sliced.

Chemistry.—Gentian root was analysed, in 1815, by Schrader;[2] in 1817 by Braconnot;[3] in 1818 by Henry;[4] in the same year by Guillemin and Fœcquemin;[5] and in 1821 by Henry and Caventou.[6] In 1837 it was examined by Leconte.[7] The constituents of gentian root, according to Henry and Caventou, are—*a volatile odorous matter, bitter crystalline matter* (*gentianin*), *fugaceous odorous principle* (*volatile oil ?*), *yellow colouring matter, green fixed oil, gum, uncrystallisable sugar, matter identical with bird-lime, a free organic acid,* and *woody fibre.* But in 1837

---

1 *Pharmakognosie.*
2 Trommsdorff's *N. Journ.* Bd. iii. S. 281.
3 *Journ. de Physiq.* lxxxiv. 345.
4 *Journ. de Pharm.* t. v. p. 97.
5 *Ibid.* p. 110.
6 *Ibid.* t. vii. p. 173.
7 *Ibid.* t. xxiii. p. 465.

H. Trommsdorff[1] and Leconte[2] showed, that under the name of gentianin two substances had been confounded,—the one crystalline and tasteless; the other bitter. The first has been called *gentisin;* the second *gentianite.* Furthermore, Leconte has shown that the substance considered by Henry and Caventou as identical with bird-lime is a compound of *wax, oil,* and *caoutchouc.*

1. OIL OF GENTIAN.—By distillation with water gentian root yields a very small quantity of a butyraceous oil, which floats on water, has a powerful odour of gentian root, and is soluble in alcohol. A few drops of the melted oil were given to a rabbit without causing any remarkable effects. I have received from Mr. Whipple two samples of this oil, the one green, the other white, like mutton·fat. Three cwts. of the root yielded only about ʒss. of oil.

Planche[3] states the distilled water of gentian caused nausea and a kind of intoxication.

2. GENTISIN, or GENTISIC ACID.—Procured by washing the alcoholic extract of the root with water, and then treating with alcohol. The tincture obtained was evaporated, and the extract treated by ether : the residue, by successive solutions and evaporations, yielded gentisin. It is pale yellow, crystallisable in needles, has a peculiar but weak smell. When cautiously heated, it gives out some yellow vapours, which are condensed on the upper part of the tube. It is scarcely soluble in water, but dissolves in alcohol. With alkalies it unites to form salts. Its saturating power is about 438. Trommsdorff says that a solution of gentisic acid is unaffected by acetate of lead, nitrate of silver, and most other tests. Chloride of iron and the salts of copper produced in the alcoholic solution the most characteristic changes.

3. BITTER PRINCIPLE OF GENTIAN (*Gentianite*).—This has not hitherto been isolated. By digesting the alcoholic extract of gentian in water, an acidulous intensely bitter solution is obtained. The acid may be thrown down by lead. When the excess of lead has been removed from the solution by sulphuretted hydrogen, a liquid is obtained, which, by evaporation, yields a sweet and very bitter extract, from which ether removes an aromatic fat, an odorous resin, and wax. The bitter matter has not been separated from the sugar.

4. PECTIN.—The existence of pectic acid (pectin) in gentian was ascertained, in 1835, by Denis.[4] To this substance is to be in part, perhaps, ascribed the gelatinisation of infusion of gentian, which, under certain circumstances, is not unfrequently observed.

5. SUGAR.—To the presence of this matter in gentian is to be ascribed the capability of the infusion of gentian to undergo the vinous fermentation, and to form an alcoholic liquor (*gentian spirit*) much admired by the Swiss.[5]

CHEMICAL CHARACTERISTICS.—The infusion of gentian is deepened in colour by the caustic alkalies. Sesquichloride of iron communicates a deep olive-brown tint. The acetate and diacetate of lead, the sulphate of copper, and the nitrate of mercury, cause flocculent or gelatinous precipitates (*metallic pectates?*).

PHYSIOLOGICAL EFFECTS.—Gentian is very properly regarded as a *pure* or *simple bitter ;* that is, as being bitter, but without possessing either astringency or much aroma. It has, therefore, the usual tonic properties of medicines of this class.

Given in full doses, it appears more disposed to relax the bowels than the

---

[1] *Berlin. Jahrbuch,* Bd. xxxvii. S. 182.
[2] *Op. supra cit.*
[3] *Bull. de Pharmacie,* t. vi. p. 551.
[4] *Journ. de Pharm.* t. xxii. p. 303.
[5] Biwald, in Pfaff's *Mat. Med.* Bd. ii. S. 29 ; and Planche, *Bull. de Pharm.* vi. 551. [The reader will find some account of this spirit, and the noxious effects produced by it, in the *Pharmaceutical Journal* for February 1853, p. 371.—ED.]

other simple bitters, and in susceptible individuals it is more apt to disorder the digestive process. In such cases, both Löseke and Voigtel[1] have seen it cause vomiting. Barbier[2] says it quickens the pulse. It is somewhat less bitter, and therefore, I presume, somewhat less powerful, than quassia. By continued use, the sweat and urine acquire a bitter taste,[3]—a sufficient proof that gentian, or its bitter principle, becomes absorbed [and is eliminated].

As some of the vegetable bitter tonics (for example, quassia and calumba) have been found to exert a specific influence over the cerebro-spinal system, and to yield preparations of a poisonous quality, we are naturally led to inquire whether any analogous facts have been made out with respect to gentian. The reply is in the affirmative. Magendie,[4] indeed, discovered no poisonous operation in *Gentianin* ; he threw several grains of this principle into the veins of an animal without any obvious effect, and swallowed two grains dissolved in alcohol, but only observed extreme bitterness, and a slight feeling of heat in the stomach. Moreover, Hartl[5] inserted two grains of the extract of gentian into the inner side of the thigh of a rabbit, without any ill effects resulting: the wound was slightly inflamed, though it soon healed. These facts prove that the bitter extractive of gentian possesses no narcotic properties. But if the narcotic principle of gentian be of a volatile nature, these experiments of Magendie and Hartl go for nothing, since, in the preparation of both the extract and the *gentianin*, this principle would be dissipated by the heat employed. Now Planche[6] has shown that the distilled water of gentian causes violent nausea, and, within three minutes, a kind of intoxication. Moreover, Buchner[7] tells us that some years ago a narcotic effect was produced in Prussia by the medicinal use of gentian root, although the presence of any foreign matter could not be detected. In the *Philosophical Transactions* for the year 1748 are mentioned some deleterious effects resulting from the use of gentian: but they were referred to a foreign root, said to have been intermixed with, and which greatly resembled, the true gentian root. All these facts, then, support the opinion of Haller (quoted by Buchner), that gentian is not so innocuous as is generally supposed.

Uses.—Gentian is adapted to most of the cases requiring the use of the pure or simple bitters. It agrees best with phlegmatic, torpid individuals, and is apt to disagree with irritable or susceptible persons. It is contra-indicated in febrile disorders and inflammatory conditions of the gastro-intestinal membrane. It is employed principally in the following cases :—

1. *In dyspepsia and other gastric disorders* attended with debility or torpidity, and unaccompanied by any marks of inflammation or irritation, or great susceptibility, of the digestive organs. Sesquicarbonate of ammonia is a very valuable adjunct.

2. *In intermittent diseases* it may be used where cinchona is admissible ; but it is much inferior to the last-mentioned substance. " Joined with galls

---

[1] *Arzneimittell.* Bd. ii. S. 359.
[2] *Mat. Méd.*
[3] Arnemann, *Prakt. Arzneimittell.* S. 188, 6te Aufl.
[4] *Formul.* p. 313, 8me édit.
[5] Quoted by Wibmer, *Wirk. d. Arzneim. v. Gifte*, Bd. ii. S. 308.
[6] *Op. cit.*
[7] *Toxikol.* S. 192.

2 s

or tormentil, in equal parts, and given in sufficient quantity, it has not failed," says Dr. Cullen,[1] " in any intermittents in which I have tried it."

3. In many other diseases marked by weakness and debility, but unattended by fever or gastro-intestinal irritation, gentian is admissible and useful; as in some forms of gout, hysteria, uterine disorders, &c. It is a constituent of the *Duke of Portland's powder for the gout.*

4. *Against worms* it has been used as if it possessed some specific influence.

5. In surgery it has been used for discutient fomentations; also, in the form of fine powder, as an application to issues, to promote their running; and as a tent, to enlarge and cleanse fistulous apertures.[2]

ADMINISTRATION.—In the form of *powder*, the dose is from grs. x. to ʒss. But the *infusion, tincture,* or *extract,* are the usual forms of exhibition.

1. INFUSUM GENTIANÆ COMPOSITUM, L. D.; *Infusum Gentianæ,* E.; *Infusion of Gentian.* (Gentian Root, sliced, ʒij.; Orange-peel, dried, ʒij.; Lemon-peel, fresh or dried, ʒiv.; Boiling Distilled Water, Oj. Macerate for an hour in a vessel lightly covered, and strain, *L.* The directions of the *Edinburgh College* are as follows :—Gentian, sliced, ʒss.; Bitter Orange-peel, dried and bruised, ʒj.; Coriander, bruised, fʒj.; Proof Spirit, ʒiv.; Cold Water, fʒxvj. Pour the spirit upon the solids; in three hours add the water, and in twelve hours more strain through linen or calico, *E.*—Gentian Root bruised, Orange Peel dried, of each ʒij.; Boiling Water, Oss. Infuse for one hour in a covered vessel, and strain. The product should measure about eight ounces, *D.*)—The infusions of the London and Dublin Pharmacopœias are very apt to spoil by keeping; but as an infusion can always be speedily procured, this is not a circumstance of much importance. However, to obviate it as much as possible, the Edinburgh College orders cold water to be used (by which less of the mucilaginous matter [pectin] is dissolved), and employs spirit to promote the solution of the bitter principle, while the quantity of gentian is much increased; so that, in fact, we have a weak tincture rather than an infusion. Besides the objections which may arise out of these deviations, a very important one is the length of time required for the maceration. Compound infusion of gentian sometimes gelatinises by keeping. This occurred in one case[3] when the infusion, instead of being strained off in an hour, had been allowed to stand forty-eight hours, and liquor potassæ had been added to it. Though this perhaps may be in part due to the action of the alkali on the pectin contained in the gentian, it is chiefly, if not entirely owing to the action of the alkali on some principle extracted by prolonged maceration from the lemon-peel[4] (see *Cortex Limonum*).

Infusion of gentian is stomachic and tonic. When prepared according to the London and Dublin Pharmacopœias, the dose is fʒj. to fʒij.; when according to that of the Edinburgh, fʒss. to fʒj.

2. MISTURA GENTIANÆ COMPOSITA, L.; *Compound Mixture of Gentian.* (Compound Infusion of Gentian, fʒxij.; Compound Infusion of Senna, fʒvj.;

---

[1] *Mat. Med.* vol. ii. p. 72.
[2] Quincy, *Dispens.*
[3] Fordred, *Pharmaceutical Journal,* vol. i. p. 229, 1841.
[4] *Ibid.* vol. i. p. 587, 1841.

Compound Tincture of Cardamoms, f℥ij. Mix.)—Tonic and cathartic. Used in dyspepsia with constipation.—Dose, f℥j. to f℥ij.

3. TINCTURA GENTIANÆ COMPOSITA, L. E. D.; *Tinctura amara; Tincture of Gentian.* (Gentian, sliced and bruised, ℥iss.; Orange-peel, dried, ℥x.; Cardamom [Seeds], bruised, ℥v.; Proof Spirit, Oij. Macerate for seven days, then press and strain, *L.* The *Edinburgh College* employs of Gentian, sliced and bruised, ℥ijss.; Bitter Orange-peel, bruised, ℥x.; Canella, in moderately fine powder, ℥vj.; Cochineal, bruised, ℥ss.; and Proof Spirit, Oij. This tincture may be more conveniently prepared by percolation, as directed for the compound tincture of cardamom, *E.* The *Dublin College* orders Gentian Root, bruised, ℥iij.; Bitter Orange-peel, dried, ℥iss.; Cardamom Seeds, bruised, ℥ss.; Proof Spirit, Oij. Macerate for fourteen days, strain, express, and filter.) — A grateful cordial tonic and stomachic. Employed as an adjunct to the infusion, effervescing draughts, bottle soda-water, &c.—Dose, f℥ss. to f℥ij.

4. VINUM GENTIANÆ, E.; *Wine of Gentian.* (Gentian, in coarse powder, ℥ss.; Yellow Bark, in coarse powder, ℥j.; Bitter Orange-peel, dried and sliced, ℥ij.; Canella, in coarse powder, ℥j.; Proof Spirit, f℥ivss.; Sherry, Oj. and f℥xvj. Digest the root and barks for twenty-four hours in the spirit; add the wine, and digest for seven days more; strain and express the residuum strongly, and filter the liquors.)—Wine of gentian is an aromatic tonic, useful in dyspepsia and anorexia. It is apt to become acetous by keeping. The dose of it is f℥ss. to f℥j.

5. EXTRACTUM GENTIANÆ, L. E. D.; *Extract of Gentian.* (Gentian, sliced, lb. iij.; Boiling Distilled Water, Cong. vj. Macerate for twelve hours in four gallons of the water, pour off the solution, and strain. Add the two gallons of water to the residue, macerate for six hours, gently press out the solution, and strain. Lastly, evaporate the solution mixed together to a proper consistence, *L.* "Take of Gentian, any convenient quantity; bruise it to a moderately fine powder; mix it thoroughly with half its weight of distilled water; in twelve hours put it into a proper percolator, and exhaust it by percolation with temperate distilled water; concentrate the liquid, filter before it becomes too thick, and evaporate in the water-bath to a due consistence," *E.* Gentian Root, in thin slices, lb. j.; Distilled Water, Oiij. Macerate the gentian in one pint and a half of the water for six hours, then strain and express. Add to the residue the remaining pint and a half of water, macerate again for six hours, strain, and express. Finally, mix the liquors, and evaporate by a steam- or water-bath to a proper consistence, *D.*)—Good gentian root yields about half its weight of extract.[1] Extract of gentian is tonic. It is usually employed as a vehicle for the exhibition of the metallic substances (especially chalybeates) in the form of pill.—Dose, grs. x. to ℥ss.

---

[1] Brande, *Dict. of Mat. Med.* p. 261.

191. OPHELIA CHIRATA, *Grisebach.*—THE CHIRETTA OR CHIRAYTA.

Agathotes Chirayita, *Don,*[1] *D. E.*—Gentiana Chirayita, *Fleming.*

Sex. Syst. Tetrandria, Monogynia.

(Herb and root, *E.*—The herb, *D.*)

HISTORY.—This plant seems to have been long in use among the natives of India. Professor Guibourt[2] thinks that it is the κάλαμος ἀρωματικός of Dioscorides.[3] Various circumstances, however, appear to me to be opposed to this opinion : one of the most conclusive is the absence of odour in the chirayta plant.[4]

BOTANY.   **Gen. Char.**—*Calyx* 5-4-parted; the segments valvate. *Corolla* withering, rotate, 5-4-parted, with glandular pits above the base. *Stamens* 5-4, inserted in the throat of the corolla; the filaments either dilated at the base, and monadelphous, or equal at the base, and free. *Ovary* 1-celled; ovules numerous, inserted on the suture. *Stigmas* 2, terminal, short, usually revolute; *style* 0, or short. *Capsule* 2-valved, septicidal, 1-celled; placentæ either spongy and sutural, or expanded near the suture. *Seeds* immersed in the placentæ, very numerous, small, and generally wingless (*Grisebach*).

Sp. Char.—Stem terete, tall, smooth, branched. Branches elongated, erect-spreading. Leaves cordate-ovate, and ovate, acuminate, sessile, smooth, 5-7-nerved. Cymes umbelliform, lax, few-flowered. Segments of the calyx sublanceolate, acuminate, shorter than the corolla; corollæ 4-parted, yellow, the segments expanded, ovate-lanceolate, acuminate; pits in pairs, oblong, distinct, fringed anteriorly by long scales; the fringes epipetalous, short, connecting the pits (*Grisebach*).

Herbaceous. Root branching. *Stem* round, jointed. *Leaves* opposite, amplexicaul, very acute, entire. *Flowers* numerous, peduncled.

Hab.—Mountains of Nepal and the Morungs.

DESCRIPTION.—The plant is pulled up by the root, about the time that the flowers begin to decay and the capsules are well formed.[5] The dried plant with the root (*herba et radix chirettæ* sive *chirayitæ*) is met with in the shops. The root is fibrous; the stem is round, smooth, not jointed, marked with the cicatrices of leaves, has a yellowish pith; the leaves are as above described. The whole plant is without odour, but has an intensely bitter taste.

COMPOSITION.—The stems of this plant were analysed by MM. Lassaigne and Boissel,[6] who obtained the following results:—*resin, yellow bitter matter, brown colouring matter, gum, malic acid [woody fibre], malate of potash, chloride of potassium, sulphate of potash, phosphate of lime, silica,* and *traces of oxide of iron.*

The BITTER MATTER is the most important constituent. No vegetable alkali has been detected in it. The substance sold as *sulphate of chirayitine* is sulphate of quina.[7]

---

[1] *Transactions of the Linnean Society*, vol. xvii. p. 522.
[2] *Journ. de Chim. Méd.* t. i. p. 229.
[3] Lib. i. cap. 17.
[4] Fée, *Cours d'Hist. Nat.* t. ii. p. 395.
[5] Roxburgh, *Fl. Ind.* vol. ii. p. 72.
[6] *Journ. Pharm.* vol. vii. p. 283.
[7] *Lond. Med. Gaz.* vol. xxi. p. 173.

PHYSIOLOGICAL EFFECTS.—Chirayita is an intensely bitter substance, and produces the before-described effects of the *simple* or *pure bitters*. In its operation, as well as by its botanical affinities, it is closely allied to gentian. It appears to possess rather a relaxing than a constipating effect.[1]

USES.—It has long been employed by the natives of India in the same class of cases in which gentian has been used in Europe. As a stomachic it is especially serviceable in the dyspepsia of gouty subjects. It strengthens the stomach, obviates flatulency, and diminishes the tendency to acidity.[2] Combined with the seeds of *Guilandina Bonduc,* it is employed with success in intermittents.[3]

ADMINISTRATION.—It may be given in *powder* in the dose of ϶j., or it may be employed in the form of *infusion, tincture* (prepared with cardamom and orange-peel, like *compound tincture of gentian*), or *extract.*

1. INFUSUM CHIRETTÆ, E. D.; *Infusion of Chiretta.* (Chiretta, ʒiv.; Boiling Water, Oj. Infuse for two hours, and strain through linen or calico, *E.* Chiretta, bruised, ʒij.; Boiling Water, ℥ixss. Infuse for one hour in a covered vessel, and strain. The product should measure about eight ounces, *D.*) —The dose of this is ℥j. to f℥ij.

2. TINCTURA CHIRETTÆ, D. (Chiretta, bruised, ℥v.; Proof Spirit, Oij. Macerate for fourteen days, strain, express, and filter.)

192. Erythræa Centaurium, *Persoon.*—Common Centaury.

Sex. Syst. Pentandria, Monogynia.

(The flowering heads, *E.*)

HISTORY.—This plant was known to the ancients, and received one of its names (*Chironia Centaurium*) from Chiron the Centaur, who is said to have lived 1270 years before Christ. But the plant which Pliny[4] says cured Chiron of a wound received by an arrow, which he dropped on his foot when examining the arms of Hercules, is supposed to be the *Centaurea Centaurium.*

BOTANY. **Gen. Char.**—*Calyx* 5-4-partite, the segments nearly flat wingless. *Corolla* funnel-shaped, naked, contorted-withering above the capsule; the tube cylindrical; the limb 5-4-partite. *Stamens* 5-4, inserted above in the tube of the corolla; anthers erect, twisted spirally, exserted. *Ovary* 1-celled or semi-2-celled in consequence of the valves being slightly inflexed; the ovules inserted at the suture. *Style* distinct, deciduous; *stigma* bilamellate or undivided and capitulate. *Capsule* bivalved, septicidal, 1-celled or semi-2-celled; the placentæ spongy and sutural. *Seeds* immersed in the placentæ, sub-globose, smooth, minute (*Grisebach*).

Sp. Char.—Stem erect, elongated, branched superiorly. Leaves elliptic-oblong, unequally acute. Flowers collected in loose heads, lateral, bibracteate. Tube of the corolla during inflorescence more than twice the length of the calyx, the tubes oval and obtuse. Capsule with the valves much inflexed, more than semi-2-celled (*Grisebach*).

Root small, tapering. *Stem* about a foot high, leafy. Radicle *leaves* obovate; the rest acute, ovate, or elliptic-lanceolate: all 3-ribbed, bright green. *Flowers* nearly sessile. *Bracts* opposite, awl-shaped. *Calyx* slender. Tube of *corolla* pale greenish; limb brilliant pink, expanded only in sunshine, closing as soon as gathered.

Hab.—Indigenous: dry gravelly pastures. Annual. Flowers in July and August.

---

[1] Baker, *Lond. Med. Gaz.* vol. ii. p. 685.
[2] Fleming, *Asiat. Researches,* vol. xi. p. 167.
[3] Johnson, *Infl. of Trop. Climates,* 3d edit. p. 58.
[4] *Hist. Nat.* lib. xxv. cap. 30, ed. Valp.

DESCRIPTION.—The herb or tops (*herba* seu *summitates* vel *cacumina centaurii minoris*) of the common or lesser centaury are without odour, but have a very bitter taste. They are collected when in flower.

COMPOSITION.—According to Moretti,[1] common centaury contains *bitter extractive, free acid, mucous matter, extractive salts,* [and *woody fibre*].

The principal constituent of common centaury is the bitter extractive, called by Dulong d'Astafort[2] *centaurin*. This, when combined with hydrochloric acid, is said to be an excellent febrifuge. Centaurin must not be confounded with *centaurite*, the bitter principle of *Cnicus benedictus*, De Cand.

PHYSIOLOGICAL EFFECTS.—Similar to those of gentian (see *ante*, p. 625), and of other simple or pure bitters.

USES.—Common or lesser centaury is rarely used by medical practitioners; yet it might be employed as an indigenous substitute for gentian.—Dose of the powder, Ɖj. to ʒj. It may also be used in infusion.

[2. ERYTHRÆA CHILENSIS, called also Chironia Chilensis, is a native of Chili and Peru. It is there called *Cochan lahuen* or *Cachen-laguen*, and has been introduced into the Spanish pharmacopœia under the name of *Canchalagua*. The plant was first made known in 1707, by Le Pas, a French physician.

PHYSIOLOGICAL EFFECTS.—According to Dr. Chapa, its effects on the body are to reduce the plasticity of the blood, to exercise a tonic influence on the digestive organs, and to excite the urinary and cutaneous excretions. It also possesses febrifuge propertics, and may be deserving of notice as a substitute for quinine.

ADMINISTRATION.—It may be given in the form of infusion or extract. A very bitter wine has been prepared by the addition of alcohol to the aqueous extract.[3]—ED.]

193. Menyanthes trifoliata, *Linn.*—Common Buckbean; Marsh Trefoil.

Sex. Syst. Pentandria, Monogynia.

(Leaves, *E.*)

HISTORY.—Sprengel[4] considers this to be the plant referred to by Theophrastus[5] under the name of μήνανθος.

BOTANY. **Gen. Char.**—*Calyx* 5-partite, the segments connected at the base so as to form a tube. *Corolla* deciduous, funnel-shaped, fleshy; the limb 5-partite, its segments naked at the margin and base, but fringed, or very rarely denuded, at the disc; no epipetalous glands. *Stamens* 5, inserted in the tube of the corolla; filaments equal at the base; anthers erect. *Ovary* surrounded by 5 hypogynous glands, 1-celled; the ovules inserted on the axis of the valves. *Style* filiform, persistent with the 2-lobed stigma. *Capsule* 1-celled, almost valveless, rupturing near the suture of the two carpella; the placenta inserted in the axis of the carpella. *Seeds* indefinite, with a shining very smooth testa (*Grisebach*).

Sp. Char.—The only species.

Rhizoma black, creeping, jointed. *Leaves* on long stalks, with broad sheathing stipules at base, ternate; leaflets nearly oval, smooth. *Scape* round, ascending, smooth. *Bracts* ovate. *Calyx* obtuse. *Corolla* white or flesh-coloured, elegant, densely shaggy. *Anthers* yellow.

Hab.—Indigenous; watery meadows, ditches, &c.; frequently cultivated in ornamental aquaria, on account of the beauty of the flowers. Perennial. Flowers in June and July.

DESCRIPTION.—The whole herb (*herba menyanthis* seu *trifolii fibrini*) is odourless, but has a very bitter taste. Its infusion strikes a green colour (*tannate of iron*) with the sesquichloride of iron. The leaves (*folia menyanthis*) are the parts usually employed.

---

[1] *Journ. de Pharm.* t. v. p. 98.
[2] *Ibid.* t. xvi. p. 502.
[3] [*Pharmaceutical Journal*, January 1855, p. 326.]
[4] *Hist. Rei Herb.* t. i. p. 82.
[5] *Hist. Plant.* lib. iv. cap. 11.

COMPOSITION.—Menyanthes was analysed by Trommsdorff,[1] who found that the fresh plant consists of 75 parts of moisture and 25 of solid matter, composed of *bitter extractive, vegetable albumen, green resin (chlorophylle), peculiar matter* precipitable by tannic acid, but soluble in water and in weak spirit, *brown gum, fecula (inulin* or *menyanthin), malic acid,* and *acetate of potash.*

The *bitter extractive* is the active principle. Brandes states that he procured a white bitter powder from menyanthes; but B. Trommsdorff[2] repeated Brandes's experiments, and procured only a yellowish-brown bitter extract.

PHYSIOLOGICAL EFFECTS.—Tonic and astringent. In large doses cathartic, and sometimes emetic.

USES.—This plant is used by the brewers of some parts of Germany, particularly Silesia and the adjacent provinces, as a substitute for hops.[3] It is rarely employed in medicine, but is applicable for the same purposes as the other bitter tonics. It has been esteemed efficacious as an antiscorbutic.[4]

ADMINISTRATION.—It may be given in *powder, infusion,* or *extract.* The dose of the powder is from Ʒj. to Ʒss.: if given to the extent of Ʒj. it generally purges. The dose of the *infusion* (prepared with Ʒss. of the dried herb, and fℨxvj. of boiling water) is fℨj. to fℨij.; of the watery *extract,* grs. x. to grs. xv.

194. Frasera carolinensis, *Walter.*

Sex. Syst. Tetrandria, Monogynia.

(Radix.)

Frasera carolinensis, Walter, Fl. Carol. 1788; *F. Walteri,* Michaux, Fl. Boreali-Americ. 1803; *American Calumba.*—A native of the southern and western portions of the United States, and very abundant in Arkansas and Missouri. The root is officinal in the Pharmacopœia of the United States. As met with in commerce, it is in transverse circular segments, about an inch in diameter, and an eighth of an inch, or more, in thickness. It contains no starch, and hence undergoes no change of colour when touched with iodine. Its infusion or decoction becomes blackish-green (*tannate of iron*) when treated with sulphate of iron, and lets fall a precipitate (*tannate of gelatine*) on the addition of a solution of isinglass. The effects, uses, and doses of Frasera are the same as those of gentian. The fresh root is said to operate as an emetic and cathartic.[5] Some years ago it was introduced into France, and sold for calumba; hence it got the name of *false calumba.* The chemical characters above given, as well as the physical properties of the root, readily distinguish it.[6]

ORDER XLVI. LOGANIACEÆ, *De Cand.*—LOGANIADS.

CHARACTERS.—*Calyx* free, 5- rarely 4-lobed. *Corolla* regular or rarely irregular, hypogynous, 5- rarely 4- or many lobed, æstivation valvate, contorted, or imbricated. *Stamens* inserted in the tube of the corolla; anthers 2-celled, dehiscing longitudinally; pollen vittate-trilobed. *Ovary* free (superior), 2- rarely 3-celled or 1-celled; ovules amphitropal, or rarely anatropal. *Style* simple; *stigma* simple or 2-lobed. *Fruit* capsular or drupaceo-baccate. *Seeds* usually peltate, sometimes winged; albumen fleshy or cartilaginous; embryo straight; radicle towards or parallel with the hilum; cotyledons 2, foliaceous.— *Shrubs, trees,* or rarely *herbs. Leaves* opposite, entire, stalked, usually with stipules. *Flowers* racemose or corymbose, rarely solitary.

PROPERTIES.—Poisonous (with some exceptions); acting on the nervous system. This

---

[1] *Ann. de Chim.* t. lxxii. p. 191.
[2] *Pharm. Central-Blatt für* 1832, p. 458.
[3] Yosy, *Origin and Progress of the Med.-Bot. Soc.* p. 12.
[4] Murray, *App. Med.* t. ii. p. 34.
[5] *United States Dispensatory.*
[6] Guibourt, *Journ. de Chim. Méd.* t. ii. p. 834.

Order contains some of the most energetic vegetable poisons. *Strychnia* and *brucia* are produced by some of the species, which in consequence excite most frightful convulsions. The medicinal species of this Order are used as spastics, anthelmintics, and tonics.

195. SPIGELIA MARILANDICA, *Linn.*—CAROLINA PINK ; PERENNIAL WORMGRASS.

Sex. Syst. Pentandria, Monogynia.

(Root, *E.*)

History.—The anthelmintic virtues of this plant were first learned from the Cherokee Indians, who became acquainted with them, according to Dr. Garden, about 1723 : they were made known to the profession about 1740.[1]

Botany. **Gen. Char.**—*Calyx* 5-partite, persistent ; the segments linear-subulate, glandular. *Corolla* gamopetalous, funnel-shaped ; the lobes 5, shorter than the tube, with a valvate æstivation. *Stamens* 5, inserted on the tube of the corolla, enclosed or rarely exserted ; filaments slender ; anthers linear, erect, 2-lobed at the base. *Ovary* 2-celled ; ovules numerous, amphitropal ; placentæ basilar, stipitate. *Style* filiform, hairy above, jointed beneath the capitate or concave stigma. *Capsule* obovoid-compressed, didymous, dicoccous, circumscissile at the base ; the cocci at length bipartite. *Seeds* few, cuneate-turbinate ; the testa scabrous-areolate ; the embryo at the base of horny albumen, small, straight (*De Cand.*)

Sp. Char.—Stem erect, simple, quadrangular, smooth. Leaves sessile, ovate-lanceolate, acute or acuminate ; the margin and nerves scabrous-hairy. Spike 3-8-flowered. Flowers sessile. Segments of the calyx four times shorter than the tube of the corolla. Anthers projecting from the tube. Lobes of the corolla lanceolate. Capsule smooth, somewhat shorter than the calyx.

Root perennial, consisting of numerous fibres, from a short cylindrical rhizome. *Stems* several, winged (from the decurrent leaves). *Leaves* decussate, entire. *Flowers* in simple one-sided spikes (or racemes). *Corolla* much longer than the calyx, of a rich carmine colour externally, paler at the base, and orange-yellow within. *Capsule* obcordate, smooth.

Hab.—Southern States of North America ; seldom found north of the Potomac.

Collection.—" It is collected by the Greek and Cherokee Indians, who dispose of it to the white traders. By these it is packed in casks, or more commonly in large bales, weighing from three hundred to three hundred and fifty pounds. That contained in casks is to be preferred, as less liable to be damp and mouldy. Owing to the imperfect manner in which the plant is dried, it seldom happens that packages of it reach the market free from dirt or mouldiness, and having the stalks of a bright colour. Some parcels have been brought free from the stalks, and have commanded more than double the price of the drug prepared in the usual way."[2]

Description.—The dried plant (*herba spigeliæ*), as usually met with in the shops, is of a greyish-green colour, has a faint odour, and a bitter taste. The root (*radix spigeliæ*) consists of numerous slender, branching, dark brown fibres, issuing from a short dark brown rhizome.

---

[1] *Essays and Obs., Phys. and Lit.,* vol. iii.
[2] *United States Dispensatory.*

COMPOSITION.—The herb and root have been analysed by Wackenroder.[1] Feneulle[2] probably analysed this plant under the name of *Spigelia anthelmintica*.

Wackenroder's Analyses.

Myricin	0·30	Fixed oil	a trace
Resin, with chlorophylle	2·40	Acrid resin, with some fixed oil	3·13
Peculiar resin	0·50	Peculiar tannin	10·56
Peculiar tannin	17·20	Bitter acrid extractive	4·89
Woody fibre	75·20	Woody fibre (which yields 16·74 of	
Malate of potash, and chloride of potassium	2·10	ashes)	82·69
Malate of lime	4·20		
Herb of Spigelia	101·90	Root of Spigelia	101·27

The decoction of spigelia strikes a dark colour with the salts of iron.

1. BITTER EXTRACTIVE.—Feneulle ascribes the activity of spigelia to a brown, bitter extractive, like that of the purgative Leguminosæ. Taken internally, it causes vertigo and a kind of intoxication. It is, I presume, identical with the *bitter acrid extractive* of Wackenroder.

2. RESIN.—This is described by Wackenroder as having an acrid, nauseous taste. It is soluble in ammonia and in oil of vitriol. It evolves ammonia when heated.

PHYSIOLOGICAL EFFECTS.—The physiological effects of this root have not been accurately determined; but the observations hitherto made, show them to be those of a local irritant (or acrid) and narcotic substance.

In the *ordinary dose* (one or two drachms for adults) it has very little sensible effect on the system, though it may act efficaciously as an anthelmintic. In *larger doses* it appears to operate as an irritant to the gastro-intestinal canal, and gives rise to purging, and sometimes to vomiting, though its effects in this way are very uncertain. In *poisonous doses* it operates as a cerebro-spinal or narcotic, giving rise to " vertigo, dimness of vision, dilated pupils, spasms of the facial muscles, and sometimes even to general convulsions. Spasmodic movements of the eyelids have been observed among the most common attendants of its narcotic action. The death of two children, who expired in convulsions, was attributed by Dr. Chambers to the influence of spigelia. The narcotic effects are said to be less apt to occur when the medicine purges, and to be altogether obviated by combining it with cathartics. The danger from its employment cannot be great, as it is in very general use in the United States, both in regular and domestic practice; and we never hear at present of serious consequences. Its effects upon the system have been erroneously conjectured to depend on other roots sometimes mixed with the genuine."[3]

USES.—Employed only as an anthelmintic. Its vermifuge properties were first made known to the profession by Drs. Lining[4] and Garden.[5] Though scarcely used in this country, it stands at the head of anthelmintics in the United States of America.

ADMINISTRATION.—The dose of the *powder*, for a child of three or four years old, is from grs. x. to grs. xx.; for an adult, ʒj. to ʒiij. This quantity

---

[1] Gmelin's *Handb. d. Chem.* ii. 1298.
[2] *Journ. de Pharm.* t. ix. p. 897.
[3] *United States Dispensatory.*
[4] '*Essays and Obs., Phys. and Lit.*, vol. i. p. 386.
[5] *Ibid.* vol. iii. p. 145.

is repeated, every morning and evening, for several days, and is then followed by a brisk cathartic. It is frequently combined with calomel.

INFUSUM SPIGELIÆ, Ph. United States; *Infusion of Pink-root.* (Spigelia Root, ʒss.; Boiling Water, fʒxvj. Macerate for two hours in a covered vessel, and strain.)—The dose, for a child of two or three years old, is fʒss. to fʒj.; for an adult, from fʒiv. to fʒviij., repeated morning and evening. A quantity of senna, equal to that of the spigelia, is usually added, to ensure a cathartic effect.

A preparation kept in the shops of the United States, and much prescribed by physicians, under the name of *worm tea,* consists of spigelia root, senna, manna, and savine, mixed together in various proportions to suit the views of different individuals.[1]

[The Pharmacopœia of the *United States* has a convenient preparation under the name of *Extractum Spigeliæ et Sennæ Fluidum.* It is prepared as follows :—Take of Pink-root, in coarse powder, lb. j.; Senna, in coarse powder, ʒvj.; Sugar, lb. iss.; Carbonate of Potash, ʒvj.; Oil of Caraway, Oil of Anise, each fʒss.; Diluted Alcohol, a sufficient quantity. Mix the pink-root and the senna with two pints of diluted alcohol, and having allowed the mixture to stand for two days, transfer it to a percolator, and gradually pour upon it diluted alcohol, until half a gallon of liquid has passed. Evaporate the liquid, by means of a water-bath, to a pint : then add the carbonate of potash, and, after the sediment has dissolved, the sugar, previously triturated with the oils. Lastly, dissolve the sugar with a gentle heat. This preparation combines the properties of an anthelmintic and a purgative, and may, from the smallness of the dose, be conveniently administered to children. Dose, ʒj. to ʒij. twice or thrice daily.—ED.]

196. Spigelia Anthelmia, *Linn.*

(Herba; Radix.)

SPIGELIA ANTHELMIA, or *Demerara Pink-root,* is a native of South America and the West India Islands. Its action is similar to that of the last-mentioned species. So poisonous has it been regarded, that in France it is called *Brinvillière,* after the Marchioness de Brinvilliers, a woman famous for poisoning in the reign of Louis XIV., and who was executed on the 16th of July, 1676.[2] Its anthelmintic properties were noticed, in 1751, by Dr. Browne.[3] This plant was analysed by Ricord Madianna.[4] In the root he found a solid fat, wax, a soft resin called *spigelin* (one grain and a half of which is sufficient to destroy a cat or dog in twenty minutes), resin, brown non-poisonous extractive, gum, ligneous fibre, albumen, and gallic acid. The stalks and leaves contained volatile oil, fat, wax, chlorophylle, blackish gummy matter, ligneous fibre, and gallic acid. Dr. Browne[5] says it procures sleep almost as certainly as opium. Dr. Bonyan[6] has recently testified to the anthelmintic efficacy of this plant, which is in great repute among the labourers of British Guiana. It is administered in the form of decoction. Two or three fresh leaves are said to be a dose.

---

[1] *United States Dispensatory.*
[2] Guibourt, *Hist. des Drog.* t. ii. p. 227.
[3] *Gentleman's Magazine* for 1751.
[4] Gmelin's *Handb. de Chem.* ii. 1297.
[5] *Nat. Hist. of Jamaica,* p. 157.
[6] *Pharmaceutical Journal,* vol. v. p. 354, 1846.

197. STRYCHNOS NUX-VOMICA, *Linn.*—THE POISON-NUT.

Sex. Syst. Pentandria, Monogynia.

(Semina Strychniæ : alkali e Nuce-vomicâ comparatum crystalli, *L.*—The seeds, *E. D.*)

HISTORY.—We became acquainted with nux-vomica through the Arabian authors. In the Latin translation of one of the works of Serapion[1] we find the word nux-vomica, but it appears to have been applied to some other substance (probably to St. Ignatius's bean). "Est nux," says he, "cujus color est inter glaucedinem et albedinem, major avellana parum et sunt in ea nodi." To which he afterwards adds, "movet vomitum ;" from which, I presume, the name of *vomic,* or *vomiting nut,* was originally derived. Mesue also mentions nux-vomica. Avicenna[2] says nux-methel "est similis nuci-vomicæ." It is probable that the *nux-mechil* of Serapion is the substance which we denominate nux-vomica.

BOTANY. **Gen. Char.**—*Calyx* 5-lobed. *Corolla* tubular, salver-shaped or funnel-shaped ; the throat naked or bearded ; limb 5-partite, the lobes valvate in æstivation, spreading during inflorescence. *Stamens* 5, inserted into the throat of the corolla ; filaments very short ; anthers subexserted. *Ovary* 2-celled. *Style* filiform ; *stigma* capitate, undivided, or obscurely subbilobed. *Ovules* indefinite, attached to fleshy placentæ, amphitropal, with an inferior micropyle. *Berry* corticated, 1-celled, many-seeded, or by abortion 1-seeded. *Seeds* nidulant in pulp, discoidal-compressed, with a ventral umbilicus ; *embryo* at the base of cartilaginous, subbilamellate albumen, excentric, straight, short ; the cotyledons sessile, foliaceous ; the radicle terete, uncertain (*De Cand.*)

Sp. Char.—Stem arboreous. No spines or cirrhi. Leaves ovate, stalked, 3-5-nerved, quite smooth. Corymbs terminal. Calyx with 5 short teeth. Corolla smooth within. Berry globose, many-seeded (*De Cand.*)

Middling-sized *tree.* *Trunk* short, often crooked, pretty thick ; the *branches* irregular ; the *wood* white, hard, and bitter. *Leaves* opposite, oval, shining, entire. *Corymbs* small. *Corolla* funnel-shaped, greenish-white. *Style* the length of the corolla. *Stigma* capitate. *Berry* round, smooth, size of a pretty large apple, covered with a smooth, somewhat hard *shell,* of a rich orange colour when ripe, filled with a white, soft gelatinous *pulp,* which is greedily eaten by many sorts of birds. *Seeds* several, immersed in the pulp of the berry, and attached to a central placenta.

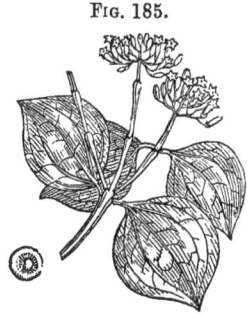

FIG. 185.

Strychnos Nux-vomica.

Hab.—Coromandel, and other parts of India ; Ceylon.

DESCRIPTION. *a.* **Of the Seeds.**—The *seeds* (*nuces vomicæ*) of commerce are round, peltate, scarcely an inch in diameter, nearly flat, or very slightly convex on the dorsal surface, and concave on the other or ventral surface, and

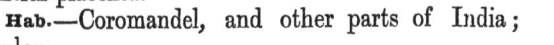

---

[1] *De Simplic. Med.* clxiii. p. 115, Argent. 1531.
[2] Lib. 2ndus, tract. 2ndus, cap. 509.

are usually surrounded by a filiform annular stria. In the centre of the ventral surface of the seed is the orbicular hilum or umbilicus. At one part of their circumference or margin there is a slight prominence, which answers to the chalaza, and to the radicle of the embryo. From this prominence to the umbilicus is a more or less obvious line, forming the raphe. From their fancied resemblance to grey eyes, as well as from their being poisonous to crows, the Germans term them *Krähenaugen* or *crows' eyes*.

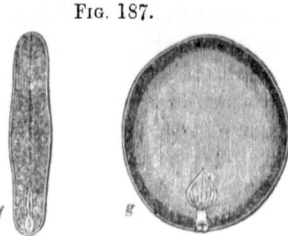

Fig. 186.

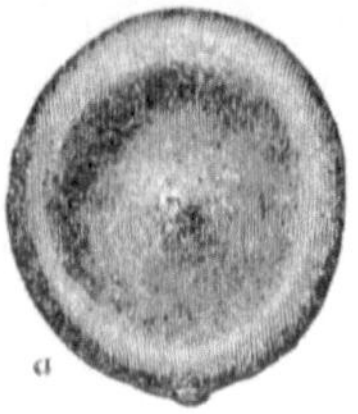

Nux-vomica.

a. The dorsal surface.
b. The ventral or concave surface.
c. Prominence indicating the chalaza and radicle.
d. Hilum or umbilicus.
e. Raphe.

Fig. 187.

Sections of Nux-vomica.

f. Transverse section of seed, showing the bipartite albumen, the cavity, and the embryo.
g. Vertical section, exposing the internal cavity, and showing the situation and figure of the embryo.

These seeds have two coats: the outer one, or *testa,* is simple, fibrous, and gives origin to short silky hairs, of an ash-grey or yellowish colour, and which are directed from the centre towards the circumference; within this is the inner coat, or *endopleura,* which is simple and very thin, and envelopes the nucleus of the seed.

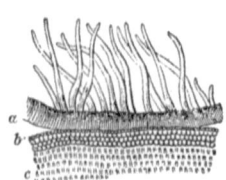

Fig. 188.

Magnified view of a portion of the Seed-coats of Nux-vomica.

a. Testa, with hairs attached.
b. Endopleura.
c. Albumen.

This nucleus is composed of two parts—namely, albumen and embryo. The *albumen* is bipartite, cartilaginous, or horny; of a dirty-white colour, of an intensely bitter taste, and has in its interior a cavity (*loculamentum verum*). Unlike that of most seeds, the albumen of nux-vomica is of a poisonous nature. The *embryo,* which is milk-white, is seated in the circumference of the seed, its locality being frequently indicated by a point somewhat more projecting than the surrounding parts. It consists of two large cordiform, acuminated, triple-ribbed, very thin cotyledons, a distinct cauliculus, and a centripetal radicle (*i. e.* a radicle directed towards the centre of the fruit).

β. **Of the Bark.**—The *bark* of the Strychnos Nux-vomica (*nux-vomica bark; cortex strychnos nucis-vomicæ; cortex angusturæ spuriæ* seu *falsæ; cortex pseudangusturæ* seu *virosæ*) occurs in quills (*pseudangustura convoluta*), in flat pieces (*pseudangustura plana*), or in pieces arched backwards and twisted (*pseudangustura revoluta*) like dried horn.

The outer or epidermic surface varies in its appearance according to the age of the bark. In the young bark it is ash-grey; and at this period has great resemblance to true angustura bark. When somewhat older, it offers numerous whitish or yellowish prominences, which were supposed by Pelletier and Caventou to be a species of lichen (*chiodecton*), but which are now known to be an epidermoid alteration or leprous exuberance.[1] At a more advanced stage of its growth, the bark is coated with a rust-coloured corky or spongy layer.   In this state it is called rusty false angustura (*pseudangustura ferruginea*), though it really has no resemblance to genuine angustura bark. The inner surface of the bark is frequently dark or blackish, but sometimes greyish-yellow.   The pieces seldom exceed four inches in length : they are compact and hard, and break with a smooth fracture.   The powder is intensely bitter, without aroma, acridity, or astringency : its colour is dirty yellow, not very dissimilar to that of jalap.

NUX-VOMICA BARK was formerly confounded with angustura or cusparia bark : hence its name of *false angustura bark.* The history of the mistake is as follows :—In 1804, Dr. Rambach, a physician at Hamburgh, observed that some specimens of angustura bark, said to be from the East Indies, acted as a powerful poison; and as repeated cases of poisoning occurred with the same substance, an order was issued forbidding the use of angustura bark.   On the 15th of October, 1815, the Commission of Health of the Grand Duchy of Baden ordered all the angustura bark in the possession of the apothecaries to be seized, and placed under a seal; the physicians at the same time receiving an intimation that they were not, in future, to prescribe this bark.   Similar ordinances were issued in Austria, Bavaria, and Wirtemberg.[2]

The origin of this bark is said by Batka to be as follows :—A quantity of it was imported from the East into England, and, not being saleable, was sent to Holland ; and as no better means of getting rid of it offered, it was mixed with, and sold as, genuine angustura or cusparia bark.[3]   Great obscurity long existed as to the tree which yielded it.   At first it was attributed to the *Brucea ferruginea* or *antidysenterica*, a native of Abyssinia, belonging to the family Xanthoxylaceæ ; but in 1831 Geiger had occasion to examine the bark of the B. ferruginea, and found that it had no resemblance to false angustura.[4]   Now the composition and effects of this bark rendered it in the highest degree probable that it was the product of some tree of the genus Strychnos ; Batka said, of the *S. Nux-vomica*, or some kindred species,—an opinion which was confirmed by my examination of the specimens of the nux-vomica plant in Dr. Wallich's collection, in the possession of the Linnean Society.[5]   In 1837, Dr. O'Shaughnessy[6] established the identity of false angustura bark and the bark of the nux-vomica tree.   Since then I have examined about 1 cwt. of the latter bark brought to this country, and find it to be identical with false angustura bark contained in my museum, and which I had purchased in Paris several years before.

Nux-vomica bark (*kuchila*) is commonly sold in Calcutta for *rohun*, the harmless bark of *Soymida febrifuga* ; and sulphate of brucia obtained from it was mistaken by Mr. Piddington[7] for a sulphate of a supposed new alkaloid, to which the name of "rohuna" was given !   By the timely discovery of the real nature of this salt by Dr. O'Shaughnessy, the dreadful consequences which might, and probably would have resulted from its employment as a febrifuge in the Indian army (to which it had been sent as a substitute for sulphate of quina), were averted.[8]

COMMERCE.—In 1838 duty was paid on 1017 lbs. of nux-vomica ; in 1839, on only 478 lbs. ; in 1840, on 550 lbs.

COMPOSITION.—The *seeds* of Strychnos Nux-vomica have been analysed

[1] Fée, *Essai sur les Cryptog. des Ecorces exot.* p. 16, 1824.
[2] Schwartze, *Pharm. Tabell.* S. 95, 2te Ausg. 1833 ; *Hufeland's Journal*, Bd. xix. St. i. S. 181.
[3] Guibourt, *Hist. des Drog.* t. ii. p. 4, 3me édit. 1836.
[4] *Pharm. Central-Blatt für* 1831, S. 477.
[5] *London Medical Gazette*, vol. xix. p. 492.
[6] *Madras Journal* for April 1837.
[7] *Trans. Med. Phys. Society of Calcutta*, vol. iv.
[8] Private information furnished me by Dr. O'Shaughnessy, and by Dr. Jackson (Apothecary-General of the Indian Army).

by Rese,[1] Desportes,[2] Braconnot,[3] Chevreul,[4] and Pelletier and Caventou.[5] The most important of these analyses is that made by the last-mentioned chemists, who also examined the *bark* of Strychnos nux-vomica, under the name of *false angustura*.[6] The leprous coating of this bark they afterwards[7] submitted to a separate examination, under the idea of its being a lichen.

Pelletier and Caventou's Analyses of the Strychnos Nux-vomica.

1. Of the Seeds.	2. Of the Bark.
Strychnic or igasuric acid.	Gallate of brucia.
Strychnia ⎫ in combination with strychnic	Fatty matter (not deleterious).
Brucia ⎭ acid.	Gum (a considerable quantity).
Wax (a small quantity).	Yellow colouring matter and alcohol.
Concrete oil.	Sugar (traces).
Yellow colouring matter.	Woody fibre.
Gum.	
Starch (a little).	Nux-vomica (false Augustura) bark.
Bassorin.	
Woody fibre.	The leprous coating was composed of a
Carbonate of lime and chloride of potassium	*greenish-yellow oil, yellow colouring mat-*
in the ashes.	*ter, reddish-yellow colouring matter,* [and
	woody fibre].
Nux-vomica seeds.	

1. STRYCHNIA.—See post.

2. BRUCIA; *Brucina; Caniramin; Vomicin;* $\overset{+}{Br}$=$C^{44}H^{25}N^2O^7$, Liebig; or $C^{46}H^{26}N^2O^8$, Regnault; Eq. Wt.=373 Liebig; or 394, Regnault.—Discovered, in 1819, by Pelletier and Caventou; exists in the bark and seeds of nux-vomica, and in St. Ignatius's bean: in the two latter substances it is associated with strychnia, and is in combination with igasuric acid; while in the bark of nux-vomica it is combined with gallic acid. The separation of brucia from strychnia is founded on its greater solubility in alcohol than the latter alkaloid. Brucia in the anhydrous form, + as obtained by fusing it, has a waxy appearance; but when combined with water, Br+8HO, it is capable of crystallising, the form of the crystals being oblique four-sided prisms; or sometimes the crystals have a pearly laminated appearance, something like boracic acid. Its taste is very bitter, though less so than that of strychnia. It is soluble in 850 parts of cold, or 500 parts of boiling water; but the presence of colouring matter, of which it is difficult to deprive it, promotes its solubility. It is very soluble in alcohol, but is insoluble in ether and the fixed oils, and is very slightly soluble only in the volatile oils. Nitric acid communicates a fine red colour to brucia; and the colour changes to violet on the addition of proto-chloride of tin; sulphuretted hydrogen and sulphurous acid destroy the colour. Chlorine communicates a red colour to brucia.[8] Bromine communicates a violet tint to the alcoholic solution of brucia. Sulphuric acid first reddens brucia, and then turns it yellow and green.

According to Dr. Fuss,[9] brucia is not a peculiar alkaloid, but a compound of strychnia and resin [yellow colouring matter]. He says that he has proved this both analytically and synthetically; and he ascribes the property of brucia to become reddened by nitric acid, and by chlorine, to the resin present. Prof. Erdmann, who examined the products of Fuss's experiments, has confirmed his statements.

The *salts of brucia* are readily formed by saturating dilute acids with brucia. They possess the following properties:—For the most part they are soluble and crystallisable, and

[1] Pfaff, *Syst. d. Mat. Med.* Bd. ii. S. 90.
[2] *Bull. de Pharm.* t. i. p. 271.
[3] *Ibid.* t. iii. p. 315.
[4] Orfila, *Toxicol. Gén.*
[5] *Ann. Chim. et Phys.* t. x. p. 142.
[6] *Ibid.* t. xii. p. 113.
[7] *Journ. de Pharm.* t. v. p. 546.
[8] Pelletier, *Journ. de Pharm.* xxiv. p. 159.
[9] *Berlinisches Jahrbuch für die Pharmacie,* Bd. xliii. S. 407, 1840.

have a bitter taste. They are decomposed by potash, soda, ammonia, the alkaline earths, morphia, and strychnia, which precipitate the brucia. They produce precipitates (*tannate of brucia*) on the addition of tannic acid. Nitric acid colours them as it does free brucia.

The effects of brucia on man and animals appear to be precisely similar to those of strychnia, though larger doses are required to produce them. Magendie[1] considers it to possess only one-twelfth of the activity of strychnia; while Andral regards it as having one-sixth the power of impure strychnia, and one twenty-fourth that of pure strychnia.— Dose, half a grain, which is to be gradually increased to five grains. It may be given in the same way as strychnia.

[3. Igasurine.—This base is stated to have been found in the concentrated mother-liquor obtained in the preparation of strychnia and brucia. Denoi, the discoverer, describes the substance as a colourless precipitate, which becomes crystalline when left in the mother-liquor. It then appears in brilliant silky needles, containing ten per cent. of water, and having a very bitter taste. It has the greatest resemblance to brucia, except in its solubility. It dissolves readily in 200 parts of boiling water, and crystallises out quickly when the solution cools. Brucia requires for its solution 500 parts of boiling water, and crystallises out again very slowly. Bicarbonate of potash or soda precipitates igasurine from solution in the presence of tartaric acid, but not brucia. The physiological action of igasurine is stated to be intermediate between that of brucia and strychnia. Its influence upon polarised light, and its behaviour with the usual reagents, are almost identical with those of brucia. This base requires further examination.[2]—Ed.]

4. Strychnic or Igasuric Acid.—Exists in the seeds of nux-vomica, St. Ignatius's bean, and snake-wood. Igasuric acid is crystallisable, and has an acid, rough taste. It is soluble in water and alcohol. The salts of iron, mercury, and of silver in solution, are unaffected by it; but those of copper are rendered green; and after some time a light green precipitate is deposited.

5. Yellow Colouring Matter.—Found in the seeds and bark of nux-vomica, in St. Ignatius's bean, and the Upas Tieuté; also in *Strychnos pseudo-quina*, Casca d'Anta, and Pareira Bark. It is soluble in water and alcohol, and is reddened by nitric acid [and by chlorine].

6. Reddish-yellow Colouring Matter.—Resides in the rust-coloured epidermoid alteration of nux-vomica bark; also in *Strychnos pseudo-quina*. It is insoluble in cold water and in ether, but dissolves with facility in alcohol. Nitric acid renders it deep green by combining with it.

7. Other Constituents.—The wax mentioned in the above analysis is probably derived from the hairs with which the seeds are invested; it enables them to resist moisture. *Resin* is probably a constituent of the seeds; for tincture of nux-vomica is rendered milky by water. An *odorous, non-acid, innocuous* principle is obtained by submitting nux-vomica and water to distillation. Meissner detected *copper* in the ashes of nux-vomica: but I have several times repeated his experiment without recognising this metal.

Chemical Characteristics.   1. Of the Seeds.—*Powdered nux-vomica* has a fallow-grey colour, a bitter taste, and a peculiar odour analogous to that of liquorice. Thrown on burning coal it inflames when the temperature is very high; but when lower, is decomposed, evolves a thick white smoke of a peculiar odour, and leaves a carbonaceous residuum. Concentrated sulphuric acid blackens it. Nitric acid communicates to it a *deep orange-yellow colour*. If the powder be digested with boiling water acidulated with sulphuric acid, the filtered liquor is turbid and slightly yellow. Nitric acid, after some minutes, reddens it; ammonia makes it brown, and precipitates blackish flocks. If the sulphuric solution be digested with finely powdered marble (to saturate the excess of acid), then evaporated to dryness, and the residue treated with boiling alcohol, we obtain a spirituous solution of sulphates of strychnia and brucia, with colouring matter. This has a bitter

---

[1] *Formulaire.*
[2] [*Pharmaceutical Journal*, December 1854, p. 280.]

taste, is reddened by nitric acid, produces convulsions when given to birds or other small animals, and forms a flocculent coloured precipitate on the addition of ammonia. Sometimes crystals are deposited from the alcoholic liquor on standing for two or three days.[1]

Ammoniacal sulphate of copper added to the *infusion* or *decoction of nux-vomica*, produces an emerald-green colour, and gradually a greenish-white precipitate (*igasurate of copper*) : ammoniacal sulphate of strychnia remains in solution. Sesquichloride of iron also produces an emerald colour, which disappears on the addition of hydrochloric acid : this colouration does not depend, according to Pelletier and Caventou, on the igasuric acid ; nor can it depend on tannic acid, for gelatin gives no indication of this substance : if the decoction be boiled with animal charcoal, it loses the power of becoming green on the addition of a ferruginous salt. Nitric acid communicates an orange-red colour to the decoction, owing to its action on the brucia and yellow colouring matter. A solution of iodine communicates a yellowish-brown tint to the decoction ; but after a few minutes the colour disappears (owing, perhaps, to the formation of the hydriodates of strychnia and brucia), and the iodine is no longer detectable by starch, without the addition of nitric acid or chlorine. Tannic acid, or infusion of nutgalls, produces in the decoction a copious precipitate (*tannates of strychnia, brucia,* and *some other vegetable matter*). Alcohol also causes a precipitate (*gum*). Diacetate of lead causes an abundant precipitate composed of *gummate and igasurate of lead, with colouring and fatty matter*).

2. Of the Bark.—An infusion of this bark reddens litmus, in consequence of the excess of acid present. Strong nitric acid added to this solution produces a red colour ; and by dropping the acid on the inner surface of the bark, a blood-red spot is produced : in both cases the effect arises from the action of the acid on the brucia and yellow colouring matter. If nitric acid be applied to the external surface of the bark, it produces a deep green colour, in consequence of the action of the acid on the yellow colouring matter (see *Strychnos pseudo-quina*, post). Infusion of galls added to the infusion of this bark occasions a white precipitate (*tannate of brucia*). Sulphate of iron colours the infusion green, from its action on the yellow colouring matter. (For other characteristics, see ANGOSTURA BARK.)

PHYSIOLOGICAL EFFECTS. **1. Of the Bark.** α. *On Animals generally.*— The experiments of Pfaff, the Vienna faculty, Emmert, Meyer, Orfila, Magendie, and Jäger,[2] have shown that it is a powerful poison to dogs, rabbits, wolves, and other animals. Thus eight, twelve, or eighteen grains of it kill dogs, the symptoms being precisely the same as those of nux-vomica, already detailed. Emmert (quoted by Christison) inferred, from experiments made on animals, that this bark acts on the spine directly, and not on that organ through the medium of the brain.

β. *On Man* it also acts as a powerful poison. Emmert[3] mentions that a boy who had taken by mistake the decoction of this bark died therefrom. His intellectual powers were unaffected ; he entreated his physician not to touch him, as violent convulsions were immediately brought on ; he was

---

[1] Orfila and Barruel, *Arch. Gén. de Méd.* viii. 22 ; R. D. Thomson, *Brit. Ann. of Med.* i. 106.
[2] Wibmer, *Wirk. d. Arzneim. u. Gift.* Bd. i. S. 182.
[3] Quoted by Wibmer, *ibid.* Bd. i. S. 188.

powerfully sweated, but did not vomit. Prof. Marc was nearly poisoned by swallowing through mistake three-quarters of a liqueur-glassful of a strong vinous infusion.[1]

2. Of the Seeds. *α. On Vegetables.*—Marcet[2] states, that a quarter of an hour after immersing the root of an haricot plant (Phaseolus vulgaris) in a solution of five grains of the extract of nux-vomica in an ounce of water, the petals became curved downwards, and in twelve hours the plant died. Fifteen grains of the same extract were inserted in the stem of a lilac tree, on July 5th, and the wound closed. In thirteen days the neighbouring leaves began to wither.

β. On Animals generally.—Nux-vomica appears to be poisonous, in a greater or less degree, to most animals. On the Vertebrata its effects are very uniform, though larger quantities are required to kill herbivorous than carnivorous animals. Thus a few grains will kill a dog, but some ounces are required to destroy a horse.[3] It occasions, in all, tetanic convulsions, increased sensibility to external impressions, asphyxia, and death.[4] The bird called *Buceros Rhinoceros* is, however, said to eat the nuts of Strychnos, and not to be subject to their noxious influence.[5]

γ. On Man.—Three degrees of the operation of nux-vomica on man may be admitted:

αα. First degree: tonic and diuretic effects.—In very small and repeated doses, nux-vomica usually promotes the appetite, assists the digestive process, increases the secretion of urine, and renders the excretion of the fluid more frequent. In some cases it acts slightly on the bowels, and occasionally produces a sudorific effect. The pulse is usually unaffected. In somewhat larger doses, the stomach not unfrequently becomes disordered, and the appetite impaired.

ββ. Second degree: rigidity and convulsive contraction of the muscles. In larger doses the effects of nux-vomica manifest themselves by a disordered state of the muscular system. A feeling of weight and weakness in the limbs, and increased sensibility to external impressions (of light, sound, touch, and variations of temperature), with depression of spirits and anxiety, are usually the precursory symptoms. The limbs tremble, and a slight rigidity or stiffness is experienced when an attempt is made to put the muscles into action. The patient experiences a difficulty in keeping the erect posture, and, in walking, frequently staggers. If, when this effect is beginning to be observed, he be tapped suddenly on the ham while standing, a slight convulsive paroxysm is frequently brought on, so that he will have some difficulty to prevent himself from falling. I have often in this way been able to recognise the effect of nux-vomica on the muscular system, before the patient had experienced any particular symptoms.

If the use of the medicine be still persevered in, these effects increase in intensity, and the voluntary muscles are thrown into a convulsed state by very slight causes. Thus, when the patient inspires more deeply than usual, or attempts to walk, or even to turn in bed, a convulsive paroxysm is brought on.

---

[1] *Journ. de Pharm.* t. ii. p. 507.
[2] *Ann. Chim. et Phys.* t. xxix.
[3] Moiroud, *Pharm. Vét.* p. 266.
[4] Orfila, *Toxicol. Gén.*
[5] Müller's *Physiology*, by Baly, vol. i. p. 478.

The sudden contact of external bodies also acts like an electric shock on him. The further employment of nux-vomica increases the severity of the symptoms; the paroxysms now occur without the agency of any evident exciting cause, and affect him even when lying perfectly quiet and still in bed. The muscular fibres of the pharynx, larynx, œsophagus, and bladder, also become affected; and Trousseau and Pidoux[1] say those of the penis are likewise influenced, and the nocturnal and diurnal erections become inconvenient even in those who, for some time before, had lost somewhat of their virility. I am acquainted with two cases of paralysis, in which the use of nux-vomica caused almost constant nocturnal erection. Females also, say Trousseau and Pidoux, experience more energetic venereal desires; and "we have," they add, "received confidential information on this point, which cannot be doubted."

The pulse does not appear to be uniformly affected; for the most part it is slightly increased in frequency between the convulsive attacks, but Trousseau says he has found it calm even when the dose of the medicine was sufficient to cause general muscular rigidity. Previous to the production of the affection of the muscles, various painful sensations are oftentimes experienced in the skin, which patients have compared to the creeping of insects (formication), or to the passage of an electric shock; and occasionally an eruption makes its appearance.

It is remarkable that in paralysis the effects of nux-vomica are principally observed in the paralysed parts. Magendie[2] states he has observed sweating confined to the paralysed parts. "I have seen," says this physiologist, "the affected side covered with an anomalous eruption, while the opposite side was free from it. One side of the tongue is sometimes sensible of a very bitter taste, which is not perceptible to the other side."

γγ. *Third degree: tetanus, asphyxia, and death.*—To illustrate this third and most violent degree of operation, I think I cannot do better than relate a case of poisoning by nux-vomica reported by Mr. Ollier.[3]

A young woman swallowed between three and four drachms of this substance in powder, and in half an hour was seen by Mr. Ollier. She was sitting by the fire, quite collected and tranquil; her pulse about 80, and regular. He left her for about ten minutes to procure an emetic, and on his return found that she had thrown herself back in her chair, and that her legs were extended, and considerably separated. She was perfectly sensible, and without pain; but seemed in alarm, laid hold of her husband's coat, and entreated him not to leave her. A perspiration had broken out on her skin, her pulse had become faint and much quicker, and she called frequently for drink. She then had a slight and transient convulsion. Recovering from it, she was in great trepidation, kept fast hold of her husband, and refused to let him go, even for the alleged purpose of getting her drink. In a few minutes after, she had another and a more violent attack, and shortly afterwards a third: the duration of these was from a minute and a half to two minutes. In them she retained her grasp; her whole body was straightened and stiffened, the legs pushed out and forced apart. I could not (says Mr. Ollier) perceive either pulse or respiration; the face and hands were livid; the muscles of the former, especially of the lips, violently agitated; and she made constantly a moaning, chattering noise. She was not unlike one in an epileptic fit, but did not struggle, though, as she was forced out, it was difficult to keep her from falling on the floor. In the short intervals of these attacks she was quite sensible; was tormented with incessant thirst; perspired; had a very quick and faint pulse; complained of being sick, and made many attempts to vomit. (I should

[1] *Traité de Thérap.* t. i. p. 515.
[2] *Formulaire*, 8me édit. p. 7.
[3] *Lond. Med. Repos.* vol. xix. p. 448.

state she had swallowed some ipecacuanha powder to evacuate the poison.) She continued to refuse to let her husband move, and to the question whether she was in pain, replied, " No—no—no !"

A fourth and most vehement attack soon followed, in which the whole body was ex tended to the utmost ; and she was rigidly stiff from head to foot, insomuch that, with al the force of the surgeon, he could not bend her thighs on the pelvis to replace her in her seat. From this she never recovered ; she fell into a state of asphyxia, and never breathed again. She now relaxed her grasp ; her discoloured hands dropped upon her knees ; her face, too, was livid ; the brows contracted ; the lips wide apart, showing the whole of the closed teeth ; and a salivary foam issued plentifully from the corners of her mouth. The expression of the whole countenance was at this time very frightful. On removal of the body, it was discovered that the urine had been discharged. She died in about an hour after taking the poison. Five hours afterwards, she was still as straight and stiff as a statue : if you lifted one of her hands, the whole body moved with it ; but the face had become pale in comparison, and its expression more placid.

POST-MORTEM APPEARANCES.—In the case just related the body was ob-served to be rigid after death, but in the lower animals the reverse is generally noticed. As in other cases where death takes place from obstructed respira-tion, venous congestion, especially in the lungs, is observed. Occasionally there is redness or inflammation of the alimentary canal, and now and then softening of the brain or spinal cord.

MODUS OPERANDI.—There are several points connected with the modus operandi of nux-vomica, which require investigation :—

1st. *Is this seed a local irritant ?*—In medicinal doses it does not usually disorder the stomach, nor is it invariably irritant in its operation, even when swallowed as a poison. In some instances, however, the pain and heat in the stomach, the burning in the gullet, and the nausea and vomiting, are evidences of its local action ; and in several cases marks of inflammation have been observed in the stomach on examination of the body after death. Strychnia also is a local irritant.

2ndly. *Does the active principle of nux-vomica become absorbed ?*—To this inquiry our answer is decidedly, Yes.

3rdly. *On what part of the body does nux-vomica exercise a specific effect ?*—The muscular contractions caused by nux-vomica arise chiefly from changes effected in the nervous stimulus, and not from alterations in the con-tractility of the muscular fibre ; for Matteucci[1] found that, in frogs poisoned by nux-vomica, when the excitability of the nerves was destroyed, and when the electric current which was applied to them no longer occasioned muscular contractions, the muscles themselves, when submitted directly to the action of the current, underwent contraction.

Every part of the nervous system is probably specifically affected by nux-vomica, though the principal manifestations of its action are in the functions of the cerebro-spinal system. The tetanic symptoms, and the absence of nar-cotism, have led to the conclusion that the spinal cord was the part principally affected,—a conclusion supported by the fact that the division of this cord—nay, even complete decollation—will not prevent the poisonous effects of nux-vomica ; whereas the destruction of the cord by the introduction of a piece of whalebone into the spinal canal causes the immediate cessation of the convul-sions ; and if only part of the cord be destroyed, the convulsions cease in that part of the body only which is supplied with nerves from the portion of

---

[1] *Traité des Phénom. Electro-Physiol. des Animaux*, pp. 241–2, Paris, 1844.

medulla destroyed. These facts, then, originally observed by Magendie, and which I have myself verified, lead to the conclusion that the abnormal influence, whatever it may be, which causes the convulsions to take place, is not derived from the contents of the cranium, but from the medulla spinalis itself. Moreover, as the motor nerves seem principally affected, it has been presumed that the disorder is chiefly seated in the anterior columns of the cord. It is probable, however, that both the posterior columns and the grey matter of the cord are affected by it.[1]

But nux-vomica affects the sensibility of the body, and heightens the sensations of touch, vision, and hearing. These effects are referable to its action on the cerebrum; though Dr. Stannius[2] considers that this increased susceptibility to external impressions arises from the action of the poison on the spinal cord. Although the intellectual functions are not usually much disordered by this drug, yet the mental anxiety commonly experienced by persons under its use, the occasional appearance of stupor, and the observations of Andral and Lallemand on the injurious effects of it in apoplexies with cerebral softening, leave no doubt that the cerebrum. is affected by this agent. Bally[3] has observed an appearance of stupor, vertigo, tinnitus aurium, sleeplessness, and turgescence of the capillaries of the face, result from the use of strychnia.

M. Flourens[4] asserted that the part of the nervous system on which nux-vomica more particularly acted, was the medulla oblongata. But MM. Orfila, Ollivier, and Drogartz,[5] in their report on a case of poisoning by this substance, particularly mention that they observed no traces of alteration in the condition of the medulla oblongata, the tuber annulare, or the crura cerebri,—which is in opposition to Flourens' opinion; for he asserted that the specific or exclusive action of each substance on each organ always left, after death, traces of its action sufficient to distinguish the affected from other organs. The cerebellum is said by some to be acted on by nux-vomica, but for the most part on hypothetical grounds; though it must be mentioned that MM. Orfila, Ollivier, and Drogartz observed the cerebellum presented more evidences of lesions than the other parts of the nervous system. Another argument which probably would be advanced by phrenologists in favour of the cerebellum by this drug is the observation of Trousseau, that the sexual feelings are usually excited by it. The ganglia also appear to be affected by nux-vomica: and hence the influence which this agent exercises over the movements of the intestinal canal and heart.

Ségalas[6] found, in his experiments on animals, that in some cases life could not be prolonged by artificial respiration, and that after death the heart could not be stimulated to contract. These and other reasons seem to show that nux-vomica exhausts the irritability of the heart. But in all probability this viscus is affected only secondarily, the essential and primary action being on the nervous system.

---

[1] The white nervous fibres are merely conductors of nervous power; the grey matter, on the other hand, is a generator or source of nervous power (see Grainger, *Struct. and Funct. of the Spinal Cord*, p. 17).

[2] *Brit. and For. Med. Rev.* vol. v. p. 221.

[3] *Ibid.* vol. vi. p. 225.

[4] *Rech. Expér. sur les Fonct. du Syst. Nerv.* 1824.

[5] *Arch. Gén. de Méd.* viii. 22.

[6] Quoted by Dr. Christison.

The nerves themselves are likewise affected; for in the last stage of poisoning by nux-vomica the nerves of frogs lose, partially or wholly, their susceptibility when submitted to the electrical current.[1]

4thly. *What kind of action does nux-vomica set up in those parts of the nervous system on which it acts?*—As the muscles receive from the nervous system a preternatural stimulus to action, it is presumed that this system (or at least certain parts of it) is in a state of excitement or irritation. In one case mentioned by Mr. Watt,[2] there was observed softening of the lumbar portion of the spinal cord; and in the case reported by MM. Orfila, Ollivier, and Drogartz, the whole cortical substance of the brain, especially of the cerebellum, was softened. Andral and Lallemand have both observed that this remedy in some forms of apoplexy produced symptoms indicating ramollissement.

5thly. *What is the reason that, in general, strychnia first displays its remarkable influence on paralytic limbs?*—No satisfactory explanation of this fact has been hitherto offered. The following are some hypotheses:—

a. According to Ségalas, the muscles of the unaffected limbs being simultaneously subject to the government of the brain and the action of the poison, are better enabled to resist the latter than paralysed muscles, which, not being under cerebral influence, are more affected by the poison. To this hypothesis, however, insuperable objections present themselves. Under the influence of strychnia paralysed parts sometimes suffer violent pain, while the healthy parts are free from it. How, asks Ollivier,[3] is this specific influence on paralysed parts only, to be explained? Does it not show, moreover, that these parts are not so entirely isolated from the influence of the nervous centres as the hypothesis of Ségalas would lead us to infer?

β. Dr. Marshall Hall[4] thus explains it:—When the paralysis is cerebral, the irritability of the muscular fibre becomes augmented, from want of the application of the stimulus of volition; and in such cases, therefore, strychnia first affects the paralysed muscles, because these are more irritable than the sound ones. But in spinal paralysis the irritability is diminished, and in such strychnia does not firstly and mostly affect the paralysed limbs. This explanation appeared to me so plausible and satisfactory, that in the first edition of this work I adopted it, believing it to present a clear and physiological elucidation of the facts before related. But in the summer of 1841 I made a number of observations on paralytic patients in the London Hospital, which convinced me that it does not correctly interpret the phenomena in question. The following is a brief abstract of one out of many similar cases:—

A middle-aged man was admitted into the hospital suffering with hemiplegia of two years' standing, and the consequence of apoplexy. He was put under the influence of the alcoholic extract of nux-vomica. In a few days the muscles of the paralysed limbs were powerfully affected by the remedy, but those of the sound side were unaffected by it. I then resolved to try the effects of voltaic electricity on the paralysed and healthy muscles. For this purpose I directed each hand to be placed in a separate basin containing a solution of salt. The two basins were then respectively connected with the electrodes of a magneto-electric machine, and a current of electricity thus simultaneously traversed the paralysed and healthy arms. To my great surprise, the muscles of the paralysed arm were comparatively but slightly affected, while those of the sound one were most powerfully convulsed. This experiment was tried repeatedly, and invariably with the same result. In this case the paralysis was undoubtedly, I think, cerebral. On Dr. Hall's hypothesis, the effects of strychnia on the paralysed limbs proved it to be so. Yet the paralysed muscles were less irritable than the sound ones, as manifested by voltaic electricity. I have observed the same effects in many other cases. Similar results as to

[1] Matteucci, *op. ante citato.*
[2] Christison, p. 183.
[3] *Traité de la Moëlle Epinière,* p. 841, Paris, 1827.
[4] *Medico-Chirurgical Transactions,* 2d series, vol. iv. Lond. 1839.

the condition of the paralysed muscles have also been obtained by Dr. Copland[1] and Dr. Todd.[2]

γ. Dr. Todd says that "the tendency of strychnine to affect the paralytic limbs before the healthy ones, is attributable to its being attracted in greater quantity to the seat of the lesion in the brain, than to the corresponding part on the other side." This hypothesis assumes that in all these cases a larger quantity of blood is "attracted" to the affected part of the brain than to the sound parts,—an assumption which cannot be admitted.

6thly. *Is any change produced in the blood-discs by strychnia?*— Müller[3] says strychnia produces no change in them; and Dr. Stannius[4] was unable to detect, by means of the microscope, any alteration in the appearance of the blood of frogs poisoned by strychnia.

7thly. *In what manner is death produced by nux-vomica?*—Frequently by the stoppage of respiration (asphyxia), in consequence of the spasmodic condition of the respiratory muscles. In other cases death seems to arise from excessive exhaustion of the nervous power (see Cloquet's case, quoted by Christison).

Uses.—The obvious indications for the use of nux-vomica, strychnia, or brucia, are torpid or paralytic conditions of the motor or sensitive nerves, or of the muscular fibre; while these agents are contra-indicated in spasmodic or convulsive diseases. Experience, however, has fully proved that when paralysis depends on inflammatory conditions of the nervous centres these agents prove injurious, and accelerate organic changes.

1. *In paralysis.*—Of all the diseases for which nux-vomica has been employed, in none has it been so successful as in paralysis; and it is deserving of notice, that this is one of the few remedies whose discovery is not the effect of mere chance, since Fouquier[5] was led to its use by legitimate induction from observation of its physiological effects. That a remedy which stimulates so remarkably the muscular system to action should be serviceable when that system no longer receives its accustomed natural stimulus, is, *à priori*, not astonishing. Paralysis, however, is the common effect of various lesions of the nervous centres, in some of which nux-vomica may be injurious, in others useless, and in some beneficial. It is, therefore, necessary to point out under what circumstances this remedy is likely to be advantageous or hurtful.

A very frequent, and, indeed, the most common cause of paralysis, is hemorrhage of the nervous centres. Blood may be effused on the external surface of these centres, into their cavities, or in their substance, the latter being by far the most common case,—in the proportion, according to Andral,[6] of 386 out of 392 instances of cerebral hemorrhage. It is almost superfluous to add that the radical cure of these cases can be effected only by the removal (that is, absorption) of the effused blood. Now the process by which this is effected is almost entirely a natural one: art can offer no assistance of a positive kind, though, by the removal of impeding causes, she may be at times negatively useful. Nux-vomica can, in such cases, be of no avail; on the contrary, it may be injurious.

The part immediately surrounding the sanguineous clot is usually much

[1] *Dict. of Pract. Medicine*, vol. iii. p. 42; *Lancet*, Dec. 20, 1845, p. 670.
[2] *Medico-Chirurgical Transactions*, 2d series, vol. xii. p. 207, 1847.
[3] *Physiology*, by Baly, vol. i. p. 107.
[4] *Brit. and For. Med. Rev.* vol. v. p. 222.
[5] Bayle, *Bibl. Thérap.* t. ii. p. 141.
[6] *Path. Anat.* by West, vol. ii. p. 722.

softened,—a condition formerly regarded as the effect of the effusion. But Lallemand has satisfactorily shown that it often, though not invariably, precedes the hemorrhage. This softening or *ramollissement* is, according to the same authority, a constant and necessary result of an acute or chronic irritation. But the facts at present known do not warrant this generalisation, since cases occur which apparently are unconnected with irritation. For this softening, art can do but little: we have, in fact, no particular or uniform treatment. If we can connect with it any increased vascular action, of course blood-letting and the other antiphlogistic means are to be resorted to; whereas, if the reverse condition of system exist, marked by great languor and debility, tonics and stimulants may be administered. Nux-vomica in these cases offers no probability of benefit; on the contrary, we might suspect that, as it irritates the spinal cord, it might probably have the same effect on the brain, and hasten the production of softening. Now experience seems to confirm our theoretical anticipations. Andral[1] relates the case of a man who was hemiplegic, in consequence of an old apoplectic attack. A pill, containing only one-twelfth of a grain of strychnia (the active principle of nux-vomica), was given to him, and it produced a strong tetanic stiffness of the paralysed members. The following day he complained of pain in the head, on the side opposite to that paralysed; his intellectual functions were weaker, and his hemiplegia was increased; in fact, he had all the symptoms characterising softening of the brain. It is, therefore, probable that the strychnia set up an inflammatory condition of the nervous substance around the apoplectic deposit, and that this condition was the precursor of ramollissement. When, therefore, nux-vomica is employed in those cases of paralysis which are connected with inflammation of the brain or spinal marrow, it is very likely to increase the evils it is intended to mitigate. Lallemand[2] reports two cases in which this drug, administered against cerebral maladies, occasioned convulsive movements, which continued until death. On opening the bodies, the cerebral substance surrounding the sanguineous clot was found disorganised and exceedingly softened. These facts suggest some useful reflections as to the use of this powerful drug in paralysis, and prevent its indiscriminate use in all cases of this disease.

But there are cases in which paralysis, arising from cerebral hemorrhage, may be advantageously treated by nux-vomica. The blood which is poured out in the apoplectic cell has at first a gelatinous consistence, some of it still remaining fluid. "Somewhat later," says Andral,[3] "twelve or fifteen days after the attack, for instance, the coagulum is found to be firmer and more circumscribed; later still, it becomes white or yellow, and is surrounded by a brownish-red fluid. The walls of the containing cavity are smooth, and lined with a delicate membrane. The surrounding cerebral substance in some cases retains its natural appearance, and in others is altered both in colour and consistence. As the interval between the effusion and the examination increases, the coagula gradually disappear." The cyst is now found to contain a serous fluid, occasionally having a few cellular bridles running from one side to the other; and nature subsequently attempts to get rid of

---

[1] Bayle, *Bibl. Thérap.* t. ii. p. 227.
[2] *Recherches anatomico-pathologiques sur l'Encephale*, p. 267, 1820.
[3] *Path. Anat.* by West, vol. ii. p. 723.

the cyst by producing adhesion of its sides, leaving only a linear cicatrix. It is well known that by long disuse of some of the voluntary muscles the power over them becomes gradually diminished; and it appears that occasionally in cerebral hemorrhage, after the absorption of the effused blood, the paralysis remains, as it were by habit. In these cases the cautious employment of nux-vomica, or of its active principle, may be attended with beneficial results, by favouring the return both of motion and sensation.

But paralysis, like some other diseases of the nervous system, may exist without our being able to discover after death any lesion of the nervous centres; and it is then denominated a functional disorder, as if there were actually no organic lesion. To me, however, the fact of the lesion of action is a strong ground for suspecting that there must have been an organic lesion of some kind, though we see nothing. "It is highly probable," says Andral,[1] "that some organic lesions do exist in such cases, although they escape our notice." Be this as it may, experience has fully established the fact that nux-vomica is more beneficial in those forms of paralysis usually unaccompanied by visible lesions of structure; such, for example, as paralysis resulting from exposure to the influence of lead and its various compounds. Thus, of ten cases of saturnine hemiplegia, treated by nux-vomica or its active principles, and which are mentioned by Bayle, three were cured, and three ameliorated.

As hemiplegia more frequently depends on cerebral hemorrhage than some other forms of paralysis, so it is, for the most part, less amenable to remedial means. Thus, while out of twenty-six cases of paraplegia nineteen were cured by nux-vomica or its active constituents, yet in thirty instances of hemiplegia only thirteen were cured. In six cases of general paralysis (that is, paralysis of both sides at once), four were cured by this remedy. In the paralysis which sometimes affects the muscles of certain organs, nux-vomica (or strychnia) has been employed with advantage. Thus a case of amaurosis, accompanied with paralysis of the eyelid, is said to have been cured by it; and several cases of incontinence of urine, depending on paralysis or diminished power of the muscular fibres of the bladder, have also been benefited by the same means. In some cases of local paralysis strychnia has been employed endermically with benefit.

2. *Paralysis of the sentient nerves.*—The good effects procured from the use of nux-vomica in paralysis of the motor nerves, have led to its employment in functional lesions of sentient nerves, characterised by torpor, inactivity, and paralysis. That benefit may be obtained in these cases is physiologically probable, from the circumstance that one of the effects of this agent is an exaltation of the susceptibility to external impressions, as I have before mentioned. Hitherto, however, the trials have not been numerous, nor remarkably successful. In *amaurosis* benefit has been obtained in some few instances; and where no organic lesion is appreciable, this remedy deserves a trial. The endermic method of using it has been preferred. Small blisters, covered with powdered strychnia, have been applied to the temples and eyebrows. The remedy causes sparks to be perceived in both eyes, especially the affected one; and it is said, the more of these, the better should be the prognosis: moreover, the red-coloured sparks are thought more favourable than

---

[1] *Ibid.* p. 709.

sparks of other colours. When the malady is complicated with disease of the brain, the remedy must be employed with extreme caution.

3. *Other affections of the nervous system.*—I have seen nux-vomica very serviceable in shaking or *tremor of the muscles* produced by habitual intoxication. A gentleman thus affected, who had for several weeks lost the power of writing, reacquired it under the use of this medicine. *Chorea* has been benefited by it.[1] In *tetanus* it has been tried at the London Hospital, without any augmentation of the convulsions. Several cases of *epilepsy* are said to have been relieved by it :[2] but, judging from its physiological effects, it would appear to be calculated to act injuriously, rather than beneficially, in this disease ; and in one case[3] the use of strychnia apparently caused paralysis and death. It has also been employed in *hypochondriasis* and *hysteria.*[4] It has also been used in *neuralgia* with good effect.[5]

4. *Affections of the alimentary canal.* — On account of its intense bitterness, nux-vomica has been resorted to as a tonic and stomachic in *dyspepsia,* especially when this affection depends on, or is connected with, an atonic condition of the muscular coat of the stomach.

In *pyrosis,* resulting from simple functional disorders of the stomach, Mr. Mellor[6] considers it to be almost a specific. Even when pyrosis is symptomatic of organic disease of the stomach, he says it is of essential service. In febrile states of the system its use is contra-indicated. Dr. Belcombe[7] has confirmed these statements, and also speaks of its good effects in *gastrodynia.* In *dysentery,* particularly when of an epidemic nature, nux-vomica has gained some reputation. Hagstrom says he has proved its value in some hundreds of cases ;[8] and his report has been confirmed by Hufeland,[9] Geddings,[10] and others. In *colica pictonum,* a combination of strychnia and hydrochlorate of morphia has been found by Bally highly successful.[11] In *prolapsus of the rectum* Dr. Schwartz[12] has recommended the use of this remedy, which he has employed for ten years, both in adults and children, with great benefit. One or two grains of the alcoholic extract are to be dissolved in two drachms of water ; and of this solution he gives to infants at the breast two or three drops ; to older children, from six to ten or fifteen drops, according to their age. In partial *borborygmi* of females I have found nux-vomica useful.

5. *In impotence.*—The excitement of the sexual feelings which Trousseau has seen produced by nux-vomica, led him to employ this remedy against impotence, and he has found it successful both in males and females. In some cases, however, its good effects were observed only while the patients were taking the medicine. A young man, twenty-five years of age, of an athletic constitution, who had been married for eighteen months without having any

---

[1] Magendie, *Formulaire.*
[2] Bayle, *Bibl. Thérap.* t. ii. pp. 135 and 230.
[3] *Ibid.* p. 233.
[4] *Ibid.* p. 134.
[5] *Lond. Med. Gaz.* Aug. 7, 1840.
[6] *Ibid.* xix. p. 851.
[7] *Ibid.* p. 964.
[8] Bayle, *op. cit.* p. 135.
[9] *Ibid.* p. 136.
[10] *Brit. and For. Med. Rev.* vol. i. p. 255.
[11] *Ibid.* vol. vi. p. 225.
[12] *Lond. Med. Gaz.* vol. xvi. p. 768.

other than almost fraternal communications with his wife, acquired his virility under the use of nux-vomica, though he again lost it soon after leaving off its employment. In spermatorrhœa it has been used with occasional benefit.

The preceding are the diseases in which nux-vomica has proved most successful. It has, however, been used in several others (as *intermittent fevers, intestinal worms*, &c.) with occasional benefit.

Administration.—Nux-vomica is used in the form of *powder, tincture*, or *extract. Strychnia* and *brucia* may be regarded as other preparations of it. The *powder* of nux-vomica is administered in doses of two or three grains gradually increased. Fouquier has sometimes increased the quantity to fifty grains.

Antidote.—Evacuate the contents of the stomach as speedily as possible. No chemical antidotes are known. Probably astringents (as infusion of galls, green tea) would be serviceable. Donné[1] regards chlorine, iodine, and bromine, as antidotes for strychnia and brucia; but further evidence is required to establish the correctness of his inferences. Emmert[2] says that vinegar and coffee increased the poisonous effects of nux-vomica (false angustura) bark. To relieve the spasms, narcotics may be employed. Sachs and others have recommended opium. As conia is the counterpart of strychnia, it deserves a trial. I applied it to a wound in a rabbit affected with tetanus from the use of strychnia: the convulsions ceased, but the animal died. In the absence of conia, the extract of hemlock should be employed. Ether and oil of turpentine have been recommended.[3] To relieve the excessive endermic operation of strychnia, acetate of morphia applied to the same spot has given relief.

1. TINCTURA NUCIS-VOMICÆ; *Tincture of Nux-vomica*. (Nux-vomica, scraped, ʒij.; Rectified Spirit, ʒviij. Macerate for seven days, and filter.)— Dose, ♏v. to ♏x. It is sometimes used as an embrocation to paralysed parts, and its good effects in this way seem to be increased by combining it with ammonia.

2. EXTRACTUM NUCIS-VOMICÆ, E.; *Extract of Nux-vomica*. ("Take of Nux-vomica any convenient quantity; expose it in a proper vessel to steam till it is properly softened; slice it, dry it thoroughly, and immediately grind it in a coffee-mill; exhaust the powder either by percolating it with rectified spirit, or by boiling it with repeated portions of rectified spirit, until the spirit comes off free of bitterness. Distil off the greater part of the spirit, and evaporate what remains in the vapour-bath to a proper consistence," *E*.)— Dose, gr. ss., gradually increased to two or three grains. The extract is given in the form of pill.

3. STRYCHNIA, L. E. D.; *Strychnine*; *Strychnina*; *Vauquelina*; *Tetanine*. In the anhydrous state its composition, according to Regnault, is $C^{42}H^{22}N^2O^4 = Sr$. Eq. Wt. = 334.—This alkaloid was discovered in 1818 by Pelletier and Caventou. It has been found in *Strychnos Nux-vomica, S. Ignatia, S. colubrina*, and *S. Tieuté*. In these plants it is frequently associated with brucia, and is always combined with an acid.

---

[1] *Journ. de Pharm.* t. xvi. p. 377.
[2] Buchner, *Toxikol.* S. 235-6.
[3] Phœbus, *Hülfsleist bei acut. Vergift.* S. 4.

In the *London Pharmacopœia* for 1850, no directions are given for the preparation of this alkaloid, which is placed in the materia medica. The directions of the *Edinburgh College* are as follows :—

"Take of Nux-vomica, lb. j.; Quicklime, ʒiss.; Rectified Spirit, *a sufficiency*. Subject the nux-vomica for two hours to the vapour of steam, chop or slice it, dry it thoroughly in the vapour-bath or hot air-press, and immediately grind it in a coffee-mill. Macerate for twelve hours in two pints of water, and boil it; strain through linen or calico, and squeeze the residuum; repeat the maceration and decoction twice with a pint and a half of water. Concentrate the decoctions to the consistency of thin syrup; add the lime in the form of milk of lime; dry the precipitate in the vapour-bath; pulverise it and boil it with successive portions of rectified spirit till the spirit cease to acquire a bitter taste. Distil off the spirit till the residuum be sufficiently concentrated to crystallise on cooling. Purify the crystals by repeated crystallisation."

In this process a decoction of nux-vomica is prepared : this contains the igasurate of strychnia with gum. This salt is decomposed by the lime, and the strychnia abstracted by rectified spirit.

In the *Dublin Pharmacopœia* for 1850, the process given is as follows :—

"Take of Nux-vomica, in powder, 1 lb.; Water, one gallon and a half; Oil of Vitriol of commerce, half a fluidounce; Slacked Lime, one ounce; Rectified Spirit, one quart; Dilute Sulphuric Acid, Solution of Ammonia, of each a sufficient quantity; Prepared Animal Charcoal, half an ounce. Macerate the nux-vomica for twenty-four hours with half a gallon of the water, acidulated with two drachms of the acid, and having boiled for half an hour, decant. Boil the residuum with a second half-gallon of the water, acidulated with one drachm of the acid; decant, and repeat this process with the remaining water and acid, the undissolved matter being finally submitted to strong expression. The decanted and expressed liquors having been passed through a filter, and then evaporated to the consistence of a syrup, let this be boiled with the rectified spirit for twenty minutes, the lime being added in successive portions during the ebullition, until the solution becomes decidedly alkaline. Filter through paper, and having drawn off by distillation the whole of the spirit, let the residuum be dissolved in the dilute sulphuric acid; and to the resulting liquid, after having been cleared by filtration, add the solution of ammonia in slight excess, and let the precipitate which forms be collected upon a paper filter, dried, and then dissolved in a minimum of boiling rectified spirit. Into this solution introduce the animal charcoal, digest for twenty minutes, then filter, and allow the residual liquor to cool, when the strychnia will separate in crystals." The weights used in this process are avoirdupoise.

[The process of the United States Pharmacopœia differs from the above. It directs of Nux-vomica, rasped, lb. iv.; Lime, in powder, ℨvj.; Muriatic Acid, ℨiij.; Alcohol, Diluted Sulphuric Acid, Solution of Ammonia, Purified Animal Charcoal, Water, of each a sufficient quantity. The first step in the operation is to convert the strychnia into a muriate by boiling with water acidulated by the acid, and repeat twice. Next decompose the muriate by the lime which separates the strychnia. Take this up by alcohol, and convert it into a sulphate by boiling with dilute sulphuric acid. Decolour by the charcoal, and finally separate the strychnia by the solution of ammonia, and dry on bibulous paper.— Ed.]

By digesting nux-vomica in water acidulated with sulphuric acid, the sulphates of strychnia and brucia are obtained. The lime decomposes these, and sets free a mixture of strychnia and brucia, which is dissolved by the spirit, and again converted into sulphates by the addition of sulphuric acid. The ammonia decomposes these sulphates; sulphate of ammonia is formed in solution, and the alkaloids are again set free, and are then dissolved by boiling alcohol. The hot alcoholic solution, being decolourised by animal charcoal, deposits, on cooling, the strychnia, the brucia being left in solution.

As a considerable quantity of mucilage is precipitated by the lime, Molyn[1] has proposed to avoid this by subjecting the nux-vomica (reduced to a coarse powder, and made into a paste with water) to the process of fermentation. Carbonic acid is evolved, the gummy and saccharine constituents are decomposed, and lactic acid is produced, which decomposes the igasurate of strychnia and brucia, and forms with these alkaloids very soluble lactates. In eighteen or twenty days the fermentation is completed.

Pure strychnia is a white, odourless, intensely bitter, crystalline substance, the form of the crystals being the octohedron or four-sided prism. When rapidly crystallised, it assumes the granular form. It is fusible, but not volatile; decomposing at a lower temperature than most vegetable bodies. Though so intensely bitter, it is almost insoluble in water, 1 part of strychnia requiring 6667 parts of water, at 50°, to dissolve it : that is, one grain needs nearly fourteen ounces of water to hold it in solution. It requires 2500 parts of boiling water to dissolve it. It is slightly soluble in boiling rectified spirit, but scarcely so in cold water. It acts on vegetable colours as an alkali, saturates acids forming salts, and separates most of the metallic oxides (the alkaline substances excepted) from their combinations with acids. In some cases, part only of the metal is precipitated, a double salt being formed in solution. Thus, when strychnia is boiled with a solution of sulphate of copper, a green solution of *cupreous sulphate of strychnia* is obtained, while a portion only of the oxide of copper is precipitated.

Strychnia is recognised by its crystallisability, its alkaline properties, its combustibility, its intense bitterness, its difficult solubility in alcohol, ether, and water, and solubility in dilute acids. A solution of bichloride of mercury added to a solution of strychnia in hydrochloric acid, causes a white clotty precipitate (composed of *bichloride of mercury* and *hydrochlorate of strychnia*). Tannic acid or tincture of nutgalls occasions a whitish precipitate in a neutral solution of hydrochlorate of strychnia. Marchand[2] has pointed out a very characteristic test for strychnia : if a small portion of strychnia be rubbed with some drops of oil of vitriol containing a hundredth part of its weight of nitric acid, no change of colour takes place (provided the strychnia be pure) : but if a minute quantity of the puce-coloured oxide (peroxide) of lead be added to the mixture, the liquid assumes a fine blue colour, which rapidly becomes violet, then gradually red, and after a few hours brownish yellow. Mack[3] has proposed to substitute peroxide of manganese, and Otto[4] bichromate of potash, for the peroxide of lead.

Commercial strychnia usually forms with strong nitric acid a red-coloured liquid, which afterwards becomes yellow. This change does not occur with pure strychnia, but depends on the presence of one or both of the two substances—viz. brucia and yellow colouring matter. As the red colour is destroyed by decolourising agents (sulphurous acid and sulphuretted hydrogen), it appears to depend on the oxidisement of the substance referred to. If potash be added to a very concentrated solution of a strychnian salt which has

[1] *Pharmaceutical Journal*, vol. vi. p. 492, 1847.
[2] *Journ. de Pharm. et de Chimie*, 3me sér. t. iv. p. 200, 1843.
[3] *Pharmaceutical Journal*, vol. vi. p. 187, 1846.
[4] *Ibid.* vol. vi. p. 479, 1847.   See also a paper by Mr. L. Thompson, in *Pharm. Journ.* vol. ix. p. 24, 1849.

been reddened by nitric acid, an orange precipitate is formed : an excess of water dissolves this precipitate.

According to the Edinburgh College, strychnia for medicinal use, which is declared to be "always more or less impure," possesses the following properties :—

Intensely bitter : nitric acid strongly reddens it : a solution of 10 grains in 4 fluidrachms of water by means of a fluidrachm of pyroligneous acid, when decomposed by one fluidounce of concentrated solution of carbonate of soda, yields, on brisk agitation, a coherent mass, weighing, when dry, 10 grains, and entirely soluble in solution of oxalic acid.

The London College (1850) gives the following characters for crystallised strychnia :—

It is dissolved in boiling alcohol. It melts by heat, and if it be more strongly urged it is totally dissipated. It tastes very bitter. Being endowed with violent powers, it is to be cautiously administered.

The *salts of strychnia,* when pure, are for the most part crystalline, white, and very bitter. They possess the following chemical characteristics :—1st, the alkalies and their carbonates occasion white precipitates in solutions of the strychnia salts ; 2dly, they are precipitated by tannic, but not by gallic acid ; 3dly, they are unchanged by the action of the persalts of iron.

The only salt of strychnia in the British Pharmacopœias is the muriate contained in the *Dublin Pharmacopœia* for 1850.

STRYCHNIÆ HYDROCHLORAS ; *Strychniæ Murias,* Ph.+Dubl. 1850 ; *Hydrochlorate* or *Muriate of Strychnia.* Formula $Sr,HCl + 2HO$. Equivalent Weight $= 389.$—The Dublin College gives the following directions for the preparation of this salt :—

" Take of Strychnia, one ounce ; Dilute Muriatic Acid, one fluidounce, or a sufficient quantity ; Distilled Water, two ounces and a half. Pour the acid upon the strychnia, and, adding the water, apply heat until a perfect solution is obtained. Let this cool, and let the crystals which form be dried upon bibulous paper. By evaporating the residual liquid to one-third of its bulk, and then allowing it to cool, an additional quantity of the salt will be obtained." The weights used are avoirdupoise.

This salt crystallises in four-sided needles, which lose their transparency in the air. It is much more soluble in water than the sulphate. When heated, it is decomposed, with the evolution of hydrochloric acid.

The *effects* of strychnia are of the same kind as those of nux-vomica, but more violent in degree. As ordinarily met with in the shops, it may be regarded as about six times as active as the alcoholic extract of nux-vomica. The following are a few examples of its poisonous operation :—

Dr. Christison[1] says, " I have killed a dog in two minutes with the sixth part of a grain, injected, in the form of alcoholic solution, into the chest : I have seen a wild boar killed, in the same manner, with the third of a grain, in ten minutes." Pelletier[2] says, " half a grain, blown into the mouth of a dog, produced death in five minutes." Half a grain, applied to a wound in the back of a dog, caused death in three minutes and a half. In all these and other instances death was preceded and accompanied by tetanus. The salts of strychnia act in the same manner. Some individuals are more sus-

---

[1] *Treatise on Poisons,* 3d edit. p. 797.
[2] *Ann. de Chim. et Phys.* x. 172.

ceptible of the action of strychnia than others. Andral[1] has seen a single pill, containing one-twelfth of a grain, cause slight trismus, and the commencement of tetanic stiffness of the muscles; while in other cases the dose may be gradually increased beyond a grain, with comparatively little effect. The largest dose I have given is a grain and a half, and this was repeated several times before the usual symptoms indicative of the affection of the system came on. Smaller doses had been previously given without any obvious effect. Subsequent experience has satisfied me that so large a dose was dangerous.[2]

The following case occurred on board the Dreadnought Hospital Ship, and was communicated to me by Mr. Cooper, surgeon :—

A Swede, aged 50—60, was admitted about the year 1833 with general paralysis, one side being more affected than the other : he was also in some degree idiotic. Strychnia was given, at first in the dose of one-eighth of a grain three times a day, which was continued for several weeks without apparent effect. The dose was then increased to one-quarter of a grain three times a day, which was also continued for some time ; and not producing any perceptible effect, the quantity was increased to half a grain twice or three times a day, and this dose was taken for many days before any influence of strychnia was manifested. But one morning, about 9 A.M., the apothecary was suddenly summoned by a message that the man was in a fit. When seen, he was insensible ; face and chest of a deep purple colour ; respiration had ceased, and the pulsation of the heart nearly so. The whole body (trunk and limbs) was in a state of tetanic spasm. Trunk extended, and shoulders thrown back : muscles of chest and abdomen hard and rigid. In a short time the rigidity became less ; the ribs could be compressed ; and artificial respiration was kept up imperfectly by compression of the thorax. Circulation was restored in some degree, and the deep purple colour of the surface went off. Spontaneous respiration returned. The man sighed, and became apparently sensible : all spasm had ceased for a minute or two ; but as soon as circulation and consciousness were in some degree restored, the spasm recurred with extreme violence, again locking up the respiratory muscles. Respiration ceased ; the surface again became purple : circulation went on, however, some time after respiration had ceased. Artificial respiration was kept up when the relaxation of the muscles would allow of it, but was this time ineffectual. The heart soon ceased to beat ; the deep purple colour was instantaneously replaced by the pallor of death ; and life was extinct.

The quick passing off of the purple colour of the surface was very remarkable ; the change appeared to commence in the face, and passed downwards like the passing of the shadow of a cloud.

This case gives some colour to the idea that strychnia, like digitalis and some other potent remedies, accumulates in the system.

A melancholy case of poisoning by strychnia occurred in 1848 : A lady swallowed a dose of a mixture containing nine grains of strychnia, which had been dispensed by mistake for salicine. It is supposed she must have swallowed between two and three grains of strychnia. She became suddenly ill, was violently convulsed, and in great agony, and died in less than two hours.[3]

The local action of strychnia is that of an irritant. Applied to the naked dermis, it causes burning and pungent pain, lasting from half an hour to an

[1] Bayle, *Bibl. Thérap.* t. ii. p. 227.

[2] [The dose here mentioned destroyed the life of a healthy young female in an hour and a half (*Lancet*, Aug. 31, 1850, p. 259). Dr. Warner, U.S., died from the effects of *half a grain* of the sulphate of strychnia in fourteen minutes. Several cases of poisoning by strychnia will be found reported in the *Medical Times and Gazette* for December 16, 1854, and April 28, 1855. In one of these a person recovered after taking a dose of four grains.—Ed.]

[3] *Pharmaceutical Journal*, vol. viii. p. 298, 1848.

hour ; and where blisters have been applied, the raw surface inflames under the use of the remedy, and affords a copious suppuration.[1]

USES.—The uses of strychnia are similar to those of nux-vomica above stated. [It has been successfully employed in paralysis of the sphincters.]

In cholera.—M. Abeille has employed this medicine in cholera, and states that it modifies advantageously and rapidly the phenomena of cholera, by its influence upon the " sensitive nerves." In the algide stage it excited re-action 19 times in 23 cases, and there were 10 recoveries. Ice should be taken after each dose, to prevent vomiting : if this take place, the dose may be repeated with safety.[2]

In incontinence of urine.—A man suffered from incontinence of urine for five months, in consequence of paralysis of the neck of the bladder, brought on by being disturbed in micturition. The urine passed from him in drops. After the fruitless administration of strychnine internally, a solution was injected into the bladder (0·50 centig. of strychnine to 500 centig. of water). The patient is stated to have recovered in thirteen days.[3]

Dr. Girard, of the Asylum at Auxerre, has applied minute quantities of sulphate of strychnine locally to the surface of the rectum in involuntary evacuation of the fæces.[4] M. Duchassay has employed this salt in the pro-lapsus ani of children. He removed a small portion of cuticle, applied one-eighteenth of a grain of the sulphate to the surface, and thereby stimulated the sphincter muscle.[5]—ED.]

The *dose* of strychnia or its *salts* (*acetate, sulphate, nitrate,* or *hydro-chlorate*) is, at the commencement, one-sixteenth or one-twentieth of a grain, which is to be very gradually increased until its effects on the muscular system are observed. Strychnia is usually given in the form of *pill* (made with common conserve of roses), or it may be dissolved in *alcohol* or *acetic acid.* The *endermic* dose of strychnia should not, at the commence-ment, exceed half a grain, and of its salts one-fourth of a grain.

[ANTIDOTE.—Chloroform vapour has been successfully employed by Dr. Mannson for the relief of the violent cramps caused by an overdose of strychnia.[6]—ED.]

198. Strychnos Tieute, *Leschinault.*

Tshettik or *Tjettek.*—A large climbing shrub, growing in Java. The aqueous extract of the bark of this tree is the poison called *Upas tieuté Tjettek,* or *Upas Radja,* and which must not be confounded with the poison of the *Antiaris toxicaria.* The Upas tieuté was analysed by Pelletier and Caventou,[7] who found it to consist of *strychnia combined with an acid* (igasuric?), *a reddish-brown colouring matter,* which becomes green when mixed with nitric acid, and a soluble *yellow colouring matter,* which is reddened by nitric acid. They could detect no brucia. The effects of this poison are precisely similar to those of nux vomica and strychnia. Thus, when applied to wounds, injected into the serous sacs or blood-vessels, or applied to the mucous membrane, it produces

[1] Ahrensen, *Brit. and For. Med. Rev.* vol. v. p. 350.
[2] [*L'Union Médicale ;* quoted in *Med. Times and Gazette,* Aug. 26, 1854.]
[3] [*Med. Times and Gazette,* Feb. 5, 1852.]
[4] [*Ibid.* July 19, 1851.]
[5] [*Ibid.* Nov. 18, 1854.]
[6] [*Pharmaceutical Journal,* Jan. 1854, p. 342.]

tetanus, asphyxia, and death. Forty drops of Upas dissolved in water, and injected into the pleura of an old horse, gave rise almost immediately to tetanus and asphyxia, and the animal died after the second attack.

199. Strychnos colubrina, *Linn.*

(Lignum.)

A large tree, a native of Silhet. In countries infested with poisonous serpents, the natives have usually some substance which is fancied to possess the power of preserving them from the bites of these poisonous animals; and thus we have various articles, seeds, roots, and wood, which have the word *snake* affixed to them.

In Asia there are several kinds of *lignum colubrinum*, or *snake-wood*, supposed to be possessed of the above-mentioned property. The specimens, however, met with in commerce, show that there are various substances to which this term is applied; some being the wood of a stem, others of a root. The most esteemed is the wood of the *Strychnos colubrina*. The *S. ligustrina* yields the ancient *lignum colubrinum of Timor*. Pelletier and Caventou[1] analysed one of these woods, and found that it had the same constituents as the bean of St. Ignatius, though in different proportions. Thus it contained more fatty and colouring matter, less strychnia, and, in the place of bassorine and starch, a larger quantity of woody fibre. Its action, therefore, is precisely similar to the before-mentioned poisons.

200. Strychnos Potatorum, *Linn.*

(Semina.)

Clearing Nut.—A large tree; a native of Silhet. The fruit is a shining berry about the size of a cherry, and, when ripe, is black. It contains 1 seed, which is about the size of a cherry-stone. These seeds, when ripe and dried, are sold in the markets of India to clear water. The mode of using them has been already pointed out. Their efficacy depends, as I have elsewhere[2] suggested, on their albumen and casein, which act as fining agents like those employed for wine and beer. If the seeds be sliced and digested in water, they yield a thick, mucilaginous, ropy liquid, which, when boiled, furnishes a coagulum (albumen), and by the subsequent addition of acetic acid, a further coagulum (casein). It is obvious, therefore, that many other seeds might be substituted for those of the Strychnos Potatorum. Almonds, beans, castor seeds, Kola nuts, &c. are used for similar purposes in some countries.

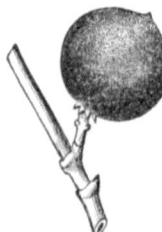

Fig. 189.

Fruit of the Strychnos Potatorum.

201. Strychnos pseudo-quina, *St.-Hilaire.*

(Cortex.)

A small tree, about 12 feet high, growing in the Brazils. The bark, called *Quina do Campo*, is employed in the Brazils as a substitute for cinchona bark. It does not possess poisonous properties. It was analysed by Vauquelin,[3] who discovered neither strychnia

---

[1] *Ann. de Chim. Phys.* x. 170.
[2] *Pharmaceutical Journal*, vol. ix. p. 478.
[3] *Mém. du Muséum*, p. 452, 1823.

nor brucia in it.   Mercadieu[1] also analysed it under the erroneous name of *copalchi*, and could not discover any vegetable alkali in it.   The internal surface of the bark (liber), touched by nitric acid, becomes red ; while the external surface becomes blackish-green.[2] In these characters, then, it agrees with nux-vomica bark.   It is employed in intermittents ; in diseases of the liver, spleen, and mesenteric glands; and in dyspepsia.[3]

202. Strychnos toxifera, *Bentham.*

(Succus.)

Strychnos toxifera, Benth., pl.; Schomburgk, in Hooker's Journ. Bot. iii. 240 ; Hooker, Icones, t. 364 and 365 ; Schomb., Ann. of Nat. Hist. vii. 411, 1841.—A poisonous tree, with a tortuous trunk, growing in British Guiana.   Its juice forms the basis of the *Ourari* or *Wourali* (also called *Urari* and *Woorara*) poison used by the savages of Guiana.   This poison causes paralysis, with convulsive movements, and death from suspended respiration: hence artificial respiration is a most important means of averting its fatal effects.[4]   Attention has been more recently drawn to its effects by Mr. Waterton.[5] It has been proposed to employ it in tetanus and hydrophobia.   Mr. Sewell conjectured that if a horse in tetanus were destroyed by poison which acts by suppressing nervous power, and life were then to be restored by artificial respiration, the nervous system, on reanimation taking place, might possibly be free of the original morbid irritation![6] Dr. Hancock[7] has used the bark of this plant as an application to foul ulcers.

203. Ignatia amara, *Linn.*

Sex. Syst. Pentandria, Monogynia.

(Semina.)

Strychnos Ignatii, Bergius, Mat. Med. 149.—A tree indigenous to the Philippine Islands, whose fruit is smooth and pyriform, and contains about 20 seeds.   These seeds, the *St. Ignatius's beans* of the shops, are about the size of olives, rounded and convex on one side, and somewhat angular on the other.   Externally they are brownish, with a bluish-grey tint.   Within the envelopes of the seed is a very hard, horny, or cartilaginous albumen, in whose cavity is contained the embryo.   These seeds have been analysed by MM. Pelletier and Caventou,[8] who found their constituents to be the same as those of nux-vomica, though in somewhat different proportions.   Their effects, therefore, are similar.

These seeds came into the Dutch shops, according to Alston,[9] about the latter end of the seventeenth century.   But there is some reason to suspect that they were known long before this, and are probably the substances which, in the Latin translation of Serapion, were denominated *nuces vomicæ*   Dale[10] gives, as one of their synonymes, "Igasur, seu Nux-vomica legitima Serapionis."

---

[1] *Journ. de Chim. Méd.* t. i. p. 236 *bis.*
[2] Guibourt, *Journ. de Pharm.* t. xxv. p. 709.
[3] Martius, *Syst. Mat. Med. Veg. Brasil.* p. 41, 1843.
[4] Brodie, *Phil. Trans.* for 1811, p. 178.
[5] *Lancet*, April 12 and 19, 1839 ; also, *Brit. and For. Med. Review*, vol. viii p. 597, 1839.
[6] Mayo's *Outlines of Physiology ;* Waterton, *op. citato.*
[7] *Lond. Med. Gaz.* vol xx. p. 281.
[8] *Ann. de Chim. Phys.* x. 147.
[9] *Lect. on the Mat. Med.* vol. ii. p. 38.
[10] *Pharmacol.* p. 328.

Order XLVII. ASCLEPIADACEÆ, *Lindley.*—ASCLEPIADS.

Asclepiadeæ, *R. Brown.*—Apocinearum pars, *Juss.*

Characters.—*Flowers* symmetrical. *Calyx* 5-partite. *Corolla* monopetalous, 5-lobed, hypogynous, deciduous, regular ; the throat naked, or furnished with glands at the sinus, or with variously formed appendages which are more or less deeply adnate to the tube of the stamens (*gynostegium*). *Stamens* 5, inserted into the base of the corolla, and alternate with its segments ; filaments usually combined so as to form a tube enclosing the pistillum (*stylostegium ; gynostegium*), rarely free ; anthers 2-celled (spuriously 4-celled) ; pollen, when the anther dehisces, cohering in masses (*pollinia*), and sticking to 5 processes of the stigmas by twos or fours, or singly. *Ovaries* 2 ; *styles* 2 ; *stigma* common to both styles, dilated, 5-cornered, with cartilaginous corpuscles at the angles which retain the pollen masses. *Follicles* 2, one of which is often abortive. *Seeds* numerous, usually comose at the micropyle, albuminous. *Shrubs*, or occasionally *herbs*, usually with a milky juice, often twining. *Leaves* entire, opposite (occasionally whorled or alternate), with interpetiolary cilia in place of stipules.

Properties.—The medicinal qualities reside in a bitter acrid juice, which possesses emetic, purgative, diaphoretic, and stimulating properties.

204. Hemidesmus indicus, *R. Brown.*

Sex. Syst. Pentandria, Digynia.

(The root, *D.*)

Periploca indica, Willd. Sp. Plant. ; *Asclepias pseudosarsa*, Roxb. Fl. Ind. ; *Ununtamul*, Hind. and Beng. ; *Nannari* or *Nannarivayr*, Tamul.—A common twining shrub in India. Its root (*radix hemidesmi indici ; rad. nannari*) is used in India under the name of *country sarsaparilla* [*Indian sarsaparilla*]. The attention of practitioners in this country was drawn to it by Dr. Ashburner in 1831 ; and again in 1833.[2] It has been called *Indian* or *scented sarsaparilla*, *nannari*, or the root of *Smilax aspera*. How this last and erroneous appellation became applied to it I cannot tell ; for I find from specimens of the root of Smilax aspera brought from the south of Europe, that no resemblance exists between the latter and the root of Hemidesmus indicus. The latter is brownish externally, and has a peculiar aromatic odour, somewhat like that of sassafras, but which has been compared to that of new hay ; and a feeble, bitter taste. It is long, tortuous, cylindrical, rugous, furrowed longitudinally, and has its cortex divided, by transverse fissures, into moniliform rings. The cortical portion has a corky consistence, and surrounds a ligneous meditullium. Mr. Garden[3] obtained from it a volatile, crystallisable acid (?), on which the taste, smell, and, probably, the medicinal properties, depend. From an erroneous notion of the origin of the root, he called the acid the *smilasperic acid*, but it may with more propriety be termed *hemidesmic acid* or *hemidesmin*. Hemidesmus indicus has been employed as a cheap and efficacious substitute for sarsaparilla in cachectic diseases ; but both its effects and uses require a more extended examination than has yet been devoted to them. Dr. Ashburner says that it increases the appetite, acts as a diuretic, and improves the general health ; "plumpness, clearness, and strength, succeeding to emaciation, muddiness, and debility." It has been used with benefit in venereal diseases. In some cases it has appeared to succeed where the sarsaparilla had failed ; and, *vice versâ*, it has frequently failed where sarsaparilla succeeds. The Tamool doctors employ it in strangury and gravel.[4] It may be administered in the form of *infusion* (prepared by steeping ℥ij. of the root in Oj. of boiling [or lime] water for twelve hours),

---

[1] *Lond. Med. and Phys. Journ.* vol. lxv. p. 1089.
[2] *Lond. Med. Gaz.* vol. xii. p. 350.
[3] *Ibid.* vol. xx. p. 800.
[4] Ainslie, *Mat. Ind.* vol. i. p. 382.

a pint of which may be given in twenty-four hours, in doses of a wine-glassful. The *decoction* may be substituted for the infusion. Carbonate of soda is frequently added to it. The *extract* is objectionable, as the heat used in preparing it must volatilise part, at least, of the hemidesmic acid. The *powder of the bark of the root* is used in India against the thrush.[1]

SYRUPUS HEMIDESMI, D ; *Syrup of Indian Sarsaparilla.* ("Take of Indian Sarsaparilla, bruised, four ounces ; Boiling Distilled Water, one pint ; Refined Sugar, in powder, as much as is sufficient. Infuse the sarsaparilla in the water for four hours in a covered vessel, and strain ; set it by until the sediment subsides, then decant the clear liquor, and, having added to it twice its weight of sugar, dissolve with the aid of a steam or water heat.")—The weights here directed to be used are avoirdupoise.

Mr. Jacob Bell[2] has given the following directions for preparing it :—Take of the Root of Hemidesmus indicus, 1 lb. avoirdupoise ; Refined Sugar, 1 lb. ; Distilled Water, about three pints. Bruise the root, separate the bark by sifting, and reject the wood. Add to the bark an equal bulk of washed sand, moisten them with water, and pack in a displacement apparatus. Macerate for four hours, and displace the liquor by the requisite quantity of water ; reserving the first six ounces. Add more water until it passes through tasteless, and evaporate it to three ounces, in which, with the addition of the first six ounces, dissolve the sugar with as moderate a heat as possible. The result is twenty ounces by measure of a syrup possessing all the aromatic qualities of the plant.

205. Calotropis gigantea, *R. Brown.*

Sex. Syst. Pentandria, Digynia.

(Radix, cortex, et succus.)

Asclepias gigantea, Willd. Sp. Pl. i. ; *Madorius,* Rumph. Amboyn. vii. t. 14, f. 1 ; *Mudar,* Hind.—A large branching shrub, a native of the East Indies ; growing in the West Indies. Stem often as thick as a man's leg or thigh. Yields, when wounded, a large quantity of an acrid milky juice. Dr. O'Shaughnessy[3] found that this milk, when dried in the water-bath, loses 75 per cent. According to the analysis of J. B. Ricord Madianna,[4] 100 parts of this [inspissated ?] juice consist of pure resin 9, fatty oil 4, solid balsam 9, cerine 12, ligneous matter from the bark of the tree 6, mucus 8, caoutchouc 45, loss by evaporation 7 = 100. The root (*radix mudaris giganteæ*), according to Ricord, is reddish, with an odour somewhat like that of horseradish. It is covered with a bark which is three or four lines thick, and which under the epidermis is white. The dried bark, such as I have received it (through the kindness of my colleague Mr. Wordsworth) from St. Kitts, is in hard, curved, or somewhat twisted pieces, which break short and smooth, and externally are whitish or greyish-yellow, and internally white. They are very amylaceous, and when examined by the microscope are seen to abound in round, hemispherical, or muller-shaped starch-grains, whose hilum is very distinct. This bark has a mucilaginous, bitter, somewhat acrid and nauseous taste. Dr. O'Shaughnessy describes it as having a heavy and very peculiar smell ; but my sample scarcely agrees with this statement. Dr. Duncan[5] obtained from the dried root-bark much starch, a white resin, and 11 per cent. of an extractive bitter principle called *mudarine* or *madarin.* This last-mentioned substance, like emetine, excites vomiting, and, according to Dr. Duncan, is the active principle of the root. Its watery solution has the remarkable property of coagulating or gelatinising by heat, and of becoming fluid again by cold. The inspissated juice, root, and bark, have been extensively used in the East for their emetic, sudorific, alterative, and purgative qualities. It has been employed in a great variety of diseases, especially obstinate cutaneous maladies, as lepra and elephantiasis, syphilis, and some spasmodic affections. Mr. Robinson[6] found it decidedly useful in a species of elephantiasis which

[1] Roxburgh, *Fl. Ind.* vol. ii. p. 40.
[2] *Pharmaceutical Journal,* vol. iii. p. 239, 1843.
[3] *Bengal Dispensatory.*
[4] *Journ. de Pharm.* t. xvi. p. 92, 1830.
[5] *Edinb. Med. and Surg. Journ.* July 1, 1829 ; *Lond. Med. Gaz.* July 18, 1829, p. 213.
[6] *Med.-Chir. Trans.* vol. x. p. 27.

Mr. Playfair[1] calls jugura or leprosy of the joints. It has also been used as a substitute for ipecacuanha. In doses of from three to seven grains the dried bark produces nausea and diaphoresis, and in this quantity has been found very efficient in some cutaneous affections. In doses of from fifteen to twenty grains it excites, in from twenty minutes to an hour, full vomiting, with much nausea. and, in some cases, purging. In very small doses it has been reputed tonic, stomachic, and expectorant. An oil of mudar is prepared by digesting 10 grains of the powdered bark in one ounce of olive oil, and pouring off the oleaginous solution from the insoluble portion. The oil may be applied, by means of a camel's hair pencil, to cutaneous ulcers.[2]   Dr. Ainslie[3] considers the dried milky juice the most efficacious preparation.

206. **Solenostemma Argel,** *Hayne.* — **Argel.**

Sex. Syst. Pentandria, Digynia.

(Folia.)

Cynanchum oleæfolium, Nectoux, Voyage dans la Haute Egypte, t. iii. p. 20, 1808; *Cynanchum Argel,* Delile, Flor. Egypt. p. 53, pl. 20, fig. 2, 1826; *Argel,* Arabicè.—A shrub; a native of Upper Egypt, Nubia, Arabia Petræa, and Ouadi Gurra. Stem 2 feet high, erect, branched. *Leaves* lanceolate, with a short petiole, leathery, veinless, whitish, wrinkled, and glaucous on the under surface. *Umbels* many-flowered. *Flowers* small and white. *Follicles* ovoid, tapering superiorly. The leaves form a portion of most samples of Alexandrian senna (see *Senna*). The plant is collected for this purpose, by the Arabs, in the valleys of the desert to the east and south of Assouan (*Delile*).

FIG. 190.

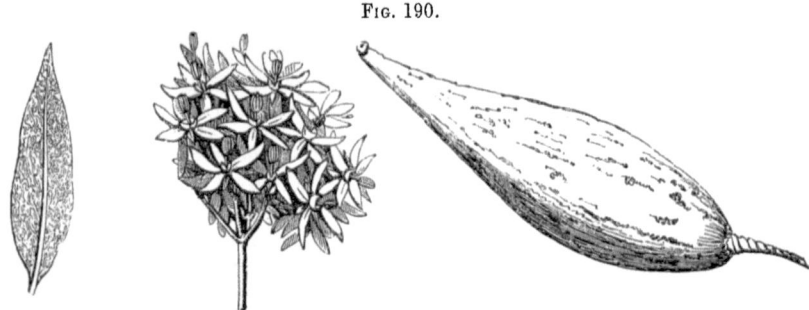

Argel Leaf, Flowers, and Fruit.

According to Dublanc, jun.,[4] the leaves consist of a *volatile oil* (to which the smell of the leaves is ascribable); a bitter, nauseous, *extractiform matter* (in which the purgative qualities of the leaves appear to reside); *chlorophylle;* a *gummy matter* analogous to bassorine; a *glutinous substance;* a *fatty matter; acetate of potash;* and *mineral salts.* According to the observations of Rouillure, Delile, Nectoux, and Puguet (quoted by Delile), the argel leaves are more active than senna leaves. Rouillure says they purge and gripe, and are used by the Arabs of Upper Egypt without the addition of senna. But more recent observations[5] appear to show that, though they occasion sickness and griping, they do not produce purging. Herberger[6] even asserts that they are harmless, because an infusion of two and a half drachms produced no effect or inconvenience. But this probably arose from the active principle of the leaves being insoluble in water.

[1] *Trans. of the Med. and Phys. Society of Calcutta,* vol. i. p. 84.
[2] Buchner's *Repertorium für d. Pharmacie,* 2te Reihe, Bd. v. p. 102, 1836.
[3] *Materia Indica,* vol. i. p. 486; vol. ii. p. 488.
[4] Mérat and De Lens, *Dict. Mat. Méd.* t. vi. p. 316.
[5] Christison, *Dispensatory.*
[6] *Pharmaceutical Journal,* vol. viii. p. 400, 1849.

ORDER XLVIII. OLEACEÆ, *Lindley.*—OLIVEWORTS.

OLEINEÆ, *R. Brown.*

CHARACTERS.—*Flowers* hermaphrodite, rarely diœcious. *Calyx* monophyllous, divided, 4-lobed or 4-toothed, persistent, inferior. *Corolla* hypogynous, monopetalous, 4-cleft, occasionally of 4 petals connected in pairs by the intervention of the filaments, sometimes absent; *æstivation* somewhat valvate. [*Fraxinus* is generally apetalous.] *Stamens* 2, alternate with the segments of the corolla or with the petals; anthers 2-celled, opening longitudinally. *Ovary* simple, without any hypogynous disc, 2-celled; the *cells* 2-seeded; the ovules pendulous and collateral; *style* 1 or 0; *stigma* bifid or undivided. *Fruit* drupaceous, berried, or capsular, often by abortion 1-seeded. *Seeds* with dense, fleshy, abundant albumen; *embryo* about half its length, straight; *cotyledons* foliaceous, partly asunder; *radicle* superior; *plumule* inconspicuous.—*Trees* or *shrubs*. *Branches* usually dichotomous, and ending abruptly by a conspicuous bud. *Leaves* opposite, simple, sometimes pinnated. *Flowers* in terminal or axillary racemes or panicles; the *pedicels* opposite with single bracts (*R. Brown*).

PROPERTIES.—Not very remarkable. The barks of some species are tonic and astringent. Manna is obtained from several species.

[207. Asclepias tuberosa, *Linn.*—Pleurisy Root; Butterfly Weed.

Sex. Syst. Pentandria, Digynia.

The stem of this plant is erect, hairy, with spreading branches; leaves oblong, lanceolate, sessile, alternate, somewhat crowded; umbels numerous, forming terminate corymbs (Beck); flowers orange-yellow. This plant is found in all parts of the United States. The portion used in medicine is the root. It is large, and formed of irregular tubers or fusiform branches; externally of a yellowish-brown colour, internally white. When recent, it has a somewhat acrid, nauseous taste; in the dried state the taste is bitter, but not unpleasant. The powder is dirty white. It yields its properties to boiling water.

The effects of this root upon the system are those of a diaphoretic and expectorant; it does not produce, however, any stimulating action. In larger doses, especially if recent, it acts upon the bowels. With a view to the effects mentioned, it is employed at the commencement of pulmonary affections; and sometimes, by its use in combination with antiphlogistics, an attack may be cut short. In rheumatism it has also proved serviceable. Dr. Chapman[1] speaks of its certainty and permanency of operation. Dr. Eberle employed it in dysentery. The dose of the powder is ℈j. to ʒj. The form of administration best adapted to produce perspiration is decoction, made by boiling ʒj. in a quart of water, and administering ʒij. every two hours.

The A. INCARNATA and A. SYRIACA have a place in the Sec. List of the *U.S. Pharm.* The roots are employed, and produce the same effects on the system as the *tuberosa*, but to a less extent. They are seldom or never used.

Two species of APOCYNUM are used for medicinal purposes in the United States.

Gen. Char.—*Calyx* very small, 5-cleft, persistent. *Corolla* campanulate, half 5-cleft, lobes revolute, furnished at base with 5 dentoid glands, alternating with the stamina. *Anthers* connivent, sagittate, cohering to the stigma by the middle. *Style* obsolete; stigma thick and acute. *Follicle* long and linear. *Seed* comose (*Nuttall*).

1. A. ANDROSÆMIFOLIUM.—Dog's bane, U.S. Secondary List.

Sp. Char.—*Leaves* ovate, smooth on both sides, cymes lateral and terminal, smooth; tube of the corolla longer than the calyx (*Beck*).

This is a common species, found in all parts of the country, from Canada to Georgia, on hill-sides, and in open woods in barren soil. It is perennial, herbaceous, generally 4 feet high, with a smooth stem, and covered with tough fibrous bark. The flowers are white, tinged with rose colour.

---

1 [*Elem. of Therap.* vol. i. p. 351.]

The part used is the root, which is large and lactescent, of a disagreeable bitter taste; of this the active portion is the bark, which forms about two-thirds of it. Its constituents are *bitter extractive, colouring principle, caoutchouc,* and volatile oil.

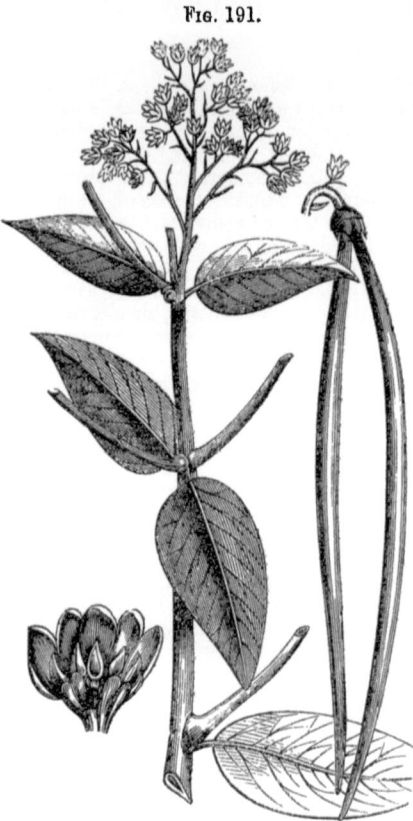

Fig. 191.

Apocynum Cannabinum.

It yields its properties to water and alcohol. Dr. Zollickoffer obtained 198 grs. of alcoholic extract, and 28 grs. of watery extract, from 3240 grains of the cortical part.

The properties of this root are emetic and diaphoretic. In doses of 30 or 40 grs. it promptly induces vomiting, with slight preceding nausea, on which account it may be used in cases where it is merely requisite to evacuate the stomach, as no relaxation is induced. It may be also used, with a view to its diaphoretic action, in doses of 5 or 10 grs. in combination with opium, but is inferior to ipecacuanha.[1] Dr. Zollickoffer states that it is tonic in doses of from 10 to 20 grs., and is "admirably calculated to improve the tone of the digestive apparatus."[2]

APOCYNUM CANNABINUM.—*Indian Hemp,* U.S. *Secondary List.*

Sp. Char. — *Stem* upright, herbaceous. *Leaves* oblong, tomentose beneath, cymes lateral, longer than the leaves.

The Indian hemp is a perennial plant, usually about 2 or 3 feet in height, having a red or brown stem, and oblong-ovate somewhat pubescent leaves. The flowers are small, and of a greenish-white colour externally, and pink internally in paniculate cymes.

This species is also found in most parts of the United States, in waste and neglected places.

The root is the portion used in medicine; it is horizontal, extending to a great distance, of a deep brown colour, becoming darker by age, and when wounded pours forth a thick lactescent juice. When fresh, it is nauseous, somewhat acrid, and permanently bitter, and possesses a disagreeable odour.

When dried it is brittle, and easily reduced to powder, which resembles that of ipecacuanha. It is composed of two portions,—an external cortical portion, which is brown without, and white within; and a ligneous cord, which is of a yellowish-white colour.

Griscom[3] found it to contain tannic acid, gallic acid (?), gum, resin, wax, fecula, bitter principle or *apocynin,* colouring matter, and woody fibre. Knapp also examined it with similar results.

The root of this plant is very potent in its effects on the animal economy. Dr. Griscom[4] states "that its first effect, when taken into the stomach, is that of producing nausea, if given in sufficient quantity, which need not be large; and if this be increased, vomiting will be the result." It also acts upon the bowels, giving rise to copious discharges. These effects are attended with a reduced frequency of the pulse. A general relaxation of the skin, and perspiration, follow these effects. In some of the cases observed by the gentleman mentioned, diuresis took place, but not so marked in some cases as others. "In three or four cases related, the urinary secretion, although somewhat increased in

[1] [Griffith, *Med. Essays,* vol. ii. p. 200.]
[2] [*Journ. of Pharm.* vol. v. p. 254; from *Am. Journ. of Med. Science.*]
[3] [*Journ. of Philad. College of Pharmacy,* vol. v. p. 136; from *Am. Journ. of Med. Science.*]
[4] [*Op. cit.*]

quantity, was not such as to be commensurate with the effect produced upon the disease by the exhibition of the medicine. In other instances its diuretic operation has been more manifest, causing very profuse discharges of urine, and in a short time relieving the overloaded tissues of their burden." The disease in which it has been found most useful, is dropsy.

When the powder is taken into the nostrils, it acts as a sternutatory.

As an emetic, the dose of the powder is from 15 to 30 grains. The best form of exhibition is in decoction, made by boiling an ounce of the root in a pint of water; the dose is ʒij. to ʒiv. two or three times daily. The watery extract will purge in doses of from 3 to 5 grains. In the treatment of cutaneous affections, the juice of the root or plant may be made use of as an application.

The bark affords a fibre which may be used in the place of hemp.[1]]

208. OLEA EUROPÆA, *Linn.*—THE EUROPEAN OLIVE.

Sex. Syst. Diandria, Monogynia.

(Oleum è fructu expressum, *L.*—Expressed oil of the pericarp, *E.*—The oil obtained from the pericarp, *D.*)

HISTORY. — Few vegetables have been so repeatedly noticed and enthusiastically described by the ancient writers, as the olive-tree. In all ages it seems to have been adopted as the emblem of benignity and peace. It is frequently mentioned in the Bible;[2] the ancient Greeks[3] were well acquainted with it; and several products of it were employed in medicine by Hippocrates.[4] Pliny[5] is most diffuse in his account of it.

Pliny[6] tells us, on the authority of Fenestella, that there were no olive-trees in Italy, Spain, and Africa, in the reign of Tarquinius Priscus, in the 173rd year from the foundation of the city of Rome; that is, 580 years before Christ. The Phœnicians are said to have introduced the olive-tree into France 680 years before Christ. Near Terni, in the vale of the cascade of Marmora, is a plantation of very old trees, and supposed to be the same plants mentioned by Pliny as growing there in the first century.[7]

BOTANY. **Gen. Char.**—*Calyx* short, campanulate, 4-toothed, rarely truncated. *Corolla* with a short tube, and a 4-partite plane spreading limb; rarely absent. *Stamens* 2, inserted in the lower part of the tube of the corolla, opposite, exserted; in the apetalous species, hypogynous. *Ovary* 2-celled. *Ovules* 2 in each cell, pendulous from the apex of the septum. *Style* short, with a bifid stigma at the apex, or subcapitate. *Drupe* berried, with oily flesh and an osseous kernel; by abortion 2- and often 1-seeded. *Seeds* inverted; albumen fleshy; embryo inverted, straight, with foliaceous cotyledons (*De Cand.*)

Sp. Char.—Leaves oblong or lanceolate, quite entire, mucronate, above smooth, beneath leprous-hoary. Racemes axillary; while flowering, somewhat erect; when in fruit, nodding. Fruit ellipsoidal (*De Candolle*).

A long-lived *tree* of slow growth. *Wood* hard; used for cabinet work. *Leaves* in pairs, shortly petioled, green above, hoary beneath. *Flowers*

---

[1] [From the American edition, by Dr. Carson.—ED.]
[2] As in *Gen.* viii. 11.
[3] Homer, *Od.* v. 477.
[4] Dierbach, *Arzneim. d. Hippokr.* p. 77.
[5] *Hist. Nat.* lib. xv. cap. 1–8 ; and lib. xxiii. cap. 34–7, ed. Valp.
[6] *Ibid.* lib. xv. cap. 1.
[7] Loudon, *Encycl. Gardening.*

small and white. *Drupe* dark bluish-green; kernel hard, with usually only one ovule. The whitish character of the foliage gives a dull and monotonous appearance to countries where the olive is extensively cultivated, as Provence and Languedoc.[1]

Fig. 192.   Fig. 193.

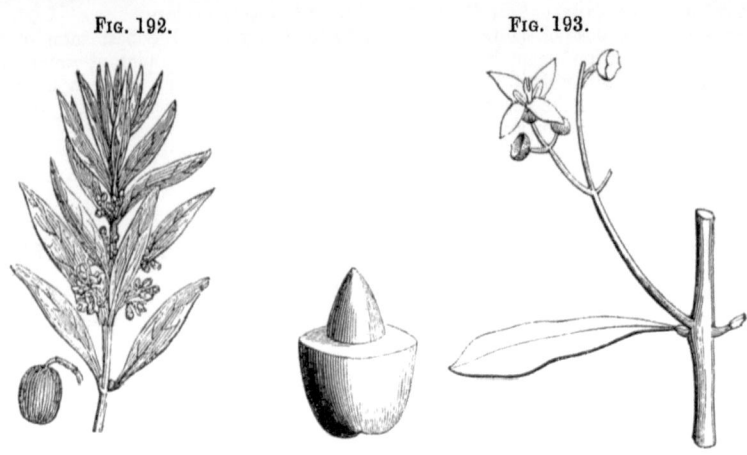

Fig. 192. *Olea europæa.*
Fig. 193. *a,* Fruit, showing the stone.

Hab.—Grows spontaneously in the East (Asia), from whence it has migrated into the South of Europe, the Mediterranean Islands, and the North of Africa, where it is extensively cultivated, and, by the dissemination of the seeds, now grows apparently wild.

Var. *α Oleaster; The Wild Olive.*—Branches more or less indurated-spinescent, and more or less quadrangular. Leaves oblong or oval. Fruit smaller.—Grows wild in the whole of the olive region, especially in rocky places.

Var. *β sativa; The Cultivated Olive.*—Branches unarmed, roundish. Leaves lanceo-late. Racemes few-fruited.—Cultivated in the whole of the olive region. There are numerous sub-varieties, with the fruit ovate, ellipsoidal, or almost spherical, obtuse at the apex, submucronate or subincurved at the apex, violet, blackish, reddish, or even white, with an austere taste, or rarely insipid, &c. &c. The sub-variety *longifolia* is cultivated in the South of France, and is said to yield the best oil. The young fruit is also most esteemed when pickled. The sub-variety *latifolia* is chiefly cultivated in Spain. Its fruit is almost twice the size of the Provence olive, or sub-variety *longifolia,* but of a strong rank flavour; and the oil is too strong for most palates.[2]

Description.—The products of the olive-tree deserving of notice are the *resiniform exudation,* the *leaves,* and the *fruit.*

1. **Resiniform exudation of the olive-tree** (*resina oleæ*).—The older writers speak of the exudation from olive-trees, described by Dioscorides[3] as the *tears of the Æthiopic olive* (*lachrymæ oleæ æthiopicæ*). In modern times it has been improperly termed *olive gum* (*gummi oleæ*) or *Lecca gum.* Pelletier[4] has analysed it, and found that it consists of *a peculiar matter* (*olivile*), *brown resin* soluble in ether, and *benzoic acid.* It was formerly employed in medicine.

[1] Sharp, *Letters from Italy,* Lond. 1768.
[2] Don's *Gardener's Dictionary,* vol. iv. 47.
[3] Lib. i. cap. 141.
[4] *Ann. de Chim. Phys.* iii. 105; li. 196.

Olivile is white, inodorous, bitter, crystallisable, very soluble in boiling alcohol and in the alkalies, but very slightly so in water and ether. The crystals consist of $C^{28}H^{18}O^{10},2HO$. By heat they lose $2HO$.

2. **Olive leaves** (*folia oleæ*).—The leaves of the olive-tree have been analysed by Pallas,[1] who found in them a bitter acid principle, a black resin, a peculiar crystalline febrifuge substance, gum, chlorophylle, tannin, gallic acid, and mineral salts. They have been employed externally as astringents and antiseptics; internally, as tonics in intermittents.[2]

[From a communication made to the *Pharmaceutical Journal*[3] by Mr. D. Hanbury, it would appear that a *decoction* of these leaves, made by boiling two handfuls in a quart of water until reduced to half a pint, has been very successfully used in the Levant in the treatment of obstinate cases of fever. Mr. Maltass, of Smyrna, states that he has found this remedy more effectual than quinine. It appears that during the Peninsular War, 1808-13, olive-leaves were used by French practitioners as a substitute for cinchona bark; and Dr. Pallas, whose analysis is above quoted by the author, observed marked beneficial effects from the use of an alcoholic extract of the bark. The crystalline febrifuge substance discovered by Pallas, and designated by him *Vauqueline*, was found to be a constituent of the *young* bark as well as of the leaves. It was associated with a bitter principle, to which the febrifuge properties are strictly due. The young bark contained more of these matters than the leaves or the old bark.

Vauqueline is a colourless, inodorous solid, crystallising either in micaceous plates, or in stellate prismatic crystals, which have a slightly sweet taste. It is readily soluble in water at all temperatures, and has a faint alkaline reaction. Boiling alcohol dissolves it, but it is precipitated as the solution cools. Young olive-bark, according to Pallas, yields nearly two per cent. of Vauqueline.

The tincture and alcoholic extract appear to be the most useful preparations. The tincture is made by digesting one part of the young bark in eight parts of rectified spirit, sp. gr. 0·867. It may be administered as Tinctura Cinchonæ. The dose of the extract is half a drachm diffused through a small quantity of water.

In the treatment of the numerous cases of fever now presenting themselves in the military hospitals in the East, it would be desirable that practitioners should give a fair trial to so easily accessible a substitute for the costly quinine.—Ed.]

3. **Fruit of the olive-trees;** *Olives* (*fructus oleæ*; *olivæ*).—The *preserved* or *pickled olives* (*olivæ conditæ*), so admired as a dessert, are the green unripe fruit deprived of part of their bitterness by soaking them in water, and then preserved in an aromatised solution of salt. Several varieties are met with in commerce, but the most common are the *small French* or *Provence olive*, and the *large Spanish olive*. Olives *à la picholine* have been soaked in a solution of lime and wood-ashes.[4] *Ripe olives* are remarkable from the circumstance of their sarcocarp abounding in a bland fixed oil.

---

[1] *Journ. de Pharm.* xiii. 604.
[2] Richard, *Elém. d'Hist. Nat.* t. ii. p. 21.
[3] [February 1854, p. 353.]
[4] Duhamel, *Traité des Arbres*, t. ii. p. 57.

EXPRESSION OF OLIVE OIL.—The process of procuring olive oil is somewhat modified in different countries, though the principle is the same in all.

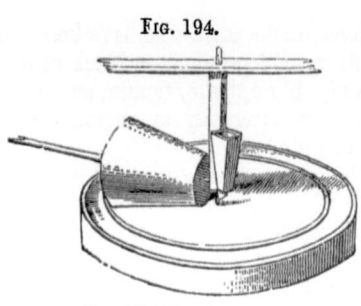

FIG. 194.

Spanish Olive Oil-mill.

In Spain the olives are pressed by conical iron rollers elevated above the stage or floor, round which they move on two little margins to prevent the kernel being injured, the oil from which is said to have an unpleasant flavour. Spanish olive oil, however, is inferior to other kinds, from the circumstance of the time which elapses between the gathering and the grinding of the olives. This arises from the number of mills not being in proportion to the quantity of fruit to be ground ; so that the olives are placed in heaps to wait their turn, and in consequence often undergo decomposition.[1]

In France the finest oil is procured by bruising the fruit in the mill immediately it is gathered, and then submitting the paste to pressure. The first product has a greenish tint, and is termed *virgin oil* (*oleum olivarum virgineum ; huile vierge*). The cake or *marc* is removed from the press, broken up with the hand, moistened with boiling water, and re-pressed. The products are water and oil of a *second quality :* these separate by standing. The cake which is left is termed *grignon,* and is employed by some as fuel ; others, however, ferment it, and, by the aid of boiling water, obtain a very inferior oil, called *gorgon,* which is employed either for soap-making or burning in lamps.[2] With the view of increasing the quantity of oil, some persons allow the olives to undergo incipient fermentation, which breaks down the parenchyma of the fruit before they are pressed ; but the quality of the oil is thereby injured. Guibourt[3] tells us that it is a yellow, but a mild and agreeable oil, and is much used for the table.

The machinery employed by the Neapolitan peasants in the preparation of the Gallipoli oil, is of the rudest kind. The olives are allowed to drop in their maturity from the tree on the ground, when they are picked up chiefly by women and children, and carried to the mill. The oil, when expressed, is sent, in sheep- or goat-skins, carried on mules, to Gallipoli, where it is allowed to clarify in cisterns cut in the rock on which the town is built. From these it is conveyed, in uteri or skins, to basins near the sea-shore ; and from these basins the oil-casks are filled.[4]

According to Sieuve,[5] 100 lbs. of olives yield about 32 lbs. of oil ; 21 of which come from the pericarp, 4 from the seed, and 7 from the woody matter of the nut (*pyrena*). That obtained from the pericarp is of the finest quality. Recently-drawn olive oil deposits, by standing, a white fibrous matter, which the ancients employed in medicine under the name of *amurca.*[6]

[1] Dillon, *Travels through Spain,* p. 343, 1782 ; Jacob, *Travels in Spain,* p. 149, 1811.
[2] Duhamel, *Traité des Arbres Fruit.* t. ii. pp. 71–2.
[3] *Hist. des Drog.* t. ii. p. 339.
[4] M'Culloch's *Dict. of Commerce.*
[5] De Candolle, *Phys. Vég.* p. 299.
[6] Pliny, *Hist. Nat.* lib. xv. cap. 3, ed. Valp.

[COMMERCE.—The quantity of this oil imported annually during a period of seven years, was as follows :—

Gallons imported.		Gallons imported.	
1844	3,770,424	1848	2,541,672
1845	3,103,380	1849	4,274,928
1846	2,150,568	1850	5,237,316
1847	2,190,384		ED.]

PROPERTIES OF OLIVE OIL.—Olive oil (*oleum olivæ* seu *olivarum ;* sweet *oil*) is an unctuous fluid, of a pale yellow or greenish-yellow colour. When of good quality, it has scarcely any smell. Its taste is bland and mild. Its sp. gr. is probably not uniform; and hence the discrepancies in the experimental results of different chemists. Saussure makes it 0·9192 at 53°·6 F., and 0·9109 at 77° F.; Heidenrich says it is 0·9176 at 59° F. In cold weather it deposits white fatty globules (a combination of elaine and margarine). At about the freezing point of water it congeals. It is soluble in about 1½ times its weight of ether; but is only very slightly soluble in alcohol. By admixture with castor oil, its solubility in rectified spirit is augmented. Pure olive oil has less tendency to become rancid by exposure to the air, than most other fixed oils; but the second qualities readily acquire rancidity. This seems to depend on the presence of some foreign matter. Olive oil is not a drying oil, and, being less apt than many oils to increase in consistence by exposure to air, is preferred for greasing delicate machinery, and especially watch- and clock-work. To prepare it for the latter application, the oil is cooled, and the more liquid portion poured off from the fatty deposit. A piece of sheet lead, or some shot, are then immersed in it, and it is exposed in a corked phial to the action of sunshine. A white matter gradually separates, after which the oil becomes clear and colourless, and is fit for use (*Brande*).

VARIETIES.—*Provence oil* (*oleum provinciale*), the produce of Aix, is the most esteemed. *Florence oil* is a very fine kind of olive oil, imported from Leghorn in flasks surrounded by a kind of net-work formed by the leaves of a monocotyledonous plant, and packed in half-chests; it is used at the table, under the name of *salad oil*. *Lucca oil* is imported in jars holding nineteen gallons each. *Genoa oil* is another fine kind. *Gallipoli oil* forms the largest portion of the olive oil brought to England; it is imported in casks. Apulia and Calabria are the provinces of Naples most celebrated for its production : the Apulian is the best. *Sicily oil* is of inferior quality; it is principally produced at Milazzo. *Spanish oil* is the worst. The foot deposited by olive oil is used for oiling machinery, under the name of *droppings of sweet oil*.

ADULTERATION.—Olive oil is liable to adulteration with some of the cheaper fixed oils; as with poppy oil, lard oil,[1] &c. Various tests have been proposed for the detection of the fraud, but none of them are very accurate, or to be absolutely relied on,—partly, perhaps, because olive oil itself is not uniform in its qualities.

The following are some of the proposed tests :—1st. Expose a few drops of the oil, in a porcelain vessel, to the heat of a lamp for a few seconds, and examine the odour of the vapour: the presence of foreign oils may be detected by their peculiar smell.[2]

---

[1] *Pharmaceutical Journal*, vol. x. p. 132, 1850.
[2] Heidenreich, *Chemical Gazette*, vol. i. p. 382, 1843.

2ndly. The sp. gr. of the oil may be determined by Gobley's *elaïometer*, whose zero is the point at which the instrument floats in poppy oil, and its 50° the point at which it floats in olive oil.[1] 3rdly. If we shake pure olive oil in a phial half filled with it, the surface of the oil soon becomes smooth by repose; whereas, when poppy oil is present, a number of air-bubbles (or *beads*, as they are termed) remain. 4thly. Olive oil is completely solidified when cooled by ice; poppy oil, however, remains in part liquid. Even two parts of olive oil to one of poppy oil will not completely congeal.[2] 5thly. Olive oil, according to Rousseau,[3] conducts electricity 675 times worse than other vegetable oils. The addition of two drops of poppy or beech-nut oil to 154½ grains of olive oil is sufficient to quadruple the conducting power of the latter. To ascertain the conducting power of oil, Rousseau used the *electrical diagometer* (from διάγω, to conduct; and μετρέω, to measure). It consists of one of Zamboni's dry piles, and a feebly magnetised needle moving freely on a pivot. The electricity developed by the pile produces a deviation in the direction of the needle; but when any substance is interposed between the needle and the pile, the deviation is less in proportion to the bad conducting power of the interposed substance. 6thly. If recently-made nitrate of mercury (prepared by dissolving 6 parts of mercury in 7·5 parts of nitric acid, sp. gr. 1·36) be mixed with twelve times its weight of pure olive oil, and the mixture strongly agitated, the whole mass becomes solid in the course of a few hours; this, however, does not occur with adulterated oil. We judge of the presence and quantity of foreign oils by the degree and quickness of solidification of the suspected olive oil.[4]

"When carefully mixed with a twelfth of its volume of solution of nitrate of mercury, prepared as for the Unguentum Citrinum, it becomes in three or four hours like a firm fat, without any separation of liquid oil."—*Ph. Ed.*

[The specific gravity of the oil will sometimes enable us to detect the adulteration. Mr. Mercer, of Liverpool,[5] has drawn up a table showing the differences in the specific gravity of olive and other oils used in pharmacy and the arts. It appears that sperm oil, if genuine, is the lightest, and castor oil the heaviest met with in commerce.

Sperm oil	·8750	Southern whale oil	·9225
Composite oil	·9152	Poppy oil	·9254
Colza oil	·9156	Cod-liver oil	·9285
Olive oil (flask)	·9158	Linseed oil	·9362
Ditto (jar)	·9171	Ditto (boiled)	·9506
Ditto (fine cask)	·9174	Castor oil	·9674
Almond oil	·9214		Ed.]

COMPOSITION.—In 1808, Gay-Lussac and Thénard[6] examined the ultimate composition of this oil. In 1815, Braconnot[7] ascertained the proximate constituents of it; and subsequently Saussure[8] examined the ultimate composition of these constituents.

PROXIMATE ANALYSIS.		ULTIMATE ANALYSES.			
Braconnot's.		*Gay-Lussac and Thénard's.*		*Saussure's.*	
Elaine (oleine)	72	Carbon	77·213	...... 76·034	.... 82·170
Margarine	28	Hydrogen	13·360	...... 11·545	.... 11·232
		Oxygen	9·427	...... 12·068	.... 6·302
		Nitrogen	0·000	...... 0·353	.... 0·296
Olive oil	100	Olive oil	100·000	Elaine 100·000	Margarine 100·000

---

[1] *Journal de Pharm. et de Chim.* 3me sér. t. iv. p. 285, 1843; *Pharmaceutical Journal*, vol. iv. p. 403, 1845.

[2] Guibourt, *Hist. des Drog.* t. ii. p. 603.

[3] *Journ. de Pharm.* t. ix. p. 587.

[4] [The reader will find some remarks on the application of this and other tests for detecting adulteration, in the *Pharmaceutical Journal* for April 1853, pp. 485 and 497; also for March 1854, p. 429.—Ed.]

[5] [*Pharmaceutical Journal*, Feb. 1854, p. 353.]

[6] *Rech. Phys. Chim.* ii. 320.

[7] *Ann. de Chim.* xciii. 240.

[8] *Ann. de Chim. et Phys.* t. xiii. p. 349.

1. ELAINE or OLEINE.—Braconnot obtained it by exposing olive oil to a temperature of about 21° F., in order to cause the congelation of the margarine. The elaine was a greenish-yellow liquid : at 14° F. it deposited a little margarine.

2. MARGARINE.—The solid matter of olive and other vegetable oils, obtained as above, is usually denominated *stearine*, but Lecanu[1] has pointed out several characters by which it is distinguished from that principle : thus it is more fusible, and is much more soluble in cold ether. In most other respects it agrees with stearine.

PHYSIOLOGICAL EFFECTS.   α. *On Vegetables.*—Olive oil, as well as other fixed oils, acts injuriously on the roots of plants, by obstructing their pores and meatus, and preventing the passage of water.[2]

β. *On Animals.*—Injected into the veins, the fixed oils prove injurious by their mechanical operation. They obstruct the circulation in the capillary vessels, and in this way cause death. Both Courten and Hertwich[3] have destroyed dogs by injecting half an ounce of olive oil into the veins.

γ. *On Man.*—The fixed oils are extremely nutritious, but they are difficult of digestion, and hence are apt to disagree with dyspeptics. Some writers (as Dr. Dunglison[4]) are of opinion, that, taken as a condiment with salad, oil promotes the digestibility of the latter ; but this notion is probably unfounded, for salad is not usually obnoxious to the digestive organs, whereas oil frequently is so. Swallowed in large doses, olive oil acts as a laxative, in general, without occasioning pain.

USES.—In England the *dietetical* uses of olive oil are very limited, being principally confined to its mixture with salads. In Spain and some other countries it is frequently employed as a substitute for butter. Dyspeptics should carefully avoid its use.

Medicinally it is not often administered by the mouth. As a *mild laxative* it may be used in irritation, inflammation, or spasm of the alimentary canal, or of the urino-genital organs. As an *emollient* and *demulcent*, it is used to involve acrid and corrosive substances, and sheathe the stomach from their action ; and taken in the form of emulsion (made with gum, albumen, or alkali) it is used to allay troublesome and spasmodic cough in pulmonary and bronchial irritation, &c. ; but in such cases almond oil is generally preferred.

As an *antidote*, it has been used in mineral, animal, and vegetable poisoning; but its operation appears to be entirely mechanical (see *Mechanical Antidotes*, Vol. i.) It envelopes the poison, sheathes the living surface, and mechanically obstructs absorption. At one time it was supposed to possess antidotal properties for arsenical poisons ; and Dr. Paris[5] tells us that the antidote on which the men employed in the copper-smelting works and tin burning-houses in Cornwall rely with confidence, " whenever they are infested with more than an ordinary portion of arsenical vapour, is sweet oil; and an annual sum is allowed by the proprietors, in order that it may be constantly supplied." Oil was formerly recommended as an antidote for cantharides; but the discovery of the solubility of cantharidin in oil has led to the suspicion that instead of alleviating it might increase the patient's danger. There is no just ground for supposing that oil, applied externally or taken internally, has

---

[1] *Ibid.* lv. 204.
[2] De Candolle, *Phys. Vég.* p. 1347.
[3] Wibmer, *Wirk. d. Arzneim. u. Gifte*, Bd. iv. S. 9.
[4] *Elem. of Hygiène*, p. 289.
[5] *Pharmacol.* 6th edit. vol. i. p. 97.

any particular influence in counteracting the operation or relieving the effects of the poison of venomous serpents, notwithstanding the high encomiums that have been passed on it. As an *anthelmintic,* olive oil is occasionally used. Olive oil is a frequent constituent of *laxative enemata,* especially in dysentery, or irritation of the bowels or of the neighbouring viscera.

Externally it is used in the form of *liniment* (as the *linimentum ammoniæ* and *linimentum ammoniæ sesquicarbonatis*). Smeared over the body, it has been recommended by Berchtold and others[1] as a safeguard against the plague. It can be beneficial only by mechanically impeding absorption. It may be employed also to relax the skin and sheathe irritable surfaces. Frictions of olive oil have been employed in ascites and anasarca.

In *pharmacy,* olive oil has been employed in the preparation of *liniments, ointments, cerates,* and *plasters.* It serves for making both a hard and a soft soap used in medicine, and is one source of *glycerine.* In *surgery,* it is used for besmearing surgical instruments, as bougies.

ADMINISTRATION.—The dose of olive oil as a laxative is from f℥j. to f℥ij.

209. FRAXINUS ORNUS, *Linn.*; et F. ROTUNDIFOLIA, *Lam.*

Sex. Syst. Diandria, Monogynia.

(Succus ex inciso cortice aëre induratus, *L.*—An exudation from this and other species constitutes the manna of commerce, *D.* — Sweet concrete exudation, probably from several species of Fraxinus and Ornus, *E.*)

HISTORY.—Although these two species of manna ash must have been known to the ancients, yet no notice is taken of the manna which they yield. It is difficult, however, to believe that they were unacquainted with it. The earliest writer who distinctly mentions it is Johannes Actuarius.[2]

It has been presumed that under the names of *honey-dew* (δροσόμελι, *mel roscidum*), *honey-air* or *aërial honey* (ἀερόμελι, *mel aërium*), and *honey-oil* (ἐλαιόμελι, *elæomeli*), the ancients included our manna.

The nature of the substance which, in our translation of the Old Testament,[3] is called manna (*man:* literally, *what is it ?*), is quite unknown. By some it has been thought to be the manna of the Tamarisk (*Tamarix mannifera*); by others, the manna of the Camel's Thorn (*Alhagi maurorum*). But neither these nor any other known sorts of manna explain the manna of Scripture, " by which abundance is stated to have been produced for millions, where hundreds cannot now be subsisted."[4]

BOTANY. **Gen. Char.**—*Flowers* polygamous or diœcious. *Calyx* 4-cleft or none. *Petals* either none or 4, usually in pairs, cohering at the base, oblong or linear. *Stamens* 2. *Stigma* bifid. *Fruit* (samara) 2-celled, compressed, winged at the apex, with 2 ovules in each cell, or by abortion 1-seeded. *Seeds* pendulous, compressed; albumen fleshy, thin; embryo longitudinal; cotyledons elliptical; radicle linear, superior (*De Cand.*)

Species. 1. FR. ORNUS, Linn.; *Ornus europæa,* Persoon; Μελία, Dioscorides, lib. i. cap. 108; *European Flowering* or *Manna Ash.*—Leaf-

---

[1] *Hufeland's Journal,* Bd. vi. S. 437; and Bd. xii. St. iii. S. 153.
[2] Friend, *Hist. of Physick,* i. 271.
[3] *Exod.* xvi. 14, 15, 31, and 33 ; *Numb.* xi. 7.
[4] Kitto's *Cyclop. of Bibl. Literature,* vol. ii. p. 293.

lets 3-4 pairs, subpetiolate, lanceolate, attenuated at both extremities, serrated at the apex, entire at the base, bearded beneath near the nerve. Buds velvety. Panicles crowded, shorter than the leaf. Fruits narrow, linear-lanceolate, obtuse, attenuated at both extremities (*De Cand.*)

A small *tree* (20-25 feet high). *Leaves* opposite, large, pinnate. *Leaflets* large. *Panicles* large and many-flowered. *Flowers* small and polygamous. *Corolla* yellowish or greenish-white. *Fruit* flat, wedge-shaped, smooth, winged.

South of Europe, in mountainous situations; especially Calabria and Sicily. De Candolle says that it rarely produces manna in Calabria.

2. F. ROTUNDIFOLIA, Lamarck; *Ornus rotundifolia,* Persoon; Μελία ὑψηλὴ καὶ εὐμήκης, Theophrastus, Hist. Pl. lib. iii. cap. 11; *Round-leaved, Flowering,* or *Manna Ash.*—Leaflets 2-4 pairs, smooth, ovate or roundish, obtusely serrate, subsessile, minutely reticulate. Petioles channelled. Buds brown externally, somewhat velvety (*De Cand.*)—A small tree (16 to 20 feet high). By some botanists considered to be a variety of the preceding species. Grows in Calabria and the East. De Candolle says that from this tree manna is chiefly obtained.

FIG. 195.

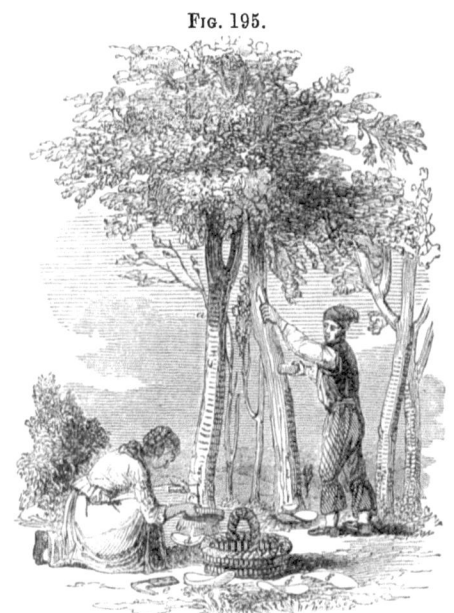

EXTRACTION OF MANNA. — Manna is obtained, both in Calabria[1] and Sicily, by incision into the stem of the trees. The mode of obtaining Sicilian manna has been described by Houel,[2] and more recently by Stettner,[3] who made his observations during the summer of 1847. In the manna districts of Capace, Cinesi, and Fabaretto, in Sicily, where the best manna is obtained, the *Fraxinus Ornus* is cultivated in separate square plantations. The trees are not tapped till they cease to produce more leaves, which happens about July or August. Cross or transverse incisions, about two inches long, are made in the stem by means of a hooked or curved knife, beginning at the lower part, near the soil, and are repeated daily in warm weather, extending them perpendicularly upwards, so as to leave the stems uninjured on one side, which is cut next year. In the lowermost sections, small leaves of the ash are inserted to conduct the juice into a receptacle formed by a leaf of Opuntia.

Extraction of Manna.

a. Stem of the tree. | c. Incision.
b. Leaf of the Ornus. | d. Leaf of the Indian fig.
e. Hooked knife.

In the right hand of each of the collectors is a box to contain the manna, which is afterwards transferred to a basket.

---

[1] Cirillo, *Phil. Trans.* vol. lx. p. 233.
[2] *Voy. Pittoresq. de Sicile,* &c. t. i. 52-3, 1782
[3] Hooker's *Journ. of Botany,* vol. i. p. 124, 1849; and *Pharm. Journal,* vol. ix. p. 283, 1849.

In this way is obtained *manna in sorts* (called *Capace* or *Gerace manna*). The *flake manna* is obtained during the height of the season, when the juice flows vigorously (*Houel*). It is procured from the upper incisions, the juice there being less fatty than that in the lower part; and, consequently, it more easily dries in tubes and flat pieces (*Stettner*). The masses left adhering to the stems after the removal of the inserted leaves are scraped off, and constitute the *cannulated manna in fragments*. Although all three kinds of manna are got from the same stem, yet the younger stems yield more of the cannulated sort, and the older ones more of the fatty kind. Dry and warm weather are necessary for a good harvest.

DESCRIPTION.—Several kinds of manna (*manna*) are described by pharmacologists.

1. The finest kind is called *flake manna*[1] (*manna cannulata* vel *m. canellata*). It is imported in deal boxes, having partitions, and frequently lined with tin-plate. It consists of pieces of from one to six inches long, one or two inches wide, and from half an inch to an inch thick. Their form is irregular, but more or less stalactitic; most of the pieces being flattened or slightly hollowed out on one side (where they adhered to the tree or substance on which they concreted), and on this side they are frequently soiled. Their colour is white, or yellowish-white; they are light, porous, and friable; the fractured surface presents a number of very small capillary crystals. The odour is somewhat like that of honey, and is to me rather unpleasant; the taste is sweet, but afterwards rather acrid.

2. Under the name of *Sicilian Tolfa manna* [?] I have received an inferior kind, corresponding to the *manna in sorts* (*manna in sortis*) of some pharmacologists. From its name I presume it is brought from Sicily, and that it corresponds in quality to Tolfa manna [?] produced near Civita-Vecchia, and which Fée[2] states is but little valued. The Sicilian Tolfa manna occurs in small pieces, which seldom exceed an inch in length : some of these present the same appearances, with respect to consistence, colour, friability, and crystalline appearance, as the flake manna; others, however, are soft, viscid, brownish, and uncrystallised, like those of the next variety.

3. The commonest kind of English commerce is called *Sicilian manna* (*manna Siciliana*). It appears to me to be the *common* or *fatty manna* (*manna pinguis*) of some writers. It consists of small, soft, viscid fragments, of a dirty yellowish-brown colour, intermixed with some few dark-coloured small pieces of the flake variety. It contains many impurities intermixed.

[Manna in sorts may be divided into various qualities, viz. :—

a. Gerace is the best of this description, because, though not always the whitest or cleanest, it is neither fat nor damp, but dry, and approaches nearest to *canellata* in fragments.[3]

b. Next to this is the quality known in commerce by the name *Capace*, which comprises not only that of the district of Capace, but also that of Cinesi and Fabaretto in Sicily. It is often collected with more care than the Gerace,

---

[1] [This variety of manna is universally preferred, and fetches everywhere a much higher price than the other sorts. The fragments are worth from one-half to two-thirds the value of the flakes, the new and white being preferred to the old and yellow.—ED.]

[2] *Cours d'Hist. Nat.* ii. 366.

[3] [Mr. Stettner says the Gerace grows in the district of Gerace, to the east of Palermo.—ED.]

and is cleaner in appearance, but it is fatty and sticky, and hard, and is less liked.

c. The *Calabrian* stands between the above two qualities, but is now seldom seen in commerce.

d. An inferior kind, known by the name of *"Manna communis,"* is obtained in the Neapolitan province Capitanata, on the declivities of Mount St. Angelo. It is not fatty, but very damp, and is chiefly consumed in Italy, or sent to the Levant. Its yearly production often exceeds 2000 cwt.[1]—ED.]

A sort of manna, called *manna foliata* or *manna de fronde*, is produced on the leaves of the manna ash by the punctures of a small hemipterous insect[2] (*Cicada Orni*, Linn. ; *Tettigonia Orni*, Fabric.) The term *manna* is also applied to several other saccharine substances obtained from plants, but which are entirely different from the manna of the shops. The following are some of them :—1st, *Manna of Briançon* (*manna brigantina*), or *manna of the larch* (*manna laricis*); 2dly, *Persian manna* (*manna persica*), or *manna of the Camel's thorn* (*manna alhagi*) [see *infrà*]; 3dly, *Tamarisk manna* (*manna tamariscina*), supposed by some to be the manna alluded to by Moses, and hence termed *manna mosaica* vel *m. Judæorum* [see *infrà*]; and 4thly, *Oak manna* (*manna quercea*).

[Dr. Landerer enumerates eight varieties of saccharine exudations known under the name of manna, and not produced by the ash. Some of these are mentioned by the author. They are—1. *Manna Laricina*, from the leaves of *Larix Europæa*; 2. *Manna Cedrina*, from the branches of *Pinus Cedrus*. This variety is brought from Mount Lebanon, and has great repute in Syria. 3. *M. Celastrina*; 4. *M. Quercina*; 5. *M. Australis*, produced by Eucalyptus resinifera; 6. *M. Cistina* sive *Labdanifera*, a rare variety met with in Greece. This is derived from several species of *Cistus*, and is called Cistus manna. 7. *M. Alhagnia*, the exudation of *Hedysarum Alhagi*, a plant indigenous to Arabia, and growing also in the maritime districts of Greece. This manna is supposed to exude from the Hedysarum, which covers extensive plains in Arabia and Palestine, as a result of the wounds produced on the plants by the browsing of sheep and goats. It is used as nutriment by the Arabs, as well as by those who form the caravans which cross the Desert. According to Landerer, it is this variety, and not the product of the ash, which corresponds to the *mel ex aëre* of Pliny, and the *humor melleus* of Theophrastus. 8. *M. Tamariscina*, called also *Manna Israelitarum*, and believed by Landerer to be the manna mentioned in the Old Testament. He informs us that this exudation is produced through the puncture of *Coccus manniferus*, an insect inhabiting the trees of the *Tamarix mannifera*, which grow abundantly in the neighbourhood of Mount Sinai. The manna exudes as a thick transparent syrup, covering the smaller branches from which it flows. It is collected by the monks of the district during the month of August. The collection takes place very early in the morning, at which time, owing to the coolness of the night, the saccharine juice has become to some extent congealed. Later in the day, the solar heat causes it to drop upon the ground. It is usually stored away in large earthen vessels, which are preserved in cellars during the entire year. This tamarisk manna is sold in little vessels of tinned iron to persons who visit the monasteries of Sinai. Landerer purchased one of these of a pilgrim, and he found the manna to consist of a yellowish granular syrupy mass, very sweet, and intermixed with the small leaves of the tamarisk. It was soluble in water and alcohol, and the aqueous solution readily underwent fermentation. The alcohol obtained by the distillation of this fermented liquid had a peculiar odour resembling that derived from the fruit of *Ceratonia Siliqua*, which contains butyric acid. The saccharine principle of this manna must, therefore, be a sugar, and not mannite (see *post*). The tamarisk manna is eaten in Palestine, and in the district of Sinai, as a delicacy, and is reputed to be efficacious in diseases of the chest.[3]—ED.]

ADULTERATION.—In 1842, more than a ton of fictitious manna was

---

[1] [We are informed that Tolfa manna is unknown to our best drug-merchants, and that no manna from the Roman States is now brought into commerce.—ED.]

[2] De Candolle, *Physiol. Végét.* t. i. p. 238 ; Brandt u. Ratzeburg, *Med. Zoologie*, Bd. ii. p. 211. [See *Pharmaceutical Journal*, March 1854, p. 412.]

offered for sale in Paris. It appears to have been potato sugar. It was distinguished from genuine manna by its general appearance; its granular fracture; its taste, which was that of caramelised sugar, followed by a slight bitterness; its non-inflammability in the candle; its more marked fermentation when its aqueous solution was mixed with yeast, and the residual liquor not yielding mannite; its containing sulphate of lime; and its property of circular polarisation.[1]

COMMERCE.—Manna is imported into this country principally from Palermo and Messina. It is also occasionally brought from other ports of Sicily; viz. Licata, Girgenti, Catania, Terra Nova, and Marsala. Furthermore, Naples, Leghorn, Trieste, Genoa, and Marseilles, are other places of shipment of it.

COMPOSITION.—Manna was analysed in 1809 by Bucholz,[2] and in 1845 by Leuchtweiss.[3]

BUCHOLZ'S ANALYSIS.		LEUCHTWEISS'S ANALYSES.			
	Manna canelata.		M. cane- lata.	M. canel. in fragmentis.	M. Calabr.
Mannite	60·0	Mannite	42·6	37·6	32·0
Fermentable but uncrystallisable sugar with colouring matter (purgative bitter matter?)	5·5	Sugar	9·1	10·3	15·0
		Mucilage, with some mannite, resinous and acid matter, and a small quantity of a nitrogenous			
Sweetish gum	1·5	substance	40·0	40·8	42·1
Gummy extractive	0·8	Insoluble matter	0·4	0·9	3·2
Fibro-glutinous matter	0·2	Water	11·6	13·0	11·1
Water and loss	30·0	Ashes	1·3	1·9	1·9
	98·0		105·0	104·5	105·3

1. MANNITE (*Mannitum*); *Manna Sugar; Grenadin.* Formula $C^6H^5O^4,2HO$; Eq. Wt. 91.—It is a constituent of manna. It may also be obtained by exciting the viscous fermentation in a solution of ordinary sugar. It may be procured from beet-root, dandelion-root,[4] and sea-weeds. It is most readily and economically obtained from manna by Ruspini's process :[5]—Common manna is first prepared by melting it over the fire in distilled or rain water in which the white of egg has been previously beaten; boil and strain the solution through a linen cloth : the strained liquor solidifies on cooling. Submit the prepared manna to strong pressure, then mix it with its own weight of cold water, and again press it. Dissolve the pressed cake in boiling water, add animal charcoal, and then filter and evaporate the solution, which is then to be set aside to crystallise.—Mannite is a white, crystalline, odourless substance, which has a sweet agreeable taste. It is soluble in 5 parts of cold water, and in a smaller proportion of boiling water; it is readily soluble in boiling alcohol, but less so in cold alcohol. It is essentially distinguished from sugars strictly so called (see SUGAR) by two characters—1st, its solution does not undergo the vinous fermentation when in contact with yeast; 2dly, its solution does not possess the property of rotatory polarisation.

[According to M. Lhermite, the essential difference in the elementary composition of mannite, as compared with sugar, is in the presence of a slight excess of hydrogen. Fresh and perfectly pure manna does not undergo alcoholic fermentation, but after a lapse of some time it is liable to a peculiar alteration. It changes from a white, opaque, dry, and almost friable substance, to that of a reddish translucent and gluey substance. It is then sufficiently hygrometric to dissolve in the water which it derives from the atmosphere; and this solution, with the addition of yeast, soon becomes converted into alcohol and

---

[1] *Journ. de Pharm. et Chim.* 3me sér. t. i. pp. 58 and 154, 1842; and *Pharmaceutical Journal*, vol. iii. p. 222, 1843.
[2] *Taschenbuch für Scheidekunst*, 1809 ; and *Berlin. Jahrbuch für d. Pharm.* p. lxi. 1809.
[3] *Annal. der Chemie u. Pharm.* Bd. liii. S. 124, 1845.
[4] Messrs. T. and H. Smith, *Pharmaceutical Journal*, vol. viii. p. 480, 1849.
[5] *Pharmaceutical Journal*, vol. vi. p. 183, 1846.

carbonic acid. These facts explain why it is that sugar is found in manna. If under an oxidising influence mannite is convertible into sugar, there can be no doubt that mannite may be also produced by the action of deoxidising agents on sugar itself : it is thus that it is formed in the juice of beet-root submitted to viscous fermentation.[1]—Ed.]

Mannite has recently been imported from Italy in the form of beautiful white crystalline masses, which are totally devoid of any disagreeable flavour.[2] It is intended to be a substitute for common manna, than which it is supposed to be more purgative. But from my own observations it appears to possess but little, if any, purgative quality. Other reasons lead us also to suspect that mannite is not the purgative principle of manna : thus fresh and flaky manna has a less irritating and nauseous flavour, and a less purgative effect, than old and common or fatty manna.

2. Resin.—Manna contains a resin which has a disagreeable odour, and a nauseous, irritating, unpleasant flavour. The quantity of it, however, is very inconsiderable. Is this the *purgative principle* of manna ? It is usually accompanied by an acid, whose solution, by evaporation, is gradually converted into resin.

Physiological Effects. *α. On Animals generally.*—In moderate doses manna is nutritive, and is greedily devoured by some animals. Thus Swinburn[3] tells us that vipers and martens are very fond of it. In large doses it acts as a mild laxative. The dose for carnivorous animals is about two ounces dissolved in broth or milk.[4] It is rarely given to horses, on account of the large dose required.

β. On Man.—It has an analogous operation on man : that is, in small doses it is nutritive, and in large ones mildly laxative. It acts on the bowels without exciting vascular irritation, and is, therefore, admissible in inflammatory cases. It is apt, however, to produce flatulence and griping. The fresher and less changed the manna, the feebler are said to be its laxative powers ; and hence the Calabrians are enabled to use it frequently as an article of food. When by keeping and partial decomposition it has acquired an increase of laxative powers, it is less easily digested, and is more apt to excite flatulence. Hence, also, we are told, the commoner kinds of manna are more laxative, and more apt to disagree with the stomach, than the finer varieties. The older writers imagined that manna promoted the secretion of bile. Manna approaches tamarinds as a laxative, but it is more nutritive and less refrigerant, in consequence of possessing more mucilaginous and saccharine matter, and less free vegetable acids.

Uses.—It is employed as a laxative, partly on account of the mildness of its operation, partly for its sweet flavour, in delicate persons, as females and children. Dr. Burns[5] recommends it for new-born infants if the meconium do not come away freely. On account of its sweetness it is frequently added to flavour purgative draughts, and is used as a common laxative for children, who readily eat it.

Administration.—It may be taken in substance, or dissolved in warm milk or water. The dose for an adult is from ʒj. to ℥ij. ; for children, from ʒj. to ʒiij.

---

[1] [See *Pharmaceutical Journal*, Aug. 1852, p. 77.]
[2] *Ibid.* vol. ix. pp. 349 and 458, 1850.
[3] *Travels in the Two Sicilies*, 1785.
[4] Moiroud, *Pharm. Vét.*
[5] *Principles of Midwifery.*

ORDER XLIX. STYRACACEÆ, *Alph. DC.*—STORAXWORTS.

CHARACTERS.—*Calyx* 5- and very rarely 4-lobed ; the lobes quincuncial in æstivation. *Corolla* 5 very rarely 4- or 6-7-lobed, consisting of 5 or 4-7 petals usually but slightly connate at the base, campanulate or subrotate, sometimes an inner whorl of petals concrete to the tube of the outer, and alternating with the lobes. *Stamens* adnate to the base of the corolla, free or connate by the filaments, in 1 or many rows ; either 8-10, alternate and opposite to the lobes of the corolla, or indefinite, free, pentadelphous or monadelphous, adelphous or longer stamina alternating with the lobes of the corolla ; *anthers* 2-celled, dehiscing laterally or inwardly, shorter than the filament ; *pollen* broadly elliptical, smooth. *Nectary* 0. *Ovary* inferior or semi-inferior, rarely free, 5-2-celled ; the cells opposite the lobes of the calyx when they are of the same number ; the partitions sometimes scarcely adhering in the centre of the ovary. *Ovules* 2 or indefinite in each cell, all pendulous, or the upper ones erect and the lower pendulous, always anatropal. *Style* simple. *Stigma* somewhat capitate. *Fruit* usually baccate, rarely dry, more rarely dehiscing, surmounted by the erect lobes of the calyx, oblong or subglobose, all the cells but one with abortive ovules. *Seeds* 5-1, usually solitary, erect, horizontal or often pendulous, albuminous. *Embryo* lying in the axis of the albumen ; cotyledons flat, never longer than the radicle.—*Trees* or *shrubs*. *Leaves* alternate, simple, without stipules. *Racemes* or *solitary flowers*, axillary, with bracts (*Alph. De Cand.*)

PROPERTIES.—Storax and Benjamin, obtained from the genus *Styrax*, are well-known stimulant balsamic resins. *Symplocos Alstonia* is used at Santa-Fé as tea. The properties of the other species are but little known.

210. STYRAX OFFICINALE, *Linn.*—THE OFFICINAL STORAX.

Sex. Syst. Decandria, Monogynia.

(Planta incerta ; Balsamum liquidum, *L.*—Balsamic exudation, *E.*)

HISTORY.—Storax, as well as the tree producing it, was known to the ancient Greeks and Romans ; by the former it was called στύραξ, by the latter *styrax*. It is mentioned by Hippocrates,[1] Theophrastus,[2] Dioscorides,[3] and Pliny.[4]

BOTANY.   Gen. Char.—*Calyx* urceolate-campanulate, 5-toothed at the apex, or nearly entire. *Corolla* monopetalous, 5-partite, rarely and perhaps by monstrosity 4- or 6-7-partite, twice or thrice the length of the calyx, with lanceolate or oblong lobes, externally whitish tomentose. *Stamens* 10, rarely variable 7-12, connate to the base of the corolla, alternate and opposite to its lobes, almost equal ; *filaments* connate at the base in a short tube, distinct at the apex, hairy especially internally ; *anthers* erect, linear, continuous with the filament, 2-celled, dehiscing inwards by longitudinal slits. *Ovary* adherent at the base, ovoid, pubescent, 3-celled ; the · partitions incomplete. *Ovules* indefinite. *Style* filiform. *Stigma* almost 3-lobed. *Fruit* globose or ovoid, adnate to the base of the persistent calyx, pubescent, 1-celled, 1-seeded, rarely 2-3-seeded. *Seed* in general solitary, marked by lines caused by the impression of the walls of the pericarp ; the hilum round,

---

[1] *De Nat. Mul.* pp. 575 and 587, ed. Fœs.
[2] *Hist. Plant.* lib. ix. cap. 7.
[3] Lib. i. cap. lxxix.
[4] *Hist. Nat.* lib. xii. cap. 40 and 45, ed. Valp.

inferior and sublateral; *albumen* fleshy; *cotyledons* ovate-rounded, as long as the radicle (*Alp. De Cand.*)

Sp. Char.—Leaves oval-obovate, on the upper surface smoothish, beneath hoary tomentose. Racemes few-flowered. Pedicels longer than the abbreviated peduncle, subternate terminal, and, as well as the calyx, hoary (*Alp. De Cand.*)

A small *tree*. *Stem* about 20 feet high; bark smooth. Younger *branches* hoary. *Leaves* alternate, petiolated, usually rounded at the apex, entire. *Racemes* axillary and terminal, shorter than the leaf, of from 3 to 5 flowers. *Calyx* almost hemispherical, with 5 short marginal teeth. *Corolla* white, externally hoary, with 6-7 segments. *Fruit* (*capsule*, Nees) coriaceous, downy, usually with 1 seed.

Hab.—The Levant, Palestine, Syria, Greece. Cultivated in the southern parts of Europe.

DESCRIPTION.—In England two sorts of storax are met with in the shops, and are used in medicine : these are—*liquid storax*, and what is usually called *styrax calamita*.

1. **Styrax liquida** (*Liquid Storax*).—The following is the mode of obtaining this substance, according to Landerer :[1]—

"The storax plant, *Styrax officinale*, is found in different parts of continental Greece, as well as in some of the islands of the Archipelago. It is there only a small shrub, and does not possess the agreeable odour which botanists ascribe to it. The bark of the tree growing in Greece has not the slightest odour,—in consequence, probably, of the neglect of cultivation. It is very different, however, with the plant growing in the Turkish Islands, Cos and Rhodes, especially that cultivated by the inhabitants of Cos.—At Cos and Rhodes the plant is called βουχοῦρι. At the flowering season it fills the air with its delightful vanilla-like perfume. At the season of the collection of the bark and of the young branches which are employed in the preparation of *Buchuri-jag*—that is, of *storax oil* (oil being called in Turkish, *Jag*)—a license is obtained from the Pasha residing at Rhodes, and for which a small sum is paid as a tax. The persons who have thus been licensed, make, with small knives, longitudinal incisions, and separate the fresh pieces of bark from the stem in the form of small narrow strips. These easily stick together on account of their glutinous juice. In this way are obtained masses of one *oka* (about 2 lbs.) each, which are either preserved for the preparation of *jag*, or are immediately purchased by Rhodian merchants and sent to Rhodes.

"The preparation of *Buchuri-jag* is effected, not by boiling, but merely by pressing the above-mentioned masses in presses somewhat warmed, and which are termed *styraki*. The *jag* obtained by slight pressure has an unctuous consistence, a light grey colour, and evolves an agreeable vanilla-like odour. This is the only kind which is exported; but they also use it at Cos and Rhodes for the preparation of an agreeable-smelling mass, and for that purpose add to it finely powdered olibanum, and therewith form cakes of about the size of a small fist, which they also call *styrakia*. The preparation of this substance is exclusively effected by the monastic clergy, who mark their produce with the monastic seal. By repeated warming and greater pressure, an almost black *buchuri-jag* is obtained, and which is used by the natives for the preparation of salves and medicines. The pieces of bark which are left behind after the expression of the juice are tied together and sent in part to Constantinople, and in part to Syra, where they are used for fumigating.

"With respect to the decoction of the bark, and the adulteration of storax with turpentine, the Rhodian merchants, from whom these accounts were obtained, declared that they were ignorant of the mode of effecting it, and that the adulteration with turpentine, if discovered, carries with it the penalty of death."

I have met with two kinds of liquid storax in the shops; one which is

---

[1] Buchner's *Repertorium*, 2te Reihe, Bd. xviii. p. 359, 1839; also *Pharm. Central-Blatt für* 1840, p. 11.

opaque (*common* or *opaque liquid storax*), and another which is pellucid or transparent (*pellucid liquid storax*).

α. *Common* or *Opaque Liquid Storax; Impure* or *Coarse Liquid Storax*, Hill.—This is imported from Trieste in casks or barrels holding about 4 cwt. each. It is opaque, of a grey colour, has the consistence of birdlime, and the odour of storax, but frequently intermixed with a feeble odour of benzole or naphthaline.[1] The substance met with in the shops, and sold to perfumers under the name of *strained storax* (*styrax colatus*), is prepared from liquid storax by heating it until the water with which it is usually mixed is evaporated, and then straining it. During the process it evolves a very fragrant odour. The impurities are stones, sand, &c.

In consequence of Petiver's statement[2] already alluded to, liquid storax has been supposed to be the produce of a species of *Liquidambar,*—probably *L. Altingia* or *L. orientale*. But several reasons are unfavourable to this opinion :—1st. Its vanilla-like odour allies it to the products of *Styrax officinale*, and at the same time separates it from all authentic products of the genus *Liquidambar*. Dr. Wood,[2] for example, found the genuine juice of *L. styraciflua* very different to that of liquid storax; and the fluid resin called liquidambar which I have met with has no resemblance to it. 2dly. Marquart[4] analysed a specimen of the genuine resin of *L. Altingia*, and obtained a volatile oil somewhat like styrol, and a substance similar to styracin; but their composition he found to be entirely different,—for while styracin consists of $C^{24}H^{22}O^2$, the liquidambar resin was composed of $C^{16}H^{22}O^2$. 3dly. Landerer's account of *buchuri-jag* applies entirely to the liquid storax of the shops.

β. *Pellucid Liquid Storax ; Storax liquide pur*, Guibourt.—This substance was sold to me under the name of *balsam* or *balsam storax ;* and I was informed that it had been imported in jars each holding 14 lbs. It agrees with the *pure* or *fine liquid storax* of Hill,[5] and the *styrax liquida finissima* of Alston.[6] Professor Guibourt, to whom I sent a sample, at first regarded it as balsam of liquidambar ; but its odour has subsequently induced him to rank it among the products of *Styrax officinale*.[7] It is a pellucid liquid, having the consistence and tenacity of Venice turpentine, a brownish-yellow colour, a sweetish storax-like or vanilla-like odour entirely different to that of liquidambar. A few particles of bran or saw-dust are intermixed with it. By keeping, it yields a white and acid sublimate on the sides of the bottle which contains it.

2. **Styrax calamita ;**[8] *Styrax vulgaris ; Common Storax.*—This probably is the inferior sort of storax described by both Dioscorides[9] and Pliny[10] as

---

[1] [According to Mr. D. Hanbury, if Buchuri-jag be mixed with a small proportion of salt water, it acquires exactly the pale opaque appearance of common liquid storax. It is probable that petroleum or naphtha is sometimes mixed with common liquid storax.—ED.]

[2] *Phil. Trans.* vol. xxvi. p. 44.

[3] *United States Dispensatory.*

[4] *Jahresbericht d. Pharmacie,* p. 343, 1842.

[5] *History of the Materia Medica,* p. 712, 1751.

[6] *Lectures on the Materia Medica,* vol. ii. p. 418, 1770.

[7] *Hist. Nat. des Drogues,* 4me édit. t. ii. p. 553, 1849.

[8] *Calamita,* from κάλαμος, *a cane* or *reed*. Galen (*De antidotis*, lib. i. cap. 14) speaks of a sort of storax brought from Pamphylia in reeds (ἐν τοῖς καλάμοις). Hoffman (*Lexicon universale*) derives the term *calamita* (or, as he writes it, *calamites*) from the circumstance that the wood of the storax tree is devoured by an insect (Strabo, lib. xii.), and the stem thereby reduced to a hollow shell, like a reed,—a very improbable explanation.

[9] Lib. i. cap. 79.

[10] *Hist. Nat.* lib. xii. cap. 55, ed. Valp.

being friable and branny, and which the latter writer states becomes covered with white mouldiness, " cano situ obductus." This is imported in large round cakes, of a brown or reddish-brown colour and fragrant odour. It is brittle and friable, being very easily rubbed into a coarse kind of powder ; yet it is soft and unctuous. When exposed to the air it becomes covered with an efflorescence (cinnamic acid ?) which, to the superficial observer, looks like a whitish kind of mouldiness, and falls to powder. It appears to consist of some liquid resin mixed with fine saw-dust or bran. Boiled with rectified spirit, it yields a reddish solution, which becomes milky on the addition of water. The insoluble residue is a reddish saw-dust (of storax wood ?). It seems probable, says Lewis,[1] " that the common storax is the juice received immediately in vessels, and mixed with saw-dust enough to thicken it ; the shops requiring, under the name of storax, a solid or consistent mass, and evaporation being found to dissipate its fragrance. At least I cannot conceive for what other purpose the woody matter could be added, for it is too easily distinguishable to have been intended as an imposition."

The three following sorts are more or less allied to the *styrax calamita* of the shops, inasmuch as the body of them consists of saw-dust. The term *scobs styracina* is applicable to all four sorts.

a. Solid or *Cake Storax* (*Storax solide* ou *Storax en pain*, Guibourt).—Under this name I have received from Professor Guibourt a substance very analogous to the preceding ; but the saw-dust obtained by digesting it in spirit is not so intensely red.

β. *Drop* or *Gum Storax.*—Under this name I have once met, in English commerce, a storax which was highly valued. It was a circular cake, about a foot in diameter, and four or five inches thick. It was blackish, with a greenish tint ; had a pilular consistence, considerable tenacity, and a very agreeable odour. By keeping, it became covered with a crystalline efflorescence (of cinnamic acid ?). Boiled in rectified spirit, it gave an inky appearance to the liquid, and left a blackish saw-dust.

γ. *Hard Blackish Storax.*—Under the name of *brown storax*, I purchased in Paris a solid, heavy, compact, hard, blackish substance, having the odour of liquid storax. Boiled in rectified spirit, it yielded an almost colourless liquid and a brownish saw-dust. Is this the false storax which Guibourt[2] says is made at Marseilles ?

Besides the preceding (the only sorts of storax found in English commerce) there are several other kinds which deserve a brief notice.

3. **Storax in the Tear** (*Styrax in granis*).—Yellowish-white or reddish-yellow tears, about the size of peas. *White storax* (*styrax albus*) is formed of tears agglutinated so as to form masses somewhat resembling pale galbanum. Both sorts, however, are exceedingly rare, and are unknown to our drug-dealers. I have never met with a single specimen in English commerce. White storax is also scarce in Paris ; for Professor Guibourt, to whom I wrote for a sample, says that there was one fine specimen at a druggist's in Paris, but it was not for sale. " I discovered it (says he) with great pleasure, having established the distinction of that variety only from a scrap of one or two drachms." This probably is the sort described by Dioscorides as being a transparent tear-like gum resembling myrrh, and which was very scarce.

4. **Amygdaloid Storax** (*Styrax amygdaloides*).—It occurs in compact masses, having a very agreeable odour, analogous to that of vanilla, and a yellowish or reddish-brown colour. They are interspersed with white tears (giving the mass an amygdaloid appearance). This variety is very scarce. I had a fine sample, weighing nearly two ounces and a quarter : it cost me, in Paris,

---

[1] *Chem. Works of C. Neumann*, by W. Lewis, p. 290, 1759.
[2] *Hist. Nat. des Drog.* 4ème édit. t. ii. p. 554, 1849.

24 francs per ounce. There is (or was a few years since) a magnificent piece in the possession of a French pharmacien, who offered to sell it for 500 francs. Amygdaloid and white storax were formerly imported enveloped in a monocotyledonous leaf, under the name of *cane* or *reed storax* (*storax calamita verus*). A fine specimen (about the size and shape of half an orange) is in Dr. Burgess's collection, belonging to the Royal College of Physicians of London. Amygdaloid storax is described by Dioscorides as being the best sort. He says it is unctuous, yellow, resinous, mixed with whitish lumps, and forms a honey-like liquid when melted; it comes, he adds, from Gabala [a Phœnician city], Pisidia, and Cilicia [countries of Asia Minor].

5. **Reddish-brown Storax** (*Storax rouge-brun,* Guibourt).—This differs from the preceding in the absence of the white tears, and in the presence of saw-dust. It is reddish-brown, and has a similar, but less powerful, odour to that of the amygdaloid kind. It is not found in the London drug-houses. The Pharmaceutical Society has a large cake of storax which is somewhat intermediate between this and the amygdaloid sort. Professor Guibourt, who examined it, considered it to be *falsified brown storax.* Micaceous films or crystalline plates are formed on its surface.

6. **Black Storax.**—Under the name of *Storax noir,* I have received from Professor Guibourt a very dark reddish-brown mass, which easily softens, and has the odour of vanilla. "It appears to be formed of a balsam which has been melted and inspissated by heat with saw-dust. Its very characteristic odour leads me to consider it," says M. Guibourt,[1] "as different from storax calamita, storax liquida, and liquidambar." It is not found in the London drug-houses.

Storax Bark is supposed to constitute the *cortex thymiamatis* vel *thuris* of some pharmacologists. It is probably the νάσκαφθον of Dioscorides.[2] It is in thin, light, red, highly odorous fragments or shavings, frequently covered with an efflorescence. I am indebted for a sample of it to Professor Guibourt.

COMMERCE.—I found, on the examination of the books of a wholesale druggist, that all the storax (solid and liquid) imported into this country during seven years came from Trieste.

COMPOSITION.—Neumann[3] submitted *common storax* (*styrax calamita* offic.) to a chemical examination. More recently, Reinsch[4] analysed three kinds of *styrax calamita.* In 1830 Bonastre[5] analysed a *storax from Bogota.* The same chemist[6] examined a fluid, which he termed *liquid storax,* but which was *liquidambar.*

Liquid storax has been analysed by Simon;[7] and some of its constituents have been examined by Drs. Blyth and Hofmann,[8] by Toel,[9] by Strecker,[10] and by Scharling.[11]

[1] *Letter to the Author.*
[2] Lib. i. cap. 22.
[3] *Chem. Works,* by Lewis, p. 290.
[4] *Pharm. Central-Blatt für* 1838, S. 537 and 810.
[5] *Journ. de Pharm.* t. xvi. p. 88.
[6] *Ibid.* t. xvii. p. 338.
[7] *Ann. der Pharmacie,* Bd. xxxi. 1839; *Journ. de Pharmacie,* t. xxvi. p. 241, 1840.
[8] *Memoirs of the Chemical Society,* vol. ii. p. 334, 1845.
[9] *Chemical Gazette,* vol. vii. p. 249, 1849.
[10] *Ibid.* vol. vii. p. 272, 1849.
[11] *Ibid.* vol. vii. p. 419, 1849.

1. *Composition of Styrax calamita.*—The following are the results of Reinsch's analyses of this substance :—

REINSCH'S ANALYSES OF STYRAX CALAMITA.

	1. *Storax calamita.* Opt. 1785. Nestler.	2. *Brown granular.*	3. *Reddish compact.*
Volatile oil	?	0·5	0·4
Resin..............................	41·6	53·7	32·7
Subresin	?	0·6	0·5
Benzoic acid	2·4	1·1	2·6
Gum and extractive	14·0	9·3	7·9
Matter extracted by potash	15·0	9·6	23·9
Woody fibre	22·0	20·2	27·0
Ammonia	traces	stronger traces	strongest traces
Water	5·0	5·0	5·0
Storax calamita	100·0	100·0	100·0

The volatile oil was obtained by digesting distilled water of storax with ether. The *solid* oil was white, crystalline, and fusible; its odour was agreeable, its taste aromatic and warm. The *fluid* oil had not so penetrating an odour.

2. *Composition of Liquid Storax.*—Simon found liquid storax to consist of a *volatile oil* (called *styrole*), *cinnamic acid, styracine, a soft resin,* and *a hard resin.*

1. VOLATILE OIL OF LIQUID STORAX ; *Styrole.* Formula $C^{16}H^8$.—Obtained by submitting liquid storax to distillation with an aqueous solution of carbonate of soda. It is a colourless, extremely volatile, transparent liquid, which has a burning taste and a peculiar aromatic odour, resembling a mixture of benzole and naphthaline. Exposed to the cold produced by a mixture of ether and solid carbonic acid, it freezes into a beautiful white crystalline mass. Its sp. gr. is 0·924 at the ordinary temperature of summer. It is soluble in alcohol and ether, burns with a sooty flame, boils at about 295° F., and at a somewhat higher temperature is converted into a firm transparent solid called *metastyrole* (Simon's *oxide of styrole*), which is isomeric with, and has the same refractive power as, styrole.

2. CINNAMIC ACID ; *Cinnamylic Acid.* Formula $C^{18}H^7O^3+HO$. Eq. 148. Symbol $\overline{Ci}$, or CiO.—This acid is a constituent of the balsams of Tolu and Peru, and of the yellow resin of Xanthorrhœa, as well as of liquid storax. It is also formed by the oxidation of the hydruret of cinnamyle or oil of cinnamon. It is a colourless crystalline acid, having a feebly aromatic acrid taste, and being sparingly soluble in cold water, but readily soluble in alcohol. It is deposited from its aqueous solution in water in the form of pearly plates, but from alcohol in rhombic prisms. It fuses at about 250°, and boils at 560° F. It has some resemblance to benzoic acid, for which it was formerly mistaken ; but it may be distinguished by boiling it with a solution of chromic acid, when it gives rise to the production of oil of bitter almonds, of which benzoic acid does not yield a trace. Taken at bed-time in doses of from 80 to 90 grains, Erdmann and Marchand[1] found that, like benzoic acid, it becomes converted in the human body into hippuric acid, which passes in the urine.

3. STYRACINE.—This is found in the still after the distillation of styrole from liquid storax. It is a crystallisable substance soluble in boiling alcohol and in ether, but insoluble in water. Its formula, according to Simon, is $C^{24}H^{11}O^2$. But Toel, who regards it as a combination of cinnamic acid having a perfectly analogous constitution to the natural fats, says its composition is best expressed by the formula $C^{60}H^{28}O^6$. By distillation with caustic potash it yields a crystallisable substance called *styrone*, whose composi-

---

[1] *Chemical Gazette,* vol. i. p. 29, 1842.

tion is, according to Toel, $C^{42}H^{28}O^5$. Strecker regards styracine as a compound of cinnamic acid, $C^{18}H^8O^4$, and of styrone, $C^{18}H^{10}O^2$, but minus 2HO.

4. RESINS OF LIQUID STORAX.—These are two in number ; one soft, the other hard.

PHYSIOLOGICAL EFFECTS.—Storax produces the before-described effects of the balsamic substances. Its stimulant properties are more particularly directed to the mucous surfaces, especially to the bronchial membrane. Hence it is called a stimulating expectorant. In its operation it is closely allied to balsam of Peru and benzoin, but is less powerful than the latter. As it contains cinnamic acid, its use increases the quantity of hippuric acid in the urine.

USES.—Internally, storax has been principally employed in affections of the organs of respiration. In chronic bronchial affections, admitting of the use of stimulants, it may be used as an expectorant. It has also been employed in chronic catarrhal affections of the urino-genital membrane. Applied to foul ulcers in the form of ointment, it sometimes operates as a detergent, and improves the quality of the secreted matter.

ADMINISTRATION.—Purified storax may be exhibited, in the form of pills, in doses of from grs. x. to Ʒj.

1. STYRAX PRÆPARATA, L. ; *Extractum Styracis*, E. ; *Strained Storax.* (Dissolve 1 lb. of storax in 4 pints of rectified spirit, and strain through linen ; then distil with a gentle heat the greater portion of the spirit, and evaporate the residuum in a water-bath to a proper consistence, *L.*—The directions of the *Edinburgh College* are essentially the same, except that the evaporation is ordered to be carried on by the vapour-bath, until the product have the consistence of a thin extract.)—This process is intended for the purification of *styrax vulgaris* (*styrax calamita* offic.) ; but Mr. Brande says it is inefficient. The strained storax of the shops is usually produced from liquid storax. It is used in perfumery, and in the preparation of *tinctura benzoïni composita* and the *pilulæ styracis compositæ.*

2. PILULÆ STYRACIS COMPOSITÆ, L. ; *Pilulæ Styracis*, E. ; *Pills of Storax.* (Prepared Storax [Extract of Storax, *E.*], ʒvj. ; Opium [powdered, *L.*], ʒij. ; Saffron, ʒij. Beat them together until incorporated [and divide the mass into 60 pills, *E.*])—These pills are useful in chronic coughs, and some other pulmonary affections. They are valuable also in another point of view : they sometimes enable us to exhibit opium to persons prejudiced against its use ; the saffron and storax concealing the smell and flavour of this narcotic, while the name of the pill cannot reveal the harmless deception.—The dose is from grs. v. to grs. x.

211. STYRAX BENZOIN, *Dryand.*—THE BENJAMIN TREE.

Benzoin officinale, *Hayne.*

Sex. Syst. Decandria, Monogynia.

(Balsamum ex inciso cortice fusum aëre induratum, *L.*—Concrete balsamic exudation, *E.*—The concrete exudation ; Benzoin, *D.*)

HISTORY.—As the ancients were acquainted with so many oriental vegetable products, we should have expected, *à priori*, that benzoin would have been known to them. But this does not appear to have been the case ; at least, we are unable to identify it with any of the substances described by the old writers.[1]

BOTANY.   **Gen. Char.**—Vide *Styrax officinale.*

Sp. Char.—Branchlets whitish-rusty tomentose. Leaves oblong, acuminate, whitish tomentose beneath. Racemes compound, axillary, nearly the length of the leaves, and, as well as the flowers, horny tomentose. Pedicels one-third as long as the flower. Calyx hemispherical sub-5-dentate (*Alph. De Cand.*)

Tree. *Stem* thickness of a man's body. *Leaves* oval-oblong, entire. *Calyx* campanulate, very obscurely 5-toothed. *Corolla* grey, of 5 petals, perhaps connate at the base. *Stamens* 10. *Ovary* superior, ovate ; *style* filiform ; *stigma* simple (condensed from *Dryander*[2]).

Hab.—Sumatra, Borneo, Siam, Java.

EXTRACTION OF THE BALSAM.—Benzoin is obtained in Sumatra as follows : When the tree is six years old, longitudinal or somewhat oblique incisions are made in the bark of the stem, at the origin of the principal lower branches. A liquid exudes, which, by exposure to the sun and air, soon concretes, and the solid mass is then separated by means of a knife or chisel. Each tree yields about three pounds of benzoin annually, for the space of ten or twelve years. That which exudes during the first three years is white, and is denominated *head benzoin.* The benzoin which subsequently flows is of a brownish colour, and is termed *belly benzoin.* After the tree is cut down the stem is split, and some benzoin scraped from the wood ; but its colour is dark, and its quality bad, owing to the intermixture of parings of wood and other impurities : this sort is called *foot benzoin.* The relative values of head, belly, and foot benzoin, are as 105, 45, 18. Benzoin is brought down from the country in large cakes (called by the natives *tampangs*) covered with mats. In order to pack it in chests, these cakes are softened by heat ; the finer by exposure to the sun, the coarser by means of boiling water.[3]

DESCRIPTION.—The several sorts of benzoin (*benzoinum ; asa dulcis*) met with in commerce may be conveniently arranged under two heads ; viz. *Siam benzoin* and *Sumatra benzoin.*

1. **Siam Benzoin** (*Benzoinum Siamense*).—Crawford[4] says that the benzoin of Siam is procured from Lao. He also states that a substance resembling, and hitherto confounded with, benzoin, produced in Lao, Raheng, Chiang-mai, and La Kon, is abundantly found in Siam. The tree producing it cannot be, he thinks, the *Styrax Benzoin,* so it grows so far north as the twentieth degree of latitude.

Siam benzoin is brought to England, either direct from Siam, or indirectly by way of Singapore. It includes the best commercial sorts, or those known in commerce as *benzoin* of *the finest quality.* It occurs in tears, in irregular lumps, and in cubical blocks ; but, unlike the Sumatra sort, it never comes over enveloped in calico. It is in general distinguished from the other sorts by its warmer or richer (yellow, reddish, or brown) tints. The dealers distinguish five or six qualities, the three best sorts being included under the name of *yellow Siam benzoin,* and the two or three inferior kinds being called *red* or

---

[1] See Garcias, *Arom. Hist.* in Clusius, *Exot.* p. 155.

[2] *Phil. Trans.* vol. lxxvii. p. 308.

[3] Marsden, *History of Sumatra,* 3d edit. p. 134 ; Crawford, *Hist. of the Ind. Archipel.* vol. i. p. 518 ; and vol. iii. p. 418.

[4] *Journal of an Embassy to Siam and Cochin-China,* p. 407, 1828.

brown Siam benzoin ; the designations yellow, red, or brown, being used on account of the tint of this resin by which the tears are agglutinated. But the division is altogether arbitrary, the colours passing universally into one another. I shall, therefore, adopt another arrangement.

α. *Siam benzoin in tears* (*Benzoinum Siamense in lachrymis*); *Yellow benzoin in the tear.*—This kind seems to be identical with the *true benzoin in tears*, which Savary[1] says was brought in considerable quantity to Paris by the attendants of the Siamese ambassadors. It consists of irregular flattened pieces, some of which are angular, and the largest of them barely exceeding an inch in length. Externally these pieces are shiny, or dusty from their mutual friction, and are of an amber or reddish-yellow colour ; they are brittle, and may be easily rubbed to powder. Internally they are translucent or milky, and frequently striped : they have a pleasant odour, but little or no taste. There is an inferior sort of Siam benzoin in tears, which consists of loose drops mixed with pieces of wood and other impurities. It is worth only one-fourth of the price of clean good-sized tears or clean lump.

β. *Siam or lump benzoin* (*Benzoinum Siamense in massis*).—The finest kind consists of agglutinated tears (*white* or *yellow lump benzoin*). More commonly we find the tears are connected by a brown resiniform mass, which, when broken, presents an amygdaloid appearance, from the white tears imbedded in the mass (*amygdaloid benzoin ; benzoinum amygdaloides*).

Inferior sorts of lump benzoin are reddish (*red lump benzoin*).

γ. *Translucent Benzoin.*—From my friend Dr. Royle I received a sample of Siam benzoin, the properties of which are somewhat different from the preceding. The small masses consist of agglomerated tears, which, instead of being white and opaque, are translucent, or, in a few instances, almost transparent.

2. Sumatra Benzoin (*Benzoinum ex Sumatrâ*).—Though placed here second, this sort is the more important, being in many countries the only kind known. It is rarely imported directly from Sumatra, but in general indirectly by way of Singapore or Bombay, and now and then from Calcutta.

It occurs in large rectangular blocks, marked with the impression of a mat, and covered with white cotton cloth. When broken, we observe but few large white tears in it. The mass is generally made up of a brown resiniform matter, with numerous white, small pieces or chips intermixed, which thereby give the broken surface a speckled appearance, somewhat like that of a fine-grained granite.

The qualities of Sumatra benzoin are distinguished as *firsts, seconds,* and *thirds.*

α. The *first Sumatra sort* occurs very seldom, and only by single chests, for which £50 or more the cwt. are paid for the Russian market.

β. The *second Sumatra sort* is also marbly, but not so white, and is also mostly taken for the Russian market at £20 to £30 the cwt. Thirty chests of this sort, perhaps, are seen before one of the first quality is met with.

γ. The *third Sumatra sort* is browner, and less, or not at all, marbly. It fetches from £5 to £10 per cwt., and forms the usual commercial quality (*common* or *brown benzoin ; benzoinum commune* vel *in sortis*). Five

---

[1] Alston, *Lect. on the Mat. Med.* vol. ii. p. 403.

times as much of this quality is met with as of all the other sorts put together.

There is a very inferior sort of benzoin (*inferior Bombay benzoin*) which invariably comes by way of Bombay.[1] If it be the produce of Sumatra it is remarkable that it never comes by way of Singapore.

COMMERCE.—Benzoin is sometimes imported into England direct from Siam and Sumatra; but usually indirectly from Singapore, Bombay, Penang, Calcutta, Madras, and Batavia. The greater part is re-exported for use in the ceremonies of the Greek and Catholic churches. In 1839 only 108 cwts. paid duty. [The importation of benzoin amounted, in the ten years 1835 to 1844, to 4196 chests,—the consumption, to only 983 chests; showing an annual average consumption of 98 chests, or 150 hundredweight, per annum. On the average of the four years 1851-4, the importation was 1054 chests per annum.—ED.]

COMPOSITION.—Benzoin has been the repeated subject of chemical analysis. It was analysed in 1811 by Bucholz,[2] in 1816 by John,[3] in 1823 by Stoltze,[4] and in 1845 by Kopp.[5] It has also been the subject of chemical examination by Brande,[6] Unverdorben,[7] and others.

	Bucholz.	*John.*	*Stoltze.*		
			White.	Amygdaloid.	Brown.
Volatile oil (aroma, *John*).................	—	—	traces	traces	traces
Benzoic acid	12·5	12·0	19·80	19·42	19·70
Resin { yellow, soluble in ether } { brown, insoluble in ether } ...	83·3	84·5	{ 79·83 { 0·25	27·10 50·53	8·80 69·73
Matter like balsam of Peru	1·7	—	—	—	—
Aromatic extractive	0·5	0·50	—	0·25	0·15
Woody matter and other impurities	2·0	2·00	—	2·60	1·45
Water and loss	—	0·25	0·12	0·10	0·17
Salts (benzoates and phosphates)	—	0·75	—	—	—
Benzoin............	100·0	100·00	100·00	100·00	100·00

Kopp followed Unverdorben's method of analysis, and obtained in two different specimens the following results :—

	I.		II.
Benzoic acid	14·0	....	14·5
Resin (α) soluble in ether	52·0	....	48·0
Resin (β) soluble in alcohol only	25·0	....	28·0
Resin (γ) soluble in a solution of carbonate of soda	3·0	....	3·5
Brown resin deposited by ether	0·8	....	0·5
Impurities	5·2	....	5·5
	100·0		100·0

Wackenroder[8] obtained 9 per cent. of benzoic acid from Siam benzoin.

---

[1] [We are informed that some hundreds of chests of this inferior kind have been imported during the last three years. It has hardly any odour or flavour.—ED.]
[2] Trommsdorff's *Journ. de Pharm.* Bd. xx. ; quoted by Stoltze.
[3] *Naturgesch. d. Succins*, Cöln, 1816 ; quoted by Stoltze.
[4] *Deutsches* (Berlin) *Jahrbuch für d. Pharmacie*, Bd. x. pp. 55 and 77, 1823.
[5] *Journ. de Pharm.* 3me sér. t. vii. p. 46, 1845.
[6] Nicholson's *Journal*, x. 82.
[7] Poggendorff's *Annalen*, xvii. 179.
[8] *Pharm. Central-Blatt für* 1843, p. 336.

1. VOLATILE OIL OF BENZOIN.—Distilled with water, benzoin does not yield any essential oil; but when exposed to heat without water, benzoic acid and an essential oil are volatilised. This oil may be deprived of its empyreuma by redistillation with water, and then smells agreeably of benzoin. It may be regarded as a product of the decomposition of the resin. An oil of benzoin obtained by distillation, without any liquid, is used at Sumatra as a perfume.[1]

2. RESINS OF BENZOIN.—By digesting benzoin in alcohol, a tincture is obtained, which, on the addition of water, forms a milky fluid (formerly absurdly called *virgin's milk*). The resin thus precipitated was formerly called the *magisterium benzoës*. The acids (acetic, hydrochloric, and sulphuric) occasion a precipitate in the alcoholic solution. Sulphuric acid yields a fine red colour with the resin of benzoin; chloride of iron, a green.

a resin; Alpha-resin of benzoin. Composed of the resins β and γ. $C^{40}H^{23}O^9 + C^{30}H^{20}O^5$ $= C^{70}H^{43}O^{14}$ (Van der Vliet[2] and Mulder[3]).—Soluble in ether, but insoluble in carbonate of potash.

β resin; Beta-resin of benzoin. $C^{40}H^{23}O^9$.—Soluble in alcohol, but insoluble in ether and in carbonate of potash.

γ resin; Gumma-resin of benzoin. $C^{30}H^{20}O^5$.—Soluble in carbonate of potash, and slightly so in ether.

3. BENZOIC ACID.—See p. 687.

We may assume, observe Pelouze and Frémy,[4] that benzoin, at the instant of its secretion, contains two different liquids : one which produces the resin; while the other, by becoming oxidised, is transformed into benzoic acid.

PHYSIOLOGICAL EFFECTS.—Benzoin produces the general effects of the balsams before mentioned. Its power of producing local irritation renders it apt to disorder the stomach, especially in very susceptible individuals. Its constitutional effects are those of a heating and stimulating substance, whose influence is principally directed to the mucous surfaces, especially of the air-tube. It is more acrid and stimulant, and less tonic, than myrrh, to which some pharmacologists have compared it. It has appeared in some instances to act as a stimulant to the sexual organs. As it contains benzoic acid, it must increase the proportion of hippuric acid in the urine.

USES.—As an internal remedy, the employment of benzoin is almost wholly confined to chronic pulmonary affections, especially those of the bronchial membrane. Its stimulant properties render it improper in all acute inflammatory complaints, and its acridity prevents its employment where there is much gastric irritation. Its use, therefore, is better adapted for torpid constitutions. Trousseau and Pidoux[5] speak most favourably of the effects of the balsams in chronic laryngitis, as I have elsewhere remarked. The mode of employing benzoin in balsamic fumigations in this disease has been already noticed.

ADMINISTRATION.—Benzoin is scarcely ever administered alone.—The dose of it in *powder* is from grs. x. to ʒss.—On account of the agreeable odour evolved when benzoin is heated, this balsam is frequently employed for *fumigations,* as in the ceremonies of the Greek and Roman Catholic churches.

1. TINCTURA BENZOINI COMPOSITA, L. E.; *Balsamum Traumaticum; Compound Tincture of Benjamin ; Wound Balsam ; Balsam for Cuts ; Friar's Balsam; Jesuit's Drops ; The Commander's Balsam.* (Benzoin,

---

[1] Marsden, *Sumatra*, p. 184.
[2] *Journ. f. pr. Chem.* xviii.; *Pharm. Central-Blatt für* 1839, p. 875.
[3] *The Chemistry of Vegetable and Animal Physiology*, p. 819, 1849.
[4] *Cours de Chimie Générale*, t. iii. p. 556, 1850.
[5] *Traité de Thérap.* ii. 477.

in coarse powder, ʒiiss. [ʒiv. *E.*] [Storax, prepared, ʒiiss. *L.*; Balsam of Tolu, ʒx. [Peru Balsam, ʒiiss. *E.*]; Socotrine or Hepatic Aloes, ʒv. [East Indian Aloes, ʒss. *E.*]; Rectified Spirit, Oij. Macerate for seven days [pour off the clear liquor, *E.*], and strain.—A stimulating expectorant : administered in chronic catarrhs.—Dose, fʒss. to fʒij. It is decomposed by water. A very pleasant mode of exhibiting it is in the form of emulsion, prepared with mucilage and sugar, or yolk of egg. Tinctura Benzoini composita is occasionally applied to foul and indolent ulcers, to excite the vascular action and to improve the quality of the secreted matter. It is a frequent application to recent incised wounds. If applied to cut surfaces it causes temporary pain, and cannot promote adhesion (or union by the first intention), though, by exciting too much inflammation, it may sometimes prevent it. But when the edges of the wound have been brought together, the tincture may be carefully applied to the lint or adhesive plaster as a varnish or cement. Here it acts mechanically, excluding air, and keeping the parts in their proper position. In the same way, it may sometimes prove serviceable in contused wounds. *Court* or *Black Sticking Plaster* (*Emplastrum adhæsivum Anglicum*, Ph. Bor.) is prepared by brushing first a solution of isinglass, and afterwards a spirituous solution of benzoin, over black sarcenet.

2. PASTILLI FUMANTES ; *Fumigating* or *Aromatic Pastiles*. (Benzoin, in powder, sixteen parts ; Balsam of Tolu, Sandal Wood in powder, of each four parts ; True Labdanum, one part ; a Light [Linden] Charcoal, forty-eight parts ; Nitrate of Potash, two parts ; Tragacanth, one part ; Gum Arabic, two parts ; Cinnamon Water, twelve parts. F. S. A. a soft and ductile mass, which is to be formed into cones with a flat tripod base. Dry at first in the air, afterwards by a stove).[1]—By burning, these pastiles diffuse a very agreeable odour. They are employed to disguise or overpower unpleasant smells.

The *Species ad suffiendum*, Ph. Bor., consists of Benzoin and Amber, of each lb. ss. ; and Lavender Flowers, ʒij.

3. ACIDUM BENZOICUM, L. E. D.; *Benzoic Acid ; Flowers of Benjamin* (*Flores Benzoini*). Symbol $\overline{Bz}$ or BzO. Formula $C^{14}H^5O^3$. Equivalent 113.—The crystallised acid contains 1 equivalent of water : $\overline{Bz},HO = 122$. This acid was described in 1608 by Blaise de Vigenere ; but it seems to have been known to Alexander Pedemontanus in 1560. It is formed by the oxidisement of the volatile oil of bitter almonds (hydruret of benzule) : $C^{14}H^6O^2 + O^2 = C^{14}H^5O^3,HO$. Chloride of benzule by the action of potash is converted into the benzoate of potash : $C^{14}H^5O^2,Cl + 2KO = KO,C^{14}H^5O^3 + KCl$. Hippuric acid under the influence of acids is converted into benzoic acid and gelatine sugar : $C^{18}H^9NO^6 + 2HO = C^{14}H^5O^3,HO + C^4H^5NO^4$.

But the usual method of obtaining benzoic acid for medicinal use is from benzoin, either by sublimation or by the action of alkalies,—commonly by sublimation. Mohr's process[2] is that adopted in the *Dublin Pharmacopœia* (1850).

"Take of Benzoin, any convenient quantity : place it in a small cylindric pot of sheet iron, furnished with a flange at its mouth ; and, having fitted the pot into a circular hole

---

[1] Henry and Guibourt, *Pharm. Raison.* t. i. p. 402.
[2] Mohr and Redwood's *Practical Pharmacy*, p. 194, 1849.

in a sheet of pasteboard, interpose between the pasteboard and flange a collar of tow, so as to produce a nearly air-tight junction. Let a cylinder of stiff paper, open at one end, eighteen inches high, and having a diameter at least twice that of the pot, be now placed in an inverted position on the pasteboard, and secured to it by slips of paper and flour paste : a couple of inches of the lower part of the pot being passed through a hole in a plate of sheet tin, which is to be kept from contact with the pasteboard by the inter-position of a few corks, let a heat just sufficient to melt the benzoin (that of a gas-lamp answers well) be applied, and continued for at least six hours. Let the product thus obtained, if not quite white, be enveloped in bibulous paper, then subjected to powerful pressure, and again sublimed."

Benzoic acid, on the large scale, is usually prepared by heating benzoin in a shallow iron pot communicating with a box (or *house,* as it is frequently termed) made of pasteboard and laths, or of thin wood, and lined with loose sheets of blotting-paper. A piece of fine muslin or paper is interposed between the mouth of the subliming pot and the box, to prevent the subli-mate falling back into the pot. The vapours of the acid traverse the muslin or pores of the paper, and condense in the box.[1]

As met with in the shops, benzoic acid occurs in the form of soft, light, feathery, white crystals, or scales, which are flexible, transparent, and of a mother-of-pearl lustre, having a sour, warm taste, but no odour when pure. It readily fuses and volatilises, its vapour being exceedingly irritating to the air-passages. It is combustible, burning with a bright yellow flame. It is very soluble in about two hundred parts of cold water, dissolves in about twenty-five parts of boiling water, and is very soluble in alcohol.

Benzoic acid is readily distinguished from other acids by its light and fea-thery crystals, its fusibility, volatility, odour of its vapour, by its great solu-bility in alkalies, by its property of being precipitated by acids from its al-kaline solutions, and by the character of its soluble salts. Thus the benzoate of ammonia produces with the sesquisalts of iron a pale-red precipitate $(Fe^2O^3,3Bz)$; and with the nitrate of silver and acetate of lead, precipitates (MO,Bz). From cinnamic acid (with which it has been confounded) it is dis-tinguished by not yielding oil of bitter almonds when distilled with oxidising agents, as chromic acid or a mixture of bichromate of potash and sulphuric acid.

Good benzoic acid has the following properties :—It is colourless, and is sublimed entirely by heat (*Edinb. Pharm.*) When cautiously heated, it totally evaporates, with a peculiar odour. It is sparingly soluble in water, but plentifully in rectified spirit. It is entirely dissolved by solution of potash or lime-water, and is precipitated from its solution by hydrochloric acid.

The *local* action of benzoic acid is that of an acrid. When swallowed, it occasions a sensation of heat and acridity in the back part of the mouth and throat, with heat at the stomach. The inhalation of its vapour causes violent coughing. On the *general system* it acts as a stimulant, whose influence is, however, principally directed to the mucous surfaces, especially the aërian membrane. In its passage through the system, it abstracts the elements of glycocoll or gelatine sugar, and becomes converted into hippuric acid, which is thrown out of the system in the urine in combination with a base.

$$C^{14}H^5O^3,HO \quad + \quad C^4H^5NO^4 \quad = \quad C^{18}H^9NO^6 \quad + \quad 2HO$$

Benzoic acid.	Glycocoll.	Hippuric acid.	Water.

[1] For some practical remarks on the preparation of this acid, see Euler and Herberger, in *Pharmaceutisches Central-Blatt für* 1840, p. 166.

Mr. Alexander Ure[1] first pointed out the fact that the quantity of hippuric acid in the urine is increased by the use of benzoic acid.[2] If, an hour after a meal, a scruple or half a drachm of benzoic acid be taken into the stomach, the urine subsequently voided, within three or four hours, will be found, on adding a small quantity (about one-twelfth part) of muriatic acid, to yield a copious precipitate of rose-pink acicular crystals of hippuric acid, which weigh, after being allowed to settle for a day, from fifteen to twenty-nine grains. Mr. Ure's observations were confirmed by the experiments of Dr. Garrod[3] and Keller.[4] It was also found by Keller that the urine which yielded hippuric acid, contained the normal proportion of both uric acid and urea.

Uses.—Benzoic acid is a constituent of the *Tinctura Camphoræ composita*, but otherwise is but little employed in medicine. It is sometimes administered in chronic bronchial affections. I have repeatedly tried it, but have seldom seen benefit result from its use. I have more frequently seen it augment than relieve the cough. On account of the alteration which it effects in the quality of the urine, benzoic acid has been administered with the view of promoting the excretion of nitrogenous matter, the retention of which is the supposed cause of disease. Thus Mr. Ure employed it in the gouty diathesis to prevent the formation of the tophaceous concretions commonly called *chalk stones*, and to correct and remove certain disordered states of the urine in individuals prone to attacks of gravel. But if Keller's observations (before stated) be correct, benzoic acid does not affect the quantity of uric acid in the urine. Further experiments with it on a larger scale are desirable, in order to determine positively whether it has or has not any influence over the excretion of uric acid or urea.—Dose, gr. v. to ʒj. It may be given in the form of a *benzoate* (which has a similar action on the urine to that of the free acid). For this purpose it may be dissolved in water by the aid of a few drops of a solution of either ammonia or potash.

Order L. SAPOTACEÆ, *Endlicher.*

Characters.—*Calyx* regular, persistent, in 5- or occasionally in 4-8 divisions, which are either valvate or imbricate in æstivation. *Corolla* monopetalous, hypogynous, regular, deciduous, its segments usually equal in number to those of the calyx, seldom twice or thrice as many, imbricate in æstivation. *Stamens* arising from the corolla, in number definite, distinct, the fertile ones equal in number to the segments of the calyx, and opposite those segments of the corolla which alternate with the latter, seldom more ; *anthers* usually turned outwards. The sterile stamens as numerous as the fertile ones, with which they alternate. *Disc* 0. *Ovary* superior, with several cells, in each of which is 1 ascending or pendulous anatropal ovule; *style* 1 ; *stigma* undivided, occasionally lobed. *Fruit* fleshy, with several 1-seeded cells, or by abortion only 1. *Seeds* nut-like, sometimes cohering into a several-celled putamen ; *testa* bony, shining, with a very long scar on the inner face, where it is opaque and softer than the rest; *embryo* erect, large, white, usually enclosed in fleshy albumen ; *cotyledons*, when albumen is present, foliaceous ; when absent, fleshy and·sometimes connate; *radicle* short, straight, or a little curved, turned towards the hilum.—*Trees* or *shrubs*, chiefly natives of the tropics, and often abounding

---

[1] *Medico-Chirurgical Transactions*, vol. xxiv. p. 30, 1841; and *Pharmaceutical Transactions*, vol. i. p. 24, 1841.
[2] In 1831, Wöhler expressed his opinion that, by digestion, benzoic acid was probably converted into hippuric acid (Keller, *infra cit.*)
[3] *Memoirs of the Chemical Society*, vol. i. p. 19, 1842.
[4] Keller, *Ann. der Chem. u. Pharm.* Bd. xliii. p. 108, 1842.

in milky juice. *Leaves* alternate, or occasionally almost whorled, without stipules, entire, coriaceous. *Inflorescence* axillary. *Flowers* hermaphrodite (*Lindley*).

Properties.—The fruit of many is esteemed as an article of dessert The seeds of several yield a fatty oil. The bark of some species is bitter and astringent, and is used as a febrifuge.

212. Isonandra Gutta, *Hooker.*—The Gutta Percha Tree.

(Succus.)

Isonandra Gutta, Hooker, Lond. Journ. of Botany, 1848; and Pharmaceutical Journal, vol. vii. p. 179, 1848.[1]—A tall tree, a native of the Malayan Archipelago, especially of Singapore. Its milky juice becomes concrete by exposure to the air, and forms the substance called *gutta percha*. "A magnificent tree of 50, or more probably 100 years' growth, is cut down, the bark stripped off, and the milky juice collected and poured into a trough formed by the hollow stem of the plantain leaf; it quickly coagulates on exposure to the air; but from one tree I was told that not more than 20 lbs. or 30 lbs. are procured" (Montgomerie).[2] It is extensively imported in blocks, and is purified by "devilling" or kneading in hot water. As imported, it is a white or dirty pinkish opaque solid. Its density is 0·79.[3] Water, alcohol, alkaline solutions, muriatic and acetic acids, have no action on it. Oil of vitriol slowly chars it; nitric acid converts it into a yellow resin. Ether and coal naphtha soften it in the cold, and by the aid of heat effect an imperfect solution of it. Its best solvent is chloroform or oil of turpentine. Its most important quality, which renders it so useful in the arts, is the facility with which it softens and becomes plastic in hot water. In this state it may be readily moulded into any required shape, and joined, by pressure, to other pieces which have also been rendered plastic by heat. When it cools it resumes its original hard and tough nature.[4]—Gutta percha of commerce consists chiefly of a *peculiar substance* (gutta percha properly so called) mixed with a small quantity of *a vegetable acid, caseine* (hence the cheesy odour which it sometimes possesses), a *resin* soluble in ether and in oil of turpentine, and a *resin* soluble in alcohol.[5] The pure gutta percha is a carbo-hydrogen, analogous to caoutchouc.[6]—The uses of gutta percha in the arts are most extensive.[7] It is already the subject of numerous patents.[8] It also serves some useful purposes in medicine, surgery, and pharmacy. A solution of it in chloroform has been used by Prof. Simpson[9] as a dressing of wounds. When a thin layer of the solution is spread upon the skin or any other surface, the chloroform rapidly evaporates, and leaves a film or web of gutta percha possessing all the tenacity and other properties of that substance. A layer of it of the thickness of good writing paper has perhaps as much strength and tenacity as to hold the edges of a wound together with all the required strength and firmness of sutures. Mr. Acton[10] finds that a compound solution of caoutchouc and gutta percha may be used to form a kind of membrane to protect the skin against the action of contagious poisons. The solution is prepared by adding a drachm of gutta percha to an ounce of benzole (the volatile principle of coal naphtha), and ten grains of India rubber to the same quantity of benzole, each being dissolved at a gentle heat, and then mixed in equal proportions. It may be used to protect the hands in post-mortem examinations, to prevent excoriation of the cheek in gonorrhœal ophthalmia, and in covering parts contiguous to a sore where the water dressing is used. In the treatment of clubfoot and fractures, Mr. Lyon[11] has found it a useful mechanical agent.

---

[1] [The reader will find additional information in this Journal for May 1851, p. 546; for June 1852, p. 575; and for March 1853, p. 452.—Ed.]

[2] *Pharmaceutical Journal*, vol. vi. p. 377, 1847.

[3] [Its true specific gravity is 0·96. The lower specific gravity formerly assigned to this substance was owing to the air-bubbles not having been removed from the surface.—Ed.]

[4] See Solly, *Pharmaceutical Journal*, vol. v. p. 510, 1846.

[5] Soubeiran, *Journ. de Pharm. et de Chimie*, 3me sér. t. xi. p. 17, 1847.

[6] Maclagan, *Pharmaceutical Journal*, vol. v. p. 472, 1846.

[7] *Ibid.* vol. vi. p. 382, 1847.

[8] *Ibid.* vol. viii. p. 141, 1849.

[9] *Ibid.* vol. viii. p. 84, 1848.

[10] *Ibid.* vol. viii. p. 297, 1849.

[11] *Half-yearly Abstract of the Medical Sciences*, vol. viii. p. 150.

Fig. 196.

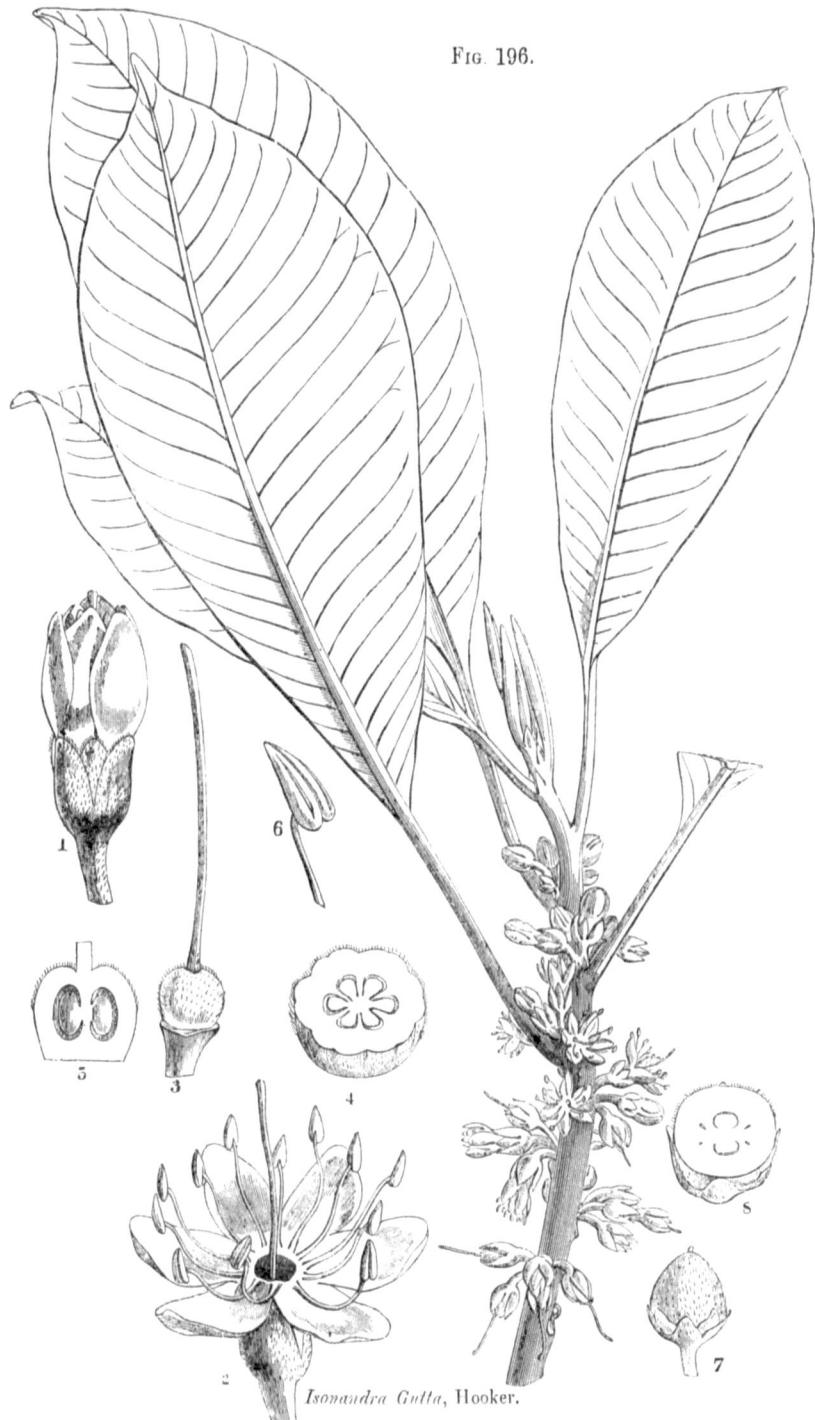

Isonandra Gutta, Hooker.

1. Flower scarcely expanded; 2, flower with the corolla expanded; 3, pistil; 4, transverse section of the ovary; 5, vertical section of the ovary; 6, anther; 7, scarcely mature fruit (natural size); 8, transverse section of ditto. (All but fig. 7, magnified.)

[The importation of gutta percha into London amounted, in 1854, to 813 tons. Of gutta percha there are three qualities imported:—

1. The fine native, in pieces of irregular shape of all sizes; it is pinkish in colour, and very hard and tough, and more or less mixed with a little bark or pulp.

2. Inferior native, in pieces of all forms and sizes, as the above, but white or grey in colour, and more porous and easily torn in pieces. It is probably the produce of a different tree.

3. The boiled sort, which is imported in oblong pieces, evidently formed in a mould. It varies in colour and toughness, but is generally pretty free from bark and pulp. It is said to consist of the above two qualities being boiled together so as to obtain an even-looking article. But the best of it, although fine in appearance, is refused by the gutta percha manufacturers, who say it becomes clammy in manufacturing it. In order to sell it, a reduction of 25 per cent. or more must be submitted to. The clamminess might probably be entirely removed by incorporating it with silicate of magnesia. India rubber is thus entirely deprived of clammy adhesiveness.—Ed.]

213. Chrysophyllum Buranheim, *Riedel*.

Sex. Syst. Pentandria, Monogynia.

(Cortex.)

Burunhem, Guaranhem, Tupin (*Mohica?*); Martius, Syst. Mat. Med. Veg. Brasil. p. 48, 1843; *Chrysophyllum glycyphlæum,* Casaretti, Journ. de Pharm. et Chim. t. vi. p. 64, 1844.—A tree growing in the Brazils near Rio de Janeiro. Its bark, which has long been in use among the Brazilians, was introduced into medicinal use a few years ago,[1] in France, under the name of *monesia* or *monesia bark* (*cortex monesiæ*). The recent bark is lactescent; but the bark such as it comes to Europe is thick, compact, heavy, very flat, brown, and hard, without any suberous or herbaceous layer. Its taste is at first sweet, afterwards astringent and bitter. It has been analysed by B. Derosne, Henry, and Payen,[2] who found it to consist of an *aromatic principle* (traces), *fat, chlorophylle,* and *wax,* 1·2; *glycyrrhisine,* 1·4; *monesine,* an acrid principle analogous to saponine, 4·7; *tannic acid,* 7·5; *red colouring matter* analogous to that of cinchona and catechu (rubinic acid), 9·2; *gum* (small quantity), *supermalate of lime,* 1·3; *salts of potash, lime,* and *magnesia, silica, oxide of iron,* &c. 3·0; *pectine* and *lignine,* 71·7 = 100. A blackish extract of the bark has been brought to Europe under the name of *extract of buranhem* or *guaranhem:* it strikes a blue colour with the salts of iron.—Monesia or Buranhem is an astringent. It is employed by the Brazilians in leucorrhœa, atonic diarrhœa, uterine hemorrhage, and chronic mucous discharges generally. It has been used in France and Germany in the same cases; but it does not appear to possess any superiority over rhatany, catechu, and other well-known astringents, and, consequently, it has now fallen into disuse.—The aqueous extract is given in doses of from a scruple to a drachm. It is soluble both in water and spirit. An ointment containing a drachm of the extract to an ounce of fatty matter has also been employed as a topical astringent. *Monesine* has also been used in medicine.[3]

---

[1] *Journ. de Chim. Méd.* t. v. 2de sér. p. 333, 1839; Guibourt, *Journ. de Pharm.* t. xxv. p. 710, 1839.

[2] *Journ. de Pharm.* t. xxvii. p. 20, 1841.

[3] For further details respecting monesia, the reader is referred to Dierbach's *Neuest. Entd. in der Mat. Med.* Bd. ii. p. 207, 1843; Dunglison, *New Remedies,* p. 438, 1846; and Mérat, *Suppl. au Dict. Univ. de Mat. Méd.* p. 175, 1846.

INDEX.

END OF PART I. VOL. II.

LONDON :
WILSON and OGILVY,
Skinner Street.

For EU product safety concerns, contact us at Calle de José Abascal, 56–1°, 28003 Madrid, Spain or eugpsr@cambridge.org.

www.ingramcontent.com/pod-product-compliance
Ingram Content Group UK Ltd.
Pitfield, Milton Keynes, MK11 3LW, UK
UKHW040618240426
470322UK00010B/189